Clinical Guide to Fish Medicine

Clinical Guide to Fish Medicine

Edited by

Catherine A. Hadfield, MA, VetMB, DACZM, DECZM (Zoo Health Management)

Seattle Aquarium
1483 Alaskan Way, Seattle, WA 98101

Leigh Ann Clayton, DVM, DABVP (Avian Practice, Reptile and Amphibian Practice), eMBA

New England Aquarium
1 Central Wharf, Boston, MA 02110

WILEY Blackwell

This edition first published 2021

Registered Offices
John Wiley & Sons, Inc., 111 River Street, Hoboken, NJ 07030, USA
John Wiley & Sons Ltd, The Atrium, Southern Gate, Chichester, West Sussex, PO19 8SQ, UK

Editorial Office
111 River Street, Hoboken, NJ 07030, USA

For details of our global editorial offices, customer services, and more information about Wiley products visit us at www.wiley.com.
Wiley also publishes its books in a variety of electronic formats and by print-on-demand. Some content that appears in standard print versions of this book may not be available in other formats.

Library of Congress Cataloging-in-Publication Data

Names: Hadfield, Catherine A., editor. | Clayton, Leigh Ann, editor.
Title: Clinical guide to fish medicine / edited by Catherine Hadfield, Leigh Clayton.
Description: Hoboken, NJ : Wiley-Blackwell, 2021. | Includes bibliographical references.
Identifiers: LCCN 2020024346 (print) | LCCN 2020024347 (ebook) | ISBN 9781119259558 (cloth) | ISBN 9781119259817 (adobe pdf) | ISBN 9781119259848 (epub)
Subjects: MESH: Fish Diseases | Fishes | Veterinary Medicine
Classification: LCC SF458.5 (print) | LCC SF458.5 (ebook) | NLM SF 458.5 | DDC 639.34–dc23
LC record available at https://lccn.loc.gov/2020024346
LC ebook record available at https://lccn.loc.gov/2020024347

Cover Design: Wiley
Cover Image: Courtesy of Catherine Hadfield

Set in 9.5/12.5pt STIXTwoText by Straive, Pondicherry, India

10 9 8 7 6 5 4 3 2 1

Contents

Preface

This is an exciting time to practice fish medicine as the field is growing rapidly, techniques and standards are evolving, and information exchange is easy and fast. Veterinary medicine for public aquariums, pet fish, aquaculture, fisheries, and research are converging as never before, allowing better care across the disciplines. Increased focus on fish welfare and sustainability is helping to refine the care of individuals and populations.

Leigh and I talked for many years about a fish medicine textbook for the busy clinical veterinarian in practice; a book that could serve as a practical reference for those starting out or already active in the field. Companion animal species have textbooks formatted to provide clinically relevant information that is easy to access during a hectic day. Why not something similar for fish vets? Eventually, we moved from talking about it to making it a reality. This is the result.

This text provides practical clinical information to help veterinarians, biologists, technicians, and students manage cases and situations effectively and efficiently. We want to help people quickly understand the information they need to consider when faced with clinical cases. We have tried to cover important topics across disciplines, with a goal of building an integrated fish health program that can be generalized to different situations. While we feel it is applicable across disciplines, we are sure it speaks most to vets working in public display facilities and pet medicine, as that is what we know best.

We are aware that despite our best intentions, we will have inevitably created an imperfect product: overlooked certain aspects of the field; missed valuable information; and suffered from our own biases. Known limitations include the constant emergence of new literature and a focus on trends in the United States. Despite these limitations, we hope this textbook can still act as a framework for integrating new information, and inspiration for others to identify and address needs as the field continues to grow. We encourage each reader to share their knowledge and shape the future of this field. In fish medicine, you are a lifelong learner.

This book is divided into three sections: A, B, and C. Section A has chapters covering clinically relevant aspects of anatomy, husbandry, and case management. Section B covers presenting problems, grouped by system, with possible differentials and suggestions on how to approach cases. Section C covers common diseases seen in clinical practice and is grouped into noninfectious diseases, viruses, bacteria, fungi and fungal-like organisms, protozoa, metazoa, myxozoa, and coccidia. Four appendices cover unit conversions, disinfectants, commercial laboratories, and veterinary training programs.

In putting this together, we relied heavily on an amazing group of contributors and reviewers, all of them experts in their field. We are indebted to every one of them. We have done all we can to ensure that the information in this text is accurate and up-to-date as of submission. If there are any mistakes in this text, the fault is with Leigh and me, not our contributors or reviewers.

To quote the indomitable Douglas Adams: "In cases of major discrepancy, it's always reality that's got it wrong."

We hope that you can use this information to improve the care provided to these amazing animals and to enjoy many more fishy cases.

Acknowledgments

This book was a collaborative effort. We would like to thank the many authors, whose brilliance, hard work, and patience are greatly appreciated: Ilana Alderman, Shane Boylan, Al Camus, Melinda Camus, Steve Divers, Rolf Gobien, Lisa Hoopes, Liz Koutsos, Stéphane Lair, Lisa Mangus, Mike Murray, Natalie Mylniczenko, Don Neiffer, Allan Pessier, Andrew Pulver, Katie Seeley, Kent Semmen, Izi Sladakovic, Andy Stamper, Jamie Torres, and Claire Vergneau-Grosset. Your contributions have greatly expanded the depth of information and discussions in this text.

We are grateful to all the additional people who contributed figures: Lance Adams, Jill Arnold, Eleanor Bailey, Pierre-Marie Boitard, Ash Bullard, Sarah Chen, Tonya Clauss, Ashleigh Clews, Andy Dehart, John Drennan, Sarah Faris, Bob George, Bartolomeo Gorgoglione, David Groman, Angie Hadfield, Sarah Halbrend, Craig Harms, Mike Hyatt, Charlie Innis, Jack Jewel, Kim Knoper, Greg Lewbart, Eva Lewisch, Chris Limcaco, Rubén López, Robert Maclean, Craig Olson, Nick Reback, Aimee Reed, Carlos Rodriguez, Sean Sheldrake, Johnny Shelley, Tianxing Shi, Amanda Slade, Brittany Stevens, Justin Stilwell, Kathy Tuxbury, Joe Welsh, Catharine Wheaton, and Li Yao. You have helped bring the concepts presented here to life.

We would also like to thank the many people who reviewed sections, including Andy Aiken, Julie Cavin, Esteban DeSoto, Ruth Francis-Floyd, Dan Fredholm, Kim Gaeta, Claudia Gili, Craig Harms, Matt Kinney, Greg Lewbart, Ken Ramirez, Drury Reavill, and Aimee Reed. Your efforts have broadened the perspectives captured here.

And a special thank you to all the staff at the National Aquarium, Seattle Aquarium, and New England Aquarium. It has been our privilege to work beside you and learn with you.

Catherine A. Hadfield and Leigh Ann Clayton

And to Leigh: I am deeply indebted to you for getting this project started and for your guidance throughout. Your leadership and friendship have shaped the vet and the person that I am.

To my cousin, Anna Feldweg: Thank you so much for all your reviews and excellent advice. Your contributions have been invaluable and I have learnt so much from you.

And I am eternally grateful to my mum and dad, Jane and Peter Hadfield, for their support and encouragement. I owe everything to them.

Catherine A. Hadfield

List of Contributors

Ilana R. Alderman
Born to Behave
Boulder, CO, USA

Shane M. Boylan, DVM
South Carolina Aquarium
Charleston, SC, USA

Alvin C. Camus, DVM, PhD
College of Veterinary Medicine, University of Georgia
Athens, GA, USA

Melinda S. Camus, DVM, DACVP
College of Veterinary Medicine, University of Georgia
Athens, GA, USA

Leigh A. Clayton, DVM, DABVP (Avian, Reptile/Amphibian), eMBA
New England Aquarium
Boston, MA, USA

Stephen J. Divers, BVetMed, DECZM (Herpetology, ZHM), DACZM, FRCVS
College of Veterinary Medicine, University of Georgia
Athens, GA, USA

Rolf P. Gobien, MD
Clinton X-Ray Specialists
Clinton, NC, USA

Catherine A. Hadfield, MA, VetMB, MRCVS, DACZM, DECZM
Seattle Aquarium
Seattle, WA, USA

Lisa A. Hoopes, MA, PhD
Georgia Aquarium
Atlanta, GA, USA

Elizabeth A. Koutsos, PhD
Koutsos Consulting, LLC
Apex, NC, USA

Stéphane Lair, DVM, DES, DVSc, DACZM
Faculté de Médecine Vétérinaire, Université de Montréal
Saint-Hyacinthe, Quebec, Canada

Lisa M. Mangus, DVM
Johns Hopkins University School of Medicine
Baltimore, MD, USA

Michael J. Murray, DVM
Monterey Bay Aquarium
Monterey, CA, USA

Natalie D. Mylniczenko, DVM, MS, DACZM
Disney's Animals, Science and Environment
Lake Buena Vista, FL, USA

Donald L. Neiffer, VMD, CVA, DACZM, MHS
National Zoological Park and
Wildlife Health Sciences, Smithsonian Institution
Washington DC, USA

Allan P. Pessier, DVM, DACVP
Washington Animal Disease Diagnostic Laboratory
Washington State University
Pullman, WA, USA

Andrew B. Pulver
National Aquarium
Baltimore, MD, USA

Kathryn E. Seeley, DVM, DACZM
Columbus Zoo and Aquarium
Powell, OH, USA

Kent J. Semmen
Disney's Animals, Science and Environment
Lake Buena Vista, FL, USA

Izidora Sladakovic, BVSc (Hons I), MVS, DACZM
Avian and Exotics Service, Northside Veterinary Specialists
Terrey Hills, New South Wales, Australia

M. Andrew Stamper, DVM, DACZM
Disney's Animals, Science and Environment
Lake Buena Vista, FL, USA

Jamie M. Torres, DVM
Audubon Aquarium of the Americas
New Orleans, LA, USA

Claire Vergneau-Grosset, DVM, IPSAV, DACZM
Faculté de Médecine Vétérinaire, Université de Montréal
Saint-Hyacinthe, Quebec, Canada

Section A

Fish Medicine Topic Reviews

Introduction

Section A contains chapters on aspects of fish care related to veterinary medicine. The focus is on practical applications to help veterinarians apply their general knowledge to fish patients. Initial topics are anatomy and taxonomy, water quality, life support systems, nutrition, and training and enrichment. These are followed by chapters on clinical examination and diagnostics, including clinical pathology, diagnostic imaging, and necropsy. Anesthesia, analgesia, surgery, and endoscopy are then discussed. The chapter on medical treatment is followed by one focused on immersion medications. This section finishes with discussions on acquisition, transport, and quarantine of fish. Readers are strongly encouraged to review the literature to develop a deeper understanding of these topics.

A1

Anatomy and Taxonomy

Natalie D. Mylniczenko

Disney's Animals, Science and Environment, Lake Buena Vista, FL, USA

Introduction

Working with patients that live in a fluid environment is both interesting and challenging. Many fish are anatomically and physiologically unique; this chapter will focus on clinically relevant anatomical features. The information will be divided into bony and cartilaginous fish (Box A1.1). The bony fish (*Osteichthyes*) consist of flesh-finned fish (lungfish and coelacanths) and ray-finned fish. The ray-finned fish group is large and includes teleosts as well as sturgeon and gars. The cartilaginous fish (*Chondrichthyes*) are divided up into elasmobranchs (sharks, skates, rays, guitarfish, and sawfish) and chimaeras. Due to the enormous variety across these groups, the level of detail will vary. Other texts provide more detail on order- or species-specific fish anatomy (Gilbert 1973; Harder and Sokoloff 1976; Ashley and Chiasson 1988; Stoskopf 1993; Hamlett 1999; Helfman et al. 2009; De Iuliis and Pulerà 2011; Farrell 2011; Carrier et al. 2012; Roberts and Ellis 2012; Jorgensen and Joss 2016; Nelson et al. 2016).

Anatomy of Bony Fish

Body Plan

Morphologic body shapes of bony fish include fusiform, laterally flattened, ventrally flattened, eel-like, ribbon-like, and spheroid (Nikolsky 1963). In these various shapes, different adaptations of common anatomical features are apparent. For example, the coelom of laterally flattened fish (e.g. sole or halibut, *Pleuronectiformes*) is situated toward the right or left of the animal, ipsilateral to the operculum. When assist-feeding these fish, the tube is oriented toward the side rather than the midline.

The coelom in most species is found along the ventrum, between the pectoral girdle cranially, vertebrae dorsally, and cloaca or anus caudally. There are exceptions, for example, in electric eels (*Electrophorus electricus*) and rainbowfish (*Melanotaeniidae*) the anus has migrated cranially to between the opercula.

Integument

The external layer of mucus is rich in mucopolysaccharides, immunoglobulins, lysozymes, and free fatty acids to create the mucosal defense system (Roberts and Ellis 2012). The epidermis consists of epithelial cells and mucous glands. It is thicker in fish that do not have scales (e.g. true eels, *Anguilliformes*) (Roberts and Ellis 2012). It differs from mammals in that it lacks keratin and all layers are capable of mitosis, including the squamous layer. The dermis includes scales in most bony fish, as well as chromatophores and mast cells. The chromatophores are clinically important, as color changes in fish can imply different physiologic states (Hoar et al. 1983). Generalized dark coloration may indicate stress or disease, color change on only one side of the body may indicate a visual problem on that side, and color change caudally can help localize the site of a spinal problem such as a vertebral fracture.

The scales are embedded within pockets of the dermal tissue and oriented toward the tail. Scales come in several types that vary in size, shape, and thickness, including placoid, cosmoid, ganoid, cycloid, and ctenoid. Cycloid and ctenoid scales are the most common in teleosts. Some scales are particularly large and thick, such as the ganoid scales of arowana (*Osteoglossidae*), arapaima (*Arapaima* spp.), sturgeon (*Acipenser* spp.), and tarpon (*Megalops* spp.). Scales can be an impediment for injections, vascular access, and

Clinical Guide to Fish Medicine, First Edition. Edited by Catherine A. Hadfield and Leigh Ann Clayton.

Box A1.1 Basic Taxonomy of Extant Fish

Class *Agnatha* (jawless fish)
- Subclass *Cyclostomata* (hagfish and lampreys)

Class *Chondrichthyes* (cartilaginous fish)
- Subclass *Elasmobranchii* (elasmobranchs)
  - *Selachimorpha* (sharks)
  - *Batoidea* (skates, rays, guitarfish, sawfish)
- Subclass *Holocephali* (chimaeras)

Class *Osteichthyes* (bony fish)
- Subclass *Sarcopterygii* (fleshy-finned fish: lungfish, coelacanths)
- Subclass *Actinopterygii* (ray-finned fish)
  - Order *Acipenseriformes* (sturgeons, paddlefish)
  - Order *Polypteriformes* (bichirs, reedfish)
  - Infraclass *Holostei* (gars, bowfins)
  - Infraclass *Teleostei* (teleosts)

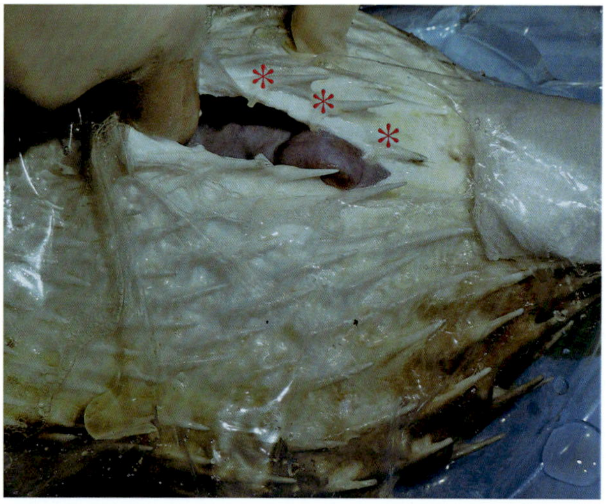

Figure A1.1 Coeliotomy in a porcupinefish (*Diodon holocanthus*) showing the cut roots of the spines (*). *Source*: Image courtesy of Catherine Hadfield, National Aquarium.

surgical incisions. During injection or venipuncture, care should be taken to pass underneath scales; if a scale is penetrated, it is removed when the needle is pulled out, which can lead to osmoregulatory problems or infections by opportunists such as oomycetes and scuticociliates. For surgical incisions, scales along the incision line may be removed to prevent contamination of the surgical site. Some fish have very fine scales, e.g. some jacks (*Carangidae*) and tuna (*Thunnini*), while others are scaleless, e.g. some jacks, true eels (*Anguilliformes*), catfish (*Ictaluridae*), and elephantfish (*Mormyridae*). Scaleless fish may be more vulnerable to toxins in the water, to medications, and to direct trauma from handling (Stoskopf 1993). Some fish have deciduous scales that are shed regularly, e.g. herring and anchovies (*Clupeiformes*) (Helfman et al. 2009).

Some fish have segmented bony plates within the dermis rather than scales, e.g. seahorses and pipefish (*Syngnathidae*), shrimpfish (*Centriscidae*), trunkfish and boxfish (*Ostraciidae*), and armored catfish or plecostomus (*Loricariidae*). In these fishes, injections and incisions should be made in softer areas to ensure success, for example on the tail of a seahorse or the peduncle of a boxfish. If plates must be cut, the area should be sealed with a wax product. Pufferfish (*Tetraodontidae*) have erectable spines derived from scales that have overlapping roots (Helfman et al. 2009); these limit the image quality on radiography and must be cut through for a coelomic incision (Figure A1.1).

Some fish produce copious mucus, including many eels (*Anguilliformes*), catfish (*Siluriformes*), and rays (*Myliobatiformes*). This can be a challenge for handling as they are quite slippery; a chamois or flannel cloth can help restraint without stripping the protective mucus layer. Parrotfish can also create a mucoid casing (cocoon) at night for protection; hand-net catches of parrotfish are much easier at night than in the daytime.

Epithelial hyperplasia is a common, nonspecific response of fish skin to irritants. This may be multifocal, e.g. the white spots caused by *Cryptocaryon irritans*. In some fancy goldfish (*Carassius auratus*), overgrowth of the head epithelium (called the wen or hood) has been genetically selected. This growth can obscure ocular and oral features to the detriment of the animal. It consists of non-ciliated epithelium with goblet cells covering a mucinous stroma. Surgical management has been described (Angelidis et al. 2009).

The lateral line lies along the body wall of fish. It is a canal within the integument that has pores along its length. In the canal are neuromasts that each have a sensory hair surrounded by gelatinous material. These organs are sensitive to water displacement and vibration (Roberts and Ellis 2012). Lateral line depigmentation (also known as head and lateral line erosion) is a common problem in teleosts.

Transparency is a feature of some fish species. The arrangement of collagen fibers allows light to pass through without reflection. An example that may be seen in the aquarium trade is the glass catfish (*Kryptopterus vitreolus*).

Bacterial luminescence is seen in the *Beryciformes* group, e.g. pinecone fish (often *Monocentris* spp.) and flashlight fish (e.g. *Anomalops katoptron*) (Hoar et al. 1983). These fish have a single species of bioluminescent bacteria (*Photobacterium fischeri*) in an organ under the eye (Morin et al. 1975). The bacteria can be obscured by being pulled into or covered by a fold of skin. The biggest clinical implication is that antibacterials can damage the bioluminescent bacteria.

Musculoskeletal System

Skeleton

Skeletal bone may be cellular or acellular. Cellular bone is more common in bony fish. Acellular bone (without osteocytes) is seen in perch-like fish (*Percidae*) and bass and sunfish (*Centrarchidae*). In both types, bones are typically solid and calcium absorption cannot occur locally; this means that fractures lack a local calcium reserve for repair. Fish lack bone marrow but there may be some vascular canals and spaces in the bone (Roberts and Ellis 2012). Hyperostosis or pachyostosis (also known as Tilly bones) has been documented in 22 fish families; the most common affected species in aquaria is Atlantic spadefish (*Chaetodipterus faber*) (Figure A1.2) (Smith-Vaniz et al. 1995). Hyperostosis is not typically considered pathologic, but if the lesions get large, they may form sequestrae with associated skin ulcerations. Removal or rongeuring the bone underneath has helped resolve signs in some patients.

Teleost skulls are a complicated series of bones; anatomy varies significantly between species. Vertebrae also vary across species. Radiographically, vertebrae usually have a prominent cross that represents the conical recesses enclosing the intervertebral pad, a neural spine, a hemal arch (or pleural ribs cranially), and a hemal spine (Roberts and Ellis 2012). Ribs are either pleural (attached to vertebrae) or intermuscular (within muscular tissue) as in salmonids (Helfman et al. 2009).

Fin shapes and locations vary between species. They may be embedded in musculature or bone. Firm fin spines are common, particularly along the dorsal fin, and present a human health hazard. Some fin spines also contain venom, e.g. lionfish (*Pterois* spp.) and stonefish (*Synanceiidae*). Some fins are modified into suckers, e.g. lumpfish (*Cyclopteridae*). The lobe-finned fish, lungfish (*Dipnoi*) and coelacanths (*Latimeria* spp.), have muscular fins with an articulating bone in their pectoral fin.

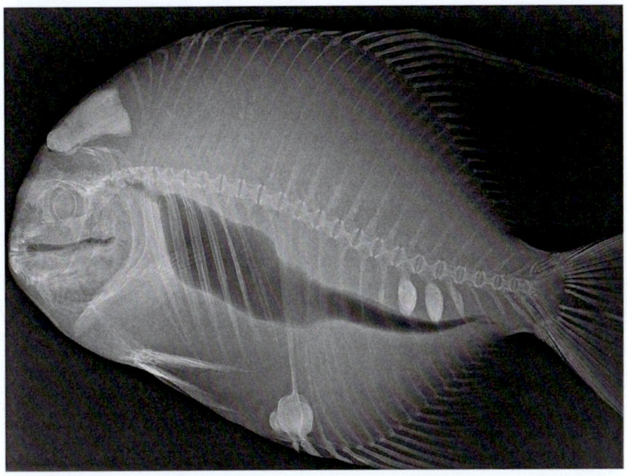

Figure A1.2 Radiograph of an Atlantic spadefish (*Chaetodipterus faber*) showing hyperostosis.

Muscle

The muscular system of fish has both red and white skeletal muscle. White (fast or twitch) muscle predominates and is important for anaerobic burst or sprint swimming (Roberts and Ellis 2012). Red (slow) muscle is associated with sustained aerobic swimming and has more blood supply; this muscle typically lies in a thin band under the skin along the lateral line and/or dorsal midline (Greek-Walker and Pull 1975). Pelagic and more active fish have a higher proportion of red muscle (Greek-Walker and Pull 1975). Drug pharmacokinetics are likely affected by muscle type although the impact is not well-known. The scup (*Stenotomus chrysops*) has pink muscle, which has less myoglobin than red muscle, and icefish in the arctic family *Channichthyidae* have yellow muscle due to a lack of hemoglobin (Helfman et al. 2009).

Fish muscle and skin are generally inelastic; therefore, injection volume and depth are important considerations. Intramuscular medications are potentially more likely to cause injection site lesions than in other vertebrate classes and volumes should be small. Leakage from injection sites is also common both immediately and once fish begin to swim after injection, which is likely to alter pharmacokinetics (Figure A1.3) (Fredholm et al. 2016).

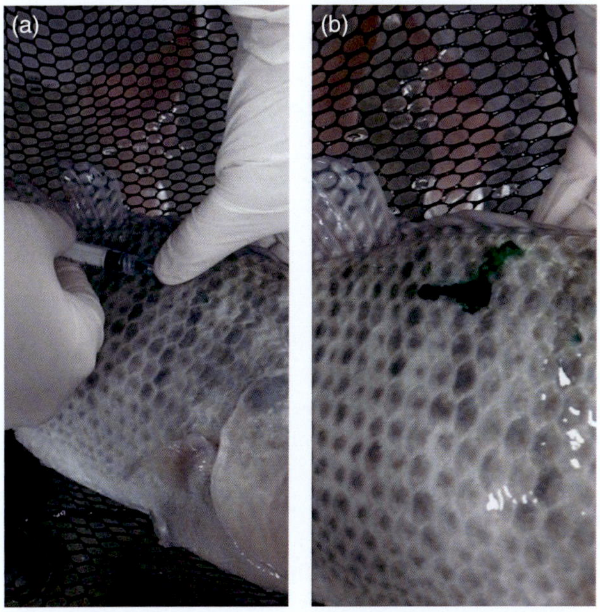

Figure A1.3 Leakage of drug with green marker following intramuscular injection in a Nile tilapia (*Oreochromis niloticus*).

Most fish are poikilothermic, with body temperature matching water temperature. A few bony fish species show regional endothermy, maintaining their body temperature above ambient, e.g. tunas (*Thunnini*), billfish (*Istiophoridae*), and one species of mackerel (*Gasterochisma melampus*). Endothermy is accomplished using retes in the brain, muscle, and viscera, and using red muscle located near the vertebral column. Endothermy improves digestion and nerve and muscle activity and is important for large predators chasing fast prey in colder waters (Block and Finnerty 1994).

Electrogeneration is possible from modified skeletal muscles in a variety of bony fish including freshwater elephantfish (*Mormyridae*), South American knifefish (*Gymnotiformes*), and electric catfish (*Malapteruridae*).

Buoyancy Organs

The swim (gas) bladder of bony fish shows extensive variations. Its primary function is buoyancy, but it can also be important in sound production and pressure reception (Roberts and Ellis 2012). It is absent in cartilaginous fish (chimaeras, skates, rays, sharks), some bottom-dwelling teleosts (e.g. flounder, *Pleuronectiformes*), weather loaches (*Misgurnus* spp.), and some highly pelagic teleosts like tuna (*Thunnini*). The swim bladder is filled with oil or fat in some bathypelagic species, e.g. lanternfish (*Myctophidae*) and orange roughy (*Hoplostethus atlanticus*) (Blaxter and Batty 1990; Phleger 1998). The volume of the swim bladder compared to body weight is typically under 5% in saltwater fish and under 7% in freshwater fish (Blaxter and Batty 1990). The gas in the bladder is composed of carbon dioxide, oxygen, and nitrogen, but not in the same percentages as air (Helfman et al. 2009).

Two types of swim bladder exist: physostomous and physoclistous. In physostomous fish, there is a pneumatic duct that connects the swim bladder to the esophagus. The gas is maintained by swallowing air. This anatomy has its disadvantages in that foreign bodies or gavaged food may enter the swim bladder (Stoskopf 1993). Common physostomous fish are salmon and trout (*Salmonidae*), catfish (*Siluriformes*), koi and goldfish (*Cyprinidae*), and tetras (*Characidae*), although some of these species also have a rete mirabile for some gas absorption.

Physoclistous fish lack a connecting duct. Inflation occurs via blood gases diffusing along one or more rete mirabile (gas glands) or vessels in the swim bladder, typically located cranially and ventrally (Figure A1.4) (Pelster 2011; Roberts and Ellis 2012). Physoclists include most marine teleosts, cichlids (*Cichlidae*), bass and sunfish (*Centrarchidae*). Some of these species also possess a capillary plexus caudodorsally (the oval or oval window) that helps resorb gases (Pelster 2011; Roberts and Ellis 2012).

Familiarity with normal swim bladder appearance is important to evaluate abnormalities on diagnostic imaging, endoscopy, coeliotomy, or necropsy. These may include hyperinflation, hypoinflation, displacement, and fluid or parasites. If injecting air to manage hypoinflation, a knowledge of normal volume is also important to prevent hyperinflation.

- One lobe is most common. It may be U-shaped (e.g. some pufferfish, *Tetraodontidae*).
- Two lobes are found in various species (Figure A1.5a), including goldfish (*Carassius auratus*) and common carp and koi (*Cyprinus carpio*), although some goldfish breeds have lost the caudal lobe.
- Three lobes are found in cod (*Gadus* spp.), channel catfish (*Ictalurus punctatus*), and some pufferfish (*Arothron* spp.) (Figure A1.5b).
- Extensions are common. The swim bladder may connect to the inner ear (e.g. herrings and anchovies, *Clupeiformes*), extend into vertebrae (e.g. freshwater angelfish, *Pterophyllum* spp.), or extend down the tail (e.g. electric eel, *Electrophorus electricus*, and arowana, *Osteoglossidae*) (Figure A1.5c).
- The swim bladder may be modified into lungs or lung-like tissues (e.g. garfish, tarpon, arapaima, and lungfish, see below).

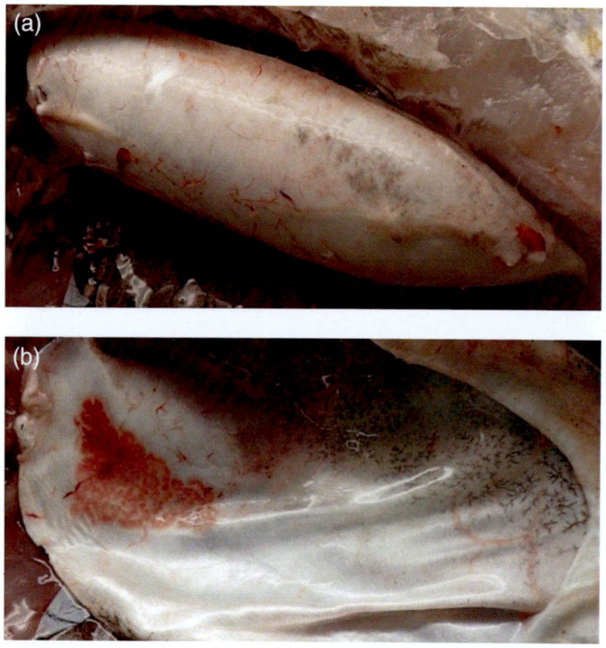

Figure A1.4 Intact (a) and incised (b) swim bladder of a bluestriped grunt (*Haemulon sciurus*) showing the rete mirabile. *Source*: Image courtesy of Carlos Rodriguez, Disney's Animals, Science and Environment.

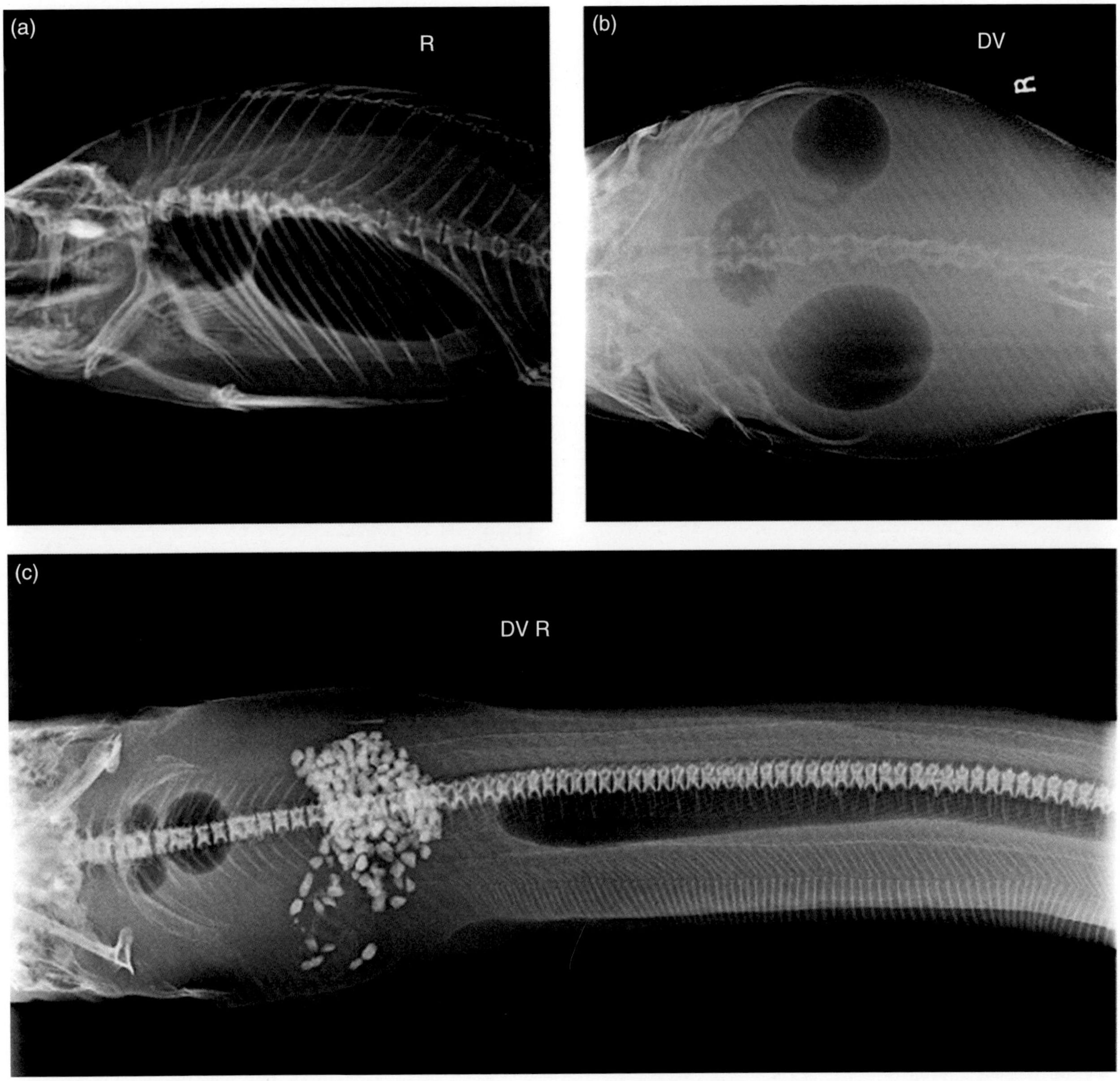

Figure A1.5 Swim bladder variations including two lobes in a spangled grunter (*Leiopotherapon unicolor*) (a), three lobes in a map puffer (*Arothron mappa*) (b), and extension down the tail in an electric eel (*Electrophorus electricus*) (c).

Adipose Tissue

Major sites of lipid deposition in bony fish are perivisceral in the coelom, within the muscle, and in the liver. In some species, lipid accumulation also occurs in the brain and under the skin (Weil et al. 2013). Coelomic fat is intended for long-term storage of lipids while liver and muscle allow easier mobilization of lipids (Sheridan 1994). Lipids in active bony fish tend to be stored in the skeletal muscle while bottom dwellers tend to store lipids in the liver (Sheridan 1988). Of the two skeletal muscle types, red muscle stores more lipids than white (Sheridan 1988).

Fat deposits fluctuate seasonally in wild animals but are less likely to change across the year in fish under human care. Over-conditioning of fish is a common problem under human care, particularly in large, mixed species habitats. Appropriate diets, targeted feeding, and suitable fasting periods can help in those situations.

Ocular Anatomy

The eyes of fish vary greatly. There are species that possess a rudimentary eye or eyespot, e.g. hagfish (*Myxinidae*), and there are eyeless fish such as the cavefish (e.g. *Astyanax mexicanus*). Fish with particularly large eyes relative to body size, e.g. some squirrelfish (*Holocentridae*) and rockfish (*Sebastes* spp.), seem more prone to ocular issues such as gas bubble disease and inflammation.

Fish do not have apposable eyelids, although many have a membrane known as the epidermal conjunctiva that covers the cornea or folds of tissue around the eye (Gelatt 2014). Some bony fish do have static eyelids to protect the eyes, e.g. salmonids (*Salmonidae*), jacks (*Carangidae*) (Figure A1.6) (Jurk 2002). Corneas in freshwater fish species are thicker than in saltwater species and some fish have two-layered corneas (Gelatt 2014). The cornea of green moray eels (*Gymnothorax funebris*) has a dermal layer (secondary spectacle) and a scleral layer (Trischitta et al. 2013) and it is common to see abnormal lipid deposition in the dermal layer. Relevant microanatomical features include the epidermal conjunctiva, a basement membrane (Bowman's membrane), and the endothelial layer (Descemet's membrane) (Roberts and Ellis 2012). In some species, there is a normal corneal iridescence or pigmentation that is likely associated with glare reduction, e.g. pufferfish (*Tetraodontidae*) (Gelatt 2014).

Most fish have a fixed pupil so there is no pupillary light reflex, but there are some exceptions e.g. true eels (*Anguilla* spp.), turbot (*Rhombus* spp.), flounder (*Pleuronectidae*), and African lungfish (*Protopterus* spp.) (Gelatt 2014). The iris can be round, pear-shaped, elliptical, or slit-like. Deep sea fish lack an iris (Stoskopf 1993). Amphibious fish such as mudskippers (e.g. *Periophthalmus* spp.) need to see above and below water and so have a flattened cornea and two pupils in each eye (Colicchia 2007). Suckermouth catfish (*Loricariidae*) have a modified iris called an "omega iris", which has a loop at the top that can expand and contract to control light exposure (Douglas and Djamgoz 2012).

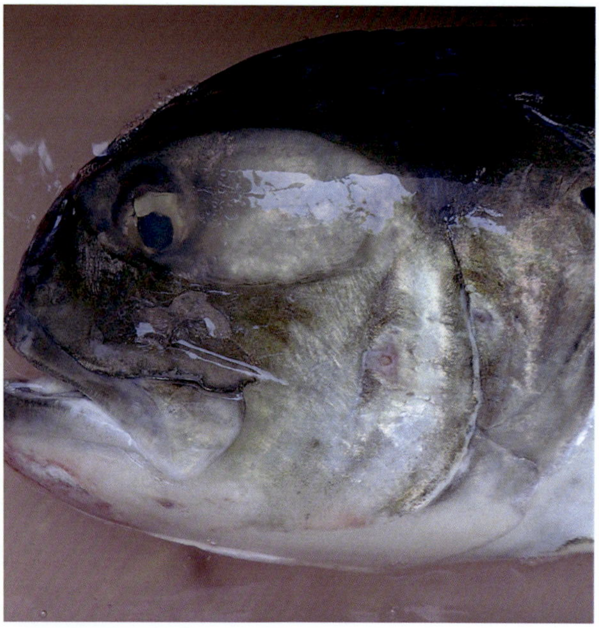

Figure A1.6 Eyelid on a crevalle jack (*Caranx hippos*). *Source*: Image courtesy of Carlos Rodriguez, Disney's Animals, Science and Environment.

Lenses are dense and spherical to compensate for the lack of refraction at the corneas and typically protrude slightly through the iris (Roberts and Ellis 2012; Gelatt 2014). There is no mechanical separation of vitreous and aqueous humor as in other vertebrates. Ciliary bodies are either absent or rudimentary and ciliary processes are absent; vitreal fluid production is not understood (Gelatt 2014).

The sclera is cartilaginous. The orbit is bony and enclosed. In some fish, a tenacular ligament anchors the globe to the orbit. Some species have scleral ossicles, e.g. sturgeon (*Acipenseridae*) (Gelatt 2014).

The retina varies significantly between species (Ali and Anctil 2012). Rods and cones are present, with more cones in diurnal species. A tapetum lucidum and fovea are present (Ollivier et al. 2004). The European eel (*Anguilla anguilla*) is the only teleost with intraretinal vascular circulation (Trischitta et al. 2013). In other teleosts, there is an organ with a vascular rete called the choroidal gland, which wraps around the optic nerve and communicates with the pseudobranch (discussed later) (Gelatt 2014). The choroidal gland is important in oxygen secretion and has been implicated in intraocular gas bubble formation (Roberts and Ellis 2012). It is also a potential source of blood loss during enucleation in teleosts.

Auditory Anatomy

The acoustic organs provide information on acoustical stimuli, gravitational forces, and linear and angular accelerations of the head. Fish make use of a labyrinth that includes semicircular canals, ampullae of the inner ear, and otoliths or otoconia (discussed in more detail under auditory anatomy of elasmobranchs) (Hoar et al. 1983). Otoliths are calcified stones that overlay sensory epithelium and are surrounded by endolymph, which facilitates their movement for sound perception and equilibrium (Roberts and Ellis 2012). In most ray-finned fish, there is a single otolith in each otic chamber, but there may be several. Otoliths can be used to age and identify bony fish. Pathology of the inner ear can lead to loss of equilibrium.

The swim bladder and other gas cavities can conduct sound using bones known as the Weberian apparatus (or ossicles) in several species, e.g. carp (*Cyprinus carpio*), bowfin (*Amia calva*), and tetras (*Characidae*) (Schulz-Mirbach et al. 2012). Fish that show a direct or indirect connection from the swim bladder to the perilymphatic system of the inner ear can perceive higher frequency sounds (e.g. up to 4000 Hz in carp and catfish, *Cyprinidae* and *Ictaluridae*) than those without (up to 520 Hz in cod, *Gadiformes*) (Roberts and Ellis 2012).

There are three methods of sound production: stridulatory (teeth, fins, spines, and bones), hydrodynamic (swimming movements), and muscle vibrations around the swim bladder (Hoar et al. 1983).

From a clinical perspective, it is difficult to evaluate these structures. Swim bladders and otoliths can be identified on radiography, computed tomography, or MRI (Figure A1.7). Animals with swim bladder disease may show reduced functional hearing. In catfish, swim bladder damage decreased the hearing frequency range (Kleerekoper and Roggenkamp 1959).

Olfactory and Gustatory Anatomy

Water-soluble chemical compounds are detected by olfaction (smell) or gustation (taste). For olfaction, teleosts have paired nares on the rostrum lined with olfactory epithelium. Hagfish and lampreys (*Agnatha*) are unique with only a single nare (Evans et al. 2004). Water passing through the nares stimulates receptors in the olfactory tracts, which send signals to the olfactory bulbs within the forebrain (telencephalon) (Roberts and Ellis 2012). Some teleosts have nasal sacs and accessory nasal sacs that actively pump water over the epithelium (coinciding with opercular movement) (Hara 1975). Some rely heavily on olfaction and have large olfactory pits extending from the rostrum to the eye, e.g. moray eels and true eels (*Anguilliformes*). Others rely on visual cues and lack nasal sacs, e.g. pufferfish (*Tetraodontidae*) (Hara 1975). In some species, males have a larger olfactory capacity (Hara 1975).

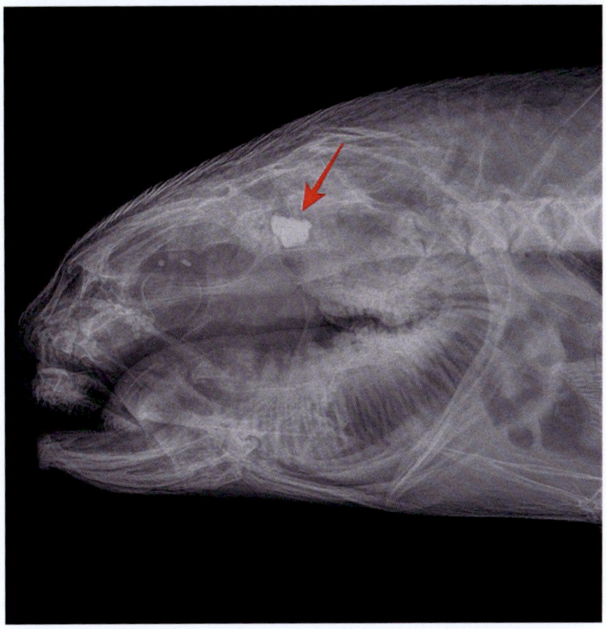

Figure A1.7 Otoliths visible on lateral radiograph of a red drum (*Sciaenops ocellatus*). *Source*: Image courtesy of Shane Boylan, South Carolina Aquarium.

Taste buds are epidermal and can be found in the oral cavity, lips, head, barbels, body wall, fins, and esophagus (Evans et al. 2004; Roberts and Ellis 2012). In some fish, the external taste buds outnumber intraoral taste buds by as much as 90% (Hara 1975). Fish have up to three anatomically different taste buds (Reutter et al. 1974). The taste cells are receptive to amino, nucleic, and organic acids (Oike et al. 2007). Fish do have aversive and preferential responses to some chemical stimuli but extensive research on gustatory preferences has not been done (Oike et al. 2007).

Oral/Pharyngeal Cavity

The oral cavity is shared by the respiratory, endocrine, and digestive systems. Feeding mechanisms are highly varied. Functionally, the mouth is for prehension of food, not chewing or predigestion. The lining of the oral cavity is thick epithelium and dermis bound to the bone or muscle (Roberts and Ellis 2012). The jaws are comprised of several fused bones and can be complex in pattern. Some fish have ornate protruding maxillary rostrums (e.g. paddlefish, *Polyodontidae*) while others, like the slingjaw wrasse (*Epibulus insidiator*), have a telescopic mouth, which protrudes for prey capture (Burgess et al. 2011). A few species have pharyngeal jaws, e.g. moray eels (*Muraenidae*) (Figure A1.8). Fish tongues have limited mobility and are simply used to propel food into the esophagus. In some species, there are teeth on the tongue to help hold prey. Buccal glands produce mucus; there are no salivary glands (Stoskopf 1993). One of the most common causes of oral masses in fish is thyroid hyperplasia (goiter), which typically presents in bony fish as a mass along the gill arches.

Dentition varies depending on feeding ecology. Teeth are acrodont with ankyloses or a fibrous attachment to the jaw

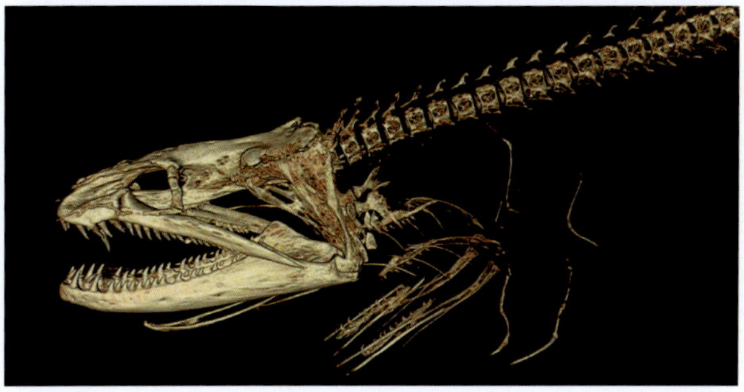

Figure A1.8 Computed tomography of the skull of a moray eel (*Muraenidae*) showing the pharyngeal jaws.

(Teaford et al. 2007). Basic tooth types are canine (Figure A1.9a), molariform, incisor, or plate-like. Dental plates are seen in lungfish (*Dipnoi*) and gar (*Lepisosteidae*) (Fishbeck and Sebastiani 2012). Pikes (*Esocidae*) have hinged teeth that are pointed backward; they bend during swallowing of prey and are erected again by elastic ligaments (Berkovitz and Shellis 2016). In parrotfish (*Scarinae*) and pufferfish (*Tetraodontidae*), the front teeth grow continuously, necessitating trimming when not fed hard food items (Roberts-Sweeney 2016). Some fish lack teeth altogether, e.g. filter feeders, seahorses and pipefish (*Syngnathidae*), sturgeon (*Acipenseridae*). Pharyngeal teeth are often present in bony fish for holding, masticating, or grinding foodstuffs (Figure A1.9b). Fish that rely heavily on pharyngeal teeth often do not have a muscular stomach (Gerking 2014).

The esophagus is a short, muscular tube. While straight in most species, it is important to be aware of differences in position and angularity when gavaging medications or food. The angle into the stomach can be dramatic (Figure A1.10) and a misplaced gavage tube can perforate the esophagus and damage the heart, liver, or swim bladder. In some fishes, the esophagus has blind diverticula (esophageal sacs) lined with calcified, esophageal teeth (Isokawa et al. 1965). In sturgeon (*Acipenseridae*), the esophagus has folds. The epithelium may have abundant mucus (esophageal) glands, particularly in carnivores, and these may be noted during gastrointestinal endoscopy (Roberts and Ellis 2012).

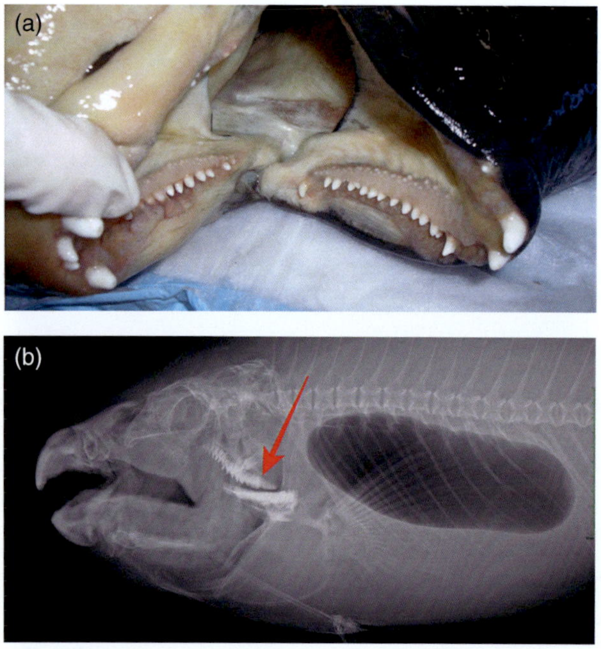

Figure A1.9 Teeth in a California sheephead (*Semicossyphus pulcher*) (a) and lateral radiograph of a rainbow parrotfish (*Scarus guacamaia*) showing pharyngeal teeth (b). *Source*: Images courtesy of Catherine Hadfield, National Aquarium.

Gastrointestinal System

The stomach varies in size depending on food items. Some species are agastric, e.g. goldfish (*Carassius auratus*), common carp and koi (*Cyprinus carpio*), and zebrafish (*Danio rerio*). The stomach becomes a grinding organ in sturgeons (*Acipenseridae*), gizzard shads (*Dorosoma* spp.), and mullets (*Mugilidae*) (Helfman et al. 2009). Histologically, the cardia consists of striated muscle and transitions to smooth muscle in the pyloric stomach. The mucosa has numerous mucus glands (Roberts and Ellis 2012). Pyloric caeca are diverticula off the stomach that are present in salmonids and many other teleosts. They increase the absorptive surface area. These organs are dissimilar to the ceca of birds and mammals as they are not fermentative (Buddington and Diamond 2016).

The intestines are variable in length and shape but fairly simple. The colon is minimal or not distinguishable (Roberts and Ellis 2012). In the lungfish (*Dipnoi*) and sturgeon (*Acipenseridae*), the intestine is spiral-shaped, similar to the elasmobranchs (Figure A1.11). A rectum is present (Roberts and Ellis 2012). Gastrointestinal emptying times are highly variable and both temperature- and volume-dependent; more details can be found in Chapter A4.

Pufferfish are unique in being able to inflate their bodies with water or air. Mouthfuls are pumped into the stomach which then expands. The pectoral girdle and head have modifications that function as a pump and the skin is very distensible; ribs are absent to accommodate inflation (Wainwright and Turingan 1997). In some species the skin has spines which stand erect on inflation.

External intestinal and urogenital openings differ among species. In most, there is a separate anus and reproductive opening or urogenital pore (Yanong 2003). In some bony fish, there is a cloaca: a common area where the intestinal, urinary, and gonadal ducts empty, e.g. lungfish and coelacanths (*Latimeria* spp.).

Liver and Gallbladder

The liver is a fairly large organ (single or bilobed) and predominantly on the left side of bony fish. It is typically orange to brown. If the liver is tan or yellow, it can indicate fatty infiltration, which may be a normal seasonal change or related to a high-fat diet. The liver is separated from the pericardial cavity by a septum (Roberts and Ellis 2012). A gallbladder is present in most species, with some exceptions, e.g. burbot (*Lota lota*) (Dutta and Datta-Mushi 1996). The gallbladder is located within or between the liver lobes

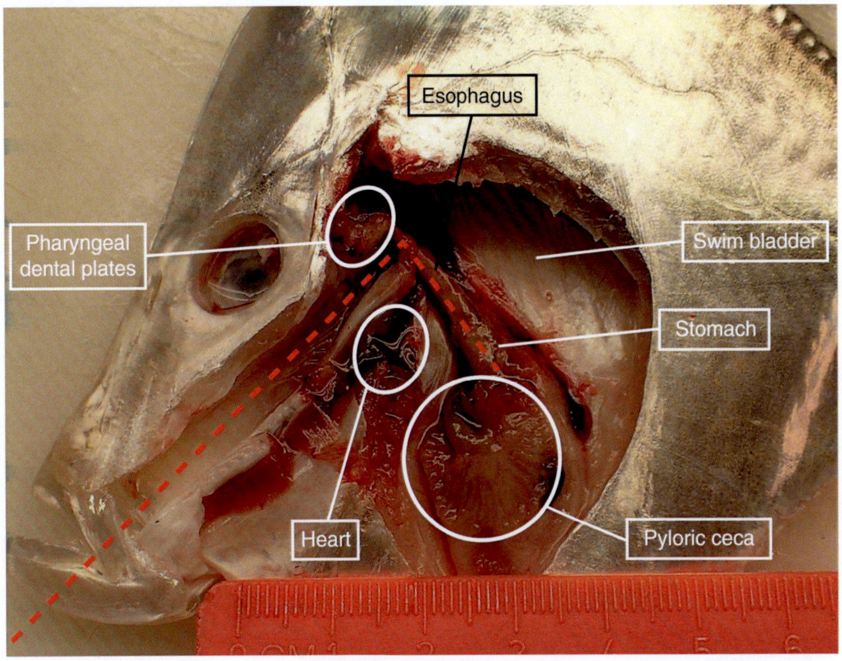

Figure A1.10 Angling of the esophagus seen at necropsy of a lookdown (*Selene vomer*), shown by the dashed red line. *Source*: Image courtesy of Carlos Rodriguez, Disney's Animals, Science and Environment.

in most fish, but lies in the caudal coelom in some, e.g. rockfish (*Sebastes* spp.). The gallbladder can become distended with anorexia (Stoskopf 1993). The bile duct enters at the stomach or small intestine. Most bile is made of bile salts and taurine conjugates of bile acids, except in carp where the principal bile salt is in the form of alcohol sulfates (Stoskopf 1993).

Respiratory System

Respiration does not involve inspiration and expiration but rather a continuous flow over the gill epithelium. Ventilatory rate reflects the muscular/opercular pumping of water over the epithelium. Gills are the primary organ for respiratory exchange in most fish; they are covered by an operculum or skin with gill slits. There are two sets of gills bilaterally which are made up of gill arches (holobranchs) with paired rows of primary gill filaments (hemibranchs) (Figure A1.12). Each primary filament has perpendicular secondary filaments. Most bony fish have four gill arches. Some gill arches also have gill rakers that function as a sieve to collect food from the water. Normal gill appearance is a uniform, dark red. In cases of anemia, the color fades to pink, light pink, or even white. This color change is also seen after death, along with autolysis. Methemoglobinemia may cause a brown discoloration. The epithelium of the gill is thin to allow gas exchange, which makes it vulnerable to pathogens and environmental toxins. Since gills have metabolic and excretory functions, damage can subject the fish to respiratory and osmoregulatory challenges (e.g. dehydration) (Hughes and Morgan 1973).

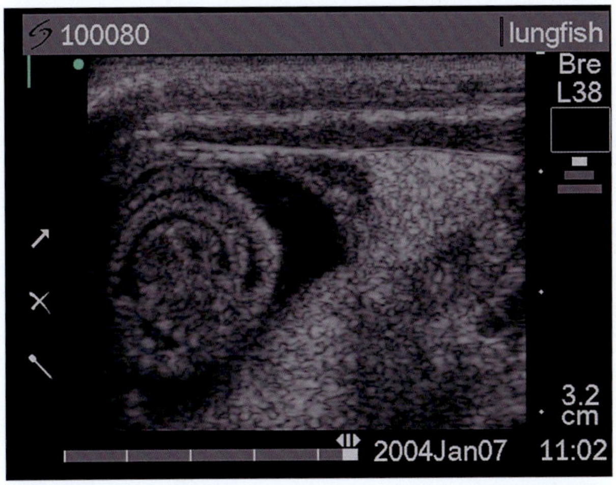

Figure A1.11 Ultrasound of the spiral intestine of an African lungfish (*Protopterus annectens*).

Gills have the capacity to regenerate, but the extent and time line are not well-characterized in all fish. It is suggested to occur within one to two weeks of an insult and take about two more weeks (Tzaneva et al. 2014).

Bilateral pseudobranchs lie dorsocranially to the gill arches in most teleosts, with the exception of the catfish (*Siluriformes*), a few eels (*Anguilliformes*), African knifefish (*Gymnarchus niloticus*), and spiny loaches (*Cobitis* spp.) (Helfman et al. 2009). There are three types: free (exposed); covered (with subtypes, see Bertin 1958); and glandular. Exposed pseudobranchs look like a partial gill arch (Figure A1.13) and have direct contact with the water;

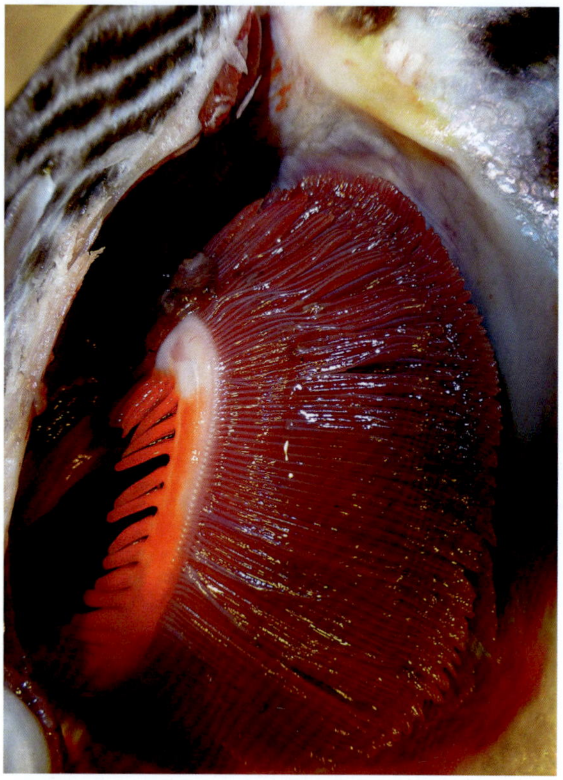

Figure A1.12 Normal gills seen during necropsy of a sweetlips (*Plectorhinchus* sp.) showing the gill rakers and primary filaments. *Source*: Image courtesy of Carlos Rodriguez, Disney's Animals, Science and Environment.

they can be seen in some perch-like fish (*Percoidei*) and many marine fish. Covered pseudobranchs resemble a gill arch but are covered with a membrane; they can be seen in cyprinids and salmonids. In the glandular type, the pseudobranch is deep within the connective tissue of the opercular cavity or buccopharynx. This is seen in some gouramis (*Anabas* spp.), snakeheads (*Channa* spp.), and featherbacks (*Notopterus* spp.) (Bertin 1958; Laurent and Dunel-Erb 1984).

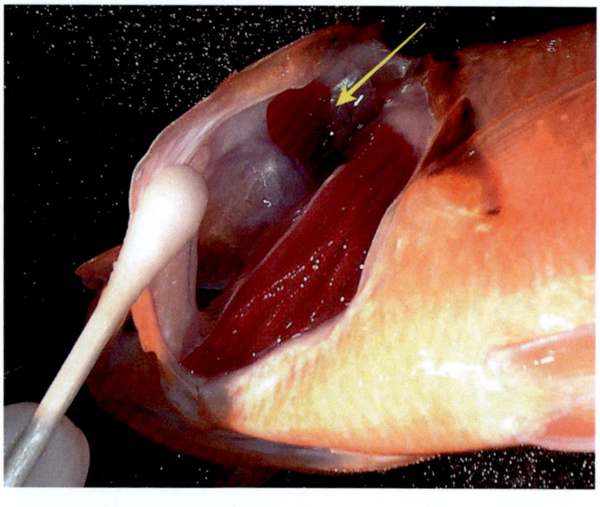

Figure A1.13 Exposed pseudobranch (arrow) in a soldierfish (*Myripristis* sp.). *Source*: Image courtesy of Catherine Hadfield, National Aquarium.

The pseudobranch delivers oxygen to the choroid of the eye via the carbonic anhydrase pathway and thus is suspected of regulating intraocular oxygen and pressure; a process that depends on hydrostatic and osmotic pressure, pH, and pCO_2 (Roberts and Ellis 2012). Some also deliver oxygen to the vascular rete of the swim bladder. There is a proposed osmoregulatory function (Na^+ and Cl^- secretion and excretion) and a glandular function that is poorly understood. Pseudobranch surgery can be performed where ocular gas is not responding to medical management. This may involve surgical removal, ablation, or cauterization (Harms and Lewbart 2000).

Most bony fish have opercula over the gills. Opercular appearance is variable, e.g. in sturgeons (*Acipenser* spp.) the operculum does not fully cover the gill filaments, while in marine angelfish (*Pomacanthidae*) the operculum has a spike that is a potential human health hazard. Opercular flaring or curling can be due to egg incubation temperature, genetics, trauma, or nutritional issues (Branson 2008). Consequences of this vary from purely cosmetic defects to gill damage. Some bony fish lack opercula with water instead flowing out from the gills through a slit in the skin. This is seen in triggerfish (*Balistidae*), eels (*Anguilliformes*), frogfish (*Antennariidae*), lumpfish (*Cyclopteridae*), and seahorses, sea dragons, and pipefish (*Syngnathidae*). This limits visibility of the gills; otoscopes or endoscopy are often needed for examination and biopsy.

Fish use pressure changes to move water over the gills from the mouth. Some fish need to swim to create the pressure gradient (e.g. pelagic sharks, tuna), and it is essential that additional ventilation is provided to these species when they are under manual or chemical restraint.

Air-breathing can occur in bony fish. This allows fish to deal with low dissolved oxygen levels in water, but it also allows a few fish species to survive brief periods out of water (as long as hydration is appropriate) or to avoid other dissolved gases such as hydrogen sulfide. Two general strategies exist: obligate and facultative air-breathing (Table A1.1). Obligate air-breathers have rudimentary gills, but do not maintain enough gas exchange across the gills for respiration without access to air (Feder and Burggren 1985; Graham 1997). If air access is restricted (e.g. if kept underwater for anesthesia), these fish cannot ventilate. Facultative air-breathers are able to maintain gas exchange across the gills and make use of air-breathing when dissolved oxygen is low. Air-breathing organs can include surfaces of the buccal/pharyngeal cavity, digestive tract, swim bladders, and lungs (Figure A1.14). The skin

Table A1.1 Obligate and facultative air-breathers.

Species	Type of air-breathing	Site of gas exchange
Gouramis, bettas (*Anabantoidei*)	Obligate	Modified epibranchial and suprabranchial chambers (labyrinth organ)
African bichirs or reedfish (e.g. *Polypterus* spp.)	Obligate	Lung (modified swim bladder)
African knifefish or aba (*Gymnarchus niloticus*)	Obligate	Swim bladder
Freshwater butterflyfish (*Pantodon buchholzi*)	Obligate	Swim bladder
Arapaima (*Arapaima gigas*)	Obligate	Lung
Electric eel (*Electrophorus electricus*)	Obligate	Pharynx
Mudskippers (e.g. *Periophthalmus* spp.)	Obligate	Skin and pharynx
Snakeheads (*Channidae*)	Obligate	Labyrinth organ
Weather loach (*Misgurnus* spp.)	Obligate	Intestine
Swamp eel (*Monopterus cuchia*)	Obligate	Pharynx
Lungfish (*Protopterus aethiopicus, Protopterus amphibius, Protopterus annectens, Protopterus dolloi, Lepidosiren paradoxa, Neoceratodus forsteri*)	Facultative in Australian lungfish (*Neoceratodus forsteri*); obligate in other species	Lung (modified swim bladder)
Arowana (*Osteoglossidae*)	Facultative	Swim bladder
Atlantic tarpon (*Megalops atlanticus*)	Facultative	Swim bladder
Gar (*Lepisosteidae*)	Facultative	Swim bladder
Alaska blackfish (*Dallia pectoralis*)	Facultative	Esophagus
Various *Siluriformes* catfish (*Clarias, Pangasius, Hoplosternum, Hypostomus, Ancistrus, Corydoras* spp.)	Facultative	Gastrointestinal tract, swim bladder, and/or labyrinth organ

Source: Graham (1997). © 1997, Elsevier.

also serves a respiratory function in many fish, including many larval stages. Air is directly absorbed across the epithelium and into the bloodstream. For a detailed review of air-breathing in fish, see Graham 1997.

Many fish species, particularly freshwater teleosts, are also able to show aquatic surface respiration (ASR). When dissolved oxygen is low, they come to the surface to skim the air/water interface because of its higher oxygen content.

Cardiovascular System

All bony fish have a two-chambered heart with four distinct anatomical regions. Blood flows through the sinus venosus into the atrium, then the ventricle, and out the bulbus arteriosus to the ventral aorta, the gills, the dorsal aorta, and the organs (Stoskopf 1993). The atrium and ventricle have partitions in the lungfish (*Dipnoi*) and coelacanth (*Latimeria* spp.). Teleosts have a pericardial sac filled with serous fluid.

Renal and hepatic portal systems are present in most fish although the proportion of blood that passes through the portal system varies by species. This may impact pharmacokinetics and toxicity if drugs that may be modified or excreted by the liver or kidneys are given in the caudal half of the body (Stoskopf 1993).

The lymphatic system is curious. In some teleosts, there is a fluid system separate from the primary circulation that is considered a lymphatic system (with leukocytes and devoid of erythrocytes). A secondary vascular system (SVS) that is not a lymphatic system has also been well-described (Steffensen and Lomholt 1992). This SVS is larger in volume than the primary circulation and has similar constituents to plasma but lacks most cellular components. Circulation rates are lower in the SVS, sometimes by hours (Roberts and Ellis 2012). Stress, hypoxia, and exercise alter the volume and cellularity in each system, most importantly resulting in a hematocrit change of the primary system (Rummer et al. 2014). The primary and secondary systems are connected with anastomoses, in contrast to other vertebrate classes. The secondary system has a role in gas and ion exchange.

Venipuncture in bony fish usually makes use of the ventral tail vessels, via a lateral or ventral approach. However, size, anatomy, or disease may necessitate other sampling sites. Other possible sites that can be used in fish are listed below.

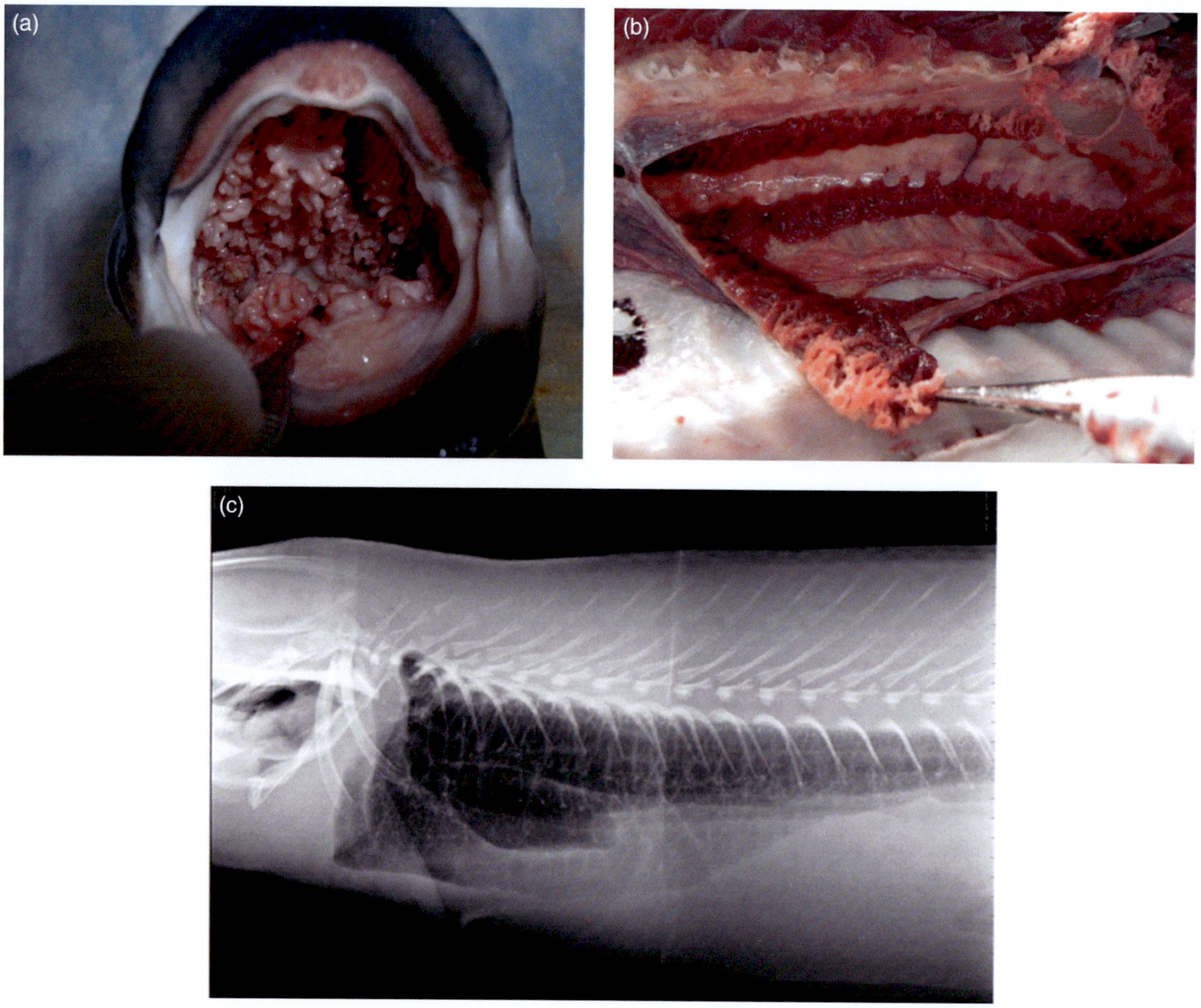

Figure A1.14 Air-breathing structures: modified pharyngeal mucosa in an electric eel (*Electrophorus electricus*) (a), modified swim bladder of a longnose gar (*Lepisosteus osseus*) (b), and a true lung seen on lateral radiograph of an African lungfish (*Protopterus annectens*) (c). *Sources*: Image (a) courtesy of Catherine Hadfield, National Aquarium. Image (b) courtesy of Carlos Rodriguez, Disney's Animals, Science and Environment.

- Gill arch (Suedmeyer 2006)
- Peduncular notch
- Retro-orbital sinus via oral cavity (Zang et al. 2013)
- Cardiac
- Cloaca superficial vessels (especially elasmobranchs)
- Dorsal fin sinus (elasmobranchs)
- Pectoral fin/radial vessels and mesopterygial vein (elasmobranchs)

Venipuncture is described in more detail in Chapter A6.

The gross appearance of blood varies in some groups. Blood and serum are blue-green due to biliverdin in humphead wrasse (*Cheilinus undulatus*) and Japanese eels (*Anguilla japonica*) (Fang and Bada 1990). The blood of icefish (*Channichthyidae*) is clear as they lack hemoglobin (Sidell and O'Brien 2006). Pale tan to brown blood can be due to methemoglobinemia, often caused by high nitrites (Mirghaed et al. 2017).

Lymphomyeloid System

Fish lack lymph nodes, Peyer's patches, and bone marrow. Hematopoiesis in bony fish occurs primarily in the spleen and the cranial kidney with some activity in the liver, thymus, and pericardium in some species (Roberts and Ellis 2012). Additional lymphoid activity occurs in the mucosa-associated lymphoid tissues (MALT). The gastrointestinal tract, gills, and skin act as pathogen barriers and contain local leukocyte populations. Another cell, the melanomacrophage, is present ubiquitously and increases in the presence of antigen stimulation. Pigmented macrophage aggregates (PMA), also known as melanomacrophage centers (MMC), are solid foci of these cells and found in high numbers in the liver, spleen, and cranial kidney (Roberts and Ellis 2012). They can be seen on wet mounts of these organs examined under direct microscopy and can increase with chronic inflammatory diseases.

The spleen is dark red to black and has sharp edges. There are multiple spleens in some fish and no distinct spleen in hagfish and lampreys (*Agnatha*).

The thymus can be very hard to find. Presence and size vary greatly among teleosts and it does not follow the mammalian involution pattern (Roberts and Ellis 2012). It may be found subcutaneously at the dorsal edge of the operculum, at the base of the gill arches, associated with pharyngeal epithelium, or within the cranial kidney (Stoskopf 1993). One pair of organs is typical, but some fish (e.g. clingfish, *Gobiesocidae*) have two pairs (Bowden et al. 2005).

Endocrine System

The endocrine system resembles that of other vertebrate classes but has some features with no mammalian counterparts such as the urophysis and the corpuscles of Stannius.

The pituitary (hypophysis) has many endocrine functions including the secretion of hormones (GnRH, TSH, vasopressin, etc.). A saccus vasculosus is associated with the hypothalamus and helps detect seasonal changes (Nakane et al. 2013). The pineal organ (epiphysis) is light-sensitive and lies between the midbrain and dorsal forebrain; it can be seen through the cartilage in young fish. The urophysis is a thickening of the caudal spinal cord and has neurosecretory cells with an osmoregulatory function (Stoskopf 1993; Roberts and Ellis 2012).

The thyroid gland is usually diffuse, with follicles along the ventral aorta, branchial arteries, pharyngeal cavity, and retro-orbital tissues. Thyroid hyperplasia (goiter) is common in fish and can cause oral or respiratory obstruction.

Pancreatic tissue (exocrine and endocrine) in bony fish is typically diffuse throughout the adipose tissue or along the portal veins (Caruso and Sheridan 2011). It is occasionally seen as white nodules (Brockmann bodies) in the mesentery around the bile ducts and portal veins (Caruso and Sheridan 2011). In some fish, the pancreas is associated with the venous system or capsule of the spleen. It is a discrete organ in the lungfish (*Dipnoi*) and some catfish (Stoskopf 1993).

In most fish, interrenal tissue is the equivalent of the mammalian adrenal cortex. It is found within the cranial kidney or around the posterior cardinal veins in teleosts. The suprarenal tissue is the equivalent of the mammalian adrenal medulla and consists of scattered chromaffin tissue within the cranial kidney (Stoskopf 1993; Roberts and Ellis 2012). In sculpins (*Cottus* spp.), the tissues are combined into a distinct adrenal organ.

Corpuscles of Stannius are endocrine cells in the caudal kidney of bony fish. They act like parathyroid glands and secrete teleocalcin (also called hypocalcin) which blocks calcium absorption across the gills (Roberts and Ellis 2012). Ultimobranchial bodies are endocrine cells located ventral to the esophagus or in the septum that separates the heart from the coelom. They also act like parathyroid glands and produce calcitonin for calcium regulation (Stoskopf 1993; Roberts and Ellis 2012)

It is reported that the pseudobranch may have some endocrine functions (see above). The gonads can also be considered part of the endocrine system as they secrete androgens and estrogens.

Urogenital System

Urinary System

The kidneys have hemopoietic, reticuloendothelial, endocrine, and excretory functions. They are located retrocoelomically and vary from parallel, paired structures to a fused single structure. Freshwater fish have larger kidneys (Helfman et al. 2009). In bony fish, kidneys are divided into a cranial (head) kidney and a caudal (excretory) kidney (Figure A1.15). Lymphoid tissue predominates in the cranial kidney; thyroid tissue may also be found (Stoskopf 1993). Excretory function is primarily in the caudal kidney. Ureters move urine from the collecting ducts to either urinary papilla or a urinary bladder where water resorption occurs. This bladder is not homologous to the mammalian bladder as it develops from the distal ureter and is not mesodermal in origin (Stoskopf 1993).

Internal body fluid composition and maintenance is complex and environmental circumstances play a huge role in how fish manage osmoregulation. Fluid exchange occurs at the gill, gastrointestinal tract, and kidney. In freshwater teleosts, osmoregulation is marked by a large influx of water from the environment and production of a large volume of dilute urine (Table A1.2). Sodium is taken up by the gills in exchange for protons in a process that is pH-dependent. Marine teleosts do drink water but do not absorb water through the gastrointestinal tract; instead

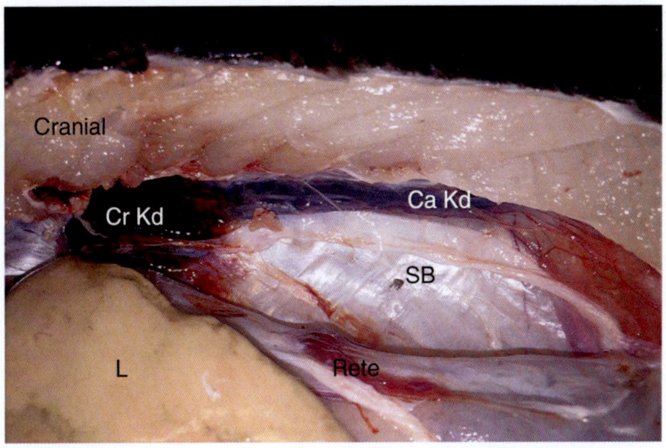

Figure A1.15 Kidneys in a deacon rockfish (*Sebastes diaconus*): cranial kidney (Cr Kd), caudal kidney (Ca Kd), opened swim bladder (SB) showing the rete, and liver (L). *Source*: Image courtesy of Catherine Hadfield, Seattle Aquarium.

Table A1.2 Fluid and electrolyte balance in freshwater and marine bony fish.

Freshwater bony fish	Marine bony fish
Hypertonic compared to the environment	Hypotonic compared to the environment
Do not drink water	Drink water
Active excretory process	Passive excretory process
Excrete large volumes of dilute urine	Excrete small volumes of urine
Ions maintained by gill and gastrointestinal uptake	Gills excrete Na and Cl. Urine is similar to plasma
	Easily become dehydrated

sodium and chloride tend to diffuse into the fish causing salt overload. The salt is mostly excreted by the gills; the kidneys are more involved in excretion of magnesium and sulfate. Marine teleosts have fewer glomeruli than freshwater teleosts and some marine teleosts are aglomerular, e.g. some seahorses (*Syngnathidae*), toadfish (*Opsanus* spp.), and goosefish (*Lophiidae*). Marine teleosts are also missing the distal segments of the nephron, including the loop of Henle. They cannot concentrate their urine above their blood osmolality and are prone to dehydration. In euryhaline species, the urinary bladder changes permeability based on environmental osmolality and regulates sodium and chloride removal. Some fish migrate between freshwater and marine environments. Fish that move from freshwater to saltwater to spawn are catadromous, e.g. true eels (*Anguillidae*). Fish that move from saltwater to freshwater to spawn are anadromous, e.g. salmonids (*Salmonidae*), sturgeon (*Acipenseridae*). For a full review, readers are directed to Hoar and Randall (1969), Hoar et al. (1983), Stoskopf (1993), and Evans et al. (2004).

Urine collection is possible but not easy. In most species, urine flow is low and continuous, limiting opportunities for collection via traditional veterinary techniques (e.g. percutaneous or catheter passage). Catheter implantation or surgically fitted collection devices are possible, but the diagnostic value of these samples is not understood (Stoskopf 1993).

Reproductive System

The reproductive system is highly variable and complex. Fish usually show separate sexes (producing sperm or ova), but hermaphroditism and parthenogenesis occur (Sloman 2011). Some bony fish show sexual dimorphism (Table A1.3). Some of the skin changes can be mistaken for pathology. Hermaphroditism is particularly common within *Perciformes*, namely parrotfish (*Scaridae*), wrasses (*Labridae*), damsels (*Pomacentridae*), and gobies (*Gobiidae*) (Sloman 2011). Hermaphroditism may be sequential or simultaneous. Sequential hermaphroditism can be divided into protandry (males become females, e.g. gilthead seabream [*Sparus aurata*] and clownfish [*Amphiprioninae*]), and protogyny (females become males, e.g. Indo-Pacific cleaner wrasse [*Labroides dimidiatus*]). Simultaneous hermaphroditism is defined by capacity to release viable eggs or sperm during the same spawning, e.g. hamlets (*Serranidae*). Parthenogenesis is less common, but examples are found, e.g. Amazon molly (*Poecilia formosa*) where all individuals are females.

Typical teleost testes are elongated, paired, and either lobular (most common) or tubular (Roberts and Ellis 2012). They are supported in the coelom by a mesorchium and surrounded by a tunica albuginea. They can be hard to differentiate grossly from ovaries in young animals, but wet mounts of the tissue can be diagnostic. The ducts can serve for both sperm transport and storage (Schulz and Nobrega 2011).

Teleost ovaries vary from clusters of follicles to a more organized organ that may be paired, fused, or coiled. They are supported within a thin mesovarium. Mature ovaries can take up a substantial amount of the coelom (up to 70%). Ovaries in bony fish are typically paired, but they are fused in some species, e.g. lampreys and hagfish (*Agnatha*), mollies and guppies (*Poecilia* spp.), and medaka (*Oryzias* sp.). There are three types of ovary (Table A1.4). In gars (*Lepisosteidae*) and most teleosts, the ovary is continuous with the oviduct, while in trout and salmon (*Salmonidae*), the oviduct is diminished or even absent and ova enter the coelomic cavity before exiting the genital pore (Helfman et al. 2009; Roberts and Ellis 2012). In live-bearing species, embryos develop in either the oviduct or the uterus (Turner 1947).

Fertilization occurs externally or internally (Table A1.5). Under human care, normal reproduction may be inhibited or altered which may result in health problems such as egg retention and oophoritis.

The reproductive systems of fish are enormously varied and important additional details can be found elsewhere (Stoskopf 1993; Farrell 2011; Wootton and Smith 2014).

Neurologic System

The teleost brain has similar components to the brain of other vertebrates: the telencephalon (forebrain); the diencephalon (epithalamus/pineal body, thalamus, and hypothalamus); the mesencephalon; and the metencephalon (cerebellum and myelencephalon or medulla oblongata). Olfactory bulbs are connected from the nares to the telencephalon. In most fish, the spinal cord extends to the tail, but it ends earlier at the urophysis in some "higher" teleosts. An exception is the ocean sunfish (*Mola mola*) whose

Table A1.3 Examples of sexual dimorphism in bony fish.

Feature	Changes	Examples
Size/shape dimorphism	Larger body in males	Discus (*Symphysodon* spp.), rainbowfish (*Melanotaeniidae*)
	Wider head in males	Channel catfish (*Ictalurus punctatus*)
	More "humped" head in males	Freshwater angelfish (*Pterophyllum scalare*)
	Large, rounded coelom in gravid females	Most species
Skin and fin changes	Brighter coloration of males during the breeding season	Zebrafish (*Danio rerio*), dwarf gourami (*Trichogaster lalius*), squarespot anthias (*Pseudanthias pleurotaenia*)
	Pearl organs or nuptial tubercles on males during the breeding season	Goldfish (*Carassius auratus*)
	Different coloration of adult males and females	Kenyi cichlids (*Maylandia lombardoi*), California sheephead (*Semicossyphus pulcher*), striped killifish (*Fundulus majalis*)
	Longer fins in males	Bettas (*Betta splendens*)
Intromittent organs	Anal fin modified into intromittent organ in males (gonopodium)	Four-eyed fish (*Anableps* spp.), guppies, mollies, mosquitofish (*Poeciliidae*)
	Ribs and pelvic bones modified into intromittent organ in males (priapium)	Priapium fish (*Phallostethus* spp.)
Urogenital changes	Urogenital pouch or patch in males	Seahorses, sea dragons, and pipefish (*Syngnathidae*)
	Rounder, larger, more concave genital papilla in females	Tilapia (*Tilapia*, *Oreochromis* spp.), carp and koi (*Cyprinus carpio*)

Source: Lodé (2012). © John Wiley & Sons.

spinal cord is shorter than its brain (Helfman et al. 2009). There are 10 cranial nerves, as with other vertebrates (Roberts and Ellis 2012).

There is a blood–brain barrier, but it is not well-characterized. The blood–brain barrier shows lower permeability in most bony fish than in elasmobranchs (Jeong et al. 2008). An exception is sturgeon (*Acipenseridae*), which are similar to the elasmobranchs (Bundgaard and Abott 2008).

Electric Organs

Some species are able to generate electric charges using electrocytes within electric organs. These are disc-like modified muscle cells. When stimulated, ions rush across cell membranes and create a small electric current. Stacks of cells essentially create batteries in series and produce an additive effect. These organs are innervated by the spinal cord and the potential voltage and frequency depend on fish species, activity level, and size (Kramer 1996; Helfman et al. 2009). Interestingly, these animals usually suffer no ill effects themselves from the electricity. It is unknown why, but reasons may include their body size, the directionality of the current, adipose under the skin, and structural proteins which provide electroprotection.

Anatomy of Cartilaginous Fish

This section highlights the differences between cartilaginous fish and bony fish (Box A1.1).

Table A1.4 Ovarian types in fish.

	Definition	Examples
Cystovarian	Ova released into oviduct	Most bony fish
Gymnovarian	Ova released into coelom, then ostium, then oviduct	Lungfish (*Dipnoi*), sturgeon (*Acipenseridae*), bowfin (*Amia calva*), cartilaginous fish
Semicystovarian (secondary gymnovarian)	Ova released into coelom, then through urogenital pore	Salmonids (*Salmonidae*)

Source: Stoskopf (1993). © 1993, Elsevier.

Table A1.5 Example of reproductive modalities in bony fish.

	Definition	Examples
Ovuliparity	Ova expelled externally, then fertilized	Salmonids (*Salmonidae*), sticklebacks (*Gasterosteidae*)
Oviparous	Internal fertilization, then ova expelled externally	Most teleost species
Ovoviviparous	Internal fertilization, retention of ova in body for embryo development, live births	Some rockfish (*Sebastidae*)
Viviparous (histotrophic or lecithotrophic)	Embryo development in body, nutrients provided by body: glandular, oophagy, adelphophagy	Guppies, mollies (*Poecilidae*)
Viviparous (hemotrophic or matrotrophic)	Embryo development in body, nutrients provided by body: pseudoplacentation or placentation	Four-eyed fish (*Anablepidae*), cusk-eels (*Ophidiidae*), some blennies (*Clinidae*), some rockfish (*Sebastidae*), splitfins (*Goodeidae*), halfbeaks (*Hemiramphidae*)

Source: Lodé (2012). © John Wiley & Sons.

Body Plan

Pelagic sharks share a similar, hydrodynamic body shape, e.g. requiem sharks (*Carcharhinidae*) and ground sharks (*Triakidae*). Epibenthic, benthic, and demersal sharks typically have large heads, more caudal dorsal fins, and lower tail angles, e.g. carpet sharks (*Orectolobiformes*). The batoids (skates [*Rajiformes*] and rays [*Myliobatiformes* and *Torpediniformes*]) and sawfish and guitarfish (*Rhinopristiformes*) show dorsoventral flattening of the body and enlarged pectoral fins. Chimaeras (*Holocephali*) show lateral compression and undulate their pectoral fins rather than their axial body.

Integument

Elasmobranchs produce placoid scales, also known as dermal denticles. These give the sandpaper feel to shark skin as well as focal areas in the skin of batoids. These denticles are formed like teeth with a calcified layer, dentin, and enamel (Moss 1977). This skin represents an abrasion risk to human handlers and exposed skin should be protected. In silky sharks (*Carcharhinus falciformis*), the denticles are minute which makes the skin softer compared to other sharks (Camhi et al. 2008). In blue sharks (*Prionace glauca*), females have a significantly thicker skin to withstand mating trauma (Camhi et al. 2008). Many rays have few to no scales e.g. whiptail rays (*Dasyatidae*), eagle rays (*Myliobatidae*), mantas and mobulas (*Mobulidae*). These species tend to have a significant mucus layer which can affect water quality during prolonged restraint. Porcupine rays (*Urogymnus asperrimus*) and some other rays have "armor" on their dorsum complicating ultrasounds from the dorsal aspect. In many batoids and some sharks, sharp spines can develop. A venomous spine or barb is present in most rays, with the exception of mantas, mobulas, and porcupine rays (Meyer and Seegers 2012). The barbs are covered by integument which includes cells where venom is created. Several barbs can be present. Chimaeras (*Holocephali*) are scaleless (except in juvenile stages) and are very sensitive to skin trauma (Didier 2004).

Elasmobranch skin has visible, symmetrical epithelial pores known as pit organs and ampullae of Lorenzini (Figure A1.16) (Hueter et al. 2004). Pit organs are free neuromasts which use sensory hair cells to detect water motion. Ampullae are gel-filled tubular structures that allow elasmobranchs to detect electric fields for navigation, prey and predator detection, and mating (Meyer and Seegers 2012). Clinicians should note that electric fields can exist in aquarium systems, especially where equipment is worn or corroded, and these impact elasmobranchs.

Musculoskeletal System

The entire elasmobranch endoskeleton is cartilaginous. It is made up of a hyaline cartilage-like core supported by mineralized tesserae (Omelon et al. 2014). Bone does exist in the form of teeth and denticles. While calcification can occur in the vertebrae and jaws, true bone is not found in those areas (Moss 1977). The centrum of the vertebral cartilage is used for aging elasmobranchs (Dean and Summers 2006). If elasmobranch cartilage is fractured, it does not heal fully but rather forms a fibrous "bandage" (Ashhurst 2004).

Many studies have examined elasmobranch skull anatomy, with particular reference to capturing prey. Three modes of prey capture occur (sometimes in combination): biting, ram feeding, and suction feeding (Wilga and Lauder 2004). Clinical relevance comes from the

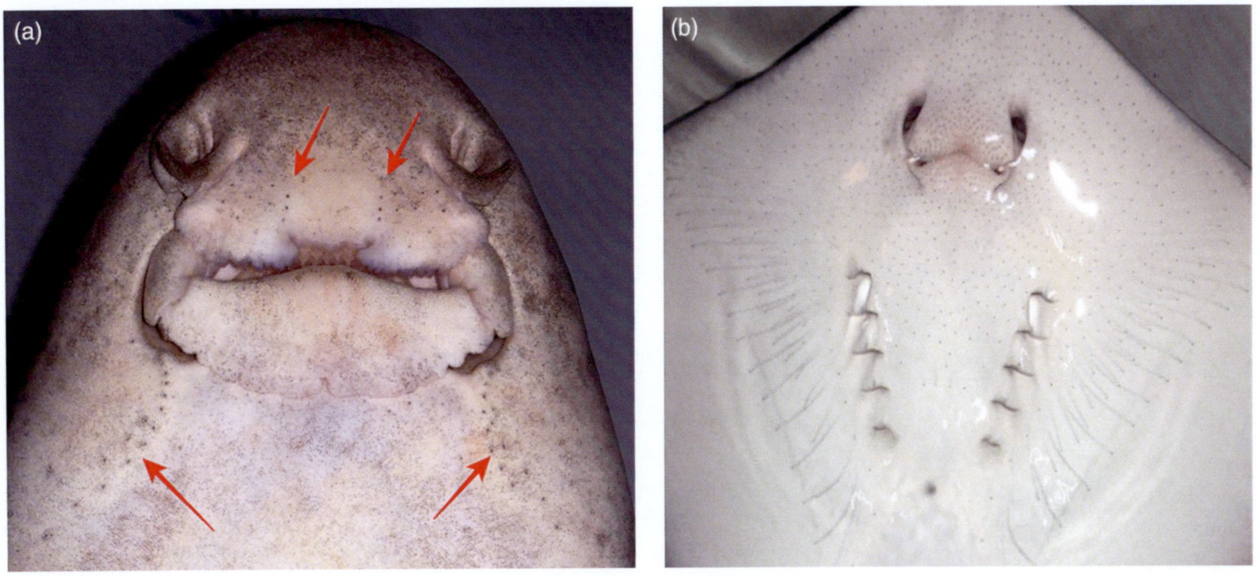

Figure A1.16 Ampullae of Lorenzini in a bamboo shark (*Chiloscyllium* sp.) (arrows) and across the ventrum of a blue-spotted stingray (*Neotrygon kuhlii*).

importance of the jaw protrusion capacity. Permanent jaw protrusion is reported to be associated with spinal deformity in sand tiger sharks (*Carcharias taurus*) (Anderson et al. 2012).

Musculature is similar to teleosts, with red and white skeletal muscle (Figure A1.17). Most elasmobranchs are poikilothermic, but regional endothermy has been described in some lamniform sharks such as makos (*Isurus* spp.), white sharks (*Carcharodon carcharias*), salmon and porbeagle sharks (*Lamna* spp.), and thresher sharks (*Alopias* spp.) (Goldman 1997; Bernal et al. 2012; Shadwick and Goldbogen 2012).

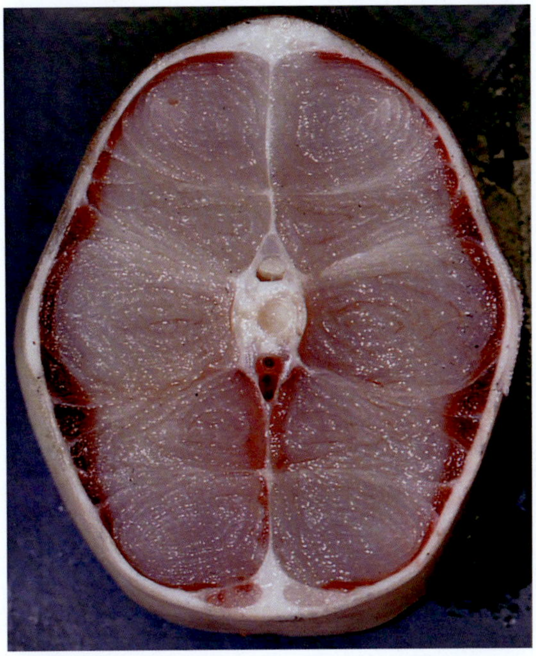

Figure A1.17 Cross-section through the peduncle of a blacktip reef shark (*Carcharhinus melanopterus*) showing red and white skeletal muscle.

Buoyancy

In cartilaginous fish, buoyancy is attributed to the cartilaginous skeleton, the large, lipid-dense liver, and urea and methylamine oxides in the blood (Withers et al. 1994; Shuttleworth 2012). No cartilaginous fish have swim (gas) bladders. The sand tiger shark (*Carcharias taurus*) typically shows a gas shadow in the stomach on imaging as it swallows air for additional buoyancy.

Ocular Anatomy

Eye anatomy in elasmobranchs is diverse. Eyelids are usually fixed, but are mobile in some species, e.g. nurse sharks (*Ginglymostoma* spp.) and catsharks (*Cephaloscyllium*), and there is a blink reflex. There is a third eyelid or nictitating membrane in some, e.g. requiem sharks (*Carcharhinidae*). Pupil type and shape are characterizing features of some species. In rays, the upper iris is modified into an operculum pupillare which covers the iris during light adaptation (Figure A1.18). The pupillary light response is highly variable: diurnal sharks exhibit rapid constriction, nocturnal sharks have an intermediate response, and batoids show the slowest response. Dilation can be produced using topical acetylcholine

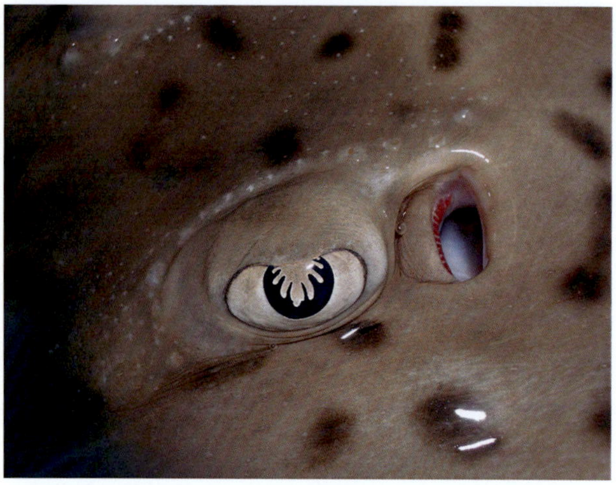

Figure A1.18 Modified iris of a clearnose skate (*Raja eglanteria*); the spiracle is visible caudal to the eye. *Source*: Image courtesy of Catherine Hadfield, National Aquarium.

(Kuchnow 1971). The sclera is thick with a cartilaginous layer. The cornea has the same layers as other vertebrates. Many sharks have a partially or totally occlusible tapetum, meaning that melanophores can migrate over the retina and block photophores to adapt to light. Some species have a fixed tapetum, e.g. catsharks and deep-sea sharks (Gruber 1977). The retina is avascular and there is no choroid gland (Gelatt 2014). Many elasmobranchs are able to pull their globes back into their eye sockets using extraocular muscles (Jurk 2002; Hart and Collin 2015). They also possess an optic pedicle which is a cartilaginous structure connecting the globe to the cranium (Gelatt 2014). The scleral cartilage, optic pedicle, and the size of the optic nerve, vessels, and muscles make enucleation much more challenging than in teleosts.

In addition to the eyes, the pineal organ/eye (epiphysis) is well-developed in most elasmobranchs, although absent in some of the electric rays (*Torpediniformes*). The photoreceptors are located superficially on the dorsal aspect of the chondrocranium (Gruber 1977).

Auditory Anatomy

The ears of elasmobranchs are similar to other vertebrates and respond to acoustical, vibrational, and gravitational forces. They are located in cartilaginous otic capsules just caudal to the large optic capsules; the only external indication of their position is tiny paired endolymphatic pores (<1 mm diameter) on the dorsal chondrocranium near the medial line (Tester et al. 1972). Each ear has an inner ear labyrinth (utriculus, sacculus, and lagena) but none of the accessory organs seen in teleosts. Within the endolymphatic duct, instead of an otolith, there is an otoconial paste of calcium carbonate granules in gel that functions like the otoliths in teleosts (Mulligan and Gauldie 1989; Popper et al. 2005). Patches of sensory epithelium known as the macula neglecta are used for vibration detection in many species (Shuttleworth 2012). Audiograms show sharks hear frequencies from 50 to 1500 Hz with greatest sensitivity at 400–600 Hz (Popper 2000; Myrberg 2001). Clinicians should recognize sensitivity of elasmobranchs to pumps and filtration equipment that produce vibration and sound in enclosed spaces.

Olfactory and Gustatory Anatomy

Olfactory bulbs are located within the rostrum and are a part of the forebrain (telencephalon); they are well-developed in elasmobranchs. The bulbs detect amino acids, bile salts, and pheromones (Evans et al. 2004). Meningitis occurs in elasmobranchs and a possible entry route is via the nares or the endolymphatic pores. Taste buds occur in the oropharyngeal cavity as with other vertebrates (Hueter et al. 2004).

Olfaction is used for feeding, particularly within 3–15 m of a prey item, while vision becomes more important at closer range (<3 m) (Hart and Collin 2015). One study showed that sharks become conditioned to the odors from normal, healthy fish within the same system. Fish can produce different odors when frightened, stressed, or excited that can stimulate predation (Tester 1963).

Oral/Pharyngeal Cavity

The types of teeth or dental plates are dictated by the feeding strategy (biting, crushing, shearing, filter feeding, etc.) and can often be used to speciate animals (Kemp 1999). The teeth or plates erupt and roll out continuously, with the caudal-most gradually replacing the front; this is polyphyodont dentition. Teeth are lyodont (embedded in the oral mucosa, not ankylosed to the jaw) and consist of dentine and enameloid. Tooth replacement rates vary among species, from 8 to 10 days per row up to 5 weeks per row (Motta 2004). If animals that normally eat crustaceans and hard-bodied prey are not provided with these foodstuffs, overgrowth of the plates can occur. Gingival hyperplasia and neoplasia have been described in sand tigers (*Carcharias taurus*) (Borucinska et al. 2004).

Denticles are present in the pharynx of most sharks (except carpet sharks, *Orectolobiformes*) and some other elasmobranchs such as guitarfish (*Rhinobatidae*). This may decrease drag for ram ventilators, prevent trauma from prey, and improve predation success (Atkinson and Collin 2012).

Gastrointestinal System

The gastrointestinal (GI) tract is short and simple, essentially a slightly S- or J-shaped tube. The ileum includes a spiral or valvular intestine that significantly increases surface area for absorption. This structure is colloquially referred to as a spiral colon but is not technically colonic tissue. The valvular intestine has four distinct variations: a spiral winding around a central column, cones directed caudally or cranially, and scroll-shaped (Hamlett 1999). The valvular intestine empties into a short tube interchangeably termed the colon and rectum (Wood et al. 2007; Theodosiou and Simeone 2012). A few elasmobranch species have a pyloric cecum or ceca, e.g. deepwater dogfish (*Somniosus* spp.) (Hamlett 1999).

The rectal gland is a unique intestinal appendage located caudal to the valvular intestine at the colon/rectum (Figure A9.7). It has an osmoregulatory function and the fluid secreted contains sodium and chloride at concentrations almost twice those of the plasma; this is in contrast to elasmobranch urine which is not concentrated (Shuttleworth 2012). The rectal gland is significantly reduced in freshwater elasmobranchs (Evans et al. 2004).

There are bilateral coelomic (abdominal) pores in the cloaca suspected to have an excretory function (Figure A6.6). They provide a possible access point for catheterization or endoscopy of the coelom.

Liver and Gallbladder

The liver is the primary lipid storage organ in elasmobranchs, which helps maintain neutral buoyancy. A large volume of lipid must be stored in the liver, and the size and density are critical in maintaining position in the water column. As the primary energy storage organ, the liver is also an indicator of general health and caloric intake, although size may fluctuate with the reproductive cycle or age (Hamlett 1999; Hussey et al. 2009). A hepatosomatic index (HSI), the ratio of liver weight to body weight, has been identified for many species as a "fitness" indicator (Sherman and Gilliam 1996; Hoffmayer et al. 2006). Grossly the liver should be tan-colored, fill a large percentage of the ventral coelom (Figure A1.19), and float in formalin; if it does not, there are inadequate lipid reserves. Normal elasmobranch livers may easily be misinterpreted as hepatic lipidosis on histology. The gallbladder is dynamic and appears to increase in size with inappetence.

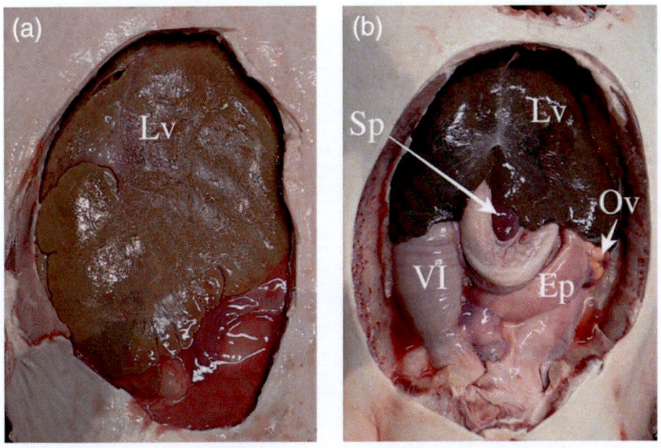

Figure A1.19 Gross appearance of a normal liver (a) and a small liver (b) at necropsy of a southern stingray (*Hypanus americanus*). The open coelom shows the liver (Lv), spleen (Sp), valvular intestine (Vl), ovary (Ov), and epigonal organ (Ep).

Respiratory System

There are usually five gill arches in elasmobranchs, although there may be up to seven. They consist of a hemibranch cranially (with one row of filaments) and holobranchs for the remaining arches (with two rows of filaments). The interbranchial septum extends to form gill slits on the external surface of the animals. The cranialmost gill slit is modified into a spiracle in some species (Figure A1.18). These are well-developed on the dorsal surface of skates and rays and they are present in some slow-moving sharks (Butler 1999). The spiracle is absent in the more pelagic sharks.

Damage to the gills can affect gas exchange as well as other physiological needs. In saltwater species, gills play an important role in acid–base balance and in freshwater species, gills are important in salt regulation. Gills are also critical for urea retention, particularly in some species like the spiny dogfish (*Squalus acanthias*) (Ballantyne and Robinson 2010).

The oral cavity is divided into orobranchial and parabranchial cavities. In species that show buccopharyngeal pumping, these areas have a double pumping action which delivers oxygenated water through the mouth or the spiracles to the gills. In ram-ventilating species, where water continually flows over the gills, the mandibular muscles control the opening of the mouth to manage the water flow (Shuttleworth 2012).

Cardiovascular System

The heart lies in a rigid pericardial chamber surrounded by a large volume of pericardial fluid. The pericardial lumen communicates with the coelomic cavity via a pericardiocoelomic canal, which is usually closed unless the pericardial fluid pressure exceeds that in the coelomic cavity. The fluid in the pericardial cavity is reported to be different from the plasma and coelomic fluid (Tota 1999; Shuttleworth 2012). The elasmobranch heart is sometimes considered four-chambered although that is a misnomer as it is not equivalent to the mammalian model. The heart consists linearly of the sinus venosus, atrium, ventricle, and conus arteriosus (similar to the bulbus arteriosus of teleosts). The sinus venosus is thin-walled and very compliant. The atrium is flaccid with a volume larger than the ventricle, the thickest of the myocardial tissues. The conus arteriosus is tubular and thick with prominent valvular structures. Detailed circulatory anatomy of elasmobranchs is available (Hoar et al. 1983; Muñoz-Chápuli and Satchell 1999). There is often a synchrony noted between respiratory and cardiac beat, but this is inconsistent and has no obvious clinical consequence (Shuttleworth 2012). Electrocardiograms are similar to other vertebrates with the exception of a V-wave (depolarization of the sinus venosus) prior to the PQRS (Shuttleworth 2012).

There is a secondary vascular system (SVS) in elasmobranchs that has different blood values than the primary system (Muñoz-Chápuli and Satchell 1999; Mylniczenko et al. 2006).

Hematopoetic and Immunologic System

Lymphomyeloid tissues of cartilaginous fish are the epigonal organ, Leydig organ, thymus, meninges of the brain, eye orbit, spleen, and gut-associated lymphoid tissue (GALT) (Rumfelt 2014).

The epigonal organ is physically associated with the gonads. In some species, the gonads are enclosed within the epigonal organs, e.g. common guitarfish (*Rhinobatos rhinobatos*) and dogfish (*Squalus* spp.), and in others the two are attached, e.g. stingrays (*Hypanus* and *Aetobatus* spp.). Generally, where there is a prominent epigonal organ, the Leydig organ is unapparent or absent.

The Leydig organ is a lymphomyeloid organ found in some species; it differs from the Leydig gland which is involved in sperm maturation. It is sometimes identifiable as a lighter-colored area within the dorsal (and occasionally ventral) submucosa of the esophagus. The area may be raised. Species with recognizable Leydig organs include skates, some rays, guitarfish, and some shark species, e.g. velvet belly lanternshark (*Etmopterus spinax*) (Rumfelt 2014).

All elasmobranchs have a bilateral thymus located dorsally near the gills (Luer et al. 1995; Rumfelt 2014). In some species, like the catsharks (*Scyliorhinus* spp.) and nurse sharks (*Ginglymostoma cirratum*), involution occurs with age and it cannot be found in adulthood. In others, it remains visible albeit small through life, e.g. bullhead sharks (*Heterodontus* spp.) and some rays (Rumfelt 2014).

The spleen is dark red and strap-like to oval in shape. Unlike mammals, it lacks marginal zones and germinal centers, likely because there is no true lymphatic system. There are melanomacrophages in the spleen and liver, but they do not aggregate as they do in teleosts (Rumfelt 2014).

Endocrine System

Elasmobranch endocrinology is complex, but the organs, stimuli, and targets of action are similar to other vertebrates.

The pituitary is similar to teleosts, with slight anatomical variations. It produces growth, thyroid, reproductive, and vasopressin-like hormones (Anderson 2015). The hypothalamus (within the diencephalon) is a well-developed organ. It is important for feeding, reproduction, aggression, and likely migration (Hofman 1999).

The interrenal gland (equivalent of the mammalian adrenal cortex) is grossly visible as a section of yellow tissue between each kidney. It is long, thin strip in sharks and a smaller oval in skates and rays (Figure A1.20). The chromaffin cells of the suprarenal bodies are separate and located on the dorsal kidneys near the dorsal aorta (Anderson 2015). The hypothalamo-pituitary-interrenal axis is considered the endocrine stress axis, although this has not been fully characterized in elasmobranchs (Shuttleworth 2012).

The single thyroid gland is encapsulated and varies in size and shape across species. In batoids, the thyroid is usually located ventral to the pharynx near the bifurcation of the ventral aorta. In sharks, it is under the commissure of the mandible. The ultimobranchial bodies produce calcitonin, similar to the mammalian parathyroid system although the actions of calcitonin in cartilaginous fish are less well-understood (Anderson 2015). In batoids, the ultimobranchial bodies are paired and found in the caudal wall of the pericardial cavity. In sharks, they are only on the left side of the body on the dorsal wall of the pericardial cavity (Stoskopf 1993).

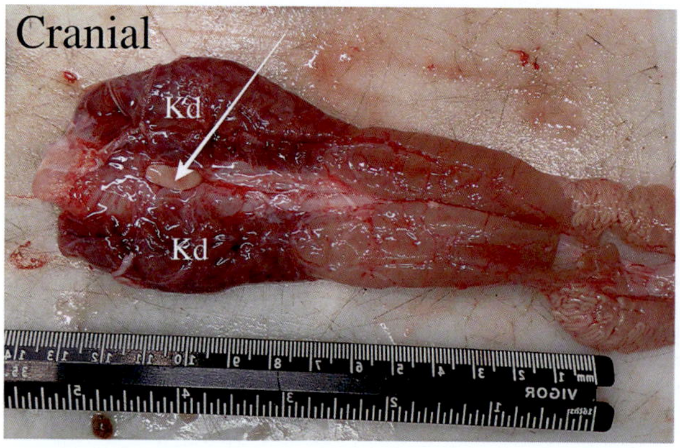

Figure A1.20 Interrenal gland (arrow) between the kidneys removed from a southern stingray (*Hypanus americanus*). *Source*: Image courtesy of Catharine Wheaton, Disney's Animals, Science and Environment.

The bilobed pancreas and gastrointestinal tract produce the expected hormones, though detail on their function and activity are limited. The heart and kidney can also be considered endocrine glands as they produce several natriuretic peptides and have a renin–angiotensin system which regulates the renal and cardiovascular systems (Anderson 2015).

The pineal organ and gonads also have endocrine functions.

Urogenital System

Urinary System

The urinary system manages osmotic and ionic regulation. Marine elasmobranchs maintain a high plasma osmolality due to high levels of sodium, chloride, urea, and methylamine oxides. They are slightly hyperosmotic to their environment, which results in an uptake of water that balances fluid lost in the urine. In contrast to marine teleosts, drinking is negligible. The gills, kidney, and rectal gland are important for maintaining homeostasis, and the kidney is the main site for urea regulation (Lacy and Reale 1999). In freshwater elasmobranchs, urea, electrolytes, and osmolality are much lower; the kidneys are microscopically simpler; and the rectal gland is significantly reduced in size and function.

The kidneys are paired and firmly attached to the dorsal wall of the caudal coelom under a thick capsule. In sharks, they lie midway in the coelomic cavity and widen as they reach caudally. In skates and rays, they are more caudal in the coelomic cavity and more lobulated. In males, the ureters leave the kidneys medially and travel along the midline to meet the seminal vesicles and sperm sacs caudally and exit through a single (or sometimes double) urogenital pore or papilla. A small urine sample may be obtained by passing a catheter past the reproductive tract; large volumes are not possible since urine production is low. A semen sample can be collected more distally and where the sacs or ampullae are.

The kidneys of marine elasmobranch are unable to produce a concentrated urine; ionic concentrations cannot be higher than those of the plasma. Glomerular filtration rates (GFRs) vary from 0.2 to 4.0 mL/kg/h, higher than seawater teleosts but similar to freshwater teleosts. Exposure to dilute environments increases the urine flow rate and decreases reabsorption of urea. Freshwater stingrays have a GFR of 8–10 mL/kg/h. Details of renal function in elasmobranchs can be found elsewhere (Evans et al. 2004; Shuttleworth 2012).

Reproductive System

The reproductive anatomy and biology of elasmobranchs are diverse. The mode of reproduction is generally split by oviparity or viviparity and fetal nutrition (Table A1.6).

Synchrony (seasonal aggregation) is important for breeding activity in some species. Gestation varies from 4.5 months to 2 years (or up to 3.5 years if you include egg cases) (Hamlett et al. 2005). Embryonic diapause has been confirmed in three species but may be more common: Australian sharpnose sharks (*Rhizoprionodon taylori*), bluntnose stingrays (*Hypanus say*), and common stingrays (*Dasyatis pastinaca*) (Waltrick et al. 2012). Parthenogenesis is a phenomenon of many elasmobranch species. Polyandry (multiple paternity) also occurs.

Sperm storage occurs in both male and female elasmobranchs. Females of many shark species store sperm in the oviducal gland. Storage time varies but may be weeks to over a year. Males store sperm in the ampullae of the distal epididymis. Storage time is weeks to months, sometimes longer (Hamlett et al. 2005).

Fertilization is internal in elasmobranchs. All males have external paired claspers (intromittent organs) that are a part of the pelvic fins. As animals mature, these get larger and become internally calcified and able to rotate.

Internal paired organs include the testes (three types: diametric, radial, and compound); genital ducts; Leydig glands which produce sperm maturation substances; and alkaline glands (Marshall's glands) in skates which produce a seminal fluid. The genital ducts (efferent ductules, epididymis, ductus deferens, and seminal vesicle) are embedded in the dorsal abdominal wall and covered by coelomic membrane. Epigonal organs can embed the testis, incorporate the caudal end, or can be distinctly separate. At copulation, sperm ejaculate through the urogenital papilla(e) and travel to the dorsal groove of each clasper. Batoids have clasper glands with many proposed functions (Hamlett et al. 2005). There are subdermal siphon sacs in sharks that are either meant for propulsion of sperm or to wash rival sperm from a female's tract. These can be prominent on ultrasound.

Surgical amputation of the claspers has been performed when necessary. This may not impact reproductive capacity as it is a transmission organ and sperm would still be active and available at the cloaca.

Ovaries in elasmobranchs are typically paired but may be single. When single, or where one is much larger than the other, the left ovary is dominant in batoids and the right in viviparous sharks. The ovaries are attached to the dorsal wall of the body cavity by a mesovarium. Ovaries have developing follicles of various sizes, follicles undergoing atresia, and corpora lutea-like tissue, all embedded together in connective tissue. The ovary can be within or separate from the epigonal organ (Hamlett et al. 2005). Hormones and functionality of the organs are highly varied and often differ from the mammalian model; see other references for details (e.g. Awruch 2016).

Table A1.6 Reproductive methods of elasmobranchs

	Reproductive method	Nutrition	Examples
Single: one egg per oviduct	Oviparous	Lecithotrophic	Bullhead sharks (*Heterodontiformes*), most skates (*Rajidae*), chimaeras (*Holocephali*)
Multiple: several eggs in oviduct	Oviparous	Lecithotrophic	Some catsharks, e.g. *Halaelurus* spp.
Yolk-sac (ovoviviparous)	Viviparous	Lecithotrophic	Most sharks
Limited (mucoid) histotrophy	Viviparous	Matrotrophic	Dogfish and lanternsharks (*Squaliformes*), angelsharks (*Squatiniformes*), sawsharks (*Pristiophoriformes*)
Lipid histotrophy	Viviparous	Matrotrophic	Rays (*Myliobatiformes*)
Oophagy (ovatrophy)	Viviparous	Matrotrophic	Some ground sharks, e.g. *Gollum, Pseudotriakis* spp. White, mako, and mackerel sharks (*Carcharodon, Isurus, Lamna* spp.)
Embryotrophy	Viviparous	Matrotrophic	Tiger sharks (*Galeocerdo cuvier*)
Adelphotrophy	Viviparous	Matrotrophic	Sand tiger sharks (*Carcharias taurus*)
Placental (placentotrophy)	Viviparous	Matrotrophic	Higher requiem sharks (*Carcharhiniformes*)

Sources: Hamlett et al. (2005) and Castro et al. (2016).

Each oviduct is differentiated into an ostium (that receives the ovum), oviducal (nidamental or shell) gland, and isthmus (in some species) which then leads to the uterus, cervix, and a common urogenital sinus. The uterus can be single or paired. When single, it is usually located on the left side of the body. In oviparous species, the uterus hardens the egg capsules and holds them until oviposition. In yolk-sac viviparous species, the uterus creates an intrauterine milieu, supplying oxygen, water, and nutrients to the embryo and regulating wastes. The uterine wall is vascularized and folded. In stingrays, there are secretory cells within uterine trophonemata (large villous projections) that also produce a milieu (histotroph) which provides nutrients. All placental species also have a limited histotrophic stage after absorption of the yolk sac and before placental implantation where the uterus provides nutrients (Hamlett et al. 2005). Since placentation is a complex subject, the reader is directed elsewhere (Hamlett et al. 2005).

Neurologic System

The elasmobranch cranium encloses the brain, olfactory bulbs, and optic and otic organs. Similar to bony fish, the brain is composed of the telencephalon (forebrain); diencephalon (epithalamus, thalamus, and hypothalamus); and mesencephalon (with the cerebellar body and auricles and the medulla) (Northcutt 1977; Hofman 1999; Shuttleworth 2012).

The brains of elasmobranchs vary widely in shape and size. Some groups show an obvious asymmetry within the cerebellum, including rays (*Myliobatiformes*), requiem sharks (*Carcharhinidae*), and hammerhead sharks (*Sphyrnidae*). This asymmetry is notable on gross examination and should not be assumed to be pathological (Northcutt 1977). Cranial nerves are similar to other vertebrates.

The choroid plexus forms the cerebrospinal fluid (CSF); there is a large space rostral to the brain where this fluid can be collected. The electrolyte composition of CSF and plasma is different and regulated independently. The blood–brain barrier is different from other vertebrates in that the endothelium is permeable but there are tight junctions between glial cells (Bradbury 1979; Shuttleworth 2012).

Electric Organs

Electric (torpedo) rays (*Torpediniformes*) have large electric organs (electroplaques) on either side of the gill arches derived from branchial musculature that can produce moderate electric discharges (Shuttleworth 2012). Skates (*Rajiformes*) can produce weak electric discharges from small bilateral electric organs in the tail (Smeets et al. 2012). Both groups are capable of intermittent and focused discharges (Sisneros and Tricas 2002). As with teleosts capable of electric discharges, the co-ordination of this discharge originates in the medulla (Sisneros and Tricas 2002; Smeets et al. 2012). The relatively low amplitude of 20–40 mV from skates contrasts with 30–60 V from electric rays (Sisneros and Tricas 2002).

Taxonomy

There is limited literature in the veterinary field on fish taxonomy, yet taxonomy relates directly to the anatomy, physiology, and disease susceptibility of these species. The following is a brief description of some of the more important fish orders and their key features. Details on classification can be found elsewhere; this section will focus on attributes that may impact clinical interpretation of disease processes and diagnostic findings. See Nelson et al. (2016) or Helfman et al. (2009) for additional details.

Taxonomy of Bony Fish (*Osteichthyes*)

Acipenseriformes (Sturgeons, Paddlefish)

Sturgeons and paddlefish are large, long-lived, freshwater fish. They have a heterocercal fin with a large dorsal lobe similar to sharks and a reduced or absent preopercle (part of the operculum) such that some of the gills are grossly visible. They have spiracles, similar to some elasmobranchs. The skeleton is mostly cartilaginous. They have a spiral valvular intestine. Gills are often brown in color and this should not be mistaken for methemoglobinemia. Paddlefish have gill rakers. Their skin is largely scaleless although sturgeons have solid dermal plates. They have a prominent pneumatic duct to the swim bladder, so care should be taken when passing a gavage tube. They have a single, simple swim bladder that is asymmetrical and positioned on the right side of the body (Helfman et al. 2009; Nelson et al. 2016).

Amiiformes (Bowfin)

The bowfin (*Amia calva*) is the only extant species of this order. They are freshwater predatory fish with long, sharp teeth, and two protruding tube-like nares. They have spiracle remnants and their skeleton is predominantly cartilaginous. They are physostomous and the swim bladder can function as a lung. There is a rudimentary spiral valvular intestine. Scales are cycloid rather than the ganoid scales typical of similar "primitive" fish. Kidney tubules open directly into the coelomic cavity. They are often mistaken for burbot (*Lota lota*) or snakeheads (*Channidae*) (Helfman et al. 2009; Nelson et al. 2016).

Anguilliformes (Eels)

Most eels are within the *Anguilliformes*. Important families include freshwater eels (*Anguillidae*) and moray eels (*Muraenidae*). Some freshwater eels are important food fish, e.g. European eel (*Anguilla anguilla*), short-finned eel (*Anguilla australis*), Japanese eel (*Anguilla japonica*), and American eel (*Anguilla rostrata*). These have complicated life cycles including freshwater and marine life stages (catadromous, moving from freshwater to saltwater to spawn) and long migrations. Some moray eels are common in display aquaria, e.g. green morays (*Gymnothorax funebris*) and zebra morays (*Gymnomuraena zebra*). They lack a pelvic girdle and most also lack a pectoral girdle. Scales are typically absent, but if present, they are cycloid and embedded. Moray eels have two sets of jaws: oral and pharyngeal (Figure A1.8). Eels can inflict a painful bite on handling. The gill opening is narrow and visualization of gills is difficult without endoscopy. The swim bladder has a single lobe (Trischitta et al. 2013). Radiographs have been used for diagnosis of swim bladder nematodes in *Anguillidae* (Palstra et al. 2007).

Beryciformes (Soldierfish, Squirrelfish, Pinecone Fish, Flashlight Fish)

These marine fish often have deep bodies and large eyes. They are prone to ocular disease, specifically gas bubbles. They tend to be nocturnal or cave dwellers. Soldierfish and squirrelfish are often dark red in color. Pinecone (*Monocentridae*) and flashlight fish (*Anomalopidae*) have bioluminescent bacteria (*Photobacterium fischeri*) in pockets of skin or in light organs near the eyes. The bioluminescent bacteria are susceptible to antibacterials. Some species have spinoid scales, where the trailing edges of scales have spines (Hoar et al. 1983; Nelson et al. 2016).

Characiformes (Piranha, Tetras, Hatchetfish)

Of these, tetras and hatchetfish are common in public and home aquariums, e.g. neon tetras (*Paracheirodon innesi*). *Characiformes*, along with *Cypriniformes*, *Siluriformes*, and *Gymnotiformes* have a Weberian apparatus (bones which connect the swim bladder to the inner ear). They have ctenoid or ctenoid-like scales, apart from the naked tetra (*Gymnocharacinus bergii*) which lacks scales. Feeding specializations of this group are diverse, including detritivory, herbivory, planktivory, predatory; some have well-developed teeth (Helfman et al. 2009).

Clupeiformes (Herrings, Anchovies)

This group includes some of the most important forage and food fish. They tend to be silvery with a consistent body plan. They have an unusual swim bladder that extends from the inner ear (otophysic) to the anus and into the lateral lines. This increases sensitivity to low-frequency sounds from other fish (Helfman et al. 2009). They are schooling and may be seen in aquaria as "balls" of fish.

Cypriniformes (Carp, Goldfish, Koi, Minnows, Zebrafish, Algae-Eaters, Loaches)

This large group of mostly freshwater fish includes several species that are common in the home aquarium or pond including goldfish (*Carassius auratus*) and common carp (*Cyprinus carpio*), of which koi are a subspecies (*Cyprinus carpio koi*). Carp are also important foodfish. Zebrafish (*Danio rerio*) are common aquarium and research animals.

The mouth, jaws, and palate are toothless but there are pharyngeal teeth in most (except algae-eaters) with a basioccipital grinding pad or "carp stone" on the dorsal pharynx. These stones are shed periodically and are often noted by owners. Algae-eaters, loaches, and suckers have oral modifications that allow them suck onto rocks and scrape algae. There is no stomach; the esophagus appears to go straight into the intestine. They have a Weberian apparatus. They are physostomous with two-chambered swim bladders, although many fancy goldfish have lost the caudal lobe (Roberts and Ellis 2012; Nelson et al. 2016; Roberts-Sweeney 2016).

Elopiformes (Tarpon, Ladyfish)

Elopiformes have an upturned mouth with a long gular plate between the lower jaws. Scales are cycloid and particularly large and thick in tarpon (*Megalops* spp.), making phlebotomy and injections difficult (Helfman et al. 2009). The swim bladder is lung-like and tarpon are facultative air-breathers. Tarpon have additional cranial outgrowths of the swim bladder that contact the auditory region and are partially enclosed in bony bullae, which presumably improve their sense of hearing (Fletcher and Crawford 2001).

Gobiiformes (Gobies, Mudskippers)

Previously classified within *Perciformes*, gobies are predominantly marine and benthic or burrowing. They lack swim bladders. Mudskippers are amphibious fish. Adaptations include a thickened epidermis with mucus cells, large gill chambers that can hold water, modified fins to allow terrestrial locomotion, and air-breathing across the cutaneous and pharyngeal epithelium. They are also able to simultaneously see out of water as well as in water.

Lepisosteiformes (Gars)

These are large, carnivorous, predominantly freshwater fish. The body and jaws are long with mouths that have needle-like teeth. They have heavy rhomboid, interlocking ganoid scales. The swim bladder is heavily vascularized for air-breathing (Figure A1.14) (Nelson et al. 2016). The vertebral centra are opisthocoelous (concave on their caudal surface, convex on the cranial, creating a ball-and-socket joint) rather than the amphicoelous centra of most other fish (concave on both surfaces) (Helfman et al. 2009).

Lophiiformes (Frogfish, Anglerfish)

This group shows a specific feeding mechanism where the first dorsal spinous process is modified into a line/rod and lure/bait (illicium and esca) to capture prey. The illicium and esca can be regenerated if damaged. Their bodies are stocky with large upward-pointed mouths to accommodate surprisingly big prey. They lack an operculum and instead have an opening behind the pectoral fins which facilitates propulsion. The swim bladder is physoclistous in some and missing in other species (Pietsch 1984; Nelson et al. 2016). Under managed care, they can be particularly hard to convert onto frozen-thawed foods and many individuals will only feed on live foods.

Osteoglossiformes (Arowana, Arapaima, Freshwater Butterflyfish, Elephantfish, Knifefish)

Known as the "bony tongues", they have well-developed teeth on the tongue and roof of the mouth that provide a shearing bite. The intestine curls around to the left of the esophagus and stomach; in most fish, it passes to the right (Nelson et al. 2016). They possess one or two pyloric ceca.

Arapaima (*Arapaima* spp.) are some of the largest freshwater fish in the world and have large, corrugated scales which complicate venipuncture and injections. They are obligate air-breathers.

Freshwater butterflyfish (*Pantodon buchholzi*) have greatly enlarged pectoral fins just dorsal to their large pelvic fins. They have a swim bladder and are obligate air-breathers. They are not related to marine butterflyfish.

Elephantfish (*Mormyridae*) have a proboscine snout. Many generate weak electric fields to locate objects and for communication (up to 10 V at low frequency) (Roberts 2011). The electric organ is derived from muscle and located in the peduncle. Their cerebellum is large and they show excellent learning skills. They have an otic gas-bladder that is separate from the swim bladder. Eyes are small and show adaptations to low light, including small reflective cups on the retina. There is only a left gonad. Uniquely, the sperm have no flagellum (Hopkins et al. 2007).

The African and Asian knifefish (*Notopteridae*) lack many fins (anal, caudal, and pelvic) but have one long dorsal fin. They also generate weak electric fields. They have small eyes and poor eyesight (Nelson et al. 2016). They are not related to the South American or neotropical knifefish (*Gymnotiformes*).

Perciformes (Perch-Like Fish)

This is the largest order of fish with a high level of diversity and confusing taxonomy (see Helfman et al. 2009; Nelson et al. 2016). These are "typical fish". Species that may be commonly seen in display aquariums and aquaculture include the following:

- *Acanthuridae*: tangs, doctorfish, surgeonfish. These have one or more scalpel-sharp spines bilaterally on the tail that can present a significant hazard during restraint.
- *Anabantidae*: gouramis, bettas. This group uses a suprabranchial organ as the primary breathing apparatus;

they need an air space to survive. Males create bubble nests as part of their reproductive strategy. The lips have horny teeth used for scraping algae.

- *Blenniidae*: blennies, cleaner wrasse. These animals often bury. They create water flow over the gills while buried using branchiostegal membranes that form small gill openings and function as a ventral pump, rather than the lateral opercular pumping of other fish. They also have finger-like projections that keep sand out of the gills.
- *Carangidae*: jacks, dolphinfish, cobia, remoras, look-downs. Remoras lack a swim bladder and have a unique disc on their head for adhering onto other animals. In some jacks, the swim bladder extends to the end of the peduncle.
- *Chaetodontidae*: marine butterflyfish. These have a spine at the angle of the preopercle. The gastrointestinal tract is coiled many times. The swim bladder has two cranially directed processes.
- *Cichlidae*: cichlids, freshwater angelfish, discus, tilapia. Tilapia are important foodfish (*Oreochromis* spp.). These fish have a single nare on either side of the face, unlike the paired, rostral nares of most species. These fish have unique and highly organized breeding activities and may be mouthbrooders or substrate brooders. Female discus secrete a milk-like substance from the skin to feed their fry.
- *Pomacanthidae*: marine angelfish. These have a spine at the angle of the preopercle that can be a hazard during handling (Figure A1.21).
- *Scorpaeniformes*: gurnards, scorpionfish, stonefish, rockfish, lionfish, sculpins. Most lack scales, but scales are ctenoid when present. The swim bladder is absent in some genera (*Plectrogenium* and *Sebastolobus* spp.). The gurnards (*Triglidae*) have huge pectoral fins which expand as they walk along the substrate using their pelvic fins. Most have spines projecting from the head including a caudally directed spine derived from a bone below the eye. In scorpionfish (*Scorpaenidae*, which includes the lionfish *Pterois* spp.) and stonefish (*Synanceiidae*), there are venomous spines along their dorsal, anal, and pelvic fins. Lumpfish (*Cyclopteridae*) are round with bony tubercles arranged in rows around their body and a sucking disc made up of modified pelvic fins. Most show internal fertilization and some show live births (e.g. *Sebastes* spp.) (Helfman et al. 2009; Nelson et al. 2016).

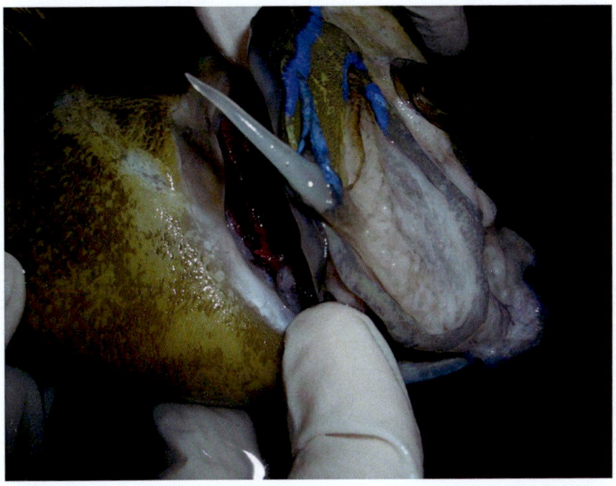

Figure A1.21 Preopercular spine on a marine angelfish. *Source*: Image courtesy of Catherine Hadfield, National Aquarium.

Pleuronectiformes (Flounder, Sole, Halibut)

Flatfish start their lives with a typical fish body plan (laterally compressed and bilaterally symmetrical) but as they mature, one eye migrates to the top of the skull and the body becomes dorsoventrally compressed. The most typical orientation is dextral (both eyes on the right side, lying on the left side) but even within the same species, sinistral orientation can occur. The eyeless side is ventral and light-colored while the side with eyes is pigmented. The dorsal fin extends onto the head at the neurocranium in most species, except spiny turbots (*Psettodes* spp.). There is no swim bladder. Other adaptations include the asymmetrical location of the mouth and protrusible eyes.

Salmoniformes (Salmon, Trout, Char)

Extant species are all within the family *Salmonidae*. Salmonids are important in aquaculture and fisheries. They are physostomous with small cycloid scales. They have pyloric ceca. There is obvious sexual dimorphism in mature adults, with modified jaws (kypes) seen in mature males (Figure A1.22). Many species migrate between freshwater and saltwater, although not all rely on migration, e.g. rainbow trout (*Oncorhynchus mykiss*) typically remain in freshwater but some populations, known as steelheads, migrate back to freshwater after spending two to three years in saltwater.

Siluriformes (Catfish)

This group lacks scales but some have bony plates or tubercles. They can produce abundant mucus which is used for cutaneous respiration (Bruton 1996). They have small eyes and up to four pairs of barbels that are chemosensory and tactile (Helfman et al. 2009). In some catfish, the spine-like rays at the front of the dorsal and pectoral fins have glandular cells that secrete a toxin with variable levels of potency. The pancreas is visible as white nodules (Brockmann bodies). They are physostomous with a bilobed swim bladder, but they are generally negatively buoyant due to the small swim bladder and heavy skull. Males in some families have an anal fin modified into an intromittent organ (Melo et al. 2011). Electric catfish (*Malapteruridae*) have bilateral electric organs in the skin that can emit up to 300 V at high frequency (Johnels 1956; Helfman et al. 2009).

Syngnathiformes (Seahorses, Sea Dragons, Pipefish, Trumpetfish, Shrimpfish)

These were historically classified within the *Gasterosteiformes*. The seahorses, sea dragons, and pipefish are within the family *Syngnathidae*. They have thick dermal scutes or plates. Seahorses have prehensile tails and lack caudal fins. Gills are unique with lobate gill filaments and a spherical appearance; there is a small opening on the top of the head instead of an operculum, limiting access to the gills. The oral cavity is a tube with an upturned mouth. The esophagus makes a sharp curve downward at the neck which requires gentle manipulation to get past when gavaging. Some species are aglomerular, others have some glomeruli (Stoskopf 1993; Koldewey 2005). The male maintains the brood in a pouch or on a patch at the base of the tail (Helfman et al. 2009). In the male, the elongated genital opening caudal to the anal fin represents the opening to the brood pouch; the anal opening is cranial to the anal fin. In females, no patch or pouch is present and the reproductive and anal openings are both cranial to the small anal fin.

Tetraodontiformes (Pufferfish, Triggerfish, Filefish, Ocean Sunfish)

The order is named for the four "teeth" in the outer jaws of pufferfish; these teeth are actually sharp-edged jaw bone. They lack ribs. The skin is thick, tough, and covered by scales that are modified into spines, bony plates, or ossicles. The first dorsal spine is prominent, particularly in the triggerfish and filefish. The base of the second spine fits into a groove in the first spine, locking it. They can create grunting noises via vibration of the swim bladder by the pectoral spines. The eyes can rotate independently. Puffers can inflate their bodies with water (or air, if exposed) as a defense. They also have toxins in their tissues (tetrodotoxin).

The ocean sunfish (*Mola mola*), seen in some commercial aquariums, have a unique shape thanks to the clavus that replaces the caudal fin. They also lack pelvic fins and a swim bladder, which is unique for this order. They have more cartilage than other teleosts, particularly in the skull and fin girdles. The spinal column has fewer vertebrae than any other fish. Females produce the most eggs of any vertebrate (>300 million) (Helfman et al. 2009; Nelson et al. 2016).

Sarcopterygii (Coelacanths, Lungfish)

These are the lobe-finned fish. Coelacanths (*Latimeria* spp.) are rarely seen and were considered extinct until a specimen was discovered in the 1930s. Lungfish (*Dipnoi*) species come from Australia, Africa, and South America. In all species, the pectoral and pelvic fins are on fleshy stalks extending from the body from a type of humerus or femur similar to the teleost model of multiple bones. Lungfish have electrosensory ampullae over the head and trunk. They have tooth-plates and teeth that are on the interior jaw bones rather than the margins. There is a spiral valve distal to the duodenum, except in Australian species where the valve starts at the esophagus. The atrium and ventricle are partly divided by a partition which more closely resembles the tetrapod four-chambered heart than typical fish hearts (Jorgensen and Joss 2016).

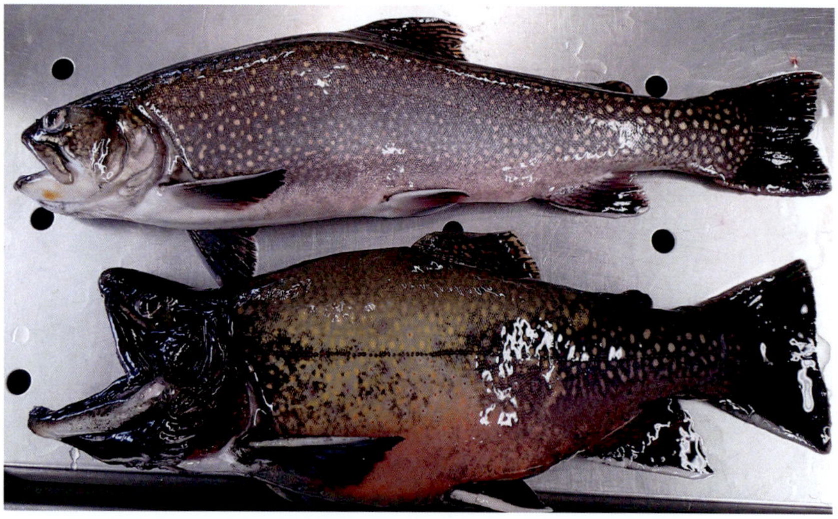

Figure A1.22 Sexual dimorphism in brook trout (*Salvelinus fontinalis*); a female is at the top of the image. *Source*: Image courtesy of Catherine Hadfield, National Aquarium.

Australian lungfish (*Neoceratodus forsteri*) are the largest, with well-developed tooth-plates. Scales are cycloid, large, and thick. Four gill arches are present. They are facultative air-breathers. There is a single lung. Sexual maturation occurs at 15–20 years and longevity is 65–70 years, with some living beyond this time frame.

African lungfish (*Protopterus* spp.) have pectoral and pelvic fins that are thinner and more filamentous. Their scales are small. The gilled lungfish (*Protopterus amphibius*) are most easily identified as they retain three large external gills on the sides of the head; otherwise only larvae have external gills. Six gill arches are present. They are obligate air-breathers with paired lungs (Figure A1.14). They are known for their ability to estivate in dry habitats for remarkable periods of time (seven to eight months, up to four years experimentally). Aestivation involves constructing a burrow which is filled with mucus that dries to form a cocoon. When estivating, the animal breathes air, its heart rate drops, and body proteins are metabolized.

South American lungfish (*Lepidosiren paradoxa*) have small scales and thin, filamentous fins. They have five gill arches, with external gills as larvae. They are obligate air-breathers with paired lungs as adults. Estivation occurs in burrows but is poorly documented (Helfman et al. 2009; Jorgensen and Joss 2016; Nelson et al. 2016)

Taxonomy of Cartilaginous Fish (*Chondrichthyes*)

The cartilaginous fish are divided into the chimaeras (*Holocephali*) and elasmobranchs (sharks (*Selachimorpha*) and skates, rays, guitarfish, and sawfish (*Batoidea*)). We will highlight the more popular aquarium species in taxonomic groups.

Chimaeriformes (Chimaeras, Ratfish, Ghost Sharks)

Chimaeriformes have a cartilaginous skeleton like elasmobranchs, but the upper jaw with grinding tooth-plates is fused to the cranium. There is one gill opening (a small operculum) over the gills; they lack a spiracle except as embryos. The eyes cannot regulate the light going onto their retinas, so exposure to bright lights is a concern. Additionally, a condition termed "bloody eye" has been reported that is a result of handling-induced damage to the pseudobranchial artery (Tozer and Didier 2004). The skin is scaleless except for denticles over the pelvic claspers and tenaculum (a club-like clasping organ on the head). The dorsal spine is venomous and can cause moderate discomfort to humans. They lack a stomach, ribs, epigonal and Leydig organs; there is a spiral intestine and a rectal gland. There are separate anal and urogenital openings, unlike the cloaca of elasmobranchs. Males have claspers and fertilization is internal (Honma et al. 1984; Tozer and Didier 2004; Nelson et al. 2016).

Carcharhiniformes (Ground Sharks)

This is the largest order of sharks. There are two dorsal fins in most and an anal fin, five gill slits, a nictitating membrane, and the mouth extends behind the eyes. They can be oviparous, ovoviviparous, or viviparous. Relevant families include the requiem sharks (*Carcharhinidae*), catsharks (*Scyliorhinidae*), hound sharks (*Triakidae*), and hammerhead and bonnethead sharks (*Sphyrnidae*).

Requiem sharks look like the "typical shark". There is an internal nictitans and spiracles are absent. The intestine has a scroll valve. Catsharks have rudimentary nictitans, small spiracles, and a spiral valve. Hound sharks have spiracles and a spiral valve. The hammerheads and bonnetheads have lateral extensions to their heads (cephalofoil) with eyes perched on the lateral aspects. Spiracles are absent and they have a spiral valve (Nelson et al. 2016).

Lamniformes (Mackerel Sharks, White Sharks, Sand Tigers)

There have two dorsal fins and an anal fin. Five gill slits are present that are broad and extend beyond the base of the pectoral fin. Sand tiger sharks (*Carcharias taurus*) differ in that the gills are in front of the pectoral fin. Spiracles are present behind the eyes but are small. The eyes lack a nictitating membrane. The mouth extends behind the eyes. They have a ring-type spiral intestine. This group is unique in its practice of oophagy or adelphotrophy (uterine cannibalism) (Nelson et al. 2016). Some members of this group practice endothermy, e.g. white (*Carcharodon carcharias*) and mako sharks (*Isurus* spp.).

Squaliformes (Dogfish, Gulper Sharks)

Two dorsal fins are present which may have spines; anal fins are absent. There are five gill slits and spiracles. A small nictitating membrane is present in the lower lid (Nelson et al. 2016). The spiny dogfish (*Squalus acanthias*) has been a common species in research studies.

Orectolobiformes (Carpet Sharks, Wobbegongs, Bamboo Sharks, Nurse Sharks)

These have two dorsal fins and an anal fin. Five gill slits with spiracles are close to the eyes. There is no nictitating membrane and eyes are dorsolateral on the head. Most have prominent nasoral grooves with barbels. Wobbegong sharks (*Orectolobidae*) have a dorsoventrally flattened head and body, rostral mouths, and fang-like teeth. Bamboo (*Hemiscyllidae*) and nurse sharks (*Ginglymostomatidae*) are some of the most frequently kept species in aquaria. This group also includes the whale sharks (*Rhincodon typus*); these are plankton feeders and the largest fish in the world (Nelson et al. 2016).

Rajiformes (Skates)

Skates are dorsoventrally compressed with enlarged pectoral fins that are continuous with their heads. They have a caudal fin and no anal fins; some have dorsal fins. The tail has no barbs. They are oviparous. The skin frequently has thorns. Some animals in the group have weak electric organs (Ebert and Sulikowski 2008; Nelson et al. 2016).

Myliobatiformes (Cownose Rays, Stingrays, Manta Rays)

These animals include the typical stingrays. These show dorsoventral compression with enlarged pectoral fins that are continuous with their heads. The five gill openings are ventral. Eyes and spiracles are on the dorsal surface and water is pulled in through the spiracles for respiration. The jaws are protrusible and do not articulate with the neurocranium (Nelson et al. 2016). There is no nictitating membrane and the cornea attaches directly to the skin around the eyes. The cranial vertebrae are fused with the pectoral girdle (synarcual). There is no anal fin. Most have one or more venomous spines (barbs) along the tail. Some key aquarium families are listed below.

- *Aetobatidae*, *Myliobatidae*, *Mobulidae*, *Rhinopteridae*: eagle rays, mobulids, cownose rays. These have a small dorsal fin on the base of the tail. The head is elevated above the pectoral fins and the eyes and spiracles are lateral on head. Tooth-plates are made up of six-sided teeth in a horizontal arrangement. They are capable of leaping into the air. The mobulids, which include manta rays (*Manta* spp.), have cephalic lobes that are cranial extensions of the pectoral fins and assist in feeding. These animals also have gill rakers. Mobulids lack venomous barbs.
- *Dasyatidae*: whiptail stingrays. These inhabit freshwater and saltwater habitats. They have a long and slender tail.
- *Potamotrygonidae*: river stingrays. These are all freshwater species and show a reduced rectal gland. Their venom is more potent than saltwater species.

Torpediniformes (Electric Rays)

These are rays with strong electric organs derived from branchial musculature. They are dorsoventrally flattened with rounded pectoral fins. They are slow-moving, and do not use their pectoral wings much for locomotion. The skin is soft with no denticles or thorns. Their eyes are very small. There is a well-developed caudal fin (Nelson et al. 2016).

Pristiformes (Guitarfish and Sawfish)

Guitarfish (*Rhinobatidae*) have a stout tail, with two dorsal fins, and a caudal fin without a barb. Bowmouth guitarfish (*Rhina ancylostoma*) are similar but their tail is bilobed and their rostrum is unique. The sawfish (*Pristidae*), also known as carpenter sharks, have a rostrum shaped like a flat blade with non-replaceable "teeth" (modified dermal denticles) embedded on the sides (Nelson et al. 2016). The mouth and nares are ventral. Oral dentition varies but teeth are mostly blunt-edged "cobblestones" in rows. Spiracles are prominent. There are no anal fins.

Acknowledgments

Many thanks go to individuals who were instrumental in the management of this document: Carlos Rodriguez, Charlene Burns, Kevin Maxson, Shane Boylan, Jennifer Dill-Okubo, and Catharine Wheaton.

References

Ali, M.A. and Anctil, M. (2012). Retinas of Fishes: An Atlas. New York: Springer Science and Business Media.

Anderson, G. (2015). Endocrine systems in elasmobranchs. In: Physiology of Elasmobranch Fishes: Internal Processes, vol. 34B (eds. E. Shadwick, A. Farrell and C. Brauner), 457–530. Amsterdam: Elsevier, Inc.

Anderson, P.A., Huber, D.R., and Berzins, I.K. (2012). Correlations of capture, transport, and nutrition with spinal deformities in sandtiger sharks, *Carcharias taurus*, in public aquaria. *Journal of Zoo and Wildlife Medicine* 43: 750–758.

Angelidis, P., Vatsos, N.I., and Karagiannis, D. (2009). Surgical excision of skin folds from the head of a goldfish *Carassius auratus* (Linnaeus 1758). *Journal of the Hellenic Veterinay Medical Society* 58: 299–305.

Ashhurst, M.E. (2004). The cartilaginous skeleton of an elasmobranch fish does not heal. *Matrix Biology* 23: 15–22.

Ashley, L.M. and Chiasson, R.B. (1988). Laboratory Anatomy of the Shark. California: W.C. Brown Co. Publishers.

Atkinson, C.J. and Collin, S.P. (2012). Structure and topographic distribution of oral denticles in elasmobranch fishes. *The Biological Bulletin* 222: 26–34.

Awruch, C.A. (2016). Reproduction strategies. In: Fish Physiology, vol. 34A (eds. A.P. Farell and C.J. Brauner), 255–310. Amsterdam: Elsevier, Inc.

Ballantyne, J.S. and Robinson, J.W. (2010). Freshwater elasmobranchs: a review of their physiology and biochemistry. *Journal of Comparative Physiology B* 180 (4): 475–493.

Berkovitz, B.K. and Shellis, R.P. (2016). The Teeth of Non-mammalian Vertebrates. Amsterdam: Academic Press, Elsevier, Inc.

Bernal, D., Carlson, J.K., Goldman, K.J., and Lowe, C.G. (2012). Energetics, metabolism, and endothermy in sharks and rays. In: Biology of Sharks and their Relatives, 2e (eds. J.C. Carrier, J.A. Musick and M.R. Heithaus), 211–237. Boca Raton, FL: CRC Press.

Bertin, L. (1958). Organes de la respiration aquatique. In: Traité de Zoologie, vol. XIII (ed. P. Grassé), 1301–1341. Paris: Masson Publishing.

Blaxter, J.H.S. and Batty, R.S. (1990). Swimbladder "behaviour" and target strength. *Rapports et Proces-verbaux des Réunions du Conseil International pour l'Exploration de la Mer* 189: 233–244.

Block, B.A. and Finnerty, J.R. (1994). Endothermy in fishes: a phylogenetic analysis of constraints, predispositions, and selection pressures. *Environmental Biology of Fishes* 40: 283–302.

Borucinska, J.D., Harshbarger, J.C., Reimschuessel, R., and Bogicevic, T. (2004). Gingival neoplasms in a captive sand tiger shark, *Carcharias taurus* (Rafinesque), and a wild-caught blue shark, *Prionace glauca* (L.). *Journal of Fish Diseases* 27: 185–191.

Bowden, T.J., Cook, P., and Rombout, J.H.W.M. (2005). Development and function of the thymus in teleosts. *Fish & Shellfish Immunology* 19: 413–427.

Bradbury, M. (1979). Why a blood-brain barrier? *Trends in Neurosciences* 2: 36–38.

Branson, E.J. (ed.) (2008). Fish Welfare. Ames, IA: Wiley.

Bruton, M.N. (1996). Alternative life-history strategies of catfishes. *Aquatic Living Resources* 9: 35–41.

Buddington, R.K. and Diamond, J.M. (2016). Aristotle revisited: the function of pyloric caeca in fish. *Proceedings of the National Academy of Sciences* 83: 8012–8014.

Bundgaard, M. and Abbott, N.J. (2008). All vertebrates started out with a glial blood-brain barrier 4-500 million years ago. *Glia* 56: 699–708.

Burgess, S.C., Wang, J., Etoundi, A. et al. (2011). A functional analysis of the jaw mechanism in the sling-jaw wrasse. *International Journal of Design & Nature and Ecodynamics* 6: 258–271.

Butler, P. (1999). Respiratory system. In: Sharks, Skates, and Rays: The Biology of Elasmobranch Fishes (ed. W.C. Hamlett), 174–197. Baltimore, MD: JHU Press.

Camhi, M.D., Pikitch, E.K., and Babcock, E.A. (eds.) (2008). Sharks of the Open Ocean: Biology, Fisheries & Conservation. Ames, IA: Blackwell Publishing.

Carrier, J.C., Musick, J.A., and Heithaus, M.R. (eds.) (2012). Biology of Sharks and Their Relatives II: Biodiversity, Adaptive Physiology, and Conservation. Baton Raton, FL: CRC Press.

Caruso, M.A. and Sheridan, M.A. (2011). Pancreas. In: Encyclopedia of Fish Physiology: From Genome to Environment (ed. A.P. Farrell), 1286–1293. Amsterdam: Academic Press, Elsevier, Inc.

Castro, J.I., Sato, K., and Bodine, A.B. (2016). A novel mode of embryonic nutrition in the tiger shark, *Galeocerdo cuvier*. *Marine Biology Research* 12: 200–205.

Colicchia, G. (2007). Vision of fish in air. *Physics Education* 42: 1876–1883.

De Iuliis, G. and Pulerà, D. (2011). The Dissection of Vertebrates: A Laboratory Manual, 2e. Amsterdam: Academic Press, Elsevier, Inc.

Dean, M.N. and Summers, A.P. (2006). Mineralized cartilage in the skeleton of chondrichthyan fishes. *Zoology* 109: 164–168.

Didier, D.A. (2004). Phylogeny and classification of extant Holocephali. In: Biology of Sharks and Their Relatives, 1e (eds. J.C. Carrier, J.A. Musick and M.R. Heithaus), 115–138. Boca Raton, FL: CRC Press.

Douglas, R. and Djamgoz, M. (eds.) (2012). The Visual System of Fish. New York: Springer Science and Business Media.

Dutta, H.M. and Datta-Mushi, J.S. (1996). Fish Morphology. Baton Raton, FL: CRC Press.

Ebert, D.A. and Sulikowski, J. (2008). Biology of Skates, vol. 27. New York: Springer Science and Business Media.

Evans, D.H., Piermarini, P.M., and Choe, K.P. (2004). Homeostasis: osmoregulation, pH regulation, and nitrogen excretion. In: Biology of Sharks and Their Relatives, 1e (eds. J.C. Carrier, J.A. Musick and M.R. Heithaus), 247–267. Boca Raton, FL: CRC Press.

Fang, L.S. and Bada, J.L. (1990). The blue-green blood plasma of marine fish. *Comparative Biochemistry and Physiology Part B: Comparative Biochemistry* 97: 37–45.

Farrell, A.P. (ed.) (2011). Encyclopedia of Fish Physiology: From Genome to Environment. Amsterdam: Academic Press, Elsevier, Inc.

Feder, M.E. and Burggren, W.W. (1985). Cutaneous gas exchange in vertebrates: design, patterns, control and implications. *Biological Reviews* 60: 1–45.

Fishbeck, D.W. and Sebastiani, A. (eds.) (2012). Comparative Anatomy: Manual of Vertebrate Dissection. Englewood, CO: Morton Publishing Company.

Fletcher, L.B. and Crawford, J.D. (2001). Acoustic detection by sound-producing fishes (Mormyridae): the role of gas-filled tympanic bladders. *Journal of Experimental Biology* 204: 175–183.

Fredholm, D.V., Mylniczenko, N.D., and Kukanich, B. (2016). Pharmacokinetic evaluation of meloxicam after intravenous and intramuscular administration in Nile tilapia (*Oreochromis niloticus*). *Journal of Zoo and Wildlife Medicine* 47: 736–742.

Gelatt, K.N. (2014). Exotic animals: ophthalmic diseases and surgery. In: Essentials of Veterinary Ophthalmology (ed. K.N. Gelatt), 485–543. Ames, IA: Wiley.

Gerking, S.D. (2014). Feeding Ecology of Fish. Amsterdam: Elsevier, Inc.

Gilbert, S.G. (1973). Pictorial Anatomy of the Dogfish. Seattle, WA: University of Washington Press.

Goldman, K.J. (1997). Regulation of body temperature in the white shark, *Carcharodon carcharias. Journal of Comparative Physiology B: Biochemical, Systemic, and Environmental Physiology* 167: 423–429.

Graham, J.B. (1997). Air-Breathing Fishes: Evolution, Diversity, and Adaptation. Amsterdam: Academic Press, Elsevier, Inc.

Greek-Walker, M. and Pull, G.A. (1975). A survey of red and white muscle in marine fish. *Journal of Fish Biology* 7: 295–300.

Gruber, S. (1977). The visual system of sharks: adaptations and capability. *American Zoologist* 17: 453–469.

Hamlett, W.C. (ed.) (1999). Sharks, Skates, and Rays: The Biology of Elasmobranch Fishes. Baltimore, MD: JHU Press.

Hamlett, W.C., Kormanik, G., Storrie, M. et al. (2005). Chondrichthyan parity, lecithotrophy and matrotrophy. In: Reproductive Biology and Phylogeny of Chondrichthyes (ed. W.C. Hamlett), 45–81. Boca Raton, FL: CRC Press.

Hara, T.J. (1975). Olfaction in fish. *Progress in Neurobiology* 5: 271–335.

Harder, W. and Sokoloff, S. (1976). Anatomy of Fishes. Stuttgart: Schweizerbart Science Publishers.

Harms, C.A. and Lewbart, G.A. (2000). Surgery in fish. *Veterinary Clinics: Exotic Animal Practice* 3: 759–774.

Hart, N.S. and Collin, S.P. (2015). Sharks senses and shark repellents. *Integrative Zoology* 10: 38–64.

Helfman, G., Collette, B.B., Facey, D.E., and Bowen, B.W. (2009). The Diversity of Fishes: Biology, Evolution, and Ecology. Hoboken, NJ: Wiley.

Hoar, W.S. and Randall, D.J. (1969). Fish Physiology Volume 1: Excretion, Ionic Regulation, and Metabolism. Amsterdam: Academic Press, Elsevier, Inc.

Hoar, W.S., Randall, D.J., and Donaldson, E.M. (1983). Fish Physiology Volume 3: Reproduction and Growth, Bioluminescence, Pigments, and Poisons. Amsterdam: Academic Press, Elsevier, Inc.

Hoffmayer, E.R., Parsons, G.R., and Horton, J. (2006). Seasonal and interannual variation in the energetic condition of adult male Atlantic sharpnose shark *Rhizoprionodon terraenovae* in the northern Gulf of Mexico. *Journal of Fish Biology* 68: 645–653.

Hofman, M.H. (1999). Nervous system. In: Sharks, Skates, and Rays: The Biology of Elasmobranch Fishes (ed. W.C. Hamlett), 273–299. Baltimore, MD: JHU Press.

Honma, Y., Okabe, K., and Chiba, A. (1984). Comparative histology of the Leydig and epigonal organs in some elasmobranchs. *Japanese Journal of Ichthyology* 31: 47–54.

Hopkins, C.D., Lavoué, S., and Sullivan, J.P. (2007). Mormyridae. In: The Fresh and Brackish Water Fishes of Lower Guinea, West-Central Africa, vol. 1 (eds. M. Stiassny, G.G. Teugels and C. Hopkins), 219–334. Paris: IRD.

Hueter, R.E., Mann, D.A., Maruska, K.P. et al. (2004). Sensory biology of elasmobranchs. In: Biology of Sharks and Their Relatives, 1e (eds. J.C. Carrier, J.A. Musick and M.R. Heithaus), 325–368. Boca Raton, FL: CRC Press.

Hughes, G.M. and Morgan, M. (1973). The structure of fish gills in relation to their respiratory function. *Biological Reviews* 48: 419–475.

Hussey, N.E., Cocks, D.T., Dudley, S.F. et al. (2009). The condition conundrum: application of multiple condition indices to the dusky shark *Carcharhinus obscurus. Marine Ecology Progress Series* 380: 199–212.

Isokawa, S., Kubota, K., Kosakai, T. et al. (1965). Some contributions to study of esophageal sacs and teeth of fishes. *The Journal of Nihon University School of Dentistry* 7: 103–111.

Jeong, J.Y., Kwon, H.B., Ahn, J.C. et al. (2008). Functional and developmental analysis of the blood-brain barrier in zebrafish. *Brain Research Bulletin* 75: 619–628.

Johnels, A.G. (1956). On the origin of the electric organ in *Malapterurus electricus. Journal of Cell Science* 3: 455–463.

Jorgensen, J.M. and Joss, J. (eds.) (2016). The Biology of Lungfish. Baton Raton, FL: CRC Press.

Jurk, I. (2002). Ophthalmic disease of fish. *The Veterinary Clinics of North America. Exotic Animal Practice* 5: 243–260.

Kemp, N.E. (1999). Integumentary system and teeth. In: Sharks, Skates, and Rays: The Biology of Elasmobranch Fishes (ed. W.C. Hamlett), 43–68. Baltimore, MD: JHU Press.

Kleerekoper, H. and Roggenkamp, P.A. (1959). An experimental study on the effect of the swimbladder on hearing sensitivity in *Ameiurus nebulosus nebulosus* (Lesueur). *Canadian Journal of Zoology* 37: 1–8.

Koldewey, H. (2005). Seahorse husbandry in public aquariums. ZSL, London, UK. www.intaquaforum.org/hg_FAI_Syngnathid05.pdf (accessed 9 September 2018).

Kramer, B. (1996). Electroreception and communication in fishes. In: Progress in Zoology, vol. 42 (ed. W. Rathmayer), 1–119. Stuttgart: Fischer.

Kuchnow, K.P. (1971). The elasmobranch pupillary response. *Vision Research* 11: 1395–1406.

Lacy, E.R. and Reale, E. (1999). Urinary system. In: Sharks, Skates, and Rays: The Biology of Elasmobranch Fishes (ed. W.C. Hamlett), 353–397. Baltimore, MD: JHU Press.

Laurent, P. and Dunel-Erb, S. (1984). The pseudobranch: morphology and function. *Fish Physiology* 10B: 285–325.

Lodé, T. (2012). Oviparity or viviparity? That is the question. . .. *Reproductive Biology* 12: 259–264.

Luer, C.A., Walsh, C.J., Bodine, A.B. et al. (1995). The elasmobranch thymus: anatomical, histological, and preliminary functional characterization. *Journal of Experimental Zoology* 273: 342–354.

Melo, R.M.C., Arantes, F.P., Sato, Y. et al. (2011). Comparative morphology of the gonadal structure related to reproductive strategies in six species of neotropical catfishes (Teleostei: Siluriformes). *Journal of Morphology* 272: 525–535.

Meyer, W. and Seegers, U. (2012). Basics of skin structure and function in elasmobranchs: a review. *Journal of Fish Biology* 80: 1940–1967.

Mirghaed, A.T., Ghelichpour, M., Hoseini, S.M., and Amini, K. (2017). Hemolysis interference in measuring fish plasma biochemical indicators. *Fish Physiology and Biochemistry* 43: 1143–1151.

Morin, J.G., Harrington, A., Nealson, K. et al. (1975). Light for all reasons: versatility in the behavioral repertoire of the flashlight fish. *Science* 190: 74–76.

Moss, M.L. (1977). Skeletal tissues in sharks. *American Zoologist* 17: 335–342.

Motta, P.J. (2004). Prey capture behavior and feeding mechanics of elasmobranchs. In: Biology of Sharks and Their Relatives, 1e (eds. J.C. Carrier, J.A. Musick and M.R. Heithaus), 165–202. Boca Raton, FL: CRC Press.

Mulligan, K.P. and Gauldie, R.W. (1989). The biological significance of the variation in crystalline morph and habit of otoconia in elasmobranchs. *Copeia* 4: 856–871.

Muñoz-Chápuli, R. and Satchell, G.H. (1999). Circulatory system: anatomy of the peripheral circulatory system. In: Sharks, Skates, and Rays: The Biology of Elasmobranch Fishes (ed. W.C. Hamlett), 198–218. Baltimore, MD: JHU Press.

Mylniczenko, N.D., Curtis, E.W., Wilborn, R.E., and Young, F.A. (2006). Differences in hematocrit of blood samples obtained from two venipuncture sites in sharks. *American Journal of Veterinary Research* 67: 1861–1864.

Myrberg, A.A. Jr. (2001). The acoustical biology of elasmobranchs. In: The Behavior and Sensory Biology of Elasmobranch Fishes: An Anthology in Memory of Donald Richard Nelson (eds. T.C. Tricas and S.H. Gruber), 31–46. New York: Springer Science and Business Media.

Nakane, Y., Ikegami, K., Iigo, M. et al. (2013). The saccus vasculosus of fish is a sensor of seasonal changes in day length. *Nature Communications* 4: 2108.

Nelson, J.S., Grande, T.C., and Wilson, M.V. (eds.) (2016). Fishes of the World. Ames, IA: Wiley.

Nikolsky, G.V. (1963). The Ecology of Fishes. Neptune, NJ: TFH Publications.

Northcutt, R.G. (1977). Elasmobranch central nervous system organization and its possible evolutionary significance. *American Zoologist* 17: 411–429.

Oike, H., Nagai, T., Furuyama, A. et al. (2007). Characterization of ligands for fish taste receptors. *Journal of Neuroscience* 27: 5584–5592.

Ollivier, F.J., Samuelson, D.A., Brooks, D.E. et al. (2004). Comparative morphology of the tapetum lucidum (among selected species). *Veterinary Ophthalmology* 7: 11–22.

Omelon, S., Georgiou, J., Variola, F., and Dean, M.N. (2014). Colocation and role of polyphosphates and alkaline phosphatase in apatite biomineralization of elasmobranch tesserae. *Acta Biomaterialia* 10: 3899–3910.

Palstra, A.P., Heppener, D.F.M., Van Ginneken, V.J.T. et al. (2007). Swimming performance of silver eels is severely impaired by the swim-bladder parasite *Anguillicola crassus*. *Journal of Experimental Marine Biology and Ecology* 352: 244–256.

Pelster, B. (2011). Swimbladder function and buoyancy control in fishes. In: Encyclopedia of Fish Physiology: From Genome to Environment (ed. A.P. Farrell), 526–534. Amsterdam: Academic Press, Elsevier, Inc.

Phleger, C.F. (1998). Buoyancy in marine fishes: direct and indirect role of lipids. *American Zoologist* 38: 321–330.

Pietsch, T.W. (1984). The genera of frogfishes (family Antennariidae). *Copeia* 1: 27–44.

Popper, A.N. (2000). Hair cell heterogeneity and ultrasonic hearing: recent advances in understanding fish hearing. *Philosophical Transactions of the Royal Society of London B: Biological Sciences* 355: 1277–1280.

Popper, A.N., Ramcharitar, J., and Campana, S.E. (2005). Why otoliths? Insights from inner ear physiology and fisheries biology. *Marine and Freshwater Research* 56: 497–504.

Reutter, K., Breipohl, W., and Bijvank, G.J. (1974). Taste bud types in fishes. *Cell and Tissue Research* 153: 151–165.

Roberts, H.E. (ed.) (2011). Fundamentals of Ornamental Fish Health. Ames, IA: Wiley.

Roberts, R.J. and Ellis, A.E. (2012). The Anatomy and Physiology of Teleosts. Hoboken, NJ: Wiley.

Roberts-Sweeney, H.E. (2016). Anatomy and disorders of the oral cavity of ornamental fish. *The Veterinary Clinics of North America. Exotic Animal Practice* 19: 669–687.

Rumfelt, L.L. (2014). Shark reproduction, immune system development and maturation a review. In: Immunobiology of the Shark (eds. S.L. Smith, R.B. Sim and M.F. Flajnik), 51–77. Baton Raton, FL: CRC Press.

Rummer, J.L., Wang, S., Steffensen, J.F., and Randall, D.J. (2014). Function and control of the fish secondary vascular system, a contrast to mammalian lymphatic systems. *Journal of Experimental Biology* 217: 751–757.

Schulz, R.W. and Nobrega, R.H. (2011). Anatomy and histology of fish testis. In: Encyclopedia of Fish Physiology: From Genome to Environment (ed. A.P. Farrell), 611–626. Amsterdam: Academic Press, Elsevier, Inc.

Schulz-Mirbach, T., Metscher, B., and Ladich, F. (2012). Relationship between swim bladder morphology and hearing abilities–a case study on Asian and African cichlids. *PLoS One* 7: e42292.

Shadwick, R.E. and Goldbogen, J.A. (2012). Muscle function and swimming in sharks. *Journal of Fish Biology* 80: 1904–1939.

Sheridan, M.A. (1988). Lipid dynamics in fish: aspects of absorption, transportation, deposition and mobilization. *Comparative Biochemistry and Physiology Part B: Comparative Biochemistry* 90: 679–690.

Sheridan, M.A. (1994). Regulation of lipid metabolism in poikilothermic vertebrates. *Comparative Biochemistry and Physiology Part B: Comparative Biochemistry* 107: 495–508.

Sherman, R.L. and Gilliam, D.S. (1996). Hepato-somatic indices and lifestyles in some batoid elasmobranchs. *Florida Scientist* 59: 275–278.

Shuttleworth, T.J. (2012). Physiology of Elasmobranch Fishes. New York: Springer Science and Business Media.

Sidell, B.D. and O'Brien, K.M. (2006). When bad things happen to good fish: the loss of hemoglobin and myoglobin expression in Antarctic icefishes. *Journal of Experimental Biology* 209: 1791–1802.

Sisneros, J.A. and Tricas, T.C. (2002). Neuroethology and life history adaptations of the elasmobranch electric sense. *Journal of Physiology-Paris* 96: 379–389.

Sloman, K.A. (2011). The diversity of fish reproduction: an introduction. In: Encyclopedia of Fish Physiology: From Genome to Environment (ed. A.P. Farrell), 613–615. Amsterdam: Academic Press, Elsevier, Inc.

Smeets, W.J., Nieuwenhuys, R., and Roberts, B.L. (eds.) (2012). The Central Nervous System of Cartilaginous Fishes: Structure and Functional Correlations. New York: Springer Science and Business Media.

Smith-Vaniz, W.F., Kaufman, L.S., and Glowacki, J. (1995). Species specific patterns of hyperostosis in marine teleost fishes. *Marine Biology* 121: 573–580.

Steffensen, J.F. and Lomholt, J.P. (1992). The secondary vascular system. *Fish Physiology* 12: 185–213.

Stoskopf, M. (1993). Fish Medicine. Philadelphia, PA: WB Saunders, Inc.

Suedmeyer, W.K. (2006). A new(er) method for fish phlebotomy. *Proceedings of the American Association of Zoo Veterinarians*: 70–71.

Teaford, M.F., Smith, M.M., and Ferguson, M.W. (eds.) (2007). Development, Function and Evolution of Teeth. Cambridge University Press.

Tester, A.L. (1963). The role of olfaction in shark predation. *Pacific Science* 17: 145–170.

Tester, A.L., Kendall, J.I., and Milisen, W.B. (1972). Morphology of the ear of the shark genus *Carcharhinus*, with particular reference to the macula neglecta. *Pacific Science* 26: 264–274.

Theodosiou, N.A. and Simeone, A. (2012). Evidence of a rudimentary colon in the elasmobranch, *Leucoraja erinacea*. *Development Genes and Evolution* 222: 237–243.

Tota, B. (1999). Heart. In: Sharks, Skates, and Rays: The Biology of Elasmobranch Fishes (ed. W.C. Hamlett), 238–272. Baltimore, MD: JHU Press.

Tozer, H. and Didier, D.D. (2004). Husbandry of spotted ratfish, *Hydrolagus colliei*. In: The Elasmobranch Husbandry Manual: Captive Care of Sharks, Rays and their Relatives (eds. M. Smith, D. Warmolts, D. Thoney and R. Hueter), 487–491. Columbus, OH: Ohio Biological Survey.

Trischitta, F., Takei, Y., and Sébert, P. (eds.) (2013). Eel Physiology. Baton Raton, FL: CRC Press.

Turner, C.L. (1947). Viviparity in teleost fishes. *Science Monthly* 65: 508–518.

Tzaneva, V., Vadeboncoeur, C., Ting, J., and Perry, S.F. (2014). Effects of hypoxia-induced gill remodelling on the innervation and distribution of ionocytes in the gill of goldfish, *Carassius auratus*. *Journal of Comparative Neurology* 522: 118–130.

Wainwright, P.C. and Turingan, R.G. (1997). Evolution of pufferfish inflation behavior. *Evolution* 51: 506–518.

Waltrick, D., Awruch, C., and Simpfendorfer, C. (2012). Embryonic diapause in the elasmobranchs. *Reviews in Fish Biology and Fisheries* 22: 849–859.

Weil, C., Lefèvre, F., and Bugeon, J. (2013). Characteristics and metabolism of different adipose tissues in fish. *Reviews in Fish Biology and Fisheries* 23: 157–173.

Wilga, C.A. and Lauder, G.V. (2004). Biomechanics of locomotion in sharks, rays, and chimeras. In: Biology of Sharks and their Relatives, 1e (eds. J.C. Carrier, J.A. Musick and M.R. Heithaus), 139–164. Boca Raton, FL: CRC Press.

Withers, P., Hefter, G., and Pang, T.S. (1994). Role of urea and methylamines in buoyancy of elasmobranchs. *Journal of Experimental Biology* 188: 175–189.

Wood, C.M., Kajimura, M., Bucking, C., and Walsh, P.J. (2007). Osmoregulation, ionoregulation and acid-base regulation by the gastrointestinal tract after feeding in the elasmobranch (*Squalus acanthias*). *Journal of Experimental Biology* 210: 1335–1349.

Wootton, R.J. and Smith, C. (2014). Reproductive Biology of Teleost Fishes. Ames, IA: Wiley.

Yanong, R.P. (2003). Necropsy techniques for fish. *Seminars in Avian and Exotic Pet Medicine* 12: 89–105.

Zang, L., Shimada, Y., Nishimura, Y. et al. (2013). A novel, reliable method for repeated blood collection from aquarium fish. *Zebrafish* 10: 425–432.

A2

Water Quality

Catherine A. Hadfield

Seattle Aquarium, Seattle, WA, USA

Introduction

Fish health is dependent on the aquatic environment; appropriate management of water parameters is critical. The term "water quality" is commonly used when discussing these parameters. At a minimum, water quality management typically encompasses temperature, salinity, nitrogenous wastes, pH, hardness, alkalinity, and dissolved gases. Other critical parameters include additional anions and cations, chlorines, heavy metals, turbidity, and the microbiome. These values are interdependent and should be evaluated together, along with the history and observation of the system and animals.

The goal of this chapter is to provide a concise review of major parameters, including common sampling and testing methods, target values, and major interactions. Values should be compared to the known requirements for the species in the system; it is important to bear in mind that the preferences of different species held in the same habitat may vary. The parameters change over time and both recent values and historical trends need to be considered. Rapid changes are more likely to negatively impact health than slow changes, and are more likely in smaller volumes of water. Management options for water quality problems (e.g. low dissolved oxygen or high ammonia) are covered in Chapter C1.

Water Source

Water source can typically be divided into municipal water (tap water), surface water (ponds, streams, rivers, lakes, or seas), or ground water (wells, springs, or aquifers). Each source presents common advantages and disadvantages (Table A2.1). These impact the treatments required, e.g. incoming municipal water often requires treatment to remove chlorines and chloramines, while incoming surface water often requires filtration and disinfection to reduce particulates and pathogens. Any source water may require temperature correction.

Dissolved Oxygen

Dissolved oxygen (DO) is critical to support animal and microbial respiration. Low DO is a common cause of acute morbidity and mortality in fish, although species sensitivity varies (see Chapter C1). Adequate microbial respiration is essential for the biological filtration within a life support system. Since low DO can damage the microbial population supporting biological filtration, it can lead to increases in toxic nitrogenous wastes.

Frequency of testing: DO should be assayed routinely where possible (e.g. daily). DO may be monitored continuously in intensive aquaculture systems or with sensitive species. At a minimum, baseline values should be obtained for each system. DO can vary across the year, particularly for surface water, so baselines should be established across all seasons. DO should be checked prior to and during any immersion treatment, restraint, or transport.

Sampling: DO must be measured on site in the system. The result represents only that moment in time and values can change rapidly. DO should be measured in multiple locations, as it will vary with depth, water flow, and surface water agitation.

Testing: DO is measured using DO meters (Figure A2.1). Most consist of an oxygen-permeable membrane and use an oxygen-dependent chemical reaction; polarographic or galvanic electrodes measure the electric current produced. Polarographic models require the probe to be moved through the water. Fiber-optic units measure the effect of oxygen on fluorescence. Calibration is required each time a

Clinical Guide to Fish Medicine, First Edition. Edited by Catherine A. Hadfield and Leigh Ann Clayton.

Table A2.1 Common advantages and disadvantages of different water sources.

	Advantages	**Disadvantages**
Municipal water	Availability Consistency Low risk of pathogens Usually high DO Usually low H_2S and CO_2	High chlorines and chloramines May have high nitrates, phosphates, or heavy metals Cost
Surface water	Good conditions for endemic species Usually low H_2S and CO_2	Need to be physically close to the source Variable quality; changes may be seasonal High risk of pathogens High risk of toxins (e.g. harmful algal blooms, pesticides) High risk of turbidity
Ground water	Consistency Low risk of pathogens Low risk of environmental pollutants Low risk of organic matter	Variable availability Often low DO and supersaturated with N_2 Often low pH and high CO_2 Often low temperature Potentially high H_2S and Fe

CO_2: carbon dioxide; DO: dissolved oxygen; Fe: iron; H_2S: hydrogen sulfide; N_2: nitrogen.

meter is turned on. Most units are calibrated against moist room air, but the instructions in the user manual should be followed. The membrane should be replaced periodically and must be changed if there are tears or bubbles.

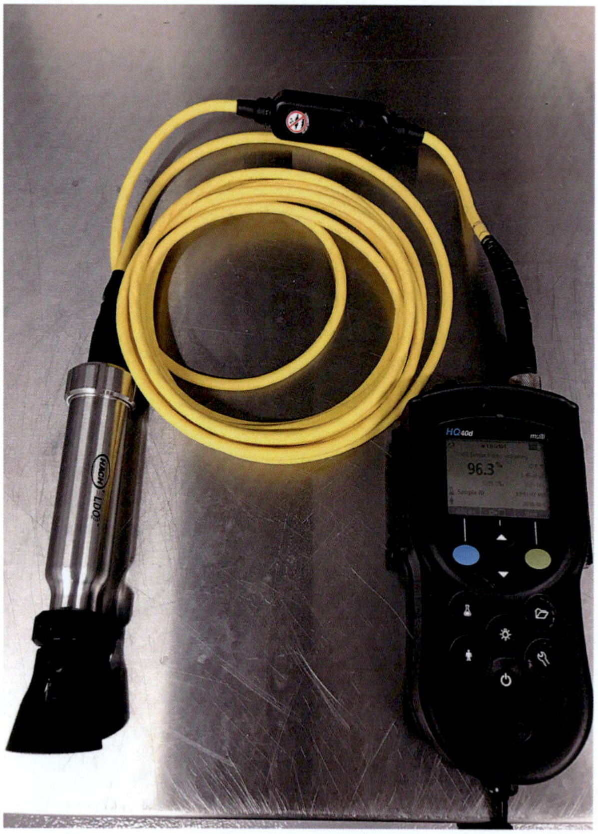

Figure A2.1 Dissolved oxygen meter.

Units: Oxygen is measured in milligrams per liter (mg/L), equivalent to parts per million (ppm). It is simultaneously reported as percentage saturation (%). This is because the amount required to saturate water varies with temperature and salinity. For example, at 10°C (50°F) in freshwater, 100% saturation is at 11.29 mg/L while at 20°C (68°F) at 20 g/L salinity, 100% saturation is at 6.19 mg/L.

Target values: Target DO is typically 6–15 mg/L or >90% saturation (Table A2.2); even if fish can tolerate lower levels, the nitrifying bacteria in biological filters require >80% saturation. Values <2–4 mg/L are likely to cause morbidity and mortality in most species.

Practical considerations:

- Low DO is a common cause of morbidity and mortality in fish. It is often due to poor water flow (e.g. because of a pump failure or in a closed transport container), reduced photosynthesis, and high organic loads. It is more problematic in warm water, because of lower solubility, and for pelagic and reef fish, because of higher oxygen demands.
- High DO is rarely a problem, although oxygen toxicity and gill damage are theoretical concerns. A safe upper limit may be 120–140%, although much higher levels are commonly used during commercial fish transports.
- DO can vary significantly across the day, particularly when vascular plants, algae, or phytoplankton are present, as these produce oxygen during daylight through photosynthesis but consume oxygen overnight. In these systems, DO values are lowest at dawn (Figure A2.2). Further discussion of low DO is provided in Chapter C1.

Table A2.2 Possible water quality parameters for some common species and groups.

	Units	Koi, goldfish, or similar freshwater species	Tropical marine fish and elasmobranchs	Tropical marine fish and corals
Dissolved oxygen	%	>90	>95	>95
Total gas pressure	%	<100–105	<100–105	<100–105
Temperature	°C	15–22	22–28	22–28
Salinity	g/L	<0.5	28–35	32–35
Unionized ammonia	mg/L	<0.02	<0.02	<0.02
Nitrite-nitrogen	mg/L	<0.1	<0.1	<0.1
Nitrate-nitrogen	mg/L	<50	<50	<15
pH	—	6.5–7.5	8.0–8.5	7.5–8.5
Alkalinity	mg/L of $CaCO_3$	50–150	>200	>200
Hardness	mg/L of $CaCO_3$	50–150	150–300	200–400
Chlorine	mg/L	<0.03	<0.03	<0.01
Iodide	mg/L	—	0.03–0.06	—

Total Gas Pressures

Total gas pressures (TGP, or total dissolved gases, TDG) include the partial pressures of oxygen, nitrogen, carbon dioxide, and argon in the water. The solubility of each gas depends on its properties as well as temperature, salinity, and total pressure. High total gas pressures (supersaturation) occur when the total of the partial pressures is greater than the atmospheric pressure. Supersaturation can cause gas emboli and associated pathology in the vasculature, eyes, or subcutaneous spaces in fish (Smiley et al. 2011). While all gases can show increased partial pressures, nitrogen is the most likely to cause gas emboli because its insolubility makes it more likely to come out of solution within the fish.

Frequency of testing: It is useful to obtain baseline gas pressures for every system; this provides a comparison if issues are seen. Gas pressures may be monitored continuously in intensive aquaculture systems.

Sampling: Gas pressures must be measured on site in the system and represent only that moment in time.

Testing: TGP meters, also known as saturometers, are used (e.g. Point Four™ Tracker, Pentair Aquatic Eco-Systems, Cary, NC). TGP meters must be kept in the water for >30 minutes as it takes time for the gases to diffuse across the membrane and produce an accurate result; the initial results need to be discarded (Figure A2.3). It is most useful to track results over at least a 24-hour period to look for transient increases.

Units: TGP is provided in milligrams per liter (mg/L). It is simultaneously reported as percentage saturation (%) relative to atmospheric pressure of air at the water surface.

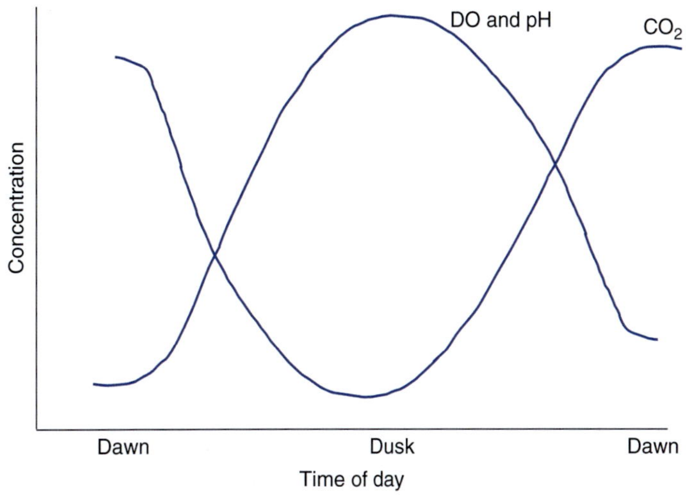

Figure A2.2 Changes in dissolved oxygen (DO), carbon dioxide (CO_2), and pH across the day due to respiration and photosynthesis.

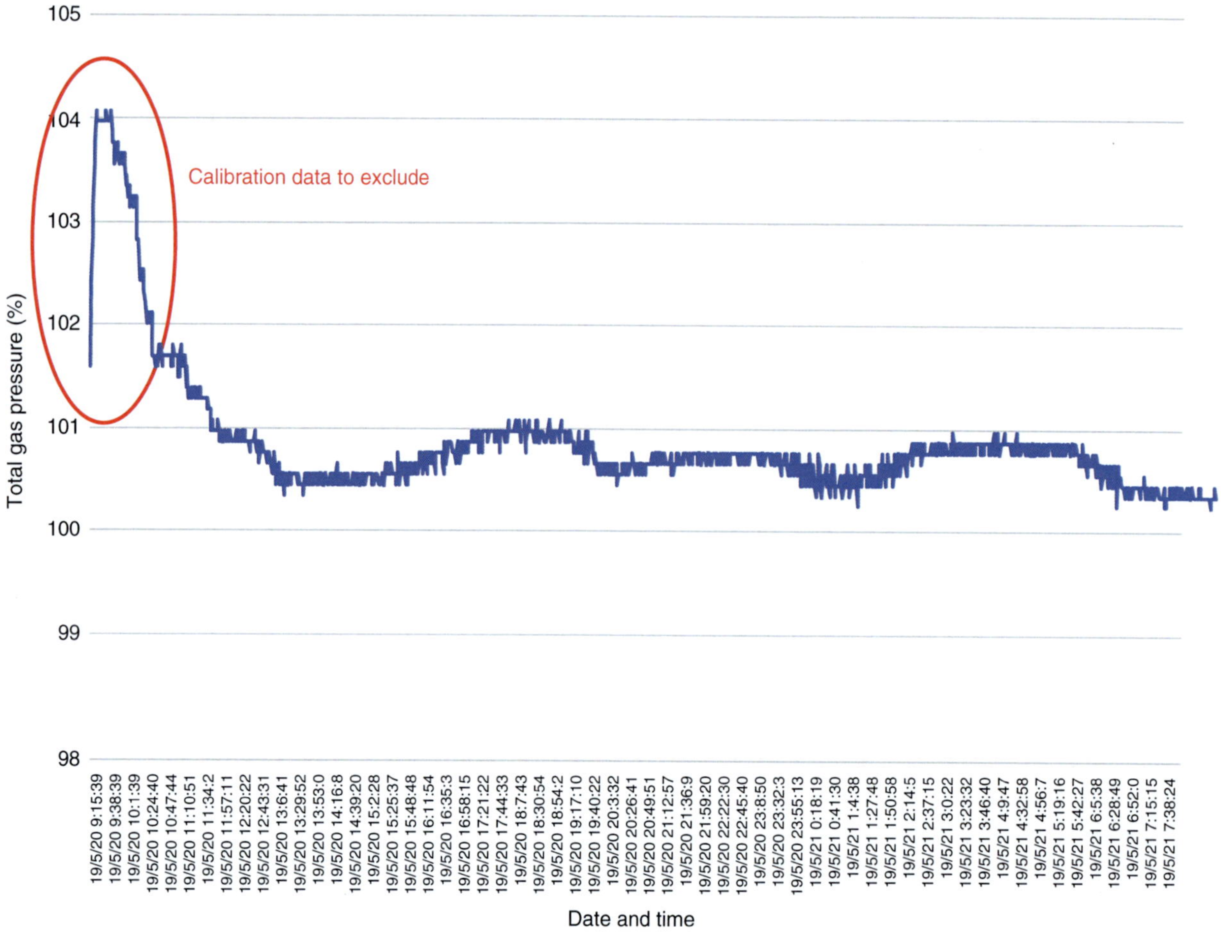

Figure A2.3 Total gas pressure meter readings from a fish system showing the initial values that are related to calibration and should be discarded.

Target values: TGP should ideally be 90–100%, but <105% is a common target (Table A2.2). Values >110% are likely to cause pathology.

Practical considerations:

- High TGPs are problematic as they can cause gas emboli in fish.
- High TGPs are often due to entrainment of air into a pump or valve due to a crack or leak upstream, turbulent water flow (particularly when at depth), or poorly designed gas-exchange towers (e.g. poor water distribution, poor selection of gas-exchange media, flooded gas-exchange media, or air entrainment leaving the tower).
- Single TGP values are less useful than serial monitoring over time (e.g. over 24 hours); supersaturation events can be transient and may be missed with a sporadic sampling schedule. The impact of corrective action is also assessed using serial monitoring.
- Low TGPs are unusual. They may be associated with low dissolved oxygen or low water flow and warrant investigation.

Further discussion of gas supersaturation is available in Chapter C1.

Temperature

Most fish are poikilothermic and have preferred temperature ranges. Water temperature impacts all aspects of metabolism, behavior, appetite, water chemistry, disease dynamics, drug pharmacokinetics, and sensitivity to toxins. Because cooler water is heavier than warmer water, steep temperature gradients (thermoclines) can develop in deep habitats.

Frequency of testing: Temperature should be assayed continuously or at least daily. It should be measured when fish are moved between bodies of water to identify any temperature differentials; these may affect acclimation needs. It should be measured during restraint and ideally during transport.

Sampling: Temperature must be measured on site in the system.

Testing: A variety of thermometers are available, both independent and integrated into heat exchangers. They may be contact or noncontact (e.g. infrared thermometers). The meters should be certified (e.g. by the National Institute of Standards and Technology [NIST] in the United States) with minimum and maximum temperatures also reported. Accuracy and precision should be checked for each thermometer as quality can vary widely.

Units: Temperature is reported in degrees Celsius (°C) or Fahrenheit (°F).

Target values: Species preferred temperature zones vary, but some approximate guidelines are:

- Tropical reef fish: 22–28°C (72–82°F).
- Goldfish (*Carassius auratus*), koi (*Cyprinus carpio koi*), similar temperate species: 15–22°C (59–72°F).
- Atlantic salmon (*Salmo salar*), rainbow trout (*Oncorhynchus mykiss*), and other similar cold-water species: 7–18°C (45–64°F).

Practical considerations:

- Water temperature needs to be within the preferred range for all animals in the system. This can be difficult with populations that include species with different preferred ranges, e.g. bonnethead sharks (*Sphyrna tiburo*) are often housed in large tropical reef systems at 23–24°C (73–75°F); while this suits many tropical teleosts, bonnetheads often do better at slightly higher temperatures.
- Temperature problems are most likely when the water temperature differs significantly from the ambient temperature (e.g. cold-water aquarium in a warm room). These animals are at high risk if there is a mechanical failure of the life support system and the water temperature becomes closer to ambient temperature.
- Temperature changes within a system are often due to inadequately sized heat exchangers, heat exchanger malfunctions (e.g. loss of power), water additions (e.g. rainfall, cold tap water), or changes in ambient temperature (e.g. during shipping or severe weather).
- Rapid changes are more likely to negatively impact fish health than slow changes. In general, water temperature should not change by >2°C/h or 5°F/h, although sensitivity varies. The most common event that might expose fish to rapid water temperature changes is when they are moved between water systems without an acclimation period.
- Handling fish under chemical or manual restraint when ambient temperature differs significantly from water temperature is another consideration. The temperature of the water for ventilating and moistening fish can easily change through the procedure and this should be monitored and managed.
- If water temperature increases in a system with high ammonia or heavy metals, their chemical equilibrium shifts to the more toxic forms and morbidity and mortality become more likely.

Further discussion of temperature stress is available in Chapter C1.

Salinity and Salt Composition

Salinity is the concentration of dissolved ions in water. The main ions in seawater are sodium and chloride, with calcium, magnesium, sulfur, potassium, and many other inorganic elements. The total salinity and the concentration of each ion affect behavior, physiology, disease dynamics, drug pharmacokinetics, and sensitivity to toxins. Since ions increase the density of water and make it easier to conduct an electric current, specific gravity and electrical conductivity can be used to indirectly measure salinity.

Marine and brackish water aquariums make use of natural or artificial seawater. Artificial seawater is typically made from dechlorinated municipal freshwater with salt mixtures added. These mixtures may be commercial (e.g. Instant Ocean®, Blacksburg, VA) or customized (Bidwell and Spotte 1985). For commercial mixes, sodium chloride alone and products with anticaking agents should be avoided. For proprietary mixes, the salts should be food-grade or reagent- and analytical-grade to reduce the risk of contaminants. Phosphates are rarely required in salt mixes for established aquariums as levels accumulate from the food fed. Bromides are less common in salt mixes now, as they do not appear to be required at the levels seen in natural seawater and can form harmful residual oxidants with ozone disinfection. Salts should be mixed in freshwater or brine in a dedicated, off-exhibit tank and then tested, at least for salinity; salts should not be added directly to an aquarium system. Salt mixtures are often a significant part of the cost of marine aquariums.

Freshwater aquariums may use municipal, surface, or ground water. Some freshwater fish do best in low-ion water; in these cases, ions may be removed from freshwater by deionization, reverse osmosis, or distilling.

Frequency of testing: Salinity should be assayed regularly; this often includes testing incoming water routinely or with each production batch, and testing each system every two to four weeks if stable. A full cation analysis (e.g. concentrations of Na^+, Ca^{2+}, Mg^{2+}, and other ions) should be considered periodically, both as quality control for artificial salt water and in long-established closed systems to check the ion balance and allow correction if needed. Salinity of transport water should be measured prior to acclimation to identify differences from the destination water; this may affect acclimation needs. For high-risk fish transports, a full cation comparison is recommended prior to transport.

Sampling: Standard sampling is described in Box A2.1. Samples can be stored for a few days at room temperature or weeks when refrigerated or frozen.

Testing: The simplest test uses a refractometer or hydrometer to measure specific gravity; this measurement of density reflects total dissolved solids rather than true salinity, but gives a quick approximation of salinity. Refractometers need to be calibrated prior to each use and some require temperature correction. Handheld conductivity meters provide more accurate indirect measurements of salinity in salt water and total dissolved solids in freshwater. Ion-exchange chromatography is used for cation analysis.

Units: Salinity in aquariums is usually measured in grams per liter (g/L), equivalent to parts per thousand (ppt). Other units include psu (practical salinity units), which are roughly equivalent to g/L values. If specific gravity is used, the results are between 1.005 and 1.030; conversion tables are available for temperature correction, if needed. In freshwater systems, electrical conductivity may be reported, typically in μSiemens per centimeter (μS/cm) or an older unit (μmho/cm); these units are equivalent.

Target values: The salinity of natural seawater is often 32–35 g/L (with a specific gravity of ~1.021–1.024 depending on temperature); many aquariums use a target range of 28–35 g/L. Freshwater salinity is typically <0.5 g/L or a conductivity of 60–2000 μS/cm (Table A2.2).

Practical considerations:

- Inappropriate salinity or rapid changes in salinity are both problematic. Effects are more severe in stenohaline species (e.g. reef species, most pelagic sharks).
- Low salinity in salt water may be seen due to freshwater contamination (e.g. rainfall, contamination from freshwater lines), insufficient salt additions, or crystallization of salts on the lids or life support system components ("salt creep").
- High salinity in freshwater or salt water may be seen due to evaporation or contamination by salts or salt water.
- Rapid changes are more likely to cause problems than slow. Rapid changes are most common when fish are moved between water systems without acclimation or during freshwater or saltwater dips for ectoparasite diagnosis and treatment.

Box A2.1 How to Collect a Water Sample for Later Analysis

1) Use a clean polyethylene or polypropylene bottle with a screw cap for most sampling (borosilicate glass can be used for pesticides).
2) Rinse the bottle in the system with the water to be tested.
3) Select an area of concern or an area with sufficient mixing to be representative of the system.
4) Dunk the bottle underwater and fill completely.
5) Cap the bottle while still under water.
6) Dry the outside of the bottle and label with system, time, and date.
7) Refrigerate or keep the sample on ice.
8) Most analyses should be run within a few hours; some analyses are still reliable after freezing and thawing.

Nitrogenous Wastes (Ammonia, Nitrite, Nitrate)

Nitrogenous wastes are produced through protein metabolism by animals and decay processes (e.g. of excess food or dead plant matter). The waste products build up rapidly in closed or recirculating systems and are toxic to fish and invertebrates. The nitrogen cycle describes the conversion of ammonia into nitrite and then nitrate (Figure A2.4).

Ammonia exists as ionized ammonium (NH_4^+) and unionized ammonia (NH_3, known as UIA). Combined, these make up total ammonia nitrogen (TAN). The unionized form (UIA) is much more toxic to fish as it can diffuse across the gills. The proportion of each depends on temperature, pH, alkalinity, salinity, and DO. More of the ammonia is in the toxic form (UIA) at high pH, high water temperature, and low salinity (e.g. a freshwater pond after a hot day). Ammonia is converted into nitrite by ammonia-oxidizing bacteria (AOB). These include Betaproteobacteria and Gammaproteobacteria (e.g. *Nitrosomonas*, *Nitrosospira*, *Nitrosolobus*, *Nitrosovibrio*, *Nitrosococcus* spp.). Nitrite can

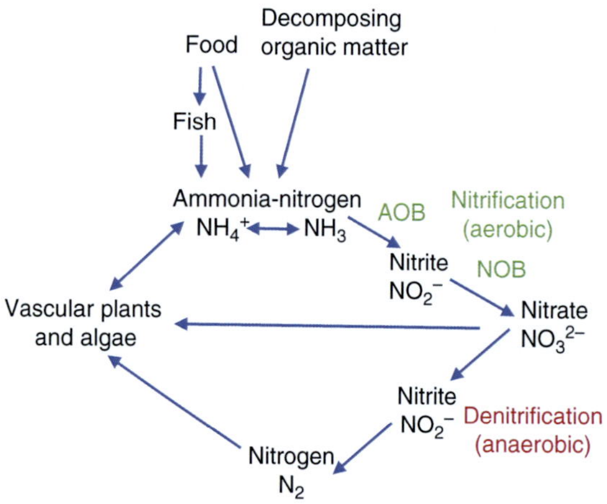

Figure A2.4 A simple schematic of the nitrogen cycle.

be toxic to fish in freshwater systems (Lewis and Morris 1986). Nitrite is converted into nitrate by nitrite-oxidizing bacteria (NOB). These include *Nitrobacter*, *Nitrococcus*, *Nitrospina*, and *Nitrospira* spp., among others. Nitrate is a stressor and endocrine disruptor (Hrubec et al. 1996; Camargo et al. 2005; Morris et al. 2011). These nitrifying bacteria (AOB and NOB) exist on all surfaces within the habitat, but are concentrated where surface area is highest (e.g. sand filters and undergravel filters). The nitrification process uses oxygen and alkalinity and produces carbon dioxide via bacterial respiration. Nitrate is removed from the system through water changes, algal or vascular plant use, and denitrification systems. With immature biological filtration, increases in ammonia, nitrite, and nitrate tend to follow each other (Figure A2.5).

Frequency of testing: Ammonia and nitrite should be assayed routinely on all systems. This may be daily on a new system, following the addition of new fish, or following an immersion treatment in order to evaluate the efficacy of the biological filtration. It may be every one to two weeks in stable systems. Ammonia should also be assayed during or following transport or restraint. Nitrate testing is often less frequent and may be done every one to two months.

Sampling: Standard sampling is described in Box A2.1. Samples for ammonia and nitrite can be stored for a few hours at room temperature, and up to 24 hours if refrigerated or 48 hours if frozen. Nitrate is more stable and samples can be stored for longer.

Testing: Commercial test kits for ammonia use one of two approaches. The Nessler method is rapid and reliable in freshwater, but is less accurate in salt water and may be falsely elevated within 24–72 hours of treatment with formalin or ammonia-locking compounds, as these often contain formalin. The test also includes mercury

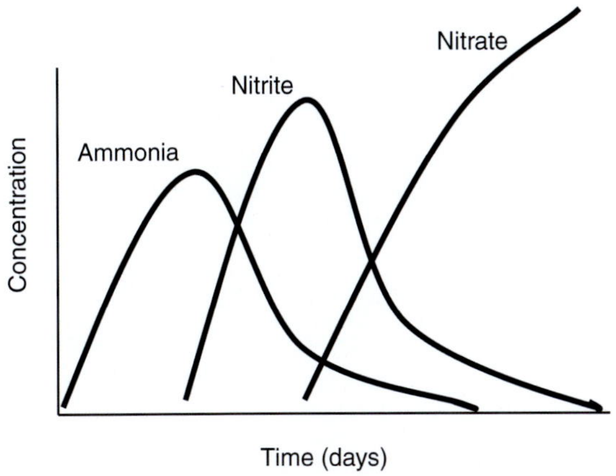

Figure A2.5 Sequential increases in ammonia, nitrite, and nitrate as the nitrifying bacteria in the biological filtration mature over time.

which must be disposed of as hazardous waste. The ammonium salicylate method is more accurate in salt water when the modifying reagent developed by Kingsley (2014) is used. This test produces sodium nitroferricyanide; while regulations may differ, this often requires disposal as hazardous waste. The ammonium salicylate method is not affected by the presence of formalin. The test is more expensive and slightly slower. Ammonia can also be measured using ion-specific electrodes. It is important to know water temperature, pH, and salinity to be able to assess ammonia results, since they affect the proportion of the more toxic UIA. Nitrite and nitrate tests are colorimetric (assayed by colorimeter or more accurately by spectrophotometer); commercial test kits are readily available.

Units: Ammonia tests report TAN in milligrams per liter (mg/L). UIA can be calculated from TAN using a conversion factor based on temperature, pH, +/− salinity. Tables are available on most test kits and conversion calculators are available on-line (Table A2.3). If nitrite tests only report nitrite-nitrogen in mg/L, multiply this by 3.3 to get the nitrite ion level. If nitrate tests report only nitrate-nitrogen in mg/L, multiply this by 4.4 to get the nitrate ion level.

Target values: Targets vary depending on species, but some potential values are listed below and in Table A2.2:

- UIA <0.02 mg/L.
- Nitrite-nitrogen <0.1 mg/L.
- Nitrate-nitrogen <50 mg/L for most fish and <15 mg/L for many invertebrates.

Practical considerations:

- Fish health concerns are associated with high ammonia, nitrite, or nitrate, although ammonia is the most toxic of the three, and nitrite is primarily a concern in freshwater.
- High ammonia, followed by high nitrite, is often seen in newly established recirculating systems in the first few weeks after animal additions, until there are sufficient nitrifying bacteria to handle the bioload. During this time, careful control of stocking density, monitoring, water changes, and other mitigation methods are essential to minimize fish exposure to the toxins while allowing the biological filtration to mature. Similar changes are also seen due to other animal additions, high stocking densities or organic load, inadequate water flow or low DO in biological filters, and environmental changes or medications that have damaged the bacteria in the biological filters.
- High nitrate is often seen in long-established recirculating systems without denitrification or adequate water changes or following contamination of a system (e.g. with nitrogenous fertilizer).

Table A2.3 Fraction of the total ammonia nitrogen (TAN) that is present as unionized ammonia (UIA) at various temperature–pH combinations. Multiply TAN (mg/L) by this conversion factor to obtain UIA (mg/L).

Temperature		pH						
Celsius	Fahrenheit	6.0	6.5	7.0	7.5	8.0	8.5	9.0
0	32	0.0001	0.0003	0.0008	0.0026	0.0082	0.0255	0.0764
1	34	0.0001	0.0003	0.0009	0.0028	0.0089	0.0277	0.0825
2	36	0.0001	0.0003	0.0010	0.0031	0.0097	0.0300	0.0890
3	37	0.0001	0.0003	0.0011	0.0034	0.0105	0.0325	0.0960
4	39	0.0001	0.0004	0.0012	0.0036	0.0114	0.0352	0.103
5	41	0.0001	0.0004	0.0013	0.0040	0.0123	0.0380	0.111
6	42	0.0001	0.0004	0.0014	0.0043	0.0134	0.0411	0.119
7	45	0.0001	0.0005	0.0015	0.0046	0.0145	0.0444	0.128
8	46	0.0002	0.0005	0.0016	0.0050	0.0157	0.0479	0.137
9	48	0.0002	0.0005	0.0017	0.0054	0.0169	0.0516	0.147
10	50	0.0002	0.0006	0.0019	0.0059	0.0183	0.0556	0.157
11	52	0.0002	0.0006	0.0020	0.0063	0.0197	0.0599	0.168
12	54	0.0002	0.0007	0.0022	0.0068	0.0213	0.0644	0.179
13	55	0.0002	0.0007	0.0024	0.0074	0.0230	0.0692	0.190
14	57	0.0003	0.0008	0.0025	0.0080	0.0248	0.0743	0.202
15	59	0.0003	0.0009	0.0027	0.0086	0.0267	0.0797	0.215
16	61	0.0003	0.0009	0.0029	0.0093	0.0287	0.0854	0.228
17	63	0.0003	0.0010	0.0032	0.0100	0.0308	0.0914	0.241
18	64	0.0003	0.0011	0.0034	0.0107	0.0331	0.0978	0.255
19	66	0.0004	0.0012	0.0037	0.0115	0.0356	0.105	0.270
20	68	0.0004	0.0013	0.0040	0.0124	0.0382	0.112	0.284
21	70	0.0004	0.0014	0.0043	0.0133	0.0410	0.119	0.299
22	72	0.0005	0.0015	0.0046	0.0143	0.0439	0.127	0.315
23	73	0.0005	0.0016	0.0049	0.0154	0.0470	0.135	0.330
24	75	0.0005	0.0017	0.0053	0.0165	0.0503	0.144	0.346
25	77	0.0006	0.0018	0.0057	0.0177	0.0538	0.153	0.363
26	79	0.0006	0.0019	0.0061	0.0189	0.0575	0.162	0.379
27	81	0.0007	0.0021	0.0065	0.0203	0.0615	0.172	0.396
28	82	0.0007	0.0022	0.0070	0.0217	0.0656	0.182	0.412
29	84	0.0008	0.0024	0.0075	0.0232	0.0700	0.192	0.429
30	86	0.0008	0.0025	0.0080	0.0248	0.0746	0.203	0.446

Values for °F are rounded off to the closest integer. *Source*: Modified from Emerson et al. (1975), reprinted with permission. © John Wiley & Sons.

- Increases are more likely to be problematic in warm water and freshwater systems because more of the ammonia is in the unionized, toxic form.
- Low levels are never a concern for fish, although vascular plants and algae need nitrate for healthy growth.

Further discussions of ammonia, nitrite, and nitrate toxicity are available in Chapter C1.

pH

Water pH represents the concentration of hydrogen ions (H^+) on a logarithmic scale. Because it is a logarithmic scale, a change in pH from 8 to 7 represents a 10-fold increase in [H^+] and from 8 to 6 represents a 100-fold increase; small changes in pH represent large changes in

[H^+]. Water pH affects behavior, physiology, disease dynamics, drug pharmacokinetics, and sensitivity to toxins.

Frequency of testing: Assays of pH should be performed routinely; this often consists of testing the incoming water regularly or with each production batch, and testing stable systems every two weeks. Testing frequency may be increased if there is a high risk of pH fluctuations (e.g. a low alkalinity system). pH should also be assayed in transport water and prior to the addition of fish to buffered tricaine methanesulfonate (MS-222).

Sampling: Standard sampling is described in Box A2.1. Samples should be assayed within a few hours; samples cannot be frozen and assayed later.

Testing: Colorimetric tests are common, but often have an accuracy of ±0.5 (Baird et al. 2017). Handheld pH meters that use electrometric or potentiometric methods are more accurate and readily available; they must be calibrated prior to each use.

Units: The scale ranges from 0 to 14, with no units; a pH of 7 is neutral, lower values are acidic and higher values are alkaline.

Target values: In freshwater systems, target pH may be between 5.5 and 7.5. In saltwater systems, target pH may be between 7.5 and 8.5 (Table A2.2). Some species have specific needs, e.g. African Rift Lake cichlids (*Cichlidae*) prefer high pH, while discus (*Symphysodon* spp.) and freshwater angelfish (*Pterophyllum* spp.) prefer low pH.

Practical considerations:

- pH needs to be within the target range for all animals in the system. While preferences are similar for most marine species, preferences of freshwater species vary widely. For example, many commonly available tropical freshwater fish are kept together at a neutral pH but prefer high pH (e.g. guppies, *Poecilia reticulata*) or low pH (e.g. neon tetras, *Paracheirodon innesi*). If a specific ecology has been targeted (e.g. Lake Victoria or Rio Negro), the life support system should be designed to replicate that pH.
- pH changes in either direction can be problematic to animals and nitrifying bacteria.
- Problems are often due to changes in buffers (such as carbonates and bicarbonates), carbon dioxide or other acids in the systems, gas exchange in the system, or the pH of the source water. New concrete can also leach materials that affect pH.
- Rapid changes are more likely to cause problems than slow changes and are more likely with low alkalinity.
- If pH increases in a system with ammonia or heavy metals, the proportion of the toxic forms increases and morbidity and mortality become more likely. This scenario is most clinically relevant with closed transport containers: when closed plastic bags are opened post-transport, the accumulated CO_2 escapes, water pH increases, and the high levels of ammonia in the transport water become more toxic. Acclimation (the slow addition of the new water) should start as soon as possible after opening closed containers.
- pH can vary significantly across the day because of diurnal changes in animal and plant respiration and photosynthesis, particularly in heavily planted systems like many outdoor ponds. pH values are lowest at dawn (Figure A2.2).

Further discussion of pH stress is available in Chapter C1.

Alkalinity and Hardness

Alkalinity is the concentration of anions or bases in water (particularly bicarbonate [HCO_3^-] and carbonate [CO_3^{2-}], but also hydroxide [OH^-], borate [BO_3^{3-}], and phosphate [PO_4^{3-}]). These act as buffers and alkalinity is a measure of the buffering capacity of the water. High alkalinity helps to limit rapid changes in pH. Hardness is the concentration of divalent cations (particularly calcium [Ca^{2+}] and magnesium [Mg^{2+}], but also strontium [Sr^{2+}], ferrous iron [Fe^{2+}], and manganese [Mn^{2+}]). These are best considered essential cations that support biological processes in fish and invertebrates (particularly corals). High alkalinity is often associated with high hardness and high pH, but that relationship does not always hold (e.g. sodium bicarbonate contributes to alkalinity but not hardness). The relationship is complex; Boyd et al. (2016) provides a good summary of the inter-relationships.

Frequency of testing: Alkalinity and hardness should be assayed routinely; this may involve testing the system every two to four weeks. Alkalinity should be assayed prior to copper sulfate immersion treatment, since low alkalinity increases the risk of toxicity. Hardness should be closely monitored in rearing systems as inappropriate hardness can affect egg hatchability and fry survival.

Sampling: Samples can be stored for a few days at room temperature or a few weeks when refrigerated.

Testing: Commercial colorimetric test kits are available. EDTA titration and atomic absorption spectrometry tests are available. Spectrophotometric testing for specific anions or cations may be considered in some systems, e.g.:

- Calcium in hard coral and egg- or larval-rearing systems.
- Ferrous iron in well water.
- Phosphates in hard coral systems, outdoor ponds where increases (e.g. from fertilizer) can cause algal blooms, and long-established closed systems where phosphates from food items build up over time.

Units: In the United States, hardness and alkalinity are reported as milligrams per liter (mg/L) of $CaCO_3$, often reported as just mg/L. They can also be reported as milliequivalents per liter (mEq/L) of $CaCO_3$. Conversion of mg/L and mEq/L depends on the molecular weight and ionic charge. In the case of $CaCO_3$, multiply the mEq/L value by 100 to get mg/L of $CaCO_3$. Hardness may also be reported as the German or French degree of hardness (dH or °f respectively).

Target values: Freshwater may be soft (hardness 40–75 mg/L or 2–4 dH) or hard (hardness 75–150 mg/L or 4–8 dH) and with an alkalinity of 50–200 mg/L. Salt water usually has a high hardness (150–300 mg/L or 8–16 dH) and high alkalinity (>200 mg/L) (Table A2.2). A possible target range for free calcium is 25–100 mg/L.

Practical considerations:

- Alkalinity and hardness need to be within target ranges for all animals in the system.
- The most common problem is a gradual decrease in alkalinity (and to a lesser extent hardness) in closed systems as these ions are used by the animals. When managing closed systems, buffers and salts are routinely added to compensate for this decline.
- Alkalinity and/or hardness are also affected by the addition or removal of salts, e.g. oyster shell ($CaCO_3$), calcitic limestone ($CaCO_3$), dolomitic limestone ($MgCO_3$ and $CaCO_3$), hydrated/slaked lime/limewater ($Ca(OH)_2$), sodium bicarbonate ($NaHCO_3$), sodium carbonate/soda ash (Na_2CO_3), and calcium chloride ($CaCl_2$). These salts may be part of the substrate (e.g. crushed coral), décor, or enclosure walls (e.g. concrete).
- Low alkalinity increases the risk of rapid changes in pH, and low alkalinity and hardness increase the dissolution and absorption of heavy metals. Copper sulfate treatment is contraindicated in low alkalinity water for these reasons.

Carbon Dioxide

Carbon dioxide (CO_2) is very dynamic in water as it is highly soluble, produced by animal and microbial respiration and decay processes, and used during photosynthesis. CO_2 reacts with water to form carbonic acid (H_2CO_3) which dissociates to bicarbonate (HCO_3^-), then carbonate (CO_3^{2-}) and hydrogen ions (H^+), depending on alkalinity, pH, salinity, and (to a lesser extent) temperature.

Frequency of testing: Testing is not common and is usually done in high-risk situations (e.g. intensive aquaculture or incoming well water).

Sampling: CO_2 should be measured on site and within about 30 minutes of sampling.

Testing: Commercial colorimetric tests are available. CO_2 can also be estimated based on pH and alkalinity using standard curves available on-line and in Hargreaves and Brunson (1996). Because of the narrow range of pH in salt water (e.g. 7.5–8.5), a low pH in salt water may indicate high levels of CO_2. A crude estimate of CO_2 can be made by collecting water from the system in an open-topped container, measuring the pH, vigorously aerating the water for about 60 minutes, and measuring the pH again. If the pH increases by more than one unit due to off-gassing of CO_2, the CO_2 may be too high.

Units: CO_2 is reported in milligrams per liter (mg/L).

Target values: Less than 20 mg/L is a common target.

Practical considerations:

- High CO_2 is problematic for fish because it affects pH and oxygen availability.
- High values are common in intensive aquaculture systems with limited off-gassing, closed transport containers, well water, and following an algal or phytoplankton die-off.
- Low levels are not a health concern for fish, but vascular plants, algae, and phytoplankton need CO_2 for photosynthesis.
- CO_2 is inversely related to pH and is a component of alkalinity, which affects pH stability.
- CO_2 can vary significantly across the day because of diurnal changes in respiration and photosynthesis; values are highest at dawn (Figure A2.2).

Chlorines and Chloramines

Chlorines and chloramines can be toxic to fish and invertebrates. Chlorines (Cl_2, OCl^-, and HOCl) should not be confused with chloride (Cl^-); chlorines are oxidants that are highly reactive, chlorides are salts that are essential to fish. Chloramines are chlorines bound to ammonia.

Chlorines and chloramines are frequently used as disinfectants in municipal water and can be present in tap water at levels that can be toxic to fish (0.5–3.0 g/L). These must be removed from the water prior to use in fish systems. Chlorine can also come from accidental exposure to bleach or similar disinfectants. Ozone disinfection can convert chlorides (and bromides) in the water into strong oxidants and oxidative by-products. These should be confined to the ozone contact chamber and not released into the fish habitat.

"Free chlorine" is the sum of the active oxidants (Cl_2, OCl^-, and HOCl). "Total chlorine" is the sum of free chlorine and combined chlorine (e.g. chloramines). There is no direct test for chloramines.

Frequency of testing: Chlorines should be assayed where they are considered a risk. Incoming municipal freshwater should be tested before and after carbon filtration or other treatment to ensure chlorines have been removed. With ozone disinfection, system water should be tested for residual oxidants, including free and total chlorine (and free and total bromine). Regular testing is more useful than individual results, because of the error margin inherent in many of the test methods.

Sampling: Standard sampling is described in Box A2.1. It is particularly important that the bottles are properly cleaned prior to use; any tap-water contamination will artificially increase the results.

Testing: Free and total chlorines are measured by colorimetry (based on the amine DPD) or potentiometry. Handheld meters are available (e.g. Pocket Colorimeter™ II, Chlorine, Hach, Loveland, CO). The error margin for many of these tests is ± 0.02 mg/L. Gel standards that simulate specific chlorine values can be used for a quick check of instrument performance and accuracy, but they cannot be used to calibrate instruments or assess technique (e.g. contamination of bottles).

Units: Free and total chlorines are reported in milligrams per liter (mg/L).

Target values: Total chlorines should be <0.03 mg/L for most fish and <0.01 mg/L for sensitive species (Table A2.2).

Practical considerations:

- The main health concern is high levels of chlorines or chloramines, as they are toxic to fish.
- High levels are most often from untreated municipal water or failure of dechlorination methods (e.g. exhausted activated carbon, miscalculation of thiosulfate to inactivate chlorine).
- Management typically consists of water changes, aeration, the addition of activated carbon filters, or treatment of the water with sodium thiosulfate, ultraviolet light, or binding products such as AmQuel® and AmQuel Plus™ (Kordon LLC) and AMMO-LOCK® (API).
- Low levels are not a concern.

Further discussion of chlorine and chloramine toxicity is available in Chapter C1.

Iodide and Iodate

Iodine (I_2) is an essential micronutrient. It exists in water primarily as iodide (I^-), iodate (IO_3^-), and dissolved organic iodine. Iodide and dissolved organic iodine are considered bioavailable. Iodide and dissolved organic iodine can be oxidized to iodate, which is not available to fish. Deficiencies are associated with goiters, particularly in elasmobranchs.

Frequency of testing: Iodide and iodate should be assayed routinely in elasmobranch systems, particularly where ozone disinfection is used.

Sampling: Standard sampling is described in Box A2.1. Samples can be stored for a few days at room temperature or weeks when refrigerated or frozen.

Testing: Iodide can be assayed using high-performance liquid chromatography (Parkinson et al. 2018). Iodide can be hard to measure accurately if nitrate levels are high.

Units: Typical units are milligrams per liter (mg/L), equivalent to parts per million (ppm). Other units are micromoles per liter (μmol/L).

Target values: In salt water with elasmobranchs, iodide should be ~0.03–0.06 mg/L (Table A2.2).

Practical considerations:

- The primary health concern is the potential for goiters in elasmobranchs due to low iodide. This is particularly common in long-established recirculating systems with ozone disinfection, as ozone converts iodide to iodate (Sherrill et al. 2004).
- It is unknown if excess iodide in the water is a problem for fish; in other classes, excess can also lead to thyroid dysfunction and levels should likely be kept at <0.1 mg/L.

Further discussion of goiters is available in Chapter C1.

Heavy Metals

Heavy metals are potentially toxic to fish. They are particularly common where surface or ground water is used. Potential toxins include copper, zinc, lead, mercury, manganese, and arsenic.

Frequency of testing: Heavy metals are usually tested based on a risk analysis. For example, the well-water source for a pond may be assayed routinely for iron, while a tropical saltwater system on treatment with copper sulfate should be assayed daily for copper ions.

Sampling: Standard sampling is described in Box A2.1. Samples can be stored for weeks or months if frozen.

Testing: Commercial colorimetric tests are available for some heavy metals (e.g. copper, iron); accuracy varies and results are best assessed using a spectrophotometer. Most other tests for heavy metals rely on atomic absorption spectrophotometry.

Units: Heavy metal concentrations are typically reported in milligrams per liter (mg/L), equivalent to parts per million (ppm), or in micrograms per liter (μg/L), equivalent to parts per billion (ppb). It is important to differentiate between the free/ionic concentration (the more toxic form) and total concentration (free and combined or chelated).

Target values: This can be hard to determine, because toxicity depends on factors such as species, life stage, pH, hardness, alkalinity, temperature, and the presence of other stressors. In general, values should be <0.03 mg/L for most heavy metals.

Practical considerations:

- While some metals are considered essential ions, the main health concern is high levels of heavy metals, particularly in the free/ionic form.
- Common causes are copper sulfate treatment, contaminated source water, drip contamination of the system, or leaching from décor, substrate, enclosure walls, or water lines.
- Toxicity is more likely at low pH, hardness, and alkalinity, and at high water temperature.

Further discussion of heavy metal toxicity is available in Chapter C1.

Turbidity/Suspended Solids

Turbidity and total suspended solids (TSS) are a measure of the suspended material in the water column, which can interfere with respiration and light penetration.

Frequency of testing: Turbidity may be tested routinely where indicated (e.g. to assess effectiveness of mechanical filtration) or in response to an upcoming treatment (e.g. copper sulfate immersion).

Sampling: Testing is usually done on site in the affected system.

Testing: In ponds and other slow-moving surface water, a black and white Secchi disk can be lowered into the water to record the depth at which the pattern cannot be seen (typically based on an average of two readings). Nephelometric tests measure the scatter from a focused light beam. Handheld probes are available.

Units: Secchi depth is reported in centimeters or inches; a low value is equivalent to high turbidity. Nephelometric tests are reported in nephelometric turbidity units (NTU), Formazin turbidity units, or a variety of other units depending on the meter.

Target values: Target for ponds may be Secchi depth of >50 cm (18 in) or turbidity <1-10 NTU.

Practical considerations:

- High turbidity can be an issue for fish because it can affect gill function, dissolved oxygen, feeding, fecundity, light penetration, and aesthetics. The particulates can also cause clogging of fine mechanical filters.
- High turbidity may be due to phytoplankton or bacterial blooms, insufficient mechanical filtration, disturbance of the substrate, or contamination (e.g. runoff).
- Low turbidity may be a concern for species that have evolved in brown or black pond or river systems.

Microbiome and Bacterial Testing

Aquatic systems are rich in microbes, including bacteria, archaea, protists, fungi, and microalgae such as diatoms. This microbiota is found within the water column and attached to all surfaces. On wet surfaces, this microbiota creates a sheltered scaffold known as the biofilm. Assessment of this microbiome in aquarium systems is in its infancy, including the relationship to fish health and biological filtration.

Bacterial indicator tests use selective bacterial media designed to look for point sources of human fecal contamination in surface water. Various commercial tests are available (e.g. total coliforms and fecal coliforms on Colilert, or *Enterococcus* spp. on Enterolert, both by Idexx, Westbrook, ME). In-house testing relies on either membrane filtration or multiple-tube fermentation methods with results available one to two days later as number of colony-forming units (CFU)/100 mL for membrane filtration and most probable number (MPN)/100 mL for multiple-tube fermentation; these results are equivalent. In the United States, targets are often extrapolated from state or US-EPA regulations for swimming beaches or USDA regulations for marine mammal habitats. These tests likely have value when assessing open systems with human access where point contamination with human sewage is possible (e.g. swim with ray programs in outdoor lagoons). However, these bacterial indicator tests are problematic in most fish systems because of a high risk of false positives (e.g. growth of plant-based *Enterococcus* spp. or nonselected genera such as *Vibrio* spp.) and because they may not have any relation to pathogen load (Pisciotta et al. 2002; Culpepper et al. 2016). Rather than a measure of potential fish morbidity, these tests may be most useful in determining if disinfection needs have changed over time: once a baseline has been established for the system, higher values may suggest a change in bacterial load in that system. However, the tests only represent a very small proportion of the total microbiome.

A more complete view is possible using fluorescent microscopy. This can directly determine populations of micro-organisms, including a wider variety of bacteria as well as viruses. To determine the types of micro-organisms, DNA analysis is required (microbiomics). This involves extracting, amplifying, and sequencing genomic DNA. Microbiome analyses have been reported for closed aquarium systems and have shown changes in bacterial diversity and evenness following routine maintenance such as water changes

(Van Bonn et al. 2015; Patin et al. 2018). Further information and resources are available at the Aquarium Microbiome Project (www.aquariummicrobiomeproject.org).

Water Quality Testing Options

There are a wide variety of test methods available; a description of a possible water quality testing kit for fish veterinarians is provided in Box A2.2. Commercial test kits are available from various distributors (e.g. API, CHEMetrics, Hach, Seachem, Tetra). Handheld or system-mounted meters are available from various commercial suppliers (e.g. Fisher Scientific, Hach, LaMotte, Oxyguard International, Pentair, YSI Inc.). Some methods, such as spectrophotometry, high-performance liquid chromatography, and ion-exchange chromatography may be limited to zoo and aquarium laboratories, and commercial, state, or federal aquatic animal health laboratories; the assays may be available to the public.

Factors to consider when selecting water quality test methods include accuracy, sensitivity (detection limits), calibration and maintenance requirements, ease of use, cost of purchase and maintenance, durability, reliability in working conditions, and associated disposal requirements (e.g. reagents).

When building a water quality testing program for an institution or practice, it is helpful to start with target ranges for each of the systems (based on the needs of the species and the life support equipment used), the expected ranges for the source water, and targets for disposal of the discharge water. This can be followed by a risk assessment of the most likely issues:

- Source water (e.g. low dissolved oxygen, inappropriate temperature, incorrect composition of salt mixes, high chlorines in municipal water, high iron in well water).
- System water (e.g. high nitrogenous wastes, pH change in low-pH systems, temperature change in tropical fish systems, oxidative by-products and low iodide in systems with ozone disinfection, drug assays). It may be useful to divide systems based on age (e.g. newly established/newly stocked versus stable) or use (e.g. quarantine systems).
- Discharge water (e.g. drug residues, temperature, salinity, pathogen load).
- Transport water (e.g. low dissolved oxygen, high ammonia, inappropriate temperature).

Consideration can also be given to potential research topics. These analyses can be used to guide decisions on type of testing, frequency of testing, and hardware, space, and staffing requirements.

Box A2.2 Minimum Water Quality Testing Kit

- Thermometer for temperature
- Refractometer or conductivity meter for salinity
- Colorimetric tests for ammonia, nitrite, nitrate, alkalinity, copper, chlorine, +/- calcium, phosphate, iodide
- pH meter
- Dissolved oxygen meter
- +/− Total gas pressure meter

Conclusion

Water quality parameters are more complicated than this chapter might suggest, but in general, acute changes should be avoided, and long-term monitoring should be used to identify gradual changes. Parameters should meet the needs of all the animals and vascular plants or algae in the system and allow for seasonal changes that match the natural history of the species. The goal is to create balanced systems that show resilience.

Additional details are available in a number of excellent references, including Mohan and Aiken 2004; Noga 2010; Stamper and Semmen 2012a, b; Baird et al. 2017.

References

Baird, R.B., Greenberg, E., Eaton, A.D., and Rice, E.W. (eds.) (2017). Standard Methods for the Examination of Water and Wastewater, 23e. Baltimore, MD: United Book Press.

Bidwell, J. and Spotte, S. (1985). Artificial Seawaters, Formulas and Methods. Boston, MA: Jones and Bartlett.

Boyd, C.E., Tucker, C.S., and Somridhivej, B. (2016). Alkalinity and hardness: critical but elusive concepts in aquaculture. *Journal of the World Aquaculture Society* 47: 6–14.

Camargo, J.A., Alonso, A., and Salamanca, A. (2005). Nitrate toxicity to aquatic animals: a review with new data for freshwater invertebrates. *Chemosphere* 58: 1255–1267.

Culpepper, E.E., Clayton, L.A., Hadfield, C.A. et al. (2016). Coliform bacteria monitoring in fish systems: current practices in public aquaria. *Journal of Aquatic Animal Health* 28: 85–90.

Emerson, K., Russo, R.C., Lund, R.E. et al. (1975). Aqueous ammonia equilibrium calculations: Effect of pH and temperature. *Journal of Fisheries Research Board of Canada* 32: 2379–2383.

Hargreaves, J. and Brunson, M. (1996). Carbon dioxide in fish ponds. SRAC publication No. 468. https://tal.ifas.ufl.edu/extensionoutreach/extension-publications/ (accessed 7 July 2019).

Hrubec, T.C., Robertson, J.L., Smith, S.A., and Tinker, M.K. (1996). The effect of temperature and water quality on antibody response to *Aeromonas salmonicida* in sunshine bass (*Morone chrysops* x *Morone saxatilis*). *Veterinary Immunology and Immunopathology* 50: 157–166.

Kingsley, E. (2014). Development of nitrate and total ammonia testing procedures at the Monterey Bay Aquarium. *Presented at the Aquality II Conference*, Atlantis, Bahamas.

Lewis, W.M. and Morris, D.P. (1986). Toxicity of nitrite to fish: a review. *Transactions of the American Fisheries Society* 115: 183–195.

Mohan, P.J. and Aiken, A. (2004). Water quality and life support systems for large elasmobranch exhibits. In: The Elasmobranch Husbandry Manual: Captive Care of Sharks, Rays and their Relatives (eds. M. Smith, D. Warmolts, D. Thoney and R. Hueter), 69–88. Columbus, OH: Ohio Biological Survey, Inc.

Morris, A.L., Hamlin, H.J., Francis-Floyd, R. et al. (2011). Nitrate-induced goiter in captive whitespotted bamboo sharks *Chiloscyllium plagiosum*. *Journal of Aquatic Animal Health* 23: 93–99.

Noga, E.J. (ed.) (2010). Fish Diseases. Diagnosis and Treatment. Ames, IA: Wiley-Blackwell.

Parkinson, L., Noblitt, S.D., Campbell, T., and Sladky, K. (2018). Comparison of two iodine quantification methods in an artificial seawater system housing white-spotted bamboo sharks (*Chiloscyllium plagiosum*). *Journal of Zoo and Wildlife Medicine* 49: 952–958.

Patin, N.V., Pratte, Z.A., Regensburger, M. et al. (2018). Microbiome dynamics in a large artificial seawater aquarium. *Applied and Environmental Microbiology* 84: 1–17.

Pisciotta, J.M., Rath, D.F., Stanel, P.A. et al. (2002). Marine bacteria cause false-positive results in the Colilert-18 Rapid Identification Test for *Escherichia coli*. *Applied and Environmental Microbiology* 68: 539–544.

Sherrill, J., Whitaker, B.R., and Wong, G.T.F. (2004). Effects of ozonation on the speciation of dissolved iodine in artificial seawater. *Journal of Zoo and Wildlife Medicine* 35: 347–355.

Smiley, J.E., Drawbridge, M.A., Okihiro, M.S., and Kaufmann, R.S. (2011). Acute effects of gas supersaturation on juvenile cultured white seabass. *Transactions of the American Fisheries Society* 140: 1269–1276.

Stamper, M.A. and Semmen, K.J. (2012a). Basic water quality evaluation for zoo veterinarians. In: Zoo and Wild Animal Medicine: Current Therapy (eds. R.E. Miller and M.E. Fowler), 177–186. St. Louis, MO: Elsevier, Saunders.

Stamper, M.A. and Semmen, K.J. (2012b). Advanced water quality evaluation for zoo veterinarians. In: Zoo and Wild Animal Medicine: Current Therapy (eds. R.E. Miller and M.E. Fowler), 195–201. St. Louis, MO: Elsevier, Saunders.

Van Bonn, W., LaPointe, A., Gibbons, S.M. et al. (2015). Aquarium microbiome response to ninety-percent system water change: clues to microbiome management. *Zoo Biology* 34: 360–367.

A3

Life Support Systems

Kent J. Semmen and M. Andrew Stamper

Disney's Animals, Science and Environment, Lake Buena Vista, FL, USA

Introduction

The condition of the water is the single most critical aspect in managing fish health. This focus on environmental factors is often the hardest learning step for veterinarians transitioning from terrestrial to aquatic animal care. It impacts all aspects of their life, including growth, reproduction, stress-resilience, and health. The life support system (LSS) is the collection of equipment used to maintain and improve the condition of the water through managing its physical, chemical, and biological properties. Ensuring good water quality represents the ultimate preventive medicine challenge for the veterinarian working with aquatic systems, as there is both a science and an art to managing water in fish systems. This chapter will focus heavily on large, closed, recirculating systems as these are the most technically complex and are fairly common in public display aquariums. The concepts discussed can readily be "scaled down" or generalized to other systems.

Bacteria and Other Microorganisms

Aquatic systems are rich in microbes, including bacteria, archaea, protozoa, fungi, and microalgae such as diatoms. This microbiota is found within the water column and attached to all surfaces. On wet surfaces, this microbiota creates a sheltered scaffold known as the biofilm.

The bacteria can be autotrophic or heterotrophic. Autotrophic bacteria synthetize energy through photosynthesis or chemosynthesis using carbon from an inorganic source, such as carbonate. Heterotrophic bacteria get their energy from other organisms and therefore play important roles in both biodegradation and pathology. Both types have species that are anaerobic, aerobic, and facultatively anaerobic (preferring oxygen, but able to derive energy from other sources, like nitrate, when oxygen is in short supply).

The microbiota has a profound impact on animal health and water quality and should be considered part of the life support system.

System Type

Systems are often categorized as open, semi-open, or closed. Open systems have continuous water input and discharge, usually from a natural body of water. Examples include pens in natural waterways, raceways, and aquariums where water flows through each system. Semi-open systems also have a mechanism to recirculate some or all of the water. Closed systems do not have continuous water input or discharge. Examples of closed systems include home aquariums, intensive aquaculture systems, ponds, and most transport containers. While closed systems can be managed using a "dump and fill" approach, where some or most of the water is occasionally removed and replaced, it is more common for closed systems to be managed with recirculation through life support equipment. For this reason, the terms closed and recirculating are often used interchangeably.

Closed systems are the most complex as they are completely dependent on equipment and management practices to condition the water and sustain life. In closed systems, predictable changes occur to the water due to natural biological processes. These changes, if not countered by the LSS, will endanger fish. They include:

- Dissolved oxygen is used and carbon dioxide is produced through respiration.

Clinical Guide to Fish Medicine, First Edition. Edited by Catherine A. Hadfield and Leigh Ann Clayton.

- Nitrogenous wastes such as toxic ammonia, nitrites, and nitrates are produced from animal waste, uneaten food, and detritus.
- pH fluctuates as buffers are used or added and carbon dioxide is produced.
- Particulate and dissolved organic carbon (DOC) build up.
- Anions and cations like carbonates and calcium are used.
- Pathogen load may increase.

The LSS is used to manage and maintain appropriate levels of dissolved gases, nitrogenous wastes, and pathogens. This may involve gas exchange, mechanical, physicochemical, and biological filtration, and ultraviolet (UV) or ozone disinfection.

In all three system types, life support equipment may also be needed to process and manage incoming and discharged water to ensure suitable water condition.

The scale of LSSs varies enormously. For smaller aquariums, there are standard, off-the-shelf components readily available. As system size increases, LSSs often require more design and construction effort to help support fish health and system management. For the largest aquarium systems, engineers are often involved in the design and maintenance of the LSS.

Most of the filtration methods currently used for LSSs have their basis in municipal wastewater, drinking water, and swimming pool industries. These have very different goals from living systems, such as high levels of disinfection. Newer approaches are incorporating the natural stabilizing processes of wild aquatic systems. This understanding may provide more efficient and cost-effective life support for aquatic animals in the future.

Oxygenation and Gas Exchange

Maintaining an appropriate balance of dissolved gases in fish systems is critical to support animal respiration, support microbial respiration within the biological filtration, maintain pH, and prevent gas supersaturation. The most critical dissolved gases are oxygen, nitrogen, and carbon dioxide. Based on individual gas solubility, their natural ratio in water is 1:2:4 respectively. The ratio and actual gas concentration depend on atmospheric pressure, water temperature, salinity, pH, biological activity, and gas exchange at the surface. The larger the surface area:volume ratio of an aquarium, pond, filter, or sump, the more potential there is for gas exchange. Movement at the water surface (e.g. air columns, pump returns at the surface, and surface skimmers) enhances gas exchange at the surface. Surface skimming action is particularly important, as it prevents accumulation of a film of surfactant material at the air/water interface that reduces gas exchange.

The primary components that maintain adequate gas exchange include:

- Air/oxygen diffusers, e.g. air stones connected to ambient air or compressed oxygen (Figure A3.1a).
- Air/oxygen exchange towers, e.g. degas towers (Figure A3.1b).
- Surface skimmers that remove the surface water.
- Air/oxygen venturis that suck in air or oxygen.

Supersaturation can occur whenever gas gets into a system at high pressure. The most common causes are compromised plumbing on the suction side of a pump, excessive deep-water aeration, or supersaturated incoming water. The percentage of supersaturation (delta P) is equal to the total dissolved gases (TDGs) compared to the barometric pressure of the air at the water's surface. This is measured using TDG meters (also known as saturometers). A delta P greater than 10% can cause gas emboli in fish (see Chapter C1).

Water Flow

Water flow should be suitable for the species and provide adequate exposure to the components of the LSS. Appropriate water flow (velocity and direction) directly impacts animal health and welfare:

- Promotes gas exchange at the surface and prevents anoxic or stagnant pockets of water.
- Promotes healthy-system bacteria in biofilms and reduces fouling bacteria in the sediment.
- Helps transfer nutrients and waste products and reduces sediment buildup.
- Reduces turbidity in the water column.
- Prevents thermal stratifications (layers) in the water column.
- Ensures correct flow through the LSS.
- Reduces pathogen loads, particularly ectoparasites.
- Affects animal behavior and feeding; these behavioral effects can be used to improve visibility of fish in display aquariums.

Water flow is typically achieved using water or air pumps. The most common is a centrifugal water pump (Figure A3.2). This is a very simple machine that imparts energy to the water by "slinging" water out of its impeller with centrifugal force, resulting in flow. They come in a variety of types and sizes. Power is reported as flow per unit time (e.g. gallons per minute). It is important to note that pumps produce noise, vibration, and heat. The effects of these on fish systems should be mitigated where possible (e.g. rubber mounts for pumps).

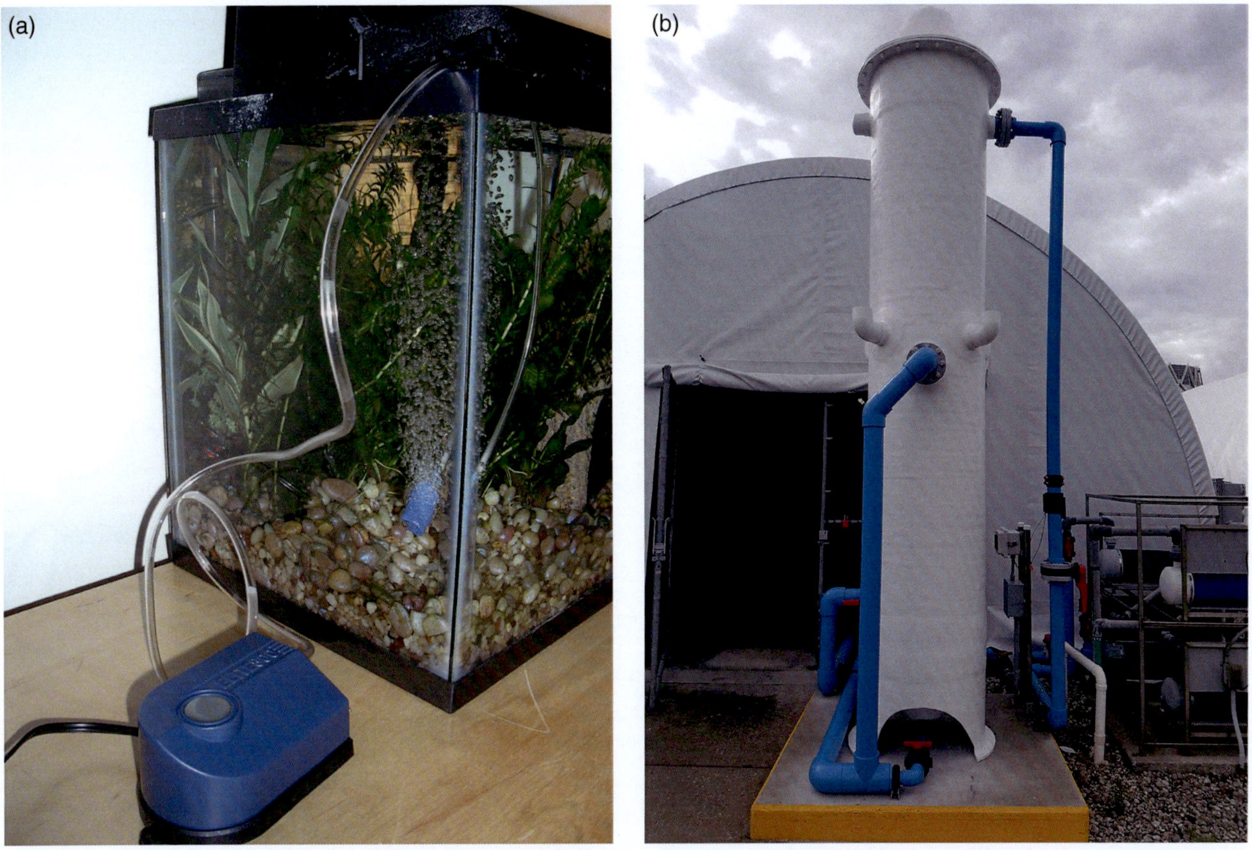

Figure A3.1 Gas exchange using an air stone (a) and a degassing tower (b). *Source*: Image (a) courtesy of Catherine Hadfield.

When designing an LSS, pump size is a critical consideration. Pumps affect the rate and pressure at which water moves through the individual LSS components, controlling their efficacy and efficiency. LSS components often have flow rate and pressure specifications they must operate under to perform adequately. The desired rate of flow is also dependent on the size of the LSS components relative to the amount of organic material (e.g. animal waste, uneaten food, detritus). Exposed outdoor systems typically have a water flow and LSS that is twice the size of an indoor system of similar size and population to help deal with external inputs such as leaves and other debris.

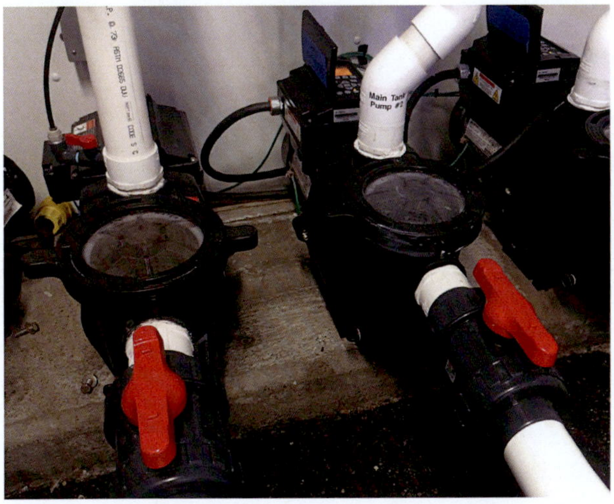

Figure A3.2 Centrifugal pumps for water flow. There are mechanical filters (known as basket filters) upstream of the pumps to reduce the risk of debris getting into the pump and ball valves to control water flow. *Source*: Images courtesy of Catherine Hadfield, Seattle Aquarium.

In some cases, all the water will go through life support equipment (batch-treatment). In other cases, some water may be diverted through life support equipment (side-stream), e.g. passing a percentage of the water through ozone disinfection.

The turnover rate is the time the total water volume of the system might take to go through the LSS; this has a profound impact on water quality. Theoretically, an aquarium with a system volume of 6300 gallons flowing through a canister filter at 30 gallons/min has a turnover rate of ~3.5 hours. However, not all water in the system will be treated in the 3.5 hours, as the water mixes in the enclosure itself. So the actual water going from the main enclosure to the LSS filters is always a mixture of different filtration histories. This mixing is described by Gage and Bidwell's Law of

Dilution. Gage and Bidwell conducted experiments on how many turnovers it actually takes to filter all of the water in a pool using calibrated soil additions and measurements of turbidity. They determined that only ~40% of a pool's water actually gets filtered in one so-called turnover, and that it takes about four turnovers to filter 98% of the water. As a result, achieving four turnovers in a day or a six-hour turnover rate became the accepted norm for large swimming pools. More than 30 years ago when large aquarium systems became more common, LSS engineers reasoned that a higher turnover rate was likely needed for living systems and modern systems are typically designed with turnover rates of an hour or less.

There are a variety of flowmeters on the market that can be used to monitor critical flow rates. Common types are mechanical, magnetic, and ultrasonic. Mechanical flowmeters measure the speed of rotation of an impeller or paddle wheel within a pipe. They are the simplest and least expensive, but are less accurate than the other two and the internal parts are vulnerable to damage or obstruction. Magnetic flowmeters work according to Faraday's formula, where flow of a conductive liquid medium (the water) is proportional to the strength of a magnetic force passing through it, measured in volts. Magnetic flowmeters come in both insertion probe or in-line styles that can be mounted anywhere, and one- or two-beam (for better accuracy) types. They are low-maintenance, show better accuracy, provide minimal to no obstruction to water flow, and have no moving parts, but are more expensive. Finally, strap-on ultrasonic flowmeters bounce high-frequency sound off solids and bubbles in the water to create a frequency shift that is directly proportional to flow rate (Doppler type), or use two bursts of sound, one in the direction of water flow (which moves faster) and one against it (which moves slower) (transit time type) to calculate flow rate. They are very easy to use, very accurate, highly portable, and can work on a wider range of water types, since they do not work off of the conductivity of the water, but they do need a run of pipe equal to or more than 10 pipe diameters ahead of them and 5 after and are the most expensive.

Mechanical and Physicochemical Filtration

The goal of mechanical filtration is to physically remove particulate waste (e.g. animal waste, uneaten food, detritus). Particulate size, in this context, extends from easily visualized material to soluble and insoluble organics. Mechanical filtration helps to physically remove large, medium, and fine particulates, nitrogenous wastes, phosphates, and some soluble and insoluble organics. Physicochemical filtration uses both physical and chemical processes to remove dissolved contaminants such as in foam fractionation, granular activated carbon, and flocculation treatments.

Surface Skimming

In most systems, it is good to have skimming to remove oils and other floating debris that produce a film on the surface. This is important since, in addition to being organic waste, these materials inhibit gas exchange and light penetration at the water's surface. Skimming is usually the first step in filtration. As the water exits the tank, skimmers at the surface divert the materials at the surface to a waste stream. Surface skimming flow rate is dependent on the surface-to-volume ratio of the tank but should be ~50–100% of the total system flow rate.

Prefilters

Large particulates can be removed using prefilters. These are often screens, for example basket screens in skimmers, sock filters, or large rotating drum screens (Figure A3.3). Size of particulates trapped depends on the mesh size, typically reported in micrometers. With smaller mesh sizes, more particulate is trapped but more labor is required to clean the filters and avoid clogging. The mesh size should be such that water will still flow when the prefilter is saturated.

Sand/Canister/Bead Filters

Medium particulates can be removed by sand, canister, or bead filtration (Figure A3.4). Sand filters (also called pressure sand filters or mixed-bed filters) use various grades of gravel and sand (decreasing in size from the bottom up) to trap particulates. Water flows through the filter from the top down, with larger to smaller particulates being removed as it flows through. Water pressure builds as material gathers in the filter, plugging the channels of water flow. When the filters reach a predetermined pressure, water flow is reversed and the contents are flushed to municipal sewer outlets; this is known as a back-flush or back-wash. Canister filters contain a variety of filter media within cartridges or bags that are easy to remove for servicing. A cartridge may consist of pleated filter media. Bead filters use buoyant polyethylene beads that are electrostatically charged to attract negatively charged particulates as the water flows through them from the bottom up. Backwashes can be driven by propeller or bubbles to dislodge the filtrate from the media and send it to municipal sewer outlets; this may be automated or done manually.

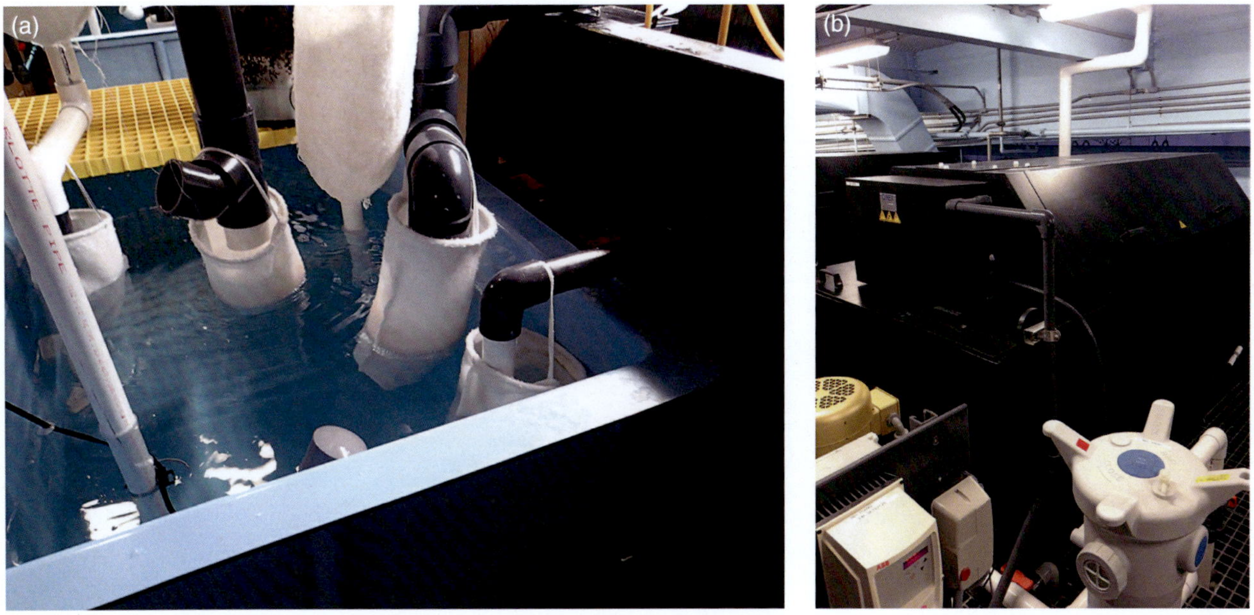

Figure A3.3 Sock filters (a) and a rotating drum filter (b).

Settling/Sedimentation Tanks

Settleable particles have a relatively high specific gravity compared to the water they are in, so they tend to settle to the bottom. Suspended particles have a specific gravity the same as, or slightly higher than, the water they are in, so they tend to stay in suspension and will only drop out slowly. A settling or sedimentation tank is designed to minimize turbulence and allow suspended particles to settle out of the system water as it flows (Figure A3.5). They can then be removed by a bottom drain or by suctioning them off the bottom at regular intervals.

Foam Fractionators

Foam fractionation (also known as protein skimming or protein fractionation) is a process that mimics the natural process of wind and wave movement on the ocean surface – this mixing of air with seawater creates a thick foam of surfactant materials, known as spindrift, which blows up onto the shore and so is taken out of the aquatic system. In a foam fractionator, this is accomplished by pushing microbubbles through a venturi injector into the base of a tall cylindrical column. System water flows through the column from top to bottom, countercurrent to the bubbles rising in

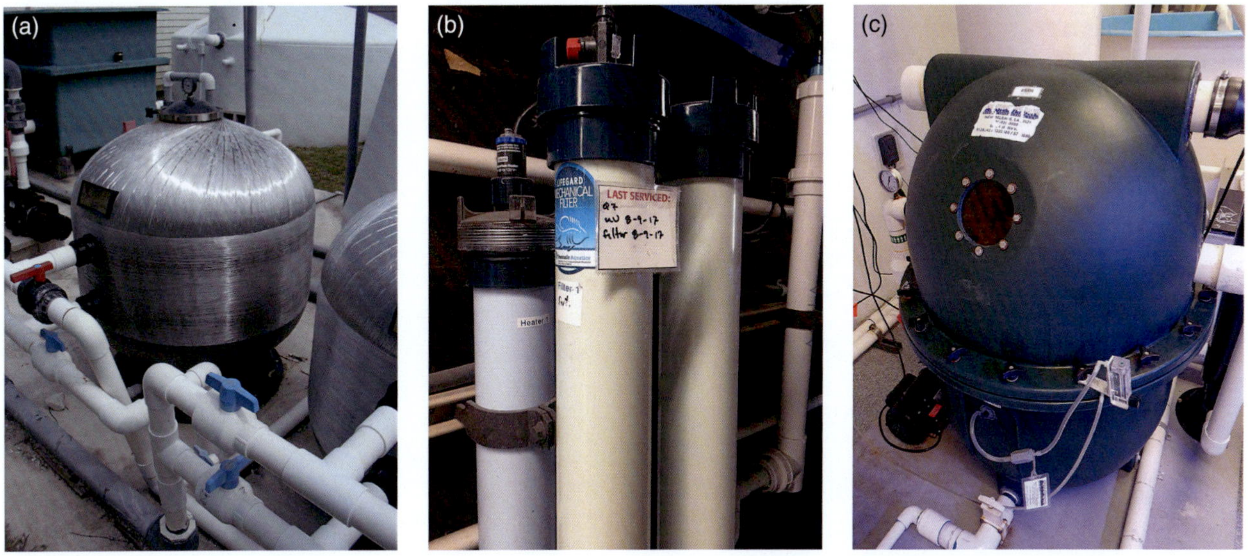

Figure A3.4 Sand filter (a), canister filter (b), bead filter (c). *Source*: Image (b) courtesy of Catherine Hadfield, Seattle Aquarium.

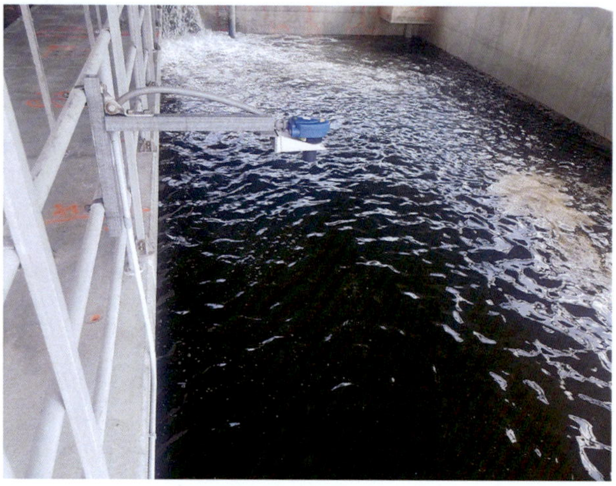

Figure A3.5 Settling tank.

the column. As the bubbles rise, long-chained organic molecules stick to them. As the bubbles contact the surface, they coalesce into a thick film, releasing air that then burps the foam up and out of an inverted funnel collection device (Figure A3.6). This collection device is usually auto-rinsed with potable water to municipal sewer on a regular cycle. When applied correctly, this provides continuous removal of proteins, amino acids, and lipids from the decomposition of organic waste in the aquarium. In addition, this sticky surfactant waste tends to also carry secondary waste products that include trace metals and bacteria through adsorption, coagulation, and microflocculation. Foam fractionators also increase aeration of the system water. Foam fractionators have to be closely managed to maintain the correct flow for efficient operation. They are not effective in freshwater; they typically require a salinity of >15 g/L to provide the necessary surfactant pressure.

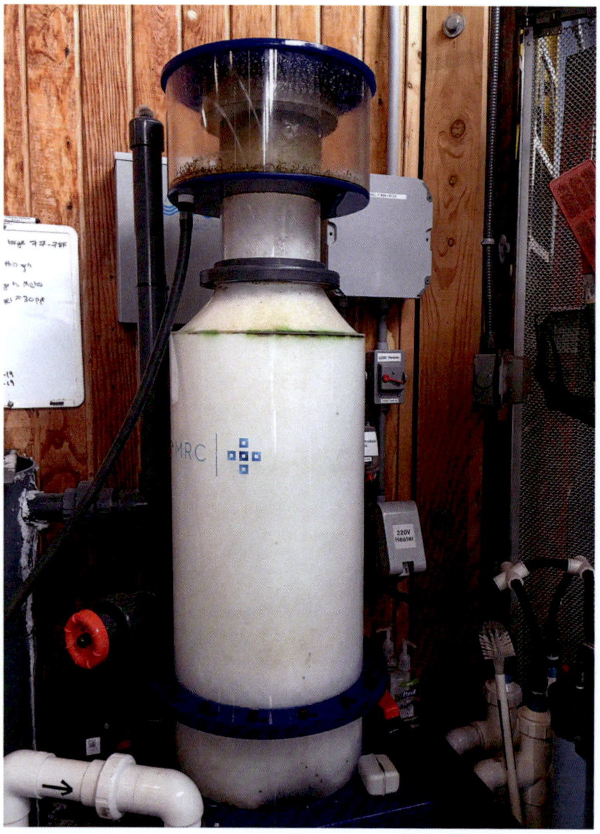

Figure A3.6 Foam fractionator. *Source*: Image courtesy of Catherine Hadfield, Seattle Aquarium.

Relatively small doses of ozone enhance the removal of organics and provide disinfection. This is typically on a side-stream equivalent to about 20% of the main filtration rate but is fed directly from the aquarium for optimum performance. This combination of foam fractionation and ozone provides increased pH, increased dissolved oxygen concentration, increased oxidation reduction potential (ORP), improved water clarity, and reduced dependency on turnover rate, sand filters, and other traditional LSS components.

Activated Carbon

Granular activated carbon (GAC) is a highly porous carbonaceous, crystalline, granulated material with a tremendous surface area-to-volume ratio (Figure A3.7). It is made by heating a carbon-based material to very high temperatures and then opening up its crystalline pore structure with steam or acid. Carbon sources include bones, coal, nut shells, peat, petroleum residues, sawdust, sugarcane pulp, wastewater sludge, and wood. Lignite coal-based carbons have a pore size ideally suited for water treatment. GAC physically adsorbs heavy metals (e.g. copper) and dissolved substances (e.g. medications, organic carbon). In aquarium systems, GAC filters are commonly used to deal with the gradual yellowing of water due to the buildup of humic and fulvic acids (Spotte 1991). GAC filters adsorb these organic materials and improve water clarity.

GAC also removes oxidants such as ozone and chlorine by oxidation on its outer surfaces (not within its pore structure).

GAC can be part of the main-stream filtration, used on a side-stream, or plumbed as an auxiliary device which allows it to be turned on and off to manage water clarity or for short-term removal of a target compound (e.g. praziquantel). Pulse-treatment is often preferred, as there are concerns that critical organics and nutrients can be depleted by its overuse. It is most efficient when placed in-line after mechanical and biological filtration.

GAC filters can easily perform chemical, mechanical, and biological water treatment but are exhausted once the binding sites are filled. Bacteria readily utilize the GAC as a growth surface, which also decreases its efficiency over time. GAC filters must be replaced when exhausted.

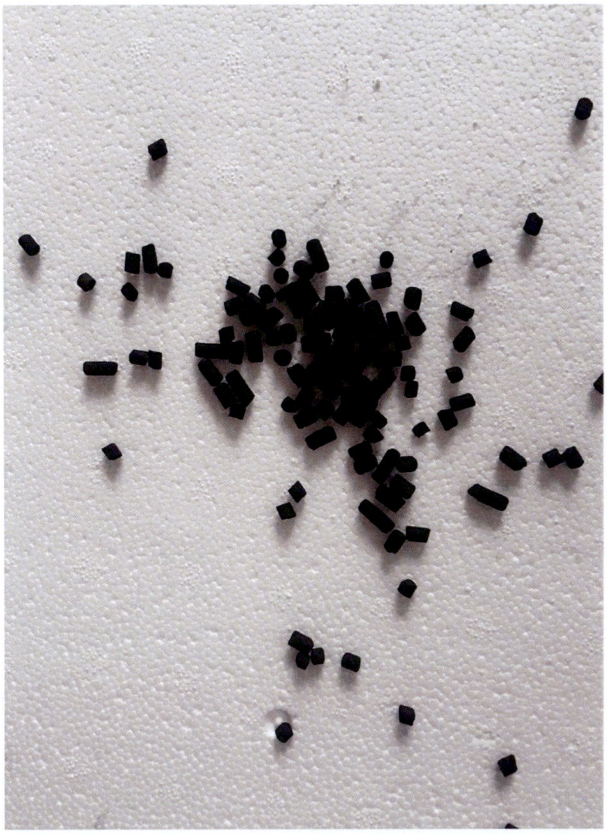

Figure A3.7 Granular activated carbon. *Source*: Image courtesy of Catherine Hadfield, Seattle Aquarium.

This may be carried out when there is increased yellowing of the water or when post-filtration levels of target substances (e.g. chlorine) are outside of acceptable ranges.

Flocculation

Flocculation uses chemicals to bind particulates in order to make them bigger and easier to remove. It focuses on dissolved organic carbon. Common flocculants used in freshwater include aluminum sulfate (alum) and natural and synthetic polymers (cationic polyelectrolytes). These act by reducing surface charges on dissolved or suspended particles, allowing them to collide and coagulate. They are most effective at $pH < 7.5$. The effects on fish and invertebrate species are not fully known and they should be used with caution, especially where other techniques are available.

Mechanical and Physicochemical Filtration Troubleshooting

Common problems include:

- Inadequate size for the organic load: The filtration should be designed to handle the highest organic load that might be found in the system.
- Inappropriate positioning: Most mechanical filters should be positioned between the system and dedicated biological filters, heat exchangers, and disinfection. Some form of mechanical filtration should be found upstream of water pumps.
- Biofouling/clogging: There should be constant, even flow through filter media. Signs of increased pressure, obvious channeling of water, or bypassing of the filter media should be investigated.

Problems with mechanical filtration often reduce water flow and/or allow the buildup of nitrogenous wastes. Short-term solutions to problems with mechanical filtration include: back-washing filters; changing some of the filter media; siphoning animal waste, uneaten food, and detritus; increasing water changes; and temporarily reducing feeding.

Biological Filtration: Nitrification and Mineralization

Biological filtration (biofiltration) involves heterotrophic and autotrophic bacteria. In some cases, archaea may also be involved or even dominate the process, especially in freshwater systems (Sauder et al. 2011). Many species of heterotrophic bacteria use available organic compounds as energy sources, degrading them into simpler and simpler compounds until they are reduced to inorganic minerals (termed mineralization). However, many of these same bacteria can also feed on living organisms including other bacteria, invertebrates, and fish, crossing over from being beneficial to detrimental. For example, many *Aeromonas* and *Vibrio* spp. can behave like this. Autotrophic bacteria use carbon from an inorganic source, such as carbonate, so they are not associated with biodegradation or pathology.

Aquatic animals release nitrogenous organic waste from the breakdown of proteins, and other metabolic waste in the form of ammonia, urea, or uric acid. Nitrification is an aerobic two-step process in which specific genera of primarily autotrophic nitrifying bacteria convert ammonia (NH_3 and NH_4^+) to nitrate (NO_3^-). Billions of aerobic bacteria on substrate and surfaces exposed to ammonia-rich water use ammonia for energy and transform it to nitrite during this process (nitrification step 1) $NH_4^+ + 1.5O_2 \rightarrow NO_2^- + H_2O + 2H^+$. Billions of other aerobic bacteria, living on the same surfaces, use toxic nitrite for energy, transforming it into the relatively nontoxic nitrate (nitrification step 2) $NO_2^- + 0.5O_2 \rightarrow NO_3^-$.

The actual species that become established in a system will vary based on the environmental conditions and the species' competitive edge. They all require sufficient oxygen. Necessary nutrients are primarily carbon (as carbonate and bicarbonate), nitrogen (as ammonia and nitrite), phosphorus (as phosphates), and sulfur. Other critical elements include calcium, iron, manganese, and molybdenum. These are primarily supplied by the solids in the water, so animal feeding and waste have direct effects on the bacterial population. It is important to note that the bacteria require complex organic foods, but only use simple sugars and small amounts of amino acids and micronutrients. Very little of the nitrogen, phosphorus, and sulfur in animal feeds or waste is used by the bacteria. The leftover dissolved organic wastes accumulate in a closed-system aquarium and can reach levels that are harmful to aquatic organisms. That is why rapid uptake of solid wastes using high flow rates through efficient mechanical filtration is so important in closed-system aquariums.

While biofiltration bacteria are on all surfaces, filters have been designed to specifically support them:

- *Sand filters* (Figure A3.4a): These filters are often a preferred location for these bacteria if the source water is rich in oxygen and nitrogen-rich organic waste. The substrate provides abundant surface area. A secondary benefit is that the biofilm aids in the filtration of organic particulates, heavy metals, and pathogenic bacteria.
- *Undergravel filters* (Figure A3.8): These consist of a perforated plate covering the bottom of the environment with an appropriate medium, ranging from fine sand to coarse gravel, on top of the plate. Air-driven uplift tubes draw the water from the space below the plate to near the surface. As a result, water is pulled downward through the media where the nitrifying bacteria exist, thus performing mechanical and biological filtration simultaneously.
- *Reverse flow undergravel filters*: In these, mechanically filtered water is introduced underneath the filter plate, making them dedicated biological filters.
- *Foam/sponge filters* (Figure A3.9): Water is drawn through a block of open-celled polyurethane foam or sponge (serving as the biological medium) by an air-driven uplift tube. These combine mechanical and biological filtration. These are particularly good for quarantine and hospital systems, since they can be easily replaced.
- *Trickle filters/biotowers* (Figure A3.10): These use a container above the water line filled with biological medium (e.g. bioballs). Prefiltered water is evenly distributed across the top of the medium via a spray bar or a perforated diffuser plate. Water then drips evenly down through the exposed medium, mixing with the air, and eventually collecting in a sump below to be pumped back into the system. These provide biological filtration and gas exchange.
- *Biowheel filters or rotating biological contactors (RBC)* (Figure A3.11a): These consist of discs or cylinders of rigid biofilter medium positioned half in and half out of the water. They rotate slowly, exposing all surfaces intermittently to water and air. These provide biological filtration and gas exchange.
- *Fluidized beds or fluidized sand bed filters* (Figure A3.11b): These consist of a tube through which the system water flows from the bottom upward through a suitable biological medium, usually a fine quartz silica sand. The upwelling water expands the sand bed as it passes through it, allowing any particulate waste to pass through and preventing plugging of the bed, and then exits out the top to return to the system. These provide highly efficient biological filtration.

The process of bacterial selection and growth within these filters can be slow, often taking several weeks. With immature filters, animal additions to the system should be very slow, allowing the biological filtration to catch up prior to further animal additions. The process may be accelerated by feeding or seeding immature filters. Filters may be fed with ammonium chloride, ammonium sulfate, or urea to allow for some bacterial selection, prior to adding fish or invertebrates. Alternatively or in combination, filters can be artificially seeded with nitrifying bacteria. These may be purchased commercially, but the contents of the mixtures are unregulated. Alternatively, bacterial media from systems with similar environmental parameters may be transferred over to accelerate colonization of the biological filters. It seems very likely that this could also transmit pathogenic bacteria, viruses, and parasites from the source system. The risk of disease transfer should be assessed. A great option for immature biological filters, and a safeguard in case of filter damage, is to manage a "biofarm" of filter media, fed artificially (without any animals), which can be used to seed systems as needed.

Biological filtration does have its challenges as well. Aquarium environments create unnaturally large populations of relatively few species of nitrifying bacteria. Any limiting factor (e.g. low dissolved oxygen, low alkalinity, low phosphate, reduced feed amounts) or any environmental change (e.g. temperature, pH, salinity, antibacterials) can have dramatic effects on these bacteria. This can destroy their ability to oxidize toxic ammonia and nitrite. The bacterial biofilm can also foul the mechanical filtration (clogging). Also, biofiltration bacteria produce by-products such as nitrate, phosphate, carbon dioxide, silicate, and biologically inert organic compounds which can lead to excess algae growth and yellowing of aquarium water. They also compete with the fish and invertebrates for dissolved oxygen and trace elements. And if deprived of oxygen (e.g. due

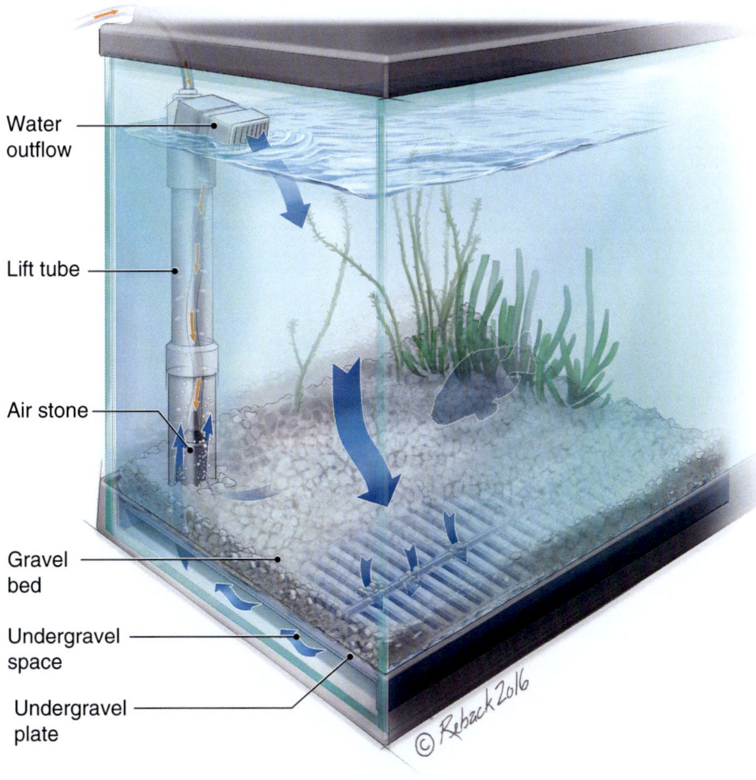

Figure A3.8 Undergravel filter showing the direction of water flow (blue arrows) and air flow (orange arrows). Some gravel has been removed to show the filter plate. *Source*: Image courtesy of Nicholas Reback, copyright reserved.

to poor water flow, deep substrate, or pump failure), they can create toxic hydrogen sulfide within the system.

Biological Filtration Troubleshooting

Common problems with biological filters include:

- Sudden reductions in nutrient availability: Biological filters require oxygen, carbonates, phosphates, and steady amounts of ammonia and nitrite. Changes in these can have major effects on nitrification.
- Changes in environmental conditions: Recent changes in environmental parameters such as temperature, pH, or salinity (e.g. from a large water change with colder water) can have dramatic impacts on nitrification. A variety of immersion medications also have antibacterial activity that can damage nitrifying bacteria (e.g. formalin, chloroquine, enrofloxacin, copper).
- Inadequate size for the organic load: Size calculations are based on the amount of food protein fed per day. If needed, biofilter manufacturers should be able to help with size estimates.
- Biofouling/clogging/channeling: With any biological filter, signs of increased pressure, obvious channeling of water, or bypassing of the filter media should be investigated. Sand filters and trickle beds are particularly prone to clogging.

In the event of problems with biological filters, short-term solutions can include: back-washing filters; changing some of the filter media; siphoning animal waste, uneaten food, and detritus; increasing water changes; and temporarily reducing feeding. Bacterial recovery takes time. Additional biological filtration can be seeded from other suitable systems, but this will not help if there are nutrient limitations.

Denitrification

Nitrifying bacteria produce nitrate. Even though nitrate is not known to be directly toxic to fish, it does act as a stressor, has endocrine-disrupting activity, and leads to algal and bacterial blooms.

Nitrates are most simply removed through water changes. They are also used by plants in the system. Where water changes are not feasible or nitrates cannot be reduced to target levels, biological denitrification is required. This is the process of turning nitrates into nitrogen through anaerobic microbial action. This involves heterotrophic, autotrophic, and/or anammox (autotrophic anaerobic ammonium oxidizing) bacteria.

Denitrification filters are technically challenging, labor-intensive, and often costly. They can also produce toxic elements that can be released into the main water system. For

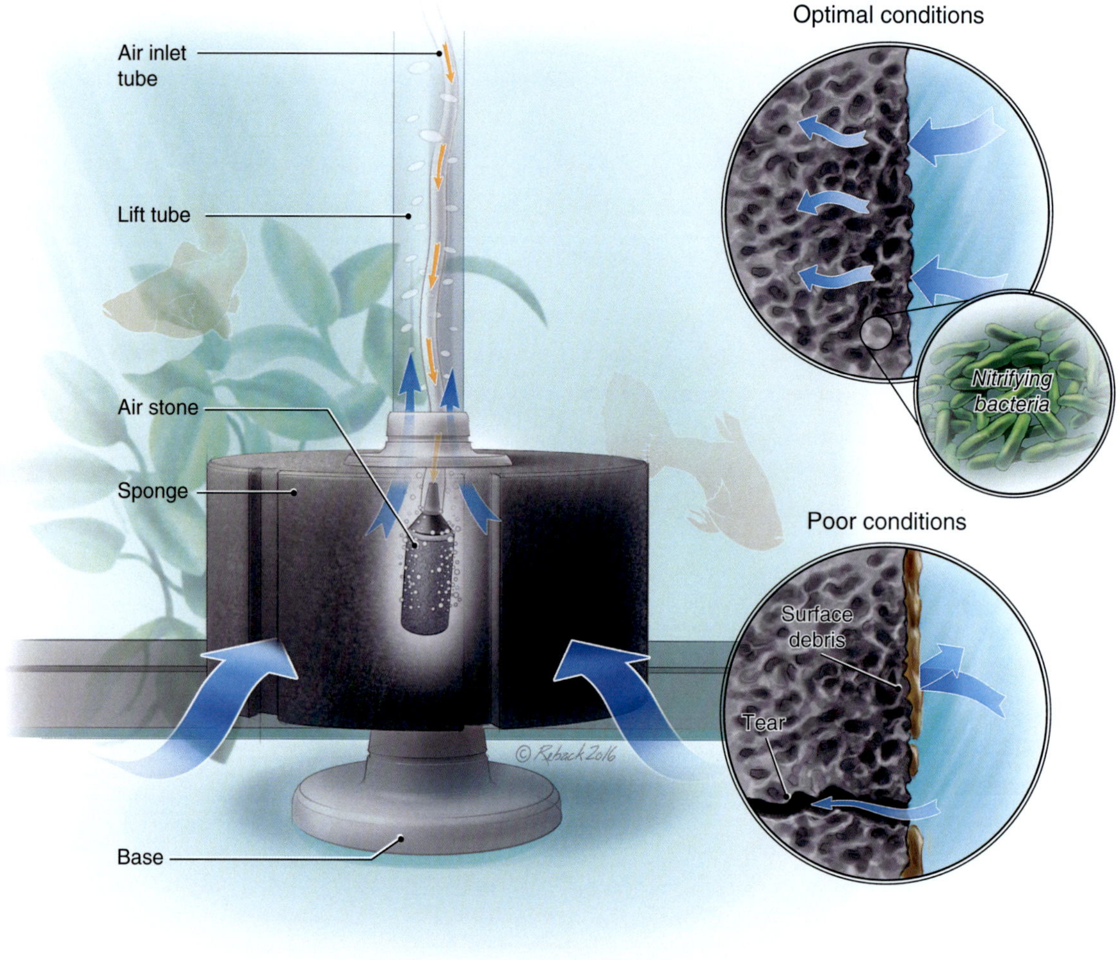

Figure A3.9 Foam/sponge filter showing the direction of water flow (blue arrows) and air flow (orange arrows) along with the position of the air stone. Inserts show how cracking of the sponge leads to channeling of the water, bypassing the filter media. *Source*: Image courtesy of Nicholas Reback, copyright reserved.

these reasons, denitrification should not be attempted without experienced staff.

Denitrification filters use a carbon source and anaerobic conditions to grow bacteria that can convert nitrate to nitrogen (or in some cases, nitrite). They are done on a side-stream off the main system LSS. Historically, a heterotrophic process using a variety of bacteria and a constant input of an organic food source (often methanol, CH_3OH) has been common. For safety, the concentration of methanol at all points in the process requires daily analyses, constant adjustment, and many fail-safes to assure that methanol residual does not build up in the water, as this can trigger a bacterial bloom resulting in rapidly falling dissolved oxygen. Bacterial blooms and reduced activity can result if the system is taken off-line for any reason; this can take days to recover from.

In recent years, a sulfur-oxidizing autotrophic process has become popular (Figure A3.12). In this case, the bacteria live and derive their food from a sulfur media. This is much less labor-intensive, requiring monitoring of outside inputs (e.g. flow rate, temperature, and organic debris), regular back-washing, and the addition of more sulfur every 6–12 months. *Thiobacillus denitrificans* was believed to be the primary bacteria in this process, but recent research has demonstrated that it is a diverse community of anaerobes that typically carry out the process (Burns et al. 2018). This denitrification process works best in tropical water (>24°C, 75°F), and the bacteria tend to establish very rapidly upon startup (e.g. two to three days at 25°C, 77°F), even with new sulfur media and no bacterial seeding. The top of the bed is established with the aerobic heterotrophic bacteria necessary to remove oxygen for the anaerobic denitrification process deeper in the bed. A buffering reactor filled with calcareous material such as scallop shell or magnesium oxide/calcite media should follow the acidifying denitrification process. Additional buffer may be needed to

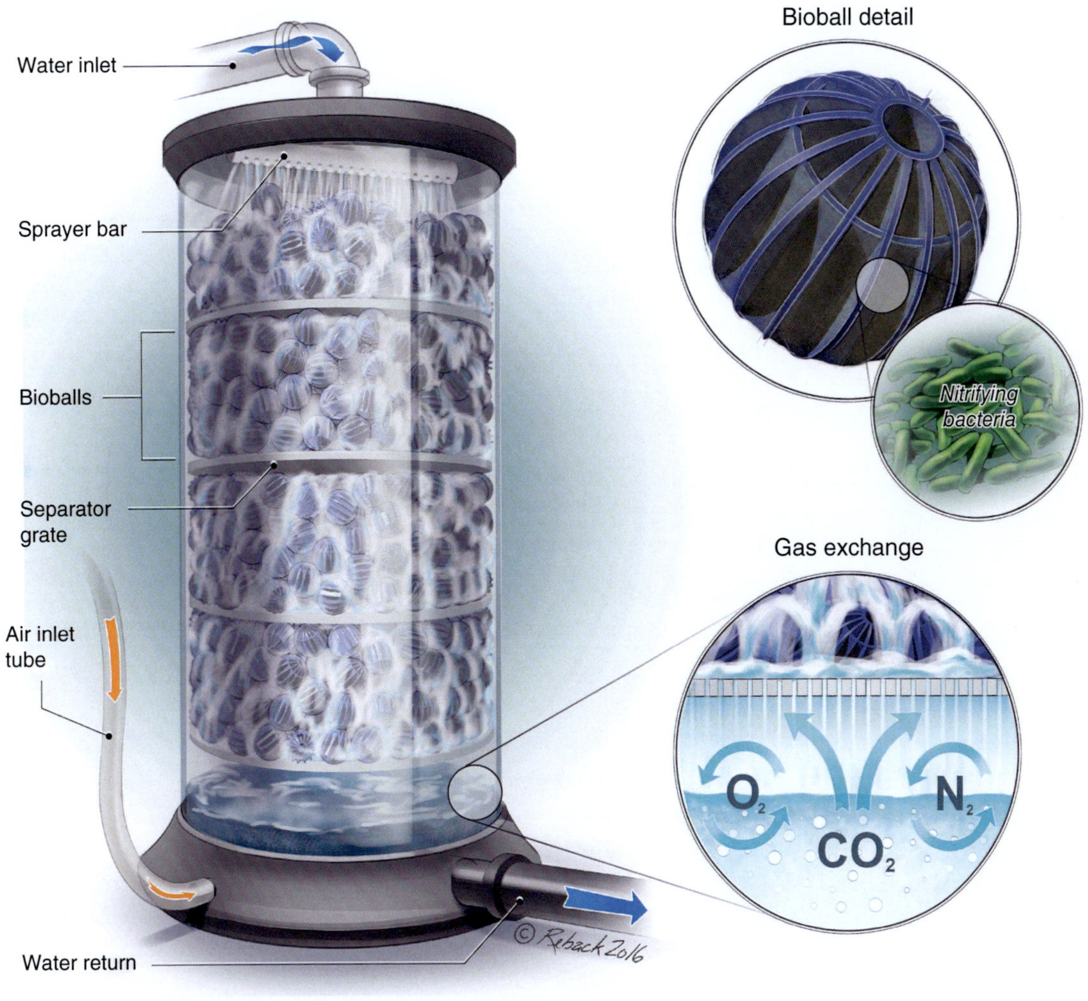

Figure A3.10 Biotower showing the direction of water flow (blue arrows) and air (orange arrows). The top insert shows one type of bioball. *Source*: Image courtesy of Nicholas Reback, copyright reserved.

manage the system pH, such as a sodium carbonate, sodium bicarbonate, or sodium hydroxide. Heavy backwashing of the media is required at regular intervals to prevent biofouling. Possible nitrite and hydrogen sulfide in the return stream must be monitored for safety. Fouled filters must be taken off-line for maintenance.

Deep sand bed filtration is used in some marine aquariums, typically within the main enclosure. A deep sand bed is designed to cultivate anaerobic bacteria in bottom layers of sand, converting nitrate to nitrogen. The filter usually consists of a bed of fine sand (0.05–1 mm grain size) with a minimum depth of 10–15 cm; this ensures that a portion of the sand at the bottom will not be exposed to water circulation. Eventually, the bed becomes established with bacteria, algae, and other marine organisms such as worms, crabs, snails, and sea stars. The animals burrow and overturn the top 5–7 cm of sand in search of food, which causes water to circulate deeper in the sand than it would if the animals were not present. This helps prevent the production of anoxic substances that would be toxic to the fish, and provides a naturally balanced microecology.

Anammox-related microorganisms were identified in both marine and freshwater aquaculture recirculating systems by Tal et al. (2003, 2004). Bacteria of the order *Planctomycetales* were shown to eliminate nitrogen by combining ammonia and nitrite to produce nitrogen gas, thereby providing an alternative approach to denitrification (van de Graaf et al. 1995). Its application has the potential to provide significant oxygen and energy savings due the oxidation of only half of the ammonia produced in the system. It is possible that the "passive denitrification" or nitrogen loss observed in recirculating systems is the result of this anammox activity. Processes to promote this special type of autotrophic bacteria (currently being tested in industry) could result in simpler and safer denitrification methods than using methanol or sulfur.

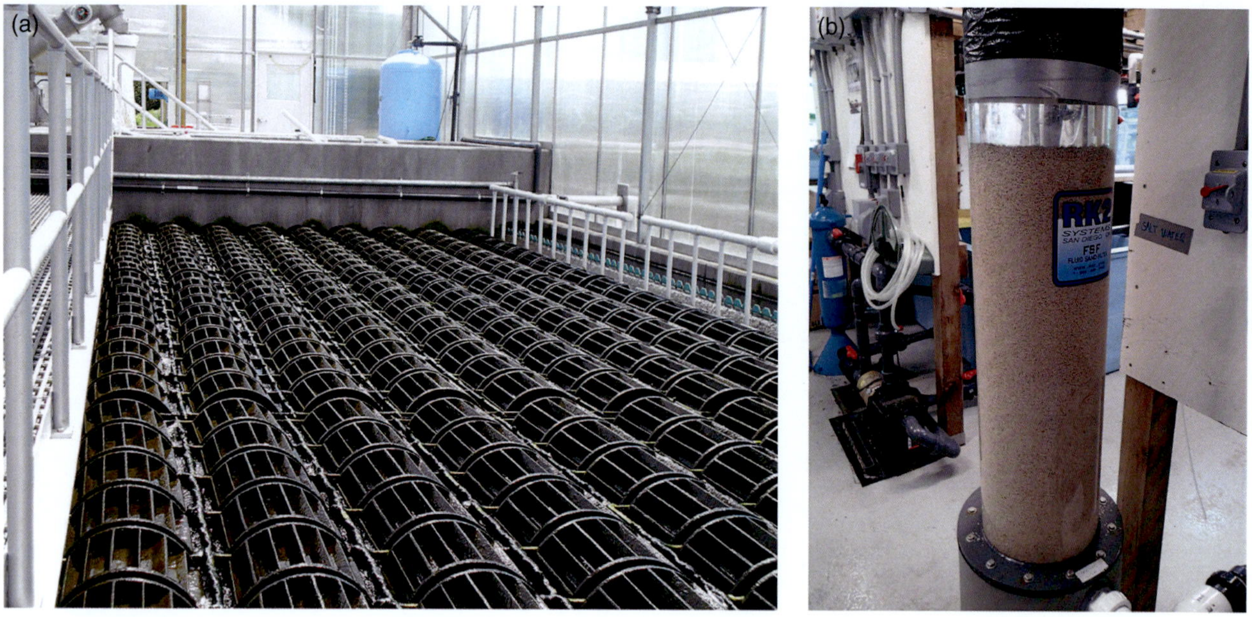

Figure A3.11 Biowheel filter (a) and fluidized bed (b). *Source*: Image (a) courtesy of Chris Limcaco, Algaewheel Technologies, LLC, and (b) courtesy of Catherine Hadfield, National Aquarium.

Ecological Scrubbers

In natural systems, bacteria break down organics rapidly to supply algae and plants with nutrients to grow. As a result, nutrients typically do not accrue in natural systems (without outside inputs like nitrogenous fertilizer). In artificial systems, when algae and plants are discouraged to grow, organic and inorganic end products build up. Biological filtration is the process in which unnaturally large populations of relatively few bacteria species convert organic waste products. Ecological filtration is the natural process centered on using balanced, diverse populations of vascular plants, algae, microorganisms (bacteria, archaea, protozoa), and/or macroinvertebrates to form an environment that cycles and/or removes waste products in the aquarium while balancing water chemistry. These organisms can also provide a rich source of nutrition for herbivores and omnivores. This type of living refugium filtration is simple to design and operate, and is usually inexpensive compared with traditional methods. This holistic approach may improve animal health, habitat operations, and aesthetics.

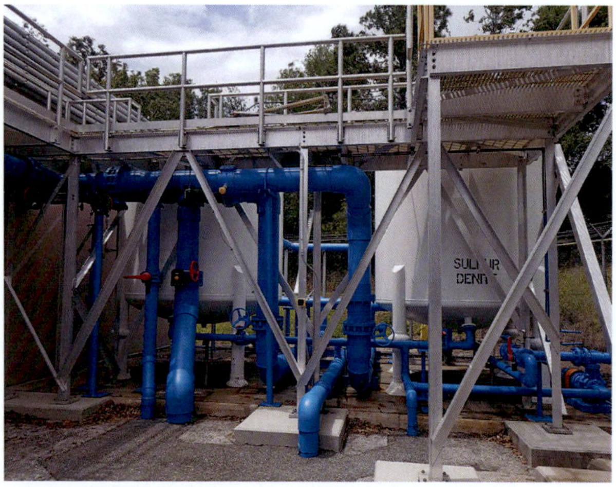

Figure A3.12 A sulfur denitrification system.

Refugium filtration based on the previously described deep sand bed filters and the use of live rock have become common in tropical reef aquariums where living corals are the predominant animals. Live rock consists of rock and aragonite originally formed by corals or other calcareous organisms and is heavily colonized by a host of micro- and macro-organisms that live in and on it. These organisms perform anaerobic and aerobic types of biological filtration in an ecologically balanced way. There are many artificially established varieties of live rock available on the market today; these reduce the need to harvest from the ocean environment.

Algae-based refugium filters are often called algal turf scrubbers or algal scrubbers. They consist of a shallow trough or raceway or rotating wheels connected in-line with the main system (Figure A3.13). They often have screens to increase the surface area. They need to be well-lit by light emitting diodes (LEDs), high-intensity metal halide, or very high-output (VHO) fluorescent lamps with ample levels of photosynthetically active radiation (PAR) in a cycle opposite to that of the main habitat (Adey and Loveland 2011). Natural sunlight to augment treatment

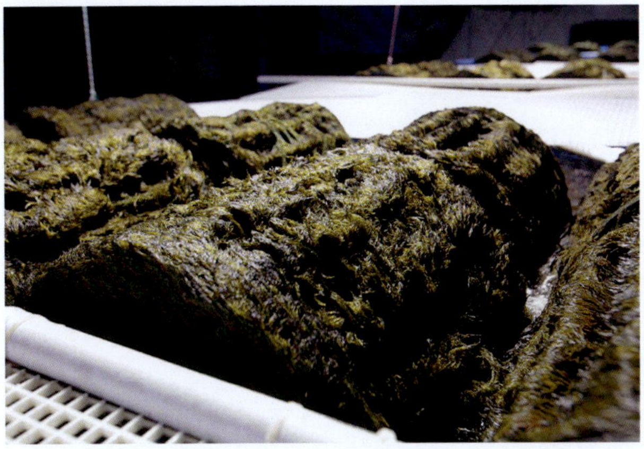

Figure A3.13 Algal scrubber wheels. *Source*: Image courtesy of Chris Limcaco, Algaewheel Technologies, LLC.

during the day can also be used, if access to unfiltered sunlight is possible. The balanced nature of these filters should provide a robust and diverse microbiome to naturally compete with potential pathogens, rather than serving as a "pathogen reservoir".

In tropical seawater, red and blue-green algae and diatoms usually dominate. With high-intensity lighting, diatoms will colonize the turf first, followed by the blue-green algae. Green and brown algae are always present, but in smaller numbers. Once the algal turf matures, it must be continually grazed (e.g. by amphipods or chironomid insects living in these systems) or it goes through succession and produces a less productive macroalgal forest (Adey and Loveland 2011). Periodic human intervention to manually harvest the algae with a tool like a plastic putty knife is occasionally needed.

In the past, aquarists have tried to force the ecological scrubbers to grow edible algae such as *Caulerpa* spp. While this appears to be a good idea, it has resulted in collapse and the sudden release of nutrients and metals as the plants decay. Ecological scrubbers should by managed with what naturally grows and evolves as this will lead to a much more stable system.

Water Disinfection

After mechanical and biological filtration, other materials such as color-producing organics and infectious agents (primarily bacteria and viruses) need to be addressed through disinfection. Point contact disinfection is a process whereby water is diverted in a side-stream fashion to be in contact with a sterilizing agent (e.g. UV or ozone) and then recycled back to the system. To improve water quality, the rate of side-stream treatment must exceed the rate of system contamination (i.e. bacterial growth in the region holding the animals). UV can have an additive or synergistic effect when used with ozone in series, reducing the required applied dose of each. Bulk-fluid disinfection is a process whereby a residual oxidant (e.g. liquid chlorine, chlorine dioxide, hydrogen peroxide, or sodium hypochlorite) is added to the main system. This should never be used with fish and aquatic invertebrates.

Ultraviolet Light Disinfection

UV light in the 254 nm range irradiates pathogens and proteinaceous material, physically destroying them. It requires adequate bulb output (measured in mJ/cm^2 or mWs/cm^2) and an appropriate contact time and flow rate (Figure A3.14). This technique is most effective when used in flow-through systems, with irradiation of the incoming water. It is less effective in closed and semi-closed systems, since the effect is localized and may not control the microbial density nearest the animal. The efficiency of UV varies and it should be continuously monitored. Target organism kill rates can be established based on contact time and flow rate. UV quality deteriorates over time and tubes need to be changed regularly (e.g. at least every six months). The quartz sleeves around the bulbs may need to be wiped down as frequently as daily or weekly to reduce biofouling.

Ozone Disinfection

Ozone (O_3) is a very strong oxidizer, which is useful for disinfection and water clarification but carries high risks and high equipment and operational costs. Ozone oxidizes therapeutics, color-producing organics, ammonia, nitrite, and micro-organisms, and it reduces turbidity through a process of microflocculation (Johnson 2000; Overby 2002). To work efficiently and safely, ozone disinfection needs:

1) Suitable ozone gas generation.
2) Appropriate gas-to-liquid mass transfer (mixing).
3) Adequate contact time for reaction (often ~10 minutes).
4) Destruction of residual ozone and oxidation by-products.

Ozone is created by exposing dry O_2 to high AC voltage across a discharge gap (Figure A3.15a). Ozone must be generated on site since it is labile. Ozone is injected into a side-stream contact chamber with system water flowing through it; this is where the oxidation occurs. The contact chamber may be a dedicated ozone chamber, trickle filter, or foam fractionator; use of a foam fractionator improves the efficiency (Figure A3.15b).

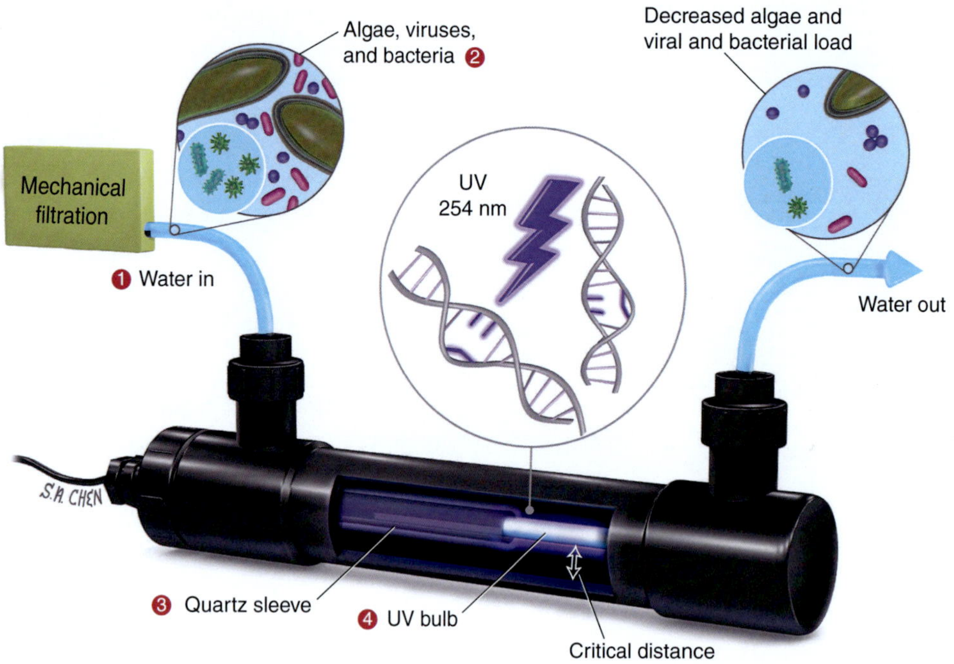

Figure A3.14 Diagram showing ultraviolet light disinfection. *Source*: Image courtesy of Sarah Chen, copyright reserved.

Ozone exposed to salt water can create residual oxidative by-products (particularly hypobromous acid and hypochlorous acid that can generate trihalomethanes), which can travel out into the main system and kill fish. Once the water flows out of the contact chamber, it should be passed through either a biological filter, and/or activated carbon, UV, or intense heat to remove residuals; these may be known as ozone destruct units. Packed column aeration is another technique for removing residuals from the water, particularly trihalomethanes. In this process, the water is trickled down a tower filled with inert material as a fan blows air upward into the tower. Most residuals are volatile and are released into the air. Ozone is short-lived, so many residuals can also be limited by simply increasing contact time in the contact chamber. Residuals can also be reduced by creating salt mixes that are low in bromides.

Ozone needs to be carefully monitored to ensure animal and human safety. This may include:

1) Monitoring ozone generation (often 0.3–0.5 mg/h/gallon) or actual ozone dose (often 0.01–0.50 mg/L).
2) Monitoring oxidation-reduction potential (ORP) in the contact chamber and in the aquarium (Figure A3.15c and d). This is often 700–800 mV for optimum disinfection in ozone contact chambers but should be <200–350 mV in the fish habitat. The trend in aquarium systems is to try to reduce this to avoid dosing above demand.
3) Monitoring residual oxidants, particularly total and free bromine. These should be very low in fish systems (HOBr < 0.02 mg/L).
4) Testing for ambient ozone leaks.
5) Testing turbidity.
6) Monitoring bioload in the system and changes in feeding and cleaning schedules.
7) Monitoring plastic, rubber, and metals as these deteriorate more rapidly in the presence of ozone.

Temperature Control

Temperature is a core factor whose importance is underestimated in the aquarium world. Animals have thermal preference zones and many ectotherms behaviorally regulate their body temperature. Thermal refuges are difficult to achieve in the aquarium setting because of the high thermal conductive nature of water. That being said, this is an ideal that the aquarium professional should strive for as technology evolves.

Currently, water temperature is controlled in bulk using heaters, chillers, heat exchangers, and insulation. Smaller systems may have independent heaters or chillers to sustain water temperatures within the thermal preference range of the species and to limit wide temperature fluctuations. Larger systems typically have heat exchangers (Figure A3.16). Heat exchangers should be placed last in-line before water returns to the aquarium or pond. Heat exchangers should be sized correctly for the temperature range of the species being maintained, the ambient temperature range, and the size, flow rate, and thermal characteristics of the sys-

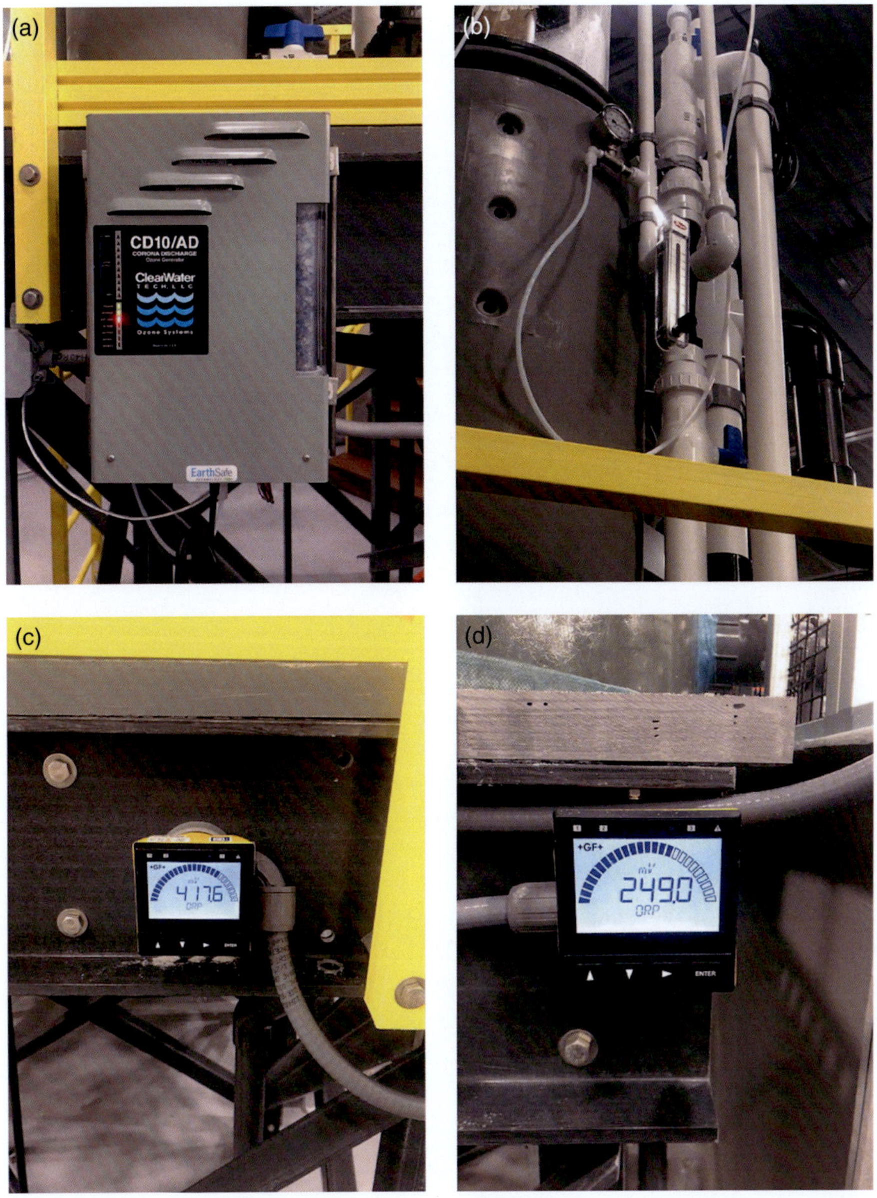

Figure A3.15 Ozone disinfection system showing the ozone gas generator (a), ozone injection into the foam fractionator contact chamber (b), and oxidation-reduction potential (ORP) reading (in mV) from the contact chamber (c) and the aquarium habitat (d). *Source*: Images courtesy of Ashleigh Clews, National Aquarium.

tem. It is important to remember that the heat exchangers themselves generate heat, which can impact aquariums in enclosed spaces. Heat exchangers should be constructed from materials that will not contaminate the system (e.g. heavy metals); titanium heat exchangers are usually the best choice, especially for saltwater aquariums.

Heaters and chillers (as well as pumps) can easily cause electrical issues if not grounded properly. These should be checked immediately if stray current is suspected.

Noise and Vibration

Noise can be an underappreciated stressor for fish and invertebrates in human care, affecting health, growth, and reproductive success (Anderson et al. 2011). Hearing sensitivities vary widely, but tend to be in the lower frequency range, particularly for vibrations intercepted by the lateral line system. Noise and vibrations can be generated from many areas, but common sources are pumps and water running through pipes that come in contact with the sides of the aquarium. Abrupt noises can be an intense source of

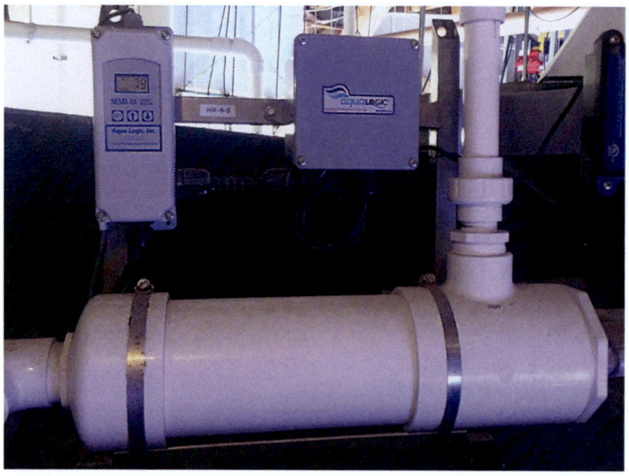

Figure A3.16 Heat exchanger. *Source*: Image courtesy of Catherine Hadfield, Seattle Aquarium.

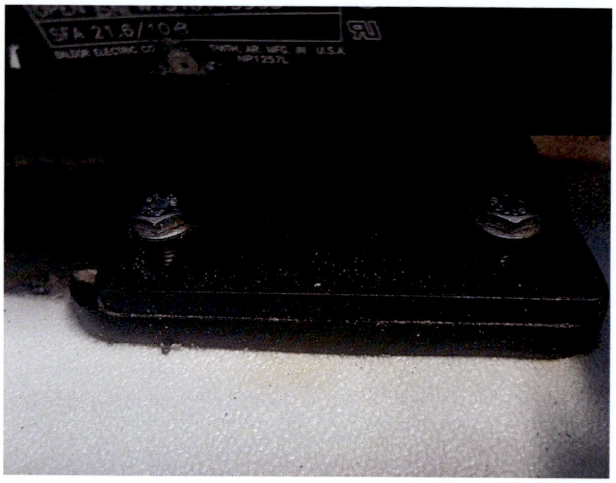

Figure A3.17 Rubber bushings for mounting of pumps to minimize noise and vibration.

distress since they are stochastic and unpredictable. Examples include nearby construction or someone tapping the sides of the aquarium. Construction noises from other areas (even across a street) can find their way into a system through acoustical conduits. Animals should be monitored for startle reflexes or repetitive swimming behavior; behaviors such as these should trigger an analysis of the situation. Large aquariums or culture facilities might consider investing in hydrophone monitoring equipment.

There are many ways to minimize noise and vibration. Pumps may be mounted on rubber bushings (Figure A3.17). Pipes resting against systems can be lifted using neoprene or closed-cell foam to limit sound transfer. Background natural sounds can be used to mask unexpected noises.

Lighting

Light intensity, spectrum, and photoperiod are important parts of the life support system. Lighting impacts feeding, reproduction, and behavior. A review of 38 species of Hawaiian fish demonstrated the great variety of visual sensitivities. Spectrums varied between 347–376 nm (ultraviolet) and 439–498 nm (blue light) and vision was affected by the lenses, corneas, and humors (Losey et al. 2003). It is important to understand the spectral needs of the fish species being housed to maximize welfare. Excess light intensity can lead to sunburn and cataracts. Scala et al. (2016) found retinal neoplasms in hybrid striped bass (*Morone saxatilis*) and pajama cardinalfish (*Sphaeramia nematoptera*) housed in systems with high-energy blue light produced by metal halide lamps. And some fish show bioluminescence or phosphorescence that is strongly impacted by lighting. Not only does one have to consider animal welfare, but lighting also has aesthetic effects that are particularly important in display aquariums.

Water filters the light spectrum, absorbing red light within the first few centimeters. The aquarium professional tries to recreate natural environments through manipulation of lighting, e.g. high intensity for shallow tropical reefs, blue for deep-water habitats, or infrared for complete darkness. With mixed species habitats, it is hard to target lighting to each species.

The need for full spectrum lighting for fish has been a topic of debate. In particular, the need for UVB remains controversial. UVB penetration depth is mainly influenced by water turbidity and the number of photons contacting the water. In the ocean, only ~10% of surface UVB can penetrate down to 35 m at full sunlight with minimal total organic carbon in the water (Aas and Højerslev 1999). A major challenge for large aquariums is the permeation of light using artificial bulbs. Bulbs have a high energy output and lose light intensity with distance due to the inverse square law of light (light intensity is inversely proportional to the square of the distance from the source point). The longer the distance, the less intense the light.

Results of UVB application to aquatic systems have been mixed. Three 160-W UVB heat lamps (T-Rex® Active UV Heat) placed 91 cm above the water surface produced a UVB intensity of $0.1 \pm 0.05\,mJ/cm^2$ or mWs/cm^2 but only over a surface area of 3.8 cm diameter directly below each lamp, despite observing a larger light footprint. A 50% variation in UVB intensity was also observed between each bulb. Additionally, light intensity degraded rapidly within the normal six-month replacement cycle (Purgley et al. 2009). A similar study involved a Mega-Ray® 275 watt Self-Ballasted Flood UVB Lamp placed 61 cm above a tank with a diameter of 305 cm and depth of 183 cm. This produced a UVB intensity ~0.015–0.050 mJ/cm^2 over a quarter of the tank and caused dermatitis in fish cohabitating with sea turtles after eight hours of exposure (Boylan pers. comm.).

A critical aspect of light is photoperiod. At a minimum, fish should be exposed to relatively steady photoperiods without sudden changes. This can be difficult in display aquaria where there is often demand for exhibit lighting during evening events. And to mimic natural diurnal cycles and prevent startling, periods of lower intensity at the start and end of the light period should be used to mimic dawn and dusk. Ideally, photoperiod should mimic natural seasonal changes for the species. Species-appropriate light refuges should be provided to allow inhabitants choice.

Other Life Support Equipment

Some other life support equipment may be found on aquarium systems or to treat incoming water.

Ion-exchange filters are deionization units that can be used to treat incoming freshwater. These use two types of synthetic resins to remove positively charged ions (cations) such as calcium, magnesium, and sodium, and negatively charged ions (anions) such as chloride, sulfate, and bicarbonate. In addition to conventional deionization, ion-exchange filters can contain resins or adsorbent media that are selective for specific contaminants such as silica, ammonia, phosphate, nitrate, and heavy metals. Many have color indicators that change color as the resins become exhausted. Products suitable for aquarium use are preferable as they have very low levels of toxic leachables. Some freshwater resins can be regenerated using warm salt water. Some saltwater resins can be regenerated on site, but they typically require strong acids or strong bases to do so and the hazardous chemical handling usually makes ion-exchange filtration impractical in saltwater systems. Expended resins should be discarded through appropriate hazardous waste. These differ from conventional ion-exchange water softeners, which produce high levels of sodium or potassium and are not designed for fish systems.

Reverse osmosis systems can remove ions from incoming freshwater. They use a semipermeable membrane to remove 90–99% of impurities such as chlorines, chloramines, nitrates, phosphates, pesticides, and heavy metals. Reverse osmosis does not remove as much as deionization, but in practical terms the resultant freshwater is similar for both processes. Deionized or reverse osmosis water may be used in systems containing fish that prefer soft, low-pH water and in the cleaning of sensitive equipment.

Carbon dioxide (CO_2) scrubbers, injectors, or reactors can remove or add CO_2. These may be found on high-density aquaculture systems and low-pH fish systems. Carbon dioxide is produced through respiration. The amount of CO_2 in aquarium water affects the pH and alkalinity, since it becomes carbonic acid when dissolved in water. Too much carbonic acid lowers system pH, while too little increases pH.

If CO_2 is too high, it can be addressed with increased aeration (e.g. air diffusers, packed column aerators), addition of calcium hydroxide or sodium hydroxide solution, or use of a CO_2 scrubber. This is a device installed on the ambient air intake of an aeration device (e.g. air blower or foam fractionator) that contains an oxide or hydroxide media that absorbs CO_2 from the air before it is drawn into the system. A color indicator is used to determine when the media is exhausted. The media is not usually considered hazardous waste, but it can be exhausted rather quickly, which can become costly to manage on larger systems.

If CO_2 is too low, CO_2 injectors or reactors can be used to supplement CO_2 into the system. An injector typically uses a fine-bubble diffuser to dissolve CO_2 directly into the water from a pressurized source such as a cylinder or dewar (vacuum flask). A reactor pre-dissolves the pressurized gas into the system water in a reaction vessel outside of the aquarium. Both methods should use a CO_2 controller with pH as the control parameter.

Calcium injectors can inject calcium directly into a system in the form of calcium hydroxide solution. These are typically found on systems that house hard corals. Calcium reactors supplement calcium by separating calcium ion from carbonic acid in calcium carbonate media (like aragonite). This is done by bubbling pressurized CO_2 into it within a reaction vessel outside of the aquarium. Both methods should be pH-controlled.

Pond Life Support

One of the biggest issues with outdoor ponds is phosphates and sunlight causing algal and bacterial blooms. These are particularly dangerous when the biological oxygen demand (BOD) is high (e.g. in a heavily stocked system or at night when photosynthesis is not active). In these situations, a bloom can lead to life-threatening hypoxic events. These can be minimized using shade and by controlling phosphates and potentially nitrogen and iron levels. Phosphates and nitrogen build up through the introduction of food and other organics into the system. Input can be limited by regular removal of decaying matter (e.g. leaves), covering with nets in the fall, and only feeding to appetite. In the system, they can be managed with chemical flocculation (e.g. precipitation with lime, lanthanum chloride, aluminum sulfate, or iron salts). Metallic flocculants work well, but some (e.g.

lanthanum salts) produce flocs that must be prevented from entering the pond as they can disrupt gill function in fish. Aluminum sulfate is one of the most commonly used, but care should be taken when applying as it will decrease pH.

Coral Reef Life Support

Compared to fish-only marine aquariums, coral reef aquariums require more intense lighting of the correct spectrum, turbulent water movement, and more stable water chemistry. Biological filtration for reef aquariums usually comes from the use of live rock from around existing reefs or from aquaculture. Foam fractionation and deep sand beds are also often used. Calcium injectors and reactors are often used to maintain proper pH, alkalinity, and calcium and magnesium levels that are critical for stony corals to maintain their calcium carbonate skeletons. Dedicated computers with electronic water quality monitoring capabilities may be used to control water chemistry parameters in complex systems.

Conclusion

In nature, aquatic organisms are an integral part of the natural environment that sustains them. Aquariology is the science of doing the best we can to model the environmental parameters needed for the species we have selected to keep in artificial environments. We cannot duplicate all of the natural processes that govern the ecological parameters that support the life of our animals in nature, but we should always endeavor to provide the best care we can.

For further reading, see studies by Carlson (1999), Overby (2002), Spotte (1991), Van der Toorn (1987), and Watson and Hill (2006), and the website of the Aquatic Animal Life Support Operators (http://aalso.org).

References

Aas, E. and Højerslev, N.K. (1999). Analysis of underwater radiance observations: apparent optical properties and analytic functions describing the angular radiance distribution. *Journal of Geophysical Research* 104: 8015–8024.

Adey, W.H. and Loveland, K. (2011). *Dynamic Aquaria: Building Living Ecosystems*. Amsterdam: Elsevier, Inc.

Anderson, P.A., Berzins, I.K., Fogarty, F. et al. (2011). Sound, stress, and seahorses: the consequences of a noisy environment to animal health. *Aquaculture* 311: 129–138.

Burns, A.S., Padilla, C.C., Pratte, Z.A. et al. (2018). Broad phylogenetic diversity associated with nitrogen loss through sulfur oxidation in a large public marine aquarium. *Applied and Environmental Microbiology* 84: e01250-18.

Carlson, B.A. (1999). Organism responses to rapid change: what aquaria tell us about nature. *American Zoologist* 39: 44–55.

Johnson, J.V. (2000). Application of ozone in marine parks and large aquariums. *Bulletin de l'Institut Océanographique* 20: 131–137.

Losey, G.S., McFarland, W.N., Loew, E.R. , Zamzow, J.P., et al. (2003). Visual biology of Hawaiian coral reef fishes. I. Ocular transmission and visual pigments. *Copeia* 2003: 433–454.

Overby, J.M. (2002). In the aquarium with ozone: a matter of living clearly? *Water Conditioning and Purification* 44: 60–62.

Purgley, H., Jewell, J., Deacon, J.E. et al. (2009). Vitamin D3 in captive green sea turtles (*Chelonia mydas*). *Chelonian Conservation Biology* 8: 161–167.

Sauder, L.A., Engel, K., Stearns, J.C. , Masella, A.P., et al. (2011). Aquarium nitrification revisited: Thaumarchaeota are the dominant ammonia oxidizers in freshwater aquarium biofilters. *PLoS One* 6: e23281.

Scala, C., Lair, S., and Marvin, J. (2016). Clusters of retinal neoplasms in aquarium-housed Atlantic striped bass (*Morone saxatilis*) and pajama cardinalfish (*Sphaeramia nematoptera*). *Proceedings of the International Association for Aquatic Animal Medicine*, Virginia Beach, VA.

Spotte, S. (1991) Disinfection of marine mammal pool waters: theoretical and health considerations. U.S. Department of Agriculture, Animal and Plant Health Inspection Service, Technical Bulletin No. 1797.

Tal, Y., Watts, J.E.M., Schreier, S.B., Sowers, K.R., et al. (2003). Characterization of the microbial community and nitrogen transformation processes associated with moving bed bioreactors in a closed recirculated mariculture system. *Aquaculture* 215: 187–202.

Tal, Y., Yechezkel, E., van Rijn, J. et al. (2004). Characterization and abundance of anaerobic ammonia oxidizing (anammox) bacteria in biofilters of recirculated aquaculture systems. *Proceedings of the International Conference on Recirculating Aquaculture, Cooperative Extension/Sea Grant*, Blacksburg, VA.

Van de Graaf, A.A., Mulder, A., de Bruijn, P. , Jetten, M.S.M., et al. (1995). Anaerobic oxidation of ammonium is a biologically mediated process. *Applied and Environmental Microbiology* 61: 1246–1251.

Van der Toorn, J.D. (1987). A biological approach to dolphinarium water purification: I. Theoretical aspects. *Aquatic Mammals* 13: 83–92.

Watson, C.A. and Hill, J.E. (2006). Design criteria for recirculating, marine ornamental production systems. *Aquacultural Engineering* 34: 157–162.

A4

Nutrition and Nutritional Support

Lisa A. Hoopes[1] *and Elizabeth A. Koutsos*[2]

[1] *Georgia Aquarium, Atlanta, GA, USA*
[2] *Koutsos Consulting LLC, Apex, NC, USA*

Introduction

Proper nutrition is a cornerstone of good health and a key component of preventative medicine programs. Poor nutrition impacts animal welfare and immune function and can tip the balance between health and disease. Understanding nutritional requirements is integral to the long-term management of species under human care and fish are no exception. Good nutrition of fish can prevent diseases, reduce the severity of clinical signs, speed recovery, and help individuals overcome environmental stressors. The goal of this chapter is to summarize the nutritional requirements of fish and to review feeding, supplementation, and nutritional support.

Natural History

An appropriate diet for fish consists of essential nutrients (proteins, lipids, carbohydrates including fiber, vitamins, and minerals), in a suitable formulation that is often similar to the wild diet, and adapted to the life stage and conditions under which the animal is managed. Most studies on fish nutrition have focused on species that are routinely cultured for food (e.g. salmon, trout, tilapia, and catfish), where the goal is often rapid growth and efficient production. Little information exists on the nutrient requirements of fish kept in zoos and aquariums and in the home, where the goal is to optimize health to enhance longevity and reproductive success. In the absence of information on nutrient requirements, understanding the wild diet and foraging ecology, metabolism and energetics, and anatomy can help in choosing appropriate items to feed.

Wild Diet and Foraging Ecology

Fish can be broadly grouped into simple trophic categories based on the types of food consumed: carnivore, omnivore, herbivore, and detritivore. However, it should be noted that while a carnivore is well-defined (consumer of animal prey), what constitutes an omnivorous, herbivorous, or detritivorous fish varies widely. Most fish species are primarily carnivorous or omnivorous; only 5% of fish families include herbivorous species (Bone and Moore 2008).

Carnivory is seen in all elasmobranchs (as predators or filter feeders) and some bony fish (often pelagic species and ambush predators). Omnivory is common in bony fish found in zoos and aquariums. Herbivorous fish include both freshwater and marine bony fish that consume vascular plants, micro- and macroalgae, detritus, and even wood in some species of catfish (German and Bittong 2009). Herbivorous fish that are commonly displayed or cultured include most parrotfish (*Scaridae*) and some tilapia (*Oreochromis* and *Tilapia* spp.). Detritivorous fish include many species of mullet (*Mugilidae*), some surgeonfish (*Acanthuridae*), and some aquaculture species including smallscale yellowfin (*Plagiognathops microlepis*).

Nutritionally appropriate diets for carnivorous and omnivorous fish can be based on known prey items. However, designing nutritionally appropriate diets for herbivorous grazers and browsers can be challenging, as they often feed on a complex mixture of plants, algae, and detritus.

In addition to the types of foods that fish eat in the wild, understanding normal feeding patterns and seasonal changes in the diet and environment are important in determining diets for fish under human care.

Clinical Guide to Fish Medicine, First Edition. Edited by Catherine A. Hadfield and Leigh Ann Clayton.

Metabolism and Energetics

Intake needs can be estimated using predictive equations of the energy requirements of a species and the estimated or determined energy content of a food item. Energetic requirements are regulated by various factors including body weight (BW). Requirements are usually expressed in units of metabolic weight, allowing scaling for a variety of body sizes. For fish, metabolic weight is generally defined as body weight $(kg)^{0.80}$ (NRC 2011). This scaling means that smaller fish should be fed at a higher percentage of body weight than larger fish. Other factors also affect energetic requirements, particularly activity level (e.g. feeding, breeding, or changes in water flow) and water temperature, with relatively linear increases in energy expenditure with increasing water temperature (NRC 2011).

There are several published equations to calculate maintenance energy requirements of fish, but they vary dramatically by species and water temperature (NRC 2011). For example, the estimated maintenance energy requirements of rainbow trout (*Oncorhynchus mykiss*) vary from 4.54 to 17.93 $kcal/kg^{0.80}$ (NRC 2011). With few energetic requirement equations available, and differences based on species, body size, activity level, and water temperature, these estimates of intake needs should be used as a guide only. Animals should always be fed to appropriate body condition.

Anatomy and Digestion

The gastrointestinal (GI) tract anatomy of fish differs based on evolutionary, dietary, and environmental constraints. The stomach in most species is a simple sac. There is no stomach in the jawless fish, e.g. hagfish and lamprey (*Agnatha*). The stomach has been secondarily lost in disparate teleost lineages, including members of the families *Cyprinidae* (goldfish, carp, and koi), *Labridae* (wrasses), and *Gobiidae* (gobies) (Day et al. 2011). This loss does not appear to impose dietary constraints, as stomachless fish cover the entire trophic spectrum, including carnivory, omnivory, herbivory, and detritivory (Horn et al. 2006; German et al. 2010). Intestinal length is variable in fish, but carnivorous fish generally have shorter intestines than herbivorous species. Many fish possess pyloric caeca. These are finger-like diverticula of the intestine at the posterior end of the stomach which secrete digestive enzymes and increase the absorptive surface area. Pyloric caeca are better developed in carnivorous than herbivorous fish (Clements and Raubenheiner 2006; Ballantyne 2014). Elasmobranchs and non-teleost ray-finned fish (bowfin, gar, sturgeon, and lungfish) have a spiral valve. This is a distal section of intestines with multiple layers in conical, scroll, or ring shapes, which increase the absorptive surface area.

Gut passage rates in fish are dependent on species, animal size, gut morphology, temperature, food type, meal size, and feeding rate. In general, gut emptying times range from <10 hours for most herbivores to 10–158 hours for teleost carnivores (Horn 1989). Elasmobranchs have slower gut passage times than similarly sized teleost carnivores at comparable water temperatures, with reported values of one to eight days (Cortés and Gruber 1992; Wood et al. 2007). Gut passage times in carnivorous teleosts and elasmobranchs are affected by the type of prey. For example, gastric emptying in sandbar sharks (*Carcharhinus plumbeus*) varied by as much as 20 hours between crab and teleost prey (Medved 1985).

Assimilation efficiency assesses how efficiently animals convert ingested food into energy. Assimilation efficiency is high in adult fish (80–90%), with a wider range in larval fish (67–99%) (Govoni et al. 1986). Food type, ration size, and gut morphology likely play a role in some of these differences. For example, Atlantic herring larvae (*Clupea harengus*) fed high rations of brine shrimp nauplii (*Artemia* spp.) defecated live nauplii, suggesting that large rations may result in low assimilation efficiency, especially in larvae with straight alimentary canals (Werner and Blaxter 1980). Assimilation efficiency in elasmobranchs has been studied in a single species (lemon shark, *Negaprion brevirostris*) and was comparable to that measured in teleosts (73%) (Wetherbee and Gruber 1993).

As in other vertebrates, the GI tract of fish provides habitat for a diverse ecosystem of micro-organisms that play an important role in the health and nutrition of the host. Information on gut microflora and microbial enzyme activity in fish GI tracts is lacking. It is well-known that terrestrial vertebrate herbivores have populations of symbiotic micro-organisms that play a key role in breaking down plant fiber (cellulose and hemicellulose) into short-chain fatty acids (SCFAs, primarily acetate, butyrate, and propionate). Gut micro-organism diversity has been studied in some freshwater and marine herbivorous fish. Work by Mountfort et al. (2002) identified the contribution of gut microbiota to energy metabolism and fermentation in the hindgut of three species of temperate marine herbivorous fish, finding that microbial fermentation is an important source of energy in these fish. Thus, establishing and maintaining appropriate GI tract microbial populations is integral to maintaining appropriate nutrition.

Nutrient Requirements

Despite great diversity in food types, all fish require the same nutrients at a cellular level. Understanding the proper nutrient requirements for fish is complicated by the fact that fish can accumulate some nutrients (e.g. minerals) directly from the water. Nutrients accumulated from the water and diet can have different physiological effects and fates, which makes balancing nutrient intake and availability a challenge.

Sources of Energy

Energy is obtained from the metabolism of protein, lipid, and carbohydrates. Fish are more efficient at using protein as an energy source than birds or mammals, since ammonia synthesis does not require energy, unlike uric acid and urea (Wright and Land 1998). However, protein is very costly and the resulting ammonia excretion can be problematic for water quality. Carbohydrates may serve as an energy source either via endogenous metabolism (e.g. absorbed glucose) or via microbial fermentation producing volatile fatty acids, but the ability to use carbohydrates varies greatly by species. Carbohydrates are generally less preferred as an energy source for carnivores compared to omnivores and herbivores, and in marine fish compared to freshwater fish. Lipids are often a preferred energy source in commercial fish feeds, as they can spare the cost of protein and are used efficiently by fish. Efforts in commercial aquaculture to use lipids as an energy source and spare protein for muscle accretion have resulted in significant improvements in growth efficiency of aquaculture species (Hixson 2014). However, there is a limit to this effect; excessive energy relative to protein can reduce total feed intake (and so limit intake of essential nutrients) and can increase body lipid deposition, which may not be optimal for fish health.

The energy of a food item may be defined based on different types of measurement. Gross energy (GE) is the total energy released upon combustion of a food item and does not necessarily represent the amount of energy available to the animal. However, this is the easiest measure of energy to determine. On average, GE values for carbohydrate, protein, and lipids for fish are 4.11, 5.64, and 9.44 kcal/g, respectively (NRC 2011). Digestible energy (DE) is based on the amount of energy in a food minus the amount of energy excreted in feces after that food is consumed and is generally 10–30% less than GE (NRC 2011). Metabolizable energy (ME) is based on the digestible energy of a food minus the energy to excrete any waste products via urinary and gill losses and generally reflects another 3–6% loss of energy (NRC 2011). When evaluating the energy needs or status of an animal, it is critical that the same units are considered. For example, if the requirements are predicted in units of ME, then the diet items should be considered in similar units or adjusted based on the assumptions described above.

Protein

There are 20 amino acids. Ten are essential and cannot be produced by fish. The remainder can be synthesized by the animal, assuming there is enough dietary nitrogen. Thus, dietary sources must provide both essential amino acids and additional nitrogen. The level of dietary protein that is required by fish has been well-documented for fast-growing aquaculture species and ranges from 29 to 42% digestible protein (Table A4.1). This requirement has not been well-documented for other species or other life stages. However, for larval fish, free amino acids may be more important as some lack the enzymatic capability to digest intact protein (Rønnestad and Fyhn 1993).

Essential amino acids for fish include arginine, histidine, isoleucine, leucine, lysine, methionine, phenylalanine, threonine, tryptophan, and valine (NRC 2011). Arginine requirements are quite high compared to terrestrial mammals or birds, due to low activity of urea cycle enzymes. Tyrosine and cysteine are considered semi-essential because they can be synthesized from phenylalanine and methionine, respectively. Taurine, an aminosulfonic acid, appears to be essential for some life stages, notably larval fish (NRC 2011). The relative ratios of amino acids that have been determined to be required by fish are generally proportional to the optimal dietary protein level. However, it is important to note that amino acid requirements have historically been determined with body weight gain as the predictive variable. The use of other functional end points (e.g. optimal immune function) may change the requirement. For example, recent work examining histidine requirements in Nile tilapia (*Oreochromis niloticus*) found that lowering histidine below previously published requirements improved weight gain, muscle fiber quality, and efficiency of protein utilization (Michelato et al. 2017). This type of refinement of nutrient requirements will continue to improve fish nutrition as well as the impact of excessive feeding on water quality and the environment.

Fish-based protein sources most closely match the nutritional requirements of fish. However, with sustainability concerns, efforts have been made to identify other protein sources for commercial fish diets, such as marine by-catch, terrestrial animals, plants, and microbes. Terrestrial animal protein sources lack some essential fatty acids and may be high in fat. Plant-based protein sources may be less expensive but often lack many essential amino acids and may contain anti-nutritional factors (discussed below).

As a final caveat, it is important to consider the energy content of the diet for which protein requirements have been determined. The ratio of protein:energy is important as amino acids serve as energy precursors in fish. For most species studied, the optimal ratio of digestible

Table A4.1 Approximate diet composition for some model fish species.

Model species	Common carp, tilapia, channel catfish, rohu	Hybrid striped bass	Rainbow trout, Atlantic salmon, Pacific salmon, European bass	Asian seabass, cobia, Japanese flounder, grouper, yellowtail
Habitat	Fresh or slightly brackish water	Freshwater	Marine or freshwater	Marine
Water temperature	Temperate	Temperate	Cold	Temperate
Feeding strategy	Omnivore	Carnivore	Carnivore	Carnivore
Digestible protein (%)	29–32	36	36–40	36–42
Crude fat (%)	<10%		15–21	
Calcium (%)	0.45–0.70			
Phosphorus (%)	0.33–0.70	0.50	0.6–0.8	0.6–0.8
Sodium (%)	0.06–0.15			
Copper (ppm)	3–5		3–5	5
Iodine (ppm)	1.1		1.0–1.1	
Iron (ppm)	30–150		30–60	
Manganese (ppm)	2.4–12.0		10–12	
Selenium (ppm)	0.25	0.25	0.15	0.70
Zinc (ppm)	15–20	37	15–37	20
Ascorbic acid (ppm)	15–45	22	20	15–54
Thiamine (ppm)	0.5–1.0		1–10	11
Vitamin E (IU/kg)	50–132	28	50–60	115–119

The values are for production animals with the goal of rapid growth. All values are on an as-fed basis. *Source:* NRC (2011).

protein:digestible energy ranges from 84 to 105 g/Mcal (NRC 2011).

Protein waste products and undigested feed can negatively impact water quality. Nitrogenous waste can be minimized by providing optimal levels of amino acids and reducing the digestible protein:energy ratio such that nitrogen retention efficiency is high (McGoogan and Gatlin 1999).

Lipid

Lipid levels from 10 to 20% of the dry weight of the diet (~20% for juveniles, 10% for adults) are usually considered sufficient for many fish to use protein without depositing excess lipid (Sargent et al. 2002). Excessive fat levels or inappropriate levels of fatty acids can lead to fatty infiltration of the liver, a common chronic health problem in aquarium fish.

Essential lipids can include cholesterol, phospholipids, inositol, and fatty acids (NRC 2011). Some fish can synthesize cholesterol endogenously. Phospholipids, the general term for lipids containing phosphorus, includes sphingomyelin, phosphatidyl-choline, -ethanolamine, -serine, and -inositol. Dietary phospholipid inclusion can improve survival and growth in larval and juvenile fish. Optimal requirements can be as high as 6% of diet dry matter for larval fish (NRC 2011). Inositol (which may also be categorized with vitamins) is a component of phosphatidylinositol in cell membranes. Inositol can be synthesized endogenously, but often not at high enough levels to meet needs. Young fish, particularly larval fish, appear to require higher levels than older fish. Fishmeal is a rich source of inositol, so diets containing fish or fishmeal generally do not require additional supplementation (NRC 2011).

Fatty acids are the preferred energy source in fish and play a key role in yolk sac and larval development, maintaining cellular membranes, and modulating immune responses (Tocher 2003). All fish species studied are known to require linoleic acid (18:2n6; an omega-6 fatty acid) and linolenic acid (18:3n3; an omega-3 fatty acid) (NRC 2011). These requirements can generally be met with terrestrial animal- and plant-based lipid sources. Many freshwater fish species are able to produce polyunsaturated fatty acids (PUFAs), including eicosapentaenoic acid (EPA, 20:5n3) and docosahexaenoic acid (DHA, 22:6n3) (Hixson 2014). However, many carnivorous and benthivorous marine fish require dietary long-chain omega-3 PUFAs and higher omega-3:omega-6 ratios (Ahlgren et al. 2009; Hixson 2014). In general, cold-water species are thought to have higher requirements for omega-3 PUFAs compared to warm-water species (NRC 2011). Omega-3 PUFAs are generally provided from marine-based sources such as fish meal and fish oils, but also can be found in algae. Vegetable oils are generally poor sources of these fatty acids, although bioengineered algae may prove useful in the future. Another PUFA, arachidonic acid (AA, 20:4n6), may also be required or recommended for optimal performance in fish. It has been shown to improve egg quality and survival, larval growth and survival, and adaptation to different salinities in several fish species (Bell and Sargent 2003).

Total lipid content and fatty acid profiles of food items vary considerably with species, life stage, and diet, but values for common seafood items are reported in Table A4.2. The same variability is seen in zooplankton, which is commonly raised for feeding larval fish, with large amounts of EPA in wild water fleas (*Daphnia* spp.), and large amounts of DHA in wild marine copepods (Ahlgren et al. 2009). These levels can be manipulated through the diet.

Carbohydrates

Carbohydrates (sugars, starches, and fiber) are poorly digested by most fish but they can be mobilized to meet energy demands. They play the largest role in the nutrition of herbivorous fish. Carbohydrates in the form of starch are generally present in commercial fish diets at 5–25% (Hua and Bureau 2009).

Starch digestibility is variable in fish but is usually low. In general, cold-water carnivorous fish appear to have the lowest capacity to digest starch, while warm-water herbivorous or omnivorous fish are more capable of starch digestion (Hemre et al. 2002). Digestibility is routinely improved by heat and pressure treatment of the starch which results in gelatinization; this occurs during commercial diet production or heating of food items prior to feeding (Kumar et al. 2006; Hua and Bureau 2009). The carnivorous Hong Kong grouper (*Epinephelus akaara*) showed reduced growth rates when fed >8% dietary carbohydrate (non-gelatinized) (Wang et al. 2016), while herbivorous blunt-snout bream (*Megalobrama amblycephala*) were able to adapt to diets containing as much as 42% carbohydrate (dextrin) (Li et al. 2016). Due to the wide variation in digestibility, it is probably advisable to limit dietary starch whenever practical, particularly for cold-water carnivorous fish.

Non-starch polysaccharides (NSPs) are relatively indigestible by fish and can lead to alterations in digesta viscosity such that nutrient absorption is impaired (Sinha et al. 2011). Carbohydrase enzymes can be added to diets to hydrolyze these NSPs, which can improve growth rates and feed use when carbohydrates are fed (Castillo and Gatlin 2015).

Fermentable carbohydrates are likely to be important substrates for microbial fermentation in the caudal GI tract in herbivorous, omnivorous, and planktivorous fish. In three species of herbivorous fish, microbial fermentation in the posterior portions of the GI tract resulted in short-chain fatty acid (SCFA) synthesis at rates that were equivalent to terrestrial vertebrates and marine reptiles, despite colder environmental temperatures (Mountfort et al. 2002). It is likely that most of the carbohydrates used for microbial fermentation are hemicellulose and cellulose (Mišurcová et al. 2010; Templeton et al. 2012). The microbial communities found in the piscine GI tract are likely critical for proper health and nutrition and should be considered when designing proper nutrition programs.

Vitamins

Vitamins serve as cofactors, hormones, and regulators of cellular differentiation. They are generally required from the diet in trace amounts. Vitamins may be categorized as fat-soluble (vitamins A, D, E, K) or water-soluble (B vitamins including thiamine [B1], riboflavin [B2], niacin [B3], pantothenate [B5], pyridoxine [B6], biotin [B7], folate [B9], cobalamin [B12]; vitamin C [ascorbic acid]; choline). Requirements are affected by size, age, growth rates, environmental factors, and inter-relationships with other nutrients (NRC 2011). Larval fish nutrition presents some unique concerns related to vitamin nutrition and is discussed in more detail later. Estimated vitamin requirements are presented in Table A4.3. As with other nutrients, these recommended levels are generally determined for optimal performance of aquaculture species and so should be used as a guideline rather than an instruction.

Fat-soluble vitamins A, D, E, and K may be supplemented in diets, but present a higher risk of toxicity since they are stored in liver and adipose and are harder to excrete in excess.

Vitamin A is involved in cellular differentiation and vision. Deficiency in larval fish is associated with incomplete eye migration, abnormal pigmentation, and skeletal abnormalities, while in juvenile fish, skin and liver hemorrhages, exophthalmos, and twisted gill opercula have been described (NRC 2011; Hamre et al. 2013). Carotenoids are pro-vitamin A compounds (and pigments) that occur naturally in many wild-type food items. Carotenoids are generally considered less toxic since the conversion of carotenoid to retinol is regulated in response to body vitamin A levels. In several freshwater and saltwater fish species, β-carotene, astaxanthin, and canthaxanthin can be converted to vitamin A, although their conversion seems most efficient when vitamin A levels are low (Moren et al. 2002). The use of astaxanthin and canthaxanthin as precursors to vitamin A is somewhat unique – most birds and mammals studied are not able to convert these carotenoids to vitamin A (Goodwin 1986).

Table A4.2 Total lipid and fatty acid composition of seafood items commonly fed to fish.

	Pacific herring, fillet (*Clupea pallasii*)	**Atlantic mackerel, fillet** (*Scomber scombrus*)	**Menhaden, whole** (*Brevoortia tyrannus*)	**Coho salmon, fillet** (*Oncorhyncus kisutch*)	**Lake herring** (*Coregonus artedii*)	**Rainbow trout** (*Oncorhyncus mykiss*)	**Lake whitefish** (*Coregonus clupeaformis*)	**Blue crab** (*Callinectes sapidus*)	**Littleneck clam** (*Protothaca staminea*)	**Pacific oyster** (*Crassostrea gigas*)
Tissue lipid content (%)	12.8	3.2	15	7.5	2.5	2.5	2.2	2.1	0.5	2.5
Lipid fatty acid composition (%)										
16:0 palmitic acid	15.1	28.2	28.9	10.2	17.7	8.2	10.5	15.2	23.8	21.4
18:1n9 oleic acid	16.9	19.3	19.3	18.6	18.1	19.8	27.2	17.6	10.8	8.5
18:2n6 linoleic acid	1.6	1.1	1.1	1.2	4.3	4.6	5.5	1.9	1.4	1.2
18:3n3 linolenic acid	0.6	1.3	1.3	0.6	3.4	5.2	3.7	1.2	1.6	1.6
20:5n3 EPA	8.6	8.6	7.1	12	5.9	5	6.4	13.4	10	21.5
22:6n3 DHA	7.6	7.6	10.8	13.8	13.3	19	8.8	11	14.5	20.2
Calculated fish fatty acid content (%)[a]										
16:0 palmitic acid	1.9	0.9	4.3	0.8	0.4	0.2	0.2	0.3	0.1	0.5
18:1n9 oleic acid	2.2	0.6	2.9	1.4	0.5	0.5	0.6	0.4	0.1	0.2
18:2n6 linoleic acid	0.2	0.0	0.2	0.1	0.1	0.1	0.1	0.0	0.0	0.0
18:3n3 linolenic acid	0.1	0.0	0.2	0.0	0.1	0.1	0.1	0.0	0.0	0.0
20:5n3 EPA	1.1	0.3	1.1	0.9	0.1	0.1	0.1	0.3	0.1	0.5
22:6n3 DHA	1.0	0.2	1.6	1.0	0.3	0.5	0.2	0.2	0.1	0.5

All values are on an as-fed basis.

EPA: eicosapentaenoic acid; DHA: docosahexaenoic acid.

[a] Calculated fish fatty acid content represents the proportion of the fatty acids relative to total fat content. *Source*: Gruger et al. (1964).

Table A4.3 Dietary vitamin requirements for teleosts and elasmobranchs.

	Juvenile teleost	Larval teleost	Broodstock teleost	Elasmobranchs
Ascorbic acid (ppm)	28 (15–54)	(25–2500)	(25–50)	(100–1100)
Biotin (ppm)	0.58 (0.06–1)			(0.1–1.5)
Choline (ppm)	811 (400–1500)			(600–3000)
Folate (ppm)	1.3 (1.0–2.0)			(5–10)
Niacin (ppm)	40 (10–150)			(20–200)
Pantothenate (ppm)	23 (10–36)			(12–50)
Pyridoxine (ppm)	7 (3–15)	Required		(3–20)
Riboflavin (ppm)	7 (4–11)			(4–20)
Thiamine (ppm)	5 (1–11)			(1–10)
Vitamin B12 (μg/kg)	35 (20–50)			(10–20)
Vitamin A (IU/kg)[a]	5854 (1667–18 667)	(16 665–103 323)	(1000–4000)	(2000–2500)
Vitamin D (IU/kg)[a]	820 (360–1600)	19 000	(500–2400)	2400
Vitamin E (IU/kg)[a]	60		(50–190)	(30–50)
Vitamin K (mg/kg)	<10			(5–10)

All values are on a dry matter basis and represent the mean (range) from published literature.
[a] Vitamin conversions: vitamin A: 1 mg retinol = 3333 IU; 1 mg retinyl acetate = 2906 IU; 1 mg retinyl palmitate = 1818 IU; vitamin D: 1 μg cholecalciferol = 40 IU; vitamin E: 1 mg D-α-tocopherol = 1.49 IU; 1 mg D,L-α-tocopherol = 1.1 IU; 1 mg D-α-tocopheryl acetate = 1.36 IU; 1 mg D,L-α-tocopherol acetate = 1 IU. *Sources*: Janse et al. (2004), Fernández-Palacios et al. (2011), NRC (2011), and Hamre et al. (2013).

Vitamin D functions in calcium homeostasis and is important for the development of skeletal tissues and cellular differentiation (NRC 2011). Vitamin D can be sourced from plants (ergocalciferol or vitamin D2) and animals (cholecalciferol or vitamin D3). Of these, D3 is significantly more effective than D2. Larval requirements for vitamin D seem to be significantly higher than those of juvenile fish. Toxicity can result in vertebral deformities, so further research is warranted before recommendations of high intakes for larval fish are made (Hamre et al. 2013).

Within the family of vitamin E molecules, α-tocopherol is the most biologically active form of the tocopherols and tocotrienols. These serve as antioxidants, stabilize membranes, affect eicosanoid signaling and cellular proliferation, and modulate immune responses. Efficacy of vitamin E as an antioxidant is dependent on levels of other antioxidants such as vitamin C and selenium-based glutathione systems. When the latter are low, vitamin E can become a pro-oxidant (Hamre 2011). As an antioxidant, vitamin E protects PUFAs at an approximate ratio of 1 molecule vitamin E:1000 molecules PUFA, with higher levels of unsaturation requiring more protection (Schwarz et al. 1988; Hamre 2011). This is why nutrient requirements for vitamin E are often described in relation to the PUFA content of the diet. This is particularly critical for fish, where diets are often rich in PUFA. Vitamin E requirements in most experiments are determined based on maximal growth rates. When other parameters are used (e.g. red blood cell fragility, immune responses), higher requirements are predicted. For example, Malabar grouper (*Epinephelus malabaricus*) required 60–100 mg D,L-α-tocopheryl acetate/kg diet for growth and up to 800 mg/kg for better nonspecific immune parameters (Lin and Shiau 2005). Requirements may increase further during disease (Durve and Lovell 1982). Commercially prepared larval fish feeds may require higher vitamin E due to the large surface area, higher risk of lipid oxidation, and high level of omega-3 PUFAs, particularly for marine fish (Hamre 2011). Very high levels of dietary vitamin E (5000–10 000 IU/kg) have been shown to promote oxidation and damage erythrocytes (NRC 2011).

Little work has been conducted on vitamin K in fish. Existing research has been inconsistent in showing a dietary requirement or GI microbial synthesis of vitamin K in fish (NRC 2011).

Water-soluble vitamins pose a lower risk of toxicity and are frequently supplemented at high levels to ensure optimal levels are met. Research has focused primarily on defining minimal requirements. Of the water-soluble vitamins, vitamin C receives the most attention. It is considered an essential or semi-essential dietary nutrient for teleosts, as there is evidence that some cartilaginous fish can synthesize ascorbic acid de novo (Cho et al. 2007). However, it is unclear if de novo synthesis is adequate to meet needs in all life stages and environmental conditions, and it has been demonstrated that supplemental vitamin C improves immune responses in some species with de novo synthesis (Xie et al. 2006). So it is advisable to supplement vitamin C in the diet of all fish species. Signs of vitamin C deficiency include lordosis, scoliosis, cartilage and collagen defects, petechial hemorrhaging, and fractures of the spine (Halver et al. 1975; Sandnes et al. 1992). These have been reported within weeks of feeding a vitamin C-deficient diet (Halver et al. 1975; Sandnes et al. 1992). Minimum requirements for growth are often much lower than the requirements for optimal immune function (Ai et al. 2004). While minimum requirements for fish are ~50 mg/kg diet, much higher doses (190–1000 mg/kg diet) often result in significant improvements in immune function, notably antibody production, complement activity, and survival after disease challenge (Navarre and Halver 1989; NRC 2011; Hamre et al. 2016). Vitamin C needs are increased during reproduction and larval fish growth (NRC 2011). Since vitamin C is heat labile, stabilized forms should be used for supplementation, e.g. L-ascorbyl-2-polyphosphate. The requirement for vitamin C is related to the level of vitamin E in the diet, as vitamin C or vitamin E can counteract the signs of deficiency of the other nutrient to some extent (Wahli et al. 1998; Sealey and Gatlin 2002).

Work on B vitamins in fish is limited. Thiamine (B1) is of concern for any fish-eating species, as thiaminases in fish tissues are activated upon death and rapidly destroy available thiamine. Thiaminase activity is particularly high in clupeids such as alewives (*Alosa pseudoharengus*) and capelin (*Mallotus villosus*), and cyprinids such as feeder goldfish (*Carassius auratus*). Any frozen/thawed fish should be supplemented with thiamine (Fitzsimons et al. 2005). Thiaminase activity has also been demonstrated in insects, blue-green algae (*Microcystis aeruginosa*) and bacteria (Honeyfield et al. 2002). Pyridoxine (B6) may be needed in the diet during larval development, as levels in the yolk sac are depleted rapidly (Hamre et al. 2013; Saha et al. 2016).

Choline, a vitamin-like nutrient, is an important component of phospholipids and a precursor of the neurotransmitter acetylcholine. Most fish cannot synthesize sufficient choline and it is a common supplement in cultured fish diets, usually as choline chloride (Wilson and Poe 1988). Additionally, choline may reduce excessive lipid accumulation and the development of fatty liver, although studies have produced mixed results (Halver 2002). Some species have shown a negative correlation between dietary choline and liver lipid levels (channel catfish *Ictalurus punctatus*, hybrid striped bass *Morone saxatilis* x *M. chrysops*, barred knifejaw *Oplegnathus fasciatus*), while others have shown a positive correlation (hybrid tilapia) or no correlation (rainbow trout, yellow perch *Perca flavescens*, Siberian sturgeon *Acipenser baerii*) (Wilson and Poe 1988; Rumsey 1991; Griffin et al. 1994; Shiau and Lo 2000; Twibell and Brown 2000; Yazdani-Sadati et al. 2014; Khosravi et al. 2015). Further studies are needed to understand the potential benefits of supplementing dietary choline.

Minerals

Minerals in the diet are often subdivided into:

- Macrominerals (calcium [Ca], phosphorus [P], sodium [Na], potassium [K], magnesium [Mg]).
- Trace minerals or microminerals (copper [Cu], zinc [Zn], iron [Fe], manganese [Mn], selenium [Se]).
- Ultra-trace minerals (iodine [I], cobalt [Co], chromium [Cr], molybdenum [Mo]).

Some minerals can be acquired by fish from the water, including Ca, Cu, Fe, K, Mg, Na, Se, and Zn (Terech-Majewska et al. 2016). It is generally assumed that Ca, K, Mg, and Na requirements can be met by the water, particularly seawater, although low pH does restrict absorption (Terech-Majewska et al. 2016). However, most commercial fish diets also meet minimum requirements. As with other nutrients, these recommended levels are generally determined for optimal performance of aquaculture species and should be used as a guide only (Table A4.4). Finally, many trace minerals interact with each other and with vitamins or other elements in the water, making it hard to determine their bioavailability to fish.

Phosphorus is likely the most discussed mineral in fish as dietary sources are required, and because of the variability in bioavailability and the environmental impact of excreted phosphorus. Phosphorus may be present in the diet from plant, animal, or chemical sources. Plant-based forms are often complexed with phytic acid (e.g. phytate-P) which generally has very low bioavailability to fish. A notable exception is Nile tilapia which can digest some phytate-P (Kumar et al. 2012). Undigested phytate-P can form complexes with other nutrients (e.g. Zn), reducing their bioavailability, and can contribute to algal blooms when excreted. Efforts to improve phytate-P digestibility have been a focus of extensive research in fish nutrition. Exogenous phytase enzymes may be provided in the diet to improve phytate-P digestibility, although efficacy varies. For example, agastric species such as the common carp (*Cyprinus carpio*) have a higher GI pH and most phytase enzymes have little effect unless dietary acidifiers or neutral pH-active phytase enzymes are used (Kumar et al. 2012; Lemos and Tacon 2016).

Selenium is a trace mineral involved in antioxidant and housekeeping functions. Deficiencies of selenium reduce antioxidant function and can result in vitamin E or vitamin

Table A4.4 Dietary mineral requirements for teleosts and elasmobranchs.

Nutrient	Juvenile teleost	Larval teleost	Elasmobranchs
Calcium (%)	0.87 (0.34–2.00)		0.5
Phosphorus (%)	0.61 (0.33–0.80)		0.70
Sodium (%)	0.11 (0.06–0.15)		(0.1–0.3)
Magnesium (%)	0.05 (0.04–0.06)		0.05
Potassium (%)	0.53 (0.26–0.80)		(0.1–0.3)
Chloride (%)	0.16 (0.15–0.17)		(0.1–0.5)
Copper (ppm)	4.3 (3.0–5.0)		(1–4)
Iodine (ppm)	1.1 (1–1.1)		(100–300)
Iron (ppm)	88 (30–150)		(50–100)
Manganese (ppm)	9 (2–12)	40	(20–50)
Selenium (ppm)	0.34 (0.15–0.70)	(1.4–3.0)	(0.15–038)
Zinc (ppm)	23 (15–37)		(15–100)

All values are on a dry matter basis and represent the mean (range) from published literature. *Sources*: Janse et al. (2004), NRC (2011), and Hamre et al. (2013).

C based pro-oxidation (Hamre et al. 2016). Deficiencies may be seen in captive-bred larval fish, as rotifers and other common aquarium food items have much lower levels than wild food items (Hamre et al. 2008; Penglase et al. 2010). Selenium can also be toxic; excess can reduce growth rates and increase mortality and has been associated with renal calcinosis (NRC 2011).

Iodine is important for all fish and functions as a component of thyroid hormones. The requirements of elasmobranchs for iodine are well-described and deficiency is a common cause of goiters (Janse et al. 2004). Ozone filtration reduces the bioavailability of water-based iodine (iodide) due to oxidation to the unavailable iodate (IO^{3-}). Additionally, high nitrate levels or other goitrogenic compounds can reduce iodide uptake (Morris et al. 2011).

Mineral (and vitamin) requirements of elasmobranchs are not well-defined. Few comprehensive studies have examined the vitamin and mineral content of their wild prey. A recent study of lemon shark prey items found that the daily Zn intake exceeded the minimum requirements for teleosts, while daily intake of Fe, Cu, and Mn was much lower than the minimal requirements for teleosts (Pettitt-Wade et al. 2011). Daily intake was calculated as a percentage of total diet at 6.6% Ca, 1.1% Na, 1.0% K, 0.3% Mg, 0.008% Zn, 0.005% Fe, 0.0007% Cu, and 0.0001% Mn.

Other Additives

Other dietary compounds can modulate animal health or performance in fish. Work in fish has demonstrated benefits from immune stimulants, probiotics, and prebiotics.

Immune stimulants are naturally occurring compounds that can increase resistance to disease. Most, if not all, essential nutrients influence disease resistance, particularly vitamins C and E (Blazer and Wolke 1984; Verlhac and Gabaudan 1994). Within non-nutrient compounds, β-glucans are the most commonly reported immune stimulants. When fed at low levels (<0.2% of the diet), β-glucans can modulate fish immune responses and improve survival following subsequent disease challenge, particularly for extracellular bacterial infections (Sinha et al. 2011; Hixson 2014). Other examples of immune stimulants include garlic and propolis (Sforcin 2007; Lee and Gao 2012). Short-chain fatty acids such as propionate may also modulate immune responses in fish (Hoseinifar et al. 2016). Further information on immune stimulants is available in Chapter A12 and reviews such as Lall and Tibbetts (2009), Nayak (2010), Verhlac-Trichet (2010), and Kiron (2012).

Probiotics are cultures of micro-organisms intended to colonize or influence intestinal flora (Nayak 2010). Numerous microbes have been identified as probiotics in fish (*Lactobacillus*, *Lactococcus*, *Leuconostoc*, *Enterococcus*, *Carnobacterium*, *Shewanella*, *Bacillus*, *Aeromonas*, *Vibrio*, *Enterobacter*, *Pseudomonas*, *Clostridium*, and *Saccharomyces* spp.). Many help feed conversion efficiency and growth, modulate the immune response, and confer protection against pathogens (Burr et al. 2005; Nayak 2010; De et al. 2014). Stability in the diet and efficacy are both concerns and more research is needed.

Prebiotics are nondigestible food ingredients that benefit the host by stimulating established microbial activity in the

GI system (Yousefian and Amiri 2009). They are usually carbohydrates that are resistant to gastric acidity, hydrolysis, and fermentation. Prebiotics include oligofructose, transgalactooligosaccharides (TOS), inulin, and lactulose. They have shown similar benefits to probiotics in feed efficiency, growth, and immune function, but more research is needed (Yousefian and Amiri 2009).

Nutrient Choice

There is some evidence that fish can select for certain nutrients when given dietary choices, particularly for macronutrients such as protein (da Silva et al. 2016). When fish could self-select between protein (from casein and gelatin), lipid (from fish oil/soybean oil mix), and carbohydrate (from dextrin), selection varied by wild-type feeding strategy. More carnivorous species selected for higher protein intake of 55–62% protein, 16–23% carbohydrate, and 16–22% lipid (Sánchez-Vázquez et al. 1999; Rubio et al. 2003; Almaida-Pagán et al. 2006). More omnivorous species selected lower protein intake levels: Nile tilapia ~45% protein, 32% carbohydrate, and ~22% lipid; and goldfish ~22% protein, 45% carbohydrate, and ~32% lipid (Sánchez-Vázquez et al. 1998; Fortes-Silva et al. 2011). Selection of lipid sources has also been demonstrated: tilapia selected flaxseed or fish oil-based diets (sources of omega-3 fatty acids) in preference to soybean oil-based diets (omega-6 fatty acids) (Fortes-Silva et al. 2010). There is less evidence of selection for appropriate nutrient intake of vitamins or minerals in fish. An important caveat is that low quality food items may not allow for selection to occur, because of an inability to modify intake levels to meet nutrient needs (e.g. low-protein diet), a net loss of nutrients (e.g. increased synthesis of microbial protein resulting in a net protein loss), and/or ingestion of toxins that may limit intake. An excellent discussion of these factors and the dietary choices of the herbivorous butterfish (*Odax pullus*) is presented by Baker et al. (2016).

Feeding

Diet Selection and Formulation

Diets should be palatable, free from contamination, and of sufficient quantity and quality. They should mimic wild diets where possible and provide variety and enrichment. Consideration should be given to the species, life stage, size, body condition, reproductive state, and/or disease state of each individual.

Diet formulation involves matching food items with the specific requirements of the animal, where known. Many diet formulation software programs are available to assist with calculations, although consultation with an animal nutritionist is recommended for interpretation. However, most of the research has been on commercially important cultured teleosts. Research on the nutrient requirements of marine teleosts and elasmobranchs is lacking. It is likely that aquarium diets for fish can be greatly improved through more published research.

Food Types

Typical diet items for fish in aquariums include a variety of commercial pellets and flake foods, gel diets, harvested fish and aquatic invertebrates, plants and algae, and live foods. Nutritional analyses for common food items fed to fish are presented in Tables A4.5–A4.8.

Animal-based diets, particularly fish-based diets, often show higher digestibility and better fatty acid and protein profiles for fish, but there may be concerns about high total fat content, cost, and sustainability (Cho and Bureau 2001). Efforts have been made to increase the use of plant-based fish diets. However, plant-based diets may contain antinutritional factors (e.g. phytate, non-starch polysaccharides (NSPs), protease inhibitors). These can reduce digestibility and impair fish health, depending on adaptations to these diets, processing of the ingredients, and enzyme additions (e.g. phytase) (Kumar et al. 2012; Lemos and Tacon 2016).

Undigested feed can negatively impact water quality in the facility and after water is released. The major concerns with fish are solid wastes, nitrogen, and phosphorus, which can contribute to eutrophication (Cho and Bureau 2001). Nitrogen tends to be of greater concern in seawater, whereas phosphorus tends to be of greater concern in freshwater, as they are essential for algal growth in the respective environments. Most of these wastes come from the diet, so improving food types can reduce environmental impacts. Nitrogenous waste can be minimized by providing optimal levels of amino acids and reducing the digestible protein:energy ratio (McGoogan and Gatlin 1999). Phosphorus waste may be the result of variable P digestibility, and/or from phytate-bound phosphorus in plant-based ingredients. In the latter situation, the addition of phytase enzymes may reduce phytate-P excretion by fish species which digest little to no phytate-P autoenzymatically (Papatryphon and Soares 2001; Hua and Bureau 2010).

Pellet and Flake Foods

Commercial pellets and flakes are generally formulated with a mixture of animal-based and plant-based ingredients. Commercial diets have several benefits beyond convenience.

Table A4.5 Nutrient parameters of seafood items commonly fed to fish.

	Capelin (*Mallotus villosus*)	**Pacific herring** (*Clupea pallasii*)	**Atlantic mackerel** (*Scomber scrombus*)	**Silverside** (*Menidia menidia*)	**Anchovy** (*Engraulis mordax*)	**Lake smelt** (*Osmerus mordax*)	**Sardine** (*Sardinops sagax*)
Dry matter (%)	20.3	31	27.5	25.1	29.7	17.6	28.3
Energy (kcal/100 g)	630.3	676.5	589.2	590.8	635.9	573.2	452.3
Protein (%)	60.4	50.9	71.0	61.4	52.5	74.6	76.5
Fat (%)	30.8	43.2	20.4	26.3	38.2	15.3	5.9
Ash (%)	9.35	7.25	9.49	10.22	10.89	9.58	19.47
Carbohydrate (%)[a]	0.0	0.0	0.0	2.1	0.0	0.5	0.0
Ca (%)	1.21	1.41	1.53	2.27	1.68	1.91	3.48
P (%)	1.57	1.35	1.70	2.01	1.55	1.71	2.48
Mg (%)	0.15	0.12	0.17	0.13	0.13	0.12	0.22
K (%)	1.22	1.02	1.49	1.08	0.85	1.26	1.6
Na (%)	0.833	0.519	0.543	0.389	0.547	0.274	1.409
Fe (mg/kg)	42	54	90	33	198	27	305
Zn (mg/kg)	57	49	67	95.0	52	90	76
Cu (mg/kg)	2	2	5	2.0	2	2	4
Mn (mg/kg)	2	4	2	5.0	6	7	8
Mo (mg/kg)	<0.1	0.2	<1	<1	<0.1	0.1	1.7
Co (mg/kg)	1.06	<0.01	<1	0.1	0.2	0.12	0.2
S (%)	0.80	0.71	0.95	1.01	0.69	0.95	1.02
Se (ppm)	1.20	1.41	3.19	1.93	1.22	1.76	2.88

All values are on a dry matter basis.
[a] Carbohydrate calculated by difference. *Source*: Hoopes unpublished data.

Table A4.6 Nutrient parameters of crustaceans commonly fed to fish.

	Krill, blanched (*Euphausia superba*)	**White shrimp, shell on, no head** (*Litopenaeus setiferus*)	**Blue crab, carapace removed** (*Callinectes sapidus*)	**Crayfish** (*Procambarus clarkii*)	**Ghost shrimp** (*Palaemonetes paludosus*)	**Mysid shrimp** (*Americamysis bahia*)
Dry matter (%)	19	19.4	31.4	24.3	18.6	14.6
Energy (kcal/100 g)	571.6	487.3	306.9	381.2	484.1	458.1
Protein (%)	62.1	81.4	42.1	57.8	77.6	70.4
Fat (%)	22.2	3.8	4.1	2.6	7.8	5.6
Ash (%)	16.51	15.5	42.57	29.77	14.71	15.64
Carbohydrate (%)[a]	0.0	0.0	11.2	9.8	0.0	8.4
Ca (%)	1.57	1.68	11.35	8.60	3.72	2.99
P (%)	1.37	1.32	1.36	0.92	1.78	1.55
Mg (%)	0.43	0.21	0.61	0.19	0.18	0.50
K (%)	1.25	0.75	0.75	1.21	1.58	1.50
Na (%)	3.119	3.286	1.390	0.551	0.897	1.81
Fe (mg/kg)	41	23	597	553	29	54
Zn (mg/kg)	51	83	73	81	96	60
Cu (mg/kg)	79	12	46	38	98	28
Mn (mg/kg)	2	4	546	285	19	14
Mo (mg/kg)	0.2	<0.1	0.3	<0.1	<0.1	<5.6
Co (mg/kg)	<0.01	0.11	0.41	0.89	0.55	<5.6
S (%)	1.66	0.89	0.57	0.53	0.98	ND
Se (ppm)	7.06	1.19	1.42	1.94	1.25	1.75

All values are on a dry matter basis.
ND: not determined.
[a] Carbohydrate calculated by difference. *Source*: Hoopes unpublished data.

Table A4.7 Nutrient parameters of mollusks commonly fed to fish.

	Surf clam (*Spisula solidissima*)	Scallop (*Placopecten magellanicus*)	Mussel (*Mytilus edulis*)	Squid (*Doryteuthis opalescens*)
Dry matter (%)	21.5	12.9	21.6	19.1
Energy (kcal/100 g)	481.6	465	498.2	564.7
Protein (%)	67.1	67.7	58.9	83.8
Fat (%)	3.3	3.7	7.4	9.3
Ash (%)	11.71	16.42	11.16	8.26
Carbohydrate (%)[a]	17.9	12.2	22.5	0.0
Ca (%)	0.08	0.03	0.3	0.09
P (%)	1.00	3.60	0.93	1.3
Mg (%)	0.25	0.1	0.38	0.24
K (%)	1.48	0.71	0.76	1.62
Na (%)	1.327	4.662	2.415	1.217
Fe (mg/kg)	407	27	91	14
Zn (mg/kg)	58	37	155	89
Cu (mg/kg)	8	1	6	95
Mn (mg/kg)	139	1	7	1
Mo (mg/kg)	0.6	<1	0.4	<0.1
Co (mg/kg)	2.36	<1	<0.01	0.47
S (%)	1.59	1.19	1.34	1.84
Se (ppm)	3.56	0.82	2.67	3.08

All values are on a dry matter basis.
[a] Carbohydrate calculated by difference. *Source*: Hoopes unpublished data.

Table A4.8 Nutrient parameters of other invertebrates commonly fed to fish.

	Bloodworms (*Glycera dibranchiata*)	Blackworms (*Lumbriculus variegatus*)	Earthworms (*Lumbricus terrestris*)	Crickets, adult (*Acheta domestica*)
Dry matter (%)	8.5	14	17.8	28.5
Energy (kcal/100 g)	514.3	611.6	517.4	650.4
Protein (%)	43.2	65.7	61.5	61.5
Fat (%)	6.4	14.5	4.0	26.8
Ash (%)	3.27	5.4	15.2	5.61
Carbohydrate (%)[a]	47.1	14.4	19.3	6.1
Ca (%)	0.14	0.09	1.23	0.13
P (%)	0.61	0.98	0.81	0.87
Mg (%)	0.08	0.08	0.2	0.10
K (%)	0.66	1	0.9	1.06
Na (%)	0.523	0.357	0.37	0.319
Fe (mg/kg)	544	1240	3890	57
Zn (mg/kg)	88	170	398	142
Cu (mg/kg)	14	22	14.0	34
Mn (mg/kg)	12	7	44.0	24
Mo (mg/kg)	0.2	0.2	2.7	<1
Co (mg/kg)	0.17	1.63	7.60	<1
S (%)	0.41	0.62	1.00	0.53
Se (ppm)	5.45	2.17	4.74	0.85

All values are on a dry matter basis.
[a] Carbohydrate calculated by difference. *Source*: Hoopes unpublished data.

Nutrient levels are generally formulated to meet or exceed known requirements. Water-stable forms of nutrients are generally used. Finally, these commercial diet items can be manufactured to optimize fish feeding strategies, i.e. pellets may be made to sink quickly, slowly, float, or some combination, allowing animals to eat in their preferred location in the water column.

Gel Diets

Gel diets are designed using gelatin or some other gelling agent. They can be purchased as gels or as a dry powder to which warm water is added. Gel diets offer several advantages including relatively high protein levels, particularly if gelatin is the gelling agent chosen, and high moisture levels and therefore higher palatability than dry diets. An additional benefit is the ease of supplementation: supplements to enhance nutrient consumption and oral medications can easily be added. Gel diets generally sink (with some exceptions) and once prepared should be handled like raw fish, so preparation and storage space should be considered when using these types of diets.

Harvested Fish and Invertebrates (Seafood)

Commercially harvested fish (particularly capelin, herring, mackerel, smelt, and silversides) and invertebrates (particularly mollusks and crustaceans) are commonly fed to fish in zoos and aquariums. It is essential to consider the wild-type diet and feeding ecology of the target species when making seafood choices. For example, fatty fish (e.g. herring, mackerel, sprat) should not be fed to macro-invertebrate or bottom-foraging species (e.g. dasyatid rays). Sustainability of food sources should also be considered. Commercially obtained seafood should be of a quality intended for human consumption.

It is important to offer freshwater-based food to freshwater fish and marine-based seafood to marine fish. This distinction may seem trivial, but the essential fatty acids (DHA, EPA, and AA) and the ratio of omega-3:omega-6 fatty acids of freshwater and marine fish vary greatly due to the respective phytoplankton sources at the base of the food web. For example, studies on juvenile seahorses (*Hippocampus* sp.) suggested that they have a high requirement for DHA which may not be met by freshwater mysid shrimp, compared to saltwater mysid shrimp (Chang and Southgate 2001).

It is important to avoid feeding herbivorous fish a diet containing seafood, as this can exceed their protein and lipid requirements, leading to fat deposition in muscle, around the coelomic organs, and/or in the liver.

Plants and Algae

Live plants in aquatic systems can provide a supplemental source of nutrition for herbivorous fish. Many species of freshwater plants have been used as food sources, including *Cabomba* spp. (fanwort), *Egeria* (*Elodea*) *densa* and *Elodea canadensis* (water weed, elodea), *Limnophila* spp. (ambulia), *Myriophyllum mattogrossense*, *Rotala indica* (toothcup), *Hygrophila polysperma*, *Nymphea* spp. (water lily, lotus), and *Lemna* spp. (duckweed). Consideration should be given to the substrate, lighting, and carbon dioxide levels necessary for photosynthesis and growth. Limited information is available on the nutritional value of freshwater plants, as research has primarily focused on weed control and alternative feed sources for domestic animals. Some research has looked at *Lemna* sp. as a potential high-protein feed source for cultured fish. When grown under ideal conditions and harvested regularly, it has 5–15% fiber, 35–43% crude protein, and ~5% polyunsaturated fat on a dry matter basis (Leng et al. 1995).

The largest use of microalgae (phytoplankton) in fish feeds is in aquaculture, where over 40 species are used. The most common are *Chlorella*, *Dunaliella*, *Scenedesmus*, and *Spirulina* spp. They are commonly used in marine herbivores, marine fish larvae, and fingerlings. Considerable attention has been given to the concentrations of omega-3 fatty acids in microalgae, especially EPA and DHA. Microalgae can also have a high fraction of β-1,3-glucan, which can act as an immune-stimulant in fish (Dalmo et al. 1996; Dalmo and Bøgwald 2008). Many microalgae are good sources of carotenoids, including astaxanthin in *Haematococcus* spp., β-carotene in *Dunaliella* spp., and β-carotene and zeaxanthin in *Spirulina* spp. *Spirulina* spp. are also a good source of thiamine, riboflavin, and cobalamin (Thajuddin and Subramanian 2005). However, microalgae show high variation in chemical composition depending on species and growth conditions (Ben-Amotz et al. 1985; Reitan et al. 1994). Microalgae can be fed directly, provided in commercial fish feeds, or gut-loaded into an intermediate food source such as rotifers.

Several macroalgae (e.g. seaweeds) are used as fish feed, including *Porphyra* spp. (nori, a red algae), *Gracilaria verrucosa* (ogonori, a red algae), *Undaria pinnatifida* (wakame, a brown algae), *Ulva* spp. (sea lettuce, a green algae), and *Cladophora glomerata* (a filamentous green algae). Carbohydrate and fiber content of select algae species have been reported by Mišurcová et al. (2010).

The benefits of incorporating algae into fish diets have been shown for a variety of fish: *Chlorella* or *Scenedesmus* spp. fed to Nile tilapia; *Chlorella* spp. fed to olive flounder (*Paralichthys olivaceus*); *Undaria*, *Ascophyllum*, *Porphyra*, or *Ulva* spp. fed to red seabream (*Pagrus major*); *Gracilaria* or *Ulva* spp. fed to European bass (*Dicentrarchus labrax*); *Ulva* spp. to striped mullet (*Mugil cephalus*); *Ulva* spp. fed or *Pterocladia* spp. fed to gilthead seabream (*Sparus aurata*); and *Porphyra* or a *Nannochloropsis–Isochrysis* spp.

combination fed to Atlantic cod (*Gadus morhua*), although many of these studies fail to identify the nutritional factors responsible for these benefits (Yone et al. 1986; Mustafa et al. 1995; Wassef et al. 2001; Wassef et al. 2005; Valente et al. 2006; Badwy et al. 2008; Walker et al. 2009; Walker and Berlinsky 2011; Rahimnejad et al. 2017).

The limitation of algae as feed is the digestibility of the cell wall in non-herbivorous species. Studies suggest that only 10–15% of dietary protein requirements of non-herbivorous fish can be met by algae without compromising growth. The type and quantity of extracellular polysaccharides, which are abundant in certain algae, can also interfere with nutrient absorption. Finally, some algae contain trace element concentrations that can be detrimental.

Live Foods

Ambush and highly visual predatory fish (e.g. frogfish, seahorses) generally require live foods to trigger an eating response. Other predatory fish that are not readily eating harvested food may require live foods while being converted onto a managed diet. Most larval fish also require live foods in the early stages of development.

The most popular live foods cultured in aquariums are brine shrimp (*Artemia* spp.) for brackish or marine fish and rotifers (particularly *Brachionus* spp.) for freshwater, brackish, or marine fish.

Brine shrimp are typically obtained as cysts or live cultures and reared in salt water. Cysts hatch into nauplii that develop into adults through several molts. Alternatively, cysts can be decapsulated to feed without worrying about removing unhatched cysts or shells. Post-hatch nauplii contain an internal yolk sac and, if no exogenous food is available, can survive on these yolk reserves for up to five days post-hatch (Treece 2000). However, the nutritional quality of nauplii declines rapidly as the yolk sac is consumed. Nauplii should either be fed out within 24 hours post-hatch or receive supplemental feeding and/or gut-loading. Brine shrimp are nonspecific feeders, as long as food size is small (<50 μm for nauplii and <60 μm for adults), and a variety of products can be used (e.g. algae, microparticles, omega-yeast, or marine oil emulsions, which are particularly rich in PUFAs). Products should have taurine, manganese, and omega-3 fatty acids with a DHA:EPA ratio of 2:1, as these promote growth, increase survivability, and improve stress resistance (Sargent et al. 1997, 1999; Woods 2003; Nguyen et al. 2008). Administration of probiotics to brine shrimp improved survival of larval European bass (Touraki et al. 2012).

Rotifers are typically obtained as cysts or live cultures and maintained in freshwater or brackish water, although some can be cultured in salt water. Providing supplemental feeding for two to four days and gut-loading for two to three hours prior to feeding out both improve nutrient concentrations (Romero-Romero and Yúfera 2012). These nutrients appear stable for at least eight hours after rotifers are placed in fish tanks (Dhert et al. 2014). Supplements should contain taurine, omega-3 fatty acids, vitamin C, vitamin E, manganese, zinc, iodine, and selenium (Hamre et al. 2008; Matsunari et al. 2013a, b). The levels of vitamin C and E in copepods (500 and 115 mg/kg, respectively) may provide an initial target, and these levels can be achieved in rotifers with supplementation (Kolkovski et al. 2000). The effectiveness of iodine supplementation depends on the source; sodium iodide is mostly lost within two hours of enrichment while thymol iodine is still present after 18 hours (Srivastava et al. 2012). Selenium enrichment of rotifers is also feasible, but the concentration and source must be considered to avoid toxicity concerns; inorganic selenium sources have the potential to be more toxic than Se-methionine sources (Penglase et al. 2010).

While brine shrimp and rotifers are the most common live foods, many other organisms are routinely available for purchase or culture. Other marine food items include mysids (*Mysis* spp.), copepods, amphipods, and fiddler crabs (*Uca* spp.). Other brackish or freshwater food items include water fleas (*Daphnia* and *Moina* spp.), ghost/glass shrimp (often *Palaemonetes* spp.), bloodworms (midge larvae), blackworms (*Lumbriculus* spp. oligochaetes), mosquito larvae, goldfish, swordtails (*Xiphophorus hellerii*), and guppies and mollies (*Poecilia* spp.). Many terrestrial invertebrates can also be easily cultured and fed to fish, e.g. crickets, earthworms, mealworms, grindal worms, and vinegar eel nematodes (*Panagrellus redivivus* (*Turbatrix aceti*)).

With live foods, consideration must be given to animal acquisition, transport, housing, and feeding. Live foods should always be housed and fed in a manner that meets their behavioral and physiological needs and practices should be sustainable and minimize stress to the feeder animals. How live prey are fed affects their health and their nutritional value to the end consumer. Without good feeding practices, many of these live foods are nutritionally incomplete. Gut-loading may be used to further increase their nutritional value. Gut-loading refers to the diet provided for a specific period of time prior to feeding out, with nutrients designed to fill the GI tract as opposed to being absorbed.

Live foods may carry infectious diseases that are transmissible to other fish or invertebrates. To minimize this risk, live foods are best cultured in-house and closely monitored for morbidity or mortality. Incoming live foods should go through a quarantine period prior to feeding out.

This quarantine period may include necropsy examinations to look for potential pathogens.

Further information on husbandry requirements of feeder animals can be found in Schaeffer et al. (1992), NRC (1996), and Spencer and Spencer (2006).

Vitamin and Mineral Supplementation

Most wild fish consume a varied diet that changes with location, season, and life stage. Variation of items fed to managed fish is recommended to minimize the risk of deficiencies. Additional vitamin and/or mineral supplementation may be used to compensate for potential dietary deficiencies and loss of nutrients during food storage and thawing and from leaching once in water. Many commercial supplements are available for fish, with combinations of vitamins, minerals, and fatty acids. The delivery methods range from liquids added to the water or used to soak foods, to capsules or tablets that are added to the food.

Liquid supplements can leach away before consumption, be removed by filtration, and/or negatively impact water quality. It is also hard to control the supplement dose. The efficacy of this type of delivery system for supplements is largely untested. In general, capsules or tablets are more reliable than liquid supplements. Elasmobranchs are routinely supplemented with a multivitamin and mineral tablet within their seafood, and several commercial multivitamins are available, e.g. Mazuri® Shark and Ray II tabs, Sea Tabs® for Birds, Turtles, Fish and Sharks, Vetafarm® Elasmo Tabs, International Zoo Vet Group Elasmobranch Tablets (Janse 2003; Hoopes 2017).

Since many essential vitamins are unstable in the presence of light, heat, oxygen and/or water (e.g. A, B1, C, and E), careful storage of supplements is important (Lešková et al. 2006). Independent nutritional testing is recommended to validate product labels and storage conditions. Regular evaluations of supplementation are suggested as animals, diets, and the information available change over time.

Feeding a portion of the total diet as high-quality pellet, flake, or gel may help ensure delivery of vitamins and minerals, since these products are often formulated using water- and heat-stable vitamin and mineral mixtures. This is particularly useful in species that are small and/or where it is difficult to deliver supplementation in tablet form.

Feeding Behavior, Amount, and Frequency

The feeding behavior of fish is complex. Fish possess several chemosensory systems which include gustation (taste), olfaction (smell), and chemical sensory and chemoreceptor cells, with the acceptance or rejection of food being primarily attributed to inputs from chemoreception (Lall and Tibbetts 2009). Hunger is the cue for feeding behavior in fish, with the primary stimulus being gut fullness and/or metabolite levels in the circulatory system (Jobling and Wandsvik 1983). Numerous abiotic and biotic factors affect food intake in fish including how the diet is presented, diet composition, hormonal and biological state, environmental conditions, fish health and developmental state, and system design (Lall and Tibbetts 2009).

It is generally accepted that fish feed to satisfy their energy requirements. Fish fed a diet low in energy content are forced to increase their consumption rate and gastric evacuation rate to compensate for a low-calorie diet. Correct food size is also important. Food items should be sufficiently small to be physically ingested, while large enough to be consumed without expending too much energy in the process (Lall and Tibbetts 2009). In European eels (*Anguilla anguilla*), optimal particle size was ~40–60% of mouth width (Knights 1983). Trout showed a similar optimal particle size, although particles up to 100% of mouth width could be consumed, particularly when the particle was smooth (Knights 1983).

Determining the optimal feed amount is important to maintain health and minimize nitrogenous waste, but it can be difficult. Feed requirements vary with diet, species, life history stage (e.g. juveniles require more energy per unit weight than adult fish); water quality (e.g. temperature, salinity); exercise level and habitat size; and social interactions (e.g. dominance hierarchy). In aquaculture, feed amount is calculated as a percentage of the total biomass of fish, with the percentage decreasing as the individuals grow. Rates for juvenile cultured species range from 4–11% BW, decreasing in adults to 0.5–2% BW, but this is highly species- and temperature-dependent (New 1987). In aquarium-maintained species, feed amounts can be more difficult to assess since the goal is longevity rather than production, and animals are often maintained in complex, multispecies systems. Generally, fish species in aquariums are fed at lower rates than those in aquaculture. In adult bony fish, 0.5–1% BW/day is a good starting point, as this is the average stomach volume of many bony fish. This should be reduced if the entire ration is not consumed within five minutes for individuals, or within 15 minutes for animals maintained in large groups. Food around the edges of the tank or settling on the bottom, or increases in ammonia, are signs of overfeeding and should be avoided. For adult elasmobranchs, starting food amounts have been outlined by Janse et al. (2004), with bottom-dwelling sharks (e.g. *Hemiscylliidae* and *Stegostomatidae*), bottom-dwelling rays (e.g. *Dasyatidae*), and ram-ventilating rays (e.g. *Myliobatidae*) at 4–6% BW/week; slow-swimming ram-ventilating sharks (e.g. *Odontaspididae*) at 1.0–2.5% BW/week;

and fast-swimming ram-ventilating sharks (e.g., *Carcharhinidae*) at 3–4% BW/week. Elasmobranchs with higher metabolic rates (e.g. *Mobula* spp.) or those that are more endothermic may require much higher rations than described above. Rations for juveniles should be multiplied by a factor of 1.5–3.0. Feeding amounts should be adjusted based on growth data, body weight and body condition comparisons with wild counterparts, and blood analyses where available (Janse et al. 2004).

Body Condition

Body condition scores (BCSs) are a useful way to assess the health and nutritional status of fish at a point in time. They are often designed with a 5-point scale where 3 represents optimal condition and 1 and 5 represent under- and over-conditioned animals, respectively.

Studies have evaluated body condition indices in wild and cultured fish by examining the relationship between body mass and body length (Kohler et al. 1995; Hussey et al. 2009). Visual BCS systems are more desirable in managed collections as they do not require fish handling for morphometrics. These have been published for zebrafish (*Danio rerio*) and spotted eagle rays (*Aetobatus narinari*) (Wilson et al. 2013; Kamerman et al. 2017). BCS systems for fusiform teleosts similar to koi (*Cyprinus carpio koi*), demersal rays similar to southern stingrays (*Hypanus americanus*), and pelagic sharks similar to requiem sharks (*Carcharhinus* spp.) are shown in Figures A4.1–A4.3. These are meant as a guide only, as different species will build fat and muscle in different anatomical locations.

Since body condition scores are subjective, they are best assessed by a team of people (e.g. husbandry staff, technicians, veterinarians, and nutritionists). They are particularly useful when compared across a group or across time, especially during periods of physiologic change (e.g. around breeding and growth).

Food Storage and Preparation

Appropriate food storage and handling are crucial. All aspects of the feeding program should be evaluated to ensure that offered food items are free of contamination (biological, chemical, and physical) and are stored, thawed, prepared, and fed in a manner that preserves nutritional quality.

Food Safety and Monitoring

Hazard Analysis and Critical Control Point (HACCP) programs can be applied to the entire food handling pathway from harvest, catch, or manufacturing through animal consumption (Schmidt et al. 2006). These can help ensure food safety with regard to biological (pathogenic microorganisms or parasites), chemical (natural toxins, pesticides, drug residues, manufactured chemicals), or physical contamination (foreign objects). HACCP programs involve the following steps:

1) Identify potential hazards or risks within the system.
2) Identify critical control points in the system where hazards could occur.
3) Establish critical limits for each potential hazard.
4) Establish monitoring of the control points.
5) Establish corrective measures when critical limits are exceeded.
6) Develop record-keeping and verification methods.

To ensure the best-quality diets, each facility should develop their own HACCP programs and ask their vendors to share their HACCP programs. Readers are referred to Schmidt et al. (2006) and Henry et al. (2010) for further discussions on developing and implementing HACCP programs.

Storage

High standards for food storage prevent nutrient loss and product degradation. Temperature, humidity, air exposure, and lighting can all affect food quality.

Frozen foods should be stored between −30 and −18°C (−22 and 0°F) in order minimize oxidation and thiaminase activity (Crissey 1998; Henry et al. 2010). Refrigeration at <4°C (39°F) should be used for storing vegetables, fruits, forage, and for short-term holding (<24 hours) of thawed seafood and gel foods. Some pelleted and flake foods also require refrigeration. Room temperature storage, e.g. 18–21°C (64–70°F) and 50–60% relative humidity, can be used for some dry foods. The foods should be off the ground and the area should be well-ventilated (Henry et al. 2010). Temperatures of food storage locations should be monitored and recorded routinely to ensure conditions are suitable.

It is common to purchase food in bulk and store items until use. Using sealed containers to minimize air and light exposure helps maintain nutrient content. It is important that containers are labeled with the:

- Date of catch, manufacture, or receipt.
- Date of opening.
- Date of discard.

The discard date, or shelf life, should be provided by the manufacturer for pelleted, flake, and gel foods. For frozen seafood, the discard date should be less than 12 months from catch. This may be reduced to six months for high-fat foods (e.g. mackerel and herring) but nutritional testing is a more reliable way of evaluating nutrient losses.

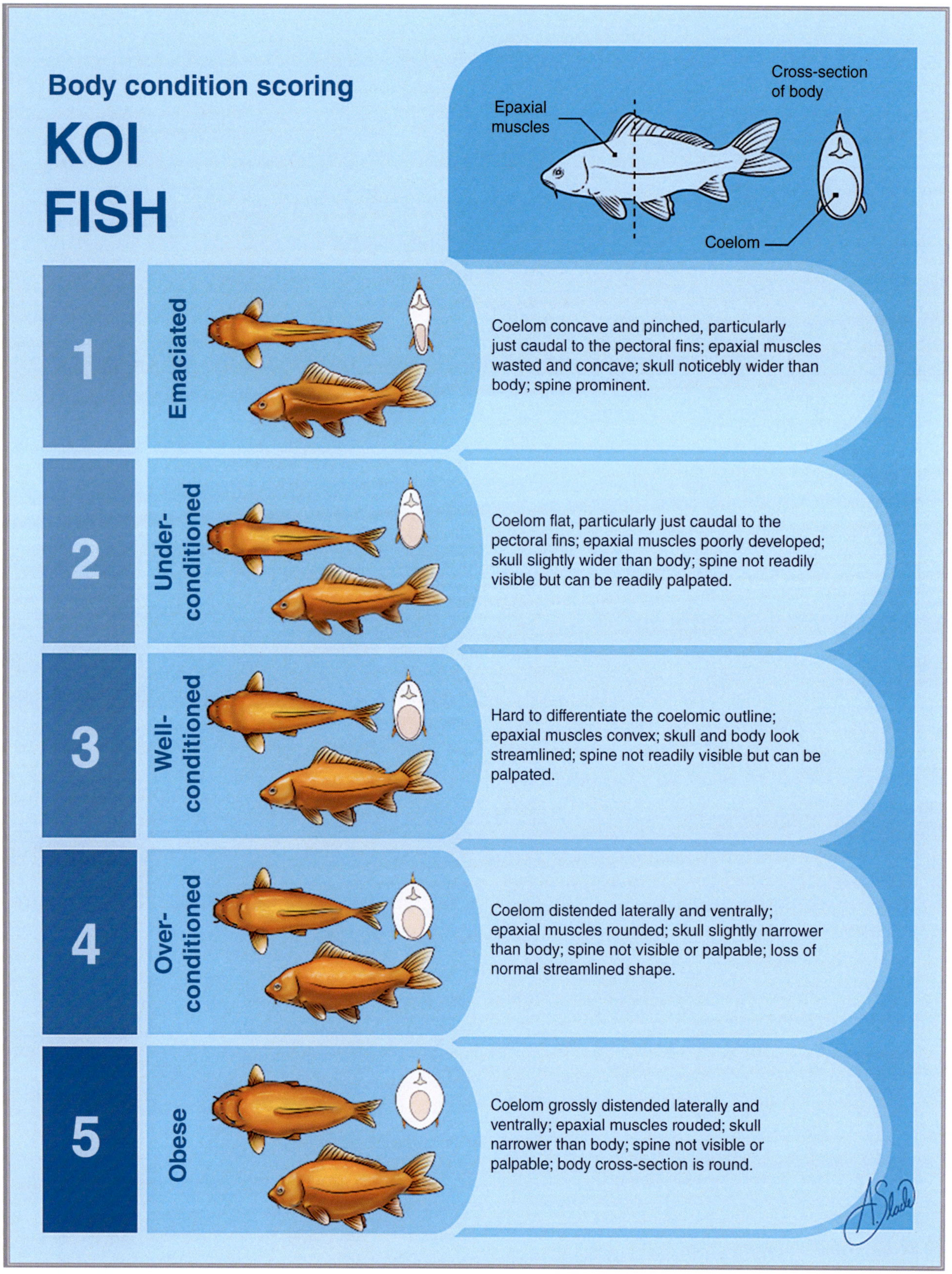

Figure A4.1 Body condition score system for koi (*Cyprinus carpio koi*) and similar fusiform fish. *Source*: Image courtesy of Amanda Slade; copyright reserved.

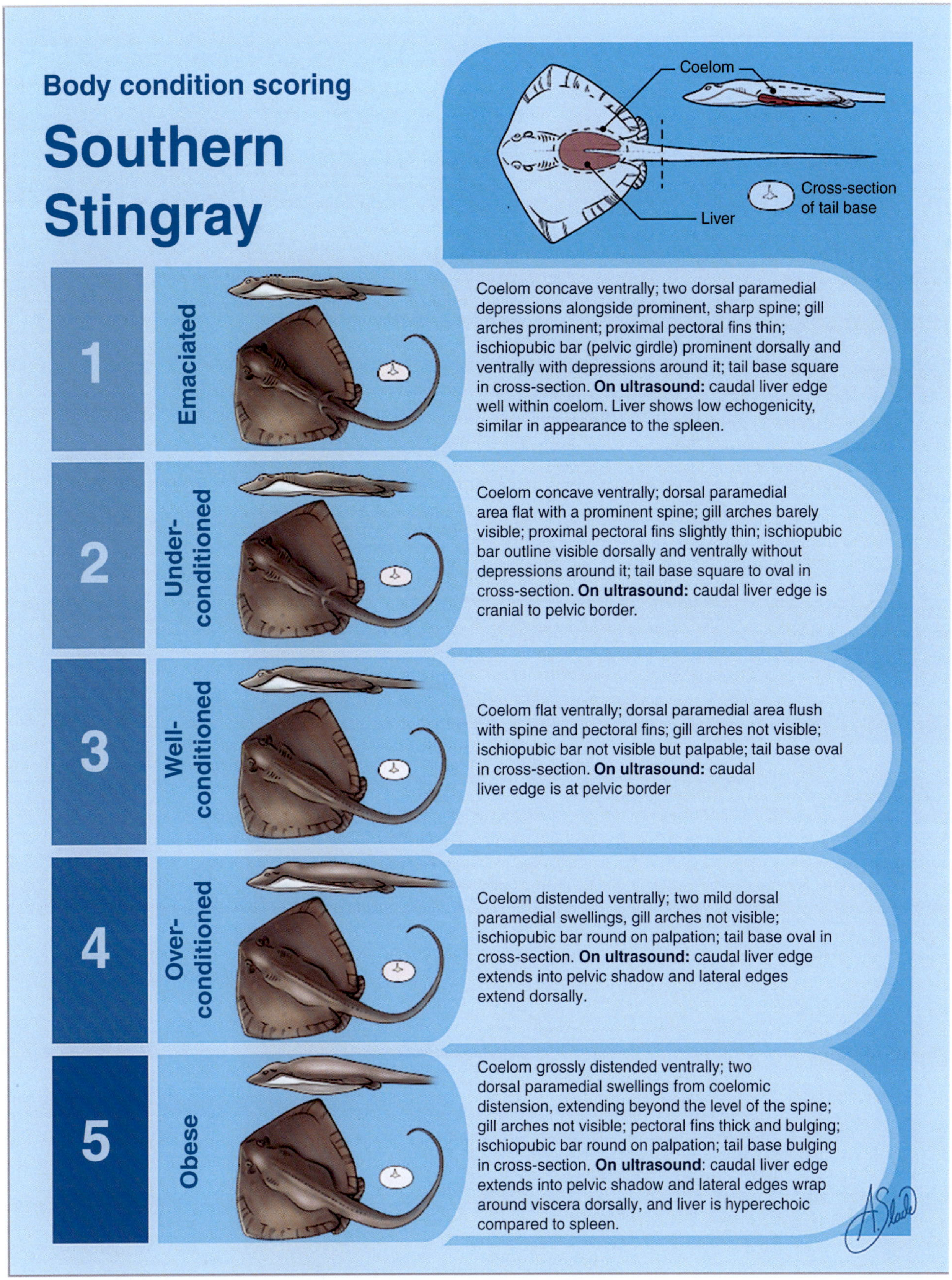

Figure A4.2 Body condition score system for southern stingrays (*Hypanus americanus*) and similar demersal rays. *Source*: Image courtesy of Amanda Slade; copyright reserved.

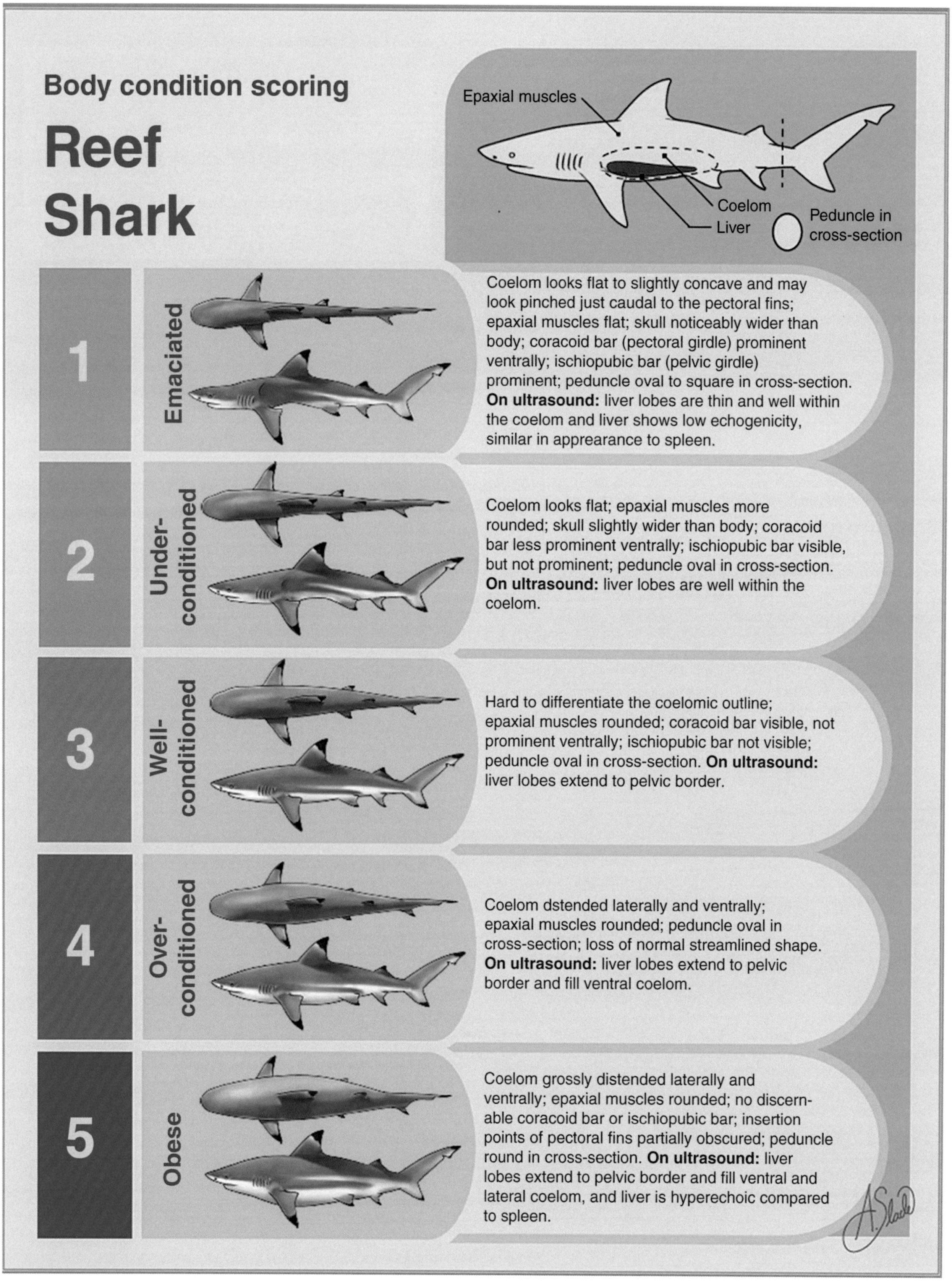

Figure A4.3 Body condition score system for reef sharks (*Carcharhinus* sp.) and similar pelagic sharks. *Source*: Image courtesy of Amanda Slade; copyright reserved.

Food Preparation

Safe food-handling procedures should be implemented for animal diets. These include washing hands before putting on gloves to handle food; washing gloves, knives, cutting boards, and other utensils between food types to prevent cross-contamination; and using properly cleaned and sanitized utensils and food containers (Henry et al. 2010). Cleaning (removal of visible food and debris) and sanitizing (reducing the number of micro-organisms on cleaned surfaces to safe levels) are separate, sequential processes. Cleaning can be done with soap and warm water. The recommended method for sanitization is a high-heat dishwasher (>71°C (160°F)). Chemical sanitization is an acceptable alternative and can include one of the following methods (Henry et al. 2010):

- 100 mg/L chlorine for >20 seconds.
- 25 mg/L iodine solution for >60 seconds.
- 200 mg/L quaternary ammonium compound for >60 seconds.
- 0.5% Virkon-Aquatic® for 10 minutes.

After the sanitizing step, dishes should be rinsed. Chlorine may be deactivated using sodium thiosulfate. Dishes should be allowed to air-dry and not towel-dried.

Seafood

Given the perishable nature of seafood, food-handling is crucial. Thawing should always be done in air under refrigeration at <4°C (39°F), never at room temperature. If rapid thawing is required, food items may be thawed in a sealed and closed container under cold running water. Incorrect thawing may result in nutrient losses, fat rancidity, microbial buildup, and loss of palatability (Crissey 1998; Henry et al. 2010).

Food should be inspected during preparation. Fresh and fresh-thawed fish should have bright red gills, clear corneas (often with lens opacities), and firm elastic flesh with no breaks in the skin. Old or thawed and refrozen fish are dull in appearance, have opaque corneas, red-bordered eyes, and soft flesh that leaves finger impressions and tears readily; these should not be fed (Crissey 1998; Henry et al. 2010).

All thawed seafood should be kept iced or refrigerated until feeding and should be used within 24 hours. Thawed food should never be refrozen. Periodic nutrient testing for quality control (see below) is encouraged, especially for fish that are high in fat.

Produce

Handling of vegetables, fruit, and forage should minimize bacterial contamination, especially in areas where other food items are prepared. Vegetables and produce should be washed and inspected for signs of spoilage, pests, and environmental damage. Individual standards should be developed for each produce or vegetable type (Henry et al. 2010).

Pelleted and Flake Feeds

Dry feeds should be inspected for foreign material, dust, mold, evidence of pests, color, smell, and product uniformity.

Gel Foods

Gel diets are generally prepared on site by mixing a dry meal base with hot water. It is critical to follow manufacturers' directions regarding ratios of dry product:water, water temperature, and mixing time to ensure proper hydration of any gelling agents and to ensure food safety (e.g. heat inactivation of micro-organisms). If a facility is using an in-house recipe, data on heat inactivation of common micro-organisms may be of use (e.g. Ericsson et al. 2002). If medications or other supplements are added to gel foods, it is important to consider the temperature to which the compound can be exposed while maintaining activity. For example, it may be preferable to inject a medication into a single piece of cooled gel food, rather than adding a medication to hot gel food during the preparation process. Once prepared, gel diets should be stored and handled as raw foods.

Quality Control

Diet analyses are an important part of monitoring the composition of food items offered to animals (Bernard and Allen 2002; Henry et al. 2010). Seafood, such as frozen or fresh fish, should be analyzed to monitor the wide fluctuations in nutrients that can occur on a seasonal, regional, or species-specific basis. Dry feeds should be analyzed due to potential inconsistencies in manufacturing. A schedule for sampling and analysis should be established, especially for items that represent a significant part of the diet. Wherever possible, primary food items, especially seafood, should be analyzed once per year or ideally with each batch. Specialty feeds that are fed to a small proportion of the collection may be analyzed less frequently. If problems are encountered, analyses may be conducted more frequently.

The types of analyses performed depend on the type of food item and the reasons for sampling. Most analyses should include proximate composition:

- Moisture (or dry matter).
- Crude protein, fat by ether extract, and ash.
- Fiber (neutral detergent fiber [NDF], acid detergent fiber [ADF], and acid lignin), particularly for plant-based or commercially prepared food items. Seafood is generally low in fiber, so this analysis is less important.

Other useful analyses include:

- Gross energy, which may be useful in understanding total calories and energy available to the animal.
- Macrominerals (Ca, P, Na, K, Mg).
- Trace and ultra-trace minerals (Cu, Co, Fe, I, Mn, Se, Zn).
- Vitamins (vitamin A, B1 [thiamine], C, D3, E as α-tocopherol, β-carotene).

Food items may also be tested for microbiological loads, toxins, organic contaminants, or pesticide residues.

When sampling feeds for analysis, the goal is to obtain a small portion that is homogeneous and representative of the entire lot (e.g. batch or harvest). Food items should be submitted to the laboratory in the form that they are prepared and consumed by the animal (e.g. fillet versus whole fish, shell removed, and supplements added). The reader is referred to Bernard and Dempsey (1999) for greater details on obtaining a representative sample and selecting an appropriate laboratory. Once the nutritional analyses are received, the results should be compared to pre-established criteria, previous analyses, "typical" nutrient composition of common food items, and the information presented in Tables A4.5–A4.8 (Dierenfeld et al. 1991; Bernard and Allen 2002; Henry et al. 2010). Consultation with a nutritionist is recommended to help identify deviations in nutrient composition.

Nutritional Support

Changes in feeding frequency or amount may be indicative of a problem such as inappropriate feeding, inappropriate environmental conditions, or disease (see Section B). Action should be taken to rule out or resolve any environmental stressors and to identify any disease issues.

Feeding can be encouraged by using food that is of the highest quality, appropriate for the species, of a size that can be processed by the individuals, and fed at appropriate times of day. This is easily confirmed if other members of the species are readily consuming the diet. Changing the feed items or delivery method may encourage feeding. This can include changing from pole feeding to toss feeding and/or changing where in the system or water column food is offered. If social stressors are a factor (e.g. tank-mate displacement), isolating individuals for directed feedings can be helpful.

Appetite Stimulants

Fish primarily detect food through olfaction and sight; however, appearance, feel, and taste are key factors in determining whether food will be consumed (Lall and Tibbetts 2009). Compounds present in the diet may act as feeding-stimulants or deterrents and will determine whether a food item is consumed or rejected.

Certain compounds in poor-quality feeds are known deterrents, including highly oxidized oils, trimethylamine (produced in decaying fish flesh), and aflatoxins (produced by molds). Improper storage leading to rancidity or mold growth depresses feed intake and can result in death if consumed in significant amounts (Lall and Tibbetts 2009).

Amino acids appear to be important feeding stimulants for fish. In omnivorous fish, betaine, glycine, alanine, and mixtures of L-amino acids are important feeding stimulants (Lall and Tibbetts 2009). In the herbivorous redbelly tilapia (*Tilapia zillii*), glutamic acid, aspartic acid, serine, and lysine are major feeding stimulants (Johnsen and Adams 1986; Adams et al. 1988). However, adding these stimulatory materials to the food has had limited practical success (Adams et al. 1988). The best practice to stimulate fish to feed is to deliver food types similar to the wild diet. For example, the feeding stimulants identified for redbelly tilapia are abundant in romaine lettuce.

Various supplements and medications have been used to encourage feeding within the hobbyist, zoo, and aquarium communities. These have included vitamin B/C/E, garlic, diazepam, mirtazapine, megestrol acetate, low-dose dexamethasone, dronabinol, capromorelin, and levothyroxine. However, the supporting literature is scarce and anecdotal reports have shown that these supplements are largely ineffective. Of these, garlic shows the most potential, although high doses can lead to oxidative damage (Ashdown and Violetta 2004; Lee and Gao 2012).

Assisted Feeding

Assisted feeding includes tube feeding (gavage) and force feeding. Deciding when to assist feed requires an understanding of the normal feeding periodicity of the species and the health, metabolic state, and history of the individual. Some species of fish exhibit normal periods of inappetence ranging from two to six months (e.g. moray eels). More metabolically active species require frequent feeds and may develop pathology without any visual decrease in body condition.

Tube Feeding (Gavage)

The prior diet of a fish (e.g. seafood, pellets, soaked flake) can often be made into a slurry or gruel for tube feeding. It is essential that gruel be well-blended and smooth, so heads, spines, fins, skin, and/or shells usually need to be removed prior to using a blender. Commercial tube-feeding formulas may also be useful (e.g. Oxbow® Carnivore Care, Mazuri®

Shark/Ray gel). The gruel or formula, or a mixture, should be blended with water or an electrolyte solution so that it is just thin enough to pass through a syringe and appropriately sized tube. It should not be any more dilute, as this will reduce the caloric concentration. A good starting point is a 60:40 ratio of food to water. This ratio can be adjusted based on the resulting gruel consistency and thickness. The volume for tube feeding will often start at 0.5–1% of fish body weight and increase to 2–3% as necessary.

Tube feeding can be performed under manual or chemical restraint. For small fish, red rubber tubes, avian tracheal tubes, or IV catheters can be used. Luer-lock syringes are useful as they hold the tubing more securely than Luer-slip syringes. For large fish (e.g. >10 kg), small or large animal gastric tubes are useful. The tubing should be cut to an appropriate length by approximating the length from the mouth to the middle of the pectoral fins (the approximate location of many fish stomachs). Beveling the leading edge of the tube and filing any rough edges may reduce the risk of trauma.

It is usually best to fill the syringe immediately before feeding to reduce the risk of clogging. Air pockets should be removed prior to feeding. Most fish are easiest to gavage in ventral recumbency, while small elasmobranchs are often easiest to gavage in dorsal recumbency and large sharks may be easiest in slight lateral recumbency. If a gag is needed, PVC tubes and syringe cases work well. The tube should be gently inserted through the mouth along the midline into the esophagus. If the tube is not centered correctly, it will emerge from one of the gill openings or the spiracle. If this happens, the tube should be retracted and replaced along the midline. It is normal to feel the pharyngeal teeth when placing a gastric tube in a bony fish. Once the resistance changes or the predetermined length has been reached, gentle pressure can be used to deliver the mixture into the stomach. Once the appropriate volume has been provided, or if any regurgitation is seen, the tube should be removed. Fish should be monitored for any subsequent regurgitation as this is common. If the syringe or tubing becomes clogged, it is usually best to remove the gavage tube and try again with a new setup. Serious problems such as gastrointestinal rupture or accidental administration into the swim bladder in physostomous fish are rare but can occur, so suitable restraint and gentle pressure are important.

When tube feeding is needed, it often needs to be repeated regularly to keep an individual on a positive nutritional plane. The frequency will depend upon the condition of the fish, its sensitivity to handing stress, practicalities of regular handling, and the animal's natural feeding periodicity. Gastrostomy tubes could be used to reduce handling requirements in some species, with one report in a green moray eel (*Gymnothorax funebris*) (Kizer 2005). Food should continue to be offered to the fish during tube feeding to encourage free feeding.

Force Feeding

For medium to large fish, whole or cut seafood may be force fed. For example, in rockfish (*Sebastes* spp.) under chemical restraint, the fish can be held in a vertical position and food gently placed into the cranial esophagus using forceps. In sharks and batoids, an appropriate-diameter PVC tube may be placed in the mouth and prey may be pushed through on a feeding pole or plunger. It is easier to force feed firm dietary items, e.g. partially thawed butterfish (*Stromateidae*).

Larval and Broodstock Nutrition

Larval fish nutrition is a relatively new area of focus for both aquaculture and conservation efforts. Larval fish grow rapidly, with reports of 30–100% growth/day in some species, and their nutrient requirements are likely different from adult and juvenile stages (Hamre et al. 2013).

The composition of the egg from which a larval fish emerges is clearly significant for long-term success. While egg composition varies dramatically between species, a few generalizations may be made based on the limited data available. Egg lipid levels tend to correlate positively with egg incubation times (Kaitaranta and Ackman 1981; Jaroszewska and Dabrowski 2011). Free amino acids, which are found in relative abundance in eggs, tend to be higher in eggs from pelagic fish than demersal fish (Jobling 2016). Larval fish usually depend on their yolk sac for three to five days post-hatch, but this period may last up to 60 days in some species (Jaroszewska and Dabrowski 2011). Appropriate egg and yolk nutrition is modulated through the broodstock. Following the yolk-sac period, larval fish transition to exogenous diet items. Mixed feeding, in which larval fish are offered food items while yolk-sac nutrition is still available, is recommended to improve overall nutrition and stimulate gut development (Jaroszewska and Dabrowski 2011).

Options for feeding larval fish include live food items and commercial diets. Diets for small fish larvae are typically based on brine shrimp nauplii and rotifers (particularly *Brachionus* spp.). They may also be fed commercial microparticulate diets with hydrolyzed protein (a source of free amino acids), as the larvae may not possess the anatomy or physiology to break down more complex food particles (Kaushik et al. 2011; Langdon and Barrows 2011). However, these are associated with several issues, including high rates of nutrient loss due to large surface area, clumping, and poor uptake by larval fish (Langdon and Barrows 2011; Hamre et al. 2013). For larger larvae, live food items may include adult brine shrimp, copepods, and a variety of commercial diets. Live foods should always be enriched prior to feeding as this can significantly improve larval survival (Hamre et al. 2008; Dhert et al. 2014).

Nutrition of the broodstock impacts larval success. For example, vitamin E supplementation improved spawning quality in several fish species, and recommended levels were >150–190 mg D,L-α-tocopherol/kg diet (165–209 IU vitamin E/kg diet) (Fernández-Palacios et al. 2011). Tryptophan also seems to be required at higher levels for reproduction than for growth (Jobling 2016). And in cod, egg fatty acid concentrations, particularly AA, DHA, and EPA concentrations, were positively correlated to hatching success (Pickova et al. 1997). The timing of critical broodstock nutrition can span a few weeks to several months, depending on when vitellogenesis occurs in the species (Fernández-Palacios et al. 2011).

In fish species that show parental care, energy requirements are likely increased due to nest defense, cleaning, and/or oxygenation (e.g. tail fanning). A reduction in food intake may also occur during parenting. The condition of the parents can have significant consequences on the success of their offspring. For example, male smallmouth bass (*Micropterus dolomieu*) show parental care and when supplemented with additional food during this period, they show lower nest abandonment and improved reproductive success compared to males with no supplemental feeding (Zolderdo et al. 2016).

New Directions in Fish Nutrition Research

Current and future areas of fish nutrition research are focused on larval and broodstock nutrition, and the use of novel ingredients in fish diets to improve performance and/or sustainability. Novel techniques including genomics, proteomics, and metabolomics are being used to better define the requirements for nutrients and to better understand the gut microbiome to improve food digestibility, gut health, and fish performance. The increasing numbers of species that are being raised in commercial aquaculture systems and in different types of environments (e.g. recirculating low-salinity rearing of marine species) will further expand our knowledge of the comparative nutrition of fish.

References

Adams, M.A., Johnson, P.B., and Hong-Qi, Z. (1988). Chemical enhancement of feeding for the herbivorous fish *Tilapia zillii*. *Aquaculture* 72: 95–107.

Ahlgren, G., Vrede, T., and Goedkoop, W. (2009). Fatty acid ratios in freshwater fish, zooplankton and zoobenthos – are there specific optima? In: Lipids in Aquatic Ecosystems (eds. M.T. Arts, M.T. Brett and M. Kainz), 147–178. New York: Springer.

Ai, Q., Mai, K., Zhang, C. et al. (2004). Effects of dietary vitamin C on growth and immune response of Japanese seabass, *Lateolabrax japonicus*. *Aquaculture* 242: 489–500.

Almaida-Pagán, P., Rubio, V., Mendiola, P. et al. (2006). Macronutrient selection through post-ingestive signals in sharpsnout seabream fed gelatine capsules and challenged with protein dilution. *Physiology and Behavior* 88: 550–558.

Ashdown, D. and Violetta, G. (2004). Using garlic as an appetite stimulant in sand tiger sharks (*Carcharias taurus*). *Drum and Croaker* 35: 59–61.

Badwy, T.M.M., Ibrahim, E.M., and Zeinhom, M.M. (2008). Partial replacement of fishmeal with dried microalga (*Chlorella* spp. and *Scenedesmus* spp.) in Nile tilapia (*Oreochromis niloticus*) diets. *Proceedings of the International Symposium on Tilapia in Aquaculture*, Cairo, Egypt.

Baker, E.J., Clauss, M., and Clements, K.D. (2016). Selection and intake of algal species in butterfish (*Odax pullus*; Labridae). *Marine Biology* 163: 1–12.

Ballantyne, J.S. (2014). Membranes and metabolism. In: The Physiology of Fishes, 4e (eds. D.H. Evans, J.B. Claiborne and S. Currie), 81–148. Boca Raton, FL: CRC Press.

Bell, J.G. and Sargent, J.R. (2003). Arachidonic acid in aquaculture feeds: current status and future opportunities. *Aquaculture* 218: 491–499.

Ben-Amotz, A., Tornabene, T.G., and Thomas, W.H. (1985). Chemical profile of selected species of microalgae with emphasis on lipids. *Journal of Phycology* 21: 72–81.

Bernard, J.B. and Allen, M.E. (2002). Feeding captive piscivorous animals: nutritional aspects of fish as food. AZA Nutrition Advisory Group Fact Sheet 005 [online]. https://nagonline.net/wp-content/uploads/2014/01/NAG-FS005-97-Fish-JONI-FEB-24-2002-MODIFIED.pdf (accessed August 2017).

Bernard, J.B. and Dempsey, J.L. (1999). Quality control of feedstuffs: nutrient analyses. AZA Nutrition Advisory Group Handbook Fact Sheet 010 [online]. http://nagonline.net/wp-content/uploads/2014/01/NAG-FS010-99-Quality-JONI-FEB-24-2002-MODIFIED.pdf (accessed June 2015 [August 2017]).

Blazer, V.S. and Wolke, R.E. (1984). The effects of α-tocopherol on the immune responses and non-specific resistance factors of rainbow trout (*Salmo gairdneri* Richardson). *Aquaculture* 37: 1–9.

Bone, Q. and Moore, R.H. (eds.) (2008). Biology of Fish, 3e. New York: Taylor and Francis.

Burr, G., Gatlin, D., and Ricke, S. (2005). Microbial ecology of the gastrointestinal tract of fish and the potential application of prebiotics and probiotics in finfish aquaculture. *Journal of the World Aquaculture Society* 36: 425–436.

Castillo, S. and Gatlin, D.M. (2015). Dietary supplementation of exogenous carbohydrase enzymes in fish nutrition: a review. *Aquaculture* 435: 286–292.

Chang, M. and Southgate, P.C. (2001). Effects of varying dietary fatty acid composition on growth and survival of seahorse, *Hippocampus* sp., juveniles. *Aquarium Sciences and Conservation* 3: 205–214.

Cho, C. and Bureau, D. (2001). A review of diet formulation strategies and feeding systems to reduce excretory and feed wastes in aquaculture. *Aquaculture Research* 32: 349–360.

Cho, Y.S., Douglas, S.E., Gallant, J.W. et al. (2007). Isolation and characterization of cDNA sequences of L-gulono-gamma-lactone oxidase, a key enzyme for biosynthesis of ascorbic acid, from extant primitive fish groups. *Comparative Biochemistry and Physiology Part B* 147: 178–190.

Clements, K.D. and Raubenheiner, D. (2006). Feeding and nutrition. In: The Physiology of Fish, 3e (eds. D.H. Evans and J.B. Claiborne), 47–82. Gainesville, FL: CRC Press.

Cortés, E. and Gruber, S.H. (1992). Gastric evacuation in the young lemon shark, *Negaprion brevirostris*, under field conditions. *Environmental Biology of Fishes* 35: 205–212.

Crissey, S.D. (1998). Handling fish fed to fish-eating animals: a manual of standard operating procedures [online]. http://www.aphis.usda.gov/animal_welfare/downloads/marine_mammals/mmfish.pdf (accessed August 2017).

Dalmo, R.A. and Bøgwald, J. (2008). Beta-glucans as conductors of immune symphonies. *Fish & Shellfish Immunology* 25: 384–396.

Dalmo, R.A., Bøgwald, J., Ingebrigtsen, K., and Seljelid, R. (1996). The immunomodulatory effect of laminarian [β (1,3)-D-glucan] on Atlantic salmon, *Salmo salar* L., anterior kidney leucocytes after intraperitoneal, peroral and peranal administration. *Journal of Fish Diseases* 19: 449–457.

da Silva, R.F., Kitagawa, A., and Vázquez, F.J.S. (2016). Dietary self-selection in fish: a new approach to studying fish nutrition and feeding behavior. *Reviews in Fish Biology and Fisheries* 26: 39–51.

Day, R.D., German, D.P., Manjakasy, J.M. et al. (2011). Enzymatic digestion in stomachless fish: how a simple gut accommodates both herbivory and carnivory. *Journal of Comparative Physiology B* 181: 603–613.

De, B.C., Meena, D., Behera, B. et al. (2014). Probiotics in fish and shellfish culture: immunomodulatory and ecophysiological responses. *Fish Physiology and Biochemistry* 40: 921–971.

Dhert, P., King, N., and O'Brien, E. (2014). Stand-alone live food diets, an alternative to culture and enrichment diets for rotifers. *Aquaculture* 431: 59–64.

Dierenfeld, E.S., Katz, N., Pearson, J. et al. (1991). Retinol and α-tocopherol concentrations in whole fish commonly fed in zoos and aquariums. *Zoo Biology* 10: 119–125.

Durve, V. and Lovell, R. (1982). Vitamin C and disease resistance in channel catfish (*Ictalurus punctatus*). *Canadian Journal of Fisheries and Aquatic Sciences* 39: 948–951.

Ericsson, C.D., Steffen, R., and Backer, H. (2002). Water disinfection for international and wilderness travelers. *Clinical Infectious Diseases* 34: 355–364.

Fernández-Palacios, H., Norberg, B., Izquierdo, M., and Hamre, K. (2011). Effects of broodstock diet on eggs and larvae. In: Larval Fish Nutrition (ed. G.J. Holt), 151–181. Oxford: Wiley.

Fitzsimons, J.D., Williston, B., Zajicek, J.L. et al. (2005). Thiamine content and thiaminase activity of ten freshwater stocks and one marine stock of alewives. *Journal of Aquatic Animal Health* 17: 26–35.

Fortes-Silva, R., Martínez, F.J., Villarroel, M., and Sánchez-Vázquez, F.J. (2010). Daily feeding patterns and self-selection of dietary oil in Nile tilapia. *Aquaculture Research* 42: 157–160.

Fortes-Silva, R., Martínez, F., and Sánchez-Vázquez, F. (2011). Macronutrient selection in Nile tilapia fed gelatin capsules and challenged with protein dilution/restriction. *Physiology and Behavior* 102: 356–360.

German, D.P. and Bittong, R.A. (2009). Digestive enzyme activities and gastrointestinal fermentation in wood-eating catfish. *Journal of Comparative Physiology B* 179: 1025–1042.

German, D.P., Nagle, B.C., Villeda, J.M. et al. (2010). Evolution of herbivory in a carnivorous clade of minnows (Teleostei: Cyprinidae): effects on gut size and digestive physiology. *Physiological and Biochemical Zoology* 83: 1–18.

Goodwin, T.W. (1986). Metabolism, nutrition, and function of carotenoids. *Annual Review of Nutrition* 6: 273–297.

Govoni, J.J., Boehlert, G.W., and Watanabe, Y. (1986). The physiology of digestion in fish larvae. *Environmental Biology of Fishes* 16: 59–77.

Griffin, M.E., Wilson, K.A., White, M.R., and Brown, P.B. (1994). Dietary choline requirement of juvenile hybrid striped bass. *Journal of Nutrition* 124: 1685–1689.

Gruger, E.H., Nelson, R.W., and Stansby, M.E. (1964). Fatty acid composition of oils from 21 species of marine fish, freshwater fish, and shellfish. *Journal of the American Oil Chemists Society* 41: 662–667.

Halver, J.E. (2002). The vitamins. In: Fish Nutrition, 3e (eds. J.E. Halver and R.W. Hardy), 62–143. San Diego, CA: Academic Press.

Halver, J., Smith, R.R., Tolbert, B.M., and Baker, E.M. (1975). Utilization of ascorbic acid in fish. *Annals of the New York Academy of Sciences* 258: 81–102.

Hamre, K. (2011). Metabolism, interactions, requirements and functions of vitamin E in fish. *Aquaculture Nutrition* 17: 98–115.

Hamre, K., Srivastava, A., Rønnestad, I. et al. (2008). Several micronutrients in the rotifer *Brachionus plicatilis* may be limiting for growth, survival and normal development of cod larvae. *Aquaculture Nutrition* 14: 51–60.

Hamre, K., Yúfera, M., Rønnestad, I. et al. (2013). Fish larval nutrition and feed formulation: knowledge gaps and bottlenecks for advances in larval rearing. *Reviews in Aquaculture* 5: S26–S58.

Hamre, K., Sissener, N.H., Lock, E.J. et al. (2016). Antioxidant nutrition in Atlantic salmon (*Salmo salar*) parr and post-smolt, fed diets with high inclusion of plant ingredients and graded levels of micronutrients and selected amino acids. *PeerJ* 4: e2688.

Hemre, G.I., Mommsen, T.P., and Krogdahl, Å. (2002). Carbohydrates in fish nutrition: effects on growth, glucose metabolism and hepatic enzymes. *Aquaculture Nutrition* 8: 175–194.

Henry, B., Maslanka, M., and Slifka, K.A. (2010). Quality control aspects of feeding wild mammals in captivity. In: Wild Mammals in Captivity: Principles and Techniques for Zoo Management (eds. D.G. Kleiman, K.V. Thompson and C.K. Baer), 104–117. Chicago, IL: University of Chicago Press.

Hixson, S.M. (2014). Fish nutrition and current issues in aquaculture: the balance in providing safe and nutritious seafood, in an environmentally sustainable manner. *Journal of Aquaculture Research and Development* 5: 234.

Honeyfield, D.C., Hinterkopf, J.P., and Brown, S.B. (2002). Isolation of thiaminase-positive bacteria from alewife. *Transactions of the American Fisheries Society* 131: 171–175.

Hoopes, L.A. (2017). Elasmobranch mineral and vitamin requirements. In: The Elasmobranch Husbandry Manual II: Recent Advances in the Care of Sharks, Rays and their Relatives (eds. M. Smith, D. Warmolts, D. Thoney, et al.), 135–146. Columbus: Ohio Biological Survey.

Horn, M.H. (1989). Biology of marine herbivorous fish. *Oceanography and Marine Biology: An Annual Review* 27: 167–271.

Horn, M.H., Gawlicka, A.K., German, D.P. et al. (2006). Structure and function of the stomachless digestive system in three related species of New World silverside fish (Atherinopsidae) representing herbivory, omnivory, and carnivory. *Marine Biology* 149: 1237–1245.

Hoseinifar, S.H., Zoheiri, F., and Caipang, C.M. (2016). Dietary sodium propionate improved performance, mucosal and humoral immune responses in Caspian white fish (*Rutilus frisii kutum*) fry. *Fish & Shellfish Immunology* 55: 523–528.

Hua, K. and Bureau, D.P. (2009). A mathematical model to explain variations in estimates of starch digestibility and predict digestible starch content of salmonid fish feeds. *Aquaculture* 294: 282–287.

Hua, K. and Bureau, D. (2010). Quantification of differences in digestibility of phosphorus among cyprinids, cichlids, and salmonids through a mathematical modelling approach. *Aquaculture* 308: 152–158.

Hussey, N.E., Cocks, D.T., Dudley, S.F.J. et al. (2009). The condition conundrum: application of multiple condition indices to the dusky shark *Carcharhinus obscurus*. *Marine Ecology Progress Series* 380: 199–212.

Janse, M. (2003). Considerations on the diet composition and feeding rate of demersal sharks in 15 European public aquaria. *Zoo Biology* 22: 203–226.

Janse, M., Firchau, B., and Mohan, P.J. (2004). Elasmobranch nutrition, food handling, and feeding techniques. In: The Elasmobranch Husbandry Manual: Captive Care of Sharks, Rays, and their Relatives (eds. M. Smith, D. Warmolts, D. Thoney and R. Hueter), 183–200. Columbus: Ohio Biological Survey.

Jaroszewska, M. and Dabrowski, K. (2011). Utilization of yolk: transition from endogenous to exogenous nutrition in fish. In: Larval Fish Nutrition (ed. G.J. Holt), 183–218. Oxford: Wiley.

Jobling, M. (2016). Fish nutrition research: past, present and future. *Aquaculture International* 24: 767–786.

Jobling, M. and Wandsvik, A. (1983). An investigation of factors controlling food intake in Arctic charr, *Salvelinus alpinus* L. *Journal of Fish Biology* 23: 397–404.

Johnsen, P.B. and Adams, M.A. (1986). Chemical feeding stimulants for the herbivorous fish, *Tilapia zillii*. *Comparative Biochemistry and Physiology Part A* 83: 109–112.

Kaitaranta, J.K. and Ackman, R.G. (1981). Total lipids and lipid classes of fish roe. *Comparative Biochemistry and Physiology Part B: Comparative Biochemistry* 69: 725–729.

Kamerman, T.Y., Davis, L., and Capobianco, J. (2017). Development of a body condition scoring tool for the spotted eagle ray, *Aetobatus narinari*. In: The Elasmobranch Husbandry Manual II: Recent Advances in the Care of Sharks, Rays and their Relatives (eds. M. Smith, D. Warmolts, D. Thoney, et al.), 147–152. Columbus: Ohio Biological Survey.

Kaushik, S., Georga, I., and Koumoundouros, G. (2011). Growth and body composition of zebrafish (*Danio rerio*) larvae fed a compound feed from first feeding onward: toward implications on nutrient requirements. *Zebrafish* 8: 87–95.

Khosravi, S., Jang, J.-W., Rahimnejad, S. et al. (2015). Choline essentiality and its requirement in diets for juvenile parrot fish (*Oplegnathus fasciatus*). *Asian-Australasian Journal of Animal Sciences* 28: 647–653.

Kiron, V. (2012). Fish immune system and its nutritional modulation for preventative health care. *Animal Feed Science and Technology* 173: 111–133.

Kizer, A. (2005). Percutaneous gastrostomy tube placement in a green moray eel. *Exotic DVM* 7: 31–35.

Knights, B. (1983). Food particle-size preferences and feeding behaviour in warmwater aquaculture of European eel, *Anguilla anguilla* (L.). *Aquaculture* 30: 173–190.

Kohler, N.E., Casey, C.G., and Turner, P.A. (1995). Length-weight relationships for 13 species of sharks from the western North Atlantic. *Fishery Bulletin* 93: 412–418.

Kolkovski, S., Czesny, S., Yackey, C. et al. (2000). The effect of vitamins C and E in (n-3) highly unsaturated fatty acids-enriched *Artemia* nauplii on growth, survival, and stress resistance of fresh water walleye *Stizostedion vitreum* larvae. *Aquaculture Nutrition* 6: 199–206.

Kumar, S., Sahu, N., Pal, A. et al. (2006). Studies on digestibility and digestive enzyme activities in *Labeo rohita* (Hamilton) juveniles: effect of microbial α-amylase supplementation in non-gelatinized or gelatinized corn-based diet at two protein levels. *Fish Physiology and Biochemistry* 32: 209–220.

Kumar, V., Sinha, A., Makkar, H. et al. (2012). Phytate and phytase in fish nutrition. *Journal of Animal Physiology and Animal Nutrition* 96: 335–364.

Lall, S.P. and Tibbetts, S.M. (2009). Nutrition, feeding, and behavior of fish. *The Veterinary Clinics of North America. Exotic Animal Practice* 12: 361–372.

Langdon, C. and Barrows, R. (2011). Microparticulate diets: technology. In: Larval Fish Nutrition (ed. G.J. Holt), 335–351. Oxford: Wiley.

Lee, J.Y. and Gao, Y. (2012). Review of the application of garlic, *Allium sativum*, in aquaculture. *Journal of the World Aquaculture Society* 43: 447–458.

Lemos, D. and Tacon, A.G. (2016). Use of phytases in fish and shrimp feeds: a review. *Reviews in Aquaculture* 9: 266–282.

Leng, R.A., Stambolie, J.H., and Bell, R. (1995). Duckweed-a potential high-protein feed resource for domestic animals and fish. *Livestock Research for Rural Development*, 7 [online]. http://www.fao.org/ag/aga/agap/frg/LRRD/LRRD7/1/3.HTM (accessed August 2017).

Lešková, E., Kubíková, J., Kováčiková, E. et al. (2006). Vitamin losses: retention during heat treatment and continual changes expressed by mathematical models. *Journal of Food Composition and Analysis* 19: 252–276.

Li, X.-F., Xu, C., Zhang, D.-D. et al. (2016). Molecular characterization and expression analysis of glucokinase from herbivorous fish *Megalobrama amblycephala* subjected to a glucose load after the adaption to dietary carbohydrate levels. *Aquaculture* 459: 89–98.

Lin, Y.-H. and Shiau, S.-Y. (2005). Dietary vitamin E requirement of grouper, *Epinephelus malabaricus*, at two lipid levels, and their effects on immune responses. *Aquaculture* 248: 235–244.

Matsunari, H., Hashimoto, H., Iwasaki, T. et al. (2013a). Effect of feeding rotifers enriched with taurine on the growth and survival of larval amberjack *Seriola dumerili*. *Fisheries Science* 79: 815–821.

Matsunari, H., Hashimoto, H., Oda, K. et al. (2013b). Effects of docosahexaenoic acid on growth, survival and swim bladder inflation of larval amberjack (*Seriola dumerili*, Risso). *Aquaculture Research* 44: 1696–1705.

McGoogan, B.B. and Gatlin, D.M. (1999). Dietary manipulations affecting growth and nitrogenous waste production of red drum, *Sciaenops ocellatus* I. Effects of dietary protein and energy levels. *Aquaculture* 178: 333–348.

Medved, R.J. (1985). Gastric evacuation in the sandbar shark, *Carcharhinus plumbeus*. *Journal of Fish Biology* 26: 239–253.

Michelato, M., Zaminhan, M., Boscolo, W.R. et al. (2017). Dietary histidine requirement of Nile tilapia juveniles based on growth performance, expression of muscle-growth-related genes and haematological responses. *Aquaculture* 467: 63–70.

Mišurcová, L., Kráčmar, S., Klejdus, B., and Vacek, J. (2010). Nitrogen content, dietary fiber, and digestibility in algal food products. *Czech Journal of Food Sciences* 28: 27–35.

Moren, M., Næss, T., and Hamre, K. (2002). Conversion of β-carotene, canthaxanthin and astaxanthin to vitamin A in Atlantic halibut (*Hippoglossus hippoglossus* L.) juveniles. *Fish Physiology and Biochemistry* 27: 71–80.

Morris, A.L., Hamlin, H.J., Francis-Floyd, R. et al. (2011). Nitrate-induced goiter in captive whitespotted bamboo sharks *Chiloscyllium plagiosum*. *Journal of Aquatic Animal Health* 23: 92–99.

Mountfort, D.O., Campbell, J., and Clements, K.D. (2002). Hindgut fermentation in three species of marine herbivorous fish. *Applied and Environmental Microbiology* 68: 1374–1380.

Mustafa, M.G., Wakamatsu, S., Takeda, T. et al. (1995). Effects of algae meal as feed additive on growth, feed efficiency, and body composition in red sea bream. *Fisheries Science* 61: 25–28.

National Research Council (NRC) (1996). Guide for the Care and Use of Laboratory Animals. Washington D.C.: National Academic Press.

National Research Council (NRC) (2011). Nutrient Requirements of Fish and Shrimp. Washington D.C.: National Academic Press.

Navarre, O. and Halver, J.E. (1989). Disease resistance and humoral antibody production in rainbow trout fed high levels of vitamin C. *Aquaculture* 79: 207–221.

Nayak, S.K. (2010). Probiotics and immunity: a fish perspective. *Fish & Shellfish Immunology* 29: 2–14.

New, M.B. (1987). Feed and feeding of fish and shrimp. Food and Agriculture Organization of the United Nations [online]. http://www.fao.org/docrep/s4314e/s4314e00.htm#Contents (accessed 1 August 2017).

Nguyen, V.T., Satoh, S., Haga, Y. et al. (2008). Effect of zinc and manganese supplementation in *Artemia* on growth and vertebral deformity in red sea bream (*Pagrus major*) larvae. *Aquaculture* 285: 184–192.

Papatryphon, E. and Soares, J. (2001). The effect of phytase on apparent digestibility of four practical plant feedstuffs fed to striped bass, *Morone saxatilis*. *Aquaculture Nutrition* 7: 161–168.

Penglase, S., Nordgreen, A., Van der Meeren, T. et al. (2010). Increasing the level of selenium in rotifers (*Brachionus plicatilis* 'Cayman') enhances the mRNA expression and activity of glutathione peroxidase in cod (*Gadus morhua* L.) larvae. *Aquaculture* 306: 259–269.

Pettitt-Wade, H., Newman, S.H., Parsons, K.T. et al. (2011). Dietary metal and macro-nutrient intakes of juvenile lemon sharks determined from the nutritional composition of prey items. *Marine Ecology Progress Series* 433: 245–260.

Pickova, J., Dutta, P.C., Larsson, P.-O., and Kiessling, A. (1997). Early embryonic cleavage pattern, hatching success, and egg-lipid fatty acid composition: comparison between two cod (*Gadus morhua*) stocks. *Canadian Journal of Fisheries and Aquatic Sciences* 54: 2410–2416.

Rahimnejad, S., Lee, S.-M., Park, H.-G., and Choi, J. (2017). Effects of dietary inclusion of *Chlorella vulgaris* on growth, blood biochemical parameters, and antioxidant enzyme activity in olive flounder, *Paralichthys olivaceus*. *Journal of the World Aquaculture Society* 48: 103–112.

Reitan, K.I., Rainuzzo, J.R., and Olsen, Y. (1994). Influence of lipid composition of live feed on growth, survival and pigmentation of turbot larvae. *Aquaculture International* 2: 33–48.

Romero-Romero, S. and Yúfera, M. (2012). Contribution of gut content to the nutritional value of *Brachionus plicatilis* used as prey in larviculture. *Aquaculture* 364: 124–129.

Rønnestad, I. and Fyhn, H.J. (1993). Metabolic aspects of free amino acids in developing marine fish eggs and larvae. *Reviews in Fisheries Science* 1: 239–259.

Rubio, V., Sánchez-Vázquez, F., and Madrid, J. (2003). Macronutrient selection through postingestive signals in sea bass fed on gelatine capsules. *Physiology and Behavior* 78: 795–803.

Rumsey, G.L. (1991). Choline-betaine requirements of rainbow trout *Oncorhynchus mykiss*. *Aquaculture* 95: 107–116.

Saha, H., Pal, A.K., Sahu, N.P., and Saha, R.K. (2016). Feeding pyridoxine prevents *Saprolegnia parasitica* infection in fish *Labeo rohita*. *Fish & Shellfish Immunology* 59: 382–388.

Sánchez-Vázquez, F., Yamamoto, T., Akiyama, T. et al. (1998). Selection of macronutrients by goldfish operating self-feeders. *Physiology and Behavior* 65: 11–218.

Sánchez-Vázquez, F., Yamamoto, T., Akiyama, T. et al. (1999). Macronutrient self-selection through demand-feeders in rainbow trout. *Physiology and Behavior* 66: 45–51.

Sandnes, K., Torrissen, O., and Waagbø, R. (1992). The minimum dietary requirement of vitamin C in Atlantic salmon (*Salmo salar*) fry using Ca ascorbate-2-monophosphate as dietary source. *Fish Physiology and Biochemistry* 10: 315–319.

Sargent, J.R., McEvoy, L.A., and Bell, J.G. (1997). Requirements, presentation and sources of fatty acids in marine fish larval feeds. *Aquaculture* 155: 117–127.

Sargent, J., Bell, G., McEvoy, L. et al. (1999). Recent developments in the essential fatty acid nutrition of fish. *Aquaculture* 177: 191–199.

Sargent, J.R., Tocher, D.R., and Bell, J.G. (2002). The lipids. In: Fish Nutrition, 3e (eds. J.E. Halver and R.W. Hardy), 182–259. San Diego, CA: Academic Press.

Schaeffer, D.O., Kleinow, K.M., and Krulish, L. (eds.) (1992). The Care and Use of Amphibians, Reptiles, and Fish in Research. Scientists Center for Animal Welfare. Bethesda, MD: Scientists Center for Animal Welfare.

Schmidt, D.A., Travis, D.A., and Williams, J.J. (2006). Guidelines for creating a food safety HACCP program in zoos or aquaria. *Zoo Biology* 25: 125–135.

Schwarz, F., Kirchgessner, M., Steinhart, H., and Runge, G. (1988). Influence of different fats with varying additions of α-tocopheryl acetate on growth and body composition of carp (*Cyprinus carpio* L.). *Aquaculture* 69: 57–67.

Sealey, W.M. and Gatlin, D.M. (2002). Dietary vitamin C and vitamin E interact to influence growth and tissue composition of juvenile hybrid striped bass (Morone chrysops♀× M. saxatilis♂) but have limited effects on immune responses. *The Journal of Nutrition* 132: 748–755.

Sforcin, J.M. (2007). Propolis and the immune system: a review. *Journal of Ethnopharmacology* 113: 1–14.

Shiau, S.Y. and Lo, P.S. (2000). Dietary choline requirements of juvenile hybrid tilapia, *Oreochromis niloticusxO. aureus*. *Journal of Nutrition* 130: 100–103.

Sinha, A.K., Kumar, V., Makkar, H.P. et al. (2011). Non-starch polysaccharides and their role in fish nutrition – a review. *Food Chemistry* 127: 1409–1426.

Spencer, W. and Spencer, J. (2006). Management guideline manual for invertebrate live food species. European Association of Zoos and Aquaria Terrestrial Invertebrate TAG Fact Sheet [online]. http://www.amphibianark.org/pdf/Husbandry/EAZA%20Management%20Guideline%20Manual%20for%20Invertebrate%20Live%20Food%20Species.pdf (accessed August 2017).

Srivastava, A., Hamre, K., Stoss, J., and Nordgreen, A. (2012). A study on enrichment of the rotifer *Brachionus* "Cayman" with iodine from different sources. *Aquaculture* 334: 82–88.

Templeton, D.W., Quinn, M., Van Wychen, S. et al. (2012). Separation and quantification of microalgal carbohydrates. *Journal of Chromatography A* 1270: 225–234.

Terech-Majewska, E., Pajdak, J., and Siwicki, A.K. (2016). Water as a source of macronutrients and micronutrients for fish with special emphasis on the nutritional requirements of two fish species: the common carp (*Cyprinus carpio*) and the rainbow trout (*Oncorhynchus mykiss*). *Journal of Elementology* 21: 947–961.

Thajuddin, N. and Subramanian, G. (2005). Cyanobacterial biodiversity and potential applications in biotechnology. *Current Science* 89: 47–57.

Tocher, D.R. (2003). Metabolism and functions of lipids and fatty acids in teleost fish. *Reviews in Fisheries Science* 11: 107–184.

Touraki, M., Karamanlidou, G., Karavida, P., and Chrysi, K. (2012). Evaluation of the probiotics *Bacillus subtilis* and *Lactobacillus plantarum* bioencapsulated in *Artemia* nauplii against vibriosis in European sea bass larvae (*Dicentrarchus labrax*, L.). *World Journal of Microbiology and Biotechnology* 28: 2425–2433.

Treece, G.D. (2000). *Artemia* production of marine larval fish culture. United States Department of Agriculture, Southern Regional Aquaculture Center Publication No. 702 [online]. http://citeseerx.ist.psu.edu/viewdoc/download?doi=10.1.1.212.3649andrep=rep1andtype=pdf (accessed August 2017).

Twibell, R.G. and Brown, P.B. (2000). Dietary choline requirement of juvenile yellow perch (*Perca flavescens*). *Journal of Nutrition* 130: 95–99.

Valente, L.M.P., Gouveia, A., Rema, P. et al. (2006). Evaluation of three seaweeds *Gracilaria bursa-pastoris*, *Ulva rigida* and *Gracilaria cornea* as dietary ingredients in European sea bass (*Dicentrarchus labrax*) juveniles. *Aquaculture* 252: 85–91.

Verhlac-Trichet, V. (2010). Nutrition and immunity: an update. *Aquaculture Research* 41: 356–372.

Verlhac, V. and Gabaudan, J. (1994). Influence of vitamin C on the immune system of salmonids. *Aquaculture and Fisheries Management* 25: 21–36.

Wahli, T., Verlhac, V., Gabaudan, J. et al. (1998). Influence of combined vitamins C and E on non-specific immunity and disease resistance of rainbow trout, *Oncorhynchus mykiss* (Walbaum). *Journal of Fish Diseases* 21: 127–138.

Walker, A.B. and Berlinsky, D.L. (2011). Effects of partial replacement of fish meal protein by microalgae on growth, feed intake, and body composition of Atlantic cod. *North American Journal of Aquaculture* 73: 76–83.

Walker, A.B., Fournier, H.R., Neefus, C.D. et al. (2009). Partial replacement of fish meal with laver *Porphyra* spp. in diets for Atlantic cod. *North American Journal of Aquaculture* 71: 39–45.

Wang, J., Li, X., Han, T. et al. (2016). Effects of different dietary carbohydrate levels on growth, feed utilization and body composition of juvenile grouper *Epinephelus akaara*. *Aquaculture* 459: 143–147.

Wassef, E.A., El Masry, M.H., and Mikhail, F.R. (2001). Growth enhancement of muscle structure of striped mullet, *Mugil cephalus* L., fingerlings by feeding algal meal-based diets. *Aquaculture Research* 32: 315–322.

Wassef, E.A., El-Sayed, A.F.M., Kandeel, K.M., and Sakr, E.M. (2005). Evaluation of *Pterocla dia* (Rhotophyta) and *Ulva* (Cholorphyta) meals as additives to gilthead seabram *Sparus aurata* diets. *Egyptian Journal of Aquatic Research* 31: 321–332.

Werner, R.G. and Blaxter, J.H.S. (1980). Growth and survival of larval herring (*Clupea harengus*) in relation to prey density. *Canadian Journal of Fisheries and Aquatic Sciences* 37: 1063–1069.

Wetherbee, B.M. and Gruber, S.H. (1993). Absorption efficiency of the lemon shark *Negaprion brevirostris* at varying rates of energy intake. *Copeia* 1993: 416–425.

Wilson, R.P. and Poe, W.E. (1988). Choline nutrition of fingerling channel catfish. *Aquaculture* 68: 65–71.

Wilson, C., Dunford, K., Nichols, C. et al. (2013). Body condition scoring for laboratory zebrafish. *Animal Technology and Welfare* 12: 1–7.

Wood, C.M., Kajimura, M., Bucking, C., and Walsh, P.J. (2007). Osmoregulation, ionoregulation and acid-base regulation by the gastrointestinal tract after feeding in the elasmobranch (*Squalus acanthias*). *Journal of Experimental Biology* 210: 1335–1349.

Woods, C.M.C. (2003). Effects of varying *Artemia* enrichment on growth and survival of juvenile seahorses, *Hippocampus abdominalis*. *Aquaculture* 220: 537–548.

Wright, P.A. and Land, M.D. (1998). Urea production and transport in teleost fish. *Comparative Biochemistry and Physiology Part A* 119: 47–54.

Xie, Z., Niu, C., Zhang, Z., and Bao, L. (2006). Dietary ascorbic acid may be necessary for enhancing the immune response in Siberian sturgeon (*Acipenser baerii*), a species capable of ascorbic acid biosynthesis. *Comparative Biochemistry and Physiology Part A* 145: 152–157.

Yazdani-Sadati, M.A., Sayed Hassani, M.H., Pourkazemi, M. et al. (2014). Influence of different levels of dietary choline on growth rate, body composition, hematological indices and liver lipid of juvenile Siberian sturgeon *Acipenser baerii* Brandt, 1869. *Journal of Applied Ichthyology* 30: 1632–1636.

Yone, Y., Furuichi, M., and Urano, K. (1986). Effects of dietary wakame *Undaria penatifida* and *Ascophyllum nodosum* on growth, feed efficiency, and proximate compositions of liver and muscle of red sea bream. *Nippon Suisan Gakkaishi* 52: 1465–1468.

Yousefian, M. and Amiri, M.S. (2009). A review of the use of prebiotic in aquaculture for fish and shrimp. *African Journal of Biotechnology* 8: 7313–7318.

Zolderdo, A., Algera, D., Lawrence, M. et al. (2016). Stress, nutrition and parental care in a teleost fish: exploring mechanisms with supplemental feeding and cortisol manipulation. *Journal of Experimental Biology* 219: 1237–1248.

A5

Fish Behavior

Training and Enrichment

Ilana R. Alderman[1] *and Leigh A. Clayton*[2]

[1] Born to Behave, Boulder, CO, USA
[2] New England Aquarium, Boston, MA, USA

Introduction

Professional animal care is composed of several key cornerstones that are essential for providing the best welfare for the animals, including a comprehensive medical program, a balanced nutrition program, a carefully monitored environment, an appropriate social structure, and a behavioral management program (Ramirez 2013).

Training is often neglected by aquarists and hobbyists, due to a lack of time, perceived low fish intelligence, and a poor understanding of fish behavior. However, training is a critical component of good fish care. Fish adapt their behaviors in response to changes in their environment, whether it be within a formal training session or unintentionally during routine care. Understanding how fish learn can prevent unwanted behaviors and improve their health and quality of life. This chapter will review the following:

- The benefits of training and behavioral management.
- Animal learning modalities and their application to fish.
- How to train individual fish and groups of fish housed together.
- Medical care and treatment techniques using behavioral management.
- Methods for using training to enhance environmental enrichment.
- Modification of problem behaviors.
- Applications for research, conservation, and education.
- Case studies illustrating successful uses of training in fish care.

Fish Abilities

The scientific community has historically focused little attention on the cognitive abilities of fish. However, a review of over 200 fish studies by Brown (2015) showed remarkable sensory abilities, learning, and memory. Panksepp (1998) has shown that fish have an emotional complexity that had previously not been understood. Additionally, the case studies highlighted in this chapter clearly demonstrate that fish are highly adaptable and capable of learning. The ability of fish to learn complex behaviors is not limited to one genus, family, or species.

When selecting a training method, it is important to know the natural and instinctive behavioral repertoire that each species possesses: mating, rearing of young, foraging, hunting, hiding, territoriality, social structure, and natural aggression. These behaviors vary among species, and must be taken into account, as they can affect training methods and outcomes.

Benefits of Behavioral Management

The primary benefits of a behavior management program are: improved exercise and physical fitness, co-operative care and medical treatment, mental and environmental enrichment, and modification of unwanted behaviors (Ramirez 2013).

- *Exercise and physical fitness:* Fish in human care do not need to expend much energy to pursue food or avoid

Clinical Guide to Fish Medicine, First Edition. Edited by Catherine A. Hadfield and Leigh Ann Clayton.

predators. Even the largest enclosures cannot replicate the space that fish would have in their natural habitat. Training gives fish a reason to use their muscles and bodies; this is particularly important for fish that might naturally swim many kilometers each day. Additionally, the social dynamics between large populations of fish can cause more assertive fish to gain access to more food and become overweight, while timid fish may not get enough food. Training allows for the equitable distribution of diet and helps maintain better body condition.

- *Co-operation with medical treatment and routine care:* Perhaps one of the most useful aspects of training for fish is the ability to receive medical care with less stress and at lower risk of trauma. Training can facilitate physical exams, treatments, and the removal and transfer of individual animals from a group enclosure to a treatment tank (Box A5.1). Training can also reduce stress and risk of injury during routine maintenance such as enclosure cleaning, water changes, etc.
- *Mental and environmental enrichment:* A well-designed habitat with an appropriate social structure and sufficient hiding places is enriching for most fish. However, even the most creative habitat design can become monotonous for the animals living there. In the wild, fish use their mental abilities to avoid predation, forage or hunt for food, seek a mate, and adapt to their changing environmental conditions. Training can be used to keep the fish mentally active and to assist them in acclimating to their habitats and new décor (Box A5.2). Enrichment items and food puzzles can be designed to give the fish more choices, and to make acquisition of food more challenging. Caregivers can use training to assure optimal use of enrichment (Salyers 2015).
- *Resolving behavior problems:* Training can assist in preventing and fixing behavior problems such as stereotypic behavior, aggression, and fear, among others (Collier and Schreiber 2014; Patel and Dickson 2014; Nylund et al. 2015).

In addition to the benefits listed above, which help individual animals directly, training can provide indirect benefits to the species at large by facilitating research opportunities and applications, and creating education programs and conservation projects.

Introduction to the Science of Learning

There are two modalities through which all organisms learn: respondent conditioning (often called classical conditioning) and operant conditioning (Kazdin 1994). Both types of learning take place simultaneously. Generally, when working with animals on a day-to-day basis, the authors find it more useful to follow operant methodologies. This chapter will focus on operant techniques and will refer to respondent aspects of learning when appropriate, particularly when it comes to understanding an animal's emotional state (Pierce and Cheney 2008).

Respondent behaviors are tied to an animal's emotional state, as the stimuli frequently elicit behavior that is tied to fear, nervousness, excitement, etc. (Chance 1999). These emotions can be observed in the animal's behavior. An understanding of respondent conditioning can be used to change or reduce a fear response, e.g. a fish that initially startles and flees at the approach of the caregiver will usually habituate to the approach over time. If the

Box A5.1 A Cup of Preventative Behavior

Behavior: Fish enters a cup voluntarily to allow transfer to a different aquarium.

Species: Copperband butterfly fish (*Chelmon rostratus*).

Facility: Zoological Society of London, London, United Kingdom.

Description: The aquarists at the London Zoo wanted a less stressful way to move fish from one habitat to another. The common practice of scooping the fish up with a net was easy, but it was often several days before the fish settled down and began exhibiting normal behavior again. The team decided to experiment with teaching a butterfly fish to swim into a cup. The aquarists used a large plastic cup, which they submerged underwater, and reinforced when the fish made any motion toward the cup. Very quickly the fish swam toward the cup each time it was placed in the water. Next they oriented the opening of the cup toward the fish and gradually approximated the fish into the cup. Once the fish swam into the cup, the aquarist rotated the mouth of the cup toward the surface, making it more difficult for the fish to swim out. However, if the fish moved toward the edges of the cup, the aquarist would rotate the cup to allow the fish to leave if it desired. Within a few weeks, the fish was staying inside the cup for several minutes, which then led to lifting the cup out of the water while the fish calmly waited for reinforcement. The team was able to successfully use this behavior to move the fish from one aquarium to another as often as needed (Mackie 2017).

Box A5.2 Follow the Bouncing Ball

Behavior: Teaching shy fish to change hiding places.

Species: Green chromis (*Chromis viridis*).

Facility: Private hobbyist, Nice, France.

Description: A hobbyist in France had a small population of green chromis who had established a comfortable hiding place within a group of artificial rocks in their habitat. The aquarist decided to provide the fish with new, more complex rocky hiding places with a greater variety of caverns and options, but a month later the new spaces remained unexplored. The aquarist had already established a food puzzle, a small food-stuffed ball with holes from which the fish learned to pick food. He attached the ball to a string, and as the fish fed from the ball he gave the ball slight tugs, moving the ball a few centimeters closer to the new rocky hides. He gradually increased the distance the fish were willing to travel to get food from the ball, and after three weeks the chromis had discovered and begun using the new rocky hiding place.

approach is paired with feeding, the startle response will tend to transition from a fearful fleeing behavior to an approach behavior (Pierce and Cheney 2008). The formula for respondent conditioning is written as follows: NS + US = B. A neutral stimulus (NS), approaching the fish, is paired with (+) an unconditioned stimulus (US), food, which causes the fish to orient toward the person feeding, a reflexive behavior (B).

Operant conditioning refers to the changing of behavior through its consequences in specific environmental contexts. The term operant refers to the fact that an organism operates on the environment, which produces a specific effect or consequence. Operant conditioning was first defined and studied by B.F. Skinner and is sometimes referred to as Skinnerian conditioning. Modern science uses the term operant conditioning, though there are some references to this learning modality as instrumental conditioning (Kazdin 1994).

The frequency of a behavior increases or decreases over time based on the antecedents that precede it and the consequences that follow (Skinner 1953; Pierce and Cheney 2008).

- An antecedent is a perceived stimulus that occurs before a given behavior (Kazdin 1994). Throughout the chapter, we will refer to antecedents as cues or prompts. The presence of a stimulus, such as an approaching person, a new object in the habitat, the movement of another fish, etc., will trigger a behavior. Trainers must be aware of all environmental stimuli to which the animal might be responding.
- When an animal moves, acts upon, or reacts to the environment, it is referred to as a behavior (Kazdin 1994). Training is a process designed to teach specific behaviors.
- Consequences are stimuli that affect the frequency of a future behavior in a given environmental context. Consequences fall into two categories: reinforcement and punishment. A reinforcing consequence, referred to as a reinforcer, strengthens the frequency of the behavior it follows. When a behavior is reinforced, the probability that the behavior will be repeated under similar conditions is increased. Conversely, a punishing consequence, or punisher, decreases the frequency of the behavior it follows. When a behavior is punished, the probability that the behavior will be repeated is diminished (Chance 1999).

There are two types of reinforcing consequences: positive reinforcement and negative reinforcement (Chance 1999). In positive reinforcement, a behavior is followed by the addition of a desirable stimulus, such as food. In negative reinforcement, a behavior is followed by the removal of an undesirable stimulus, such as a bright light or unpleasant sound. In both cases, the probability that the behavior will be repeated under similar conditions is increased; the behavior is reinforced. For example, if a fish pushes at a rock and uncovers a piece of food, it will likely push the rock again. When a fish hides in a rocky cave to escape a large predator, it is negatively reinforced if the predator then swims away. Positive reinforcement is the most effective and least intrusive technique to modify behavior. In this chapter, the focus is on positive reinforcement.

For training to be effective, reinforcement must be delivered immediately after the desired behavior (Kazdin 1994). One way to improve timing is through the use of a conditioned reinforcer, known as a bridging stimulus or marker signal. A conditioned bridging stimulus is one that has been repeatedly followed by a primary reinforcer, such as food, and has become reinforcing in itself (Chance 1999). For example, every time the trainer flashes a light, the fish receives food. Over time, the light will predict that food will follow, and will elicit a respondent behavior, an anticipatory approach from the fish. When such a stimulus pairing is established, it can then function to determine the exact moment the fish performs a desired behavior. The purpose of the bridging signal is to bridge the time gap between the desired behavior and the delivery of the primary reinforcer. A bridging stimulus allows the trainer to capture and reinforce behavior that occurs very quickly (such as movement to one direction or staying still for short durations of time) and capture behavior at a distance; in these cases, it is often hard to provide a primary reinforcer, such as food, at the correct time to reinforce the desired behavior.

A simple example of operant learning is seen when a trainer places an object, such as a target, in the enclosure. When the fish touches the object, it receives a food reinforcer, and is more likely to repeat the behavior of touching the object. This is often written as a formula in behavior science labs as: A → B → C. The antecedent or cue (A) is the object placed in the enclosure, which prompts the behavior of touching the object (B), which in turn is reinforced by the delivery of food (C).

Before Training Begins

Several factors must be taken into consideration before starting to train, including being familiar with the species, knowing the individual, having detailed behavioral and medical histories, and having the necessary tools on hand.

- *Understand the species:* Each species has different behavioral, environmental, and nutritional needs. Training is most effective when these needs are met. For example, giving pelagic fish sufficient space to swim, reef fish ample hiding places, and schooling fish appropriate companions will increase their comfort and set them up for success. When considering the environment, it is important to be aware of the species' sensitivities to vibrations, noises, and lights.
- *Know the individual's behavioral history:* Each fish is an individual and knowing its housing history, its past exposure to enrichment, and its previous social cohorts should be taken into account when creating a training plan. When records are unavailable or incomplete, gather the relevant information from aquarists who have worked with the individual or group.
- *Learn the medical history:* It is valuable to be informed of any previous morbidity, common diagnostics, and the frequency and type of treatments that have been required for the individual and species in that habitat. Knowing what has been tried in the past, successfully or not, is helpful in putting together a training plan.
- *Recognize that learning is always taking place:* Animals learn during every interaction they have with people (Ramirez 1999). It is important to be aware of how fish are behaving during daily routine interactions. Cleaning, or the introduction of new plants, rocks, or enrichment, can disturb the fish and cause stress. These daily interactions can inadvertently teach the fish to be fearful of people, which will slow their acceptance of training.
- *Take a behavioral and physical baseline:* A behavioral baseline will help detect improvements or problems that may occur. Knowing preferred hiding places, existing social dynamics, and regular swimming patterns will help caretakers understand the impact of training efforts. Formal behavioral ethograms are ideal (Lehner 1987); however, even a few minutes of informal observations at varied times of day over the period of a week will provide insight into what is normal in the life of the animals in the habitat (Ramirez 1999).
- *Prepare needed tools:* Determine what type of food will be used – usually a portion of the normal diet that can be delivered easily. Determine a food delivery method based on the species and whether training a single fish or a group. Determine and test the marker signal: a flashlight, clicker, finger tap on the water, or other. Write out a training plan that anticipates the steps that will be taken. An example of a potential training plan is provided in Box A5.3. It is still important to be prepared to be flexible and to change the plan as needed.

Getting Started with Training

The most commonly used techniques for training new behaviors are capturing, shaping, luring, and targeting:

- Capturing is the process of marking and reinforcing a behavior the fish does naturally, e.g. archerfish (*Toxotes* spp.) spitting water (Pryor 2009a). The behavior can then be put on cue and elicited in new contexts.
- Shaping is the process of gradually building a new behavior in small increments by capturing smaller component behaviors and approximating toward more complex behavior (Pryor 2009b). For example, if a fish is reinforced when it swims along the front of its enclosure, the trainer can gradually increase the distance the fish swims before marking and reinforcing; over time, the fish could be shaped to swim the entire perimeter of the enclosure.
- Luring means using food to guide a fish to a desired location or position (Ramirez 1999). Luring is useful as a prompt but is normally phased out over time when possible.
- Targeting is a process that teaches the fish to touch some part of its body to an object. It is used to guide the fish toward a desired behavior (Ramirez 1999).

Most training goals will require the ability to deliver reinforcers accurately, so that competition is minimized and reinforcement is delivered to the correct individual at the appropriate time. Fish are almost always housed in groups. Consequently, it can be difficult to deliver the food reinforcer to the correct individual and to avoid competition from other fish. To begin, trainers must establish a consistent feeding protocol and determine where feeding will be

Box A5.3 Possible Training Plan for Stingrays in a Touch Pool

Animal Name: Stingray group. Trainer: Ken Ramirez.

Behavior: Touch by the public.

Probable Reinforcers: Daily diet in small pieces.

Tools Needed: Food, extra helpers (to pose as guests and to make noise), camera flash, radio.

Partnerships: Aquarists, guest service staff, veterinary team, public relations team.

Anticipated Steps (each step may take multiple sessions):

1) Establish that all the rays are readily eating tossed food.
2) Begin tossing reinforcers closer to the trainer so that the rays approach the side of the habitat and get used to eating there.
3) Place one hand in the water, then drop food close to hand with other hand, eventually allowing the rays to brush against the hand in the water.
4) Wait for the rays to brush by the hand before dropping food in the water.
5) Begin to use two fingers to touch each ray briefly as it swims by, then drop food in the water.
6) Gradually increase the duration of the tactile before delivering reinforcers; increases in increments of a few seconds until achieving 15–30 seconds, or longer if possible.
7) Once rays accept tactile for >15 seconds, increase the number of trainers to guarantee all the rays are getting an opportunity to participate.
8) Gradually introduce more erratic and unpredictable movements, replicating the way guests might try to touch the rays.
9) As comfort level increases, begin to talk in gradually louder voices and include laughter, replicating the conditions the guests will create.
10) Start using the microphone at a low volume and gradually increase to realistic levels.
11) Although flash camera use is not allowed, it would be wise to prepare the animals for the inadvertent flashes that will take place. Begin using the flash from a distance and gradually bring it closer.
12) Invite small groups of staff from other departments to come in for sessions so that the rays' reaction can be evaluated and areas of concern and further training can be determined.
13) If training is going well, gradually introduce members of the public through soft opening.

Anticipated Time Frame: Two months if steps progress well.

most advantageous to long-term goals. The fish will see the trainer approach and wait in the determined location in anticipation of the food. Sufficient quantity and scattering the food over a large enough area will eliminate most competition. There are several options for individual feeding within groups.

- Poles, tongs, and tweezers (Figure A5.1).
- Feeding straws (tubes) or squeeze bottles for smaller fish or smaller types of food.
- Hand feeding by divers.

Basic Training

Common training goals for fish include stationing, targeting, physical contact or restraint, sampling, and enrichment.

Stationing is the assigning of specific locations to individuals or groups for feeding and training. Locations can be in relation to objects in the animal's environment, in relation to conspecifics, or in relation to the trainer. Stations provide a place for the animal to be between cues where it can always get reinforced and it brings the animal to a location that makes access for training easier. Stations can be taught to individuals (Box A5.4) or groups (Box A5.5).

Targeting as a behavior (rather than the process) is the term for training an animal to touch a target object. Targeting gets the attention and focus of an individual animal, and can assure that each animal receives its proper diet and its required medications or supplements. It can also be used to guide individuals from place to place. The London Zoo used a cup as a target to guide an individual fish into the cup for stress-free removal from the habitat for medical treatment (Box A5.1). The Shedd Aquarium used targeting to teach a grouper (*Epinephelus lanceolatus*) to touch a buoy at the surface of the water so that treatment of a surgical site could be accomplished with ease (Box A5.6). Disney's Seas encountered aggression toward divers from their spotted eagle rays (*Aetobates narinari*) and taught them to touch a PVC target to redirect their attention and eliminate aggression (Muraco and Stamper 2003).

Fish can be trained to accept physical restraint. For example, various species of grouper have been trained to target, accept handling and treatment application, and facilitate transport (Mullin 2006; Reierson 2014). Several facilities have trained nurse sharks (*Ginglymostoma cirratum*) and zebra sharks (*Stegostoma tigrinum*) to allow

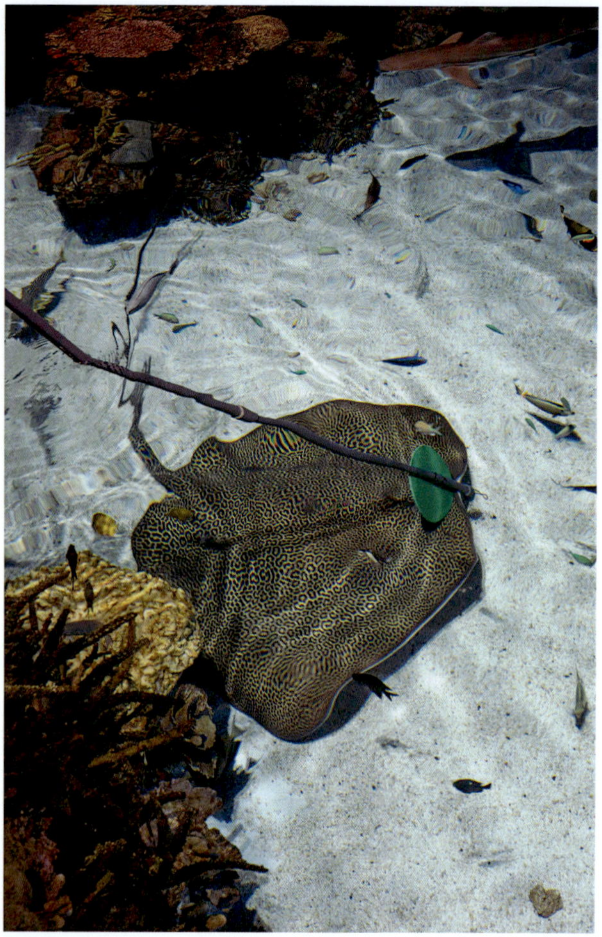

Figure A5.1 Training a reticulated whipray (*Himantura uarnak*) to feed at a specific target. *Source*: Image courtesy of Catherine Hadfield, National Aquarium.

handling for easier transport, physical examinations, ultrasound, and blood samples (Jensen and Jensen 2001; Terrel 2013; Rink and Kageno 2016; Boxes A5.7–A5.8). Successful handling has been accomplished with ram-ventilating sharks, considered to be obligate swimmers and thought to be incapable of slowing down for handling (Crostello and Bogden 2015). And as touch pools have become more popular, increasing numbers of facilities are using training to desensitize fish to touch and noise.

An important aspect of fish behavioral health is providing an enriching environment. Sometimes, individuals can be hesitant to explore or use new enrichment items. Training can assist in acclimation to these new stimuli. One technique is to place food deep within crevices of new enrichment, which encourages fish to explore and accept novel stimuli. Another technique, useful for animals not confident enough to explore new areas, is to approximate them into those areas either by placing food outside the entrance to a new area and gradually moving the food into the new space over time (Box A5.2).

Food puzzles and other enrichment encourage species-specific behavior, particularly foraging. Aquarists and hobbyists have developed several types of interactive feeders. Training can also be used to provide exercise and mental stimulation. For example, archerfish can be trained to use their natural spitting behavior to spit at targets, and stingrays to follow a line in the sand for cognitive and physical exercise (Ramirez and Krevin 1988; Boxes A5.9–A5.11).

Beyond Basic Training (Other Reasons to Train)

Training can be used to wider benefits including research, conservation, and education goals. Once training has been established, it can be used to investigate animals' abilities.

Box A5.4 A Tube for Every Eel

Behavior: Stationing in a tube at feeding time to eliminate aggression.

Species: Green moray eel (*Gymnothorax funebris*).

Facility: The Seas with Nemo and Friends, Orlando, Florida, USA.

Description: A group of five moray eels housed in a community habitat began showing aggression toward one another at feeding time. Staff taught the eels to enter individual PVC tubes when it was time to eat. At first, the tube was held with one end facing the eel, with a long pair of tongs extended through the tube to feed each eel, allowing the eels to habituate to seeing food emerge from the tube while the eels stayed safely hidden in the rocks. As each eel's comfort level increased, the food was held just inside the tube, so that the eel had to stick its head into the tube entrance to eat. Over time, staff gradually approximated the food further inside the tube. Within a few weeks, the eels were swimming through the tubes and poking their head out the other side to eat. Once all five eels had learned this behavior, a device with five PVC tubes separated by sufficient space to keep them out of each other's reach was placed in the habitat at feeding time. As soon as the PVC device was placed in the water, all five eels entered their respective tubes, and all five could be fed with no aggression. The tubes became a favorite hangout for the eels, and even after feeding time was over, several of the eels stayed comfortably in their tubes.

Box A5.5 Responding to the Dinner Bell

Behavior: Target and sound recognition to reduce competition for food.

Species: Whitespotted guitarfish (*Rhynchobatus australiae*), green sawfish (*Pristis zijsron*), zebra sharks (*Stegostoma tigrinum*), oceanic whitetip sharks (*Carcharhinus longimanus*), blacktip sharks (*Carcharhinus limbatus*).

Facility: Shedd Aquarium, Chicago, Illinois, USA.

Description: The Shedd Aquarium Wild Reef habitat includes many teleost and elasmobranch species in a 2 270 000-L habitat. To avoid competition between three species of sharks, a guitar fish, and a sawfish, each species was taught to feed from a particular location around the habitat. Each species was taught to recognize a unique symbol or name target and cued to come to that target when a specific audible sound was emitted in the water (clinking of a triangle, tapping of an iron bar, clicking of an aluminum plate, etc.). These targets, sounds, and locations were taught over a period of many months. By the time the habitat opened to the public, different species (sharks) or individuals (guitarfish and sawfish) could be fed on different days of the week, which allowed for daily public feedings without competition for food between the fish. The ability to feed one group or individual at a time reduced the need to have a large staff on hand during feedings, and daily feeding could be accomplished with one aquarist and a volunteer to assist.

The more training is integrated into fish and invertebrate care, the easier it becomes to use training for research projects. For example:

- Color discrimination in triggerfish (Ramirez 2007).
- Evaluation of dietary needs in goliath groupers (*Epinephelus itajara*) (Kittell and Ratte 2008).
- Training and learning of *Nautilus* sp. (Barod 2014).

Research projects can be tied to conservation efforts. A shark hearing study conducted in a South African facility was used to determine the safety and long-term ramifications of the use of underwater tones on sharks before the tones were approved for use in a worldwide study of global warming (Markinson 1993; Box A5.12). Well-documented studies can assist government agencies in making decisions about emerging conservation issues, such as invasive lionfish (*Pterois* spp.) elimination in the Caribbean, or adjusting fishing practices to decrease incidental bycatch (Lien 1995; Barbour et al. 2011).

Box A5.6 Bubba's Postsurgical Cancer Treatment

Behavior: Stationing and application of medication.

Species: Queensland grouper (*Epinephelus lanceolatus*).

Facility: Shedd Aquarium, Chicago, Illinois, USA.

Description: Bubba was a Queensland grouper that was donated to the Shedd Aquarium in Chicago when he outgrew a home aquarist's aquarium. Over the next 16 years, Bubba grew to nearly 70 kg. During the later years of his life, Bubba developed neoplasia and a team of veterinary oncologists removed a tumor from his forehead. Afterward, he received regular chemotherapy treatments, as well as care and treatment of his surgical site. Prior to his surgery, the aquarist team had developed a training plan that included touching a variety of targets with his head and following the target from place to place. During his postsurgical care, the targeting behavior was used to get Bubba to station in front of staff with his forehead above the water so that topical treatment could be applied twice daily (Mullin 2006).

Public aquariums use training for educational programming with a variety of fish species and there has been an increase in interactive programs such as snorkel experiences and stingray and shark encounter programs (Bogden 2006; Clews et al. 2015; Czaja and Ferraro 2015; McLaurin 2016). Additionally, educational programs have been designed using trained insect-catching archerfish demonstrations, matching to sample demonstrations, and a wide variety of feeding programs, for example with jellies, electric eels (*Electrophorus electricus*), and tarpon (*Megalops* spp.) speed demonstrations (Boxes A5.10 and A5.13).

Modifying Problem Behaviors

Stress reduction, extinction, and redirection, are the primary ways of modifying undesirable behaviors.

Stress reduction is the first step in the resolution of problem behavior. This includes providing a comfortable, safe, and healthy environment. The trainer must be aware of signs of discomfort and stress in a species and make every effort to eliminate the sources of that discomfort.

Extinction is a process of withholding reinforcement from a previously reinforced behavior (Chance 1999). Some unwanted behaviors can be extinguished through the identification and elimination of likely reinforcers. For

Box A5.7 Ready for Treatment and Travel – Shark Stretcher Training

Behavior: Stretcher training for restraint and transport.

Species: Nurse sharks (*Ginglymostoma cirratum*).

Facility: Dolphinarus, Riviera Maya, Mexico.

Description: A nurse shark at a public aquarium in Riviera Maya, Mexico had developed several lesions due to rubbing against a rocky crevice. The veterinarians determined that the lesions needed to be kept dry for 15–30 minutes and a topical treatment needed to be applied daily. Staff taught the shark to swim into a stretcher on its own. Training began by teaching the shark to follow a target to a submerged canvas stretcher. Over the course of a seven days, the shark was reliably following the target and stationing above the submerged stretcher. Over the next week, staff approximated the stretcher up from the bottom of the habitat and brought it gradually closer to the belly of the shark. As the shark's comfort level increased, staff were able to wrap the stretcher around the shark and begin to put pressure on the shark's body to simulate lifting and restraint. After four weeks of training, staff had completed the training and were able to treat the shark every day. Over the next year, staff trained seven other nurse sharks in their program to swim into stretchers (Jensen and Jensen 2001).

example, if a group of fish regularly congregate in one corner of their habitat, because it is their normal feeding location, by discontinuing feeding in that location, the fish will eventually spend less time there. In addition to using extinction, giving the fish an alternate behavior, such as feeding them from several other new locations will accelerate the desired change in their behavior. Identifying and eliminating reinforcers is not always an easy task, and even when they are withheld, behavior may not automatically disappear. The process of extinction takes time, and the absence of reinforcement can sometimes cause the behavior to increase in frequency before it eventually fades away. This phenomenon is called an extinction burst (Kazdin 1994). It is, however, important to be vigilant and aware of stimuli in the environmental that may be serving to reinforce an unwanted behavior.

Box A5.8 Shark Tickles

Behavior: Handling for physical examination, ultrasound, and venipuncture.

Species: Zebra sharks (*Stegostoma tigrinum*).

Facility: Shedd Aquarium, Chicago, Illinois, USA.

Description: Shedd Aquarium in Chicago had established a zebra shark training program to reduce feeding competition. Staff increased the amount of tactile used in training and found that the sharks stayed at station for rubbing and tickles. They continued to use food reinforcers, but the tactile reinforcers proved very powerful. Over time, each of the zebra sharks was trained to stay at station for three minutes or more, which allowed the aquarium's medical team to conduct ultrasound exams and eventually blood sampling. As the aquarium was a leader in zebra shark reproduction, these medical procedures were helpful and enhanced our understanding of this species' reproductive capabilities (Mullin 2006).

Redirection is a technique that focuses on reinforcing a desirable behavior instead of focusing on the unwanted behavior (Kazdin 1994). A useful way to approach problem-solving is to determine what behaviors would be acceptable in a situation in which the unwanted behavior is seen; if the trainer can find an acceptable alternative behavior, the fish can be reinforced for the preferred behavior, and the unwanted behavior can gradually be eliminated.

- Competition for food and aggression can be resolved through strategic feeding and stationing. The fish cannot both stay at station and chase other fish.
- Stereotypic behavior and self-injurious behaviors can be minimized through training that increases individual behavioral repertoires. A fish cannot exhibit newly trained behavior and engage in stereotypic behavior at the same time. In Castaway Key in the Bahamas, stingrays were trained to change swimming patterns on cue to relieve injuries from a repetitive swimming pattern (Box A5.11).

Conclusion

A well-executed behavioral management program will help prevent common behavior problems and set the trainer up for success when a serious problem occurs. Trainers can anticipate future needs and prepare for them, treating the problems without having to stress the fish. It is therefore wise to establish basic behaviors such as stationing, targeting, and thoughtful enrichment well in advance.

When a behavioral management program is established properly and is an integrated part of a professional husbandry program, fish receive the best care and enjoy the best welfare.

Additional references on fish behavior are presented in Box A5.14.

Box A5.9 Anchovy Calisthenics

Behavior: Exercise swims.

Species: Japanese anchovy (*Engraulis japonicus*).

Facility: Port of Nagoya Aquarium, Nagoya, Japan.

Description: The Port of Nagoya Aquarium has a large schooling fish habitat that houses thousands of Japanese anchovies. For several years, twice a day, the aquarium featured a show, set to music with colored lighting, that demonstrated the schooling ability of these fish. As the music played and the colorful lights pulsed on and off, the large group of fish would part in the center with half swimming to the audience's far right and the other half swimming to the far left. Then, on cue, the fish would come together in the center and swim as a unit in a wide circle, only to part ways again into four groups and then back together again. It was a showy spectacle that amazed the audience. How it was trained: Four large groups of fish were trained to respond to different lighted targets held above the habitat. Each group of fish consisted of over 5000 individuals; the group simply followed their specific target. The entire choreographed show consisted of one behavior, following a light target, but the end result seemed magical to the audience. Prior to implementation of the show, morbidity and mortality reports had showed an abnormal number of overweight individuals. After the show had been in place for two years, there were no obesity concerns (Soichi 2009). Following these findings, similar training was implemented for several other groups of fish, not for show but for the physical exercise it provided (Yuichiro 2014).

Box A5.10 Right on Target!

Behavior: Spitting on cue for enrichment and for educational programming.

Species: Banded archerfish (*Toxotes jaculatrix*).

Facility: Marineworld, Galveston, Texas, USA.

Description: Archerfish naturally spit water to knock insects into the water for feeding. Marineworld of Texas trained their archerfish to spit at a circular target above the water to gain access to insects. Aquarists had noted that the archerfish sometimes spit at dark spots on trees or plants, so they decided to paint a black dot on a red circle and place it above the pool's surface. Each time the archerfish spit and hit the target, the aquarists dropped an insect into the water. This behavior was reliably cued by simply placing the red target with the black dot in the center within view of the archer fish. Staff scheduled archerfish feeding demonstrations twice daily for the public to showcase the natural abilities of archerfish (Ramirez and Krevin 1988). Due to the ease of capturing this natural behavior, this type of training is commonly used in aquariums.

Box A5.11 Change Direction

Behavior: Change of swimming direction when cued to relieve self-injurious behavior.

Species: Southern stingray (*Hypanus americanus*).

Facility: Marineworld, Galveston, Texas, USA.

Description: Marineworld of Texas had a community habitat that housed 12 southern stingrays along with several dozen other species. Five of the stingrays began to develop lesions along the outer edges of their wings from rubbing against the perimeter of their habitat. The rays swam in a counterclockwise direction, irritating the lesions daily. The rays were trained to come to a diver to eat when an underwater tone was sounded. The staff devised a plan to encourage the rays to swim in the opposite direction. At the start, it required the use of three divers, each placed around the circular perimeter of the habitat. The first diver sounded a tone and reinforced them while they were swimming in a clockwise direction. Immediately, the next diver called them over with the tone, and the rays swam clockwise to be reinforced by him. Each diver repeated this in sequence until the stingrays had circled the habitat 10 times. Once the pattern of swimming during feeding was well-established, one of the divers was removed from the habitat. The trainers increased the number of rotations around the habitat to 15. Over the next several weeks, the divers approximated themselves to the surface of the water so that eventually they could deliver food from the surface without being in the water, and they increased the number of rotations to 20. After four months of training, the entire process was handled by one trainer at the surface. The trainer began varying the location of reinforcement, and sometimes a ray was allowed to swim around the habitat several times before receiving reinforcement. Six months into the project, the trainer could sound the tone and all the rays would reverse direction and maintain clockwise swimming for approximately 90 minutes. The trainer would reinforce randomly for the first 30 minutes, but once he was done, the rays continued to swim in a clockwise direction for an additional 60 minutes or longer. The sessions were conducted three times a day. One year after starting the training project the lesions were healed and did not appear again (Krevin and Ramirez 1987). An aquarium in China replicated this project with yellowfin tuna (*Thunnus albacares*) with similar results (Zhang 2009).

Box A5.12 Shark Hearing Study

Behavior: Shark trained to respond to different frequency tones as a hearing study within a conservation project.

Species: Dusky shark (*Carcharhinus obscurus*).

Facility: Bayworld, Port Elizabeth, South Africa.

Description: A global warming study required the emission of high-frequency sounds from Heard Island near Antarctica. The tones were to be emitted daily for several years while listening stations around the world would record how long the sounds took to reach each location, providing an accurate measure of global temperatures in the world's oceans. When the study was proposed, concerns were raised about the impact the sounds may have on various species of animals including dolphins, sea turtles, and sharks. The Bayworld facility implemented a study to test the hearing of dusky sharks, one of the species of sharks which inhabit the oceans closest to Heard Island. The shark was trained to swim in a tight circle whenever he heard a tone played. The spinning behavior was quickly trained using a target. Once the spin was reliable, it was put on a cue emitted from a special underwater speaker. Once the shark learned to spin on a single tone, it was taught to also spin on a second, third, and fourth tone. All tones were known to be within that species' hearing range. The research team began gradually increasing and lowering the frequency of the tones until a hearing threshold audiogram was created. After successfully training with the first shark, the project was replicated with two additional conspecifics (Markinson 1993). Although there is still much to learn about the hearing of sharks, this study was one of the first of its kind.

Box A5.13 Blue Tang Visual Match to Sample

Behavior: Visual matching to sample for educational demonstration and research project.

Species: Palette surgeonfish (*Paracanthurus hepatus*).

Facility: Osaka Aquarium, Osaka, Japan.

Description: An aquarist at the Osaka Aquarium trained a surgeonfish to do a visual matching to sample task. The fish was presented with three symbols on a tray at the bottom of the habitat, then presented with a fourth symbol just below the surface that matched one of the symbols on the tray. The fish was reinforced for touching or targeting the matching symbol on the tray. As the training progressed, the fish was able to accurately touch the correct symbol out of three options in over 80% of trials with symbols that were randomly selected from 18 possibilities. This project started as an educational presentation for the public and led to a research project that demonstrated fish capabilities that had not previously been tested (Ramirez 2007).

Box A5.14 Recommendations for General Fish Behavior Resources

He, P. (2010). *Behavior of Marine Fishes: Capture Process and Conservation*. Ames, IA: Wiley-Blackwell.

DeLoach, N. and Humann, P. (1999). *Reef Fish Behavior: Florida, Caribbean, Bahamas*. Jacksonville, FL: New World Publications.

Magnhagen, C., Braithwaite, V., and Forsgren, E. (2008). *Fish Behavior*. Boca Raton, FL: CRC Press.

Reebs, S. (2001). *Fish Behavior in the Aquarium and in the Wild*. London: Comstock-Cornell University Press.

Sloman, K. and Balshine, S. (2005). *Fish Physiology: Behavior and Physiology of Fish*, vol. 24. Cambridge, MA: Academic Press/Elsevier.

References

Barbour, A., Allen, M., Frazer, T., and Sherman, K. (2011). Evaluating the potential efficacy of invasive lionfish (*Pterois volitans*) removals. *PLoS One* 6 (5): e19666.

Barod, J. (2014). Can you teach an old nautilus (*Nautilus belauensis*) new tricks? *Proceedings of the Regional Aquatic Workshop*, Wilmington, NC.

Bogden E. (2006). Training sharks for educational interactive programs. *Proceedings of the International Marine Animal Trainers Association Regional Workshop*, Miami, FL.

Brown, C. (2015). Fish intelligence, sentience, and ethics. *Animal Cognition* 18: 1–17.

Chance, P. (1999). Learning and Behavior, 4e. Pacific Grove, CA: Brooks/Cole Publishing Company.

Clews, A., Meyers, M., and Clayton, L. (2015). A touching experience. *Proceedings of the Regional Aquatic Workshop*, Monterey, CA.

Collier, A. and Schreiber, C. (2014). Behavior modification to alleviate stereotypic behavior in a whale shark (*Rhincodon typus*). *Drum and Croaker* 45: 35–42.

Crostello, M. and Bogden, E. (2015). Training ram ventilation sharks for stationing behaviors. *Proceedings of the International Marine Animal Trainers Association Conference*, Nassau, Bahamas.

Czaja, J. and Ferraro, V. (2015). There's no stopping us right now. *Proceedings of the International Marine Animal Trainers Association Conference*, Nassau, Bahamas.

Jensen, J. and Jensen, L. (2001). Stretcher training nurse sharks (*Ginglymostoma cirratum*) for educational enhancement and husbandry purposes. *Proceedings of the International Marine Animal Trainers Association Conference*, Albuquerque, NM.

Kazdin, A. (1994). Behavior Modification in Applied Settings, 5e. Pacific Grove, CA: Brooks/Cole Publishing Company.

Kittell, M. and Ratte, M. (2008). Monitoring feed amounts in goliath groupers (*Epinephelus itajara*) using behavioral conditioning in a large mixed species exhibit. *Zoo Biology* 27: 414–419.

Krevin, J. and Ramirez, K. (1987). Behavioral modification of stereotyped swimming and resolution of self-injurious behavior in southern stingrays (*Dasyatis americana*). *Proceedings of the Fish Biology Symposium*, College Station, TX.

Lehner, P. (1987). Design and execution of animal behavior research: an overview. *Journal of Animal Science* 65: 1213–1219.

Lien, J. (1995). Conservation aspects of fishing gear: cetaceans and gillnets. *Proceedings of Workshop, Solving Bycatch: Considerations for Today and Tomorrow*. University of Alaska Sea Grant College Program, Seattle, WA.

Mackie, J. (2017). Personal communication; Jim Mackie of the Zoological Society of London.

Markinson, A. (1993). Hearing threshold in three dusky sharks (*Carcharhinus obscurus*). *Proceedings of the Biennial Bioacoustics Symposium*, Honolulu, HI.

McLaurin, L. (2016). Enriching the lives of touch tank southern cownose rays (*Rhinoptera bonasus*) at Phoenix Zoo. *Drum and Croaker* 47: 73–83.

Mullin, W. (2006). Bubba's amazing story: a life in review. *Shedd Aquarium Annual Report*. Shedd Aquarium Society, Chicago, IL.

Muraco, H. and Stamper, M. (2003). Training spotted eagle rays (*Aetobatus narinari* (Euphrasen)) to decrease aggressive behaviors towards divers. *Journal of Aquariculture and Aquatic Sciences* VIII: 88–98.

Nylund, J., Robertson, M., Serafin, R., Slagoski, A. et al. (2015). Improving animal wellness and guest experience through learning opportunities and secondary reinforcers with a goliath grouper (*Epinephulus itajara*). *Proceedings of the International Marine Animal Trainers Association Conference*, Nassau, Bahamas.

Panksepp, J. (1998). Affective Neuroscience: The Foundations of Human and Animal Emotions. London: Oxford University Press.

Patel, E. and Dickson, J. (2014). Training of marine eels: how to make feeding easier. *Proceedings of the Regional Aquatic Workshop*, Wilmington, NC.

Pierce, W. and Cheney, C. (2008). Behavior Analysis and Learning, 4e. New York: Psychology Press.

Pryor, K. (2009a). Capturing and naming behavior. *Dog Trainer Professional Program*. Karen Pryor Academy, Waltham, MA.

Pryor, K. (2009b). Efficient shaping. *Dog Trainer Professional Program*. Karen Pryor Academy, Waltham, MA.

Ramirez, K. (1999). Animal Training: Successful Animal Management through Positive Reinforcement. Chicago, IL: Shedd Aquarium Society.

Ramirez, K. (2007). Reflections on the unique training from my recent visit to Japan. *WaterShedd: The Membership Newsletter of the John G. Shedd Aquarium*, Chicago, IL.

Ramirez, K. and Krevin, J. (1988). Training an archerfish (*Toxotes jaculatrix*) to spit on cue. *Proceedings of the Fish Biology Symposium*, Galveston, TX.

Ramirez, K. (2013). Husbandry training. In: Zookeeping: An Introduction to the Science and Technology (eds. M.D. Irwin, J.B. Stoner and A.M. Cobaugh), 424–434. Chicago, IL: University of Chicago Press.

Reierson, A. (2014). The successful training, capture, and transport of a goliath grouper (*Epinephulus itajara*). *Proceedings of the Regional Aquatic Workshop*, Wilmington, NC.

Rink, L. and Kageno, E. (2016). Operant conditioning of a giant sea bass (*Stereolepis gigas*). *Proceedings of the Regional Aquatic Workshop*, New Orleans, LA.

Salyers, J. (2015). Not another octopus (*Octopus vulgaris*) enrichment talk: a quantitative approach to enrichment. *Proceedings of the Regional Aquatic Workshop*, Monterey, CA.

Skinner, B.F. (1953). Science and Human Behavior. New York: Free Press.

Soichi, T. (2009). Using exercise to reduce obesity in captive fish. *Proceedings of the Society for Chinese Ichthyology Biennial Conference*, Beijing, China.

Terrel, R. (2013). Management of *Arapaima gigas* with operant conditioning. *Proceedings of the Regional Aquatic Workshop*, Atlanta, GA.

Yuichiro, A. (2014). Personal communication and observation; consulting visit with Akune Yuichiro, Port of Nagoya Aquarium.

Zhang, S. (2009). Exercise protocol to eliminate stereotypic swimming patterns in yellowfin tuna (*Thunnus albacares*). *Proceedings of the Society for Chinese Ichthyology Biennial Conference*, Beijing, China.

A6

Clinical Examination and Diagnostic Sampling

Kathryn E. Seeley

Columbus Zoo and Aquarium, Powell, OH, USA

Introduction

The field of aquatic animal medicine is expanding, providing more opportunities for clinicians to work with fish in private households, public display aquaria, commercial aquaculture, and research facilities. This chapter is intended to cover the basic approach to a fish case, including how to take a history, perform a thorough clinical examination, and collect and process appropriate samples. The evaluation of diagnostic samples is covered in more detail in Chapter A7.

History

The first step is always to obtain a thorough history. Clients have different levels of fish experience. It is important to know this when interpreting a history and considering the differential list; clients with less experience are more likely to be dealing with common husbandry issues (particularly water quality) or common infectious diseases. It is also important to understand the client's goals, as examination and management plans may differ if the goal is to maximize production on a farm, to minimize risk to an established collection, or to maximize longevity of a pet fish.

Some parts of the history are common to all taxa, including the signalment of all affected animals, presenting signs, duration and progression of signs, previous and current diet, previous and current medications, quarantine protocols, and medical history (Table A6.1). Since fish are usually housed in groups, the health status of other animals in the system must be considered. This helps to determine early on if the problem is limited to a single individual or a group. This has significant implications for differential lists, diagnostic choices, and treatment considerations. It is helpful to discuss previous morbidity or mortality in the collection as this may highlight recurrent disease issues. It is important to always ask if any new animals or plants have been added to the system in the prior three months.

Fish health is deeply impacted by the environment, particularly the life support system and water quality. The history must include a detailed review of the environment. This should include type of system, size of system, water source, water quality, frequency of water changes or additions, management protocols, and any concerns (Table A6.1). It is invaluable to be able to assess basic water quality parameters in the clinic, particularly ammonia, nitrite, salinity, pH, copper, and chlorine. Water quality testing is discussed in Chapter A2.

Clinical Examination

Observation

After discussing the history, the next step is to observe the fish in its system, whenever possible. A great deal of information can be gleaned by simply watching and, for this reason, site visits always provide a more complete picture than bringing the fish to the clinic for evaluation. If a site visit is not possible, photographs and videos of the system should be evaluated to get a better understanding of the environment.

It is often helpful to first observe from a distance, then move closer, since human presence may affect fish behavior. Observation can provide information on all the following:

- Activity level (e.g. lethargy, hyperactivity), alertness, and responsiveness to visual or tactile stimuli and/or feeding.

Clinical Guide to Fish Medicine, First Edition. Edited by Catherine A. Hadfield and Leigh Ann Clayton.

Table A6.1 Important questions when obtaining the history of an aquatic patient.

Topic	Value	Comments/examples
System parameters	Indoor/outdoor	Outdoor systems (e.g. a pond or raceway) are exposed to weather, predators, and runoff contaminants
	Size of tank (actual enclosure) and size of system (including the water in connected tanks, sumps, and life support equipment)	Small systems have less stable environmental parameters Large systems usually receive smaller water changes, resulting in higher nitrates and depleted macronutrients, and animal access may be limited
	Substrate	Some species require substrate, e.g. wrasse (*Labridae*) Fish often ingest substrate Substrate can be a refuge for parasites Deep substrate can become anoxic
	Types and sizes of filters	Filtration affects every aspect of the environment, including oxygenation, gas pressures, nitrogenous wastes, pH, and pathogen load
	Lighting and light cycle	Fish do best with a species-appropriate light spectrum and light cycle Some common tropical ornamental fish do better with lower light intensities than seen in most aquariums (e.g. squirrelfish *Holocentridae*)
	Décor, including live plants	Most fish do better with suitable shelters Abundant décor can make it hard to see morbidity and mortalities Live plants affect dissolved oxygen, carbon dioxide, and pH
	Other individuals and species in the system and their approximate sizes	A high stocking density increases the risk of infectious disease and water quality problems Incompatibility is a common problem
	Recent introductions of plants, invertebrates, fish, amphibians, or reptiles	Recently introduced fish can transmit novel pathogens and may be exposed to new pathogens in the system Other animals and plants may be biological or mechanical vectors of pathogens and may affect the social structure
	How long the system has been running	Newly established systems are most likely to have life support and water quality problems
	Possible contaminants	Recent fertilizer around a pond or recent painting near an aquarium can expose fish to toxins
Water quality parameters	System type (e.g. closed and recirculating, semi-open with some recirculation, open/flow-through)	Recirculating systems are heavily dependent on their life support systems For open and semi-open systems, the condition of the incoming water is critical
	Water type (e.g. freshwater, natural seawater, commercial saltwater mix, proprietary saltwater mix)	Salt composition should be appropriate for all species and life stages in the system Quality control of saltwater mixes varies
	Water source	Quality and treatment of incoming water varies greatly Municipal freshwater usually requires dechlorination Surface water (e.g. natural seawater or lake water) often requires mechanical filtration and disinfection
	Frequency and percentage of water changes and date of most recent water change	Low water turnover can lead to buildup of toxins or depletion of essential ions Morbidity or mortality immediately after a water change may be due to issues in the incoming water or lines

(Continued)

Table A6.1 (Continued)

Topic	Value	Comments/examples
	Water additives – recent and historical	Recirculating systems often receive routine additions (e.g. sodium bicarbonate, potassium iodide, calcium carbonate) Morbidity or mortality after additions may be due to miscalculation or contamination
	Temperature – current and historical range	Temperature should be appropriate for all species in the system and fluctuations should be kept to a minimum
	Water quality parameters including dissolved oxygen, pH, salinity, ammonia, nitrite, nitrate, hardness, alkalinity – current and historical ranges	These should be appropriate for all species in the system and rapid fluctuations should be kept to a minimum
Diet	Food storage, preparation, and supplementation	Inappropriate or prolonged storage of foods and supplements can deplete nutrients Inappropriate thawing and soaking of foods deplete nutrients
	Food types and amounts that are offered or available	These should be appropriate for all species and life stages and allow the animals to express normal feeding behaviors
	Food types and amounts that are actually eaten – current and historical	What is eaten may differ from what is offered
	Frequency of feeding	Small and larval fish often need frequent feeding, in some cases on a continuous drip system Some fish species do best with periods of fasting
Medical history	Source and time in owner's possession	Reputable sources reduce the risk of problems Newly acquired fish are at higher risk of infectious disease
	Time in current system	A recent move means catch and transport stress and novel pathogen exposures
	Quarantine protocols	Ectoparasites are more likely in fish that did not go through an isolated quarantine Inappropriate use of medications in quarantine can lead to morbidity and mortality
	Reproductive history	Mating in some species (e.g. elasmobranchs) is a common source of trauma Bony fish that have never spawned in a system and are showing coelomic distension may be egg-bound
	Prior medical concerns in the system/species	Recurrence of diseases in the same species or system is common and previously diagnosed issues should always be considered
	Number and species of fish affected	This helps to answer the critical question of whether it is an individual or group problem
	Clinical signs, including duration and progression	This helps determine if acute, chronic, or acute on chronic
	Recent mortalities	This helps determine if acute, chronic, or acute on chronic Diagnostics may have been run on the mortalities
	Previous diagnostics	These can change the differential list, but because of effects from sample handling, processing, and laboratory choice, they should not rule out repeating the diagnostics
	Previous treatments	A variety of treatments are available over-the-counter and it is not uncommon for owners to have tried other treatments before seeking veterinary care

- Behavior, e.g. flashing (where the fish brushes itself against the bottom of the tank), congregating in areas of high water flow, displacement, schooling fish swimming alone.
- Body position and conformation, e.g. staying at the surface, lateral recumbency, spy hopping, spinal deformity, mid-water species sitting on the substrate. If a fish is positively or negatively buoyant, it is helpful to see if the fish is trying to correct its position in the water column or is showing no response to its abnormal position.
- Body condition and shape of the coelom: Most fish should look streamlined, without bulging of the muscle or coelom or obvious concavities.
- Respiratory rate and effort based on opercular or gill slit movement: A dyspneic fish will often show high respiratory rate and effort and may gasp at the surface (piping) or stay near areas of turbulence.
- Overall coloration and any skin or fin abnormalities, e.g. light or dark spots, hyperemia, ulcers, erosions, masses, visible parasites, abnormal fin movements.
- Eye abnormalities, e.g. exophthalmos, buphthalmos, discoloration.
- Cloacal or anal abnormalities, e.g. distension, prolapse, discharge.

If the clinician has not worked with the species frequently, it is helpful to review normal appearance and behavior using internet searches, comparing to normal cohorts, and through discussions with the client. It is important to use this opportunity to assess the stocking density. This is typically measured based on total length or biomass per unit volume. For example, a 20 gallon system that has 10 cardinal tetras with an average total length of 1 inch has a stocking density of 0.5 in/gallon (0.35 cm/L). In the author's experience, for ornamental fish, a stocking density of >1.5 in/gallon (1 cm/L) often increases the risk of infectious disease.

The life support system should also be assessed. A simple approach that works for many systems is listed below.

- Identify the water pumps and check that they are working and that there is flow through the system. The whole volume of water should turn over more than once per hour. Pumps are prone to fouling which reduces water flow over time, particularly ones without mechanical traps (prefilters) to stop debris from entering the pump.
- Identify the type of biological filtration (e.g. canister filter, sand filter, undergravel filter). Where possible, check that there is adequate, even water flow through the filter media. Channeling of water through gaps in the media is a common problem. At a very rough estimate, the volume of the biological filtration for most display aquariums is likely to be ~1/4–1/6th the water volume of the system.
- Identify any mechanical or physiochemical filtration (e.g. sand filter, foam fractionator, carbon filter). Where possible, check that there is adequate flow through the filters; sand filter pressures should be low (often <20 PSI). Foam fractionators should have fine bubbles skimming off at the top.
- Identify any disinfection (e.g. ozone or ultraviolet). This should follow after mechanical and biological filters. Ozone systems should have visible ORP meters that read <200–350 mV in fish systems. Well-managed UV filters should have the date that the bulb was last changed and the sleeves protecting the bulbs should be clean.
- Evaluate the water temperature and the functionality of any components that heat or chill the water.
- Evaluate the mechanism for aeration and identify any additional air supplementation (e.g. air stones) to check that these are running appropriately. For most systems, there should be visible movement of the water at the surface and in the water column with few or no microbubbles. With some experience, clinicians can also evaluate areas of gas exchange in the system to assess the probability of low or high gas pressures.
- Evaluate the type and depth of the substrate, if present. Substrate should be suitable for the species, have limited debris, and not be too deep (e.g. substrate depth of >20 cm (8 in) may be prone to anoxia).
- Evaluate the décor for suitability for the species and sufficient shelter for the animals.
- Evaluate the lighting system for suitability for the species, and check that timers and bulbs are working as expected.
- Evaluate the area around the system for noise and vibration (e.g. pumps), other disturbances (e.g. high traffic area, recent painting), and possible overhead contamination (e.g. dripping condensate from HVAC systems).

Clinicians are encouraged to get experience evaluating systems from experts in the field, as life support problems commonly contribute to morbidity and mortality in fish.

Transport Considerations

If a fish needs to be moved to a clinic for further diagnostics or treatment, there are some important transport considerations.

- The fish should be transported in water from the same system or at least 50% of water from the same system (e.g. 50% freshwater from the pond and 50% new dechlorinated freshwater).
- The container should be nonabrasive and have an escape-proof lid.
- Water temperature changes should be kept to a minimum by traveling at a suitable time of day, using a climate-controlled vehicle, and providing plenty of insulation (e.g. putting the fish bag into a cooler).

- If the container is sealed, e.g. a closed bag, it should have a ratio of 2:1 air (or oxygen) to water.
- There should be sufficient water to allow for anesthesia and recovery if needed (e.g. by bringing a second container with additional water).

A common setup that might work for a small teleost such as a goldfish (*Carassius auratus*) is a large waterproof plastic bag with 2:1 air to system water that is knotted at the top, put into a second bag in case of a leak, then put into a cooler. Suitable bags are available from any fish store. Alternatively, a clean 5 gallon bucket with a lid can be used. For larger fish, a cooler the fish can turn in often works well. Additional aeration is recommended (e.g. air stone and battery-powered pump), even for short transports. A water sample that is brought in for analysis should be kept separate from this transport water (e.g. in a clean 1 L bottle). Transport is covered in more detail in Chapter A14.

Handling Considerations

After a thorough observation of the fish and system, the next step may be to handle the fish for closer evaluation and diagnostic samples. However, handling is not always indicated. The primary diagnosis may be clear from the history and visual exam (e.g. ammonia increase following recent fish introductions or channeling through the biological filtration), in which case, handling may not be required unless additional problems are suspected. Clinical signs may also preclude handling or increase the risk of adverse effects (e.g. handling fish showing severe dyspnea can increase the risk of mortalities). In any case, handling should be done with care (e.g. appropriate net, calm capture technique, good environmental conditions) as it is an additional stressor and can damage the external mucus layer or skin.

Additionally, handling can pose risks to humans, including trauma, envenomation, and electric shock. Many fish have strong tails or peduncles and/or sharp spines, spurs, or teeth that can inflict significant damage and lead to infection. Common examples of hazards are:

- Rigid dorsal fin spines on many bony fish.
- Rigid spines on the dorsal fin and pectoral fins of many catfish (*Ictaluridae*), of which some are potentially venomous.
- Peduncle blades on most surgeonfish (*Acanthuridae*), of which some are potentially venomous.
- Teeth or dental plates, particularly in some sharks, rays (*Myliobatiformes*), moray eels (*Muraenidae*), barracuda (*Sphyraenidae*), parrotfish (*Scaridae*), and piranha (e.g. *Pygocentrus* spp.).
- Sharp denticles in the skin of sharks and in focal areas in the skin of skates (*Rajidae*) and some rays.
- Strong tail on whiptail rays (*Dasyatidae*) and strong peduncle of larger sharks and sawfish (*Pristis* spp.).

These hazards must be considered prior to handling.

For venomous species, knowing the type and location of the venom and the severity of envenomation is essential for human safety (Table A6.2). For instance, lionfish (*Pterois* spp.) have venomous spines on their dorsal, pelvic, and anal fins, whereas stingrays have a venomous spine on the dorsal aspect of the tail (Figure A6.1). Whenever venomous species are handled, a response plan should be established beforehand in case of an envenomation. For some species (e.g. lionfish, rabbitfish, scorpionfish, and stingrays) the toxins are heat labile and, after dealing with any shock or first aid needs, running the affected area under tolerable hot water (~40°C or 105°F) should inactivate the toxins (Reavill 2006). In other species, such as the stonefish (*Synanceia* spp.), envenomation is more serious and

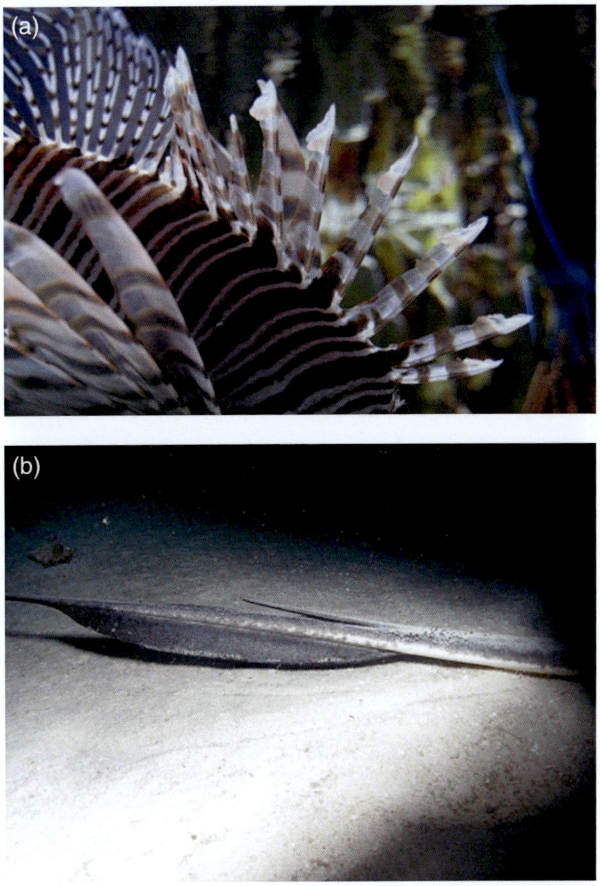

Figure A6.1 Venom is found under the epithelium of the rigid fin spines in lionfish (a) and the barb on the dorsal aspect of the tail of stingrays (b). *Source*: Images courtesy of Catherine Hadfield, National Aquarium.

Table A6.2 Common venomous fish species.

Scientific name	Common name	Site of venom
Synanceia spp.	Stonefish	Dorsal fin; venom is highly toxic
Scorpaenidae including *Pterois* spp.	Scorpionfish including lionfish	Dorsal, pelvic, and anal fins
Siganus spp.	Rabbitfish	Dorsal, pelvic, and anal fins
Plotosus lineatus	Coral catfish	Dorsal and pectoral fins
Uranoscopidae	Stargazer	Spines dorsal to their pectoral fins
Thalassophryne and *Daector* spp.	Toadfish	Opercular spines and dorsal fins; there are many nonvenomous toadfish
Chimaeriformes	Chimaeras	Dorsal fins
Hexatrygonidae *Plesiobatidae* *Urolophidae* *Urotrygonidae* *Dasyatidae* *Potamotrygonidae* *Gymnuridae* *Myliobatidae*	Stingrays	Base of tail or mid-tail spines

specific antivenins are needed. Venomous fish should not be confused with toxic fish that can cause toxicity when ingested.

For electrogenic fish, knowledge of the potential size of the electric charge is important. Of fish that are often seen in display aquariums, the electric eel (*Electrophorus electricus*), electric catfish (*Malapterurus* spp.), and electric rays (particularly *Torpedo* spp.) have the potential to generate sufficient charge to injure a human. They should be handled using gloves rated for high-voltage electric work. There are many more species that can generate mild electric charges that are unlikely to be felt by humans.

Another important consideration prior to handling is how to meet the environmental needs of the patient. This usually includes sufficient water from the original system, supplemental aeration (e.g. air stone and air pump or oxygen cylinder and regulator), a plan for monitoring and maintaining water temperature, and providing additional water flow if needed (e.g. suitable power head or large syringes). Monitoring water quality (e.g. temperature, dissolved oxygen, pH, and ammonia) helps to ensure suitable conditions. Time spent out of the water should be kept to a minimum, and if the examination requires it, there must be a way to provide ventilation and keep the skin wet.

Gloves should be worn when handling fish. This helps to protect the external mucus layer of the fish and reduces the risk of zoonotic disease transmission. Zoonotic diseases of fish are more typically acquired through ingestion of raw, undercooked, or inadequately processed seafood, however some can be transmitted through contact and inoculation into wounds (Table A6.3). Depending on the animal and procedure, clean work gloves or new latex, vinyl, or nitrile examination gloves may be most suitable. Gloves should be rinsed prior to use to remove any fine dust that may be present.

All equipment needed for the examination should be ready prior to handling. A list of equipment that may be used for examination and diagnostic sampling is listed in Box A6.1.

Manual Restraint

The method of handling varies depending on the species, size, type of procedure, equipment available, the fish's handling history, and personal experience. In some cases, brief manual restraint in a suitable net or stretcher may be sufficient. It is advisable, when possible, to use plastic/vinyl nets instead of the more traditional mesh nets (Figure A6.2). This reduces the risk of damage to the skin and prevents the fish from becoming entangled, which is especially common for species with firm fin rays or denticles.

Manual restraint is often used for short, noninvasive procedures in nonvenomous bony fish (e.g. for a visual examination, skin scrape, or intramuscular injection). Bony fish may be restrained within the catch net or a gloved hand. Some species are particularly easy to manually restrain because their movement is solely reliant on fins rather than body movement, e.g. seahorses, pipefish, and seadragons (*Syngnathidae*), trunkfish and cowfish (*Ostraciidae*). Invasive procedures in these species must still be carried out using suitable anesthesia and analgesia.

Box A6.1 List of Equipment Needed for Clinical Examination of Koi (*Cyprinus carpio koi*) or Similar-Sized Fish

Water quality testing
- Thermometer
- Refractometer for salinity
- Colorimetric tests for ammonia, nitrite, nitrate, alkalinity, copper, chlorine, +/− calcium, phosphate, iodide
- pH meter
- Dissolved oxygen meter
- +/−Total gas pressure meter

Restraint
- Suitable nets, stretchers, and containers
- Aerator stone, air line, and air pump or oxygen bottle and regulator
- Anesthetic (e.g. MS-222, sodium bicarbonate, pH pen)
- Water pump(s), large syringes
- Doppler ultrasound
- +/− Recirculating anesthesia system
- +/− Plastic or foam padding

Physical exam and routine diagnostics
- Suitable scale(s); often a gram scale for drugs and small fish and a larger scale for large fish
- Measuring tape or calipers
- Flashlight/headlight
- Small towels
- Powder-free gloves
- Mouth gags, e.g. rubber dog bones, tongue depressors
- Needles (25–20 ga)
- Syringes (1–60 mL)
- Red rubber catheters (5–12 Fr)
- Heparin blood tubes, heparin solution to heparinize syringes
- Plain blood tubes
- Culturettes and blood culture vials
- PCR swabs and viral transport media
- Whirl-paks and cryovials
- Labeled vials with 10% neutral buffered formalin
- Slides and cover slips
- Scalpel blades
- Scissors (small iris, Mayo, and Metzenbaum)
- Atraumatic forceps
- Fluorescein stain
- Slit lamp, ophthalmoscope
- Benchtop microscope

Treatments
- Common medications (e.g. ceftazidime, florfenicol, amikacin, methylprednisolone, formalin 37%, praziquantel, copper sulfate, fluids, sodium thiosulfate)
- Suitable gavage food options
- Small surgical pack and absorbable monofilament suture (3/0–5/0) on tapered needles

Manual restraint is often used for a greater range of procedures in elasmobranchs, but this requires experienced handlers. Some elasmobranchs will enter a state of tonic immobility in ventrodorsal recumbency that allows for safe collection of a variety of diagnostics, including blood (Henningsen 1994).

With positive reinforcement training, animals can become voluntary participants in husbandry care. For example, animals can be trained to move into nets, stretchers, or tubs to facilitate catch and transport or allow ultrasound examination or diagnostic sampling. This training significantly reduces the stress associated with handling and should be considered wherever possible.

Chemical Restraint

Anesthesia is indicated for invasive procedures, active fish, and fish that present human health hazards. Immersion anesthesia is most common in fish. It should always be done in water from the fish's system, although source water can be used in an open system. The most common fish anesthetic is tricaine methanesulfonate by immersion (MS-222, Syndel USA (formerly Western Chemical), Ferndale, WA) (Neiffer and Stamper 2009; Carter et al. 2011). MS-222 is strongly acidic, so it should always be buffered (e.g. with sodium bicarbonate). Eugenol-based products are also used, particularly clove oil after initial dissolution in ethanol (Javahery et al. 2012). Many injectable protocols have been reported, but results have been variable (Flemming et al. 2003; Neiffer and Stamper 2009). Depth of anesthesia is typically assessed based on voluntary movement, righting reflex, and opercular or gill slit movement and frequency. A Doppler or other ultrasound device or ECG can be used to monitor heart rate (Neiffer and Stamper 2009). Further details regarding anesthesia and anesthetic monitoring are covered in Chapter A10.

Components of the Physical Examination

As with any other patient, a physical examination should be complete and systematic. One approach is to go from head to tail. The oral cavity should be examined, but care needs to be taken as many fish have teeth that can inflict damage (Figure A6.3). Appropriately sized bite blocks may be needed to safely examine the oral cavity. Common abnormalities detected on oral examination include erosions, dental disease, foreign bodies, and masses (Roberts-Sweeney 2016).

Table A6.3 Zoonotic diseases that may be acquired from fish or water through contact or inoculation.

Disease	Most likely clinical signs in humans	Probability of zoonotic transmission
Aeromonas spp.	Local wound infection that can become severe or systemic	Very low; most likely from ingestion
Edwardsiella spp.	Local wound infection that can become severe or systemic	Very low; most likely from ingestion
Erysipelothrix spp.	Local wound infection that can become severe or systemic	Very low; more likely from processing pork products
Mycobacterium spp. (atypical species)	Local, nonhealing wound	Low
Vibrio spp.	Local wound infection that can become severe or systemic	Very low; most likely from ingestion

Transmission by ingestion of raw or undercooked seafood or contamination of food sources is much more common but not covered in this table.

A slit lamp and ophthalmoscope are useful to evaluate ocular structures. Most fish do not show a pupillary light reflex and the lens normally protrudes slightly through the pupil (Figure A6.4). If ulceration or other corneal defects are suspected, fluorescein stain can be applied to evaluate the integrity of the epithelium. The stain strip can be added to an electrolyte solution (e.g. sterile artificial tears) and then applied to the affected eye while it is out of water. The cobalt blue light setting on a slit lamp is the most effective way to look for uptake. Tonometry can be used to measure intraocular pressure, although this technique is not commonly reported in fish. Common ocular abnormalities include corneal edema, corneal ulceration, lens luxation, cataracts, uveitis, exophthalmos, and buphthalmos. Distension may be due to gas, fluid, or soft tissue.

The gills must be visually inspected. In most fish, this is possible by gently lifting the operculum or gill slits, although access is limited in some species, e.g. seahorses, pipefish, skates, rays, moray eels, blennies (*Blenniidae*), and lumpsuckers (*Cyclopteridae*). In these cases, the gills can be evaluated more fully using a small laryngoscope, endoscope, or otoscope. Normal gills should be dark red with distinct lamellae of even length (Figure A6.5a). Common grossly visible gill abnormalities include pallor (e.g. due to anemia), grey or brown discoloration, petechiation, congestion, edema, clumping, blunting, irregular lengths or margins, and grossly visible parasites (Figure A6.5b).

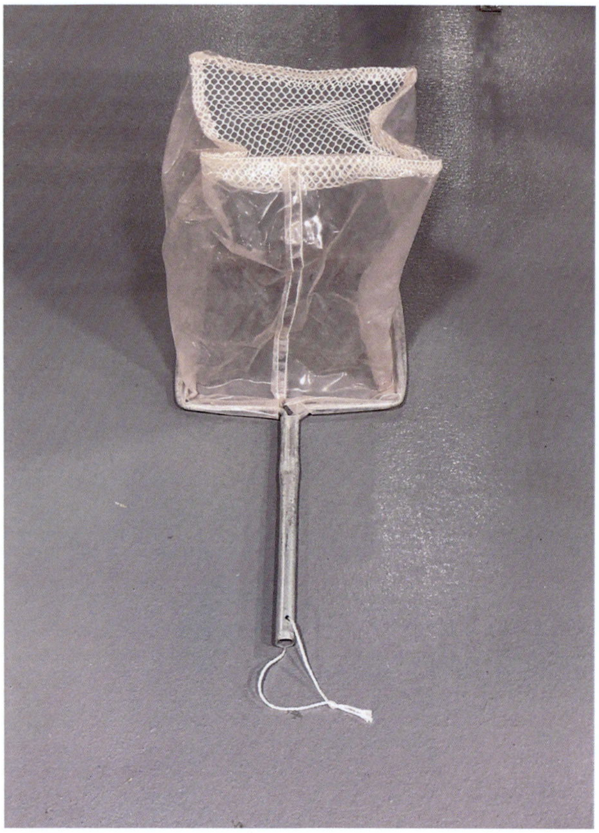

Figure A6.2 Plastic nets that are suitable for catching and restraining fish. *Source*: Image courtesy of Ashleigh Clews, National Aquarium.

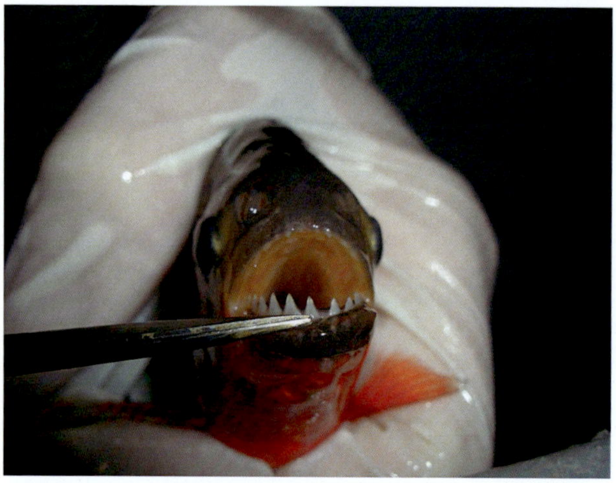

Figure A6.3 Cutting/shearing teeth on a piranha (*Pygocentrus nattereri*). *Source*: Image courtesy of Catherine Hadfield, National Aquarium.

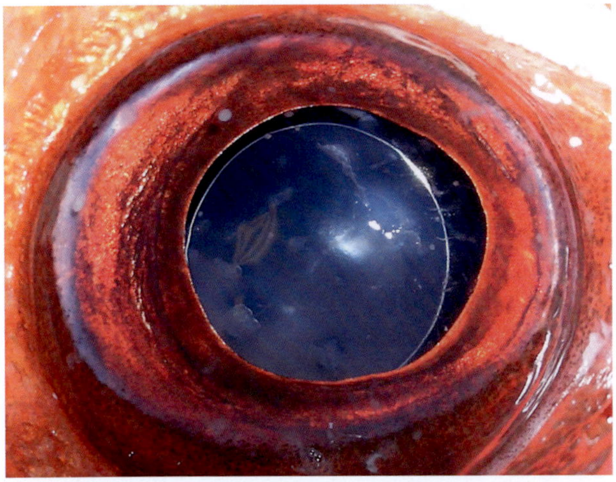

Figure A6.4 Normal eye of a squirrelfish (*Holocentrus* sp.). *Source*: Image courtesy of Catherine Hadfield, National Aquarium.

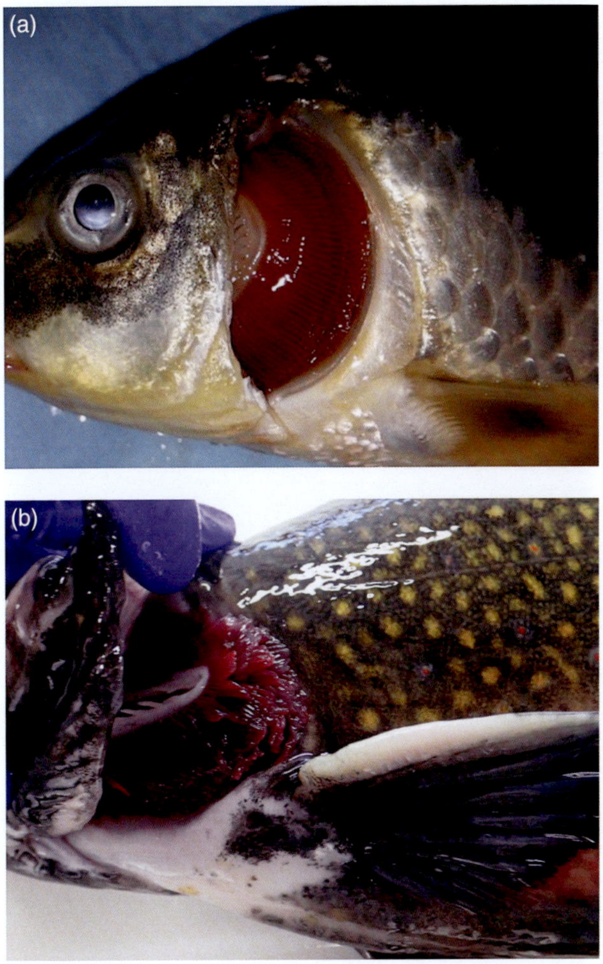

Figure A6.5 Normal gills of a koi (*Cyprinus carpio koi*) (a). Irregular, congested, and edematous gills of a brook trout (*Salvelinus fontinalis*) (b). *Source*: Images courtesy of Gregory Lewbart, North Carolina State University.

The skin and fins should be assessed fully for any color change, spots, or plaques (which may be white, tan, brown, black, or red), visible mucus, hyperemia, petechiae, ulcers, erosions, lacerations, edema, masses, or visible parasites. Each fin should be fully extended to look for lesions.

The epaxial muscles should be palpated to assess tone, which should be firm and even. The coelomic cavity should be palpated for masses or distension and any asymmetry should be noted. The cloaca or vent area should be evaluated for any distension, prolapse, or discharge. Elasmobranchs have several unique anatomical features that should be evaluated. The abdominal or cloacal pores on either side of the cloaca should be evaluated for any discoloration or discharge (Figure A6.6). The claspers (in males) should be evaluated for size, rotation, and skin changes (Figure A6.7). In large elasmobranchs, it is possible to do a digital cloacal examination to check the mucosal surfaces, urinary papilla, and cervix (in females).

Body weights provide important clinical and growth information and allow for accurate dosing of oral or parenteral medications. For small individuals, a weight can be obtained by placing the patient in an atraumatic plastic container (Figure A6.8). For large patients, a stretcher and hoist system that accommodates a hanging scale is often the best option.

Other measurements may include:

- Total length (Figure A6.9).
- Snout-to-vent length.
- Disc width (curved dorsal surface or straight ventral surface) in skates, rays, guitarfish.
- Girth, often just caudal to the pectoral fins.
- Precaudal length in sharks.
- Clasper length in male elasmobranchs (from cranial cloaca to tip of one clasper).

It is helpful to record details of the method used so that measurements are easily repeatable.

Individual Identification

Individual identification allows tracking of clinical signs, diagnostics, treatments, and outcomes during case management. Individual identification also helps provide long-term information on health trends (e.g. life span, sequelae). Identifiers may not be needed when a fish is the only one of its species or will always be visibly distinct from its conspecifics, or where only group management is desired.

There are several ways to distinguish individual fish. External features, ideally using photographic identification, are often the most useful for daily management. Colored implants, clear implants that are only visible under UV light, and a variety of fin tags are available for

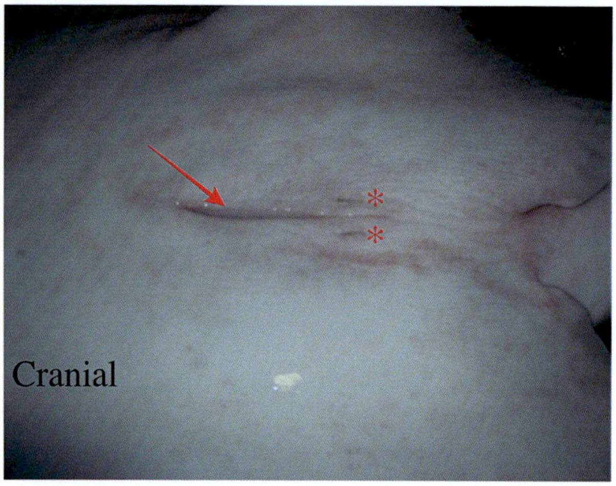

Figure A6.6 Normal abdominal pores in a female stingray (*Hypanus* sp.) (*) either side of the cloaca (arrow). *Source*: Image courtesy of Catherine Hadfield, National Aquarium.

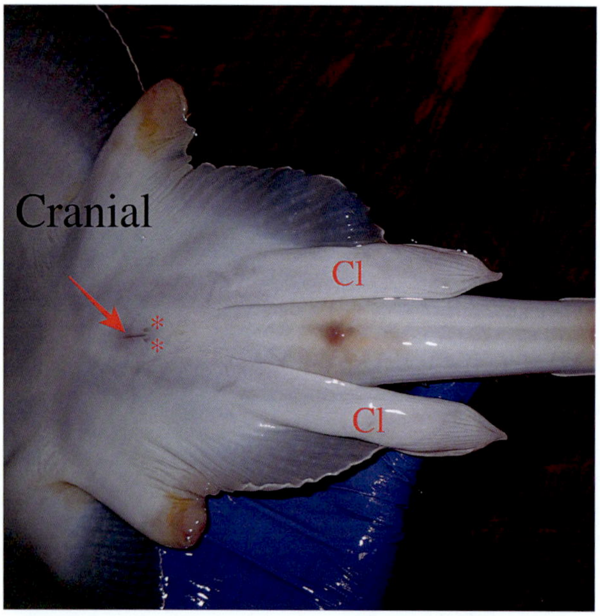

Figure A6.7 Claspers (Cl) in a male little skate (*Leucoraja erinacea*) with ventral ulcers; the abdominal pores (*) and cloaca (arrow) are also marked. *Source*: Image courtesy of Catherine Hadfield, National Aquarium.

external identification (e.g. Floy® tags, Petersen discs) (Figure A6.10). Temporary external identification can be achieved using distinct notches in the fins, but these may not be easy to see unless under chemical restraint. Passive internal transponders (PIT tags) do not typically allow external identification while animals are free-swimming but are the best permanent identification available. They are usually placed in the left epaxial muscles using routine PIT tag injection systems; no skin preparation is required. They should be considered for most large, ornamental fish to allow tracking of individual animal health history.

Diagnostic Sampling

Fish often present with nonspecific clinical signs. If the diagnosis has not been reached based on the history and visual and physical examinations, or if secondary diseases are suspected, further diagnostics are needed. Lists of common infectious diseases for different taxa are provided to help narrow the differential list (Boxes A6.2–A6.8) (Matthews 2004; Noga 2010; Francis-Floyd 2011; LePage et al. 2015). The diagnostic samples taken and how they are collected and processed can affect the results, so it is important to record details of the techniques used.

Skin Scrapes

One of the most useful, minimally invasive diagnostics in bony fish is a skin scrape. Depending on the size and activity of the fish, this can often be done without sedation. A clean coverslip or slide is placed at a ~45° angle to the skin and scraped in a cranial-caudal direction (Figure A6.11). The most common places to sample are under the pectoral fins, at the base of the dorsal fins, and across any visible lesions. Enough pressure should be applied to remove the external mucus layer and sometimes a few scales, but not enough to create lacerations or a deeper ulcer. The sample can then be gently smeared onto a slide with a drop of system water or water of similar salinity and temperature. Water of different salinity and temperature can affect

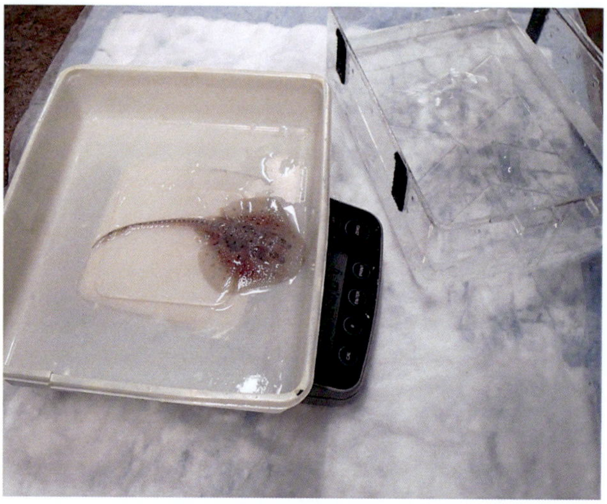

Figure A6.8 Obtaining a weight on a little skate (*Leucoraja erinacea*) under anesthesia. *Source*: Image courtesy of Catherine Hadfield, National Aquarium.

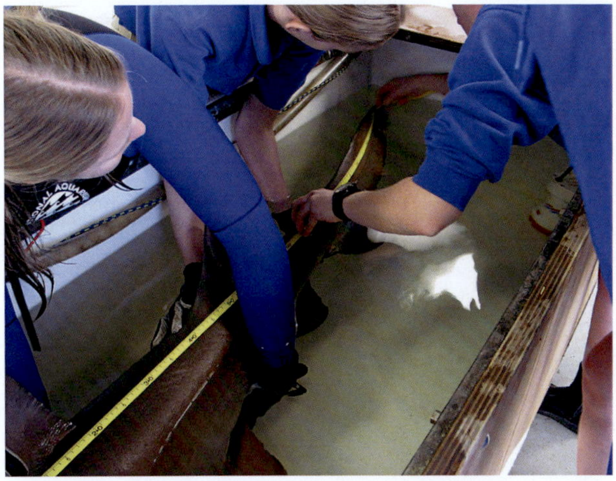

Figure A6.9 Measuring the total length on a sand tiger shark (*Carcharias taurus*) under manual restraint. *Source*: Image courtesy of Catherine Hadfield, National Aquarium.

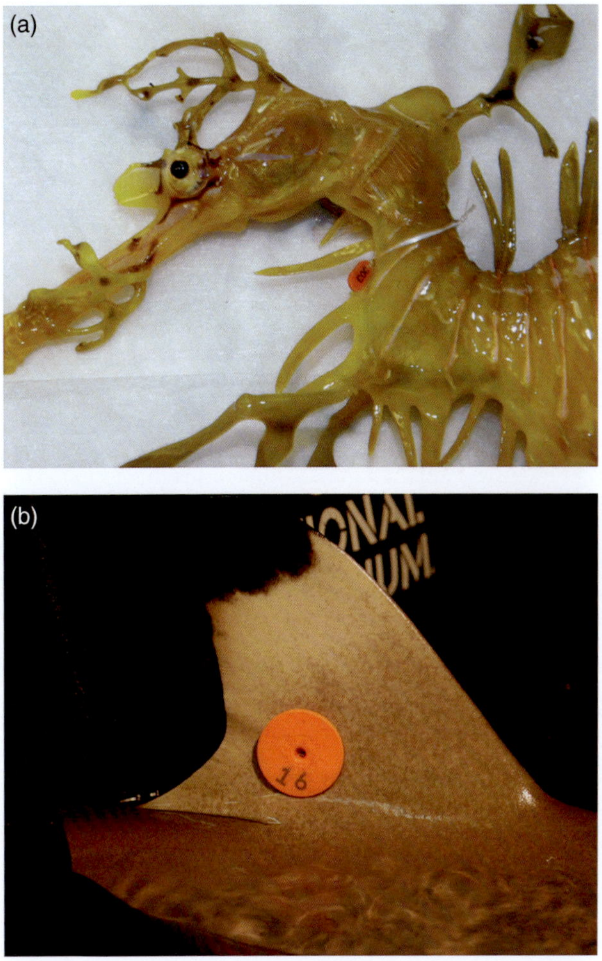

Figure A6.10 External tag tied loosely onto a leafy seadragon (*Phycodurus eques*) (a) and in the first dorsal fin of a blacktip reef shark (*Carcharhinus melanopterus*) (b). *Source*: Images courtesy of Catherine Hadfield, National Aquarium.

parasites and reduce diagnostic sensitivity and specificity. For larger parasites (e.g. copepods, leeches, and some monogeneans) it is often more practical to pull off a few parasites with forceps and put them onto a slide for identification. The slides should be examined as soon as possible under direct microscopy, beginning at low magnification (×4 objective = ×40 total magnification) and moving to high magnification (×40 objective = ×400 total magnification). It is important that the microscope condenser is low for direct cytologies (see Figure A9.1).

Normal findings are scant mucus and epithelial cells. Common abnormalities include increased mucus, ectoparasites (e.g. ciliates, dinoflagellates, monogeneans), abundant or abnormal bacteria (e.g. *Flavobacterium* spp.), oomycetes, fungal hyphae or spores, and abnormal cells (e.g. large cells typical of lymphocystis). A simplified key to common fish parasites is provided in Box A9.2 in Chapter A9. Common artifacts include air bubbles, pollen, diatoms or other algae, and salt crystals.

Gill Biopsies

Gill biopsies should be assessed in most sick fish. They should be collected under chemical restraint to minimize the risk of hemorrhage and ensure that a diagnostic sample is obtained. To collect the sample, the operculum or gill slit should be lifted to visualize the gills. Using clean fine scissors (e.g. iris scissors), a small section (1–3 mm) of the tips of three to five primary lamellae from one gill arch can be excised and placed on a slide (Figure A6.12). For species where the operculum or gill slit is not large enough to allow

Box A6.2 Common Infectious Diseases of Koi and Goldfish (*Cyprinidae*)

- Carp edema virus (CEV)
- Herpesviruses (carp pox, goldfish hematopoietic necrosis virus, koi herpesvirus)
- Lymphocystivirus
- Spring viremia of carp (SVC)
- Opportunistic bacterial infections, e.g. *Aeromonas*, *Flavobacterium* spp.
- Oomycetes
- Ciliates, e.g. *Ichthyophthirius multifiliis*, *Chilodonella* spp., *Heteropolaria* (previously *Epistylis*) spp.
- Monogeneans, e.g. *Dactylogyrus*, *Gyrodactylus* spp.
- Copepods, e.g. *Ergasilus*, *Lernaea* spp.
- Leeches
- Branchiurans, e.g. *Argulus* spp.
- Myxozoans, e.g. *Hoferellus carassii* (polycystic kidney disease)

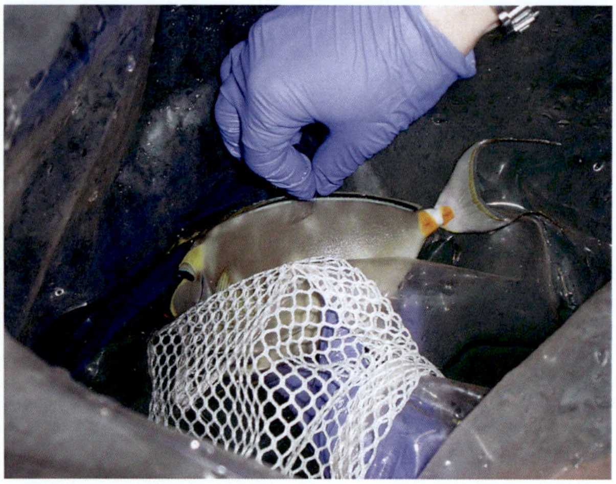

Figure A6.11 Skin scrape on a sedated orangespine unicornfish (*Naso lituratus*). *Source*: Image courtesy of Catherine Hadfield, National Aquarium.

sampling as described above, an endoscope, laryngoscope, or otoscope can be inserted into the gill cavity to guide forceps or long-handled scissors for a gill biopsy. In some fish, the opercular slit is too small to allow a gill biopsy without cutting the skin (e.g. seahorses, some blennies, and lumpsuckers). Once collected, a coverslip is useful to slide the filaments from the scissors onto a slide. A drop of system water (or water of similar salinity and temperature) and a coverslip should be added. The sample should be examined as soon as possible under direct microscopy, beginning at low magnification and moving to higher magnification. Oil immersion magnification may be needed to visualize small organisms like flagellates, microsporidia, and bacteria (×100 objective = ×1000 total magnification). It is important that the microscope condenser is low for direct cytologies. There may be bleeding from the gill biopsy site; this typically resolves without intervention, although it may be more severe in elasmobranchs.

Box A6.3 Common Infectious Diseases of Salmon and Trout (*Salmonidae*)

- Infectious hematopoietic necrosis virus
- Infectious pancreatic necrosis virus
- Infectious salmon anemia virus
- Salmonid alphavirus
- Viral hemorrhagic septicemia
- Piscine reovirus
- *Aeromonas salmonicida* (furunculosis and atypical)
- Motile aeromonad septicemia
- *Flavobacterium* and *Tenacibaculum* spp.
- *Francisella noatunensis* subsp. *noatunensis*
- *Piscirickettsia salmonis*
- *Renibacterium salmoninarum* (bacterial kidney disease)
- *Vibrio* and *Photobacterium* spp.
- *Weissella* spp.
- *Yersinia ruckeri* (enteric redmouth)
- Ciliates, e.g. *Ichthyophthirius multifiliis*
- Monogeneans, e.g. *Gyrodactylus* spp.
- Copepods, e.g. *Lepeophtheirus*, *Caligus* spp.
- Freshwater myxozoans, e.g. *Myxobolus cerebralis*, *Tetracapsula bryosalmonae*, *Ceratomyxa shasta*
- Saltwater myxozoans, e.g. *Kudoa thyrsites*, *Chloromyxum truttae*, *Henneguya salminicola*

Normal findings are uniform, dark red lamellae with straight cartilaginous supports and scant bacteria. Erythrocytes and some leukocytes are often seen coming from the cut surfaces. Common abnormalities include pallor, edema, hyperplasia, fusion, petechiation, telangiectasia (dilated blood vessels), increased mucus, ectoparasites (e.g. ciliates, dinoflagellates, monogeneans), endoparasites (e.g. nematodes, encysted parasites, blood flukes), gas emboli, granulomas, abundant or abnormal bacteria, oomycetes, fungal hyphae or spores, cartilage damage, and abnormal cells. A simplified key to common fish parasites is provided in Box A9.2.

Fin Biopsies

Fin biopsies are less common but should be done whenever fin lesions are noted in teleosts. A wedge-shaped biopsy is cut from the distal end of a translucent fin using suitable scissors. The tissue should be placed flat on a slide with a drop of system water (or water of similar salinity and temperature) and a coverslip. It should be examined immediately under direct microscopy, beginning at low magnification and moving to higher magnification. Oil immersion may be needed to visualize small organisms like flagellates and bacteria.

A normal fin biopsy in a bony fish shows translucent fin and fin rays with stellate chromatophores (Figure A9.4). Common abnormalities include increased mucus, erosions, ectoparasites (e.g. ciliates, dinoflagellates, monogeneans), gas emboli, abundant or abnormal bacteria, oomycetes, and fungal hyphae or spores. A simplified key to common fish parasites is provided in Box A9.2.

Fecal Collection

Fecal examination should be considered for fish in quarantine and fish with abnormal fecals, anorexia, coelomic distension, or pruritus. Fecal material can be collected from the water using a fine-mesh net or syringe. Fish will often defecate when caught or handled, so it is useful to look for fecal material in transport and restraint containers. If fecal material cannot be collected from the water, a cloacal or rectal wash can be done (Figure A6.13). An appropriately sized red rubber catheter (e.g. 3–5 Fr catheter for small fish, up to 10 Fr for large fish) should be attached to a syringe and loaded with 0.9% sterile saline at a volume of ~0.5 mL/kg. The tube should be lubricated then gently advanced into the anus and the saline gently infused, then withdrawn. If there is no visible material in the fluid, it is rarely worth evaluating. If there is visible particulate or fecal material, direct evaluation can identify parasites and cytologies can be used to assess enteric flora. Flotation techniques have not been evaluated in fish, but silver nitrate float solutions are likely to work for many metazoan ova.

Normal fecal material has undigestible food components (e.g. crustacean exoskeletons), scant bacteria, and rare protozoa. Common abnormalities include bacterial overgrowth (particularly when collected post-mortem), parasites (particularly flagellates and nematodes), and increased leukocytes or erythrocytes.

Diagnostic Imaging

Radiography in fish is particularly useful for evaluating dental and skeletal structures and swim bladders. Radiography plates should always be securely wrapped in plastic to prevent water damage. Images can be taken by removing the anesthetized fish from the water and placing it directly on the plate. In rare cases, radiographs may be taken of the fish in water (e.g. if anesthesia and handling are contraindicated). This can be done with a vertical beam and the fish in a shallow container of water, or with a horizontal beam with the fish in a narrow container (e.g. Ziplock®). However, shooting through water attenuates the signal and the images have less detail. Contrast studies can be carried out using barium or iodine compounds. More details are covered in Chapter A8.

Ultrasonography in fish is useful for evaluating coelomic structures (particularly the liver and reproductive tract) and any coelomic effusion. It is also useful for evaluating structures such as the heart and thyroid tissue in large fish, and the siphon sacs and clasper glands in male elasmobranchs. Image quality is usually excellent in elasmobranchs and scaleless teleosts, and ultrasound should be considered with every physical examination. Image quality is more variable in teleosts due to differences in scale anatomy. The choice of probes depends on the species being examined, but a 5–8 MHz transducer will provide sufficient penetration for most species. Water is an excellent conductor and ultrasound gel is only needed where water cannot be used. A plastic rectal sleeve or examination glove can be used to cover the probe to protect it from the effects of salt water and spines or scales. Gel can be placed within the glove to improve conduction. More details are covered in Chapter A8.

Box A6.4 Common Infectious Diseases of Ictalurid Catfish (*Ictaluridae*)

- Channel catfish virus (CCV)
- Motile aeromonad septicemia
- *Clostridium botulinum*
- *Edwardsiella ictaluri* (enteric septicemia of catfish), *E. tarda*, *E. piscicida*
- *Flavobacterium columnare*
- *Yersinia ruckeri*
- Oomycetes
- Branchiomycosis
- Ciliates, e.g. *Ichthyophthirius multifiliis*, trichodinids, *Ichthyobodo* spp.
- Monogeneans, e.g. *Dactylogyrus* spp.
- Digenes, e.g. *Bolbophorus* spp.
- Copepods, e.g. *Ergasilus*, *Lernaea* spp.
- Branchiurans, e.g. *Argulus* spp.
- Myxozoans, e.g. *Henneguya ictaluri* (proliferative gill disease)

Blood Collection

Our understanding of fish clinical hematology and biochemistry is in its infancy. It is most useful diagnostically when comparison values are available (e.g. same individual over time or from cohorts in the same habitat). Extrapolating across species, different environmental conditions, and different techniques should be done with caution.

The volume of blood taken should be <1% of the total body weight. In anemic or compromised fish, less should be taken. There is typically no skin preparation in fish to avoid damaging the mucus and skin, but a single swipe with a sterile 70% alcohol or 0.9% saline gauze may be used in elasmobranchs and a saline flush may be used in any fish.

The best site for blood collection depends on the species and animal size. In most bony fish, the ventral tail vessels are recommended. These can be accessed from a ventral or lateral approach. The size of the needle depends on the fish and the site, e.g. a 25 ga 1 in (2.5 cm) needle and 1 mL syringe will work for most fish <100 g, while a 19 ga 1.5 in (3.8 cm) needle may be needed for a teleost >5 kg. If using a ventral approach, the needle is inserted into the ventral midline of the caudal peduncle and advanced until it hits the ventral aspect of a vertebra or vertebral process (Figure A6.14a). If there is no blood in the hub, the needle is "walked" along the vertebrae using small movements

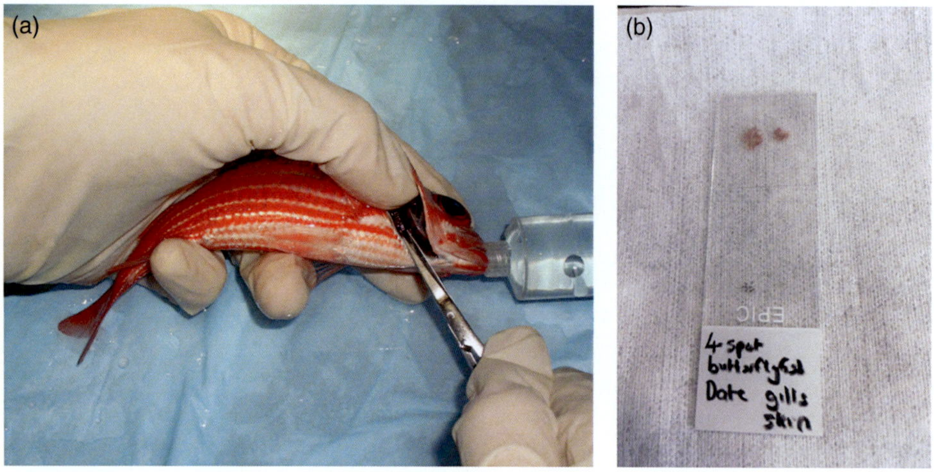

Figure A6.12 Gill biopsy being taken from a squirrelfish (*Holocentrus* spp.) (a) and skin and gill samples on a slide (b). *Source*: Images courtesy of Catherine Hadfield, National Aquarium.

until a flash of blood appears. If using the lateral approach, the needle should be inserted just below the lateral line at a 45° angle. The needle should be advanced until it hits the ventral surface of the vertebrae, it may need to be "walked" cranially/caudally or dorsally/ventrally to find a vessel. This method is often better for large bony fish with laterally compressed peduncles, because the depth needed for the ventral approach can be prohibitive. Other possible sites in bony fish include the gill arch (Figure A6.14b), the dorsal aorta within the oral cavity (Figure A6.14c), the cloaca, the retro-orbital sinus, or the heart, which can be accessed from the ventral midline (Figure A6.14a) or from the opercular space, although cardiac puncture is often reserved for terminal procedures. For small bony fish, blood flow can be slow and it is often useful to heparinize the syringe prior to obtaining the sample, although this may affect hematology results (Johnson et al. 2014).

In elasmobranchs, the ventral tail vessels are recommended as hematology and blood gas results are likely to be more reliable (Mylniczenko et al. 2006; Naples et al. 2012). This site is typically accessed with the animal in dorsal recumbency, although for rays with long tails, it may be possible to curl the tail up gently to access the vessel. When approaching the ventral tail artery/vein, the needle needs to be at a 90° angle on the ventral midline (Figure A6.15a, b, e, f). In skates and rays, the needle needs to be advanced through cartilage prior to reaching the vessel. In species where the ventral tail may be inaccessible, such as large sharks, rays, and sawfish, the sinus caudal to the dorsal fin or the pectoral fin/radial vessels can be used. The dorsal fin sinus runs paramedial and is most accessible at the caudal insertion point of the dorsal fins. The needle should be at a 30° angle and redirected while applying negative pressure until blood is obtained (Figure A6.15c, d). The pectoral fin vessels can be approached dorsally or ventrally (Figure A6.15g, h). In batoids, they run parallel to the lines of cartilage. The needle is inserted at a 90° angle between the pectoral fin cartilages, to half the depth of the pectoral fin, then walked cranially to caudally while applying negative pressure. This site is used in whale sharks (*Rhincodon typus*) under human care by swimming alongside a free-swimming shark (Ueda et al. 2017). Butterfly needles or extension sets are particularly useful for the dorsal fin sinus and pectoral fin vessels (Cusack et al. 2016).

Box A6.5 Common Infectious Diseases of Tilapia (*Oreochromis*, *Tilapia* spp.)

Tilapia Lake virus
Betanodaviruses
Motile aeromonad septicemia
Flavobacterium columnare
Francisella noatunensis subsp. *noatunensis*
Streptococcus iniae, *S. agalactiae*
Oomycetes
Ciliates, e.g. *Ichthyophthirius multifiliis*, trichodinids, *Ichthyobodo* spp.
Monogeneans, e.g. *Dactylogyrus* spp.
Copepods, e.g. *Ergasilus*, *Lernaea* spp.
Branchiurans, e.g. *Argulus* spp.

Box A6.6 Common Infectious Diseases of Zebrafish (*Danio rerio*)

Opportunistic bacterial infections, e.g. *Aeromonas*, *Pseudomonas*, *Flavobacterium* spp.
Mycobacterium spp.
Microsporidians, e.g. *Pseudoloma neurophila*, *Pleistophora hyphessobryconis*
Dinoflagellates, e.g. *Piscinoodinium* spp.
Nematodes, e.g. *Pseudocapillaria tomentosa*
Myxozoans, e.g. *Myxidium* spp.

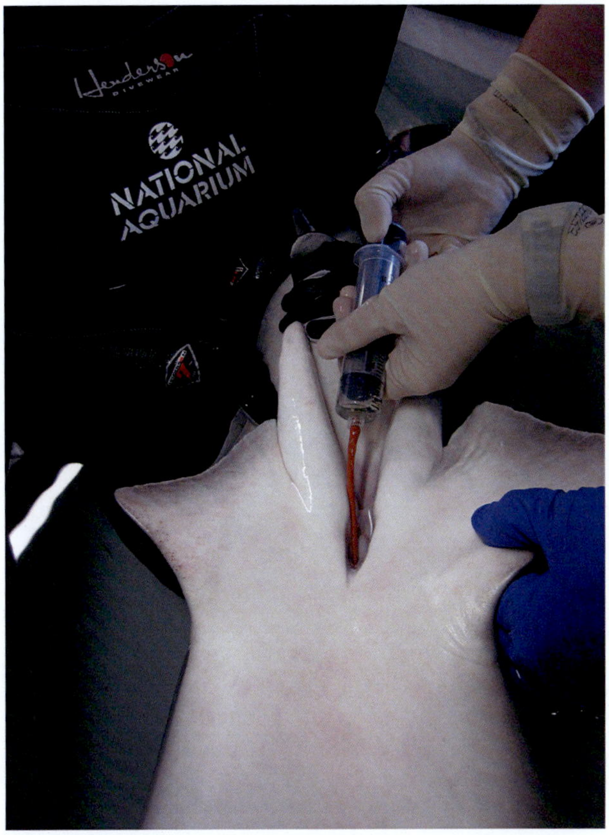

Figure A6.13 Cloacal wash on a male sandbar shark (*Carcharhinus plumbeus*). *Source*: Image courtesy of Catherine Hadfield, National Aquarium.

A new site has recently been reported for rays: the mesopterygial vein along the ventrolateral aspect of the metapterygium cartilage adjacent to the coelomic cavity (Westmoreland et al. 2019).

Careful handling of fish blood is required to ensure accurate results. If blood cultures are indicated, a blood sample without anticoagulant should be placed in suitable media first. Blood gas analyses should be run next. Several blood smears should be made swiftly, before the rest of the blood is put into microhematocrit and anticoagulant tubes. EDTA and heparin are both effective, but EDTA can lyse cells if ratios are incorrect and can affect the viscosity of stingray blood, so heparin is the more common anticoagulant. Chemistries should be run as soon as possible after collection. If it is not possible to run the sample within six hours, it should be separated and the plasma frozen at −80°C (−112°F). Hematology should also be run soon after collection. A Natt–Herrick stain is recommended for a complete blood count in bony fish; this can be modified for the high osmolality of marine elasmobranchs (Arnold 2005). Even in anticoagulant, fish blood samples cannot survive overnight shipping to a hematology lab. If hematology cannot be run within six hours, samples can be preserved in 10% neutral buffered formalin (NBF) at a 1:5 ratio (e.g. 50 μL of heparinized blood and 200 μL of 10% NBF); hematology samples can then be stored at room temperature for prolonged periods (Arnold et al. 2014). Hematological and biochemical parameters are reviewed in Chapter A7.

Musculoskeletal Impression Smears, Aspirates, or Biopsies

Cutaneous and musculoskeletal masses are common in fish. As with terrestrial species, diagnosis is often based on aspirates or biopsy for cytology, cultures, and histology.

Impression smears can provide valuable diagnostic information, particularly if the mass has ruptured or ulcerated. A clean slide is pressed directly onto the mass or lesion and lifted without smearing the sample, then allowed to air-dry. Multiple samples can be obtained for various cytology preparations.

A fine-needle aspirate of a mass can be done using an appropriately sized needle on a 3–6 mL syringe. There is usually no skin preparation, but a sterile 0.9% saline flush may be used (Sladsky and Clarke 2016). One technique is

Box A6.7 Common Infectious Diseases of Tropical Marine Teleosts

Lymphocystivirus
Opportunistic bacterial infections, e.g. *Vibrio*, *Pseudomonas* spp.
Ciliates, e.g. *Cryptocaryon irritans*, *Brooklynella hostilis*, *Amyloodinium ocellatum*, scuticociliates
Monogeneans, e.g. *Neobenedenia*, *Gyrodactylus* spp.
Digenes
Turbellaria

Box A6.8 Common Infectious Diseases of Seahorses, Pipefish, and Sea Dragons (*Syngnathidae*)

Opportunistic bacterial infections, e.g. *Vibrio*, *Aeromonas*, *Tenacibaculum* spp.
Mycobacterium spp.
Exophiala spp.
Fusarium spp.
Microsporidians, e.g. *Glugea heraldi*
Dinoflagellates and flagellates, e.g. *Ichthyobodo necator*, *Cryptobia*, *Amyloodinium* spp.
Ciliates, e.g. scuticociliates
Monogeneans, e.g. *Gyrodactylus* spp.
Apicomplexans, e.g. *Cryptosporidium* spp.

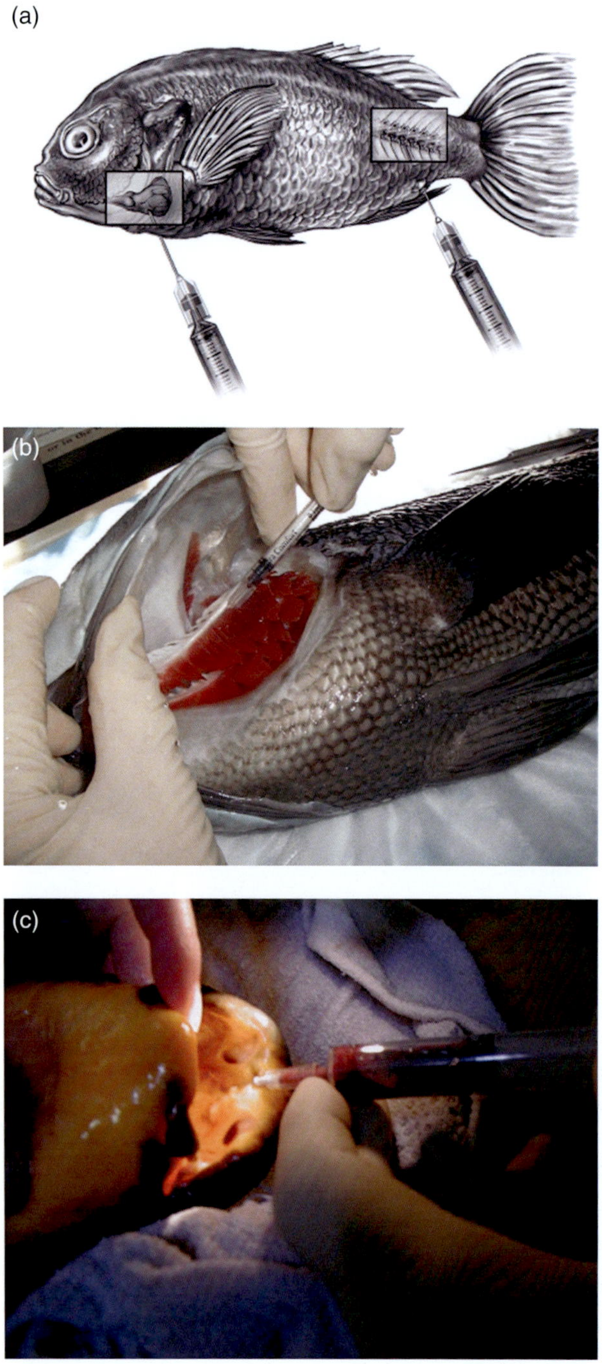

Figure A6.14 Sketch of venipuncture from the ventral tail vein and heart (a) and image of venipuncture from the gill arch (b) and dorsal aorta (c). *Source*: Image (a) courtesy of Sarah Faris; copyright reserved. Other images courtesy of Catherine Hadfield, National Aquarium, and Natalie Mylniczenko, Disney's Animals, Science and Environment.

to insert the needle into the lesion alone, then move it in multiple directions to obtain cells. After the needle is removed, a syringe is used to push air through the needle and expel the cellular material onto a slide. It should be gently smeared using perpendicular movement against a second slide prior to air-drying. Another option is to insert the needle while attached to the syringe and apply intermittent suction to remove cellular material. The syringe can then be used to expel the contents of the mass onto a slide prior to smearing and air-drying.

Routine Romanowsky stains (e.g. Dif-quik) can provide information on the cellular composition and presence of bacteria, fungi, or parasites. Gram stains are useful in characterizing bacteria (Table A9.1). Acid-fast stains, such as Ziehl–Neelsen, are commonly used in fish because of the frequency of disease due to acid-fast positive organisms such as *Mycobacterium* and *Nocardia* spp., myxozoans, and microsporidians (Table A9.2). When evaluating stained impression smears on microscopy, high magnification is required (100× oil objective = 1000× magnification) and the condenser should be high.

A biopsy is often needed to obtain a definitive diagnosis for a mass. A complete excisional biopsy is preferred since it has the potential to be both diagnostic and curative. However, where excision is not possible, an incisional biopsy can be performed for diagnosis. Biopsies should be taken under anesthesia and the site should be prepared as described above. Depending on the location, options include a punch biopsy, tru-cut biopsy, or standard surgical biopsy. Margins should be included where possible. Sections can be fixed in 10% formalin, electron microscopy fixative, and frozen at −80°C (−112°F). Biopsy sites in fish are typically left to heal by second intention.

Box A6.9 Polymerase Chain Reaction (PCR/RT-PCR) Tests That Are Often Commercially Available for Fish

Epizootic hematopoietic necrosis virus
Infectious hematopoietic necrosis virus
Infectious pancreatic necrosis virus
Infectious salmon anemia virus
Koi herpesvirus
Largemouth bass virus
Red seabream iridoviral disease
Salmonid alphavirus
Spring viremia of carp virus
Viral hemorrhagic septicemia
Clostridium tetani
Flavobacterium psychrophilum
Mycobacterium spp.
Renibacterium salmoninarum (bacterial kidney disease)
Yersinia ruckeri (enteric redmouth)
Aphanomyces ulcerans (epizootic ulcerative syndrome)
Loma salmonae
Myxobolus cerebralis (whirling disease)

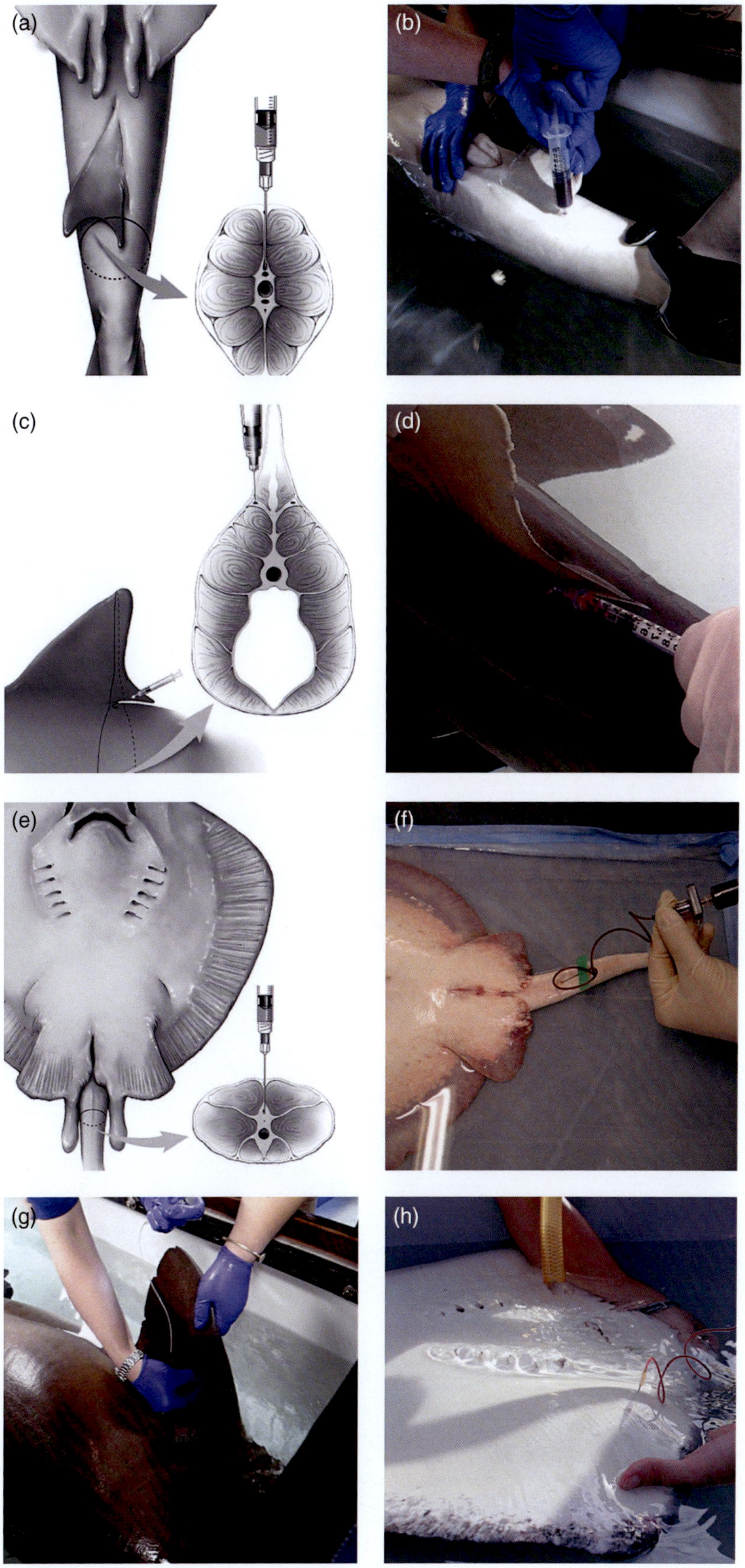

Figure A6.15 Venipuncture options in elasmobranchs: ventral tail vessel in a shark (a, b); dorsal fin sinus in a shark (c, d); ventral tail vessel in a ray (e, f); and pectoral fin/radial vessel in a shark (g) and ray (h). *Source*: Images (a, c, e) courtesy of Kimberly Knoper, copyright reserved. Other images courtesy of Catherine Hadfield, National Aquarium.

Coelomic Aspirates or Biopsies

If coelomic effusion is suspected, a coelomic aspirate is recommended to determine the type of fluid and look for pathogens. Ultrasound guidance is recommended, but the procedure is commonly done without. An appropriately sized butterfly needle (e.g. 25–22 ga) can be inserted at the dependent portion of the coelom, often paramedial and cranial to the vent; the left is recommended for elasmobranchs to avoid the spiral valve. If the amount of sampled material retrieved is too small to be diagnostic, a coelomic wash can be performed. Sterile saline, up to 5 mL/kg body weight and at patient temperature, can be introduced and then aspirated. Fluid can be evaluated on direct microscopy and stained cytologies, and a refractometer and urine dipstick can be used to obtain specific gravity and protein estimates. The fluid can be characterized as inflammatory, noninflammatory, hemorrhagic, or neoplastic, and may show bacteria, fungi, or parasites (e.g. *Eimeria* spp.).

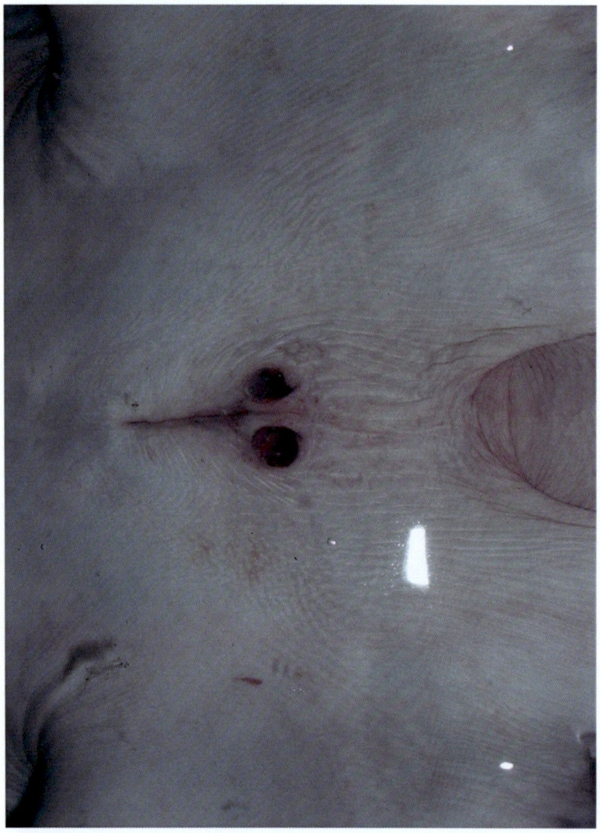

Figure A6.16 Inflamed abdominal pores in a southern stingray (*Hypanus americanus*). *Source*: Image courtesy of Catherine Hadfield, National Aquarium.

In elasmobranchs, it is possible to sample coelomic effusion by passing a red rubber catheter through the abdominal pores and aspirating the coelomic fluid. Indications include coelomic effusion and inflammation of the pores (Figure A6.16). It is not known if this method causes any physiological problems and it should probably be used with caution if there are no clinical signs.

If coelomic masses or organomegaly are suspected, aspirates or biopsies are often indicated. These can be percutaneous, endoscopic, or surgical. Details are covered in Chapter A11.

Swim bladder aspirates are common in bony fish in response to hyper- or hypoinflation of the swim bladder. Ultrasound or radiographic guidance is recommended, but the procedure is commonly done without. A lateral approach is used, typically at the widest part of the body, just ventral to the lateral line. Needle size should be suitable for the likely depth (e.g. most 2 kg perch-like fish need a 2 in (5 cm) needle). Negative pressure should be maintained until air is reached. The procedure can be used diagnostically and therapeutically.

Periocular and Ocular Aspirates

Ocular disease is common in bony fish, particularly exophthalmos and buphthalmos. It can be useful to collect aspirates of the retrobulbar or intraocular space to evaluate and treat the distension. Aspirates should be obtained under sedation to avoid damaging ocular structures. The area should be prepped by rinsing with sterile artificial tears or 0.9% saline. To obtain a retrobulbar sample, a 25 ga needle or butterfly needle on a 1–6 mL syringe can be inserted into periocular tissue, avoiding the globe. To obtain an intraocular aspirate from the anterior or posterior chamber, a 27–25 ga needle on a 1–3 mL syringe can be inserted into the chamber, avoiding the iris, lens, and retina. Iatrogenic vitreous hemorrhage may be seen following aspirates from the posterior chamber. The material aspirated may be air, fluid, or cellular material. These aspirates can be evaluated under direct microscopy and stained cytologies. Abnormalities include leukocytes, neoplastic cells, bacteria, and parasites.

Cerebrospinal Fluid Collection

Cerebrospinal fluid (CSF) collection is reported in elasmobranchs, as the cranial vault is cartilaginous and the CSF volume is large. Indications include central neurologic signs (e.g. circling, dullness). A suitably sized needle can be inserted in the dorsal midline, slightly rostral to the eyes, and perpendicular to the skin. Ultrasound-guidance may be effective in some species. Normal CSF in elasmobranchs is slightly serosanguinous. Abnormalities include abundant leukocytes, bacteria, and parasites.

Egg or Sperm Collection

Eggs (roe) and sperm (milt) are collected commonly from cultured teleosts in a process known as stripping. This is generally done under anesthesia. The cloaca or urogenital opening should be rinsed and dried prior to stripping as anesthetic can damage the gametes and water can activate the semen, shortening the life span of the sperm. One hand is used to apply pressure to the coelom in a cranial to caudal direction, which results in expulsion of the gametes if the fish is at the correct reproductive stage. Environmental changes and hormone protocols can be used to help induce spawning (Mylonas and Zohar 2000; Islami et al. 2017). Sperm collection has been reported in some sharks, rays, and skates following catheterization of the urogenital papilla (Daly and Jones 2017). While assisted reproductive techniques in elasmobranchs are in their infancy, they play an important role in our expanding conservation programs.

Commercial Laboratories

The choice of diagnostic laboratory is important. Laboratories that specialize in fish are more likely to have suitable media, temperature protocols, cell lines, and molecular tests than high-throughput domestic animal laboratories. Equipment and quality control also vary across laboratories, and results from one may not be comparable with results from another.

Common tests offered by commercial fish laboratories include bacterial and fungal culture, virus isolation, histology, fluorescent antibody tests, and polymerase chain reaction (PCR) tests. These are typically aimed at major pathogens in cultured species (Box A6.9). Diagnostic techniques for noninfectious diseases are often extrapolated from other species (e.g. hematology, total thyroxine). However, a laboratory with experience in fish medicine will try to adapt techniques for the relevant taxa.

It is important to check with the laboratory prior to sampling to discuss the case, differentials, and their sampling recommendations. Some of the laboratories in the United States with expertise in fish can be found in Appendix 3: *Fish Diagnostic Laboratories.*

References

Arnold, J.E. (2005). Hematology of the sandbar shark, *Carcharhinus plumbeus*: standardization of complete blood count techniques for elasmobranchs. *Veterinary Clinical Pathology* 34: 115–123.

Arnold, J.E., Matsche, M.A., and Rosemary, K. (2014). Preserving whole blood in formalin extends the specimen stability period for manual cell counts for fish. *Veterinary Clinical Pathology* 43: 613–620.

Carter, K.M., Woodley, C.M., and Brown, R.S. (2011). A review of tricaine methanesulfonate for anesthesia of fish. *Review of Fish Biology and Fisheries* 21: 51–59.

Cusack, L., Field, C.L., Hoopes, L. et al. (2016). Comparison of pre- and postquarantine blood chemistry and hematology values from wild-caught cownose rays (*Rhinoptera bonasus*). *Journal of Zoo and Wildlife Medicine* 47: 493–500.

Daly, J. and Jones, R. (2017). The use of reproductive technologies in breeding programs for elasmobranchs in aquaria. In: *Elasmobranch Husbandry Manual II: Recent Advances in the Care of Sharks, Rays and their Relative*, 2e (eds. M. Smith, D. Warmolts, D. Thoney, et al.), 255–262. Columbus: Ohio Biological Survey, Inc.

Flemming, G.J., Heard, D.J., Floyd, R.F., and Riggs, A. (2003). Evaluation of propofol and medetomidine-ketamine for short-term immobilization of Gulf of Mexico sturgeon (*Acipenser oxyrinchus desotoi*). *Journal of Zoo and Wildlife Medicine* 34: 153–158.

Francis-Floyd, R. (2011). Mycobacterial infections in fish. *Southern Regional Aquaculture Center* 4706: 1–12.

Henningsen, A.D. (1994). Tonic immobility in 12 elasmobranchs: use as an aid in captive husbandry. *Zoo Biology* 13: 325–332.

Islami, M.F., Sudrajat, A.O., and Carman, O. (2017). Induction of maturation and ovulation of red fin shark fish *Epalzeorhynchos frenatus* in non-spawning season. *International Journal of Fisheries and Aquatic Studies* 5: 418–424.

Javahery, S., Nekoubin, H., and Moradiu, A.H. (2012). Effect of anesthesia with clove oil in fish (review). *Fish Physiology and Biochemistry* 38: 1545–1552.

Johnson, J.G., Nevarez, J.G., and Beaufrère, H. (2014). Research effect of manually preheparinized syringes on packed cell volume and total solids in blood samples collected from American alligators (*Alligator mississippiensis*). *Journal of Exotic Pet Medicine* 23: 142–146.

LePage, V., Young, J., Dutton, C.J. et al. (2015). Diseases of captive yellow seahorse *Hippocampus kuda* Bleeker, pot-bellied seahorse *Hippocampus abdominalis* (Lesson) and weedy seadragon *Phyllopteryx taeniolatus* (Lacépède). *Journal of Fish Diseases* 38: 439–450.

Matthews, J.L. (2004). Common diseases of laboratory zebrafish. *Methods in Cell Biology* 77: 617–643.

Mylniczenko, N.D., Curtis, E.W., Wilborn, R.E., and Young, F.A. (2006). Differences in hematocrit of blood samples obtained from two venipuncture sites in sharks. *American Journal of Veterinary Research* 67: 1861–1864.

Mylonas, C.C. and Zohar, Y. (2000). Use of GnRHa-delivery systems for the control of reproduction in fish. *Reviews in Fish Biology and Fisheries* 10: 463–491.

Naples, L.M., Mylniczenko, N.D., Zachariah, T.T. et al. (2012). Evaluation of critical care blood analytes assessed with a point-of-care portable blood analyzer in wild and aquarium-housed elasmobranchs and the influence of phlebotomy site on results. *Journal of the American Veterinary Medical Association* 241: 117–125.

Neiffer, D.L. and Stamper, M.A. (2009). Fish sedation, anesthesia, analgesia and euthanasia: considerations, methods and types of drugs. *Institute for Laboratory Animal Research Journal* 50: 343–360.

Noga, E.J. (ed.) (2010). *Fish Diseases. Diagnosis and Treatment*. Ames, IA: Wiley-Blackwell.

Reavill, D.R. (2006). Common diagnostic and clinical techniques for fish. *Veterinary Clinics of North America Exotic Animal Practice* 9: 223–235.

Roberts-Sweeney, H.E. (2016). Anatomy and disorders of the oral cavity of ornamental fish. *Veterinary Clinics: Exotic Animal Practice* 19: 669–687.

Sladsky, K.K. and Clarke, E.O. (2016). Fish surgery: presurgical preparation and common surgical procedures. *Veterinary Clinics of North America Exotic Animal Practice* 19: 55–76.

Ueda, K., Yanagisawa, M., Murakumo, K. et al. (2017). Physical examination, blood sampling, and sedation of large elasmobranchs. In: *Elasmobranch Husbandry Manual II: Recent Advances in the Care of Sharks, Rays and their Relative*, 2e (eds. M. Smith, D. Warmolts, D. Thoney, et al.), 255–262. Columbus: Ohio Biological Survey, Inc.

Westmoreland, L.H., Archibald, K.E., Christiansen, E.F. et al. (2019). The mesopterygial vein: a reliable venipuncture site for intravascular access in batoids. *Journal of Zoo and Wildlife Medicine* 50: 369–374.

A7

Clinical Pathology and Ancillary Diagnostics

Alvin C. Camus and Melinda S. Camus

University of Georgia, Athens, GA, USA

Introduction

Veterinarians and technical staff can gain useful diagnostic information from pre- and postmortem examinations performed on fish "in-house." These may include cytology, hematology, and biochemistry tests. In addition, fish diagnostic services are available through a number of federal and state agencies, veterinary schools, and private sources. In all cases, the information gained must be considered in association with the signalment, history (including environmental conditions and husbandry), clinical signs, and results of other diagnostic tests.

For most fish species, laboratory results from clinically healthy animals for comparison are limited. In many cases, the effects of methodology and sample handling remain poorly understood and caution should be exercised when attempting to extrapolate information from other, particularly mammalian, species. Diagnostic testing is complicated by the large numbers of agents that affect fish and idiosyncrasies of their identification or culture. Also, few fish diseases produce pathognomonic lesions, while some produce no lesions at all. Consequently, no single diagnostic modality may be adequate and a multifaceted approach is often required to make informed clinical decisions. To maximize diagnostic success and minimize costs, it is critical to understand the uses and limitations of available methodologies and technologies, as well as appropriate sample selection, processing, and preservation.

Reference Materials in Fish Medicine

There is a lack of appropriately derived reference intervals for most diagnostic tests in fish, which can be frustrating and limit the utility of laboratory data. Ideally, reference intervals are derived by the laboratory at which testing is done from a population of at least 120 members of the same species, under the same husbandry conditions, using the same instrumentation. This is virtually impossible for most fish species, due to the low number of clinically normal specimens available for testing and the small blood volumes associated with some species. The American Society for Veterinary Clinical Pathology (ASVCP) has guidelines that are helpful in deriving reference intervals that account for these limitations (Friedrichs et al. 2012).

When reference intervals are unavailable from the testing laboratory, online databases (e.g. IVIS – *International Veterinary Information Service*) or the primary or secondary literature may provide additional information. Extreme caution must be taken when using these values, as many were derived erroneously, with values from different analyzers, samples collected from animals in different life stages or husbandry conditions, and/or from a very low number of animals. When assessing the potential value of reference intervals, it is good to critically evaluate the methods from which they were derived to assess statistical analysis, treatment of outliers, the number of reference individuals, the methodology used, and the associated

Clinical Guide to Fish Medicine, First Edition. Edited by Catherine A. Hadfield and Leigh Ann Clayton.

confidence intervals. Well-constructed reference interval studies include those of Tripathi et al. for koi (*Cyprinus carpio koi*) and Hrubec et al. for striped bass (*Morone* hybrids) and tilapia (*Oreochromis* hybrids) (Hrubec et al. 1996, 2000; Tripathi et al. 2004). Where insufficient reference intervals are available, comparison with healthy animals of the same species housed in the same conditions using the same methodology, or examining trends over time, can be helpful in interpreting laboratory data (Flatland et al. 2018).

As with quantitative data, there is a paucity of information regarding the microscopic appearance of normal fish tissues and cell types in hematologic, cytologic, and histologic preparations, particularly when uncommon species are involved. The primary literature often serves as reference material for cytologic specimens, although case reports often focus on abnormal rather than normal findings. Enlisting the services of pathologists familiar with fish and their associated pathologies is advised.

Overall, it is important for clinicians to exercise good judgment when interpreting results and be fully aware of the limitations in diagnostic testing to avoid over-interpretation.

Wet Mount Examinations

Wet mounts are probably the most common diagnostic modality used in fish medicine. Wet mounts involve placing a small sample on a slide, adding a suitable solution, then compressing the sample with a cover slip for evaluation without staining (direct microscopy). The choice of solution is important, as parasites can lose motility, become distorted, or die when exposed to inappropriate salinities. It is important to use freshwater or salt water for the evaluation of freshwater and marine ectoparasites, respectively. Ideally the water would be from the system of origin and of a similar temperature, although the microscope light provides significant warming. For samples from internal organs, physiologic saline is recommended.

Although a major expenditure, a high-quality binocular microscope is an essential piece of equipment for fish diagnostics. It should be equipped with 4, 10, 20, 40, and 100× objectives, a 10× ocular, and ideally a digital camera. Evaluation of wet mounts is facilitated by lowering the microscope condenser or flipping it out of the light path if the microscope has a swing-in type (Figure A7.1). Partially closing the iris diaphragm will also improve visualization by increasing contrast between organisms and background.

Wet mounts are especially useful in the identification of parasites, particularly when the observation of motility is helpful diagnostically. Wet mounts can also provide information on the presence of other pathogens (e.g. bacteria, fungi, oomycetes), abnormal cells or cellular structures (e.g. granulomas), and tissue changes (e.g. congestion).

Several factors can increase the risk of inaccurate results and false negatives on wet mounts. In particular, fresh samples are critical to accurate diagnoses and slides should be examined immediately after collection. Certain parasites may leave a host after its death or die themselves and become grossly distorted by osmotic forces, complicating identification (Figure A7.2). Conversely, environmental saprophytes (e.g. bacteria, oomycetes, scuticociliates) can proliferate after death of the host leading to misinterpretation. Certain parasites, particularly monogeneans, preferentially inhabit specific sites on a host and can be missed unless multiple sites are sampled (Buchmann and Lindenstrøm 2002).

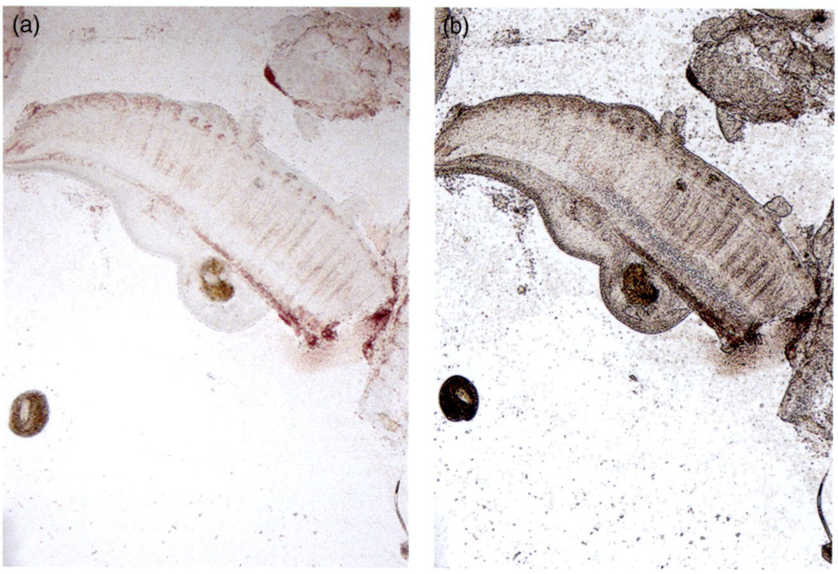

Figure A7.1 Direct microscopy of a gill clip wet mount demonstrating *Ichthyophthirius multifiliis* trophozoites in a channel catfish (*Ictalurus punctatus*) viewed with the iris diaphragm open or condenser raised (a) and with the diaphragm partially closed or the condenser lowered (b). 100×.

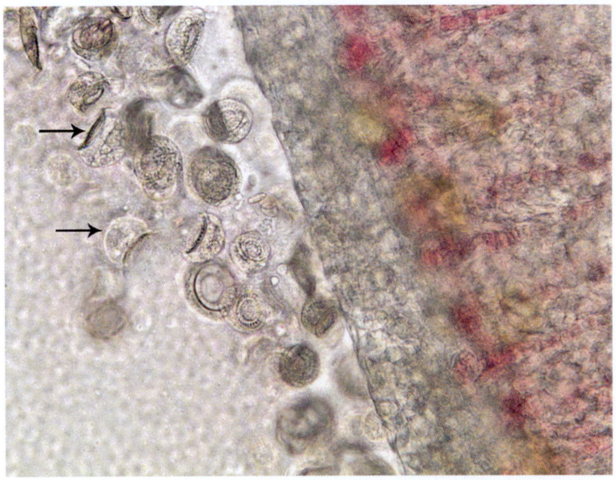

Figure A7.2 Postmortem distortion of trichodinids seen on direct microscopy of a gill clip from a channel catfish (*Ictalurus punctatus*). The protozoans have begun to die, imbibe water, and swell (arrows). 400×.

Skin Scrapes

Wet mount preparations of skin scrapes are commonly used in fish, particularly bony fish. It is important that the sample is spread out beneath the coverslip. A few scales and mucus should be collected with the scrape, but overly thick samples can obscure pathogens. Skin scrapes are particularly useful for identifying ectoparasites, which commonly include ciliates (e.g. *Cryptocaryon irritans*, *Ichthyophthirius multifiliis*, trichodinids, scuticociliates), dinoflagellates (e.g. *Amyloodinium ocellatum*, *Piscinoodinium* spp.), monogeneans, leeches, copepods, and branchiurans (e.g. *Argulus* spp.). Examples of other diseases or agents that can be tentatively identified on skin scrapes include columnaris, caused by *Flavobacterium columnare*, oomycetes (e.g. *Saprolegnia* spp.), and the hyperplastic cells characteristic of lymphocystis disease (Figure A7.3).

Gill Biopsies/Gill Clips

When preparing gill clips, distal portions of filaments should be clipped far enough from the arch to be seen separately on the microscope slide (Figure A7.4a). Do not attempt to view entire arches with filaments attached or allow filaments to lie adjacent to or on top of one other (Figure A7.4b). It is also important to avoid overly thick samples where filaments are too large to allow the solution to surround them. In normal fresh samples, gill lamellae appear as a series of sharply defined lines or plate-like structures. Interlamellar spaces should be free of tissue debris and excess mucus. In the filament, a central cartilage rod is bordered by marginal arterioles and an epithelial layer (Figure A7.5). Common pathologic changes include swelling and hyperplasia of the lamellar epithelium, which can fill interlamellar spaces resulting in clubbing of entire filaments. Other changes include congestion, hemorrhage, telangiectasia (lamellar aneurysms), excess mucus production, necrosis, and a host of parasites (e.g. sessile ciliates, Figure A7.6). It should be remembered that gill tissues deteriorate rapidly after death, particularly when fish are allowed to remain in water postmortem. The resultant autolysis can mimic many of the previously mentioned pathologic changes.

Certain cells seen on gill biopsies can be mistaken for parasites or other cell types. One example is the eosinophilic granular cell (EGC) or coarse eosinophilic granulocyte (CEG). Considered a mammalian mast cell equivalent, these cells should not be misidentified as a protozoan or an eosinophil.

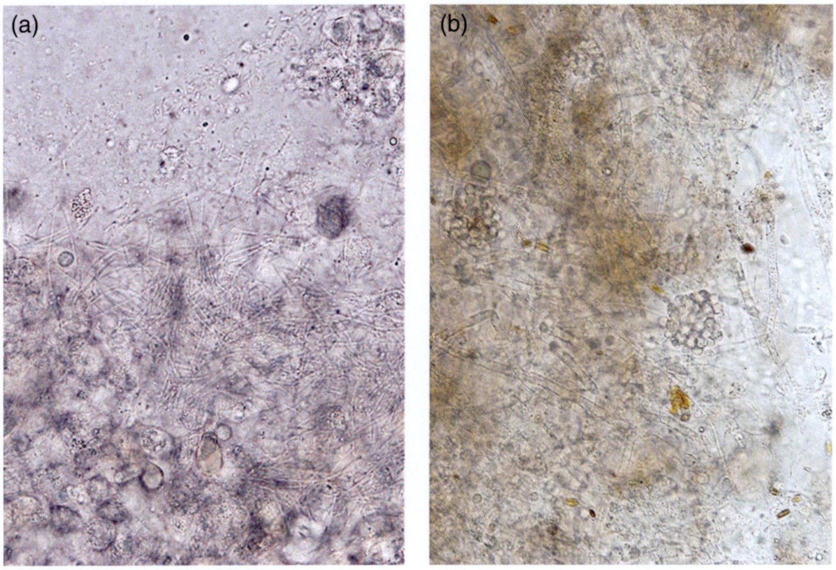

Figure A7.3 Wet mount of an ulcerative skin lesion in a channel catfish (*Ictalurus punctatus*) showing abundant long, slender bacterial rods typical of *Flavobacterium columnare* (a) and in a bluegill (*Lepomis macrochirus*) showing aseptate, branching oomycete hyphae and sporangia suggestive of *Aphanomyces invadans*.

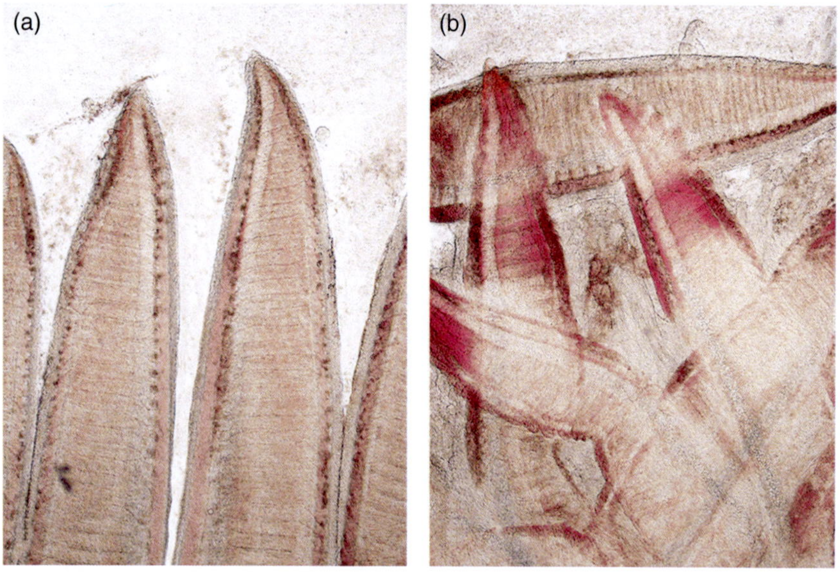

Figure A7.4 Wet mounts of gill clips that are well-made with individualized primary filaments (a), and crowded, overlapping filaments that hinder interpretation (b).

In cytologic and histologic samples, tissue-associated EGCs have abundant, large, round cytoplasmic granules and eccentric ovoid nuclei (Figure A7.7). The granules are intensely eosinophilic on cytologic and histologic stains (Reite 1997; Reite and Evensen 2006). In contrast, eosinophils are smaller cells, with smaller, less intensely staining granules. Another cell type is the rodlet cell. Encountered between epithelial cells lining tubular lumens and other sites, including the gills, these flask-shaped cells have eosinophilic, apical rods with basal bulbs and a basilar nucleus. Rodlet cells may be an inflammatory cell, possessing secretory granules (Figure A7.8) (Reite and Evensen 2006).

Fin Biopsies/Fin Clips

Fin clips should be placed flat on slides and manually spread to eliminate folds and tissue overlap. The same general considerations and pathologic criteria used to evaluate gill samples are applicable to fin clips. In addition, fin biopsy samples contain dendritic pigment cell types with branched tree-like projections (Figure A7.9). Special attention should be paid to the free margin of the fin clip, which can often appear tattered or scalloped as a result of tissue loss and necrosis.

Fecal Wet Mounts

Fecal wet mounts are most frequently used to identify endoparasites, including protozoans and metazoans (adults and eggs) (Figure A7.10). Samples may be obtained by various methods, including gastrointestinal mucosal scrapings collected at necropsy. Compared to mammals, the intestinal tracts of teleosts contain relatively few bacteria (Lumsden 2006). While high bacterial numbers can indicate enteritis, this is more commonly a reflection of postmortem autolysis. If enteritis is suspected, stained cytologic preparations should be evaluated for the presence of inflammatory cells and phagocytized bacteria. Evaluation of fecal samples can also be confounded by the presence of commensal organisms (e.g. opalines) and artifacts (e.g. pollen grains, eggs of ingested crustaceans).

Tissue Wet Mounts/Squash Preparations

Wet mounts can be made from any tissue specimen (e.g. biopsy of a mass), but are commonly performed during postmortem examinations on major organs (e.g. liver, spleen, kidney) and grossly abnormal tissues. Samples should be small (~1 mm^3) and significant pressure may be needed to produce a thin sample. Normal samples of parenchymal organs should be homogeneous and include typical components of the particular tissue (e.g. tubules and glomeruli in the caudal kidney). Commonly encountered abnormalities include granulomas (e.g. mycobacteriosis) and parasitic agents with histozoic development, including microsporidians, myxozoans, apicomplexans, and encysted larval stages of metazoan parasites (e.g. cestodes, digenes, nematodes) (Figure A7.11). Certain flagellates (e.g. *Cryptobia* spp., *Spironucleus* spp.) and ciliates (e.g. scuticociliates) that can spread systemically may also be detected. Tissue wet mounts can also be useful for sex determination and assessment of gonadal maturity.

Cytologic Examination

Cytology is the microscopic examination of host tissue cells in order to assess cell morphology and detect the pres-

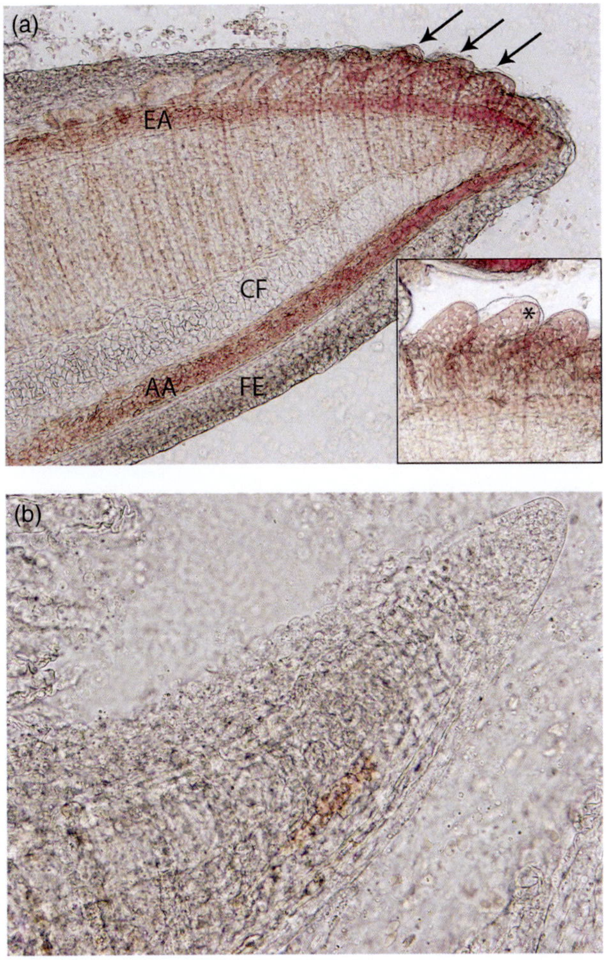

Figure A7.5 Wet mount of a fresh gill clip (a) showing filament epithelium (FE), cartilage filament (CF), afferent arteriole (AA), efferent arteriole (EA), and individual lamellae (arrows). In the inset, pillar cells within the lamellar vascular space create the speckled pattern (*). When autolyzed (b), there is loss of morphologic detail; the tissue appears granular, lamellar and vascular structures are no longer readily visible; and there is abundant cellular debris.

ence of pathogens. Commonly examined specimens in fish medicine include tissue or fluid aspirates, impression smears, and fecal samples. The cytologic stains used most commonly are Romanowsky stains (e.g. Dif-Quik®). Gram and acid-fast stains can be used along with Romanowsky-stained samples to further categorize findings.

Factors that Affect the Diagnostic Quality of Stained Cytologies

The diagnostic utility of stained cytology samples is affected by numerous factors, including composition of the tissue being sampled, collection method, staining method, slide preparation technique, and skill of the microscopist. Typically, tissues of epithelial origin (e.g. skin, gills) exfoliate better than tissues of mesenchymal origin (e.g. connective tissue, bone). For this reason, aspirates and impression smears of epithelial tissues are usually of greater cellularity than those from mesenchymal tissues, which often yield too few cells to evaluate adequately. To maximize sample cellularity, the largest needle that can be used safely should be selected for sample collection. In order to prevent breakage, minimal force and even pressure should be used when expelling samples onto slides and when spreading samples. Thin, evenly dispersed samples help prevent uneven staining.

Air-dried specimens are adequate in most cases, while heat fixation may be required to prevent loss of sample, particularly when using Gram and acid-fast stains. Staining intensity varies by sample and the amount of time the sample remains in contact with the stain components. While the staining techniques listed on the package inserts typically provide adequate cellular detail, prolonged staining times may be needed for thick samples, such as fecal swabs or gill clips.

Care must be taken to minimize precipitation of stain components by keeping them tightly closed when not in use to limit evaporation. Basophilic stain precipitate can resemble bacteria and complicate interpretation (Figure A7.12). If precipitates accumulate, the stain can be filtered using a small-bore coffee filter. Micro-organisms can also enter stain from the environment and from contaminated samples. If a stain becomes tainted with micro-organisms or excessive precipitate, it should be discarded and replaced, rather than filtered. The replacement frequency depends on the degree of usage, the type of samples, and the way in which stains are handled. In some instances, it is reasonable to have both a "clean" set of stains for use with hematology samples and most aspirates

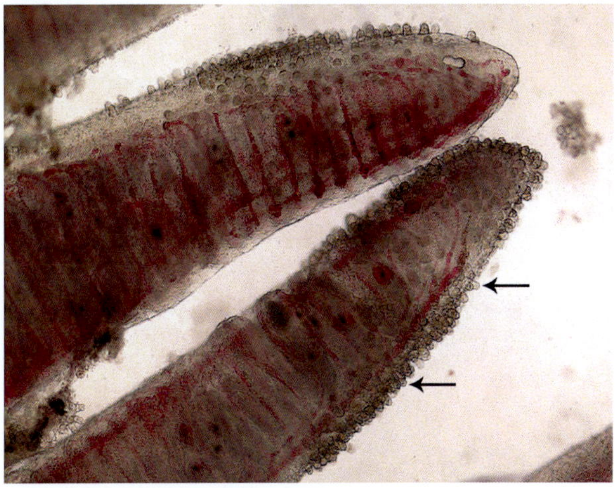

Figure A7.6 Sessile ciliates (*Ambiphrya* sp., arrows) and congestion in a gill clip from a channel catfish (*Ictalurus punctatus*).

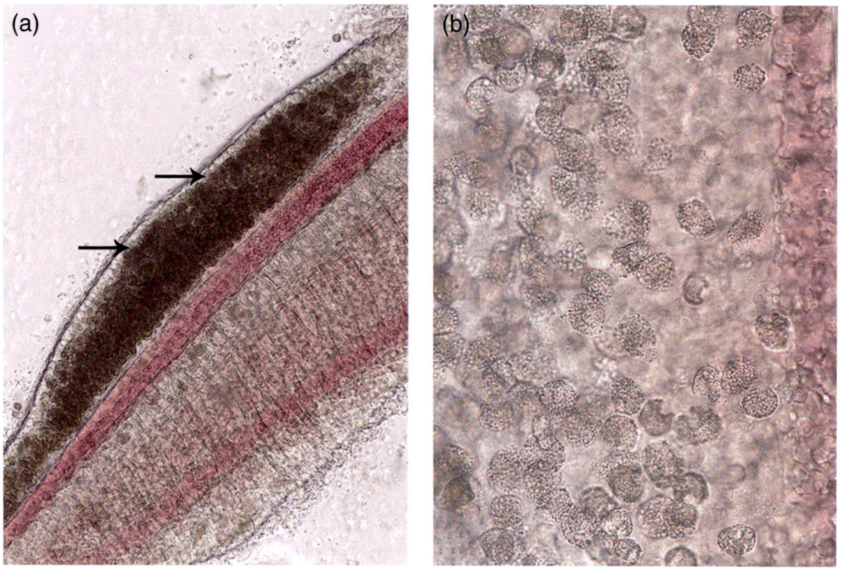

Figure A7.7 Eosinophilic granular cells (EGCs) in a gill clip from a threadfin shad (*Dorosoma petenense*) showing cellular infiltrate focally expanding the gill filament (arrows) (a) and EGCs under higher magnification (b). These should not be mistaken for organisms.

and a "dirty" set of stains to use when micro-organisms are anticipated (e.g. in fecal samples).

Tinctorial properties of stained specimens can be dramatically altered by the presence of formalin, which acts by cross-linking proteins. Slides exposed to formalin, including formalin fumes, are typically deeply basophilic and lack adequate detail for interpretation. Formalin fumes permeate most materials and, for this reason, unstained slides should not be stored or shipped in packages containing biopsy or other specimens fixed in formalin, as this often renders them inconclusive due to loss of cellular detail. Pre-staining slides prior to shipping prevents this dilemma. Examples of common cytologic artifacts are illustrated in Figure A7.13.

Cytologic Sample Evaluation

When examining stained microscopic specimens, it is critical to evaluate only intact cells and to base interpretations on adequately cellular samples with good cytologic detail (Figure A7.14). If cells are ruptured, often due to the use of excessive force when preparing slides, their cell membranes are disrupted, allowing fluid uptake within both the cytoplasm and the nucleus, imparting artifactual morphologic characteristics that are easily misinterpreted. A distinct cytoplasmic border should be visible around the entire cell in order for a cell to be included in microscopic evaluation (Figure A7.13e). Microscopists must resist the temptation to include broken cells in their evaluations,

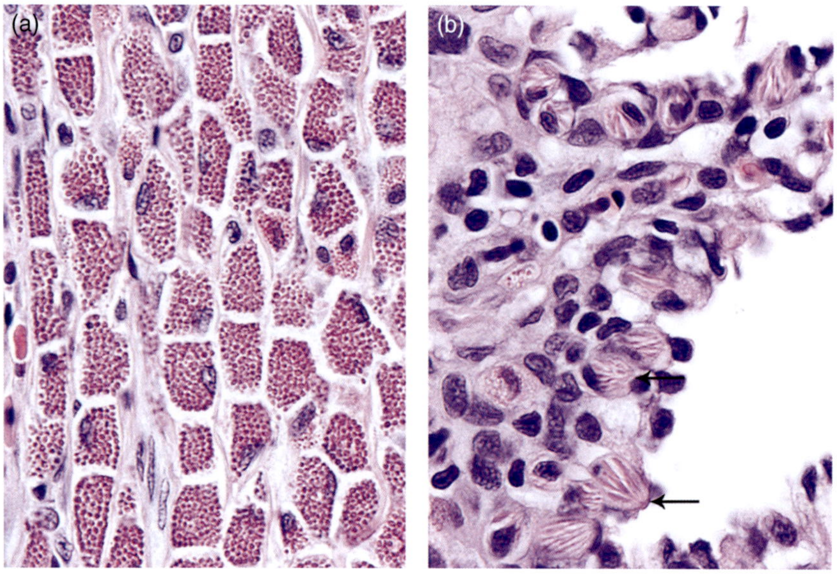

Figure A7.8 Eosinophilic granular cells (EGCs) in the intestinal submucosa of a pinfish (*Lagodon rhomboides*) (a), and rodlet cells with basal nuclei and cytoplasmic rods (arrows) in the gill epithelium of a red piranha (*Pygocentrus nattereri*) (b) H&E 1000×.

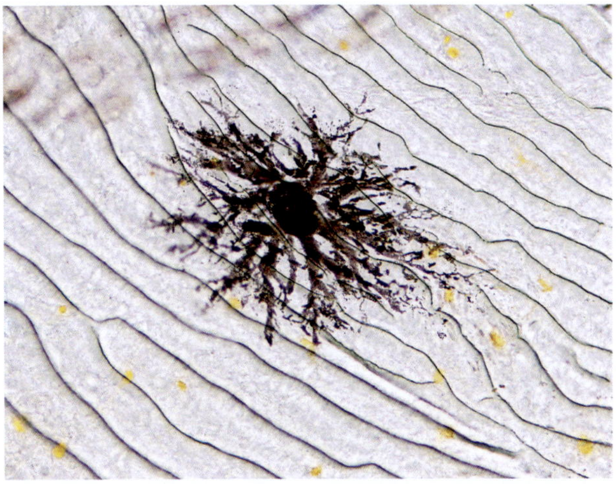

Figure A7.9 A normally occurring melanophore in a fin clip from a grass carp (*Ctenopharyngodon idella*) that should not be confused with an organism.

even if they can strongly speculate on a cell's identity. When performing a differential cell count, as is commonly done with inflammatory cells in cytologic specimens or with hematology specimens, it is important to remember that certain cell populations, particularly lymphocytes, are more prone to rupture than others. This can dramatically affect a differential percentage and subsequent interpretation derived from that percentage. Take caution to avoid including leukocytes associated with iatrogenic hemorrhage at the time of sample collection in the microscopic interpretation. Often when cells are broken and slides are prepared, nuclear material is spread across the slide in a linear fashion ("nuclear streaming") and can be mistaken for foreign material, including fungal organisms (Figure A7.13d).

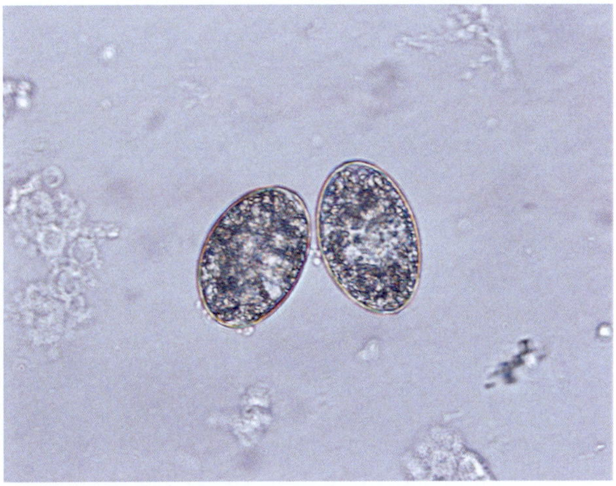

Figure A7.10 Eggs of the Asian tapeworm (*Schyzocotyle acheilognathi*) in fecal material from a koi (*Cyprinus carpio koi*).

When submitting cytologies to a diagnostic laboratory, be sure to complete the requisition form completely. Signalment, lesion location, and objective clinical findings are invaluable, as context accounts for the majority of lesion interpretation (Pinson 2014).

Romanowsky Stains

Romanowsky stains are used typically for both cytologic and hematologic specimens. These stains can be used to identify cells, examine cell morphology, and identify pathogens. They contain blue, pink, and purple components and stain proteins pink, nuclear material purple, and most bacterial organisms blue (Figure A7.12). Mycobacteria do not take up Romanowsky stains. Stains in this family include Wright's stain, which is used typically in large diagnostic laboratories, and the rapid Diff-Quik and Camco® stains. These stains are designed for use with air-dried smears and heat fixation should be limited to samples that are difficult to adhere to a glass slide.

Gram Stains

While Romanowsky stains are the primary stain for detecting bacteria in cytologic specimens, Gram stains may be helpful to further characterize bacteria to guide therapy in advance of culture results. Gram stains should be used in conjunction with Romanowsky-stained smears for concurrent evaluation of inflammatory cells to minimize over-interpreting bacterial contaminants. The presence of bacterial organisms alone is not necessarily consistent with the presence of a pathogen and should be interpreted in light of other clinical and laboratory findings.

Gram stains help characterize bacteria based on differential color reactions. Simple-to-use staining kits are commercially available and can be applied to tissue impressions, wet mount preparations, and bacterial cultures. Heat fixation of the slides is typically recommended. Gram-positive organisms (e.g. *Streptococcus* spp., *Mycobacterium* spp., *Renibacterium salmoninarum*) stain violet, while Gram-negative bacteria, which represent the majority of fish pathogens, stain red. It is important to note that the vast majority of bacterial pathogens stain blue with Romanowsky stains and should not be equated with a positive Gram stain reaction. Interpretive failures are common from over decolorization or uneven decolorization that results when suspensions to be stained are smeared too thick, preventing bacteria and tissue from dispersing on slides (Figure A7.15). Microsporidia and the polar capsules of myxozoans also stain Gram-positive, which can be useful in their identification (Figure A7.16).

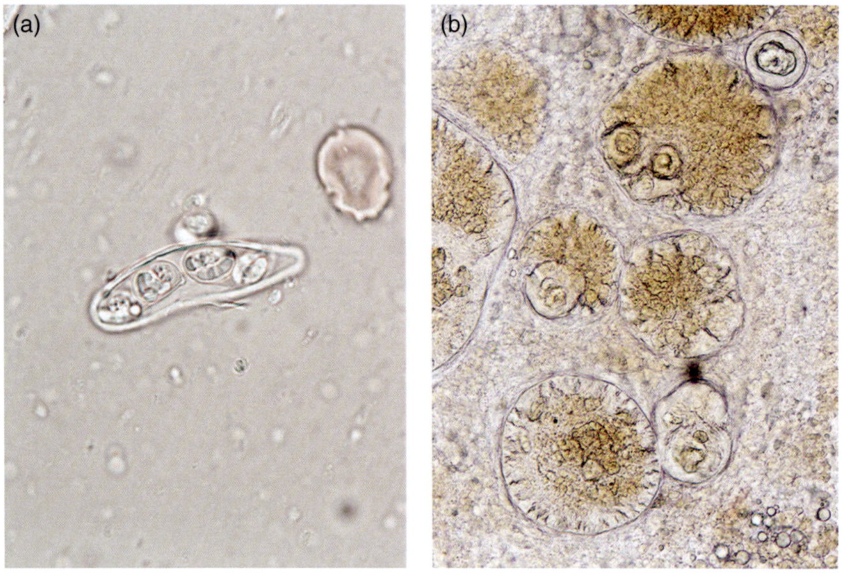

Figure A7.11 *Eimeria southwelli* oocyst, with four sporocysts each containing two sporozoites, in a serosal scraping from the liver of a cownose ray (*Rhinoptera bonasus*) (a), and granulomas in a liver wet mount from an Australian rainbowfish (*Melanotaenia fluviatilis*).

Acid-Fast Stains

Acid-fast stains (e.g. Ziehl–Neelsen, Kinyoun's, Fite's) are used primarily to detect mycobacteria in cytologic and histologic specimens. A number of staining kits are available commercially. While all use the red dye carbol fuchsin, procedures vary. The Kinyoun's stain, known as a "cold method" or as a modified Ziehl–Neelsen stain, is particularly user friendly, as no heating step is required. Acid-fast bacteria and cellular structures stain pink/red. Using Romanowsky stains, mycobacteria are "negatively" stained, appearing as linear clear spaces free or within macrophage cytoplasm. In these instances, the diagnosis can be confirmed by acid-fast staining (Figure A7.17).

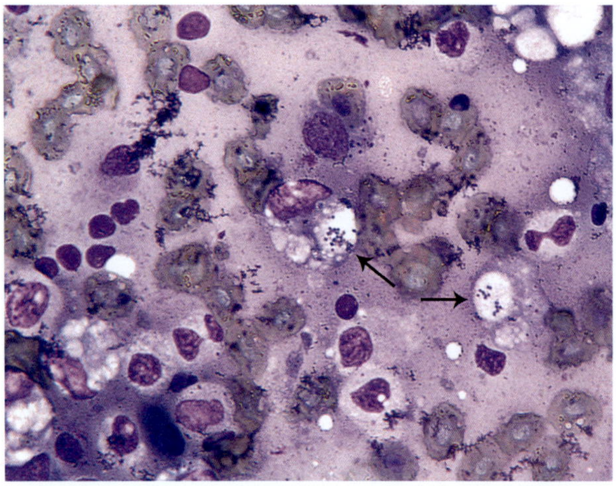

Figure A7.12 Impression smear of exudate from a channel catfish (*Ictalurus punctatus*). Uniform bacterial cocci are within a macrophage and extracellularly within a vacuole (arrows). Less distinct, more irregular, basophilic stain precipitate overlies much of the background and should not be confused with micro-organisms. Diff-Quik 1000×.

Nocardia spp. bacteria stain weakly or not at all with Ziehl–Neelsen type stains, but are strongly acid-fast positive when stained using the Fite's modification (Dill et al. 2017). Microsporidia, the shell valves of myxozoans, and coccidian sporozoites also stain acid-fast positive (Figure A7.18).

Histopathology

Histopathologic examination of biopsy or necropsy specimens can provide additional information not available through examination of wet mounts or stained cytologic specimens. When submitting samples for histology, it is recommended that the pathology laboratory be thoroughly familiar with the processing and evaluation of fish samples. Clinicians and pathologists should develop a positive working relationship regarding sample submission and ancillary testing, as well as an environment in which clinical and histologic findings can be freely discussed. This relationship begins with the submission of a thorough clinical history and should include results of any additional testing. Pathology reports should include meaningful comments that discuss the significance of negative findings and potential differential considerations when no definitive diagnosis is determined.

Tissue samples placed in an inadequate volume of formalin or that are too large to fix properly are common causes of diagnostic failure and histopathologic misinterpretation. For most general diagnostic purposes, 10% neutral buffered formalin provides adequate results. However, acid-containing fixatives, including modified Davidson's, Dietrich's, or Bouin's solutions may provide superior results for evaluation of gills, kidneys, and testes. Acid fixa-

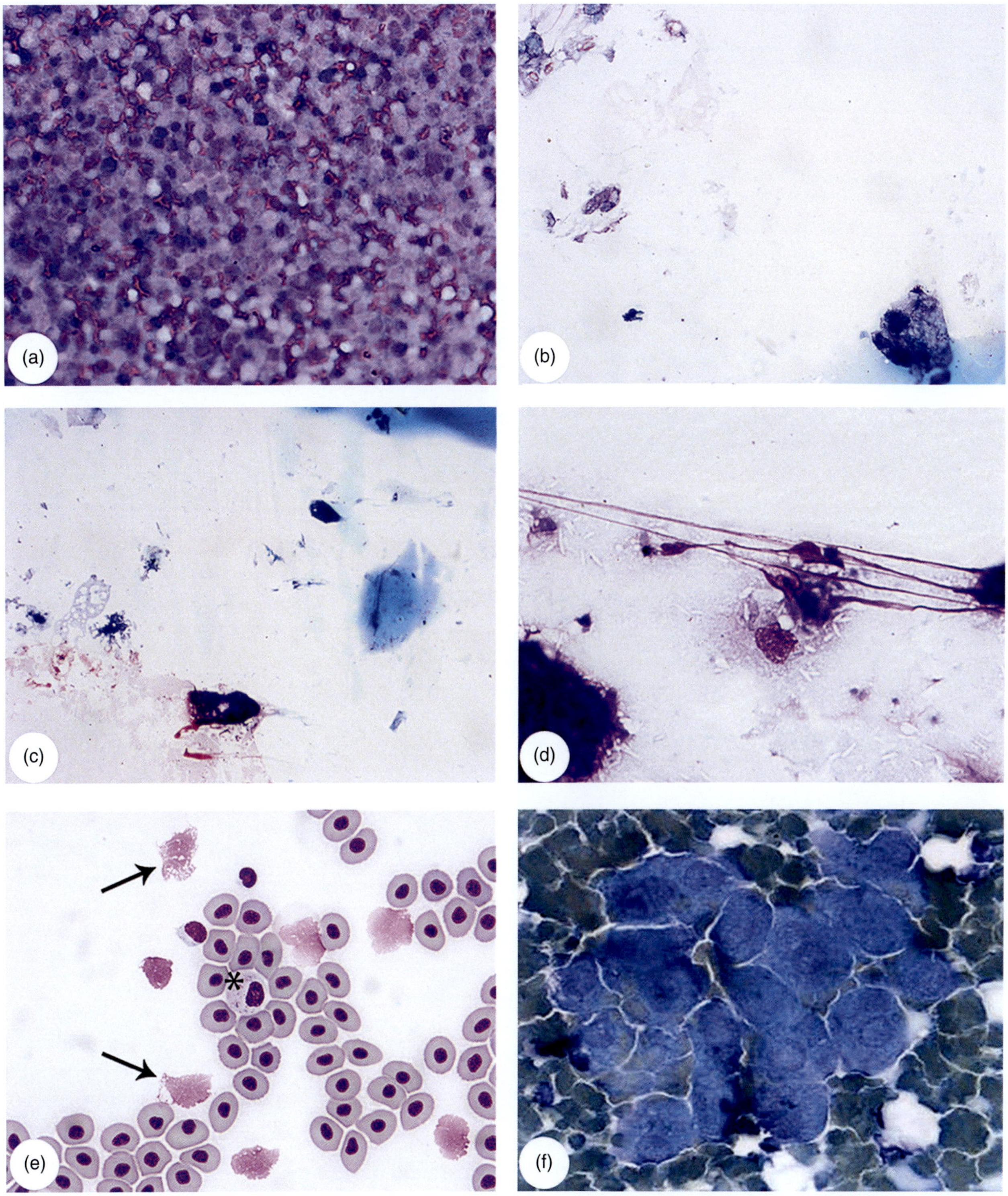

Figure A7.13 Cytologic artifacts include a sample that is too thick (a); poorly cellular, such as from this splenic aspirate (b); unevenly stained, with differences in tinctorial properties (pink, blue, and purple) across the slide (c); prepared with excess pressure, inducing nuclear streaming (d); with lysed leukocytes (arrows), as compared with an intact neutrophil (*) (e); and demonstrating formalin artifact in a liver aspirate exposed to formalin fumes (f). Erythrocytes stain bluish-green due to formalin exposure.

tives also have decalcifying properties that can speed tissue processing times (Wolf et al. 2014). To promote rapid tissue fixation, preserve morphology, and avoid bacterial overgrowth, formalin-to-tissue volumes should approximate a

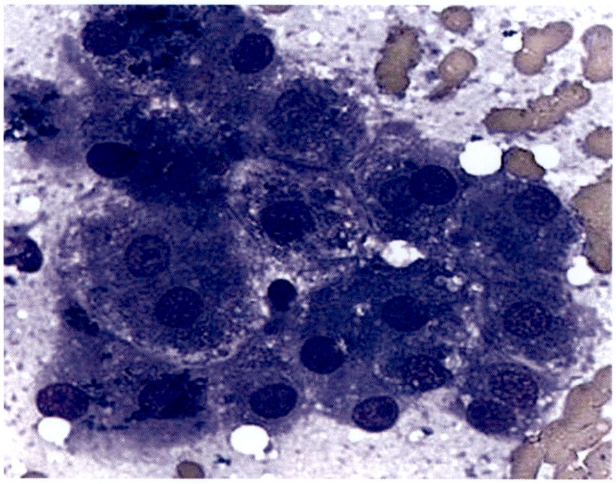

Figure A7.14 In contrast to Figure A7.13f, there is good morphologic detail in this well-stained liver aspirate. Modified-Wright's 1000×.

ratio of 10:1 or more (Figure A7.19). Samples should be less than 5–10 mm thick, although thinner sections facilitate rapid fixation. Fish less than 5–10 cm in length are best preserved whole, with their coelomic cavities incised to allow formalin permeation. Tissues should be collected using sharp dissection and samples from lesion margins should include normal and abnormal tissue. Scalpel blades produce fewer crush artifacts than scissors and forceps. In certain circumstances, important lesions or tissues should be identified with tags or placed in labeled tissue cassettes. Samples should be trimmed thin enough to prevent compression within cassettes (Figure A7.20). To avoid having to ship formalin, excess formalin can be poured off after 24 hours and the fixed samples wrapped loosely in formalin-soaked gauze or paper towels in sealed bags.

Hematology

Hematology includes the analysis of the white blood cells (leukon), red blood cells (erythron), and thrombocytes (thrombon). Hematologic analysis in fish is relatively common in clinical and academic practice, but due to a wide variety of methodologies and granulocyte nomenclature, interpreting hematologic results in fish remains a significant challenge. Hematology results should be interpreted with caution.

Hematologic Sample Processing

Blood smears should be made immediately upon sample collection, without the addition of anticoagulants. The remaining sample should be mixed with appropriate volumes of anticoagulants for accurate cell counts. EDTA works well for teleosts and most elasmobranchs, although it is known to cause red cell lysis in some species. If the sample-to-EDTA ratio is inappropriate due to underfilling of a tube containing liquid anticoagulant, dilution errors

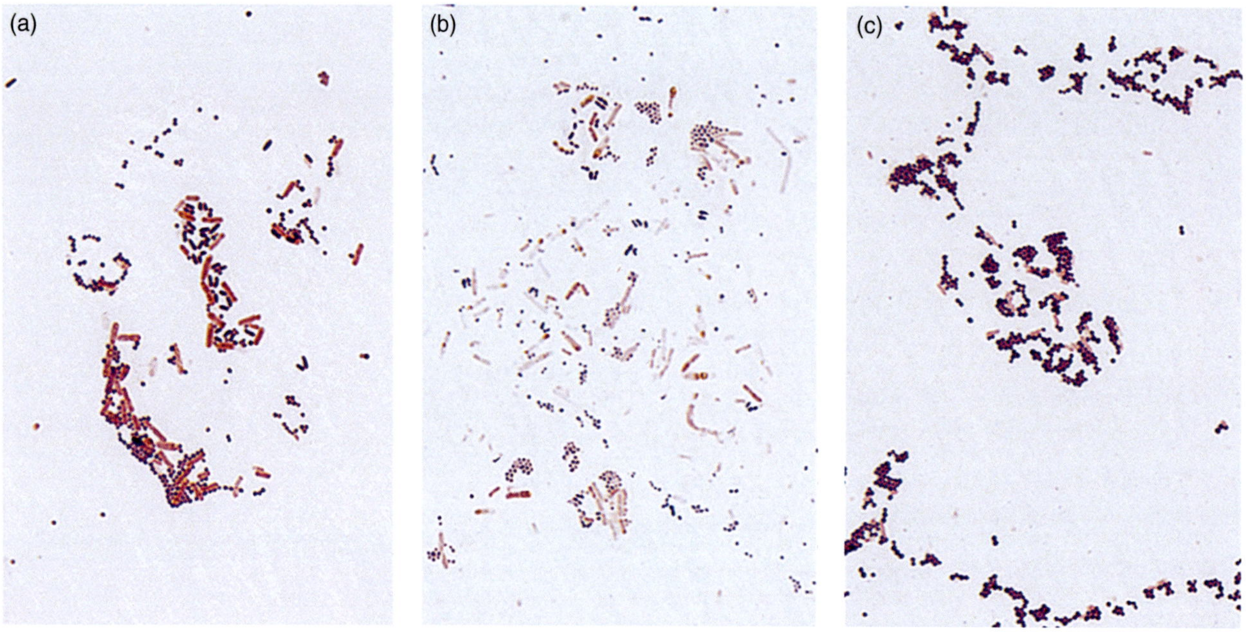

Figure A7.15 Well-executed Gram stain showing good differentiation between purple Gram-positive cocci and short rods and bright red Gram-negative rods (a); compared to a pale, overly decolorized sample that complicates interpretation (b), and an overly dense sample in which the morphology of individual bacterial types is obscured (c).

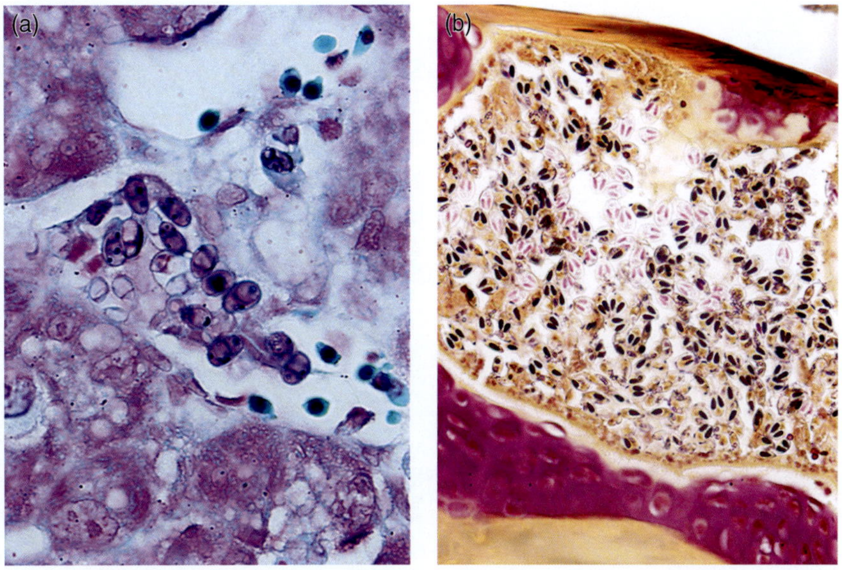

Figure A7.16 Gram-positive staining of microsporidian spores (a) and the polar capsules of myxozoans (b). 1000×.

will occur. This can be avoided using tubes containing powdered anticoagulant. In stingrays, EDTA may cause the sample to become more viscous, therefore stingray blood should be drawn into heparin. However, heparin induces thrombocyte clumping, making accurate quantitation difficult. If sufficient blood volume is available, evaluation of the erythron from a heparinized sample and evaluation of the leukon and thrombon from an EDTA sample are ideal. To avoid cell lysis, elasmobranch blood may be adjusted for its high plasma osmolality by adding urea and sodium chloride (Houston 1990).

If samples cannot be processed immediately, they can be preserved in 10% neutral buffered formalin (NBF) at a 1:5 ratio (one part blood and four parts NBF) until laboratory analysis can be completed (Arnold et al. 2014). Fixation using this method preserves the sample indefinitely. When submitting to an outside laboratory, all additives and dilutions should be noted on the submission form in order to ensure appropriate processing.

Hematologic Sample Evaluation

Fish blood requires manual hematologic evaluation due to the large, nucleated erythrocytes that cannot be differentiated from leukocytes by most automated analyzers. Quantitative evaluation of the erythron is typically limited to a spun packed cell volume (PCV). Quantitation of erythrocytes in a hemocytometer is laborious and unnecessary, since the PCV provides a quantitative measure of erythrocyte mass. The measurement of hemoglobin requires spe-

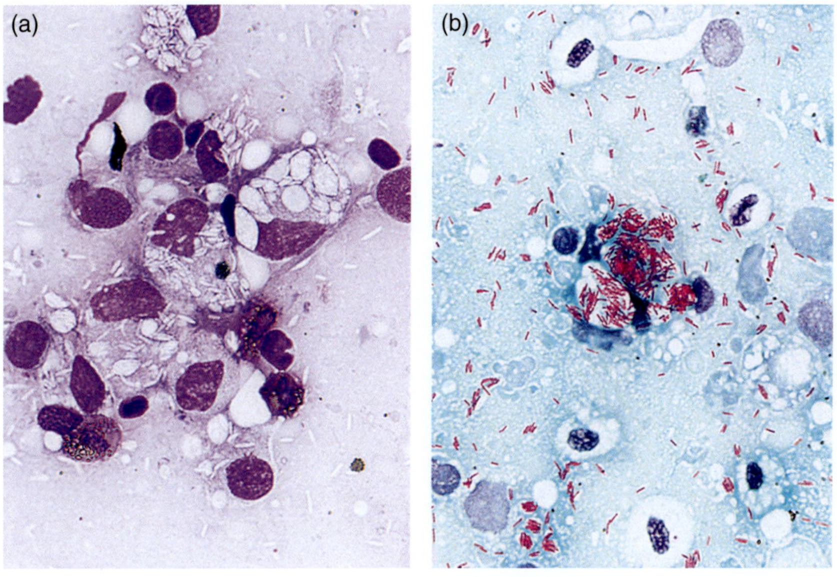

Figure A7.17 Mycobacteria are negatively staining, rod-shaped spaces in the background and within the cytoplasm of macrophages on Diff-Quik stain (a), and bright pink/red beaded rods on acid-fast stains (b). 1000×.

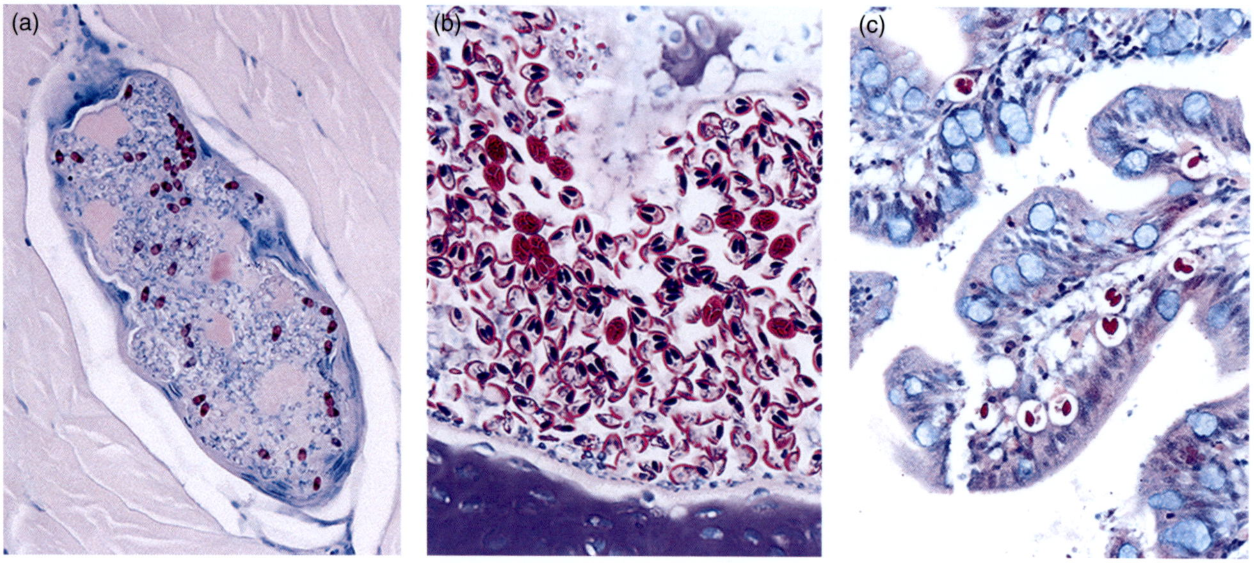

Figure A7.18 Acid-fast stains also highlight microsporidian spores (a), the shell valves of myxozoans (b), and sporozoites within developing oocysts of coccidian parasites (c). Ziehl–Neelsen 1000×.

cialized instrumentation for quantification and is typically unavailable in routine diagnostic laboratories.

It is important to note that although they are often used interchangeably, the terms PCV and hematocrit (HCT) are different. While both are used to express the percentage of blood occupied by erythrocytes, a PCV is a manual result, derived by reading a spun microhematocrit tube against a standardized scale, while a hematocrit is a value calculated by an automated hematology analyzer using the red blood cell concentration and mean cell volume (MCV). As these values are not typically available for fish, PCV is the method, and the correct term, to use for fish blood.

When performing PCVs, it is important to spin the sample for an appropriate time, based on the centrifugal force of the instrumentation used. This prevents trapping of plasma between erythrocytes, which falsely increases the

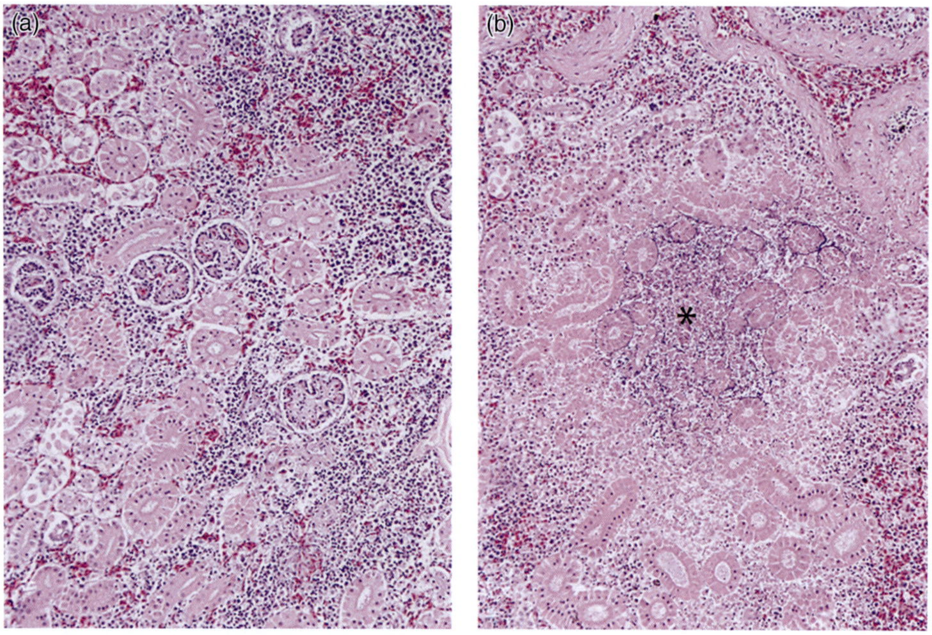

Figure A7.19 Histologic section of normal, well-fixed kidney from an electric eel (*Electrophorus electricus*). Tubules, glomeruli, and hematopoietic tissue are readily visible with differential staining of basophilic nuclei and eosinophilic cell cytoplasm (a), compared to an autolyzed section from the center of a large, poorly fixed sample with pale staining tubules, faded nuclei, and postmortem bacterial proliferation (*) (b). H&E 100×.

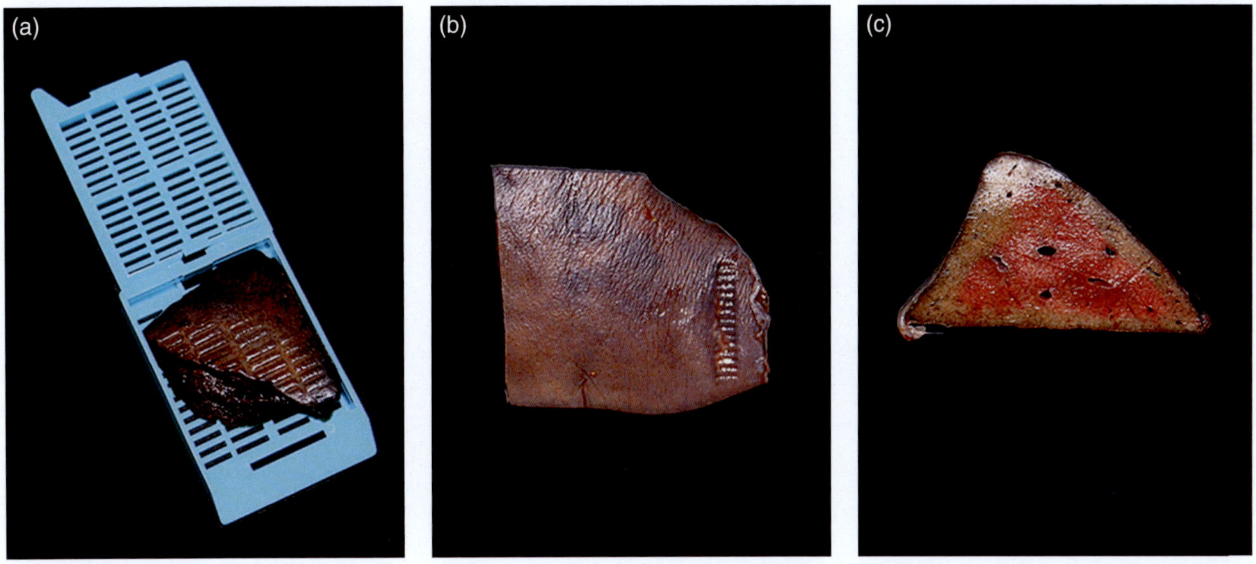

Figure A7.20 Common histologic artifacts can be caused by placing too thick of a specimen in a cassette (a), crushing tissue with instruments such as hemostats (b), and submitting sections thicker than 0.5 cm (c); despite 24 hours in formalin, the red center of this liver was not fixed.

PCV. It is also important to perform regular maintenance on the microhematocrit centrifuge using a tachometer to ensure that it is spinning at the appropriate speed. This is typically performed by an equipment calibration specialist and should be done annually. PCVs should be read at the interface between the red cell column and the leukocyte column, to prevent overestimation of the red cell percentage in the case of a profound leukocytosis (Figure A7.21).

Knowledge of both fish physiology and the impacts of environmental conditions is helpful when evaluating the erythron. For example, a low PCV may be due to hemorrhage, infectious disease, toxicity, or nutritional deficiency, but erythrocyte indices also drop with decreased water temperature. This could be the result of decreased metabolic demand for oxygen or the presence of increased dissolved oxygen at lower temperatures (Leard et al. 1998; Camus et al. 2014; Stacy et al. 2014). Elevated PCV has been associated with more active species, hemoconcentration, and handling stress (Hrubec et al. 2000; Cooke et al. 2008; Campbell 2012; Matsche 2013).

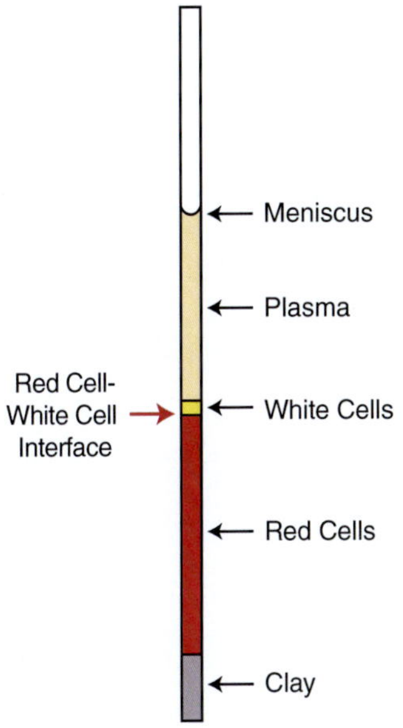

Figure A7.21 A spun PCV tube should be read at the red cell and white cell interface (red arrow).

Accurate leukocyte quantification requires manual counts via hemocytometry. Natt & Herrick's solution is the preferred stain/diluent in bony fish, as it stains all leukocytes and allows for direct, rather than calculated, leukocyte concentrations. Staining should be done as described in the diluent package insert. A modified Natt & Herrick's solution is recommended in elasmobranchs, with addition of sodium and chloride to match the osmolality of elasmobranch blood (Arnold 2005). A Neubauer counting chamber is typically recommended.

With Natt & Herrick's solutions, erythrocytes stain light pink to red (Figure A7.22). Thrombocytes are often slightly darker purple than erythrocytes and frequently have indistinct margins. Leukocytes of all types stain dark purple. It is still often challenging to distinguish thrombocytes from small lymphocytes in the hemocytometer, particularly when thrombocytes are stripped of their cytoplasm during sample processing. Accurate quantification requires microscopists specifically trained in nonmammalian hematology. In the event that distinguishing between thrombocytes and lymphocytes is impossible, both can be

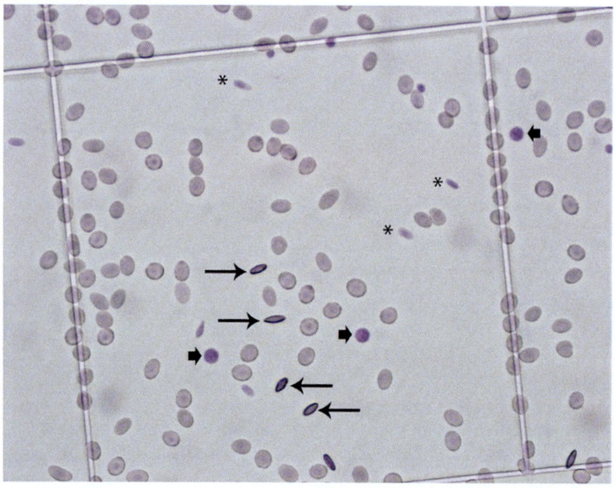

Figure A7.22 A hemocytometer with peripheral blood from a channel catfish (*Ictalurus punctatus*) showing erythrocytes, thrombocytes (*), and leukocytes (thick arrows). Care must be taken not to confuse thrombocytes with lateralized erythrocytes (thin arrows), which appear deeper pink and refractile. Natt & Herrick's 40×.

counted and the leukocyte concentration can be adjusted downward based on a differential percentage determined from corresponding blood smears (Persky et al. 2012). A variety of factors have been linked to changes in white blood cell concentration, including environmental, physiologic, and pathologic factors. Accurate interpretation of these changes requires knowledge of the leukocyte differential and should be interpreted in light of sample collection site and restraint method.

Evaluation of a blood smear is critical for a complete hematologic evaluation as it provides a qualitative leukocyte estimate, a cell differential, and information on cell morphology. Blood smears should be stained with Romanowsky stains, as described above. Leukocyte estimations from blood smears should be limited to qualitative (e.g. low/normal/high) assessments. Quantitative white blood cell estimates from blood smears are highly inaccurate and should be avoided (Camus and Pope 2012). Despite the fact that numerous estimation formulas exist, variability in microscope ocular diameter, leukocyte preservation, cell distribution, and operator training make interoperator variability too high for quantitative leukocyte counts. For the cell differential, familiarity with cell morphology is critical.

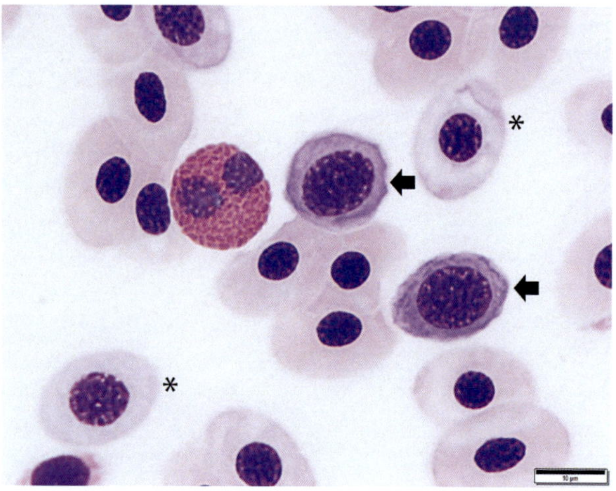

Figure A7.23 Peripheral blood from a southern stingray (*Hypanus americanus*) showing erythrocytes in various stages of maturation including early (arrows) and later maturation (*). A coarse eosinophilic granulocyte (CEG) is also visible. Diff-Quik 1000×.

Erythrocytes are round to ovoid and may be biconcave or biconvex, depending on the species (Yakote 1982). They have an elongated nucleus with condensed chromatin. Elasmobranch erythrocytes are typically larger than those of teleosts and have a lower nucleus:cytoplasm (N:C) ratio. Immature red cells are typically smaller with more open chromatin and more deeply basophilic cytoplasm. In most species, low numbers (up to 3%) of circulating erythrocytes are immature (Figure A7.23).

Fish thrombocytes are nucleated with pale, basophilic cytoplasm and are easily confused with lymphocytes (Figure A7.24). Identification of thrombocyte clumps is often helpful in elucidating thrombocyte morphology. In elasmobranchs, a subset of thrombocytes contains rod-shaped pink granules (Arnold 2009). When activated, thrombocytes can become elongated and easier to distinguish from other hematologic components.

Fish leukocytes, particularly granulocytes, can be challenging to classify. The literature varies tremendously on the nomenclature of fish granulocytes, which is partially due to perpetuation of older, description-based literature that attempts to correlate cell types with mammalian counterparts based primarily on morphology rather than function.

Teleost Leukocytes

Lymphocytes are the most numerous leukocyte in the peripheral blood of teleosts and are similar in form and function to those of mammals, birds, and reptiles. Fish lymphocytes are round with a high N:C ratio. These cells have a scant amount of lightly basophilic cytoplasm that surrounds a large, round to irregularly shaped, centrally located nucleus with condensed chromatin. Small, medium, and large lymphocytes, along with occasional plasma cells, can be found in peripheral circulation (Figure A7.25). Occasional granular lymphocytes containing distinct azurophilic granules are noted in peripheral blood (Houston 1990).

Neutrophils in teleosts have been confirmed by ultrastructure, cytochemical, and functional studies. They are the predominant granulocyte of most teleosts, although

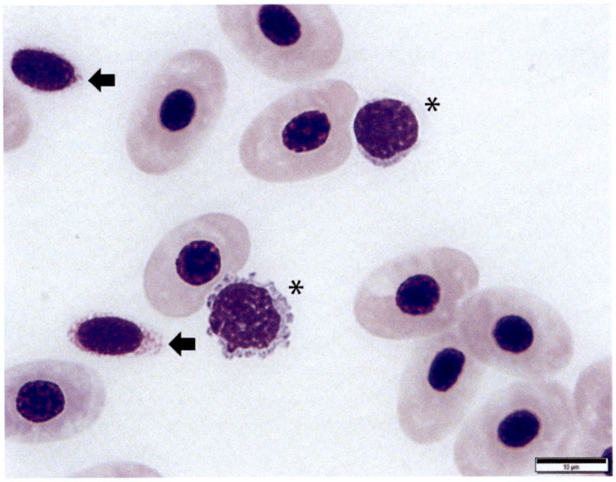

Figure A7.24 Peripheral blood from a southern stingray (*Hypanus americanus*) showing two lymphocytes (*) and two thrombocytes (arrows) among erythrocytes. Diff-Quik 1000×.

species variations exist (Ferguson 1976; Ellis 1977; Roberts and Ellis 2001; Flerova and Balabanova 2013). Nuclei are usually eccentrically placed and round or lobed, oval, or slightly reniform. Salmonid fish are an exception, where segmented nuclei reminiscent of mammalian granulocytes are present. Neutrophils are surrounded by a moderate amount of pale blue cytoplasm containing nonstaining ("neutral") granules (Figures A7.25 and A7.26). However, small red, blue, or violet granules exist in some species (Zinkl et al. 1991). A notable exception is the goldfish, which reportedly has heterophils with pink, rod-shaped intracytoplasmic granules. Fish neutrophils participate in acute inflammatory reactions and have been described as weakly or selectively phagocytic (Ainsworth 1992).

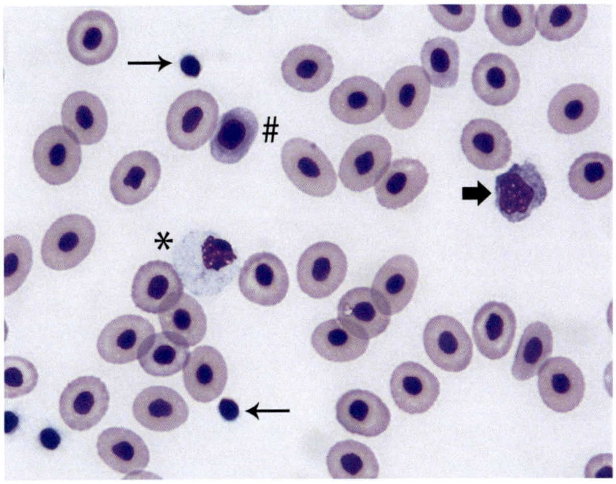

Figure A7.25 Peripheral blood from a channel catfish (*Ictalurus punctatus*) showing a neutrophil (*), lymphocyte (thick arrow), thrombocytes (thin arrows), and an early erythroid precursor (#). Modified Wright's 1000×.

Monocytes are the largest fish leukocyte and are present in low numbers in circulation. Monocytes resemble those of other animals. They are round with a moderate amount of basophilic cytoplasm that often contains discrete vacuoles and surrounds a reniform to lobulated, irregular nucleus with coarse chromatin.

The existence of teleost eosinophils and basophils is controversial, although they are described in low numbers in several species. Eosinophils are round with round to lobed, eccentrically placed nuclei. They have lightly basophilic cytoplasm filled with pink, round to rod-shaped granules. Their function is poorly understood. Basophils are round with eccentrically located round nuclei. Dark purple to magenta cytoplasmic granules often obscure the nuclei. These cells resemble tissue mast cells and are likely of the same ontogeny (Rowley et al. 1998; Flerova and Balabanova 2013).

Elasmobranch Leukocytes

Elasmobranchs have lymphocytes and monocytes resembling those of both mammals and teleosts. Sharks, unlike skates and rays, have neutrophils in peripheral blood. However, there is much discordant information regarding the classification of other elasmobranch granulocytes, including the adaptive use of avian terminology, a numeric classification system, and a descriptive system. In the descriptive system, cells containing round or lobed nuclei surrounded by cytoplasm containing slender, rod-shaped pink granules are often termed fine eosinophilic granulocytes (FEGs) and have been likened to heterophils (Arnold 2009). Leukocytes containing large round pink to red to orange granules are called coarse eosinophilic granulocytes (CEGs) and have been likened to eosinophils (Arnold 2009; Haines and Arnold 2014) (Figure A7.27). These should not be confused with the eosinophilic granular cells (EGCs) described under gill biopsies of teleosts. Basophils are abundant in stingrays but present in low numbers in other elasmobranchs. They have blue-black granules which often obscure the nucleus. Regardless of classification, microscopists should take care to identify all cellular components on a smear prior to attempting differential classification.

Special Stains for Hematology

New methylene blue (NMB) is a stain used primarily to identify immature erythrocytes in circulation, in an attempt to assess a regenerative response to anemia. Regeneration is typically associated with anemias caused by either blood loss or hemolysis, where the patient's hematopoietic system can respond to a decreased red blood cell mass. NMB is a vital stain, which means that it requires live cells to take up the dye. Therefore, it should not be applied to a

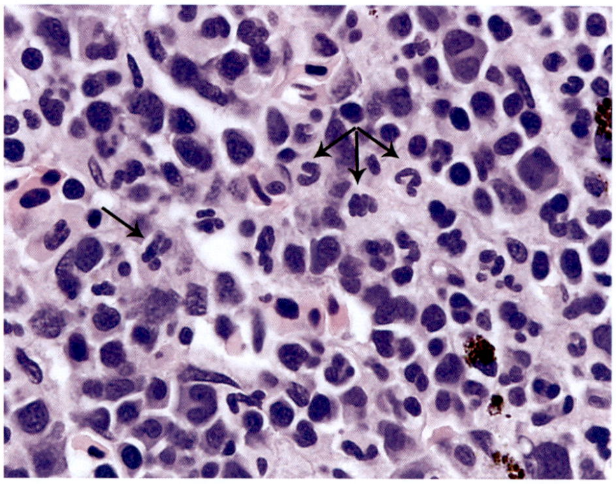

Figure A7.26 Histologic section of cranial kidney from a brown trout (*Salmo trutta*) showing numerous maturing neutrophils with band-shaped and segmented nuclei (arrows). H&E 400×.

premade blood smear. Instead, it needs a 10 minute incubation of a drop of anticoagulated blood with a drop of stain, from which a blood smear is made. In fish species, aggregated RNA (reticulin) takes up stain and must encircle the nucleus to be compatible with reticulocytes. NMB can also be used to assess the presence of denatured hemoglobin associated with oxidative damage, which can be induced by exposure to chemicals such as ozone (Fukunaga et al. 1999).

Blood Biochemistry

Blood biochemistry analysis is common in clinical and academic practice due to ready access to analyzers, but there are still significant limitations in fish. This is in part attributable to the lack of standardized collection protocols that likely affects results and complicates interpretation (Braceland et al. 2017). Few well-designed validation studies have been done in fish species to ensure that the analyte being quantified is truly the one being assayed. As in mammals, caution must also be used when interpreting samples that are hemolyzed, as hemolysis can affect most assays. When samples are analyzed using whole blood, hemolysis may not be visualized. Therefore, sample centrifugation (at least of a microhematocrit tube) is recommended to visually assess the degree of hemolysis prior to interpreting results.

Biochemistry testing is best reserved for species in which relevant, published reference intervals are available or where individual variation is monitored over time (Flatland et al. 2018). In the absence of appropriately derived reference intervals or individual animal trends, comparison with one or more control animals from the same environment, collected using the same methods and analyzed on the same instrument, can be performed.

Blood gas analysis is used to evaluate the acid–base status of animals, particularly elasmobranchs. Comparing changes over time in the same individual or group using the same methodology is particularly important for evaluating blood gases.

Biochemistry Sample Processing

Samples for biochemical analysis can be drawn into either a red top tube with no anticoagulant for serum analysis, or into a green top tube containing heparin for plasma or whole blood analysis. In fish, analysis of heparinized plasma is most common (Campbell 2012). It is important to remember that plasma contains both fibrinogen and clotting factors and will result in higher total protein concentrations than serum from the same patient. It is important to spin and separate plasma and serum as soon as possible, to prevent artifactual changes (e.g. hypoglycemia) that result from prolonged contact of erythrocytes with serum or plasma (Collicutt et al. 2015). If analysis is delayed beyond 24 hours, the plasma or serum should be frozen.

Handling stress can dramatically affect blood biochemistry results, as transmembrane electrolyte shifts occur within seconds of handling. For example, stress-induced catecholamine release can increase gill permeability, resulting in the loss or influx of sodium (Na) and chloride (Cl) ions in freshwater and marine teleosts, respectively (Campbell 2012). Additionally, lactate release from white muscle during handling can induce lactic acidosis within five minutes of capture and restraint (Campbell 2012). The resultant acidosis perpetuates electrolyte shifts, affecting many blood biochemical analytes, including Na, Cl, potassium (K), bicarbonate (HCO_3), and ammonia (NH_3) (Heming 1989). Unfortunately, attempts to minimize handling stress through chemical restraint also affect blood biochemistry values. For example, the use of tricaine methanesulfonate (MS-222) reportedly induces hyperglycemia and hyperkalemia and increases urinary electrolyte excretion in teleosts (Campbell 2012).

If blood gas analysis is clinically warranted, the most accurate results are obtained by drawing samples into glass syringes without exposure to air and processing immediately from the syringe. Use of plastic syringes for sample collection is common, but allows diffusion of oxygen through the plastic which may affect results (Rupell 2006; Wiwanitkit 2006). Similarly, exposure to room air alters the gas composition of samples, so samples should not be processed from blood tubes that have had their caps removed.

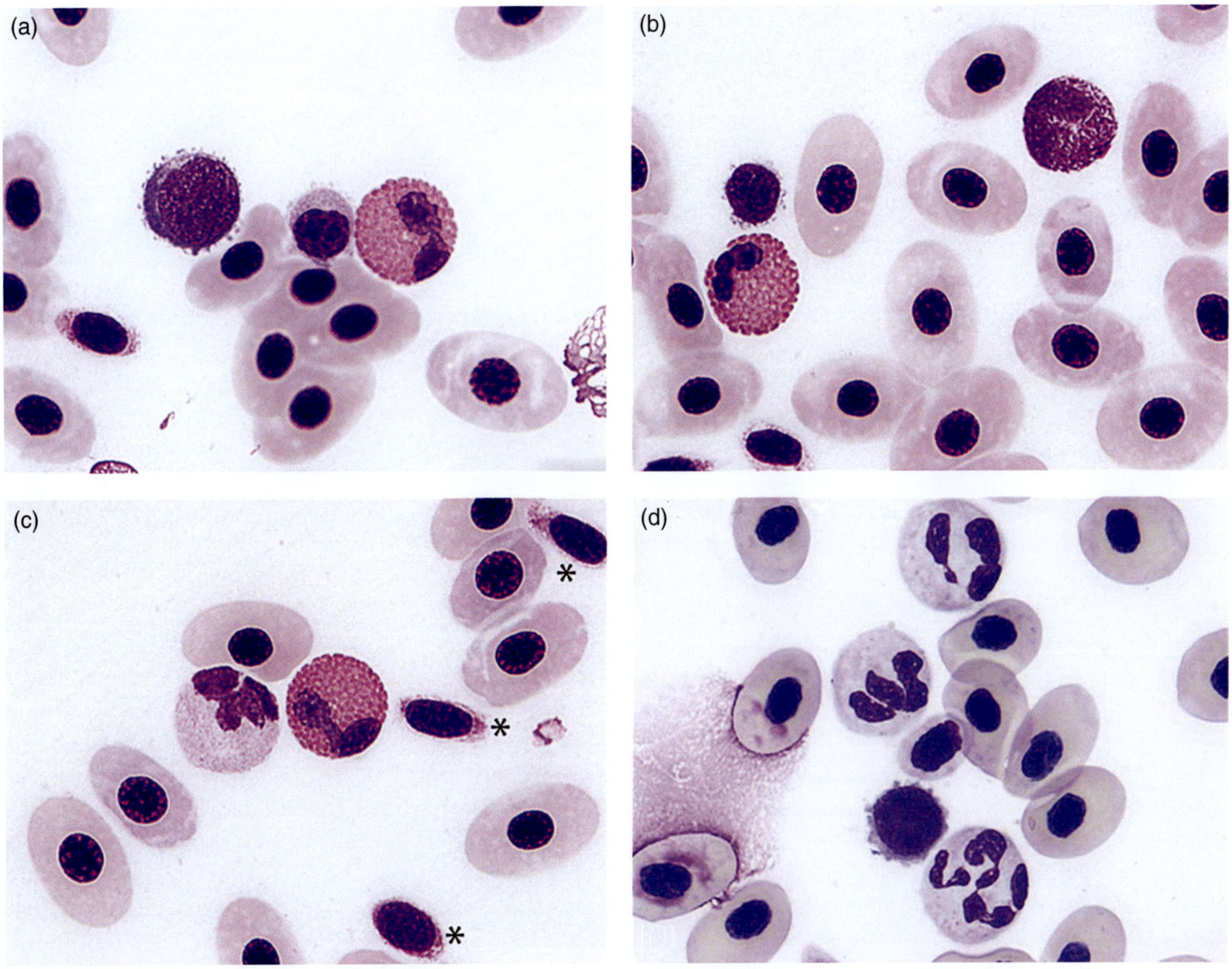

Figure A7.27 Peripheral blood from a southern stingray (*Hypanus americanus*) (a–c) and a dusky smooth-hound (*Mustelus canis*) (d) showing two lymphocytes and a coarse eosinophilic granulocyte (CEG) (a); a basophil (right) and CEG (b); fine eosinophilic granulocyte (FEG) (left), CEG (right), and thrombocytes (*) (c); and three neutrophils (d). Diff-Quik 1000×. *Source*: Image courtesy of Jill Arnold, National Aquarium.

As several blood gas parameters are temperature-dependent (pH, pCO_2, and pO_2), water temperature (presumably equivalent to patient temperature in poikilotherms) should be entered into the blood gas analyzer to allow for some temperature correction. The default temperature for most blood gas analyzers is 37°C (98.6°F) and analysis at this temperature will provide erroneous data.

Biochemistry Sample Evaluation

Fish physiology varies significantly between teleosts and elasmobranchs and between their respective freshwater and marine counterparts. While an in-depth discussion of these differences is beyond the scope of this chapter, physiology has a direct bearing on serum and plasma biochemistry values. Knowledge of the species being evaluated is critical to appropriate interpretation of laboratory values.

Marine teleosts maintain plasma osmolality values around 330 mOsmol/kg, which is approximately 33% that of seawater and slightly higher than that of freshwater teleosts (Harms et al. 2002). Sodium and chloride are the major ions in the blood of all fish and levels are similar in freshwater and marine teleosts. Sodium and chloride levels are expected to decrease in freshwater teleosts with gill disease and increase in marine teleosts with the same clinical condition.

Marine elasmobranchs have plasma osmolality slightly hyperosmotic to seawater (800–1100 mOsmol/kg), due to high levels of urea, trimethylamine oxides (TMAO), Na, and Cl. Sodium and chloride concentrations are substantially higher than those of teleosts and often exceed the linearity of most biochemistry analyzers, resulting in error messages or erroneous values (Hammerschlag 2006). Depending on the methodology of the instrument used (direct versus indirect ion-specific electrode), dilutions may be helpful in determining accurate electrolyte and urea concentrations in elasmobranchs.

Electrolyte changes can be indicators of renal disease, environmental conditions (salinity and pH), impaired gill function, and catecholamine-mediated stress responses. Potassium, which is predominantly intracellular, is less affected by changes in gill permeability and renal blood flow than Na and Cl. Decreased K concentration has been associated with loss through the gastrointestinal tract and skin. It has also been associated with nitrite toxicity. Increased K concentration is often artifactual but has been associated with muscle damage, handling stress, and hemolysis. Magnesium (Mg) can also increase up to 10-fold in hemolyzed samples, as fish erythrocytes are particularly rich in Mg. Blood calcium (Ca) is derived primarily from water via transport across the gills. Regulated excretion occurs in the kidney. Although levels are similar in freshwater and marine teleosts, regulatory mechanisms are incompletely understood. Calcium and phosphorus (P) can increase during vitellogenesis due to mobilization from scales (Guerreiro et al. 2007; Campbell 2012).

Nitrogenous wastes are excreted primarily across the gill epithelium. In teleosts, urea, uric acid, and creatinine concentrations are of minimal use in assessing renal disease. Instead, increases in urea have been linked to gill damage or dysfunction (Nelson et al. 1999). In marine elasmobranchs, urea is a primary osmolyte produced by the liver and resorbed by the kidney. Therefore, urea concentrations can decrease with hepatic disease and rise with renal disease. However, these findings are nonspecific, as other factors, including prolonged anorexia, can result in a decreased urea concentration. Creatine, which accounts for >50% of renal nitrogenous waste in most fish, may be of value but is uncommonly measured and has limited commercial availability (Campbell 2012). Blood ammonium (NH_4^+) may be affected by gill or liver disease but is seldom quantified because it deteriorates rapidly and must be measured within minutes of collection.

Assessment of enzyme activity is limited by the paucity of information on species-specific normal enzyme activity and wide variation across groups. Teleost hepatocytes contain aspartate aminotransferase (AST) and may contain alanine aminotransferase (ALT). Therefore, elevations in concentrations of these analytes may correlate with hepatocellular damage and associated leakage in some teleost species. High concentrations of AST are also found in skeletal muscle, so elevations in AST are not tissue-specific and must be correlated with clinical signs and other laboratory data. Creatine kinase (CK) is also present in fish muscle and concurrent elevation of AST and CK suggests muscle origin. However, the half-life of CK is short and levels may return to reference intervals shortly after injury, while AST may remain elevated. Lactate dehydrogenase (LDH) activity is often used to assess liver health, but is affected by temperature, pH, collection site, difficulty of capture, nutritional status, and activity levels, rendering interpretation difficult. The physiologic concentration of bilirubin versus biliverdin varies by fish species, minimizing clinical utility of bilirubin measurement (Campbell 2012). Gamma-glutamyl transferase (GGT) activity is usually below detectable limits in plasma and serum samples from healthy fish, although activity was identified in the kidneys and urine in lionfish (*Pterois* spp.) (Anderson et al. 2010).

In elasmobranchs, activity of several enzymes is often below detectable limits on most analyzers (e.g. CK, LDH, GGT, amylase).

Liver function tests are also limited in fish, as little is known regarding bile acid secretion. With decreased hepatic function, hepatic glycogen stores decrease, theoretically resulting in hypoglycemia with profound liver dysfunction. However, fish can maintain glucose concentrations during prolonged starvation (up to 150 days), suggesting that liver glycogen stores may not correlate well with peripheral glucose concentrations. Additionally, glucose levels vary tremendously with species, activity, nutrition, reproductive status, and both corticosteroid and catecholamine-mediated stress. Cholesterol concentration, often used as an indicator of mammalian liver function, is affected by diet, sex, and reproductive status. Extrapolation from human reference intervals is particularly ill-advised in fish species, as cholesterol levels in fish are typically higher than in mammals and consist primarily of high-density lipoproteins (HDLs) (Campbell 2012).

Protein differentiation should also be interpreted with care. Refractometric total protein is often used, but is a better reflection of "total solids", as any substances that induce light refraction (e.g. urea, glucose) can affect these results, typically producing erroneously high protein values. This is particularly problematic in elasmobranchs, due to elevated urea concentrations compared to teleosts. Suspected interferences with albumin quantitation using bromocresol green (BCG), as documented in birds, have been noted in some teleosts. Therefore, albumin and globulin measured on biochemistry analyzers may be invalid. Protein electrophoresis is the gold standard for protein fractionation in most species. However, these results should still be interpreted with caution in saltwater fish, as salinity has been shown to affect both albumin and globulin levels using this methodology (Peyghan et al. 2014).

Toxicologic and Nutritional Analyses

Toxicology

Collecting samples for toxicologic evaluation is often considered in the face of large-scale morbidity or mortality. These occur in both natural environments and managed care systems as a result of anthropogenic activities, equipment failures, natural events, and infectious diseases. Sudden events, particularly those affecting multiple species, suggest a water quality issue. When fish kills do occur, laypersons may be quick to suspect "poisoning", but that is relatively rare. More common water problems, such as oxygen depletion, should be excluded first.

Many chemicals do not produce pathognomonic gross or microscopic lesions and histology may only suggest toxin exposure (Meyers and Hendricks 1982) (Figure A7.28). However, histology may help rule out infectious or other causes. Most veterinary diagnostic laboratories do not offer basic water quality testing and even fish diagnostic laboratories may only offer basic parameters (pH, ammonia, nitrite, hardness, alkalinity, copper, and chlorine). The number of laboratories offering testing for chemical residues and other toxins is limited. If seeking assistance, state agriculture departments, local extension offices, and natural resource departments may provide information on how and where to submit samples, or they may be equipped to collect samples themselves, particularly when natural bodies of water are involved.

An incomplete list of potential toxins includes nitrogenous wastes, heavy metals, ozone, chlorine, hydrogen sulfide, cyanide, drugs, acids and alkalis, detergents, volatile organic compounds, harmful algal blooms, pesticides, herbicides, petroleum products, other hydrocarbons, and endocrine disrupting compounds. Clients should be informed that there is no all-inclusive screen for toxic substances and that analysis can be expensive. While technologies such as gas chromatography/mass spectrometry (GC/MS) have the potential to detect thousands of manufactured chemicals and natural toxins, a complete history is essential to narrowing the list of likely toxins and limiting analysis costs.

Interpretation of results for certain chemical analyses may be limited by a lack of baseline reference values for many fish species. This can be partially overcome by submitting water and tissue samples collected from unaffected "clean" sites for comparative purposes. It is important to note that the toxicity of individual compounds can vary across life stages, and between freshwater and marine bony and elasmobranch fish. For example, in freshwater fish, the main target of many waterborne metals is the gills, while in marine teleosts the intestines may also be affected because these species drink seawater (Grosell et al. 2003; Bielmyer et al. 2006).

If investigating a fish kill, dissolved oxygen levels and water temperature should be measured on location. Water (1 L minimum) and fresh fish, or their tissues, should be collected and submitted immediately to a testing laboratory. Due to the variety of potential toxins and associated environmental conditions, the testing laboratory should always be consulted prior to submission for specifics on acceptable samples, sample sizes, and collection and storage requirements. Polyethylene or glass containers are suitable for most water samples, but exceptions exist, for example, glass containers are preferred by many laboratories when organic chemicals are suspected. Many chemicals degrade rapidly in water or sunlight or become bound to sediments. Samples should be protected from light and chilled immediately. Carcasses or individual tissues should be wrapped in aluminum foil, placed in sealed plastic bags, and similarly chilled. If samples will not be submitted the same day or shipping is required, freezing may be necessary based on recommendation by the testing laboratory (Meyer and Barclay 1990; Sink 2015). Care should be taken not to cross-contaminate samples when handling. Personal protective measures should be taken to prevent potential human toxin exposure when handling samples.

If litigation is anticipated, many states require specific steps be followed, including written unambiguous records of collection (clinical signs, dates, times, locations, personnel involved, statements, etc.) and clear chain of custody documentation. In general, clients should not collect samples for legal cases unless supervised by a local or state official.

Vitamin and Mineral Analysis

Nutritional disease is relatively uncommon in wild fish from natural habitats and in commonly cultured species fed formulated diets. However, in other conditions, natural diets may be difficult to provide and specific nutrient requirements are often unknown (Dill et al. 2016). As a result, vitamin and mineral analyses are periodically needed to assess the nutritional and metabolic status of fish. Submission guidelines for vitamin and mineral analyses and limitations to their interpretation are similar to those for toxicologic evaluations. Methodologies vary between testing laboratories and for individual analytes. Laboratories should be consulted prior to sample submission for specific requirements regarding preferred samples

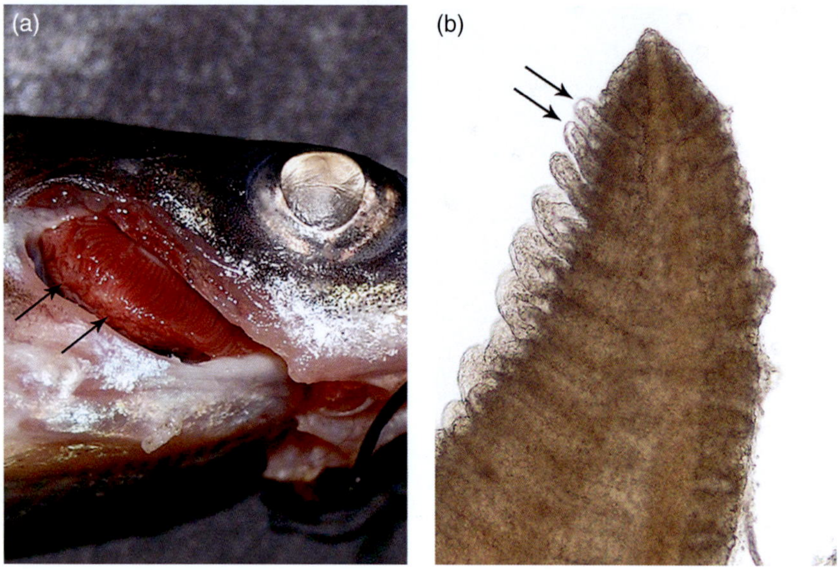

Figure A7.28 Pallor and edema in channel catfish (*Ictalurus punctatus*) gills damaged by euthanasia with unbuffered MS-222 (a), resulting in swelling of lamellar tips and lifting of their epithelial surfaces (arrows) on direct microscopy (b).

(e.g. whole blood, serum, tissue, feed), sample sizes, and preservation and shipping recommendations. For example, iron is measured in serum, while lead is measured in whole blood and is preferably collected in EDTA. The sample sizes required may be prohibitive for small fish, necessitating the pooling of samples or whole animal analyses.

Microbiology

Microbiology samples may be collected antemortem but are more often acquired during necropsies, particularly in the event of significant morbidity or mortality in a group. In such cases, a minimum of three affected fish should be evaluated, with the objective of identifying a common cause for the signs. The detection of an identical agent in multiple samples from the same patient, or within several individuals from a group of fish, greatly increases the likelihood that the agent is significant (Sontakke et al. 2009). Results should always be interpreted in relation to the history, clinical signs, other diagnostic tests, and degree of autolysis.

Normal-appearing fish collected at random frequently do not yield positive results in a group where disease prevalence is low, even though mortalities may be occurring. Assuming a 5% prevalence level of a specific pathogen in a population of 100 fish, 45 individuals would have to be sampled to be 95% confident that at least one fish was infected with the agent (AFS-FHS 2014). The best specimens for full necropsy, histopathology, and ancillary testing are living fish exhibiting signs typical of the diseased population. For postmortem testing, the animal should be euthanized, removed from water once euthanized, and examined immediately. If animals cannot be necropsied immediately, fin spines should be removed and the fish sealed individually in plastic bags with no water added. Bags should be correctly labeled and then placed in a refrigerator or on ice. Freezing is ideal when a potential need for molecular diagnostics exists and may also be suitable for bacterial or viral culture. Freezing is not acceptable for wet mounts and creates artifacts for histologic evaluation.

Bacteriology

Appropriate bacterial culture and sensitivity testing is an important component of fish medicine. Bacterial identification from culture media has traditionally relied on phenotypic traits, including Gram staining, culture and growth characteristics, and biochemical profiling. The latter has used individual "tube" media in conjunction with reagent-based tests and flow charts/dichotomous keys or commercial test systems in which test results produce a numerical code that is compared to a database (e.g. API® BioMérieux, Durham, NC) or automated systems (e.g. Sensititre™ ThermoFisher Scientific, Waltham, MA) for identification. In addition to being time-consuming and labor-intensive, it is becoming increasingly clear that phenotypic traits may not be adequate for pathogen identification, particularly for discrimination among closely related organisms. Furthermore, certain fish pathogens are not found in the databases of commercial identification systems and the databases are not regularly updated as new fish pathogens emerge.

A newer technology with the potential to replace phenotypic identification for routine culture isolates is matrix-assisted laser desorption/ionization time-of-flight mass spectrometry (MALDI-TOF-MS) (Biswas and Rolain 2013;

Calderaro et al. 2014). A sample, in some instances as little as a single bacterial colony, is mixed with an energy absorbing matrix that facilitates the ionization of organic molecules to a gaseous state using laser energy. An electric field then accelerates the molecules toward a detector based on their mass and charge. The "time of flight" required for each molecular species to reach the detector creates a recorded spectrum that can be compared to a database of bacterial species for identification (Biswas and Rolain 2013). MALDI-TOF-MS is particularly useful for identifying slow-growing or fastidious organisms that are difficult to maintain in culture. Similar to other methods, proper identification is dependent upon completeness and accuracy of the reference database.

Bacteriology Sample Submission

When submitting samples for bacterial culture, environmental contaminants and postmortem overgrowth of insignificant bacterial species are major impediments to accurate diagnoses (Figure A7.29). To avoid contamination, samples should be collected aseptically by disinfecting the body wall with 70% ethanol prior to opening the coelomic cavity or other sites and flaming instruments before contacting tissues (Plumb and Bowser 1983). It is preferable to culture individual organs using a culture loop, rather than swabbing coelomic cavities. Particularly with small fish, the use of large tip culturettes is a common source of sample contamination. Small (2–3 mm) tissue samples can also be smeared directly onto culture plates and streaked. Alternatively, entire organs from small fish or larger tissue pieces removed by sharp dissection can be placed in sterile containers, such as Whirl-Pak® bags (Nasco, Fort Atkinson, WI), for transport to a diagnostic laboratory. Aseptic technique is particularly important when blood cultures, which are easily contaminated, are collected from live animals.

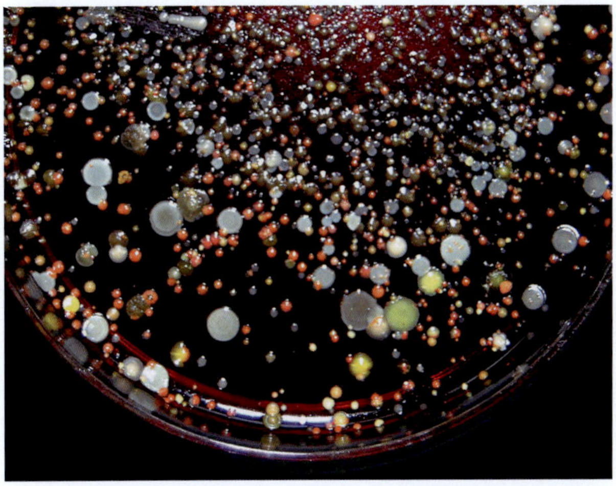

Figure A7.29 Heavy growth of various bacterial colony types following culture of a skin ulcer from a fish that was found dead.

Ulcerative skin lesions are common in fish and pose a particular culture challenge. Swabbing lesion surfaces will commonly yield ambiguous results due to the large numbers of environmental bacteria that are often present. However, the offending bacterial species frequently will be present in highest numbers along the spreading margin of a lesion. This feature can be exploited in postmortem specimens by disinfecting the lesion surface and adjacent skin with 70% ethanol, then collecting material for culture from beneath the lesion edge with an inoculating loop or tip of a scalpel blade (Plumb and Bowser 1983; Noga 2010).

Clinicians should identify laboratories familiar with fish pathogens and discuss the suspected organisms and environmental conditions of the fish with laboratory personnel prior to submission. If submitting samples to a bacteriology laboratory that primarily receives mammalian submissions and is not familiar with the culture of fish pathogens, it is important to understand potential limitations of the services they provide. Most follow standard operating procedures (SOPs) that use standard media and culture conditions (temperature and time), which may not support the growth of certain fish bacteria, such as *Flavobacterium columnare*. Commonly encountered problems include a lack of specialized media for fastidious fish pathogens and failure to provide proper culture conditions. For example, some bacterial pathogens (e.g. mycobacteria) are stimulated by carbon dioxide (Pfyffer et al. 2003). Improper incubation temperatures can also greatly influence culture results. In general, bacteria that infect warm-water fish are best cultured at 25–30°C (77–86°F) and those infecting cold-water fish are cultured at 15–20°C (59–68°F) (Plumb and Hanson 2011). Certain organisms (e.g. *Aliivibrio salmonicida*) may require even lower culture temperatures. Temperature may also influence the results of commercial identification systems, which are designed to be incubated at 37°C (98.6°F) and interpreted after a specific period of time. While accurate results may be obtainable with additional incubation time at lower temperatures, accredited veterinary diagnostic laboratories may be reluctant to deviate from manufacturer's guidelines and their established SOPs. Less commonly, laboratories unfamiliar with fish pathogens may fail to recognize the significance of certain bacteria, particularly when multiple species are isolated, and simply not report them. The use of antibiotic therapy prior to culture may also lead to negative culture results.

Common Bacterial Media and Their Uses

Many common bacterial fish pathogens will grow on general-purpose standard bacterial media, including Tryptic Soy Agar (TSA), TSA with 5% blood, and Brain Heart

Infusion Agar. However, certain fastidious organisms, such as *Flavobacterium* spp. and *Renibacterium salmoninarum* require special media. Certain intracellular pathogens, such as *Piscirickettsia salmonis*, originally isolated in cell culture can now be grown on artificial media (Makrinos and Bowden 2016). The isolation of additional bacteria can be facilitated by the modification of standard media. For example, the addition of salt may enhance the isolation of halophilic *Vibrio* spp. A few bacterial pathogens, including the agents of epitheliocystis disease in fish, have never been cultured in cell lines or on artificial media. Table A7.1 contains a partial list of commonly used bacterial media and there uses.

Antibiotic Sensitivity Testing

While basic principles of antibiotic sensitivity testing are identical for fish and mammalian bacterial isolates, standards, including interpretive criteria, are not as well-established for the testing of all fish pathogens. As a result, some veterinary diagnostic laboratories may report results with disclaimers attached. The adoption of standardized procedures is also not universal among fish diagnostic laboratories and can influence test outcomes. Differences can include how media and inoculums are prepared, incubation times and temperatures, the use of reference strains for controls, and special procedures for fastidious organisms. However, guidelines for disc diffusion susceptibility testing of certain bacterial fish pathogens have been published by the Clinical and Laboratory Standards Institute (CLSI 2006, 2014a, 2014b).

Virology

Viral diseases have historically been diagnosed using various combinations of signalment, clinical signs, histopathology, electron microscopy, and virus isolation in cell culture with observation of compatible cytopathic effect (CPE). Antibody and molecular-based diagnostics are becoming increasingly common confirmatory tests. Today, polymerase chain reaction (PCR) protocols can be found for most common and reportable fish viral diseases in the primary literature, the OIE Manual of Diagnostic Tests for Aquatic Animals, and the American Fisheries Society Fish Health Section Bluebook (AFS-FHS 2014; OIE 2018). A list of OIE reportable diseases can be found in Table A7.2.

Virus isolation involves the homogenization of suspect tissue (often ~1.5 g), centrifugation to remove cell debris, filtering to remove contaminating bacteria, and inoculation of appropriate cell lines, followed by incubation and observation for CPE. Prior to the inoculation of cell lines, samples can be stored at 4°C (39°F) for 24–48 hours. If longer storage periods are required, they should be frozen at −80°C (−112°F).

Suitable cell lines exist for commonly cultured fish species, such as salmonids and channel catfish. However, many fish viruses are relatively host-specific and their isolation has been impeded by a lack of permissive cell lines. This problem has been compounded by the increasingly long list of fish species grown in aquaculture and displayed in aquariums. Despite this, cell culture remains an important component of fish disease diagnostics. An extensive list of fish cells and their diagnostic uses can be found in Plumb and Hanson (2011). Cell lines used to detect OIE reportable viral pathogens are listed in Box A7.1.

The number of viruses and viral families identified in fish has increased dramatically in recent years. However, the great diversity that exists among viral families limits the use of generic identification approaches similar to the 16S rRNA gene widely used in bacteria. Although some PCR protocols exploit similarities between families, such as the polymerase gene of the large DNA viruses, there is no simple one-size-fits-all approach to the diagnosis of viral diseases (Hanson et al. 2006). Particularly with novel viruses, or when viral disease is suspected and cell culture is either unavailable or has failed, sequence-independent metagenomic approaches (next-generation sequencing) have great promise for the identification of viral agents. However, costs at present are too high for routine diagnostics and these techniques remain primarily research tools.

Molecular Diagnostics

Nucleic Acid Amplification Methods

PCR, qPCR, RT-PCR

Molecular assays detect and identify micro-organisms in fish and environmental samples based on the sequences of their genetic material (DNA or RNA). Offering speed, specificity, and sensitivity, the most widely used among these methods are nucleic acid amplification assays based on the polymerase chain reaction (PCR). PCR assays are particularly useful in the detection of slow-growing or fastidious organisms that require special culture conditions. They can also avoid problems resulting from contamination or the presence of multiple organisms that can plague culture-based diagnostics. Depending on the approach, PCR testing can be specific for certain organisms (e.g. conventional PCR, qPCR) or more general in nature (e.g. consensus primer PCR). Specific primer sets have been published for many important fish pathogens (AFS-FHS 2014; OIE 2018). Primer sets can also be designed from known genetic sequences. Although a lengthy review of molecular assays is beyond the scope of this chapter, a brief description of commonly used PCR methods follows.

Table A7.1 Standard and specialized bacterial media and their uses.

Bacterial media	Bacterial species	Reference
Brain Heart Infusion Agar (BHIA)	*Aeromonas* spp.	
Tryptic Soy Agar (TSA)	*Pseudomonas* spp.	
Blood Agar (BA)/TSA with 5% sheep blood	*Vibrio* spp.	
	Edwardsiella spp.	
	Streptococcus spp.	
	Yersinia ruckeri	
	Carnobacterium piscicola	
TSA with 5% sheep blood	*Weissella ceti*	AFS-FHS (2014)
	Aliivibrio salmonicida	Egidius et al. (1984)
	Photobacterium damselae subsp. *damselae* and *piscicida*	Robohm (1983)
	Mycobacterium marinum	Hawke (1996)
	Mycobacterium fortuitum	Plumb and Hanson (2011)
	Mycobacterium chelonae	
Tryptone Yeast Extract Salts Agar (TYES)	*Flavobacterium psychrophilum*	AFS-FHS (2014)
Shieh Medium	*Flavobacterium columnare*	Shieh (1980)
Cytophaga Agar	Flavobacteria	Anacker and Ordal (1959)
Modified Cytophaga Agar		Wakabayashi and Egusa (1974)
Hsu–Shotts Agar		Baxa et al. (1986)
Anaker & Ordal Agar with 70% seawater	*Tenacibaculum maritimum*	Avendaño-Herrera et al. (2006)
Hsu–Shotts with 50% seawater and antibiotics		
TSA with Coomassie Brilliant Blue	*Aeromonas salmonicida*	
Selective Kidney Disease Medium-2 (SKDM-2)	*Renibacterium salmoninarum*	Austin et al. (1983)
Shotts–Waltman	*Yersinia ruckeri*	Waltman and Shotts (1984)
BHI and TSA with 1–1.5% (or higher) NaCl	*Vibrio anguillarum*	Plumb and Hanson (2011)
	Vibrio ordalii	
	Aliivibrio salmonicida	
BHI and TSA with 2% NaCl	*Photobacterium damselae* subsp. *damselae* and *piscicida*	Hawke (1996)
Cysteine Heart Agar with Hemoglobin (CHAH)	*Francisella* spp.	Soto et al. (2009)
Thayer–Martin		
Various cysteine and iron supplemented media	*Piscirickettsia salmonis*	Makrinos and Bowden (2016)
Lowenstein–Jensen	*Mycobacterium* spp.	
Middlebrook (7H10)		
Todd Hewitt	*Streptococcus* spp.	Plumb and Hanson (2011)
Columbia CNA		

Conventional (or end-point) PCR requires the use of a thermostable polymerase, deoxynucleotides of each base, target DNA, and oligonucleotide primers designed to target a specific DNA region. After the extraction of DNA from a sample, a series of reaction cycles (denaturation, annealing, and extension) allow the target DNA to be amplified in an exponential fashion (Wittwer and Kusukawa 2007). Most laboratories use commercially available extraction kits tailored to specific sample conditions. The amplification assays are used to produce enough copies of a nucleic acid target to be visualized on an agarose gel or sequenced. On gels, a band of correct size indicates a positive test, while sequenced PCR products are compared to sequences in genetic databases such as GenBank® (National Institute

Table A7.2 OIE-listed fish diseases in 2019.

Disease and/or agent	Classification
Epizootic hematopoietic necrosis (EHN)	*Iridoviridae*; *Ranavirus*
Red sea bream iridovirus (RSIV)	*Iridoviridae*; *Megalocytivirus*
Infectious salmon anemia (ISA)	*Orthomyxoviridae*; *Isavirus*
Infectious hematopoietic necrosis (IHN)	*Rhabdoviridae*; *Novirhabdovirus*
Viral hemorrhagic septicemia (VHS)	*Rhabdoviridae*; *Novirhabdovirus*
Spring viremia of carp (SVC)	*Rhabdoviridae*; *Vesiculovirus*
Koi herpesvirus (KHV)	*Alloherpesviridae*
Salmonid alphavirus (SAV)	*Togaviridae*; *Alphavirus*
Gyrodactylus salaris	*Monogenea*
Aphanomyces invadans, epizootic ulcerative syndrome (EUS)	Oomycete

Source: OIE (2018). © John Wiley & Sons.

of Health). Genetic sequencing provides more information and is often used to discriminate between closely related organisms or to identify novel species. PCR products can also be used in fingerprinting assays, such as restriction fragment length polymorphisms (RFLP), in which the amplified product is digested by one or more restriction enzymes and electrophoresed to produce a pattern of gel bands that can be used to compare differences between organisms (Wittwer and Kusukawa 2007).

Conventional PCR provides a yes or no answer, not quantitative data, and as a result, pathogen loads cannot be assessed. This shortcoming is important to infections such as koi herpesvirus disease, where it may be desirable to differentiate an active infection from a carrier state. This problem is overcome by a rapid quantitative method known as real-time PCR, often abbreviated qPCR, to avoid confusion with reverse transcription PCR (RT-PCR). qPCR employs the same DNA amplification principles as the conventional method but uses a thermocycler that monitors the process in real time. A final gel electrophoresis step is not required. In its simplest format, fluorescent dyes, most commonly SYBR Green, are added to the initial reaction mixture. If any DNA is amplified, fluorescence increases with each reaction cycle as more dye binds to the growing number of dsDNA copies. How early a signal is detected depends on the amount of target DNA initially present, providing a systematic method of quantification. A melting curve can also be generated when fluorescence is monitored continuously as the temperature is increased. Melting analyses are used to verify the identity of the amplified products and to detect sequence variants. A second detection format uses fluorescent labeled oligonucleotide probes, in addition to PCR primers, to increase specificity (Bustin and Kessler 2014).

Box A7.1 Cell Lines Used to Test for OIE-Reportable Viral Fish Pathogens (OIE 2018)

- Epithelioma papulosum cyprini (EPC)
- Bluegill fry (BF-2)
- Fathead minnow (FHM)
- Rainbow trout gonad (RTG)
- Chinook salmon embryo (CHSE-2)
- Salmon head kidney (SHK-1)
- Atlantic salmon kidney (ASK)
- Grunt fin (GF)
- Koi fin (KF)
- *Cyprinus carpio* brain (CCB)
- Striped snakehead (SSN-1)

Reverse transcription PCR is an amplification variant used to detect RNA expression. This two-step process first uses reverse transcriptase enzymes to synthesize complimentary DNA (cDNA) from an RNA template. The cDNA can then be further amplified and analyzed using conventional and qPCR. While applicable to studies of gene expression, RT-PCR is also used diagnostically to detect RNA viruses, including the infectious salmon anemia orthomyxovirus, rhabdoviruses, salmonid alphaviruses, and betanodaviruses (OIE 2018).

Despite their advantages, PCR-based methods have limitations. Notably, PCR does not allow direct correlation of infectious agents with lesions, a major attribute of immunohistochemical (IHC) and in situ hybridization (ISH) techniques. Primer design requires some knowledge of the target sequence, limiting the identification of unknown pathogens. Other potential problems include sample contamination with exogenous nucleic acids, nonspecific primer binding to nontarget sequences, poor primer binding to intended sequences, and errors in nucleotide incorporation by polymerases into product sequences (Garibyan and Avashia 2013). Prior to formalin fixation, if PCR-based analysis is anticipated, suspect tissue samples should be frozen or fixed in 70% ethanol. Formalin fixation will limit the sensitivity of PCR. Nucleic acids in formalin-fixed tissues, particularly formalin-fixed paraffin-embedded tissues, become trapped, degraded, and fragmented. The degree of damage depends on fixation duration, fixative type, tissue type, temperature, and severity of pre-fixation autolysis (Gilbert et al. 2007; Dietrich et al. 2013). Fixation in 10% neutral buffered formalin is generally not deleterious if tissues are fixed less than 24–48 hours or DNA targets are small (less than 125 bp). Acid fixatives, such as Bouin's solution, severely compromise amplification and should not be used prior to PCR (Greer et al. 1990; Fiallo et al. 1992). RNA is more labile than DNA and requires different processing methods (Bonin and Stanta 2011).

Multiplex PCR

Multiplex PCR is an adaptation of the polymerase chain reaction in which multiple primer sets are used in a single PCR to amplify one or more possible targets. The primers must be designed such that all are optimized for the same annealing temperature and ideally produce amplicons of varying sizes that can be differentiated using gel electrophoresis. Applications include the detection of multiple pathogens common to fish in a geographic area or prevalent in a certain fish species (Tapia-Cammas et al. 2011; Itsaro et al. 2012).

Consensus PCR

A widely employed, nonspecific PCR approach to pathogen detection uses consensus primers directed against genes that are universal to the group under investigation. The primers target highly conserved portions of a gene flanking variable regions that are used for comparative purposes. If an amplicon of expected size is visualized on a gel, it is purified, sequenced, and compared in a sequence database such as GenBank, by performing a basic local alignment search tool (BLAST) inquiry (Maes et al. 2014). Amplification and sequencing of the bacterial 16S rRNA gene, or portions of it, are the best-known broad range procedure of this type (Clarridge 2004). The 18S rRNA gene and other members of the RNA gene cluster are used similarly with fungi (Khot et al. 2009). This approach is less applicable to viruses, due to the great genomic diversity among viral families.

From a clinical standpoint, 16S rRNA sequencing can expedite identification of slow-growing organisms and can identify non-culturable species or those inhibited by antibiotic therapy. It is less subjective than phenotypic testing and generally better for identifying poorly described, rarely isolated, or biochemically atypical strains. As such, it can lead to the discovery of novel pathogens and is useful for demonstrating phylogenetic relationships among bacteria (Clarridge 2004). However, 16S rRNA sequencing alone may not discriminate between strains or closely related species (Mignard and Flandrois 2006; Sontakke et al. 2009). Furthermore, only a limited number of gene sequences may be available for comparison of unusual or uncommon isolates (Sontakke et al. 2009). Additional problems can arise when searching unverified and non-peer reviewed databases, such as GenBank, that will accept any linked name and sequence and often contain errors (Clarridge 2004).

DNA Sequencing

DNA sequencing can be used to confirm the identity of suspected pathogens (e.g. 16S or 18S rRNA gene sequences) or establish entire novel genomes, particularly viral. Since its introduction in the late 1970s, DNA sequencing has evolved to include multiple methodologies and varied instrument platforms, each with advantages and disadvantages, which have catalyzed an ongoing revolution in biomedical research (Mardis 2008, 2013, 2017; Metzker 2010). Automated Sanger sequencing, often referred to as first-generation sequencing, is used for the sequencing of PCR products, for the validation of next-generation sequencing (NGS) results, and when longer reads are desirable, such as in the construction of reference genomes. However, Sanger technology requires some prior knowledge of the target sequence in order for PCR primers to be designed. NGS methods have no such requirement and are useful when unknown agents, particularly viruses, are suspected. NGS is responsible for the discovery of many new viruses in fish, including the first characterization of a viral genome from an elasmobranch (Dill et al. 2018). For large-scale genome analyses, there has also been a shift toward NGS platforms, which have dramatically increased output and decreased operating costs. All rely on basic principles of DNA replication and incorporate PCR amplification, with the exception of emerging single-molecule sequencing (SMS) technologies. Differences among platforms include the medium on which amplification occurs, e.g. glass (Illumina) versus magnetic beads (Applied Biosystems); method of nucleotide addition, e.g. synthesis (Roche/454, Illumina, Ion Torrent) versus ligation (Applied Biosystems); and sequence detection, e.g. fluorescence (Illumina, Applied Biosystems) versus pH change (Ion Torrent). However, differences in throughput capacity, error rates, and read lengths are the most important practical considerations. Sanger sequencing generates reads of 600–800 bp, while NGS reads are shorter, 50–400 bp depending on the platform used.

NGS begins with the construction of a library of DNA fragments created from a sample of interest and ligation of synthetic DNA adapters to each end that serve as priming sites to initiate PCR amplification. Since all platforms generate massive amounts of data, sophisticated computational analysis is required for sequence evaluation and assembly, which has significance to read lengths. With longer Sanger sequences, assembly is performed using shared sequence overlaps. In contrast, NGS reads are aligned to a known reference sequence or are assembled de novo (Metzker 2010). Although technologies are constantly improving, the short reads generated by NGS pose alignment problems, especially with large genomes and those with repetitive content, necessitating much higher read numbers to reduce error rates (Metzker 2010; Mardis 2017). De novo assembly is generally restricted to the smallest, primarily viral, genomes and its use is based on reference sequence availability (Metzker 2010).

With SMS, individual DNA molecules are sequenced in parallel, rather than PCR-amplified prior to sequencing. This is a more straightforward process that requires less starting material than NGS (Metzker 2010). While these platforms produce much longer and easier to assemble reads, error rates are higher. However, the Pacific Biosciences SMS platform, which can produce reads of up to 40 kb, uses computational methods to produce sequences with error rates comparable to Sanger assemblies and NGS alignments. A less expensive and increasingly feasible SMS alternative in terms of error rates is Oxford Nanopore technology (Mardis 2017).

Metagenomics and Microbiomes

The growing number of sequenced microbial genomes has enabled researchers to interpret partial sequences, such as bacterial 16S rRNA gene sequences, from environmental samples. Known as metagenomics, this growing field has demonstrated much greater biodiversity than revealed by culture in a variety of environments, including niches within the bodies of animals. Additionally, these diverse microbial communities, or microbiomes, vary with the health status of the animal (Mardis 2008). In the gastrointestinal tract, they have important effects on nutrient processing, immune and other homeostatic functions, and provide a rationale for the use of commensal organisms as therapeutic agents (Hooper and Gordon 2001).

Immunohistochemistry

Immunohistochemistry (IHC) is used as an adjunct to routine histology to visualize specific antigen presence within tissue sections (Figure A7.30). Diagnostically, the identification of an antigen within a lesion enhances its significance and, as such, IHC is used primarily to identify infectious agents (e.g. *Piscirickettsia salmonis*, infectious pancreatic necrosis virus) and to characterize neoplastic cell types (e.g. the presence of cytokeratin in squamous cell carcinomas). The basic principle exploits the ability of antibodies to react with specific antigens and other antibodies. Linking antibodies to colorimetric reporters permits localization of target molecules in cells or tissues by light or fluorescent microscopy. Reporter systems are based on enzyme– (e.g. alkaline phosphatase, horseradish peroxidase) substrate reactions triggered when antigen–antibody binding occurs. The most commonly used substrate molecules are chromogenic (e.g. DAB, AEC) or fluorogenic (e.g. TITC, FITC). As with some serologic assays, IHC protocols may be direct or indirect. In direct protocols, a labeled antibody reacts directly with an antigen in tissue. With indirect protocols, an unlabeled primary antibody is bound to the target antigen, followed by a second labeled antibody directed against the animal species from which the first antibody was derived. Sensitivity is greater with indirect assays, because the signal is amplified by the binding of multiple secondary antibodies to sites on the first (Ramos-Vara and Miller 2013).

IHC methodology is complex and ultimately dependent on qualities of the primary antibody and the antigen's ability to bind it. As with PCR, formalin fixation induces protein cross-linking that can mask antigenic sites and cause false negative results. However, this has been largely overcome by the use of antigen retrieval techniques that reverse the effects of formalin fixation on proteins. Steps must also be taken to block interference by enzymes and other endogenous substances (Ramos-Vara and Miller 2013). Consideration should also be given to the use of monoclonal versus polyclonal antibodies, as the latter have a greater likelihood of cross-reacting with other pathogens (Maes et al. 2014). Unfortunately, many commercial antibodies derived from mammalian sources do not cross react with their corresponding antigenic targets in fish. Comprehensive IHC protocols to identify specific cell types in fish are lacking and nonspecific tissue immunoreactivity has been reported. In addition, even antibodies generated in fish can show interspecies differences in reactivity (García et al. 2005; Spitsbergen et al. 2011; Paquette et al. 2015). These complicating factors make it essential that appropriate positive and negative controls be used with IHC protocols to distinguish nonspecific reactions, negative reactions, and failures of antibodies to react with fish tissue.

In Situ Hybridization

IHC and in situ hybridization (ISH) have similar applications, including the demonstration of pathogens within tissues or lesions (Figure A7.31). However, while IHC exploits antigen–antibody interactions, ISH is directed against gene sequences through the hybridization of reporter-labeled nucleic acid probes to their complementary DNA or RNA targets (Maes et al. 2014). Many technical variations exist that are appropriate to different probe types and targets. DNA probes can be generated by DNA synthesizers or conveniently produced from PCR products. RNA probes are

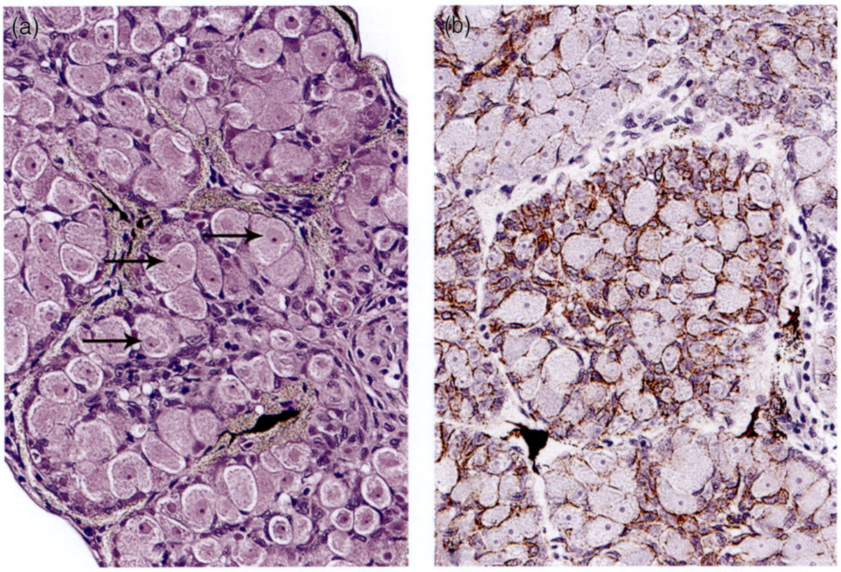

Figure A7.30 X-cell pseudotumor in a histologic section of skin from a slippery dick (*Halichoeres bivittatus*). The protozoan parasites (arrows) are not readily discernable with H&E staining (b), but are outlined using an IHC stain for cytokeratin (CK) in the host's epithelial cells. CK AE1/AE3 400×.

prepared by reverse transcription of cDNA templates. Most labeling and detection systems use biotin or digoxigenin in conjunction with chromogenic or fluorogenic reporter systems. Digoxigenin-labeled probes offer greater sensitivity and less background staining than biotinylated probes, as digoxigenin does not cross-react with animal tissues like biotin. Similar substrates as used for IHC produce color (Jin and Lloyd 1997). When fluorochromes are used, the procedure is referred to as FISH. This approach can make pathogens more readily visible when their target nucleic acid is present in only small amounts. Most protocols require two to three days to complete and include the permeabilization of cells to facilitate probe entry (e.g. with proteinase K), denaturation with heat (if target is dsDNA), hybridization of probe to target, washing, and signal detection (Brown 1998).

Advantages include the use of either generic or species-specific probes and, because mRNA synthesis precedes that of its encoded proteins, ISH can detect pathogens earlier than IHC. Used in combination with IHC, ISH can differentiate sites of productive versus nonproductive viral infection. Major shortcomings of both IHC and ISH relate to the differentiation of specific from nonspecific background labeling of tissue components (Brown 1998; Maes et al. 2014). Concerning fish diagnostics, laboratories are frequently hindered by a lack of similarly processed control tissue containing the desired target or pathogen in detectable levels (Maes et al. 2014).

Antibody-Based Testing

Antibody-based testing can be used to identify suspected pathogens or antibodies produced by an animal in response to a specific disease agent. The high specificity of antigen–antibody based interactions can be exploited to identify antibodies directed against specific agents in the blood and bodily fluids of animals. Similarly, preformed antibodies prepared against specific antigens can be used in diagnostic tests to identify specific agents in culture or clinical samples. Quantification of antibody levels, or serum titers, can provide additional information on past versus active infection. Unfortunately, the utility of immune-based assays in fish health is frequently limited by the availability of reagents, including pathogen-specific labeled antibodies, as well as fish species-specific antibodies (AFS-FHS 2014). Two of the most widely employed immune assays used in fish diagnostics are fluorescent antibody tests (FA) and enzyme-linked immunosorbent assays (ELISA). Variations of both methods include direct and indirect assays. While direct assays are technically simpler, indirect assays are more sensitive and the use of secondary antibodies avoids the expensive production of conjugated antibodies for individual antigens. Protocols for many important fish pathogens can be found in the OIE Manual of Diagnostic Tests for Aquatic Animals (OIE 2018) and the American Fisheries Society Fish Health Section Bluebook (AFS-FHS 2014).

Fluorescent Antibody Testing

With direct FA tests (DFAT), a target antigen fixed to a glass cytology or histology slide is bound by a fluorescently labeled antibody. The antigen can then be illuminated and detected using a fluorescent microscope. DFAT is useful for the rapid detection of bacteria, particularly species that are difficult to isolate in culture. With indirect FA tests (IFAT), antigen is again fixed to a slide. This is followed by the addition of a purified unlabeled antibody prepared in one animal species against the antigen. A secondary labeled

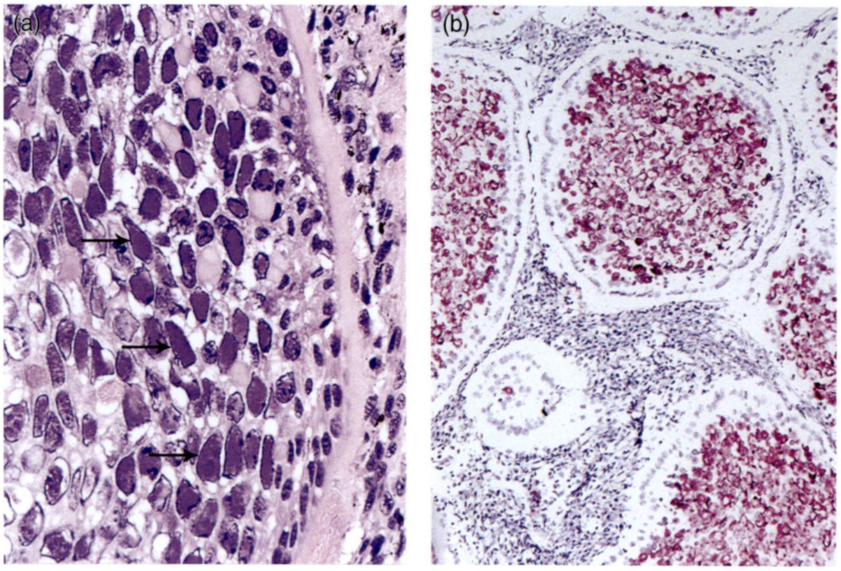

Figure A7.31 Histologic sections of skin from a giant guitarfish (*Rhynchobatus djiddensis*) showing amphophilic intranuclear inclusion bodies (arrows) in proliferative epithelial cells. H&E 400× (a). Using in situ hybridization, a virus-specific probe labeled with fast red localized viral DNA to nuclei of epithelial cells in the spinous layer. Cells of the basal layer and adjacent dermis are unaffected. 100× (b).

antibody, prepared in a second animal species against the first, is added for fluorescence detection. Alternatively, patient serum can be used as the first antibody. As an example, both direct and indirect FA tests are used to detect *Renibacterium salmoninarum*.

Enzyme-Linked Immunosorbent Assays (ELISAs)

ELISAs are similar in principle to FA testing, involving at least one antibody with specificity for a particular antigen, and they can also be modified to detect antigen or antibody. They have been widely used in the diagnosis of salmonid diseases, including the viruses of infectious pancreatic necrosis, infectious hematopoietic necrosis, and viral hemorrhagic septicemia. With ELISAs, antigen is immobilized, usually on 96-well polystyrene microtiter plates, and detection is colorimetric. Color is produced using enzyme-conjugated antibodies (e.g. horseradish peroxidase) and substrate (e.g. ABTS, OPD, TMB) reactions similar to those used in ISH or IHC. In a direct ELISA, the antigen in question is adhered to the well bottom and covered with a nonreacting protein to which the specific enzyme-conjugated antibody is added. If antigen binding has occurred, a color change results upon substrate addition. The intensity of color production is proportional to the amount of antibody bound, making it possible to quantify the assay using a spectrophotometer and comparing results to a standard curve. With an indirect ELISA, a secondary conjugated antibody is used, similar to and with the same limitations as IFAT. Sandwich ELISA tests are used to detect antigens in clinical samples, such as patient serum. Adhered antibody is used to capture a specific antigen, followed by the addition of a primary unconjugated antibody, which could be in patient serum, "sandwiching" the antigen between the two. Finally, a secondary conjugated antibody and substrate are added.

Conclusion

Fish are increasingly popular as pets and as display animals in public aquariums. Aquaculture production supplies approximately half of the world's demand for fish protein. Fish also serve as sentinels of environmental health and as important laboratory species. Since 2000, over half of the emerging pathogens identified in wildlife have come from fish (Tompkins et al. 2015). As a result, there is a growing demand for trained individuals, diagnostic services, and improved diagnostic methods in fish health that include both traditional approaches, such as hematology, biochemistry, and microscopy, as well as state-of-the art molecular techniques, like next-generation sequencing. It is critical that clinicians and diagnosticians be familiar with available testing methods, their applications, and their limitations. Diagnostic investigations and the interpretation of results should consider the unique anatomic and physiologic adaptions encountered in fish, the negative impacts created by disturbances in the quality of their varied aquatic habitats, and how these many factors influence host pathogen interactions.

References

AFS-FHS (2014). *Fish Health Section Blue Book, 2014 Edition, Suggested Procedures for the Detection and Identification of Certain Finfish and Shellfish Pathogens* [online]. http://www.afs-fhs.org/bluebook/bluebook-index.php (accessed 1 November 2018).

Ainsworth, A. (1992). Fish granulocytes: morphology, distribution, and function. *Annual Review of Fish Diseases* 2: 123–148.

Anacker, R.L. and Ordal, E.J. (1959). Studies on the myxobacterium *Chondrococcus columnaris,* I. Serological typing. *Journal of Bacteriology* 78: 25–32.

Anderson, E.T., Stoskopf, M.K., Morris, J.A. et al. (2010). Hematology, plasma biochemistry, and tissue enzyme activities of invasive red lionfish captured off North Carolina, USA. *Journal of Aquatic Animal Health* 22: 266–273.

Arnold, J.A. (2005). Hematology of the sandbar shark, *Carcharhinus plumbeus*: standardization of complete blood count techniques for elasmobranchs. *Veterinary Clinical Pathology* 34: 115–123.

Arnold, J. (2009). Hematology of fish: WBC and RBC cell morphology. *Proceedings of the American College of Veterinary Pathology*, Monterey, CA.

Arnold, J., Matsche, M., and Rosemary, K. (2014). Preserving whole blood in formalin extends the specimen stability period for manual cell counts in fish. *Veterinary Clinical Pathology* 43: 613–620.

Austin, B., Embley, T.M., and Goodfellow, M. (1983). Selective isolation of *Renibacterium salmoninarum*. *FEMS Microbiology Letters* 17: 111–114.

Avendaño-Herrera, R., Toranzo, A.E., and Magariños, B. (2006). Tenacibaculosis infection in marine fish caused by *Tenacibaculum maritimum*: a review. *Diseases of Aquatic Organisms* 71: 255–266.

Baxa, D.V., Kawai, K., and Kusuda, R. (1986). Characteristics of gliding bacteria isolated from diseased cultured flounder, *Paralichthys olivaceous*. *Fish Pathology* 21: 251–258.

Bielmyer, G.K., Tomasso, J., and Klaine, S.J. (2006). Physiological responses of hybrid striped bass to aqueous copper in freshwater and saltwater. *Archives of Environmental Contamination and Toxicology* 50: 531–538.

Biswas, S. and Rolain, J.-M. (2013). Use of MALDI-TOF mass spectrometry for identification of bacteria that are difficult to culture. *Journal of Microbiological Methods* 92: 14–24.

Bonin, S. and Stanta, G. (2011). RNA extraction for formalin-fixed paraffin-embedded tissues. In: *Guidelines for Molecular Analysis in Archive Tissues* (ed. G. Stanta), 57–61. New York: Springer.

Braceland, M., Houston, K., Ashby, A. et al. (2017). Technical pre-analytical effects on the clinical biochemistry of Atlantic salmon (*Salmo salar* L.). *Journal of Fish Diseases* 40: 29–40.

Brown, C. (1998). In situ hybridization with riboprobes: an overview for veterinary pathologists. *Veterinary Pathology* 35: 159–167.

Buchmann, K. and Lindenstrøm, T. (2002). Interactions between monogenean parasites and their fish hosts. *International Journal for Parasitology* 32: 309–319.

Bustin, S.A. and Kessler, H.H. (2014). Amplification and detection methods. In: *Molecular Diagnostics of Infectious Diseases*, 3e (ed. H.H. Kessler), 63–84. Boston, MA: Walter de Gruyter.

Calderaro, A., Arcangeletti, M.C., Rodighiero, I. et al. (2014). Matrix-assisted laser desorption/ionization time-of-flight (MALDI-TOF) mass spectrometry applied to virus identification. *Scientific Reports* 4: 6803.

Campbell, T. (2012). Clinical chemistry of fish and amphibians. In: *Veterinary Hematology and Clinical Chemistry*, 2e (eds. M.A. Thrall, G. Weiser, R.W. Allison and T.W. Campbell), 607–614. Ames, IA: Wiley.

Camus, M. and Pope, D. (2012). Explaining the uncertainties: examination of inherent inaccuracy in WBC estimates from peripheral blood smears. *Proceedings of the American College of Veterinary Pathologists*, Seattle, WA.

Camus, A., Wise, D., Khoo, L. et al. (2014). Iron status of channel catfish *Ictalurus punctatus* affected by channel catfish anemia and response to parenteral iron. *Diseases of Aquatic Organisms* 107: 241–248.

Clarridge, J.E. (2004). Impact of 16S rRNA gene sequence analysis for identification of bacteria on clinical microbiology and infectious diseases. *Clinical Microbiology Reviews* 17: 840–862.

CLSI (2006). VET03-A: Methods for Antimicrobial Disk Susceptibility Testing of Bacteria Isolated from Aquatic Animals. Wayne, PA: Clinical and Laboratory Standards Institute.

CLSI (2014a). VET04-A2: Methods for Broth Dilution Susceptibility Testing of Bacteria Isolated from Aquatic Animals, 2e. Wayne, PA: Clinical and Laboratory Standards Institute.

CLSI (2014b). VET03/VET04-S2: Performance Standards for Antimicrobial Susceptibility Testing of Bacteria Isolated from Aquatic Animals, 2nd Informational Supplement. Wayne, PA: Clinical and Laboratory Standards Institute.

Collicutt, N.B., Garner, B., Berghaus, R.D. et al. (2015). Effect of delayed serum separation and storage temperature on serum glucose concentration in horse, dog, alpaca, and sturgeon. *Veterinary Clinical Pathology* 44: 120–127.

Cooke, S.J., Suski, C.D., Danylchuk, S.E. et al. (2008). Effects of different capture techniques on the physiological condition of bonefish *Albula vulpes* evaluated using field diagnostic tools. *Journal of Fish Biology* 73: 1351–1375.

Dietrich, D., Uhl, B., Sailer, V. et al. (2013). Improved PCR performance using template DNA from formalin-fixed paraffin-embedded tissues by overcoming PCR inhibition. *PLoS One* 8: e77771.

Dill, J., Brown, C., Heym, K. et al. (2016). Lipoid liver disease, atherosclerosis and glomerular lipidosis in a Gulf flounder *Paralichthys albigutta* (Jordan and Gilbert 1882): a case report. *Journal of Fish Diseases* 40: 273–278.

Dill, J., Sanchez, S., McDermott, A., and Camus, A. (2017). Disseminated nocardiosis associated with the isolation of *Nocardia nova* in a longsnout seahorse *Hippocampus reidi* (Ginsburg). *Journal of Fish Diseases* 40: 1235–1239.

Dill, J.A., Camus, A.C., Leary, J.H., and Ng, T.F.F. (2018). Microscopic and molecular evidence of the first elasmobranch adomavirus, the cause of skin disease in a giant guitarfish, *Rhynchobatus djiddensis. MBio* 9: e00185-18.

Egidius, E., Soleim, O., and Anderson, K. (1984). Further observations on cold-water vibriosis or hitra disease. *Bulletin of the European Association of Fish Pathologists* 4: 50–51.

Ellis, A.E. (1977). The leukocytes of fish: a review. *Journal of Fish Biology* 11: 453–391.

Ferguson, H.W. (1976). The ultrastructure of plaice (*Pleuronectes platessa*) leukocytes. *Journal of Fish Biology* 8: 139–142.

Fiallo, P., Williams, D.L., Chan, G.P. et al. (1992). Effects of fixation on polymerase chain reaction detection of *Mycobacterium leprae. Journal of Clinical Microbiology* 30: 3095–3098.

Flatland, B., Camus, M.S., and Baral, R.M. (2018). Analytical quality goals: a review. *Veterinary Clinical Pathology* 47: 527–538.

Flerova, E.A. and Balabanova, L.V. (2013). Ultrastructure of granulocytes of teleost fish (Salmoniformes, Cypriniformes, Perciformes). *Journal of Evolutionary Biochemistry and Physiology* 49: 223–233.

Friedrichs, K., Harr, K., Freeman, K. et al. (2012). ASVCP reference interval guidelines: determination of de novo reference intervals in veterinary species and other related topics. *Veterinary Clinical Pathology* 41: 441–453.

Fukunaga, K., Nakazono, N., Suzuki, T. et al. (1999). Mechanism of oxidative damage to fish red blood cells by ozone. *Life* 48: 631–638.

García, D.M., Bauer, H., Dietz, T. et al. (2005). Identification of keratins and analysis of their expression in carp and goldfish: comparison with the zebrafish and trout catalog. *Cell and Tissue Research* 322: 245–256.

Garibyan, L. and Avashia, N. (2013). Research techniques made simple: polymerase chain reaction (PCR). *Journal of Investigative Dermatology* 133: e6.

Gilbert, M.T., Haselkorn, T., Bunce, M. et al. (2007). The isolation of nucleic acids from fixed, paraffin-embedded tissues – which methods are useful when? *PLoS One* 2: e537.

Greer, C.E., Peterson, S.L., Kiviat, N.B. et al. (1990). PCR amplification from paraffin-embedded tissues. Effects of fixative and fixation time. *American Journal of Clinical Pathology* 95: 117–124.

Grosell, M., Wood, C.M., and Walsh, P.J. (2003). Copper homeostasis and toxicity in the elasmobranch *Raja erinacea* and the teleost *Myoxocephalus octodecemspinosus* during exposure to elevated water-borne copper. *Comparative Biochemistry and Physiology Part C* 135: 179–190.

Guerreiro, P.M., Renfro, J.L., Power, D.M. et al. (2007). The parathyroid hormone family of peptides: structure, tissue distribution, regulation, and potential functional roles in calcium and phosphate balance in fish. *American Journal of Physiology. Regulatory, Integrative and Comparative Physiology* 292: R679–R696.

Haines, A.N. and Arnold, J.E. (2014). Elasmobranch blood cells. In: *Immunobiology of the Shark* (eds. S.L. Smith, R.B. Sim and M.F. Flajnik), 89–103. Boca Raton, FL: CRC Press.

Hammerschlag, N. (2006). Osmoregulation in elasmobranchs: a review for fish biologists, behaviourists and ecologists. *Marine and Freshwater Behaviour and Physiology* 39: 209–228.

Hanson, L.A., Rudis, M.R., Vasquez-Lee, M. et al. (2006). A broadly applicable method to characterize large DNA viruses and adenoviruses based on the DNA polymerase gene. *Virology Journal* 3: 28.

Harms, C., Ross, T., and Segars, A. (2002). Plasma biochemistry reference values of wild bonnethead sharks, *Sphyrna tiburo. Veterinary Clinical Pathology* 31: 111–115.

Hawke, J.P. (1996). Importance of a siderophore in the pathogenesis and virulence of *Photobacterium damselae subsp. piscicida* in hybrid striped bass (*Morone saxatilis* x *Morone chrysops*). Ph.D. Dissertation. Louisiana State University, Baton Rouge, LA.

Heming, T. (1989). Clinical studies of fish blood: importance of sample collection and measurement techniques. *American Journal of Veterinary Research* 50: 93–97.

Hooper, L.V. and Gordon, J.I. (2001). Commensal host-bacterial relationships in the gut. *Science* 292: 1115–1118.

Houston, A. (1990). Blood and circulation. In: *Methods in Fish Biology* (eds. C. Schreck and P. Moyle), 273–334. Bethesda, MD: American Fisheries Society.

Hrubec, T., Smith, S., Robertson, J. et al. (1996). Comparison of hematologic reference intervals between culture systems and type of hybrid striped bass. *American Journal of Veterinary Research* 57: 618–623.

Hrubec, T., Cardinale, J., and Smith, S. (2000). Hematology and plasma chemistry reference intervals for cultured tilapia (*Oreochromis* hybrid). *Veterinary Clinical Pathology* 29: 7–12.

Itsaro, A., Suanyuk, N., and Tantikitti, C. (2012). Multiplex PCR for simultaneous detection of *Streptococcus agalactiae*, *Streptococcus iniae* and *Lactococcus garvieae*: a case of *S. agalactiae* infection in cultured Nile tilapia (*Oreochromis niloticus*) and red tilapia (*Oreochromis niloticus* x *Oreochromis mossambicus*). *Songklanakarin Journal of Science and Technology* 34: 495–500.

Jin, L. and Lloyd, R.V. (1997). In situ hybridization: methods and applications. *Journal of Clinical Laboratory Analysis* 11: 2–9.

Khot, P.D., Ko, D.L., and Fredricks, D.N. (2009). Sequencing and analysis of fungal rRNA operons for development of broad-range fungal PCR assays. *Applied and Environmental Microbiology* 75: 1559–1565.

Leard, A., Wagner, B., Camp, K. et al. (1998). Seasonal values of selected blood parameters of farm-raised channel catfish (*Ictalurus punctatus*) in the Mississippi Delta. *Journal of Veterinary Diagnostic Investigation* 10: 344–349.

Lumsden, J.S. (2006). Gastrointestinal tract, swim bladder, pancreas and peritoneum. In: *Systemic Pathology of Fish*, 2e (ed. H.W. Ferguson), 168–199. London: Scotian Press.

Maes, R.K., Langohr, I.M., Wise, A.G. et al. (2014). Beyond H&E: integration of nucleic acid-based analyses into diagnostic pathology. *Veterinary Pathology* 51: 238–256.

Makrinos, D.L. and Bowden, T.J. (2016). Growth characteristics of the intracellular pathogen, *Piscirckettsia salmonis*, in tissue culture and cell-free media. *Journal of Fish Diseases* 40: 1115–1127.

Mardis, E.R. (2008). Next-generation DNA sequencing methods. *Annual Review of Genomics and Human Genetics* 9: 387–402.

Mardis, E.R. (2013). Next-generation sequencing platforms. *Annual Review of Analytical Chemistry* 6: 287–303.

Mardis, E.R. (2017). DNA sequencing technologies: 2006-2016. *Nature Protocols* 12: 213–218.

Matsche, M.A. (2013). Relative physiological effects of laparoscopic surgery and anesthesia with tricaine methanesulfonate (MS-222) in Atlantic sturgeon *Acipenser oxyrinchus oxyrinchus*. *Journal of Applied Ichthyology* 29: 510–519.

Metzker, M.L. (2010). Sequencing technologies – the next generation. *Nature Reviews/Genetics* 11: 31–46.

Meyer, F.P. and Barclay, L.A. (eds.) (1990). *Field Manual for the Investigation of Fish Kills*. U.S. Fish and Wildlife Service. Resource Publication 177.

Meyers, T.R. and Hendricks, J.D. (1982). A summary of tissue lesions in aquatic animals induced by controlled exposures to environmental contaminants, chemotherapeutic agents, and potential carcinogens. *Marine Fisheries Review* 44: 1–17.

Mignard, S. and Flandrois, J.P. (2006). 16S rRNA sequencing in routine bacterial identification: a 30-month experiment. *Journal of Microbiological Methods* 67: 574–581.

Nelson, K., Jones, J., Jacobson, S. et al. (1999). Elevated blood urea nitrogen (BUN) levels in goldfish as an indicator of gill dysfunction. *Journal of Aquatic Animal Health* 11: 52–60.

Noga, E.J. (ed.) (2010). *Fish Disease Diagnosis and Treatment*, 2e. Ames, IA: Wiley.

OIE (2018). *The World Organization for Animal Health Manual of Diagnostic Tests for Aquatic Animals* [online]. http://www.oie.int/international-standard-setting/aquatic-manual/access-online/ (accessed 1 November 2018).

Paquette, C.E., Kent, M.L., Peterson, T.S. et al. (2015). Immunohistochemical characterization of intestinal neoplasia in zebrafish *Danio rerio* indicated epithelial origin. *Diseases of Aquatic Organisms* 116: 191–197.

Persky, M.E., Williams, J.J., Burks, R.E. et al. (2012). Hematologic, plasma biochemistry, and select nutrient values in captive smoot dogfish (*Mustelus canis*). *Journal of Zoo and Wildlife Medicine* 43: 842–851.

Peyghan, R., Khadjeh, G., and Enayati, A. (2014). Effect of water salinity on total protein and electrophoretic pattern of serum proteins of grass carp, *Ctenopharyngodon idella*. *Veterinary Research Forum* 5: 225–229.

Pfyffer, G.E., Brown-Elliott, B.A., and Wallace, R.J. (2003). Mycobacterium: general characteristics, isolation, and staining procedures. In: *Manual of Clinical Microbiology*, 8e (eds. P.R. Murray, E.J. Baron, J.H. Jorgensen, et al.), 532–559. Washington, D.C.: ASM Press.

Pinson, D.M. (2014). Writing diagnostic laboratory requisition form histories. *Journal of the American Veterinary Medical Association* 244: 408–411.

Plumb, J.A. and Bowser, P.R. (eds.) (1983). *Microbial Fish Disease Laboratory Manual*. Auburn, AL: Auburn University.

Plumb, J.A. and Hanson, L.A. (eds.) (2011). *Health Maintenance and Principal Microbial Diseases of Cultured Fishes*, 3e. Ames, IA: Wiley.

Ramos-Vara, J.A. and Miller, M.A. (2013). When tissue antigens and antibodies get along: revisiting the technical aspects of immunohistochemistry – the red, brown, and blue technique. *Veterinary Pathology* 51: 42–87.

Reite, O. (1997). Mast cells/eosinophilic granule cells of salmonids: staining properties and noxious agents. *Fish and Shellfish Immunology* 7: 567–584.

Reite, O. and Evensen, O. (2006). Inflammatory cells of teleostean fish: a review focusing on mast cells/eosinophilic granule cells and rodlet cells. *Fish and Shellfish Immunology* 20: 192–208.

Roberts, R. and Ellis, A. (2001). The anatomy and physiology of teleosts. In: *Fish Pathology* (ed. R. Roberts), 17–61. Philadelphia, PA: W.B. Saunders.

Robohm, R.A. (1983). *Pasteurella piscicida*. In: *Antigens of Fish Pathogens* (eds. D.P. Anderson, M. Dorsen and P.H. Dubourget), 161–175. Lyon: Collection Foundation Marcel Merieux.

Rowley, A., Hunt, T., Page, M., and Mainwaring, G. (1998). Fish. In: *Vertebrate Blood Cells* (eds. A. Rowley and F. Ratcliffe), 29–128. Cambridge, UK: Cambridge University Press.

Rupell, G.L. (2006). Of time and temperature, plastic and glass: specimen handling in the blood-gas laboratory. *Respiratory Care* 51: 717–718.

Shieh, H.S. (1980). Studies on the nutrition of a fish pathogen, *Flexibacter columnaris*. *Microbiology Letters* 13: 129–133.

Sink, T.D. (2015). Investigating a Fish Die-Off and Submitting a Sample for Toxicology or Disease Diagnosis. Southern Regional Aquaculture Center Publication No. 472, p. 8.

Sontakke, S., Cadenas, M.B., Maggi, R.G. et al. (2009). Use of broad range 16S rDNA PCR in clinical microbiology. *Journal of Microbiological Methods* 76: 217–225.

Soto, E., Hawke, J.P., Fernandez, D. et al. (2009). *Francisella* sp., an emerging pathogen of tilapia, *Oreochromis niloticus* (L.), in Costa Rica. *Journal of Fish Diseases* 32: 713–722.

Spitsbergen, J.M., Buhler, D.R., and Peterson, T.S. (2011). Neoplasia and neoplasm-associated lesions in laboratory colonies of zebrafish emphasizing key influences of diet and aquaculture system design. *ILAR Journal* 53: 114–125.

Stacy, N., Arnold, J., and Boylan, S. (2014). Diagnostic hematology of fish: review and tips. *Proceedings of the Association of Reptilian and Amphibian Veterinarians*, Orlando, FL.

Tapia-Cammas, D., Yañez, A., Arancibia, G. et al. (2011). Multiplex PCR for the detection of *Piscirickettsia salmonis*, *Vibrio anguillarum*, *Aeromonas salmonicida* and *Streptococcus phocae* in Chilean marine farms. *Diseases of Aquatic Organisms* 97: 135–142.

Tompkins, D.M., Carver, S., Jones, M.E. et al. (2015). Emerging infectious diseases of wildlife: a critical perspective. *Trends in Parasitology* 31: 149–159.

Tripathi, N., Latimer, K., and Burnley, V. (2004). Hematologic reference intervals for koi (*Cyprinus carpio*), including blood cell morphology, cytochemistry and ultrastructure. *Veterinary Clinical Pathology* 33: 74–83.

Wakabayashi, H. and Egusa, S. (1974). Characteristics of myxobacteria associated with some freshwater fish diseases in Japan. *Bulletin of the Japanese Society of Scientific Fisheries* 40: 751–757.

Waltman, W.D. and Shotts, E.B. (1984). A medium for the isolation of *Yersinia ruckeri*. *Canadian Journal of Fisheries and Aquatic Sciences* 41: 804–806.

Wittwer, C.T. and Kusukawa, N. (2007). Nucleic acid techniques. In: *Fundamentals of Molecular Diagnosis* (eds. D.E. Burns, C.A. Burtis and E.R. Ashwood), 46–79. St. Louis, MO: Saunders.

Wiwanitkit, V. (2006). Glass syringes are better than plastic for preserving arterial blood gas for oxygen partial pressure determination: an explanation based on nanomaterial composition. *International Journal of Nanomedicine* 1: 223–224.

Wolf, J., Baumgartner, W., Blazer, V. et al. (2014). Non-lesions, misdiagnoses, missed diagnoses, and other interpretive challenges in fish histopathology studies: a guide for investigators, authors, reviewers, and readers. *Toxicologic Pathology* 43: 297–325.

Yakote, M. (1982). Blood. In: *An Atlas of Fish Histology* (ed. T. Hibya), 64–72. Tokyo: Japan Marine Products Photo Materials Association, Kodansha.

Zinkl, J., Cox, W., and Kono, C. (1991). Morphology and cytochemistry in leucocytes and thrombocytes of six species of fish. *Comparative Haematology International* 1: 187–189.

A8

Diagnostic Imaging

Shane M. Boylan[1], *Natalie D. Mylniczenko*[2] *and Rolf P. Gobien*[3]

[1] *South Carolina Aquarium, Charleston, SC, USA*
[2] *Disney's Animals, Science and Environment, Lake Buena Vista, FL, USA*
[3] *Clinton X-Ray Specialists, Clinton, NC, USA*

Introduction

Fish medicine is as complex as the nearly 30 000 species it represents. This diversity creates a significant challenge for the clinician, as understanding normal anatomy is essential for interpretation of diagnostic imaging. Radiography and ultrasonography should be part of routine diagnostics for anesthetized fish; this can improve diagnostic sensitivity and build baseline data on the species. Conventional radiography is useful for skeletal structures and gas-filled spaces such as the swim bladder. Ultrasonography allows better evaluation of soft tissue structures, particularly in elasmobranchs. Advanced imaging modalities such as computed tomography and magnetic resonance imaging provide greater resolution and are becoming more available.

Conventional Radiography

Conventional digital radiography is becoming the most common form of imaging in veterinary medicine. Digital radiography systems provide faster processing, fewer chemical discharge concerns, and improved imaging compared to conventional film radiography. The main drawback is the capital cost, particularly with expected replacement of the plate (detector) and interface every 5–10 years.

Cassette-read (CR) systems use a plate analogous to those used in conventional film radiography. The processing fluids of a developer have been replaced with a processing unit (reader) that removes, processes, cleans, and replaces the digital film within the cassette. The processing unit transfers files to designated computers using the standard DICOM format (Digital Imaging and Communications in Medicine) used for all imaging modalities. The main benefit of CR over direct-read (DR) systems is the lower cost of plate replacement should it get damaged.

With DR systems, processing occurs within the plate, which is connected directly to an interface (laptop or tablet) though a cable or wireless connection. Since there is no need for a separate processing unit, these units are portable. They are becoming more economical and their imaging quality is now comparable to CR systems. Wireless and cordless DR systems are preferred as they avoid cable hazards and allow the expensive plate to be completely sealed within waterproof bags.

In all systems, the plates must be protected from water damage. Some water-resistant plates are now available, but all should still be protected in heavy-duty watertight, radiolucent bags; fish transport bags often work well (Figure A8.1a). For additional protection, plates may be used within heavy-duty tunnels to protect them from excessive weight or damage from teeth, spines, or heavy-bodied animals (Figure A8.1b).

Radiographic Safety

Radiographic safety is paramount. Human exposure can be minimized using standard ALARA ("as low as reasonably achievable") principles. The three pillars of this system are:

1) Minimize the amount of radiation (dose, time, number of exposures).
2) Maximize the distance of personnel from the beam.
3) Appropriate use of shielding.

In order to minimize the number of exposures needed, it is important to use suitable chemical restraint and to record and assess exposure techniques for fish to create accurate exposure charts. DR and CR systems offer preset algorithms for specific views in domestic species (e.g. large

Clinical Guide to Fish Medicine, First Edition. Edited by Catherine A. Hadfield and Leigh Ann Clayton.

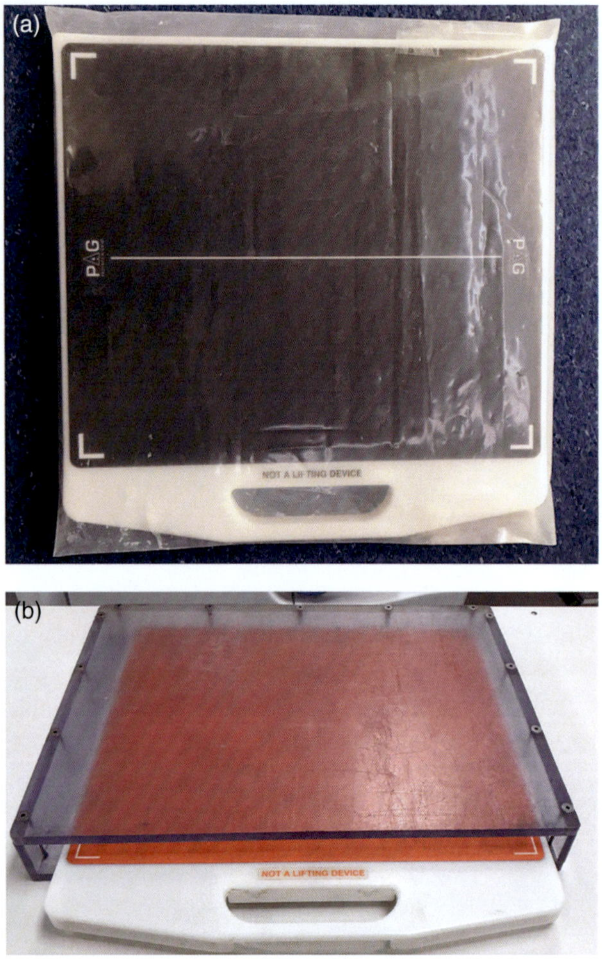

Figure A8.1 Heavy-duty plastic bag (a) and radiolucent tunnel (b) to protect a radiography plate (detector).

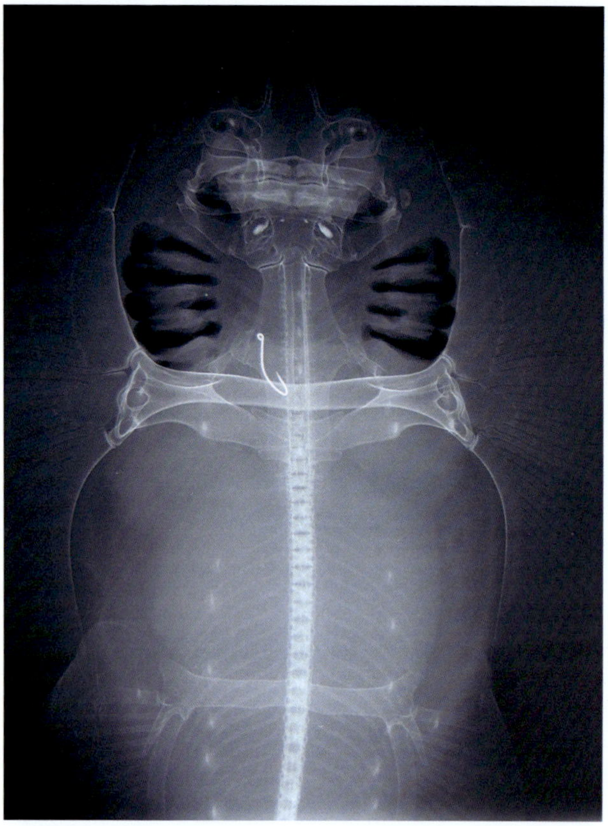

Figure A8.2 Dorsoventral radiograph of a thornback guitarfish (*Platyrhinoidis triseriata*) showing a hook foreign body. *Source*: Image courtesy of Catherine Hadfield, National Aquarium.

canine lateral thorax). With each new system, there is a certain amount of trial and error to identify which algorithms and additional settings provide the best image quality for common views in fish. These details should be recorded along with the exposure techniques.

Plain Radiography

Plain radiography is particularly useful to assess swimming and buoyancy abnormalities, as these may be due to spinal or swim bladder pathology. Some calculi and foreign bodies are readily visible on plain radiographs (e.g. fishing hooks) (Figure A8.2). Dental pathology is also easy to evaluate radiographically (Figure A8.3). Unfortunately, soft tissue contrast is limited. In bony fish with abundant coelomic fat and air–tissue interfaces, some soft tissue detail is visible (Figure A8.4a), but detail is particularly poor in elasmobranchs (Figure A8.4b). In some fish, prominent dermal plates or spines complicate interpretation of radiographs (Figure A8.5).

Survey radiographs should be considered whenever a fish is anesthetized. This provides useful diagnostic information, particularly for skeletal structures and the swim bladder (if present). The images can also be used to establish a database of reference images for the species seen at the clinic. The value of radiographs increases significantly when images of conspecifics are available, as there are few published radiographic studies of normal fish (Smith and Smith 1994; Tyson et al. 1999; Fisher et al. 2003).

Radiography should be done prior to the necropsy of any fish, even if autolyzed. Even frozen carcasses can provide valuable information about the skeletal system, with the added benefit that they can be imaged whenever it is convenient.

In most cases, fish should be anesthetized for radiography. Anesthetized fish are less likely to injure themselves or require repeat imaging due to motion artifacts. The best image quality is provided by removing the fish from water and putting it directly onto a bagged plate or tunnel. Water droplets create artifacts that can be problematic (Figure A8.6). When a fish is removed from the water, it should be tipped head down to remove water from the buccopharyngeal cavity before being placed on the plate or tunnel. The fish should be returned to water as soon as

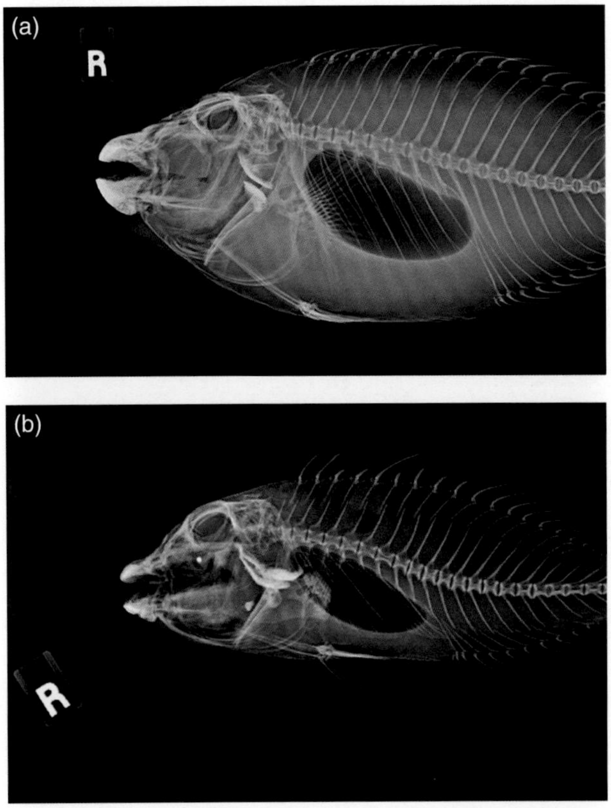

Figure A8.3 Lateral radiograph of a parrotfish (*Sparisoma* sp.) showing normal pharyngeal teeth (a) and abnormal thickening of the pharyngeal teeth due to concretions from the plaster of Paris used to produce feeding blocks (b). *Source*: Images courtesy of Catherine Hadfield, National Aquarium.

possible, although suitable ventilation with aerated water can allow more time out of the water.

In rare circumstances, fish may be radiographed while still in water. This is usually limited to cases where chemical restraint is declined or impractical. A fish may be placed in a narrow plastic bag hung beside a vertical plate using a horizontal beam (Figure A8.7a). Alternatively, a fish may be held in shallow water in a secure container on top of the plate using a vertical X-ray beam. The image quality is poor because of movement and attenuation of the signal by the water, even with high exposures (Figure A8.7b).

Radiographic evaluations of fish should include orthogonal views wherever possible.

- The lateral view typically involves a vertical beam and the fish in lateral recumbency. This "resting lateral" view rarely requires stabilization, and the spine and swim bladder (if present) are easily evaluated.
- A "standing lateral" view should be considered when there are buoyancy abnormalities or the radiolucency of the swim bladder is decreased. This view shows the fish in its natural orientation and may reveal a fluid line in the swim bladder that is not visible on the resting lateral. The fish is placed in ventral recumbency next to a vertical plate with a horizontal beam. Most fish require support for this view (e.g. clear bags, bubble wrap, plastic V-shaped troughs, or foam blocks). Small fish can be briefly placed in radiolucent plastic bags and the bags suspended adjacent to the plate. Standing laterals can

Figure A8.4 Lateral radiograph of a blue tang surgeonfish (*Acanthurus coeruleus*) showing a coelomic mass (a). Dorsoventral view of a white-spotted bamboo shark (*Chiloscyllium plagiosum*) showing the poor soft tissue contrast in elasmobranchs (b). *Source*: Image (a) courtesy of Catherine Hadfield, National Aquarium.

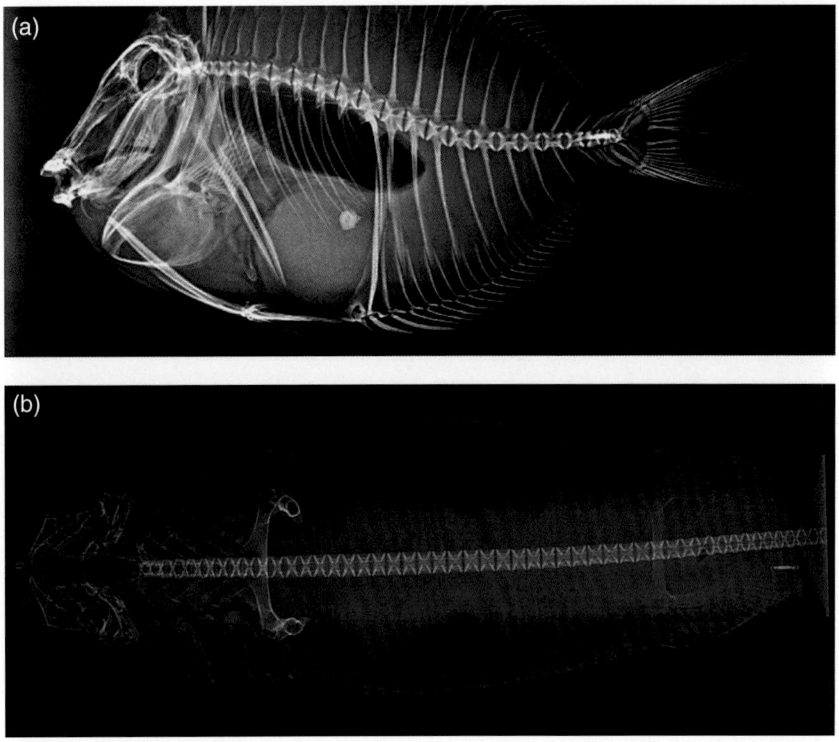

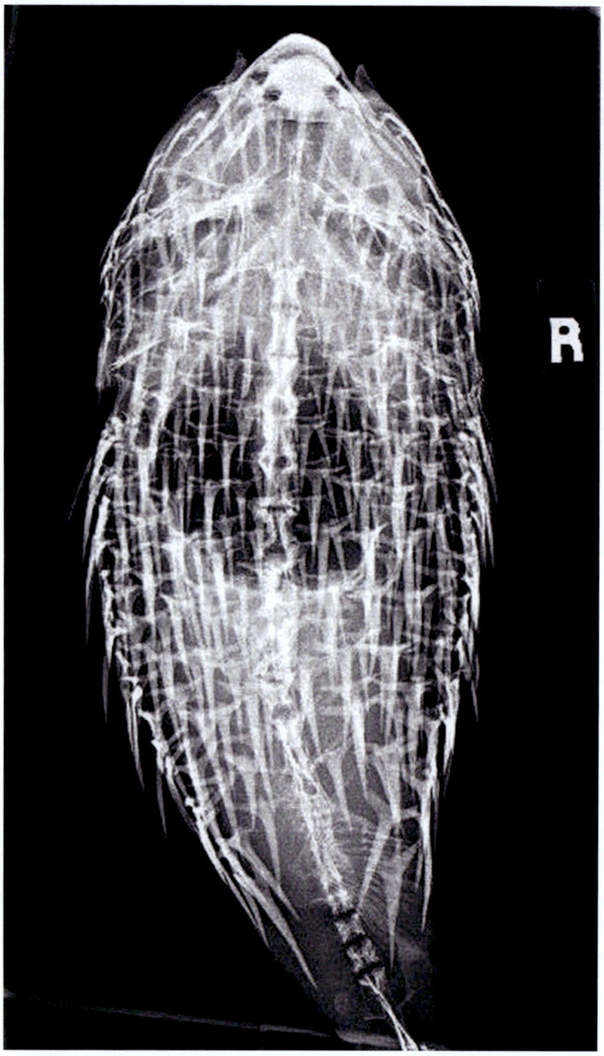

Figure A8.5 Dorsoventral radiograph of a longspined porcupinefish (*Diodon holocanthus*) showing the prominent dermal spines. *Source*: Image courtesy of Catherine Hadfield, National Aquarium.

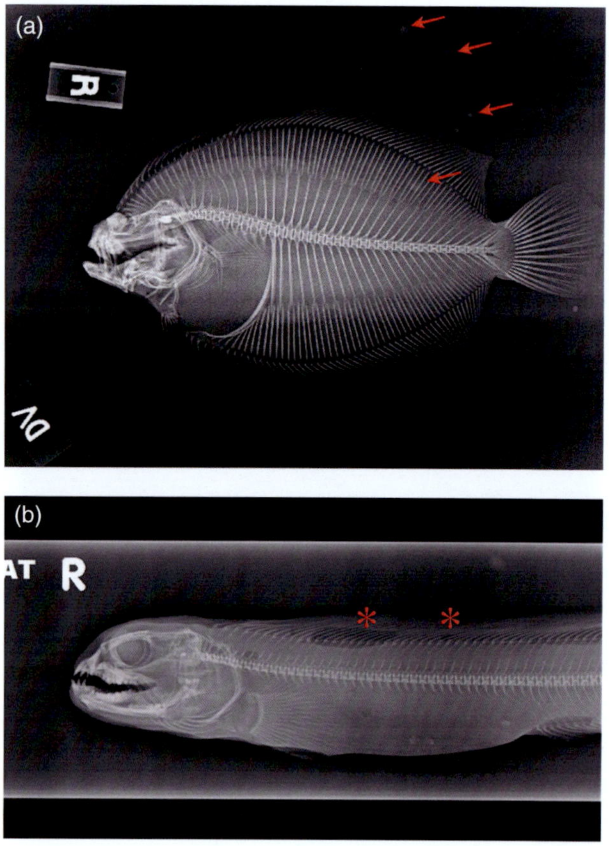

Figure A8.6 Water droplets creating artifacts (arrows) on a radiograph of a four-spot flounder (*Hippoglossina oblonga*) and gas bubble artifacts (*) on a radiograph of a wolf eel (*Anarrhichthys ocellatus*) (b). *Source*: Images courtesy of Catherine Hadfield, National Aquarium.

also be used for dorsoventrally flattened fish such as flatfish (*Pleuronectiformes*), and skates and rays (*Batoidea*) (Figure A8.8).

- The dorsoventral view should be taken when possible and is the more common view in dorsoventrally flattened fish such as flatfish, skates, and rays. This view is often less useful for individuals that are laterally compressed and <3 cm in width because of superimposition of structures.

Radiograph markers (e.g. L, R, DV) should be added to the plates to ensure that important location information is not lost.

Whenever plates are removed from wet bags, it is important to use dry hands as water/debris on the plate can be damaging to the plate as well as to the processor in a CR system.

Contrast Radiography

Contrast radiography uses positive or negative contrast agents to highlight structures not visible on plain radiography, typically the gastrointestinal or urogenital tracts (Macrì et al. 2014). It is often indicated in cases of inappetence or suspected radiolucent foreign bodies.

There are a variety of positive contrast media available. These are most commonly applied in food, by gavage, or per rectum (Figure A8.9). Barium compounds are readily available in veterinary practices, but can adhere to gills if gavaged and regurgitated, which is particularly common in elasmobranchs. Barium-impregnated spheres (BIPSs) carry less risk of gill damage if regurgitated, but may be ingested if regurgitated; if this happens in the same individual, it confuses the radiographic interpretation, and in smaller cohorts, it may represent a foreign body risk. BIPSs also do not accentuate mucosal detail. Aqueous iodine compounds are generally safer: they carry less risk of gill damage if regurgitated and less risk of coelomitis in cases of gastrointestinal perforation. Examples include diatrizoate sodium (e.g. Gastroview®, Leibel-Flarsheim, Raleigh, NC) and

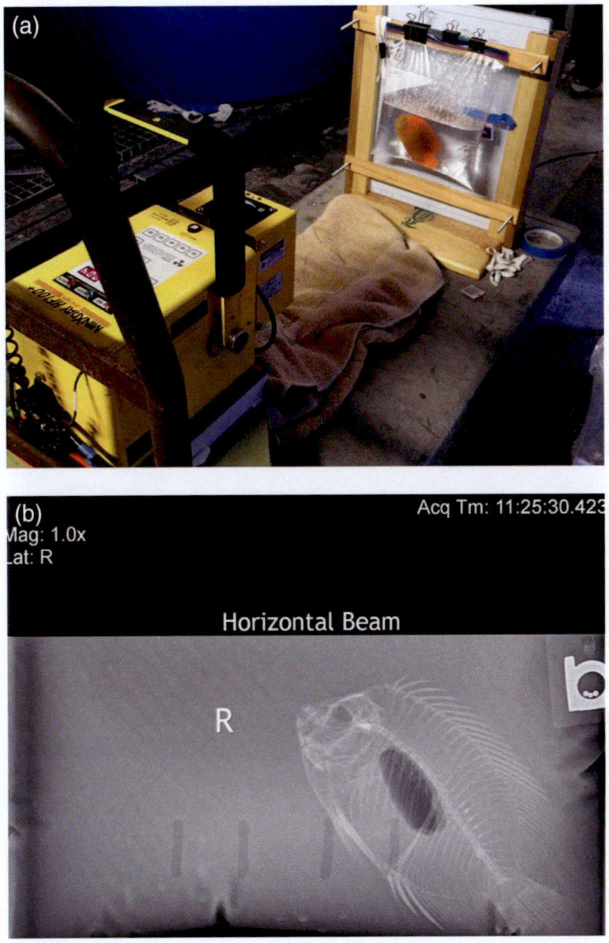

Figure A8.7 Taking a radiograph of a marine angelfish (*Centropyge* sp.) in water using a horizontal beam (a) and the resulting image showing attenuation of the X-rays (b). *Source*: Images courtesy of Michael Murray and Sarah Halbrend, Monterey Bay Aquarium.

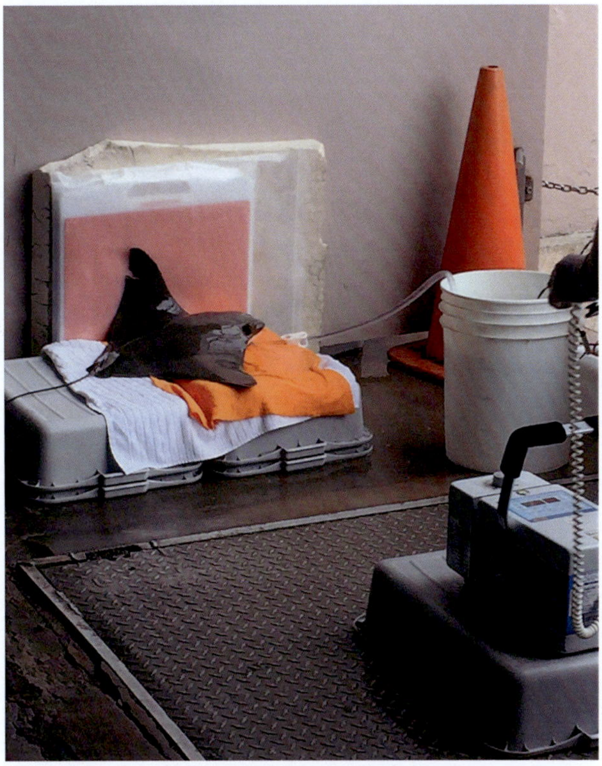

Figure A8.8 Standing lateral radiograph of a cownose ray (*Rhinoptera bonasus*); the ray is being ventilated during the radiographs.

iohexol (e.g. Omnipaque™, GE Healthcare, Waukesha, WI). The volume of contrast required depends on size and anatomy and often requires experimentation. For example, 10 mL/kg may be a starting point for a gastrointestinal contrast study in a grouper (*Epinephelus* sp.), while 3 mL/kg may be sufficient in a similarly sized koi (*Cyprinus carpio koi*) as this species lacks a true stomach. Postmortem imaging provides a good opportunity to experiment with volumes of contrast agents.

Intravenous contrast agents have limited diagnostic use in fish at this time. Perimortem and postmortem intravenous aqueous iodine agents have been instrumental in identifying vasculature for use in phlebotomy or drug delivery. Contrast studies of the dorsal fin sinus of the bonnethead shark (*Sphyrna tiburo*) shows that it communicates well with the coelomic vasculature (Figure A8.10). Iopamidol, an aqueous iodine compound available under several trade names and concentrations, has been used at 400–800 mg/kg in koi that were recovered and perimortem in other species (Brust et al. 2018). No associated pathology has been seen on subsequent histology. Similar doses of 660–990 mg/kg have been used for Iohexol-330 by one author without adverse effects.

Negative contrast agents include air and carbon dioxide. Room air can be injected into the oral cavity of living and deceased fish to define cranial gastrointestinal structures. An approximate starting volume for fish with stomachs is 5 mL/kg. Air can also be administered into the valvular intestine of elasmobranchs to help evaluate size and integrity. In antemortem cases, negative contrast should be used sparingly as trapped air will alter buoyancy unless it can be easily removed. Sand tiger sharks (*Carcharias taurus*) normally have air in their stomach to help with buoyancy, providing a natural negative contrast that helps with evaluating the overlying vertebrae (Figure A8.11). The absence of air in the stomach may indicate that the shark cannot effectively surface to gulp air. Handling can cause either regurgitation of the gas or excessive swallowing of air.

In other vertebrates, contrast radiography typically involves serial radiographs taken over several hours or days. Many fish cannot be repeatedly sedated on that schedule and strategic timing is required. One option is to provide contrast both orally and rectally, radiograph at

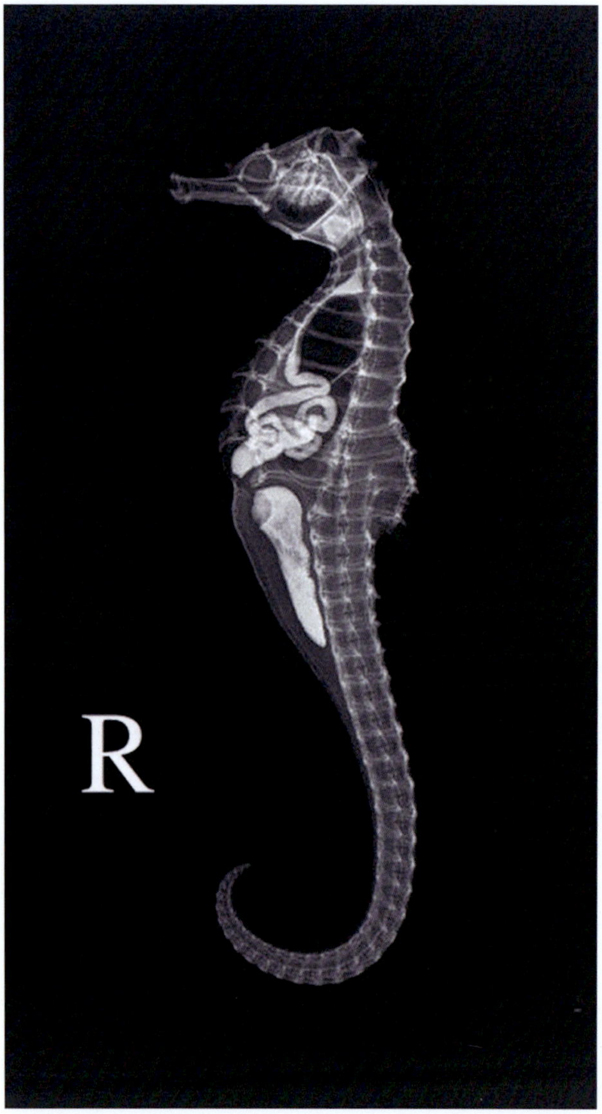

Figure A8.9 Positive contrast in the gastrointestinal tract and pouch of a male lined seahorse (*Hippocampus erectus*).

time = 0 and the following day. Partial or complete obstructions and enteroliths can be detected in this way, even in fish with much faster gastrointestinal transit times.

Interventional Radiography

Radiography can play an important role in treatment, although this is often overshadowed by its use in diagnosis. With a good understanding of anatomy, conventional radiography can be turned into interventional radiography in a number of ways. By placing radiodense markers, radiographs can direct percutaneous aspiration or biopsy of the swim bladder, masses, or organs. The markers can also be used to localize treatment, e.g. intralesional chemotherapy of a tumor or injection of blood patches into a swim bladder to seal small tears (Boylan et al. 2018).

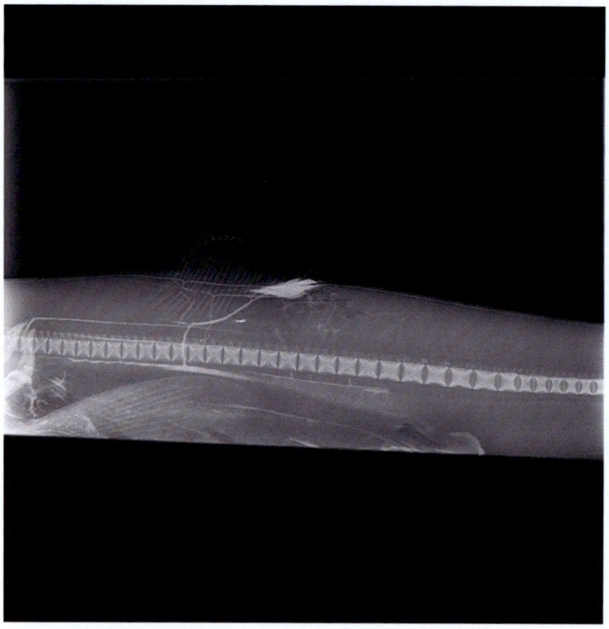

Figure A8.10 Positive contrast injected into the dorsal fin sinus of a bonnethead shark (*Sphyrna tiburo*) showing that the contrast is distributed into the dorsal aorta.

Computed Tomography

Computed tomography (CT) is becoming more accessible to aquatic veterinarians. Conventional CT uses computer processing of multiple X-rays to generate cross-sectional images (slices). Multi-slice CT systems are able to image multiple cross sections simultaneously, resulting in much shorter scan times than single-slice CT. The two-dimensional images provide better soft tissue contrast and avoid the superimposition seen with conventional radiographs. They allow for measurement of density, typically in Hounsfield units (HU) (Carr et al. 2014). The three-dimensional reconstructions can elucidate structures obscured in conventional radiography and allow volume measurements (Pees et al. 2009). Conventional CT scans are getting progressively faster, with many units requiring less than a minute.

Cone-beam CT (CBCT) technology has recently come onto the veterinary market. CBCT systems use a larger detector to acquire data from a wide X-ray beam rather than a slice. Veterinary units are mobile within a practice and have similar radiation safety requirements to traditional radiology, unlike conventional CT. Resolution is reported as higher than conventional CT technology, but there is a higher risk of motion artifacts and, at least anecdotally, diagnostic soft tissue detail might require positive contrast. A few veterinary CBCT systems are available, e.g. small-animal unit Vimago™ (Epica International, San Clemente, CA), with a capacity of approximately 90 kg (200 lb), and the equine unit Pegaso™ (Epica).

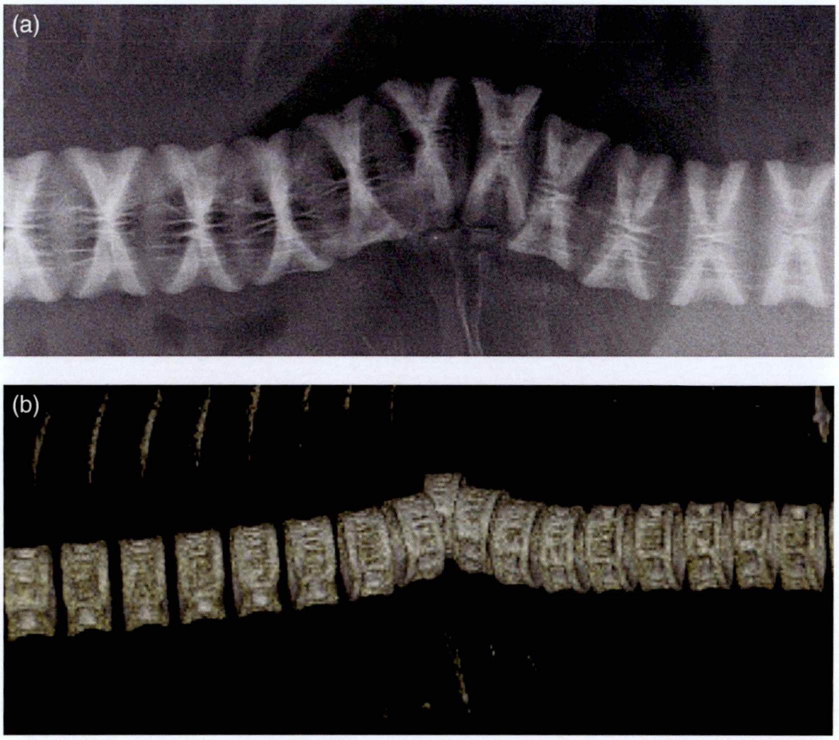

Figure A8.11 A sand tiger shark (*Carcharias taurus*) with kyphosis and scoliosis visible on a dorsoventral radiograph against the normal gas shadow in the stomach (a) and a three-dimensional CT reconstruction showing the greater resolution provided (b).

Most CT scanners are sensitive to water damage. Fish should always be sedated for scans. They may be maintained out of water for a short CT scan; however, ventilation is preferable (Boylan et al. 2017). Sedated fish can be held within a closed container (e.g. transport bag) with a small volume of water. In these cases, it is still important to provide some restraint to prevent motion (e.g. radiolucent trough). Alternatively, a sedated fish can be restrained in an open container and a pump used to provide ventilation across the gills (Figure A8.12).

CT imaging is particularly useful for identifying subtle changes in the skeleton or swim bladder, as well as gas pockets in exophthalmos or buphthalmos, gas bubble disease, and barotrauma (Figure A8.13). As technology progresses, the image quality of soft tissue structures continues to improve, particularly in cases with coelomic fat (Figure A8.14). Intravenous contrast can also be used to improve image quality of soft tissue structures. Micro-CT provides incredibly high-resolution imaging of small fish (Weinhardt et al. 2018). Some CT atlases are available, e.g. pacu (*Colossoma macropomum*) and medaka (*Oryzias latipes*) (Carr et al. 2014; Weinhardt et al. 2018).

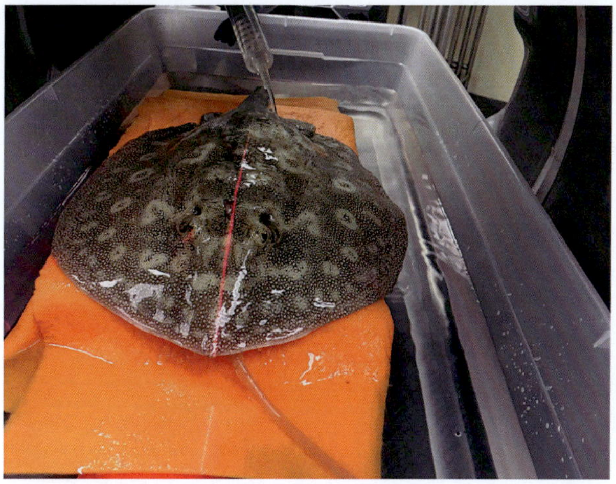

Figure A8.12 Recirculating anesthetic bath for computed tomography of a yellow ray (*Urobatis jamaicensis*). The line going to the mouth and gills is visible. The handheld syringe is used to regularly wet the surface of the animal with suitable water.

Magnetic Resonance Imaging

Magnetic resonance imaging (MRI) typically provides better soft tissue detail than CT and is used primarily for evaluation of the nervous system and other soft tissues. Unlike CT, MRI does not rely on X-rays, rather it uses magnetic fields and radio waves to generate images. It remains an uncommon imaging modality for most fish clinicians because of the lengthy duration of the scanning procedure (typically 20–60 minutes) and the high cost and limited availability of the equipment. Currently, its use is often restricted to postmortem or research studies, although case reports exist (Rogers et al. 2008; Dumonceaux et al. 2010; Wu et al. 2015). Over time, as scan times and costs come down, MRI will likely become more common in fish.

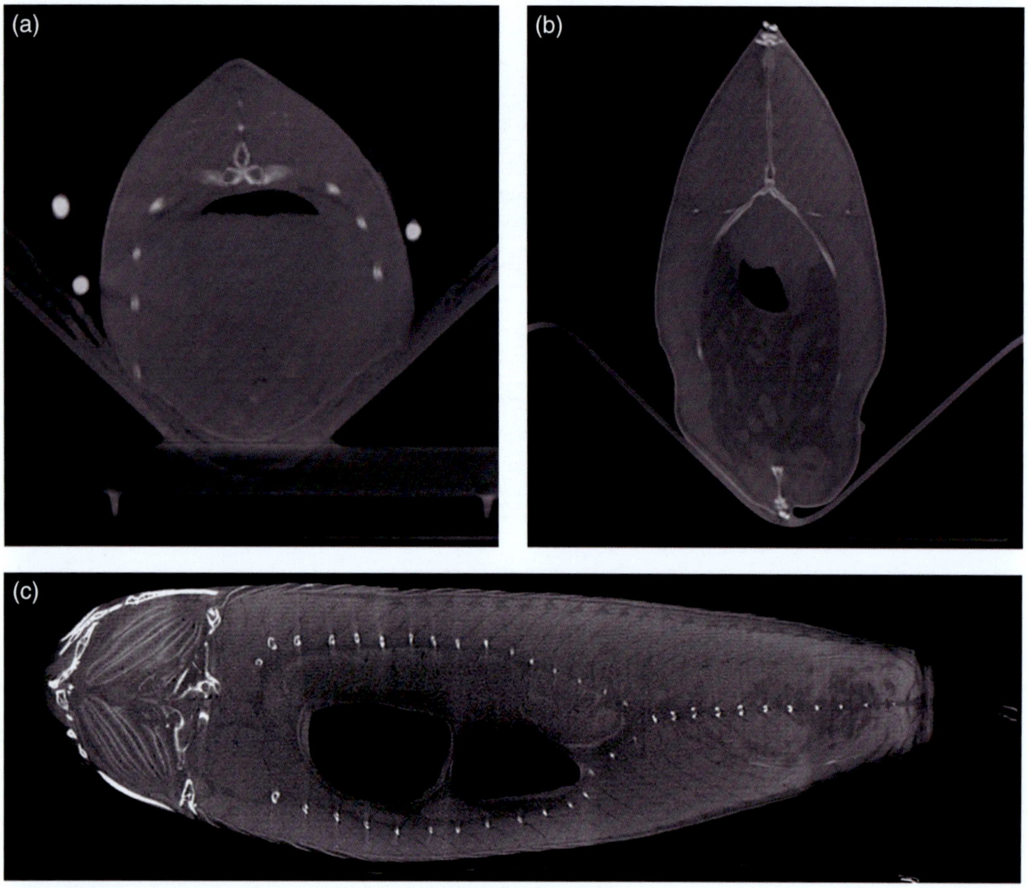

Figure A8.13 Conventional computed tomography images: transverse section showing fluid in the swim bladder of a koi (*Cyprinus carpio koi*) (a); transverse section showing a renal mass dorsal to the swim bladder in a unicornfish (*Naso* sp.) (b); and coronal section showing lateral displacement of the swim bladder in a koi (c).

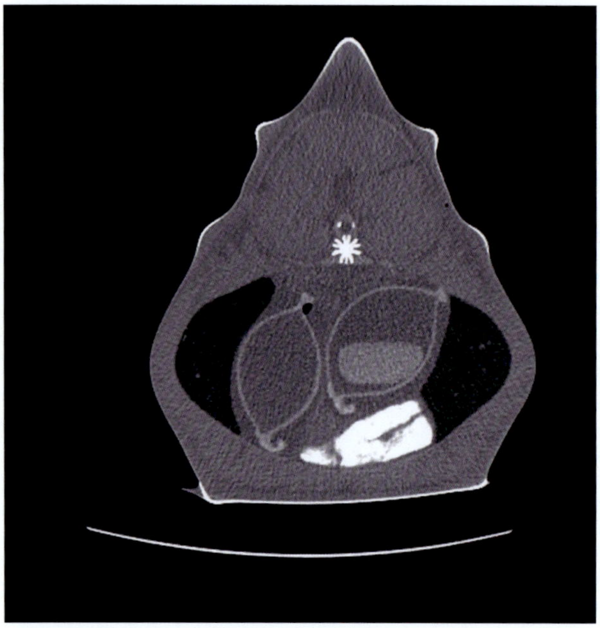

Figure A8.14 Conventional computed tomography image showing good soft tissue detail in a transverse section through a gravid zebra shark (*Stegostoma tigrinum*). *Source*: Image courtesy of Kathryn Seeley, Columbus Zoo and Aquarium.

Ultrasonography

Ultrasonography uses high-frequency sound waves to evaluate fluid and soft tissue structures. Unlike radiography, CT, or MRI, ultrasound can often be carried out at the point-of-care without removing the fish from water. In some cases, ultrasound can be done without any restraint, for example under positive reinforcement training or in stationary fish such as lumpsuckers (*Cyclopteridae*).

A variety of portable units are available. Typical transducers (or probes) are 3.5–12 MHz, with some up to 22 MHz. Higher frequencies produce greater resolution but less depth penetration. Most transducers now allow the operator to change the frequency (e.g. 3.5/5.0 MHz), although some fixed transducers are still found. Transducers may be linear or convex. Linear transducers have better resolution and are particularly useful for thin fish or thin tissues. In a practice that predominantly sees fish of the same species and sizes, careful selection of the probe can improve diagnostic quality (Jennings et al. 2005). While some new ultrasound units are rugged

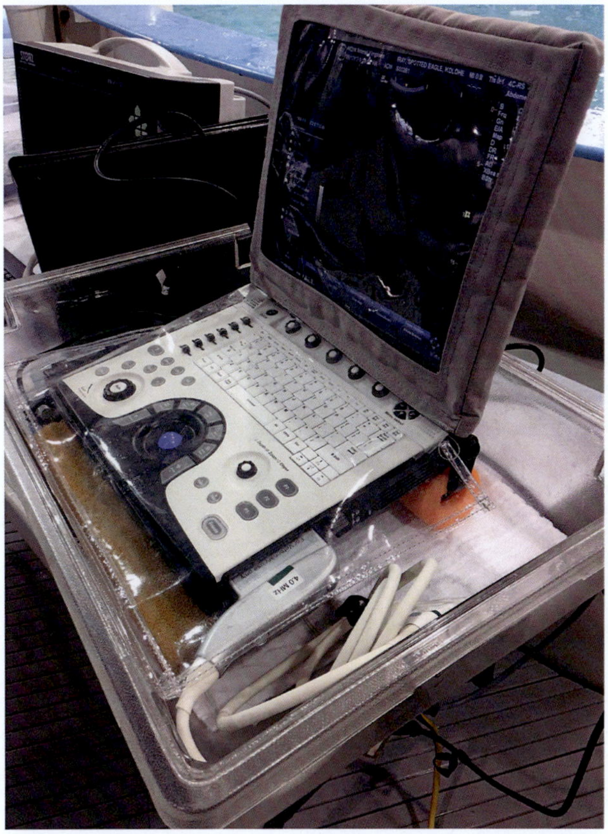

Figure A8.15 Custom-made plastic cover for a portable ultrasound machine.

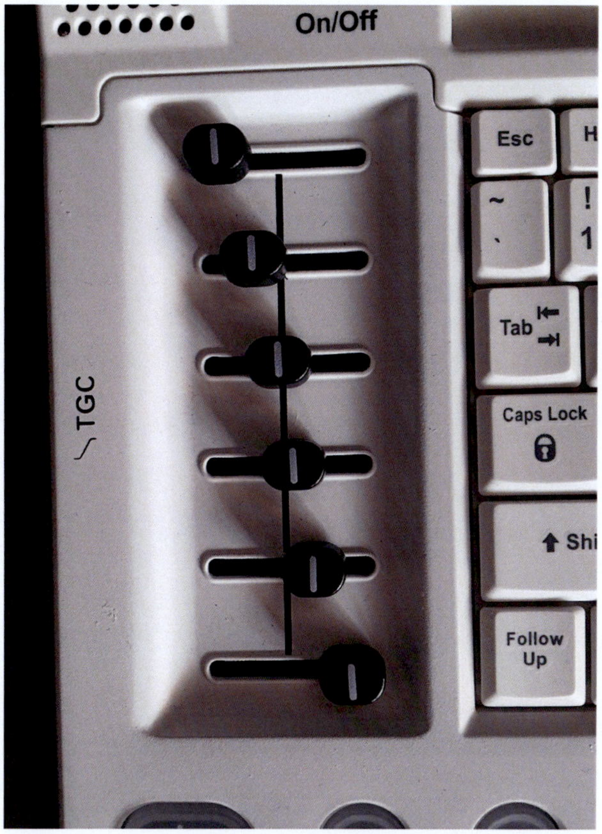

Figure A8.16 Possible arrangement of time gain compensation (TGC) to smooth gain across the field on an ultrasound unit. *Source*: Image courtesy of Catherine Hadfield, Seattle Aquarium.

and water-resistant, in general, water exposure must be avoided. To protect the unit, waterproof covers should be considered (Figure A8.15); these often need to be custom-made.

Water is an excellent conductor of ultrasound waves, so examinations are usually done with the fish underwater without any need for coupling gel. It is common to protect the transducer within a plastic glove or bag; while transducers should be waterproof, dermal structures such as spines and denticles may damage the piezoelectric crystal arrays. Some gel is required between the transducer and the inside of the plastic. The transducer may be held against the body wall or 1–3 cm away from it. Holding the probe off the body wall allows the water to act as a standoff (or spacer) in order to evaluate superficial structures or small patients. It is also useful for awake patients and where dermal structures may impede movement of the transducer on the body wall. Scales can create significant artifacts depending on the type of scale and the degree of overlap. In some species, available windows are limited to around the pectoral fins and the cloaca or anus.

The approach may be dorsal, lateral, or ventral; it depends on the species, area of interest, access, and the clinician's familiarity. However, the direction of the transducer should be consistent across studies, with the orientation marker (often a notch or ridge) always positioned cranially or to the right of the patient. Possible abnormalities should always be examined in two imaging planes (e.g. sagittal and transverse).

Depth and focal zone should be adjusted to bring the area of interest into the middle of the view. Gain and time gain compensation (TGC, also known as depth gain compensation) should be adjusted to maximize resolution of the area of interest. In older ultrasound units, it is often helpful to increase the gain in the far-field and decrease the gain in the near-field (Figure A8.16); newer units compensate for this automatically. Color flow Doppler allows imaging of blood flow that can help with vascular access, identifying vascular abnormalities, or assessing fetal viability in viviparous species.

Most ultrasound reports in the literature involve assessing the reproductive tract of bony fish (e.g. sex, maturity, fecundity, gonadosomatic index, gestational status) (Jennings et al. 2005; Newman et al. 2008; du Columbier et al. 2015; Munhofen et al. 2014; Novelo and Tiersch 2016). Other common uses in clinical practice include monitoring the heart rate during anesthesia, assessing the liver or gastrointestinal tract, evaluating effusions, and guiding fine needle aspirates or transcutaneous biopsies.

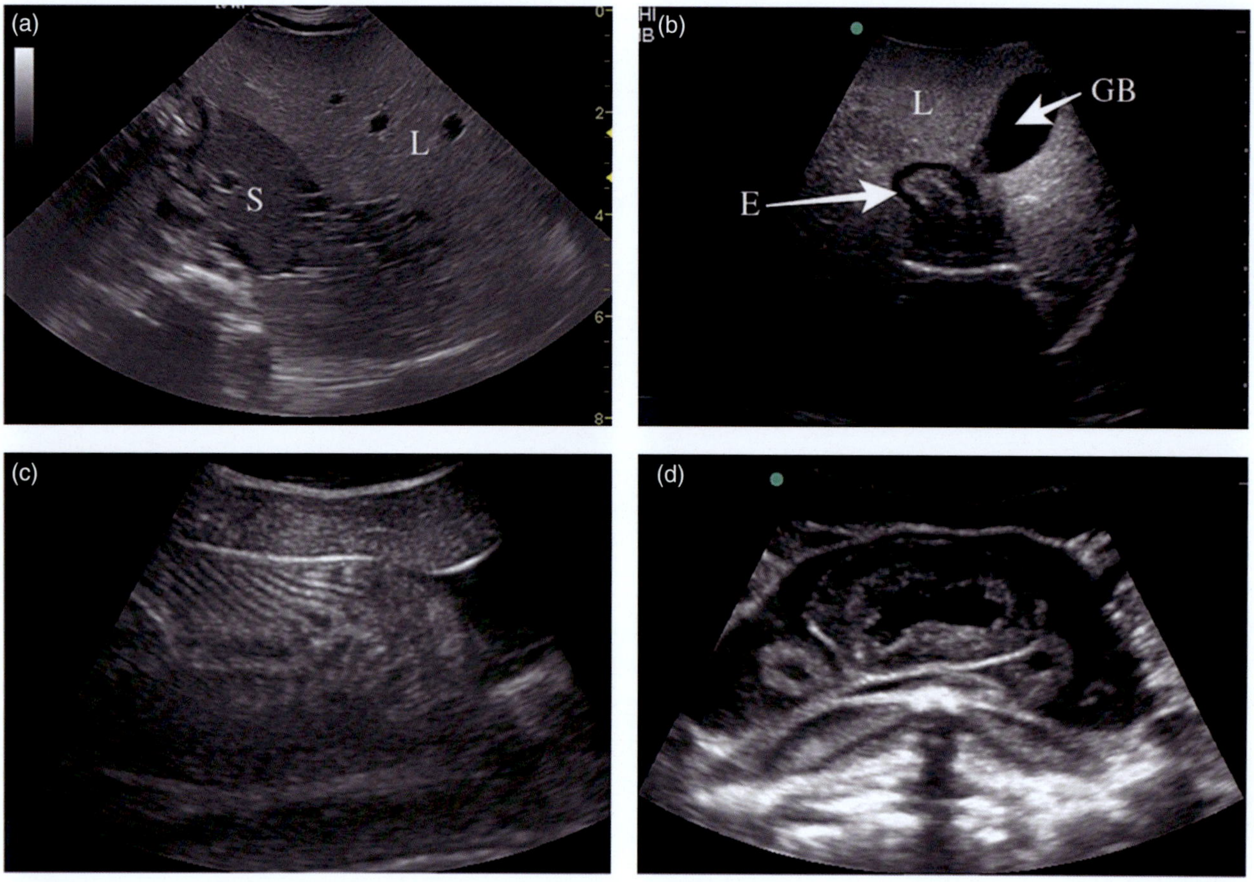

Figure A8.17 Ultrasound image of the liver (L), and spleen (S) of a southern stingray (*Hypanus americanus*); liver (L), gallbladder (GB), and esophagus (E) of a black-blotched stingray (*Taeniurops meyeni*) (b); valvular intestine of a zebra shark (*Stegostoma tigrinum*) (c); and cross section of the heart of a black-blotched stingray (d). *Source*: Images (b)–(d) courtesy of Catherine Hadfield, National Aquarium.

High-frequency transducers can also be used to examine ocular lesions (Williams et al. 2007; Rahmati-Holasoo et al. 2016). Ultrasound waves cannot travel through bone, cartilage, or air, so interpretation of skeletal structures and swim bladders is limited to their surfaces nearest to the transducer.

Ultrasound image quality is particularly good in elasmobranchs (Mylniczenko et al. 2017). Initial landmarks include the body wall/water interfaces, liver, valvular intestine, and heart.

- The liver should fill a large percentage of the ventral coelom and should be hyperechoic to the spleen (Figure A8.17a). The difference in echogenicity can be used to assess body condition (Grant et al. 2013; Mylniczenko et al. 2018). Ultrasound also allows assessment of the liver-to-coelom ratio in some ray species (distance between the pectoral girdle and caudal pole of the liver compared to the distance between the pectoral and pelvic girdles) to assess body condition (Grant et al. 2013), but this is limited to animals that are not gravid and do not have active reproductive disease. The gallbladder is an anechoic structure within the liver (Figure A8.17b).
- The gastrointestinal tract can usually be followed as the esophagus comes through the liver to the stomach, followed by the short length of intestine. The valvular (or spiral) intestine runs along the right body wall and is a useful landmark (Figure A8.17c). The rectal gland is hard to identify (Mylniczenko et al. 2017).
- Heart rate and contractility are easy to visualize and echocardiograms have been reported in elasmobranchs (Lai et al. 2004). Obvious pericardial fluid is normal (Mylniczenko et al. 2017) (Figure A8.17d).
- The reproductive tract anatomy varies enormously across species and reproductive stage. With experience, ultrasound can provide a reliable quantitative and qualitative assessment of the reproductive tract, including gonad measurements, pregnancy detection, and gestational monitoring (Carrier et al. 2003; Daly et al. 2007; Whittamore et al. 2010; Sheldon et al. 2018).

There is more interoperator variability with ultrasound than with other imaging modalities, and the diagnostic value depends heavily on the skills and experience of the operator. Ultrasonography should be included as part of each clinical examination to build experience and develop a database of normal images for species seen at the practice.

Common Abnormalities on Diagnostic Imaging

Spinal Pathology

Vertebrae are typically easy to evaluate using orthogonal radiographic views, although CT imaging is particularly useful where available. Vertebrae of bony fish are circular with pronounced dorsal and ventral processes. Vertebrae of cartilaginous fish are typically square in shape with an "X" pattern on lateral views. Most elasmobranchs and some teleost species lack ribs. Common asymptomatic abnormalities include hemivertebrae, fused vertebrae, and fractured hemal/neural spines; lesions should be considered pathologic only if clinical signs are present. Vertebral fractures and spinal curvature (kyphosis, lordosis, scoliosis), fusion, and compression are also common in fish. Possible causes include electrofishing, lightning strikes, stray voltage, physical trauma, and developmental or nutritional problems (Barlow 1993; Bakal et al. 1998; Fjelldal et al. 2018). Sand tiger sharks are particularly prone to spinal deformities and should receive regular evaluation of their spines (Preziosi et al. 2006; Anderson et al. 2012; Huber et al. 2013). Other common spinal pathology includes osteolysis due to neoplasia or osteomyelitis (Figure A8.18). Hyperostosis is a normal ageing process in some marine species (e.g. jacks, *Carangidae*). The calcified deposits in the ribs, posterior gill area (cleithrum), spines (hemal and neural bones), and supraoccipital crests are common but rarely pathogenic (Figure A8.19) (Smith-Vaniz et al. 1995).

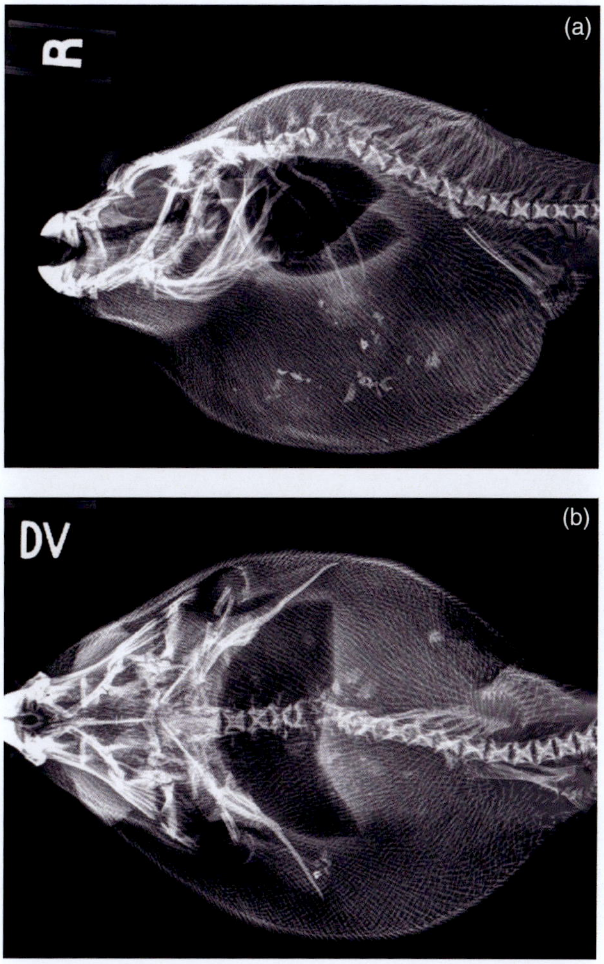

Figure A8.18 Radiographs of a map puffer (*Arothron mappa*) with a lytic spinal lesion consistent with osteomyelitis. *Source*: Images courtesy of Catherine Hadfield, National Aquarium.

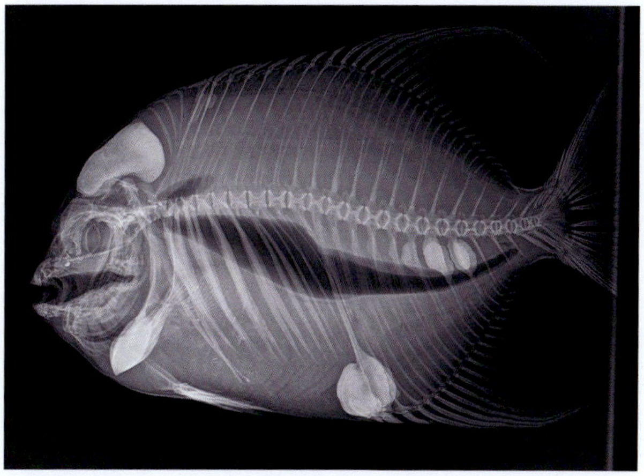

Figure A8.19 Lateral radiograph of an Atlantic spadefish (*Chaetodipterus faber*) with hyperostosis. These lesions are rarely pathogenic.

Swim Bladder Pathology

The swim bladder is the most common structure evaluated by radiography in pet fish medicine (Love and Lewbart 1997). Dorsoventral and resting and standing lateral views should be considered to properly evaluate the swim bladder (Figure A8.20). CT imaging is particularly useful where available (Pees et al. 2009).

Normal comparisons are essential, as species demonstrate a wide and often surprising array of normal swim bladder shapes and sizes. Fancy goldfish (*Carassius auratus*) show a tremendous variety, often with obvious asymmetry.

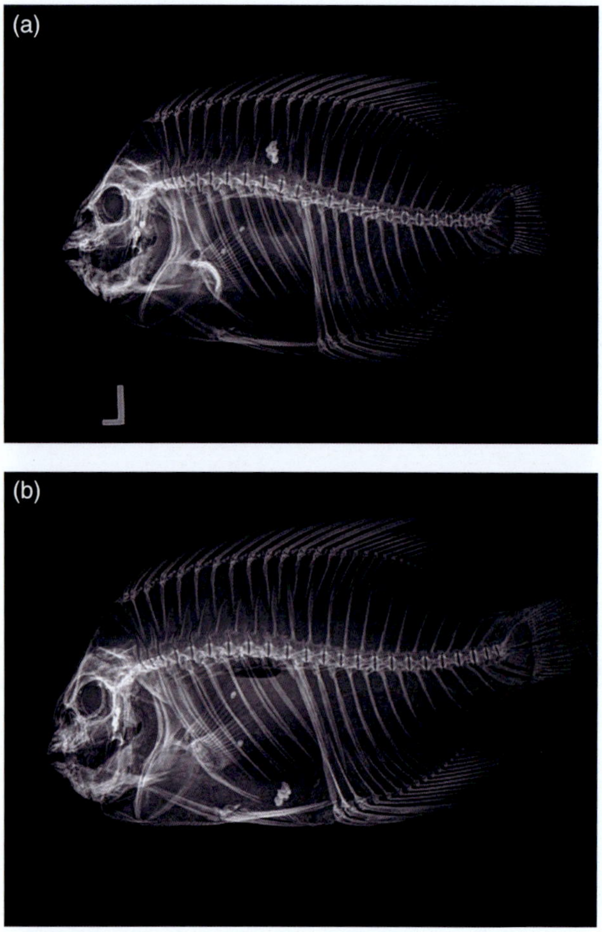

Figure A8.20 A queen angelfish (*Holacanthus ciliaris*) with negative buoyancy seen on a resting lateral radiograph (a) and a standing lateral radiograph (b); the standing lateral view shows a fluid line that was not visible on the resting lateral view.

Puffers (*Tetraodontiformes*) frequently have bilobed or trilobed swim bladders. Many fish also show connections between the swim bladder and their Weberian apparatus that improve acoustic detection (Schulz-Mirbach et al. 2012). Some teleosts lack swim bladders, including demersal teleosts such as flatfish and fish that swim constantly, e.g. mahi (*Coryphaena* spp.) and cobia (*Rachycentron canadum*). Swim bladders are not present in elasmobranchs.

Soft tissue opacities within the swim bladder can have inflammatory, infectious, hemorrhagic, or neoplastic etiologies (Pees et al. 2009). The presence and extent of swim bladder nematodes in European eels (*Anguilla anguilla*) can be assessed using radiography (Beregi et al. 1998). Swim bladder trauma can produce intraluminal hemorrhage that over time becomes a dried membrane visible on radiographs as a linear radiodensity against the background of swim bladder gas.

Hyperinflation of the swim bladder can be due to variety of causes including barotrauma, gas supersaturation, or septicemia. Gas in the coelom can be from a ruptured swim

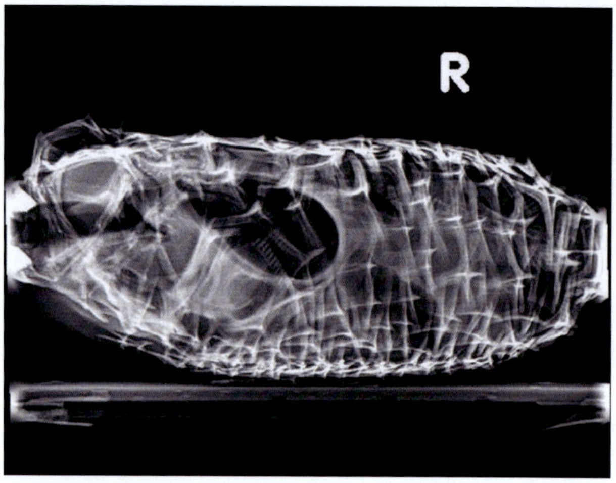

Figure A8.21 Lateral radiograph of a striped burrfish (*Chilomycterus schoepfii*) with positive buoyancy. There is gas in the caudal coelom due to a tear in the swim bladder. *Source*: Image courtesy of Catherine Hadfield, National Aquarium.

bladder due to physical trauma (e.g. penetration of fish spines), barotrauma, or iatrogenic venting of a swim bladder with a needle (Figure A8.21) (Rummer and Bennett 2005; Brown et al. 2010; Boylan et al. 2018).

Radiography can be used to provide landmarks to help with aspiration of the swim bladder or treatment of swim bladder pathology, including injection of therapeutics, blood patch treatment, and surgery (Lewbart et al. 1995; Boylan et al. 2018).

Skin and Pouch Pathology in Syngnathids

Gas can accumulate in the swim bladder, skin, or pouch (if present) of seahorses, pipefish, and seadragons (*Syngnathidae*). When kept in a single-sex population, adult male seahorses will inflate their brood pouch with oxygen released from a rete mirabile designed to aerate their eggs (Wilson et al. 2003). Without the eggs, the brood pouches inflate and the fish may become positively buoyant. Radiographs can easily diagnose a gas-distended brood pouch and the gas can be removed using a catheter or other small tube (Figure A8.22). Recurrence is common until mature females are added. With gas emphysema, radiographs can show subcutaneous gas trapped near the tail tip (typically in females) or around the brood pouch in males. Gas supersaturation is often the cause and a total gas pressure meter (or tensiometer) should be used to determine the total gas pressures.

Gastrointestinal Pathology

Plain and contrast radiography can be essential in identifying gastrointestinal abnormalities, including foreign bodies (Figure A8.23). An understanding of the normal

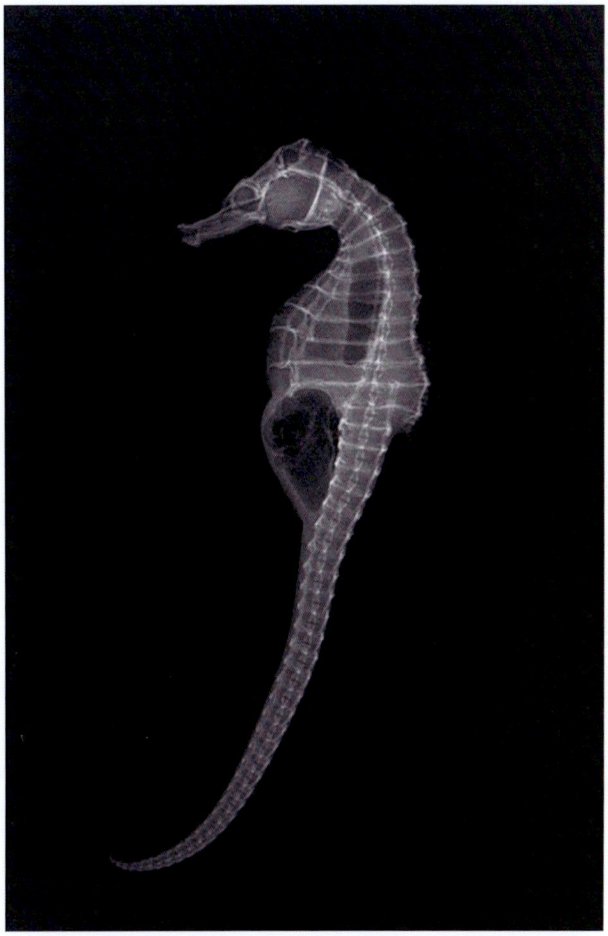

Figure A8.22 Lateral radiograph of a male lined seahorse (*Hippocampus erectus*) showing gas accumulation in the pouch. The swim bladder looks normal.

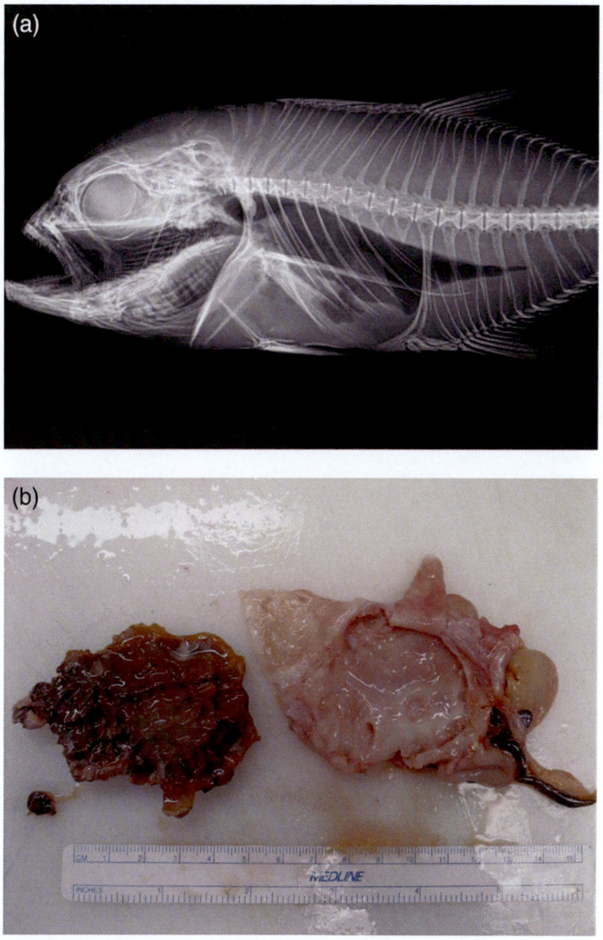

Figure A8.23 Lateral radiograph of horse-eye jack (*Caranx latus*) that had ingested tank sealant; the swim bladder's negative contrast helps to highlight the foreign body (a). Postmortem view of the ingested tank sealant removed from the stomach (b).

gastrointestinal anatomy and potential gastrointestinal transit times is helpful; that information can sometimes be found in the literature or by reviewing previous necropsies or imaging studies.

Coelomic effusion can be readily identified using ultrasound (Figure A8.24). Gastrointestinal ulcerations, perforations, dilatations, mucosal thickening, and foreign bodies may be visualized on ultrasound.

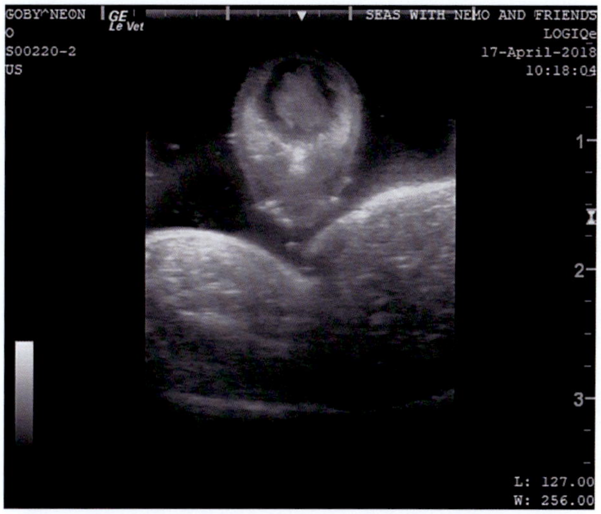

Figure A8.24 Ultrasound image of a neon goby (*Elacatinus oceanops*) in ventrodorsal recumbency, showing a cross section of the body and effusion around the coelomic viscera.

Hepatic Pathology

Hepatomegaly is a common abnormality in fish and can be diagnosed using ultrasound, particularly in some elasmobranchs (Figure A8.25a). Since the liver is the primary lipid storage organ in elasmobranchs, lipid-depletion is also visible on ultrasound – the liver becomes smaller and similar to or hypoechoic to the spleen (Grant et al. 2013; Mylniczenko et al. 2018). Other hepatic changes, such as fibrosis, cysts, or masses, can also be identified on ultrasound (Figure A8.25b). The gallbladder can have sludge or stones that can be diagnosed on ultrasound.

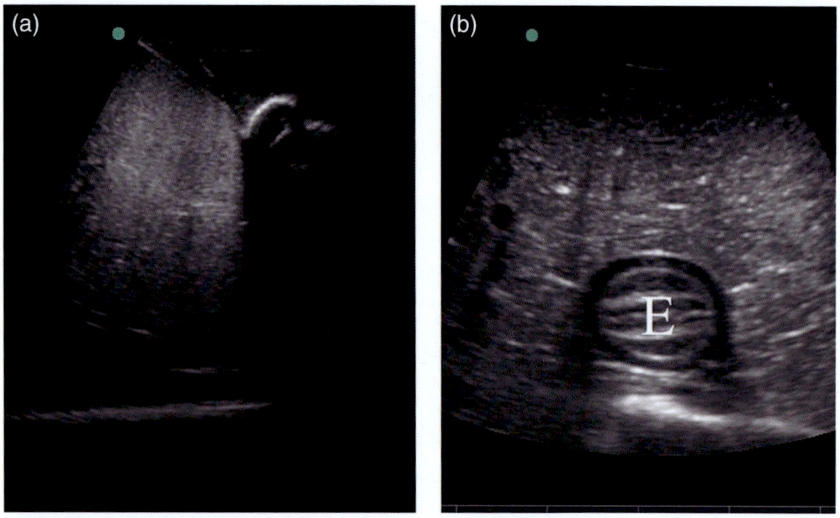

Figure A8.25 Ultrasound of a black-blotched stingray (*Taeniurops meyeni*) showing an enlarged liver that extends caudal to the pelvic girdle (a); ultrasound of a reticulated whipray (*Himantura uarnak*) showing hepatic fibrosis (b). The esophagus (E) is visible in the image. *Source*: Images courtesy of Catherine Hadfield, National Aquarium.

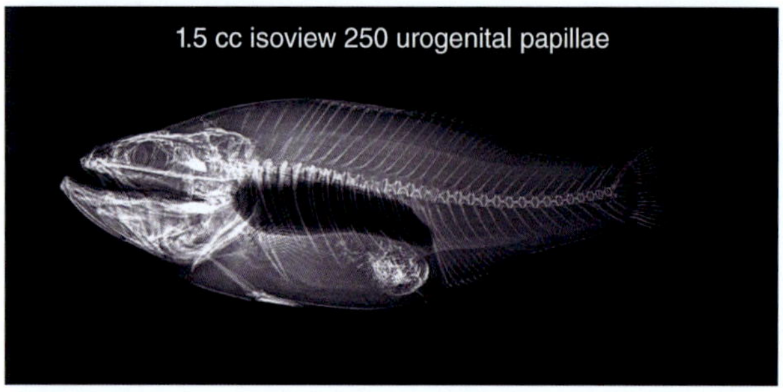

Figure A8.26 Largemouth bass (*Micropterus salmoides*) with aqueous iodine introduced into the urogenital opening highlighting the presence of eggs.

Reproductive Pathology

Ultrasound is the best imaging modality for evaluating the gonads and reproductive status of fish. Many studies still rely on postmortem evaluation for reproductive information. Endoscopy allows nonlethal assessments with higher accuracy than ultrasound, but ultrasound provides a noninvasive and rapid diagnostic (Munhofen et al. 2014). The ability to follow reproductive events using ultrasonography is an important step in the application of assisted reproductive technology for breeding under human care (Carrier et al. 2003; Daly et al. 2007; Munhofen et al. 2014). Radiography can still be useful, particularly in viviparous species, where the calcified vertebrae or otoliths can reveal the location and number of embryos and the presence of gas or fragmentation can suggest embryonic death. Introducing aqueous iodine compounds into the urogenital opening of the vent can highlight the presence of eggs using radiography if ultrasonography is unavailable (Figure A8.26).

Common reproductive pathology in fish includes egg-binding (egg retention), oophoritis, and cystic ovaries and mucometra in elasmobranchs (Mylniczenko et al. 2019). Ultrasound can provide a tentative diagnosis for each of these and a useful method of monitoring progress.

Conclusion

Diagnostic imaging should be a routine component of the physical examination of fish under anesthesia and at necropsy. Each opportunity allows the clinician to improve their understanding of the species, which can improve the value of imaging for future patients. Simple suggestions like standing lateral views and simultaneous oral and aboral contrast can improve the diagnostic value of radiography. The paucity of published images for comparison can be corrected through communication with like-minded clinicians who are building libraries of normal and pathologic images. With the decreased cost of digital radiography, ultrasonography, and CT, more clinicians will have access to noninvasive diagnostics that improve our fish patients' quality of life.

References

Anderson, P.A., Huber, D.R., and Berzins, I.K. (2012). Correlations of capture, transport, and nutrition with spinal deformities in sandtiger sharks, *Carcharias taurus*, in public aquaria. *Journal of Zoo and Wildlife Medicine* 43: 750–758.

Bakal, R.S., Love, N.E., Lewbart, G.A., and Berry, C.R. (1998). Imaging a spinal fracture in a kohaku koi (*Cyprinus carpio*): techniques and case history report. *Veterinary Radiology and Ultrasound* 39: 318–321.

Barlow, A.M. (1993). 'Broken backs' in koi carp (*Cyprinus carpio*) following lightning strike. *Veterinary Record* 133: 503.

Beregi, A., Molnár, K., Békési, L., and Székely, C.S. (1998). Radiodiagnostic method for studying swim bladder inflammation caused by *Anguillicola crassus* (Nematoda: Dracunculoidea). *Diseases of Aquatic Organisms* 34: 155–160.

Boylan, S.M., Camus, A., Gaskins, J. et al. (2017). Spondylosis in a green moray eel, *Gymnothorax funebris* (Ranzani 1839), with swim bladder hyperinflation. *Journal of Fish Diseases* 40: 963–969.

Boylan, S.M., Daniel, W., and Dale, S. (2018). Use of pleurodesis/blood patch to correct a ruptured swim bladder in a goliath grouper (*Epinephelus itajara*). *Proceedings of the Eastern Fish Health Workshop*, Chattanooga, TN.

Brown, I., Sumpton, W., McLennan, M. et al. (2010). An improved technique for estimating short-term survival of released line-caught fish, and an application comparing barotrauma-relief methods in red emperor (*Lutjanus sebae* Cuvier 1816). *Journal of Experimental Marine Biology and Ecology* 385: 1–7.

Brust, K.D., Phillips, K.L., Stevens, B.N. et al. (2018). Intravenous contrast-enhanced computed tomography anatomy in normal adult koi (*Cyprinus carpio*). *Proceedings of the International Association of Aquatic Animal Medicine*, Durban, South Africa.

Carr, A., Weber, S., Murphy, C.J., and Zwingenberger, A. (2014). Computed tomography and cross-sectional anatomy of the normal pacu (*Colossoma macropomum*). *Journal of Zoo and Wildlife Medicine* 45: 184–189.

Carrier, J.C., Murru, F.L., Walsh, M.T., and Pratt, H.L. (2003). Assessing reproductive potential and gestation in nurse sharks (*Ginglymostoma cirratum*) using ultrasonography and endoscopy: an example of bridging the gap between field research and captive studies. *Zoo Biology* 22: 179–187.

Daly, J., Gunn, I., Kirby, N. et al. (2007). Ultrasound examination and behavior scoring of captive broadnose sevengill sharks, *Notorynchus cepedianus* (Peron, 1807). *Zoo Biology* 26: 383–395.

du Columbier, S.B., Jacobs, L., Gesset, C. et al. (2015). Ultrasonography as a non-invasive tool for sex determination and maturation monitoring in silver eels. *Fisheries Research* 164: 50–58.

Dumonceaux, G., Hovland, E., and Coy, S. (2010). Magnetic resonance imaging of a white tipped reef shark (*Triaenodon obesus*) at the Florida Aquarium. *Proceedings of the International Association of Aquatic Animal Medicine Conference*, Vancouver, Canada.

Fisher, S., Jagadeeswaran, P., and Halpern, M.E. (2003). Radiographic analysis of zebrafish skeletal defects. *Developmental Biology* 264: 64–76.

Fjelldal, P.G., van der Meeren, T., Fraser, T.W. et al. (2018). Radiological changes during fracture and repair in neural and haemal spines of Atlantic cod (*Gadus morhua*). *Journal of Fish Diseases* 41: 1871–1875.

Grant, K.R., Campbell, T.W., Silver, T.I., and Olea-Popelka, F.J. (2013). Validation of an ultrasound-guided technique to establish a liver-to-coelom ratio and a comparative analysis of the ratios among acclimated and recently wild-caught southern stingrays, *Dasyatis americana*. *Zoo Biology* 32: 104–111.

Huber, D., Neveu, D.E., Stinson, C.M. et al. (2013). Mechanical properties of sand tiger shark *Carcharias taurus* vertebrae in relation to spinal deformity. *Journal of Experimental Biology* 216: 4256–4263.

Jennings, C.A., Will, T.A., and Reinert, T.R. (2005). Efficacy of a high- and low-frequency ultrasonic transducer for measuring ovary volume and estimating fecundity of striped bass *Morone saxatilis* in the Savannah River Estuary. *Fisheries Research* 76: 445–453.

Lai, N.C., Dalton, N., Lai, Y.Y. et al. (2004). A comparative echocardiographic assessment of the ventricular function in five species of sharks. *Comparative Biochemistry and Physiology A* 137: 505–521.

Lewbart, G.A., Stone, E.A., and Love, N.E. (1995). Pneumocystectomy in a Midas cichlid. *Journal of the American Veterinary Medical Association* 207: 319–321.

Love, N.E. and Lewbart, G.A. (1997). Pet fish radiography: technique and case history reports. *Veterinary Radiology and Ultrasound* 38: 24–29.

Macrì, F., Passantino, A., Pugliese, M. et al. (2014). Retrograde positive contrast urethrocystography of the fish urogenital system. *Scientific World Journal* https://doi.org/10.1155/2014/384165.

Munhofen, J.L., Jiménez, D.A., Peterson, D.L. et al. (2014). Comparing ultrasonography and endoscopy for early gender identification of juvenile Siberian sturgeon. *North American Journal of Aquaculture* 76: 14–23.

Mylniczenko, N.D., Culpepper, E.E., and Clauss, T. (2017). Diagnostic imaging of elasmobranchs: updates and case examples. In: *Elasmobranch Husbandry Manual II: Recent Advances in the Care of Sharks, Rays and their Relatives* (eds. S. Smith, D. Warmolts, D. Thoney, et al.), 303–324. Columbus, OH: Ohio Biological Survey Inc.

Mylniczenko, N.D., Penfold, L., Guttridge, T. et al. (2018). Ultrasound comparison of the liver to spleen as an evaluation of liver and body condition in elasmobranchs. *Proceedings of the American Association of Zoo Veterinarians Conference*, Prague, Czech Republic.

Mylniczenko, N.D., Sumigama, S., Wyffels, J. et al. (2019). Ultrasonographic and hormonal characterization of reproductive health and disease in wild, semiwild, and aquarium-housed southern stingrays

(*Hypanus americanus*). *American Journal of Veterinary Research* (10): 931–942.

Newman, D.M., Jones, P.L., and Ingram, B.A. (2008). Sexing accuracy and indicators of maturation status in captive Murray cod *Maccullochella peelii* using non-invasive ultrasonic imagery. *Aquaculture* 279: 113–119.

Novelo, N.D. and Tiersch, T.R. (2016). Development and evaluation of an ultrasound imaging reproductive index based on the ovarian cycle of channel catfish, *Ictalurus punctatus*. *Journal of the World Aquaculture Society* 47: 526.

Pees, M., Pees, K., and Kiefer, I. (2009). The use of computed tomography for assessment of the swim bladder in koi carp (*Cyprinus carpio*). *Veterinary Radiology and Ultrasound* 51: 294–298.

Preziosi, R., Gridelli, S., Borghetti, P. et al. (2006). Spinal deformity in a sandtiger shark, *Carcharias taurus* Rafinesque: a clinical-pathological study. *Journal of Fish Diseases* 29: 49–60.

Rahmati-Holasoo, H., Shokrpoor, S., Tavakkoli, A. et al. (2016). Liposarcoma or invasive lipomatosis in flower horn fish hybrid cichlid: clinical, radiological, ultrasonographical and histopathological study. *Journal of Fish Diseases* 39: 309–315.

Rogers, B.L., Lowe, C.G., Fernandez-Juricic, E., and Frank, L.R. (2008). Utilizing magnetic resonance imaging (MRI) to assess the effects of angling-induced barotrauma on rockfish (*Sebastes*). *Canadian Journal of Fisheries and Aquatic Sciences* 65: 1245–1249.

Rummer, J.L. and Bennett, W.A. (2005). Physiological effects of swim bladder overexpansion and catastrophic decompression on red snapper. *Transactions of the American Fisheries Society* 134: 1457–1470.

Schulz-Mirbach, T., Metscher, B., and Ladich, F. (2012). Relationship between swim bladder morphology and hearing abilities – a case study on Asian and African cichlids. *PLoS One* 7 (8): 1–13.

Sheldon, J.D., Allender, M.C., George, R.H. et al. (2018). Reproductive hormone patterns in male and female cownose rays (*Rhinoptera bonasus*) in an aquarium setting and correlation to ultrasonographic staging. *Journal of Zoo and Wildlife Medicine* 49: 638–647.

Smith, S.A. and Smith, B.J. (1994). Xeroradiographic and radiographic anatomy of the channel catfish, *Ictalurus punctatus*. *Veterinary Radiology and Ultrasound* 35: 384–390.

Smith-Vaniz, W.F., Kaufman, L.S., and Glowacki, J. (1995). Species-specific patterns of hyperostosis in marine teleost fishes. *Marine Biology* 121: 573–580.

Tyson, R., Love, N.E., Lewbart, G. et al. (1999). Techniques in advanced imaging of fish. *Proceedings of the American Association of Zoo Veterinarians*, Columbus, OH.

Weinhardt, V., Shkarin, R., Wernet, T. et al. (2018). Quantitative morphometric analysis of adult teleost fish by X-ray computed tomography. *Scientific Reports* 8: 1–12.

Whittamore, J.M., Bloomer, C., Hanna, G.M., and McCarthy, I.D. (2010). Evaluating ultrasonography as a non-lethal method for the assessment of maturity in oviparous elasmobranchs. *Marine Biology* 157: 2613–2624.

Williams, D.L., Goddard, P.J., and Brancker, W.M. (2007). Ultrasonographic examination of ocular lesions in farmed halibut. *The Veterinary Journal* 173: 456–458.

Wilson, A.B., Ahnesjö, I., Vincent, A.C., and Meyer, A. (2003). The dynamics of male brooding, mating patterns, and sex roles in pipefishes and seahorses (family Syngnathidae). *Evolution* 57: 1374–1386.

Wu, J.-L., Zhang, M.L., Zhang, J.-L. et al. (2015). Evaluation of the distribution of adipose tissues in fish using magnetic resonance imaging (MRI). *Aquaculture* 448: 112–122.

A9

Necropsy and Ancillary Diagnostics

Lisa M. Mangus[1] and Allan P. Pessier[2]

[1] *Johns Hopkins University School of Medicine, Baltimore, MD, USA*
[2] *Washington State University, Pullman, WA, USA*

Introduction

Necropsy is an essential diagnostic in fish medicine. Detailed necropsies with ancillary diagnostics provide more information than is possible premortem, are an essential component of assessing overall group health, and are invaluable in the event of morbidity and mortality in a group of fish. Fish necropsies may be carried out by pathologists, veterinarians, technicians, biologists, or students. They should be considered within a broader framework that includes a thorough history and environmental and water quality evaluations.

Specimen Selection

In the event of morbidity and mortality in a group, the ideal necropsy specimens are fish showing early clinical signs. Fish showing late clinical signs or that were found dead often have secondary diseases or other changes that complicate interpretation. The fish should be euthanized and examined rapidly, albeit more than 30 minutes after cessation of reflexes and respiration. If specimens cannot be examined that quickly, they should be refrigerated at ~4°C (39°F) or bagged and kept in ice for examination the same day or at least the following morning. In some cases, specimens must be shipped overnight to outside laboratories (Box A9.1). The sensitivity of a necropsy decreases the longer that specimens wait for examination. The time frame and effects vary across studies, but possible changes over time include loss of ectoparasites, colonization by environmental organisms, and tissue autolysis (Kvach et al. 2016). The tissues damaged most rapidly by autolysis are usually the gills, gastrointestinal tract, liver, and brain.

Where necropsy is not possible within 24 hours, it may be necessary to freeze the specimen and thaw it later for necropsy. These specimens may still allow diagnosis of gross lesions (e.g. hepatomegaly, masses, and some bacterial and viral tests) but ectoparasites and subtle lesions will be missed and cellular detail on histology tends to be poor.

The worst specimens are fish that were found dead and autolyzed. Signs of autolysis include brown- or tan-colored uneven gills, dull coloration, skin erosions, thick mucus, corneal opacities, obvious signs of predation, liquid coming from the body cavity or gathering in the corner of the container, and a sour odor. These specimens provide little useful information, although gross lesions may be visible and radiography may identify skeletal lesions.

Euthanasia of Fish

The American Veterinary Medical Association (AVMA) provides guidelines on euthanasia of fish (Leary et al. 2020). The most common method is an overdose of buffered tricaine methanesulfonate (MS-222) at more than 5–10 times the anesthetic dose. Fish must be kept in the anesthetic solution for more than 15–30 minutes after cessation of reflexes and opercular movement. At this time, the gills should have paled, confirming cessation of the heartbeat. The heart beat can also be checked using ultrasonography. Effectiveness of methanesulfonate for euthanasia varies by species and life stage; it is recommended to follow with a

Clinical Guide to Fish Medicine, First Edition. Edited by Catherine A. Hadfield and Leigh Ann Clayton.

Box A9.1 Recommendations for Shipping Dead Fish to Diagnostic Laboratories

1) Contact the laboratory to discuss the sample submission and confirm the delivery timing and any additional shipping recommendations.
2) Double-bag the fish in suitable bags (e.g. Ziploc®) with no water.
3) Place in an insulated box with ice packs.
4) Include the submission form with a full history inside a third bag.
5) Label the box clearly with shipping address, sender's address, and (in the United States) the label "Exempt animal specimen".
6) Ship same day or overnight.

secondary method (e.g. pithing, freezing, pentobarbital) to produce a two-step euthanasia (Collymore et al. 2016; Balko et al. 2018; Leary et al. 2020). In large fish and obligate air-breathers (Box A1.1), tricaine may be used to provide sedation followed by intravenous pentobarbital. More details are provided in Chapter A10.

Human Safety

Fish necropsies present similar hazards to routine fish handling, although the risk of a penetrating skin trauma (e.g. fish spine, scalpel blade) is higher. Risks include physical trauma, envenomation, and zoonotic disease transmission (e.g. mycobacteriosis, vibriosis). Necropsies should be carried out in a dedicated area. This may be as simple as a dedicated tray for small fish, but the ideal scenario is a dedicated room with negative pressure ventilation. Human food and drinks should never be in a necropsy area. Latex, nitrile, or vinyl gloves must be used for all fish necropsies. Additional barriers may be indicated for larger fish (e.g. neoprene gloves, gowns, full sleeves). The risk of envenomation should be considered (Table A6.2) and any venomous spines or barbs should be carefully removed and disposed of in a rigid, labeled box prior to starting the necropsy. Cleaning and disinfection of the work area and instruments and thorough hand-washing should be standard after fish necropsies.

Equipment Needed

Equipment needs are minimal for most fish necropsies. Common supplies for a mixed species aquarium are listed here.

- Scale, ruler, measuring tape.
- Cutting board or tray.
- Small and large scissors.
- +/− Pruning shears or bone cutters, large cutting knives, bone saw for large fish.
- Small and large forceps (e.g. DeBakey, Brown-Adson).
- Scalpel handle and blades.
- Hemostats to close hollow viscus (e.g. esophagus).
- Slides and coverslips.
- Dropper bottle with freshwater, salt water, and physiologic saline.
- Syringes and needles.
- Digital camera.
- Bright-field microscope, ideally with a mounted camera.
- +/− Dissecting microscope or head loupe for small specimens.
- Leakproof containers with 10% neutral buffered formalin (or other fixative) and appropriate labels.
- 70% ethanol or lighter for aseptic preparation.
- Culturettes and blood culture tubes.
- Rayon, polyester, or nylon-flocked swabs for PCR testing.
- Cryovials and plain blood tubes.
- +/− Stains for impression smears (e.g. Dif-Quik, Gram, and acid-fast stains).
- +/− Electron microscopy fixative (e.g. 2% glutaraldehyde in phosphate buffer).
- +/− DNA or RNA stabilizers (e.g. DNA/RNA Shield™, ViveST™).
- +/− Viral transport media.
- Recording sheet or wet-board.
- Cleaning brushes, soap, and disinfectant.
- +/− Cold-sterile solution for instruments.
- Ultrasonic cleaner and instrument milk to maintain instruments.
- Sharpening instruments for knives and shears.

Hazardous equipment (e.g. knives) and fixatives must be stored appropriately between uses.

Gross Necropsy

Ancillary Diagnostics

Anticipated ancillary diagnostics should be determined before starting a necropsy, as some samples should be collected prior to full necropsy (e.g. culture, radiographs) and some require specific equipment or procedures (e.g. consulting laboratories for viral sampling protocols). Potential ancillary diagnostics may include radiography, bacteriology, mycology, virology, parasitology, toxicology, and collecting otoliths for ageing studies.

Radiography should be considered with every necropsy, as it provides information on skeletal condition that may not be seen at necropsy. It also helps to build an image database.

Common culture sites for bacteriology and mycology include blood, liver, spleen, kidney, brain, cerebrospinal fluid (elasmobranchs), effusions, and lesions. Sample requirements should be determined prior to starting by discussing goals with the diagnostic laboratory. Samples should be collected as soon as possible and aseptically. This may involve ethanol or flame treatment of a surface prior to sterile incision for culture. Blood samples are easy to collect aseptically by prepping the skin with ethanol prior to venipuncture. Liver samples can be collected after the first ventral incision, as soon as the liver is visible. Kidney samples can be collected aseptically following a transverse cut dorsally through the epaxial muscles and spine.

Common sampling sites for virology include the gills, liver, spleen, kidney, brain, and lesions. Samples should be collected as soon as possible. Viral transport media, DNA or RNA stabilizers, or electron microscopy fixative may be required.

Parasites that cannot be identified to the required taxonomic level can be fixed for later morphological or molecular testing. Methods vary, but often require fixatives that may not be readily available. Practical options for helminths are described by Justine et al. 2012: washing with 0.9% saline, followed by fixation in near-boiling saline, followed by fixation in 95% ethanol.

For toxicology or nutritional analysis, common samples are blood, serum, liver, or muscle. Samples that may be used for toxicology or nutrient analysis can typically be frozen at −20°C (−4°F). Specific sampling and storage requirements may exist for some tests to avoid contamination; the best option is to discuss plans with the diagnostic laboratory.

More information on sampling is available in Chapter A7 and Gardner et al. 2016.

External Examination

A thorough external examination is essential. It should include an assessment of the body condition (epaxial musculature and coelomic cavity), skin, fins, eyes, oral cavity, gills, and anus and urogenital pores or cloaca. A weight and either total length or snout-vent length should be recorded. For skates and rays (*Batoidea*), disc width should be recorded. Standard photos (e.g. right and left lateral and dorsoventral views) can be useful.

Common abnormalities include poor body condition with loss of epaxial musculature and/or a pinched coelomic cavity; coelomic distension; skin or fin hyperemia or erosions; ocular inflammation, gas, or edema; cloacal (or anal or urogenital pore) inflammation or discharge; and visible ectoparasites (e.g. leeches, copepods). A simplified key to common external fish parasites is provided in Box A9.2.

Gill, Skin, and Fin Wet Mounts

Wet mounts of the gill, skin, and fin examined under direct microscopy should be standard with all fish necropsies. All wet mounts should be kept moist using suitable water to prevent damage to parasites and tissues. The water should ideally come from the fish's system, but if unavailable, water of similar salinity and temperature can be used. When examined under the microscope, the condenser should be low or out of the way (Figure A9.1); this differs from examination of stained slides, when the condenser should be high.

For gill biopsies (also known as gill clips), scissors should be used to cut three to five primary filaments (Figure A9.2a). They can be gently transferred to a slide using a coverslip. A few drops of suitable water should be added followed by the coverslip. The sample should be examined under direct microscopy on low to high power. In elasmobranchs, the thick gill cartilage in larger specimens limits the usefulness of a gill biopsy. The gill filaments can instead be scraped from base to tip, then mounted on a slide for examination under direct microscopy on low to high power. Common abnormalities in bony fish include ciliates, dinoflagellates, flagellates, monogeneans, copepods, myxozoans, cysts, oomycetes, fungal organisms (e.g. *Branchiomyces* spp.), granulomas, gas bubbles, telangiectasia (dilated blood vessels), hyperplasia, and increased mucus (Figure A9.2b–f). Typical abnormalities in cartilaginous fish include monogeneans, copepods, and increased mucus. A simplified key to common external fish parasites is provided in Box A9.2.

Skin scrapes are often carried out using a coverslip to scrape mucus from the dorsum, pectoral fin area, or any lesions, following the direction of the scales. The coverslip should be rolled onto a slide to smear the sample. A drop of suitable water may be needed to get rid of air spaces. The sample should be examined under direct microscopy on low to high power. Common abnormalities include ciliates, dinoflagellates, flagellates, monogeneans, nematodes, copepods, hypertrophied cells, abnormal bacterial load (e.g. *Flavobacterium* spp. in characteristic haystacks), oomycetes, and increased mucus (Figure A9.3). A simplified key to common external fish parasites is provided in Box A9.2.

Scissors can be used to cut a small sample of translucent fin for examination on a slide. If the sample becomes folded, it should be unfolded prior to adding the coverslip. The sample should be examined under direct microscopy on low to high power (Figure A9.4). Common abnormalities include dinoflagellates, leeches, and gas bubbles.

Box A9.2

This is a simplified key to common fish parasites found on gross examination and/or direct microscopy of the skin, fins, or gills. This is not meant as an absolute guide, but as a starting point for further investigation. There will be parasites that cannot be keyed this way, particularly unusual species within each parasite group, less common life stages, and free-living organisms that may be found on fish.

1) Visible to the naked eye and on microscopy
   a) Exoskeleton and jointed appendages present
      I) Prominent segmentation
         i) Large, dorsoventrally flattened body, often a single individual, firmly embedded – **isopod**
         ii) Laterally flattened body, abrupt, quick movements – **amphipod**
      II) Distinct body sections, but not segmented
         i) Oval or long, thin body, single simple eye spot, no compound eyes, large paired egg sacs – **copepod**
         ii) Oval body, paired compound eye spots, paired suckers that look like compound eyes – **branchiuran**
         iii) Oval, large body, four pairs of prominent limbs – **mite**
   b) Worm-like, no limbs present
      I) Segmented
         i) Long and thin, round, or flat in cross section, with anterior and posterior suckers, eye spots may be present, looping or wave-like motion – **leech**
         ii) Long and thin or leaf-shaped, flat in cross section, scolex (hooks) at the anterior end, no digestive tract, eggs may be visible in mature proglottids – **cestode**
         iii) Stout, coiled or C-shaped, round in cross section, pseudosegmentation just visible, hooks at the anterior end, nonmotile, usually found in thin-walled cysts – **pentastomid**
      II) Unsegmented
         i) Oval to long and thin body, flat in cross section.
            - Terminal attachment organ is a large haptor with hooks, four black eyespots, paired ceca, eggs may be present, move by stretching and jerking – **oviparous monopisthocotyle monogenean (e.g. dactylogyrid, capsalid, monocotylid)**
            - Terminal attachment organ is a small haptor with hooks, no eyespots, paired ceca, hooks of larvae often visible within the parasite, move by stretching and jerking – **gyrodactylid monogenean**
            - Terminal attachment organ is a small haptor with no hooks, no eyespots, paired ceca, eggs may be present, move by stretching and jerking – **microbothrid monogenean**
            - Terminal attachment organ has multiple pairs of suckers with barely visible hooks, paired ceca, eggs may be present, move slowly by stretching and jerking – **polyopisthocotyle monogenean**
            - Subterminal attachment sucker and midbody sucker, paired ceca, eggs may be visible, move by peristalsis, may be within a cyst – **digene**
            - No terminal attachment organ, cilia around the edge, paired eye spots, complete digestive tract, move with a smooth gliding motion, may be grouped within a cyst – **turbellaria**
         ii) Long and thin body, round in cross section
            - No hooks or suckers, full digestive tract with visible radially symmetrical esophagus, eggs may be visible, move by sigmoidal wriggling or thrashing – **nematode**
            - Large spiny proboscis at anterior end that may be everted or inverted, no digestive tract, often firmly anchored – **acanthocephalan**
         iii) Paired shell present – **larval freshwater mussel (e.g. *Glochidia* sp.)**
         iv) Anemone-like – **hydroid**
2) Visible on microscopy only
   a) Motile – free or attached
      I) Small protozoan
         i) Cilia present
            - Round, some are large (up to 1 mm), light gold to brown, may have a visible macronucleus, slowly rotating – ***Ichthyophthirius multifiliis* (FW), *Cryptocaryon irritans* (SW)**
            - Teardrop-shaped, small, with fast, forward motion – **scuticociliate**
            - Heart-shaped or oval with a notch, gliding motion – ***Chilodonella* sp. (FW), *Brooklynella* sp. (SW)**

- Round, symmetric, with rings of denticles and a spinning motion – **trichodinid**
- Funnel-shaped, bell-shaped, or round, small, attached by a stalk or filament that may periodically contract, with cilia visible at the opposite end – **sessile ciliate**

ii) Flagellum or flagella present producing a disjointed, tumbling motion, small (oil immersion often needed)

- Comma-shaped – ***Ichthyobodo* sp.**
- Teardrop-shaped, often on intestinal samples – ***Hexamita*, *Spironucleus*, *Cryptobia* sp.**
- In blood or effusion – ***Trypanosoma*, *Cryptobia* sp.**

b) Nonmotile

I) Thin-walled cyst or spore; after initial examination, try to rupture with gentle pressure to look at contents

i) Hooks visible, motile larva within – **larval cestode**

ii) No hooks visible, motile larva within – **larval nematode, digene, leech**

iii) Round to cigar-shaped with 2–4 round structures within, some variability in size – ***Eimeria* sp., other coccidia**

iv) Uniform, small spores with 1–7 (usually 2) symmetric polar capsules, free or within cyst-like capsules (plasmodia), acid-fast positive – ***Myxozoa***

v) Uniform, small round spores with subtle ring appearance – ***Mesomycetozoea***

vi) Uniform, very small, oval spores with a circular vacuole, Gram- and acid-fast positive – ***Microsporidia***

II) Dark brown or dark yellow, almost round structures with varying sizes and no identifiable contents – ***Amyloodinium* sp. (SW), *Piscinoodinium* sp. (FW)**

III) Ova; these are particularly hard to classify and this is a rough guide

i) Round to oval with a thin wall – **digene (except blood flukes), copepod**

ii) Round to oval with a thick wall – **cestode**

iii) Triangular, tetrahedral, spindle-shaped with one or more filaments – **oviparous monogenean**

iv) Barrel-shaped with bipolar plugs – **camallanid nematode, capillarid nematode, trichosomoidid nematode, acanthocephalan**

v) Spindle-shaped, within gill blood vessels – **blood fluke**

Many fish ectoparasites can be readily visible to the naked eye (e.g. monogeneans, leeches, copepods, branchiurans). These can be removed with forceps, mounted on a slide with a coverslip and a few drops of suitable water, and examined under direct microscopy on low to high power.

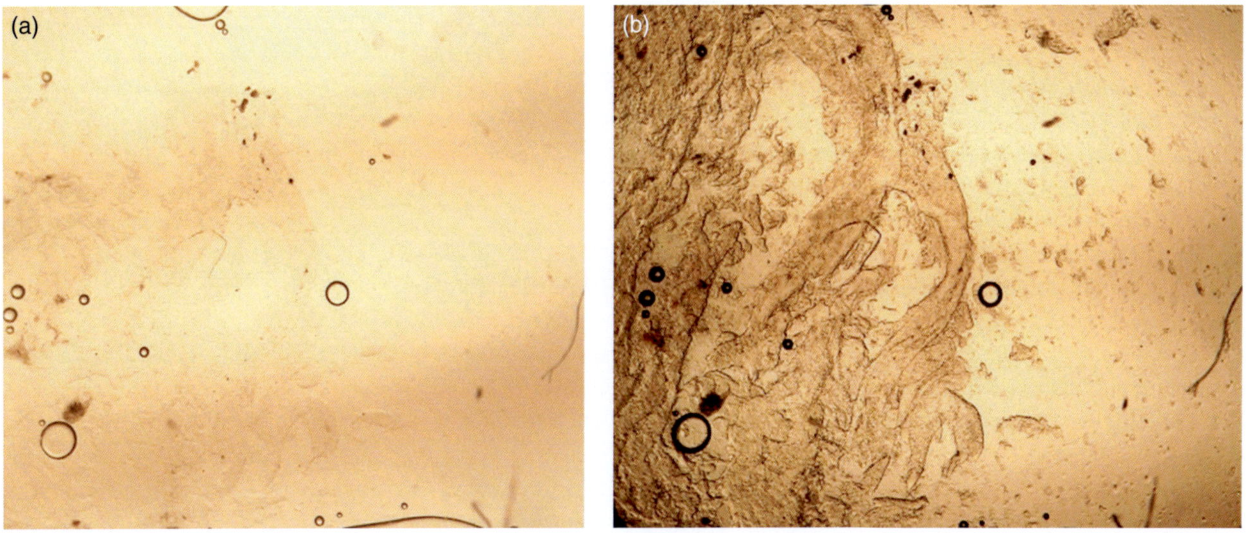

Figure A9.1 Skin scrape examined under direct microscopy showing the difference in contrast with the condenser set high (a) and low (b). *Source*: Images courtesy of Catherine Hadfield, National Aquarium.

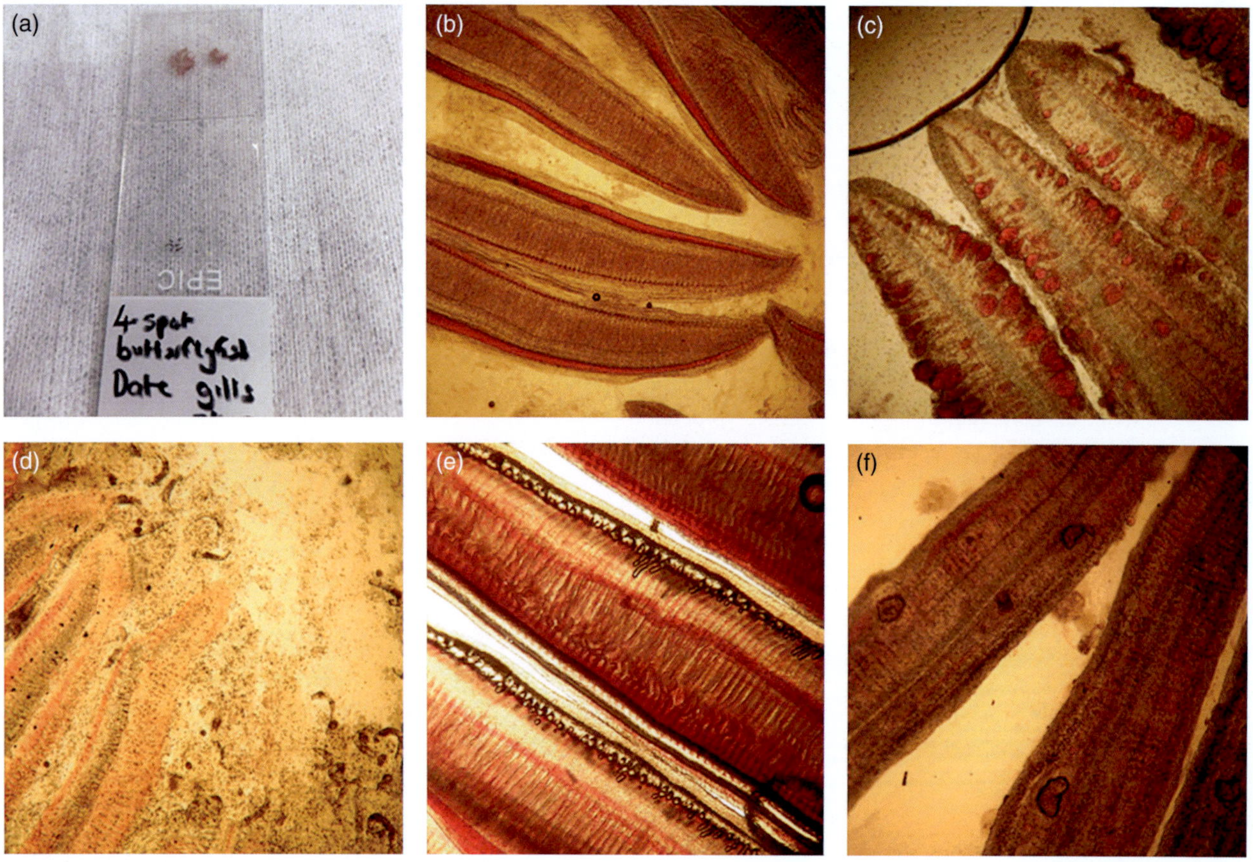

Figure A9.2 Wet mount of a gill biopsy and skin scrape (a); normal gills on direct microscopy (b); abnormal gill biopsies showing telangiectasia (c), dactylogyrid monogenean adults, ova, and mucus (d), gas bubbles (e), and granulomas (f). *Source*: Images courtesy of Catherine Hadfield, National Aquarium.

Necropsy Approach

Most fish are placed in right lateral recumbency to cut open the left body wall and operculum. The easiest approach is usually to put the tip of scissors into the cranial vent and make a single cut, then move the scissors cranially through that cut into the coelom. Scissors can then be used to cut along the ventral midline through to the base of the operculum and dorsally from the vent to either the lateral line or where the muscle gets too thick to cut readily; this usually marks the dorsal limit of the coelom. The scissors can then be used to cut cranially through the skin and hypaxial muscle to the operculum. The left operculum and left pectoral girdle should be removed to expose the gills and heart. This may require pruning shears or bone cutters in larger fish.

Some fish cannot be placed in right lateral recumbency. This includes flatfish (*Pleuronectiformes*) and some elasmobranchs. Flatfish are placed in ventrodorsal recumbency (with eyes ventrally); the position of the vent helps dictate where the incision should start. Sharks may be approached ventrally or from the left lateral aspect; dorsal fin(s) usually need to be removed to allow positioning. Skates and rays are placed in dorsal recumbency and two cavities are opened: the coelomic cavity is easily opened using a scalpel to cut around the cranial and lateral aspects of the coelom, then carefully cutting through the pelvis with scissors or pruning shears; the gills and heart are exposed using a scalpel or scissors to cut along the gill slits laterally, then across the lower jaw and the cranial aspect of the pectoral girdle (Figure A9.5).

When incisions are made, it is important to keep the blade superficial to avoid damaging underlying structures, particularly the swim bladder, if present. It is also important to identify the type and extent of any effusions as the incisions are made, as fluids often get contaminated over time.

Large fish and fish with thick dermal plates (e.g. sturgeon, *Acipenseridae*) or dermal spines (e.g. porcupinefish, *Diodontidae*) can be particularly hard to open at necropsy. Large cutting instruments are often needed and may need to be changed or sharpened during a necropsy.

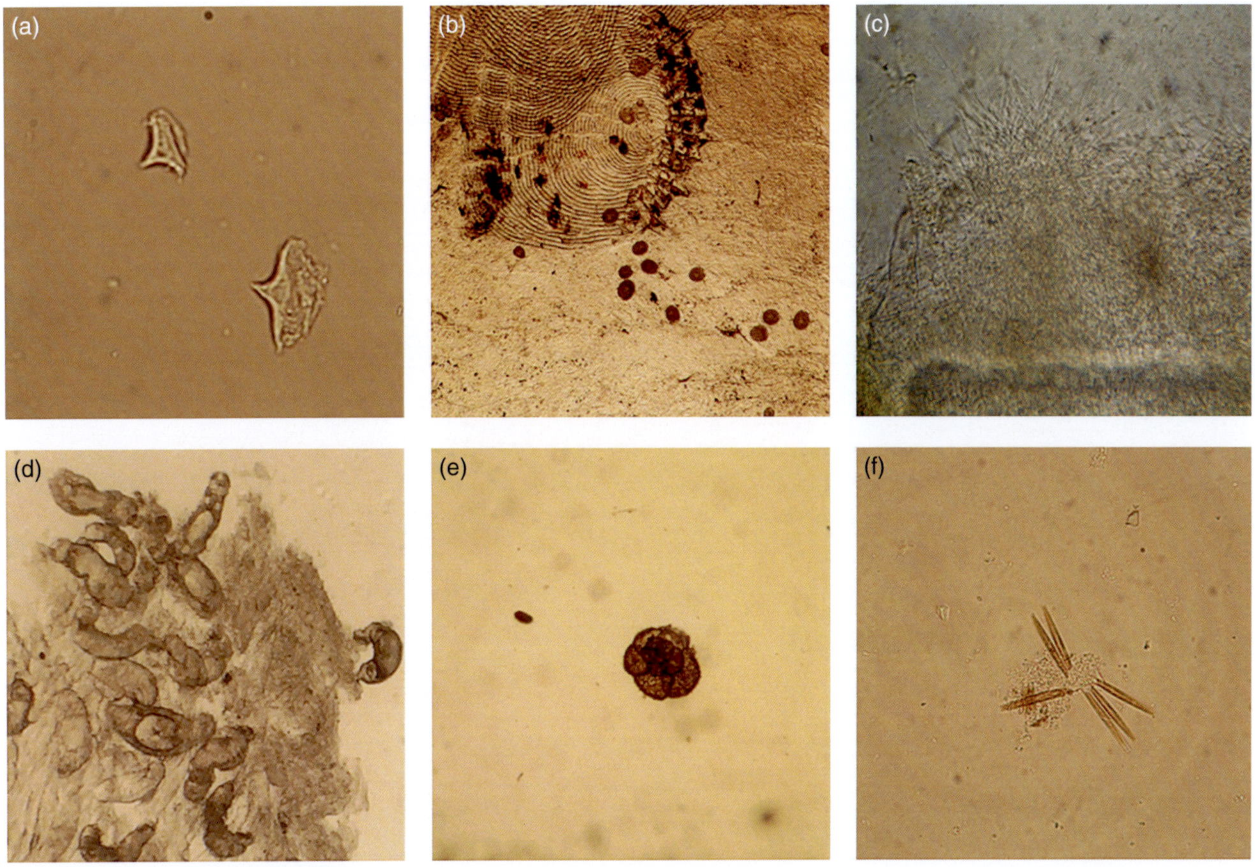

Figure A9.3 Skin scrapes examined under direct microscopy showing scales from a seahorse (*Syngnathidae*) (a) and grunt (*Haemulidae*) (b); abnormal findings include *Amyloodinium* sp. (b), the typical haystack appearance of *Flavobacterium* spp. (c), and gyrodactylid monogeneans (d); incidental findings include a foraminifer (e) and diatoms (f). *Source*: Images courtesy of Catherine Hadfield, National Aquarium.

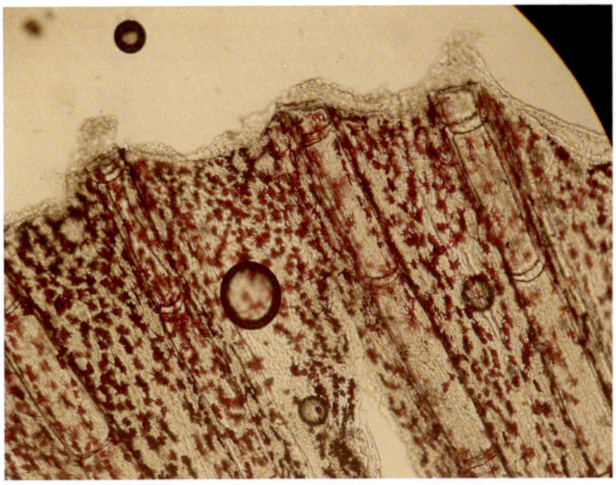

Figure A9.4 Normal fin biopsy examined under direct microscopy with some air bubbles trapped under the coverslip. *Source*: Image courtesy of Catherine Hadfield, National Aquarium.

Examination In Situ

Once opened, all tissues should be examined in situ to determine any abnormalities and decide if other ancillary diagnostics are required. A photo of the body cavity after opening is useful for later review and for comparison with conspecifics (Figure A9.6). Useful references include Fisher and Myers (2000) and Yanong (2003). Common abnormalities include effusion, congestion, organomegaly (particularly the liver, kidney, spleen, and gonads), obesity, and adhesions.

Organ Evaluation

Once examined in situ, and after collection of any aseptic samples, tissues in larger fish should be removed for detailed evaluation. The sequence will vary based on anatomy and experience. Additional evaluations may include photographs, measurements, and collection of samples.

The liver in fish varies significantly by species, condition, and diet; it is usually orange or brown but can be

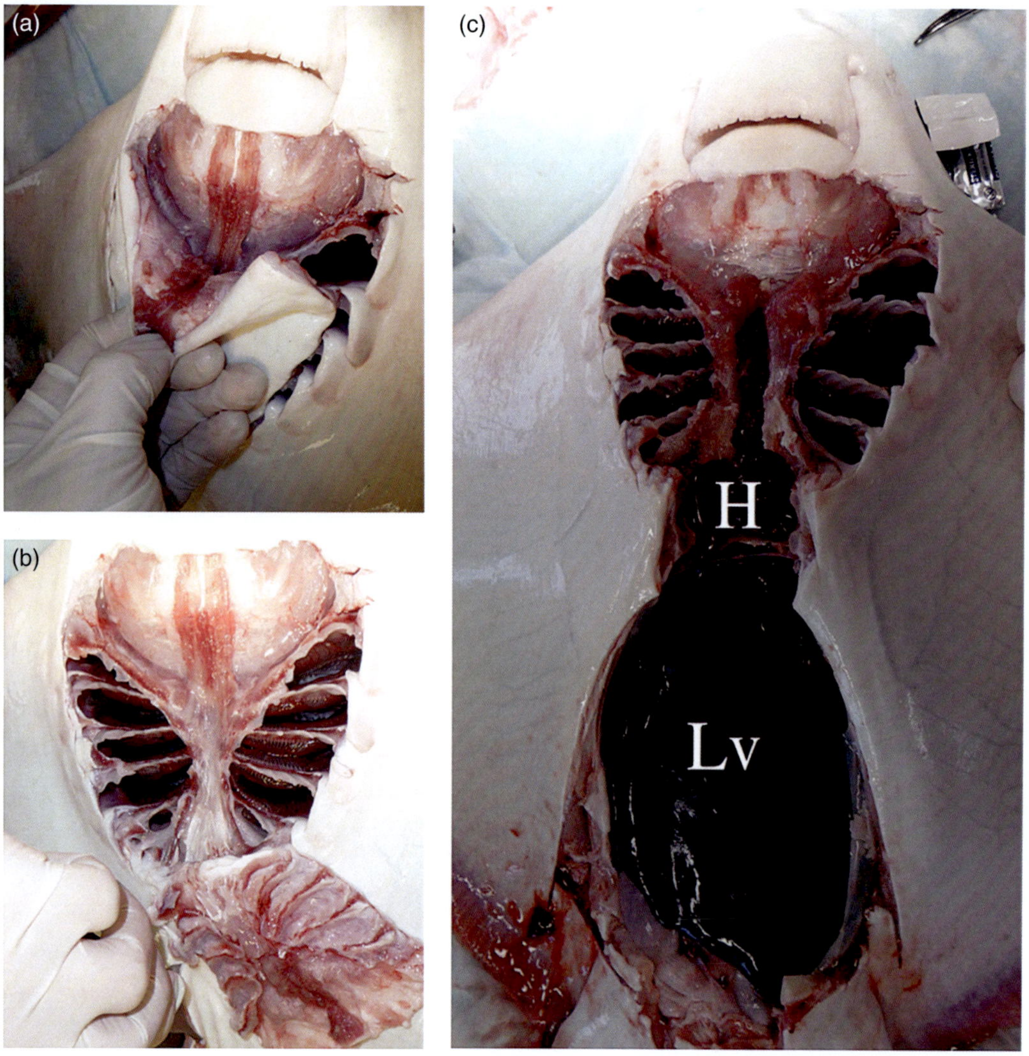

Figure A9.5 Cavities opened in a cownose ray (*Rhinoptera bonasus*) showing one method to expose the gills and heart (a, b), and a view of both cavities (c). H: heart, LV: liver. *Source*: Images courtesy of Catherine Hadfield, National Aquarium.

tan or red in color. It should have sharp edges and be soft but not be friable. It is always in the cranial coelom and has a lobulated appearance in some species (e.g. pufferfish, *Tetraodontidae*). The liver can be weighed and used to generate a liver-to-body weight ratio. Large viscera should receive serial cuts (i.e. "bread slices") to examine the entire organ. Common liver abnormalities include hepatomegaly, congestion, granulomas, cysts, and fatty infiltration. The gallbladder, when present, will often stain surrounding tissue green. Bile should be yellow to green in color and clear. The gallbladder is often large in inappetent fish. The spleen should be dark red and firm in all fish species, although the shape varies. It is usually close to the stomach. Common abnormalities include splenomegaly, granulomas, and cysts. A distinct pancreas is readily visible in elasmobranchs but not in most bony fish.

The gastrointestinal (GI) tract anatomy varies widely in fish. The stomach, if present, has a thicker wall than the rest of the GI tract. It may be intimately associated with ceca, the liver, and fat bodies. A valvular or spiral intestine is found in lungfish (*Dipnoi*), sturgeon (*Acipenseridae*), and elasmobranchs. A rectal gland is found in elasmobranchs connecting to the distal intestines (Figure A9.7a). The GI tract should be removed and opened to evaluate the contents and look for irregularities of the mucosa (Figure A9.7b).

The swim bladder, present in most bony fish, varies widely in shape, wall thickness, and position. The tissue is typically uniform, thick, and smooth. In some species, a rete is clearly visible. Common abnormalities include distension, fluid and/or soft tissue within the lumen, parasites, and congestion.

The kidneys in most fish are retrocoelomic and look red to brown with a firm to friable texture. While kidneys are

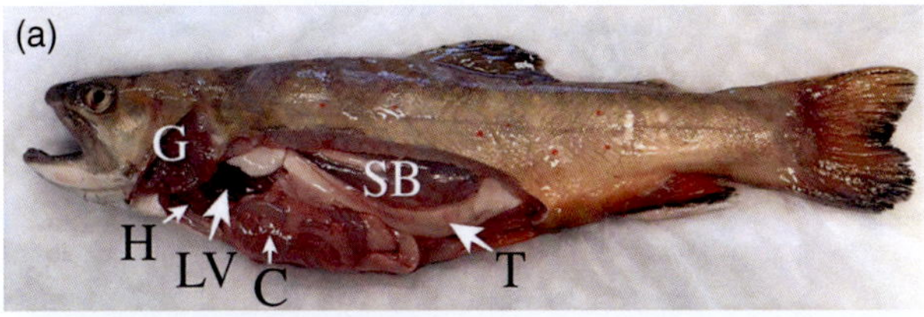

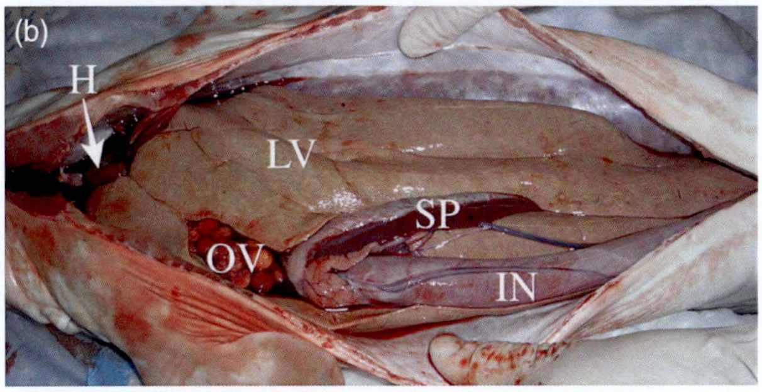

Figure A9.6 Necropsy images with organs in situ from a clinically healthy brook trout (*Salvelinus fontinalis*) (a) and bonnethead shark (*Sphyrna tiburo*) (b). H: heart, G: gills, LV: liver, SP: spleen, C: ceca, IN: intestine, SB: swim bladder, OV: ovary, T: testis. *Source*: Images courtesy of Catherine Hadfield, National Aquarium.

primarily excretory organs, the cranial kidney of most bony fish is primarily hematopoietic. Common problems include renomegaly, congestion, granulomas, and cysts. A urinary bladder is present in some species, and the tissue is usually thin and uniform.

Ovaries vary enormously in morphology and size but should be bilaterally symmetrical in most bony fish. In sharks and rays, one ovary is more prominent (Figure A9.6b). Round follicles are almost always visible in ovaries, although immature ovaries may require magnification to see the follicles. Testes are more consistent across species and are usually pale, homogeneous structures (Figure A9.6a). Sperm can be mistaken for flagellates; if suspected, a wet mount or impression smear of the testes will typically confirm the appearance of sperm. Epigonal tissue is tightly associated with the gonads of elasmobranchs. It varies greatly in size but is typically pink and homogeneous. Common ovarian problems include enlargement, congestion, granulomas, and cysts. Dystocia may be seen in viviparous species, and mucometra may be seen in elasmobranchs.

The heart has two obvious chambers but four compartments (Figure A9.8):

1) Very thin-walled, dark red sinus venosus.
2) Thin-walled, brown to dark red atrium.
3) Firm, light red ventricle.
4) Thick, white to cream-colored, conical-shaped bulbus or conus arteriosus.

Pericardial fluid is minimal in bony fish and abundant in elasmobranchs. Common problems include endocarditis.

Skeletal muscle may be red or white and should have an even, firm texture and regular striations. Common abnormalities include discoloration, edema, hemorrhage, or masses.

The brain can be particularly challenging to examine and remove. For many teleosts, the easiest approach is to remove the head, remove the gill arches, opercula, and lower jaw, then approach the brain ventrally by cutting through the foramen magnum. In some teleosts and most elasmobranchs, the easiest approach is to use a suitable blade to "shave off" the cranial vault dorsal to the brain. It is worth noting that the brain of healthy elasmobranchs sits within a large volume of cerebrospinal fluid. Common

Figure A9.7 Gastrointestinal tract and rectal gland (*) (a) and erosive lesions in the valvular intestine (b) in a southern stingray (*Hypanus americanus*). St: stomach, VI: valvular intestine, P: pancreas. *Source*: Images courtesy of Catherine Hadfield, National Aquarium.

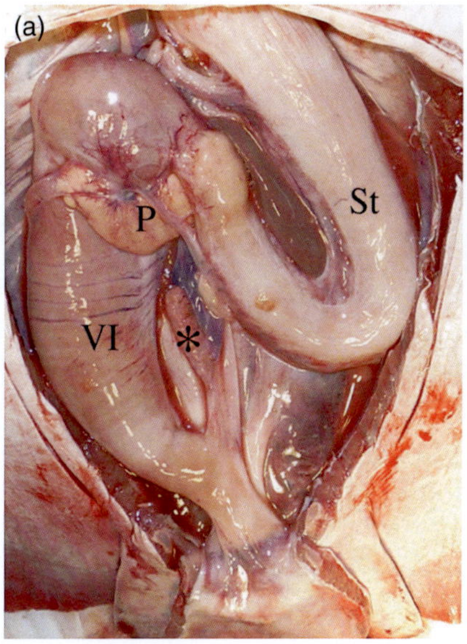

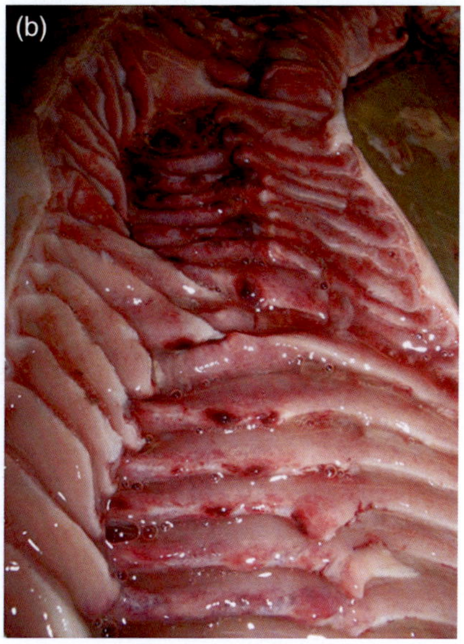

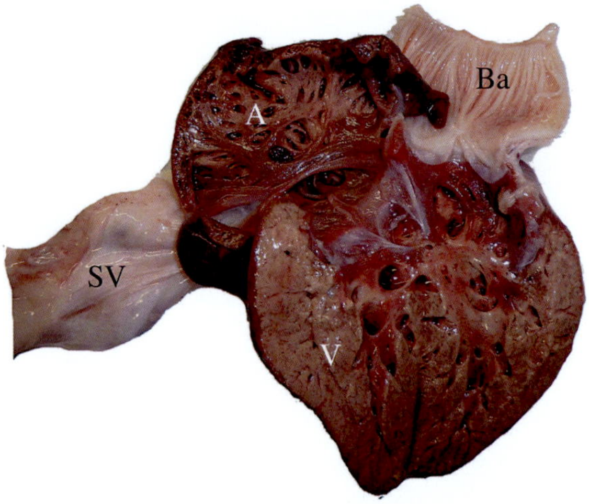

Figure A9.8 Normal teleost heart showing the four compartments. SV: sinus venosus, A: atrium, V: ventricle, Ba: bulbus arteriosus. *Source*: Image courtesy of Catherine Hadfield, National Aquarium.

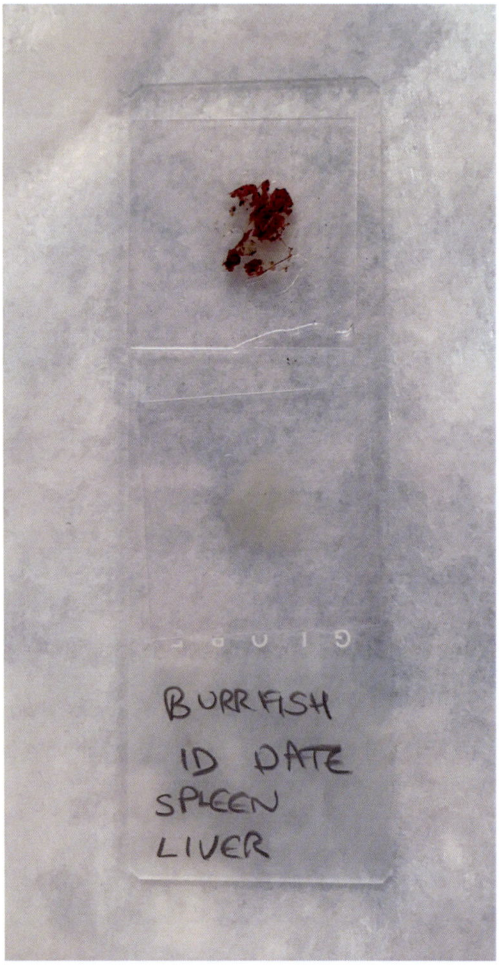

Figure A9.9 Gross image of wet mount samples of the spleen and liver under coverslips showing an appropriate size and thickness for the specimens. *Source*: Image courtesy of Catherine Hadfield, National Aquarium.

problems include inflammation, congestion, and various parasites.

Organ Wet Mounts and Impression Smears

Wet mounts examined under direct microscopy and impression smears stained in-house should be standard with necropsies, as they provide immediate results that may help with case management.

Tissue wet mounts (also known as squash preps) are often made from the liver, spleen, kidney, intestine, and gonad. A small piece of tissue (~1 mm^3) is cut and placed on a slide; a coverslip can help with transferring the sample. A drop of physiologic saline should be added, then the sample should be gently squashed using a coverslip (Figure A9.9).

Normal wet mounts of the liver, spleen, kidney, and gonad should be free of parasites, bacteria (unless autolyzed), fungi, and congestion. Liver wet mounts should be homogenous and pale (Figure A9.10a). The spleen should be homogenous and darker. The cranial kidney resembles the spleen. Wet mounts of the caudal kidney may show tubules (Figure A9.10b). Normal intestinal scrapes in a fish may show undigested food (e.g. carapaces), diatoms, bacteria, flagellates, and ciliates (Figure A9.10c). Wet mounts of gonads are particularly helpful to determine or confirm the sex in bony fish: ovaries always contain numerous round follicles (Figure A9.10e) while testes look like homogeneous parenchyma and may show sperm.

Common abnormalities on wet mounts include granulomas, congestion, increased pigmented macrophage aggregates (PMAs, previously called melanomacrophage centers), cysts, digenes, nematodes, myxozoans, microsporidians, and motile or nonmotile bacteria (Figure A9.10). Granulomas are a common sign of chronic inflammation in fish. Box A9.3 lists some of the possible causes of granulomas in fish. Box A9.4 lists some possible causes of cysts.

Impression smears are often made from the liver, spleen, and kidney. Common abnormalities include bacteria, fungi, abnormal cell morphology, and inflammatory cells (e.g. granulocytes, macrophages). A small piece of tissue (~1 mm^3) is cut, dabbed to remove superficial blood cells, then pressed several times onto several slides. These slides are air-dried, heat-fixed if needed, then stained, often with Dif-Quik, Gram, and acid-fast stains. (Figure A9.11). Dif-Quik is a type of Romanowsky stain that is useful for cellular differentiation and readily available, although Wright–Giemsa stains often provide additional cellular details. Gram and acid-fast stains provide additional categorization of bacteria and other pathogens (Tables A9.1 and A9.2). While *Mycobacterium* spp. are the most commonly reported acid-fast pathogens, many others exist and all look different on cytology.

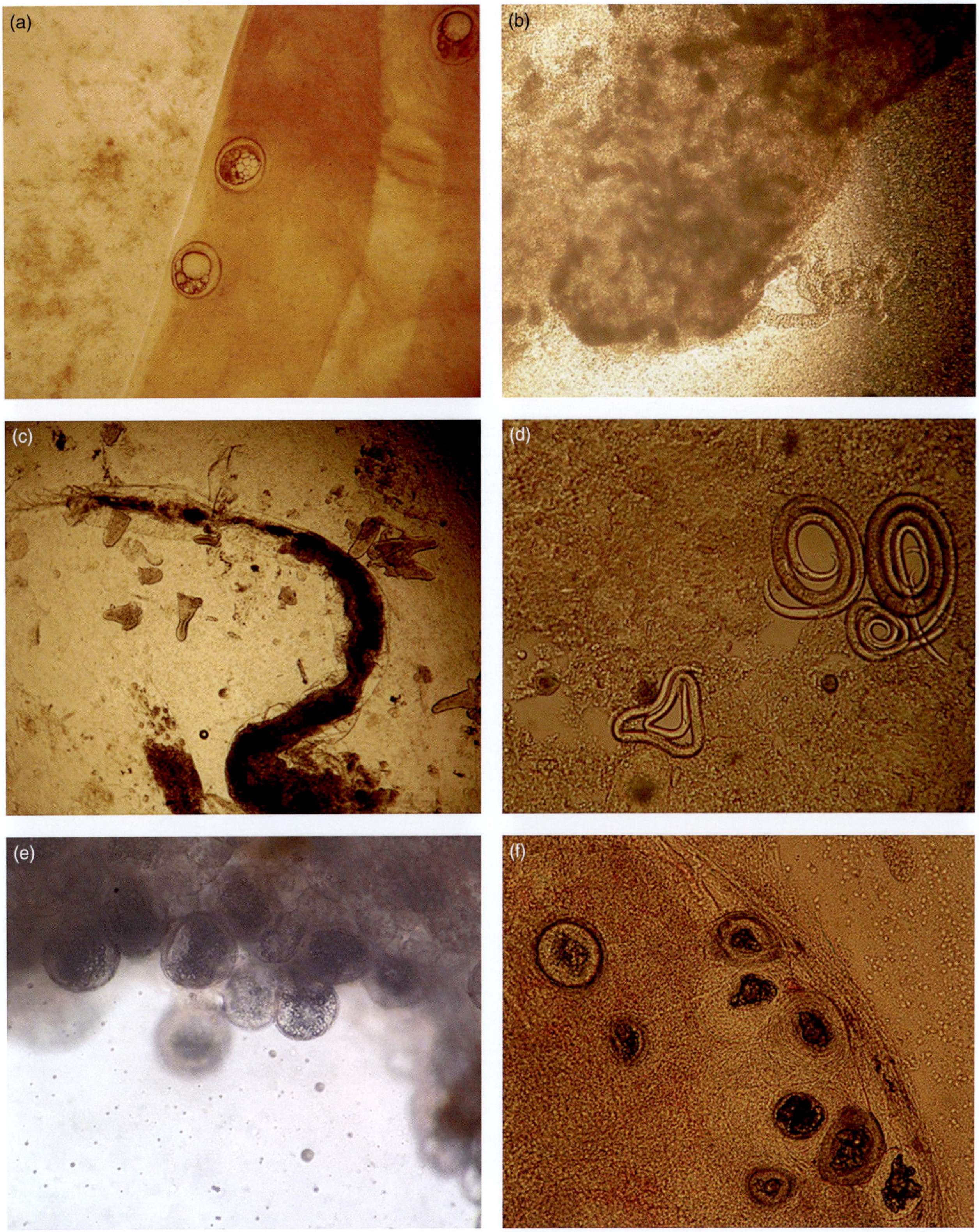

Figure A9.10 Wet mounts examined under direct microscopy: normal liver with incidental encysted digenes (a), normal caudal kidney showing tubules (b), intestinal scrape showing an ingested crustacean (c) and nematode larvae (d), ovary showing abundant follicles (e), and granulomas in a cranial kidney (f). *Source*: Images courtesy of Catherine Hadfield, National Aquarium.

Sample Storage and Bio-artifacts

In some cases, it may be beneficial to save samples for additional testing at a later date, depending on results from initial diagnostics (e.g. molecular testing if histology shows viral inclusions). Samples should be labeled and stored at appropriate temperatures in an organized fashion that will enable them to be retrieved in the future. Long-term storage of formalin-fixed tissues can lead to protein and nucleic acid degradation that limits the utility of the tissue. Samples may benefit from being transferred to an alternative solution for long-term storage, such as 70% ethanol or phosphate-buffered saline.

In educational and scientific settings, bio-artifacts may be kept for education. Samples should be properly labeled and inventoried so that sources are clear, and organizations should ensure that they maintain any required permits.

Disposal

Disposal of remaining tissues must follow all national, state, and local regulations. In the US, some states list animal waste as biomedical waste if there is any risk of infectious disease. This typically requires that the tissues are collected in a designated, labeled freezer prior to disposition through incineration through an approved biomedical waste company. In most cases, there are weight and size limits on these samples, so large specimens often need to be cut down prior to disposal.

Disposal of some necropsy supplies (particularly fixatives such as formalin and ethanol) requires careful review of the relevant legislation, as these are often considered hazardous waste.

Box A9.3 Possible Causes of Granulomatous Inflammation in Fish

- Infectious
  - Bacteria: *Mycobacterium, Nocardia, Edwardsiella, Francisella, Streptococcus, Photobacterium, Renibacterium* spp., *Flavobacterium psychrophilum*, piscirickettsial-like organisms
  - Fungi or fungal-like: atypical oomycetes, *Exophiala, Fusarium* spp., *Mesomycetozoea*, microsporidians
  - Protozoa: *Cryptobia, Spironucleus, Hexamita, Amyloodinium* spp.
  - Metazoa: Encysted digenes, cestodes, nematodes
  - Myxozoa
  - Apicomplexa: *Cryptosporidium* spp.
- Foreign bodies (e.g. suture material, fiberglass)
- Xanthomas
- Calculi (e.g. nephroliths, calcinosis cutis)

Histology

Fixatives

Ten percent neutral buffered formalin (NBF) is by far the most commonly used histologic fixative. It is relatively inexpensive and readily available. Although NBF fixation is suitable for the vast majority of diagnostic cases, fixatives that contain a mixture of formalin and acid, such as Bouin's and Davidson's solutions, can provide superior morphologic detail for certain fish tissues (e.g. gills, testes, kidneys), (Fournie et al. 2000; Wolf et al. 2015). These acid-containing fixatives have the added benefit of softening bony and cartilaginous structures, which makes them good alternatives for fixing entire, small fish that will be processed whole. Because long-term storage in acid-containing solutions can result in tissue degradation and altered staining properties, it is recommended that tissues be thoroughly rinsed after 24–48 hours, at which time they can be transferred to 70% ethanol for storage.

Table A9.1 Gram-stain characteristics of common fish bacteria.

Gram stain	Typical motility on wet mount	Bacterial genera
Gram-negative bacilli	Motile or nonmotile	*Aeromonas* *Citrobacter* *Edwardsiella* *Moritella* *Photobacterium* *Pseudomonas* *Vibrio* *Yersinia*
Gram-negative bacilli	Nonmotile	*Francisella* Chlamydia-like organisms Piscirickettsial-like organisms
Gram-negative, long, thin bacilli	Motile	*Flavobacterium* *Tenacibaculum*
Gram-positive bacilli	Nonmotile	*Mycobacterium*[a] *Nocardia*[a] *Renibacterium*
Gram-positive cocci	Nonmotile	*Streptococcus* *Lactococcus* *Vagococcus* *Enterococcus*

This is a simplified table that describes typical characteristics, but many genera show pleomorphism (e.g. *Vibrio*, *Francisella* spp.) and variable motility.

[a] Often with weak and/or nonuniform staining.

Box A9.4 Possible Causes of Cysts in Fish

- Digenes
- Nematodes
- Cestodes
- Leeches
- Turbellaria
- Myxozoans
- Microsporidians

Samples

Small fish, <30 g, are often best fixed with all tissues in situ after opening the coelomic cavity. In medium-sized fish (up to ~100 g), it can be helpful to fix the liver, gastrointestinal tract, spleen, and gonads together (i.e. the "pluck"), while leaving the kidneys and swim bladder attached to the spine.

For larger fish, tissue samples should be less than 5–10 mm thick, although thinner sections facilitate rapid fixation. With larger samples, only the outside of the tissues may fix, leading to autolysis of the deeper tissues. Samples should be collected without crushing the tissue; scalpel blades and fine forceps are usually preferable to scissors and rat-tooth forceps. Samples of abnormal tissues should include normal tissue at one margin for orientation and comparison. Even normal samples may benefit from being collected at margins to help with orientation (e.g. collecting esophagus and stomach together at the margin). Samples that are small, from a specific location (e.g. left ovary), or may be hard to identify following fixation (e.g. masses) are best submitted in labeled cassettes. Heavy pencils (e.g. 2B) or China pencils should be used to write on cassettes. Cassettes should be large enough to prevent crushing. A final volume of 1 part tissue to 10 parts fixative is recommended to provide sufficient fixative. Large amounts of non-fixative fluids in the sample container (e.g. blood, lipid, GI contents) can dilute the fixative solution and result in inadequate fixation; it is recommended to change out fixative that has become obviously discolored or cloudy during the collection process. Placing tissue jars on a laboratory rocker or orbital shaker for the first 24 hours following necropsy can also help to achieve thorough, even fixation.

Typical samples from a large bony fish include the following:

- Gill arch (not the lateral gill arch, as that will have received more physical trauma).
- Fin.
- Body wall and skin.
- Liver.

Table A9.2 Organisms that may stain acid-fast positive.

	Appearance of acid-fast structures
Cryptosporidium spp.	3–5 μm round oocysts with distinct walls and content
Cyclospora spp.	8–10 μm round to oval oocysts with distinct walls and content
Isospora, *Cystoisospora* spp.	20–30 μm round to oval oocysts; may be 1–2 within a sporoblast
Microsporidians	1–6 μm oval spores with a lighter staining vacuole at one end
Mycobacterium spp.	Short beaded rods typically <10 μm in length
Myxozoans	8–24 μm bilaterally or radially symmetrical spores with 1–7 (typically 2) polar capsules
Nocardia spp.	Long branching rods up to 20 μm in length

This is a simplified table that describes typical characteristics, but pleomorphism is common.

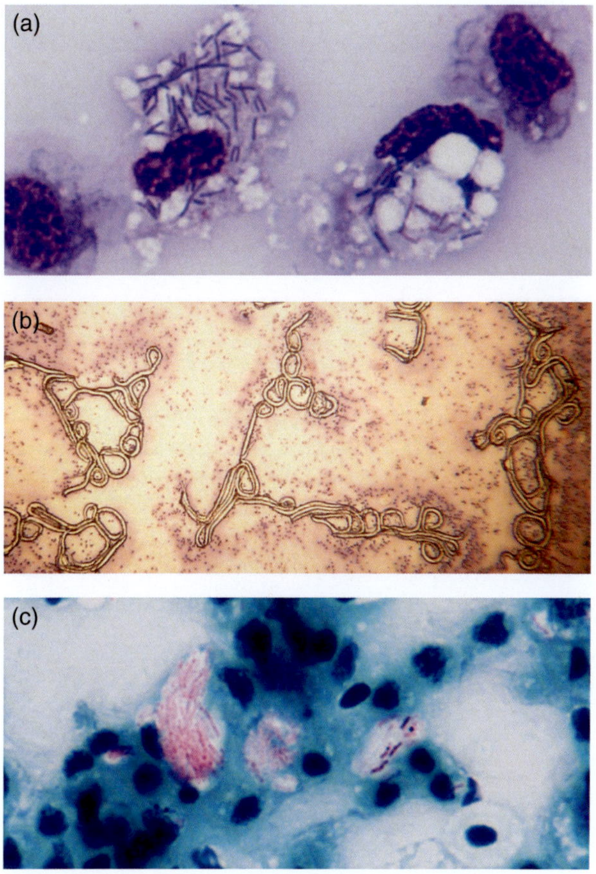

Figure A9.11 Abnormalities seen on impression smears: intracellular bacteria on Dif-Quik stain (a), nematode larvae on Dif-Quik stain (b), and acid-fast beaded rods consistent with *Mycobacterium* spp. on an acid-fast stain (c). *Source*: Images courtesy of Catherine Hadfield, National Aquarium.

- Gallbladder.
- Spleen.
- Cranial kidney.
- Caudal kidney, often together with swim bladder, vertebrae, and spinal cord.
- Esophagus, stomach, pyloric ceca (if present), intestines, anus/cloaca.
- Coelomic fat.
- Gonad and other reproductive structures.
- Urinary bladder (if present).
- Swim bladder, typically at the rete if present.
- Heart, including the bulbus arteriosus.
- Both eyes.
- Brain, either excised or submitted within the cranial vault for later decalcification.

Typical samples from an elasmobranch may include the following:

- Gill section.
- Heart.
- Thyroid.
- Body wall and skin.
- Liver.
- Gallbladder.
- Spleen.
- Pancreas.
- Esophagus, stomach, intestines, rectal gland, cloaca.
- Gonad, epigonal tissue, oviducts.
- Kidney.
- Both eyes.
- Brain, typically excised.

Shipping

If samples need to be shipped, international, national, state, and local legislation must be followed. Tissues or samples that may represent a human health hazard fall under specific restrictions. Several fixatives (e.g. formalin and >70% ethanol) are considered hazardous materials in the United States, and specific regulations apply to shipping them. In some cases, fixed specimens without the fixative are considered exempt, as long as they are packaged and labeled correctly.

Processing and Stains

Upon arrival to the lab, fixed tissues are examined by a prosector who collects representative sections and transfers them into labeled tissue cassettes, a process referred to as trimming. Samples of bone from teleosts need to be placed into a decalcifying solution before they are soft enough to trim. This can take hours to days depending on the size and density of the sample. In addition to bone, histologic sections of gills from large fish, scales, eyes, and grossly mineralized lesions are often improved by a brief decalcification step prior to trimming.

Before fixed tissues can be embedded in paraffin wax, all water and fixative must be removed from the samples using a technique known as tissue processing. In most labs, processing is automated. The tissues are first dehydrated by incubating the cassettes in increasing concentrations of alcohol (e.g. 70, 95, and 100% ethanol). This is followed by a clearing step in which tissues are incubated in an organic solvent solution, most commonly xylene, and finally by infiltration of the tissue by paraffin wax. The paraffinized tissues are then manually transferred into molds containing molten paraffin. These harden to form blocks that are sectioned using a microtome. A common thickness for diagnostic histopathology is 5 μm, but thinner or thicker sections may be used for specific tissues or studies. Once cut, sections from the microtome are carefully floated in a warm-water bath, scooped onto microscope slides, and allowed to dry prior to staining. A variety of stains may be used for histology in fish to identify certain materials and organisms (see Table A9.3).

Histopathologic Interpretation

The enormous diversity among fish species can make it challenging to differentiate between normal histology, artifacts, and true lesions. It is important to work with pathologists who have extensive fish experience, even when it is not the most convenient option (Groff 2004; Wolf et al. 2015). A comprehensive collection of normal microanatomy for all fish species is naturally beyond the scope of any single publication, but some excellent reference materials for normal fish histology and common histopathologic changes are available (Ferguson 2006; Menke et al. 2011; Garner 2013; Wolf et al. 2015; Frasca et al. 2018; Stedman and Garner 2018; Terio et al. 2018). For rare fish species, submitting specimens without obvious gross lesions can be valuable for establishing normal baseline histology.

Common sites for lesions in fish include the gills, liver, kidneys, and gonads; however, this may reflect biased sample submission as some tissues (e.g. brain, eyes, bone) are not always submitted for histology.

In addition to being one of the more common sites for histopathologic changes in fish, the gills are also one of the most difficult tissues to interpret. Gill filaments have a complex three-dimensional structure, making them prone to sectioning artifacts that can easily be misinterpreted as fusion, blunting, and loss of the secondary lamellae (Figure A9.12a). Therefore, evaluation of gill morphology should be limited to areas where secondary lamellae appear

Table A9.3 Commonly used cytology and histology stains.

Stains	Uses (and positive color)
Romanowsky (e.g. Wright, Giemsa, Wright–Giemsa, Wright–Leishman, May–Grunwald, Dif-Quik)	Cellular differentiation – cytology
Hematoxylin and eosin (H&E)	Cellular differentiation – histology
Gram	Gram-negative bacteria (pink); Gram-positive bacteria and myxozoans (blue)
Acid-fast (e.g. modified Ziehl–Neelsen, Fites, Kinyouin)	*Mycobacterium*, *Nocardia*, myxozoans, microsporidians, *Cryptosporidium* spp. (pink/red)
Luna stain	Microsporidians, Negri bodies (red)
Periodic acid–Schiff (PAS)	Glycogen and other carbohydrates, fungi, lipofuscin (pink)
Gomori methenamine silver (GMS)	Fungi (excluding *Basidiobolus* spp.) (black)
Lactophenol	Fungi (blue)
Prussian blue	Iron (blue)
Oil red O	Lipids (red)
Sudan black stain	Lipids (black)
Congo red	Amyloid (pale green under polarized light)
Toluidine blue	Mucopolysaccharides (blue)
Macchiavello or Gimenez	Chlamydials and rickettsials (red)

symmetrical and full-length (Figure A9.12b). Fusion of secondary lamellae occurs due to lamellar epithelial hyperplasia (LEH), a nonspecific response to gill damage or irritation, which manifests histologically as infilling of the interlamellar space by thickened respiratory epithelium (Figure A9.12c). Lamellar blunting or loss is actually an uncommon finding that will affect scattered lamellae rather than long stretches or an entire side of the filament, as can be seen with sectioning artifact (Wolf et al. 2015). Gills undergo rapid autolysis due to their high metabolic rate, creating another interpretive challenge for pathologists. Autolyzed gill tissue exhibits widespread sloughing of the lamellar epithelium and diffuse nuclear pyknosis, which can be confused for antemortem inflammation and necrosis (Figure A9.12d). Collections of mature lymphocytes are frequently found along the gill arch and lower portions of filaments in fish without any other signs of gill inflammation, and likely represent normal resident lymphoid populations rather than an active inflammatory response.

The histologic appearance of the normal fish liver can vary greatly depending on many factors including species, sex, nutritional condition, and reproductive status. Hepatocytes of well-nourished, aquarium-housed teleosts typically contain low to moderate amounts of lipid in the form of round, clear, sharply demarcated vacuoles (Figure A9.13). Since this does not necessarily reflect a pathologic change or underlying disorder of lipid metabolism, the term "lipidosis" should be avoided unless there is evidence of accompanying liver damage such as hepatocellular necrosis, inflammation, or fibrosis. Hepatic lipid content is even more striking in elasmobranch species, where the liver is the primary site of fat storage. Normal elasmobranch liver tissue floats in formalin and is microscopically characterized by large, coalescing lipid vacuoles that would be interpreted as severe hepatic lipidosis in other species (Figure A9.14a). Chronically ill or malnourished elasmobranchs often have reduced hepatic lipid stores (Figure A9.14b). The liver is a common site for granuloma formation in fish with mycobacteriosis and other chronic infections. Granulomas in fish may take the form of nonencapsulated aggregates of epithelioid macrophages or discrete, circumscribed nodules of amorphous necrotic debris surrounded by few, concentric layers of flattened macrophages. Both types of granulomas in can be seen in the same fish, and even the same organ (Figure A9.15).

The cranial and caudal kidneys of teleosts normally contain large numbers of hematopoietic cells in the interstitium that should not be mistaken for interstitial nephritis (Figure A9.16a). Inflammatory responses in the kidney typically take the form of discrete or nonencapsulated granulomas, similar to those seen in the liver, or less commonly, granulocytic infiltrates. Hematopoietic elements in the kidneys undergo increased proliferation in response to increased demand, as in the setting of blood loss or systemic inflammation, resulting in expansion of volume of the interstitium relative to the tubular components. However, because the proportion of hematopoietic tissue to nephrons varies widely among fish species, by sex, and along the length of the kidneys, a diagnosis of hematopoietic tissue hyperplasia is difficult to make without carefully matched control tissues. Autolyzed or suboptimally fixed kidney tissue often exhibits changes such as nuclear pyknosis and separation of tubular epithelial cells from the basement membranes, which may be misinterpreted as necrosis (Figure A9.16a). True renal necrosis is easiest to appreciate in samples from freshly euthanized fish and frequently manifests as disruption of tubular architecture and/or replacement of normal hematopoietic cells by eosinophilic and karyorrhectic debris (Figure A9.16b). As in other organs, pigmented macrophages aggregates (PMAs) are often numerous in fish kidneys (Figure A9.17). Their color on histologic sections can vary from light golden-brown to dark black, and they occasionally contain

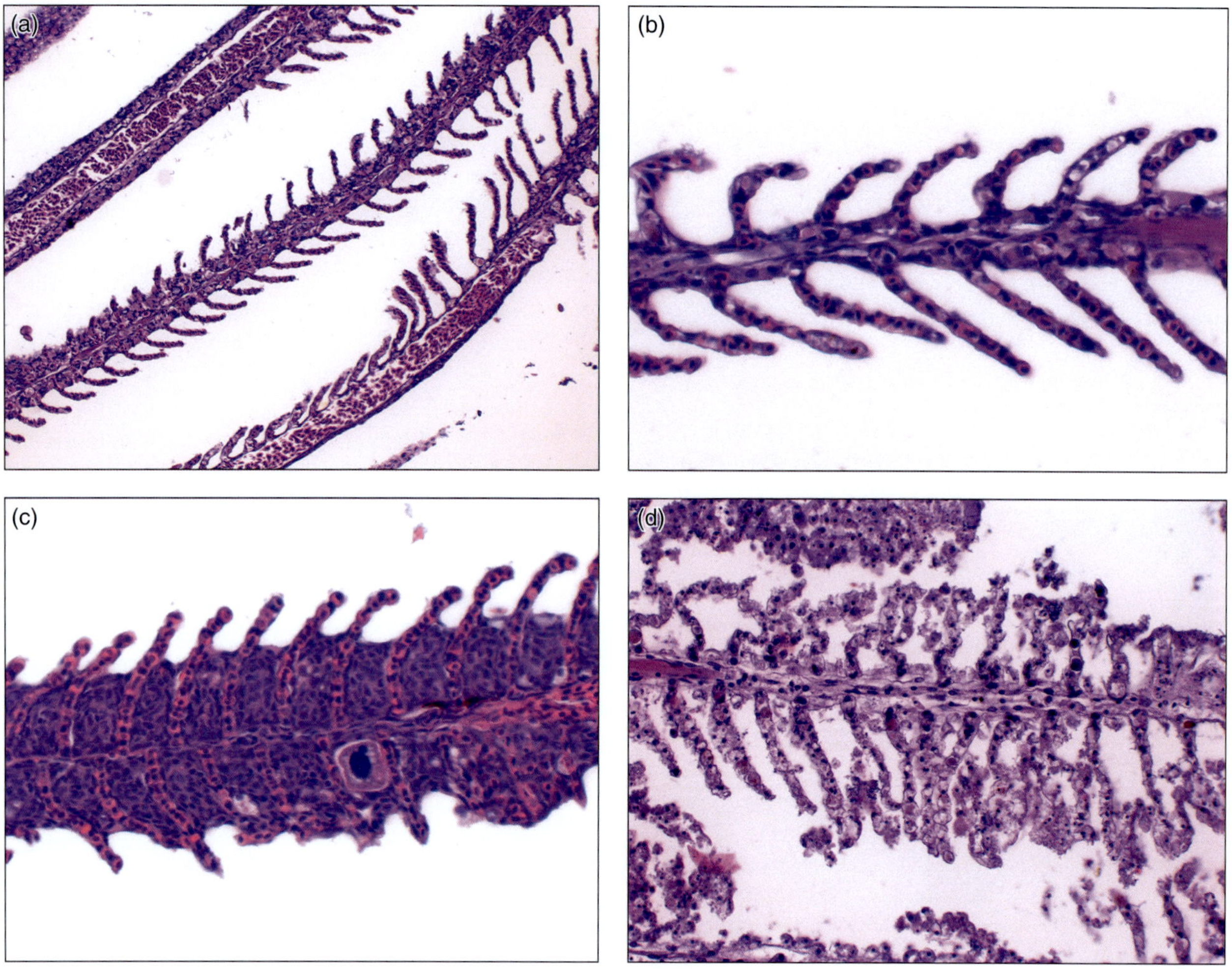

Figure A9.12 Normal gills from a sheepshead minnow (*Cyprinodon variegatus*) euthanized immediately prior to necropsy; sectioning artifact has resulted in areas where secondary lamellae appear shortened or lost (a). Interpretation should be limited to areas where secondary lamellae are symmetrical and full-length (b). Gills from a glass knifefish (*Eigenmannia virescens*) with lamellar epithelial hyperplasia and true lamellar blunting and fusion due to *Ichthyophthirius* sp. (c). Autolyzed gills from a sheepshead minnow that was found dead (d). H&E.

discrete, encapsulated granulomas in fish with granulomatous disease. Although the number and size of PMAs are thought to increase with age and chronic disease (i.e. PMA or melanomacrophage hyperplasia), this should be interpreted cautiously as there is also broad species variation in PMAs among healthy fish.

The kidneys of elasmobranchs do not contain hematopoietic elements. Rather, hematopoietic cells are found in the thymus, spleen, and two organs that are unique to elasmobranchs: the epigonal glands, located adjacent to the testes or ovary, and the Leydig organ, located in the wall of the esophagus. The epigonal glands and Leydig organ normally contain large numbers of maturing granulocytes that could be confused for intense granulocytic inflammation (Figure A9.18).

Common gonadal lesions include chronic oophoritis in females and seminomas in males (Figure A9.19). Chronic oophoritis is frequently encountered in animals with a clinical history of egg retention (also known as egg binding) and may be sterile or associated with bacterial infection. Seminomas are often invasive and may mimic round cell tumors such as lymphoma.

Bacterial and fungal infections are common histologic findings in fish submitted for necropsy, but are often inapparent without the aid of special stains (Figures A9.15 and A9.20). When bacteria and fungi are present in autolyzed specimens, attempts should be made to differentiate antemortem infection from postmortem overgrowth of commensal and/or environmental organisms. Findings consistent with postmortem overgrowth include lack of

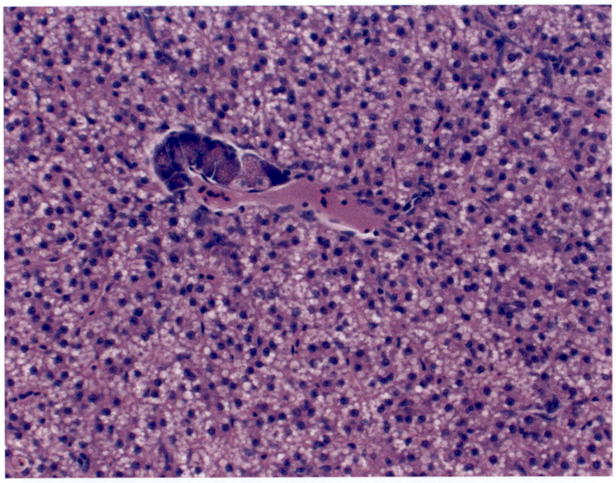

Figure A9.13 Normal liver from a banded killifish (*Fundulus diaphanus*) showing hepatocytes with moderate numbers of small, lipid-type vacuoles. Exocrine pancreatic cells containing brightly eosinophilic zymogen granules can be seen adjacent to a small blood vessel. H&E.

associated inflammation, diffuse or random distribution throughout tissues, and a predominance of large, Gram-variable bacilli. However, these clues are not full-proof as stressed, immune-compromised fish may have impaired inflammatory responses with florid growth of organisms. Thus, the relevance of bacteria and fungi seen on histology should be interpreted in the context of the fish's clinical history, the overall postmortem condition, and other histopathologic findings. Diagnosis of viral infection by routine histology is typically made on the basis of identifying viral inclusion bodies (Figure A9.16b) or specific cytopathic changes. While highly diagnostic when present, these changes are often transient (i.e. only apparent during early stages of infection) and can be obscured in autolyzed samples. Ancillary diagnostics, such as PCR and virus isolation, are recommended when there is a high index of suspicion for viral disease.

A variety of protozoan and metazoan parasites may be seen on histology (Figure A9.21). References providing detailed descriptions and images of parasites in histologic section are available (Gardiner et al. 1998; Bruno et al. 2006; Gardiner and Poynton 2006). In practice, identification is often limited due to degeneration/distortion of the organisms or absence of defining morphologic features in the examined sections (Figure A9.21c). Special stains such as Gram, acid-fast, PAS, and Luna can be helpful for highlighting internal and external structures, particularly with myxozoans and microsporidians (Figure A9.21d, e). Definitive identification often requires direct microscopy (i.e. wet mounts), or morphological or molecular assessment of fixed specimens.

Conclusion

Necropsy and ancillary diagnostics are essential components of a preventive medicine program and for managing disease in fish. Many causes of morbidity and mortality in fish can be identified on necropsy with wet mounts and cytologies. These findings can guide quick responses to emerging diseases to limit further morbidity and mortality. Histology and other diagnostics can provide additional information, particularly to help with long-term assessments of collection health.

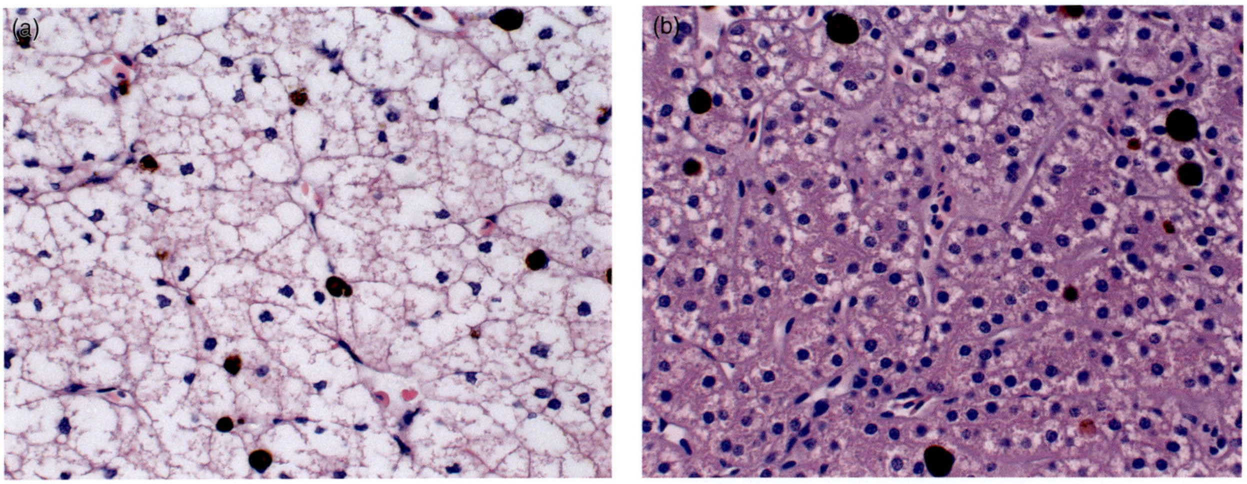

Figure A9.14 Abundant lipid vacuoles in a normal liver from a horn shark (*Heterodontus francisci*) (a) and depleted lipid stores in an epaulette shark (*Hemiscyllium ocellatum*) in poor nutritional condition (b). H&E.

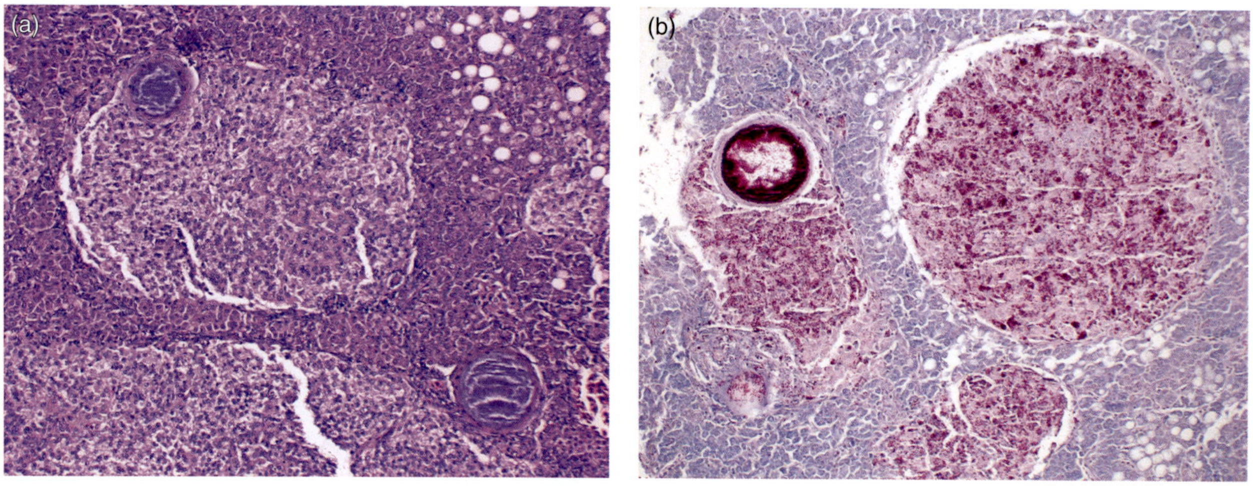

Figure A9.15 Granulomas in the liver of a rosyside dace (*Clinostomus funduloides*) with mycobacteriosis on H&E stain (a) and Ziehl–Neelsen acid-fast stain (b).

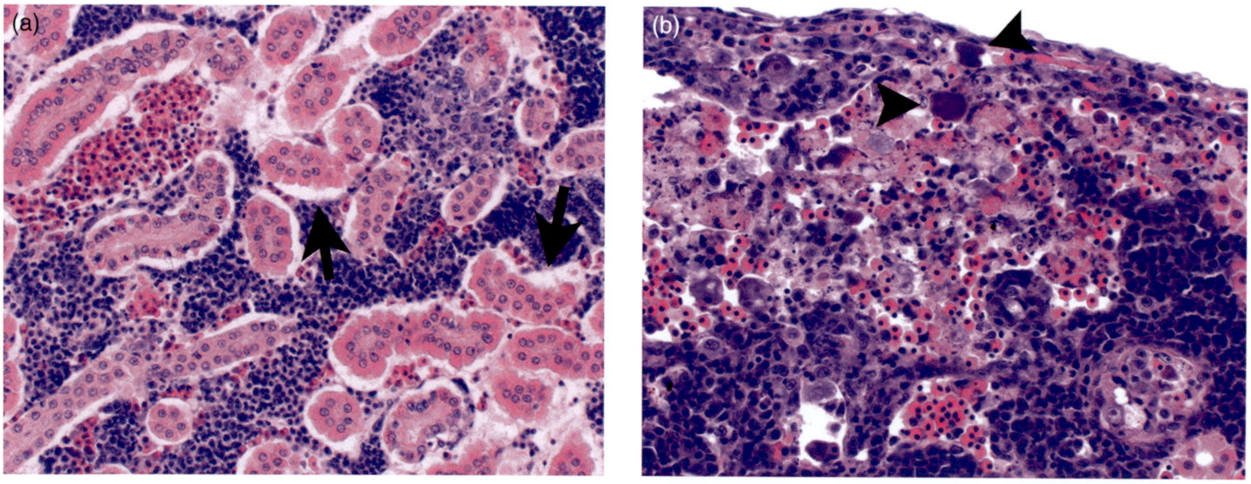

Figure A9.16 Normal kidney from a three-spot angelfish (*Apolemichthys trimaculatus*) with large numbers of hematopoietic cells in the interstitium (a). Separation of the tubular epithelial cells from the basement membrane is an artifact of suboptimal fixation (arrows). True renal necrosis in a blackcap basslet (*Gramma melacara*) due to megalocytivirus infection (b). Large, basophilic viral inclusion bodies (arrow heads) can be seen within an area of eosinophilic and karyorrhectic cellular debris. H&E.

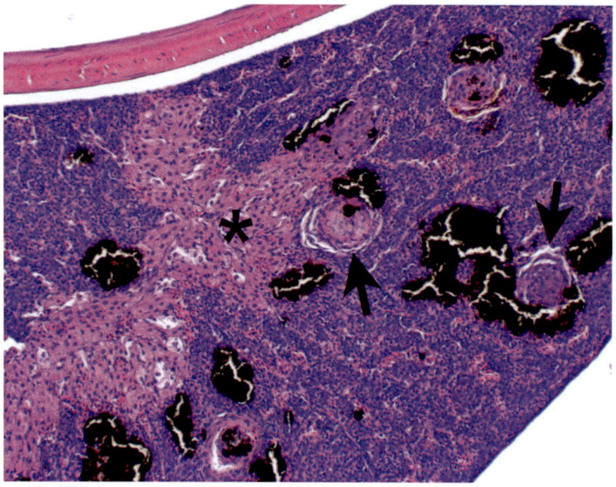

Figure A9.17 Anterior kidney from a glass knifefish (*Eigenmannia virescens*) showing several dark-black pigmented macrophage aggregates and few small, chronic granulomas (*). The aggregated brightly eosinophilic, polygonal cells are interrenal cells (arrows), analogous to the mammalian adrenal cortex. H&E.

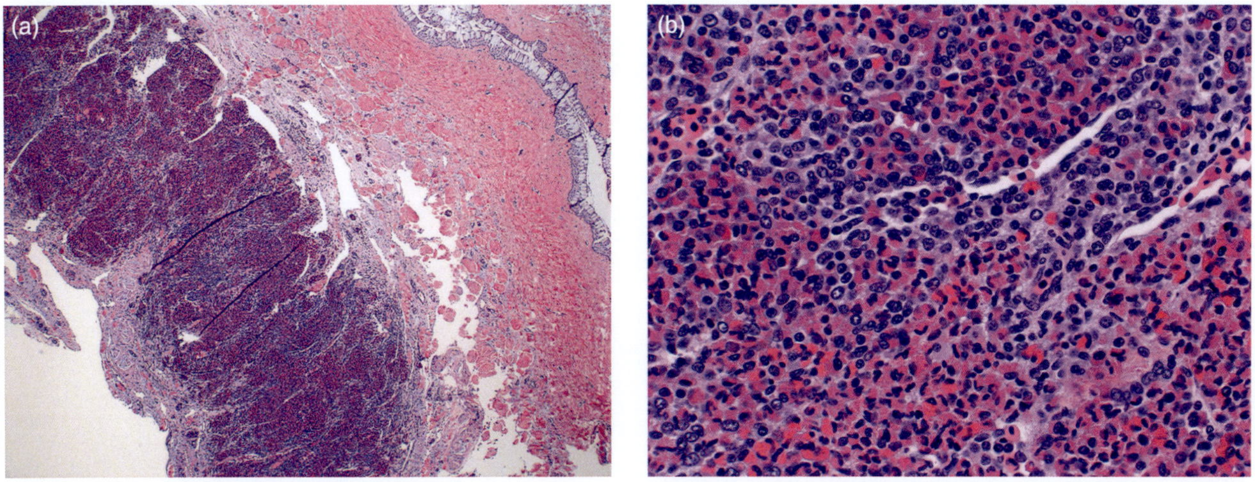

Figure A9.18 Low (a) and high (b) magnification images of a normal Leydig organ in the esophagus of a southern stingray (*Hypanus americanus*). H&E.

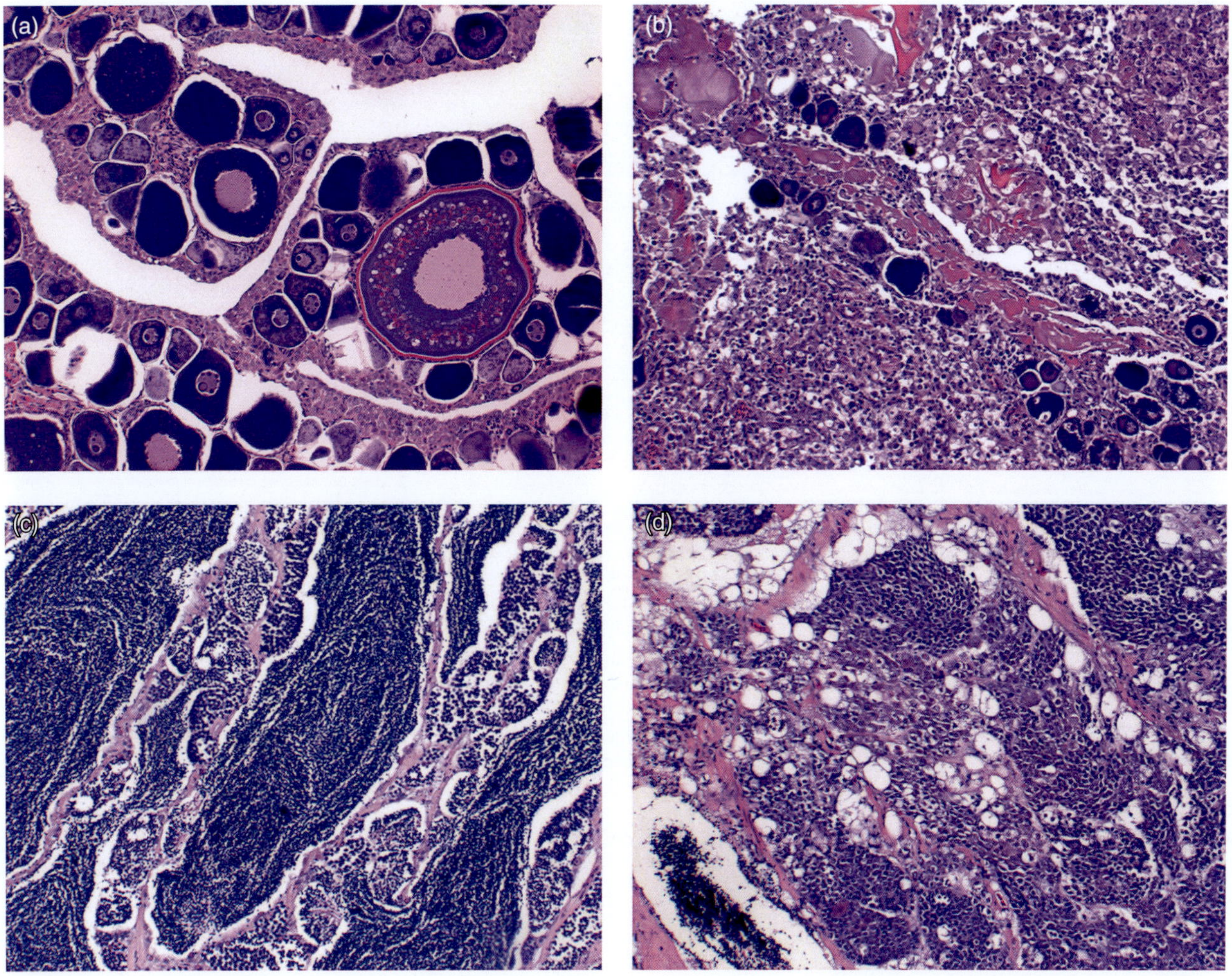

Figure A9.19 Normal ovary from a black grouper (*Mycteroperca bonaci*) (a) and ovary from a doctorfish (*Acanthurus chirurgus*) with chronic oophoritis (b); the ovarian interstitium is expanded by large numbers of macrophages and degenerate yolk material. Normal testis (c) and seminoma (d) in a sooty grunter (*Hephaestus fuliginosus*); in the seminoma, normal testicular architecture is effaced by sheets of neoplastic germ cells. H&E.

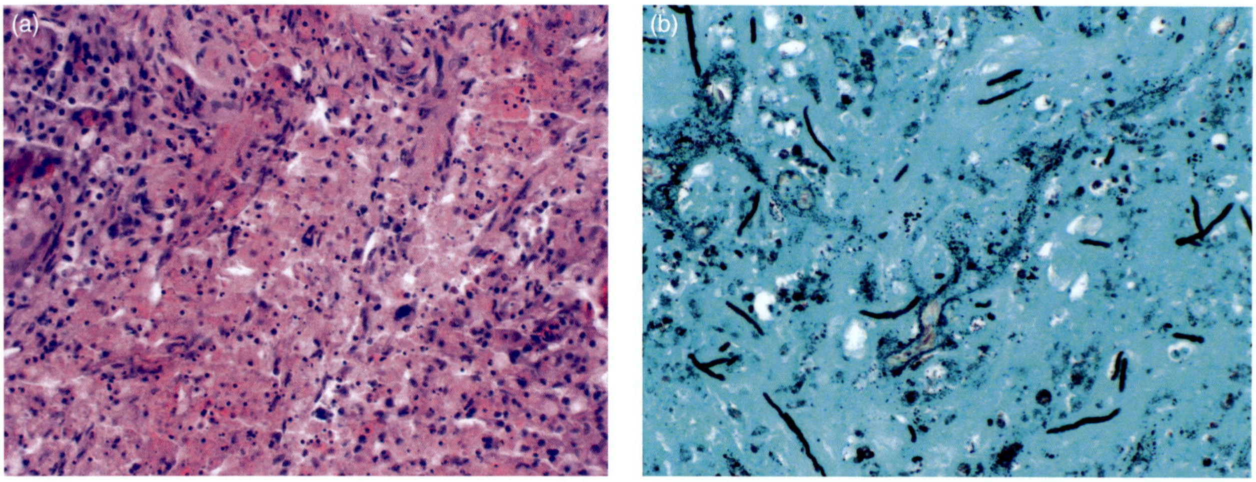

Figure A9.20 Cutaneous phaeohyphomycosis in a four-spot flounder (*Hippoglossina oblonga*). Fragments of lightly pigmented fungal hyphae are barely visible within necrotic cellular debris on H&E (a), but readily apparent on Gomori methenamine-silver stain (b).

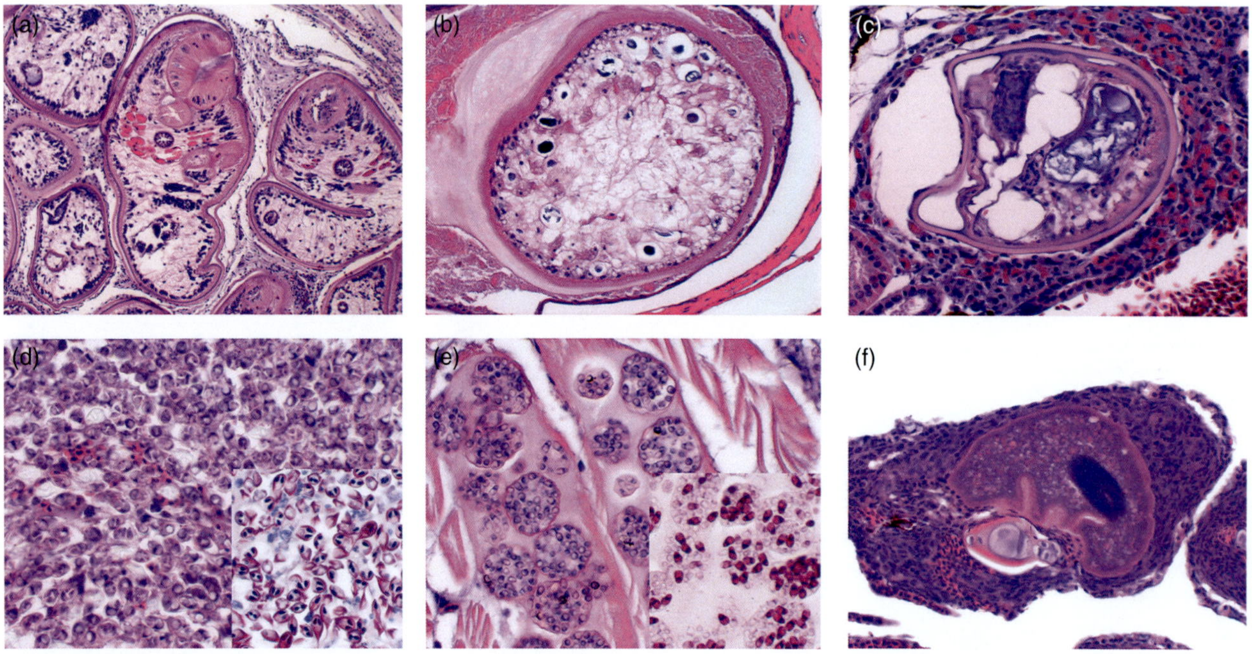

Figure A9.21 Fish parasites in histologic section. Digenes in the ganglia of a black rockfish (*Sebastes melanops*) on H&E (a). Cestode in the mesentery of a harvestfish (*Peprilus paru*) on H&E (b); the darkly basophilic, ovoid calcareous corpuscles are unique to cestodes. An unidentified, degenerate metazoan in the kidney of a banded killifish (*Fundulus diaphanus*) on H&E (c). Numerous myxozoan spores in the blood vessel of a doctorfish (d); morphology is indistinct on H&E but with a Ziehl–Neelsen acid-fast stain (inset), the paired polar capsules of mature spores appear dark blue and the outer spore capsules appear bright pink. Developing microsporidial spores in the skeletal muscle of a rummy-nose tetra (*Hemigrammus rhodostomus*) on H&E (e); the Ziehl–Neelsen acid-fast stain (inset) highlights the typical clog-like morphology of the spores. A ciliate (consistent with an *Icthyophthirius multifiliis* trophont) embedded within hyperplastic lamellar epithelium in the gills of a glass knifefish (*Eigenmannia virescens*) on H&E (f).

References

Balko, J.A., Oda, A., and Posner, L.P. (2018). Use of tricaine methanesulfonate or propofol for immersion euthanasia of goldfish (*Carassius auratus*). *Journal of the American Veterinary Medical Association* (12): 1555–1561.

Bruno, D.W., Nowak, B., and Elliot, D.G. (2006). Guide to the identification of fish protozoan and metazoan parasites in stained tissue sections. *Diseases of Aquatic Organisms* 70: 1–36.

Collymore, C., Banks, E.K., and Turner, P.V. (2016). Lidocaine hydrochloride compared with MS222 for the euthanasia of zebrafish (*Danio rerio*). *Journal of the American Association of Laboratory Animal Science* 55: 816–820.

Ferguson, H.W. (ed.) (2006). Systemic Pathology of Fish, 2e. Scotian Press.

Fisher, J.P. and Myers, M.S. (2000). Fish necropsy. In: Handbook of Experimental Animals – The Fish (ed. G.P. Ostrander), 543–556. London: Academic Press.

Fournie, J.W., Frol, R.M., and Hawkins, W.E. (2000). Fixation of fish tissues. In: Handbook of Experimental Animals – The Fish (ed. G.P. Ostrander), 569–577. London: Academic Press.

Frasca, S., Wolf, J.C., Kinsel, M.J., Camus, A.C., et al. (2018) Osteichthyes. In: Pathology of Wildlife and Zoo Animals (Eds. Terio, K.A., MacAloose, D., and St. Leger, J.). Academic Press, London, 945–994.

Gardiner, C.H. and Poynton, S.L. (2006). An Atlas of Metazoan Parasites in Animal Tissues. Washington, D.C.: Armed Forces Institute of Pathology.

Gardiner, C.H., Fayer, R., and Dubey, J.P. (1998). An Atlas of Protozoan Parasites in Animal Tissues. Washington, D.C.: Armed Forces Institute of Pathology.

Gardner, I.A., Whittington, R.J., Caraguel, C.G.B. et al. (2016). Recommended reporting standards for test accuracy studies of infectious diseases of finfish, amphibians, molluscs and crustaceans: the STRADAS-aquatic checklist. *Diseases of Aquatic Organisms* 118: 91–111.

Garner, M.M. (2013). A retrospective study of disease in elasmobranchs. *Veterinary Pathology* 50: 377–389.

Groff, J.M. (2004). Histological and histopathological examination of elasmobranchs. In: The Elasmobranch Husbandry Manual: Captive Care of Sharks, Rays, and their Relatives (eds. M. Smith, D. Warmolts, D. Thoney and R. Hueter), 433–439. Columbus, OH: Ohio Biological Survey.

Justine, J.-L., Briand, M.J., and Bray, R.A. (2012). A quick and simple method, usable in the field, for collecting parasites in suitable condition for both morphological and molecular studies. *Parasitology Research* 111: 341–351.

Kvach, Y., Ondračková, M., Janáč, M., and Jurajda, P. (2016). Methodological issues affecting the study of fish parasites. I. Duration of live fish storage prior to dissection. *Diseases of Aquatic Organisms* 119: 107–115.

Leary, S., Underwood, M., Anthony, R. et al. (2020). AVMA Guidelines for the Euthanasia of Animals: 2020 Edition. https://www.avma.org/sites/default/files/2020-01/2020-Euthanasia-Final-1-17-20.pdf (accessed August 2020).

Menke, A.L., Spitsbergen, J.M., Wolterbeek, A.P.M., and Wourtersen, R.A. (2011). Normal anatomy and histology of the adult zebrafish. *Toxicologic Pathology* 39: 759–775.

Stedman, N.L. and Garner, M.M. (2018). Chondrichthyes. In: Pathology of Wildlife and Zoo Animal (eds. K.A. Terio, D. MacAloose and J. St. Leger), 995–1010. London: Academic Press.

Terio, K.A., McAloose, D., and St. Leger, J. (2018). Pathology of Wildlife and Zoo Animals. Amsterdam: Elsevier, Inc.

Wolf, J.C., Baumgartner, W.A., Blazer, V.S. et al. (2015). Nonlesions, misdiagnoses, missed diagnoses, and other interpretive challenges in fish histopathology studies: a guide for investigators, authors, reviewers, and readers. *Toxicologic Pathology* 43: 297–325.

Yanong, R.P.E. (2003). Necropsy technique for fish. *Seminars in Avian and Exotic Pet Medicine* 12: 89–105.

A10

Anesthesia and Analgesia

Donald L. Neiffer

National Zoological Park, Washington DC, USA

Introduction

There is increasing evidence of pain perception in fish, and although that debate continues, it is accepted that fish display robust neuroendocrine and physiologic stress responses to noxious stimuli (Huntingford et al. 2006; Braithwaite and Boulcott 2007; Neiffer and Stamper 2009; Posner 2009; Sneddon 2009). Consequently, anesthetic and analgesic drugs should be used for fish restraint to reduce handling trauma and physiologic changes (Kumlu and Yanar 1999; Myszkowski et al. 2003; Small 2003; Bressler and Ron 2004; Cooke et al. 2004; Small and Chatakondi 2005; Ross and Ross 2008). In addition, chemical restraint increases safety for the handler.

Anesthetic agents in fish are typically provided in the water (immersion/bath). Other potential routes include intramuscular or intravenous injection. Oral administration is rare. Regardless of route, it is essential that fish are provided with appropriate water quality (dissolved oxygen, salinity, pH, ammonia, and temperature) and adequate water flow throughout induction, maintenance, and recovery.

It is important to note that the term "fish" represents a paraphyletic "catch-all" for over 30 000 species belonging to one of four typological classes of the subphylum *Vertebrata* (Bond 1996). A consummate fish species (e.g. rainbow trout, *Oncorhynchus mykiss*) is not much more related to a bull shark (class *Chondrichthyes*) than to a bull terrier (class *Mammalia*). This complicates comparisons and generalizations across species. Unfortunately, the literature does not reflect this diversity and the clinician often has to extrapolate from published data on a limited number of species, primarily teleosts that are common in aquaculture. Additionally, most studies involve adult fish, requiring extrapolation to different life stages (Harms and Bakal 1995; Stetter 2001; Ross and Ross 2008). Online search engines are useful sources of peer-reviewed literature. Search terms such as "anesthesia", "anatomy", "physiology", "site fidelity", and "fecundity" will often identify studies that required chemical restraint. Secondary literature (e.g. texts) and other data sources (e.g. websites, listserves) also provide useful information, but the clinician should be cautious of anecdotal information. Regardless of the source, the anesthetic regimen for an unfamiliar species should be tested through to recovery using one or a small group of fish before applying it to a larger number of fish.

Anatomical and Physiological Considerations

Respiratory Systems

All fish have gills. For most fish species, gas exchange relies on forcing water over the gill surface through rhythmic movements of the mouth, lower jaw, and opercula or gill slits. Some species (e.g. tuna, pelagic sharks) use ram ventilation, with water moved over the gills by forward propulsion of the body; failure to perfuse the gills during anesthesia of these species may result in hypoxia (Bushnell and Jones 1994). A few other species rely minimally on gill tissue with gas exchange occurring primarily within outpouchings of the alimentary tract or modified swim

Clinical Guide to Fish Medicine, First Edition. Edited by Catherine A. Hadfield and Leigh Ann Clayton.

bladders (Table A1.1). A number of these species are obligate air-breathers and "drowning" will occur if they are not given access to atmospheric air or oxygen (Ishimatsu and Itazawa 1993; Graham 1997; Bassi et al. 2005). These species usually require much higher concentrations of immersion anesthetic agents.

Many freshwater fish species that evolved to survive in hypoxic environments perform aquatic surface respiration (ASR), positioning their mouths to skim the air/water interface (Ishimatsu and Itazawa 1993; Graham 1997; Rantin et al. 1998). Examples include pacu (*Piaractus mesopotamicus*), bettas and gouramis (*Anabantiformes*), and snakeheads (*Channidae*). This behavior can be problematic for the clinician as the fish, responding to confinement, gill irritation, and/or low dissolved oxygen, may use ASR which will reduce its exposure to immersion anesthetics (Hseu et al. 1997).

The skin also serves a respiratory function in many fish, accounting for up to 30% of oxygen uptake in some species (Bruecker and Graham 1993). This is most common in marine fish, young fish, and scaleless or fine-scaled species (Ishimatsu and Itazawa 1993; Oikawa et al. 1994; Myszkowski et al. 2003). Immersion anesthesia in these species or life stages may require lower dosages compared to freshwater species or similarly sized, but heavily scaled, species.

Skin and Muscle

Most fish have scales, but there is marked variation in distribution and design of these dermal structures. In species with large scales or protective denticles, intramuscular and intravenous injections may be difficult or impossible without restraint or initial sedation/anesthesia using immersion agents.

Most fish have aerobic, slow-oxidative muscles (red muscle) and anaerobic, fast-twitch muscles (white muscle). Highly oxygenated slow-oxidative muscle is usually found running along the dorsal midline of the body. Injection of anesthetic agents into this region may result in more rapid induction and clearance compared to agents administered into white muscle (Totland et al. 1981; Williams et al. 2004).

Temperature and Metabolism

As most fish species are ectothermic, lower water temperatures are usually associated with longer induction and recovery times than higher temperatures (Gelwicks and Zafft 1998; Stehly and Gingerich 1999; Gomes et al. 2001; Peters et al. 2001; Detar and Mattingly 2004). Some fish (e.g. tuna, some laminid sharks) are endothermic; these species are able to elevate tissue temperature above the ambient temperature through the conservation of metabolic heat (Bushnell and Jones 1994; Blank et al. 2004). Clinicians working with these species may note an increased rate of anesthetic uptake and a need for higher anesthetic dosages.

Water Quality Considerations

Dissolved Oxygen and Temperature

Dissolved oxygen (DO) and water temperature are critical factors for fish anesthesia. Anesthetic induction is usually associated with hypoventilation (i.e. decreased buccal or opercular movement) and reflex bradycardia. These changes, along with low DO, can contribute to hypoxia and put the fish at risk (Rantin et al. 1998; Ross and Ross 2008). As water temperature increases, tissue oxygen demand increases while DO in the water decreases. Consequently, hypoxia is more likely to occur during anesthesia at high water temperatures (Harms 2003). Tropical marine fish are most at risk, as they have few adaptations for hypoxic environments (Rothwell et al. 2005). Clinicians must ensure a constant flow of aerated water across the gill surface of anesthetized fish and ideally monitor DO levels during any fish anesthesia.

pH and Nitrogenous Waste

The significance of pH in fish is often overlooked. Many fish species come from environments with narrow pH ranges, particularly marine species where the range is often 8.0–8.3. The pH scale is logarithmic and small numeric changes correspond to large changes in pH. For example, water with a pH of 5 is 10 times more acidic then water with a pH of 6. Consequently, abrupt changes in pH should always be avoided.

A drop in pH is common with immersion anesthetics, particularly unbuffered tricaine methanesulfonate (MS-222). This causes metabolic acidemia and physiologic stress and reduces anesthetic efficacy because of drug ionization (Ross and Ross 2008). To address these issues, buffering agents (e.g. sodium bicarbonate, sodium carbonate) are added to neutralize the pH. Many sources state that salt water, with its greater natural buffering capacity compared to freshwater, may not require the addition of buffering agents (Oikawa et al. 1994; Harms and Bakal 1995; Ross and Ross 2008). This has not been the experience of the author, however, and it is recommended to check the pH level of all anesthetic baths prior to addition of any fish and ideally to monitor pH throughout procedures.

Ammonia builds up in recirculating anesthetic systems, particularly during prolonged procedures, with small water volumes, and when several fish are anesthetized in the same water. Ammonia is directly toxic to the fish. Any exposure can damage gills and may affect uptake and clearance of immersion anesthetics and compromise oxygen uptake. The risk of ammonia toxicity is greater in marine or brackish systems because the higher pH favors the presence of the more toxic unionized ammonia (UIA; NH_3). Monitoring nitrogenous compounds prior to and during anesthetic procedures is advisable. Ammonia is easy to measure with tank side kits, although more sensitive colorimetric laboratory tests are available. Ammonia testing will not be accurate for the few species that excrete primarily urea (e.g. Gulf toadfish, *Opsanus beta*) (Gilmour et al. 1998). Clinicians should also use visual indicators of deteriorating water quality such as surface foam formation or mucus in the water. Prevention of toxicity can be as simple as exchanging 20–50% of the water in the anesthetic chamber with suitable water.

Ionic Balance

Water chemistry is far more complex than we often consider. Samples with identical pH and salinity may differ wildly in ionic and organic compounds. Immediately transferring fish from one to the other can result in physiologic challenges. The best way to ensure limited changes in the water chemistry is to use the source water for induction, maintenance, and recovery, with additional 20–50% water changes as needed. For the same reason, when fish are returned to their source system after anesthesia, they should be acclimated slowly to the new water chemistry, even if temperature is the same. The one exception to this may be if the water has become badly fouled or the dissolved oxygen is too low and cannot be corrected; in these cases, fish should be transferred rapidly to more suitable water.

Anesthetic Techniques and Drugs

Human Safety

Fish can present hazards to humans. These include sharp and blunt force trauma, particularly from teeth and spines, as well as electric shocks. Some species are venomous. Zoonotic disease transmission must also be considered, and suitable powder-free gloves should always be worn when working with fish to reduce exposure to zoonotic diseases and medications. A respiratory mask may be appropriate when measuring out powdered anesthetics. Handling and safety considerations are reviewed in more detail in Chapter A6.

Preanesthetic Preparation

Baseline behavioral parameters (i.e. ventilation, color, caudal fin stroke rate, position in the water column, and activity level) should be recorded prior to anesthesia. In some cases, the client can be asked to record this information prior to removing fish from their system for transport.

Food may be withheld for 12–24 hours before anesthesia to limit the risk of regurgitation as this can foul gill tissue and increase ammonia levels (Harms and Bakal 1995; Stetter 2001). However, fasting is not typically recommended for young or small fish that are fed frequently.

Whenever possible, water from the fish's tank should be used for transport, induction, maintenance, and recovery. Each container should have adequate water, with enough available for potential water changes. Physical (e.g. temperature) and chemical (e.g. pH, salinity) variables of the anesthetic water should match those of the fish's source water and be determined prior to anesthesia. Dissolved oxygen should be maintained at >5 mg/L with 6–10 mg/L or 95–100% saturation considered ideal (Harms 1999; Stetter 2001). It is important to determine how aeration will be supplemented if needed. Clinicians must be ready to provide supplemental ventilation (e.g. suitable pump or syringes). A plan to prevent drying of the skin, fins, and eyes during out-of-water procedures should be in place. Coverage of the fish with clear plastic drapes and regular rinsing of tissues with water from a bulb syringe or a small portable atomizer is usually effective (Harms 1999; Ross and Ross 2008).

Anesthetic Drug Administration and Agents

Immersion Anesthesia

Immersion is the most common method used for fish anesthesia. To be effective, immersion drugs must either be water-soluble or combined with a water-soluble solvent. Anesthetic agents dissolved in solution enter the bloodstream through the gills, accessory respiratory organs, and/or skin. Once taken into the circulation, the drugs are passed rapidly to the central nervous system. As both the gill tissue and skin contain abundant lipid, efficiency of uptake is related to lipid solubility. For example, MS-222 has a relatively high lipid solubility and uptake is rapid. As mentioned previously, the skin of scaleless or fine-scaled fish favors drug uptake (Ferreira et al. 1984).

Anesthetic induction can be accomplished by transferring the fish to an aerated container with the desired concentration of dissolved drug. Alternatively, the anesthetic solution can be added directly to the water containing the fish, but it is often better to mix the water and test the pH prior to adding the fish. When immersion in a container is impractical (e.g. large fish in a large system) or dangerous to handlers, drugs in solution may be applied directly to the gills using a syringe, pump sprayer, or similar device. These individuals can then be worked on in their habitat or transferred to another container for administration of maintenance anesthesia. Since some immersion agents decrease water pH, the pH should be checked and buffer must be added if needed prior to contact with fish (Harms 1999; Ross and Ross 2008).

Spontaneous ventilation is often reduced during immersion anesthesia, particularly during longer anesthetic events or at greater anesthetic depth. Artificial ventilation may simply involve the use of a bulb or other syringe to flush water regularly over the gills (Figure A10.1a). Another option for out-of-water procedures is a simple gravity-driven delivery system whereby an aerated container holding anesthetic water feeds water over the gills via tubing (e.g. IV fluid bag with a drip set attached). Alternatively, a submersible pump may be used to provide continuous flow. The addition of a bifurcation from the pump allows one line to be placed in the mouth to ventilate the gills and a second line to keep the skin and eyes wet, or for lines to be directed toward both sets of gills (Figure A10.1b). Regardless of the technique used, flow should follow the normal direction of water movement over the gills to maximize gas and anesthetic exchange.

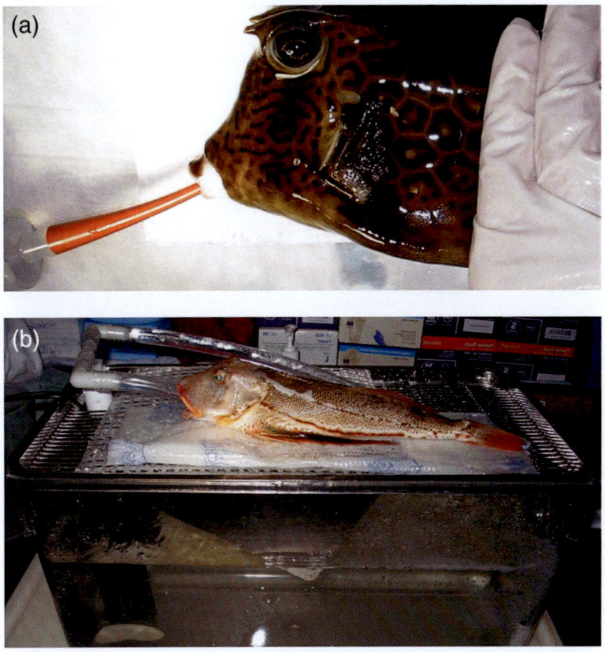

Figure A10.1 Fish anesthesia using a syringe and red rubber catheter (a) and using a recirculating pump system (b). *Source*: Images courtesy of Catherine Hadfield, National Aquarium.

Non-recirculating anesthetic water, whereby the water crossing the fish's gills or skin is not reused, is suitable for short procedures in small- to medium-sized fish. For longer procedures involving large fish or where anesthetic drug cost and wastewater concerns exist, recirculating systems are more appropriate. With this type of system, anesthetic water is delivered from a reservoir to the gills but the effluent is recycled either by syringe or a submersible pump (Figure A10.1b). This system requires close monitoring of dissolved oxygen and ammonia (Harms 1999; Stetter 2001; Ross and Ross 2008).

The drug concentration of immersion agents needs to be changed during all but the shortest immersion anesthetic events. Maintaining a fish for a prolonged period of time (e.g. >15 minutes) at an induction dose will likely result in excessive anesthetic depth. Several options exist:

- Prepare multiple anesthetic solutions at different concentrations in separate bags or reservoirs for use in either recirculating or flow-through systems.
- Measure specific volumes of unmedicated water and additional anesthetic and buffer to be able to increase or decrease the dose by a specific amount, e.g. having 2 gallons of unmedicated water available to reduce the drug concentration of a 10-gallon anesthetic system by ~20%.
- Deliver anesthetic-free water directly to the gills using a bulb or syringe, without disconnecting the fish from the maintenance system.
- If hand-ventilating using a bulb or syringe, adjust the dose by mixing the solutions within the syringe, e.g. using a 1:1 ratio of induction agent and unmedicated water.

Along with drug concentration, flow rate can be used to regulate anesthetic depth. While a minimum effective flow rate during fish anesthesia has not been determined, 1–3 L/min/kg is typically recommended. Any evidence of gastric dilatation likely indicates flow rates that are too high while lack of fluid exiting both opercula supports rates being too low with resultant poor gas exchange (Harms 1999; Stetter 2001; Ross and Ross 2008). Increasing the flow rate of medicated water can increase anesthetic depth, while increasing the flow rate of unmedicated water can speed recovery time.

It is imperative that all staff recognize the fragility of gill tissue. Unnecessary manipulation, inadequate perfusion with water, and prolonged exposure to immersion agents, particularly those that are inadequately buffered, can all lead to gill damage.

During recovery from immersion anesthesia, the fish is placed in unmedicated water where it excretes most drugs or drug metabolites primarily via the gills. The accessory respiratory organs, skin, and kidneys may assist with elimination (Walsh and Pease 2002; Ross and Ross 2008). It is important to remember that excreted drugs may be reabsorbed (Oikawa et al. 1994). Recovering the fish in flow-through systems or changing out some of the water during the recovery process may improve the quality and rate of recovery and should be seriously considered if recovering multiple fish in the same system.

MS-222 (Tricaine Methanesulfonate) MS-222 is the most common anesthetic agent used in fish. It is a derivative of benzocaine and is available as a white powder. Many clinicians maintain stock solutions (10 g/L) for efficiency and to reduce human exposure to the powder. The shelf life of stock solutions is largely unknown, and a conservative approach would be to prepare fresh stock solutions after 30 days. Both the drug and stock solutions should be protected from light. Black/gray speckling within the white powder or stock solution is not uncommon and most clinicians continue to use the product without issues. However, stock solutions should be discarded if oily residues or a change in color is noted.

MS-222 reduces water pH and buffer should be used for animal safety and to improve drug absorption. Sodium bicarbonate (baking soda) is the most commonly used buffer, although others such as sodium carbonate (soda ash) may be used. Many aquarists and veterinarians have been taught that combining one part MS-222 to two parts sodium bicarbonate by weight will limit or prevent acidification of water. This assumption may lead to unexpected pH changes. A better approach is to start with a 1:2 ratio (MS-222:sodium bicarbonate) followed by pH measurement of the resulting solution. It is very likely that more buffer will need to be added incrementally to reach the starting pH of the source water. Sodium carbonate is a much more potent buffer and the starting ratio may be closer to 2.5:1 (MS-222:sodium carbonate), with pH measurements as the buffer is added in increments. In general, stock solutions should not be buffered as the pH will continue to change in the solution and pH measurement and adjustment in either direction is often still required prior to use (e.g. with sodium bicarbonate or low pH water).

MS-222 has a wide safety index in fish and can often be used to effect. Typical doses for induction are 60–120 mg/L, buffered to an appropriate pH. However, there are some important considerations. As a general rule, freshwater species require higher concentrations of MS-222 compared to brackish and marine species (Oikawa et al. 1994; Harms and Bakal 1995; Davis and Griffin 2004). Higher doses are usually needed for obligate and facultative air-breathing fish species (Table A1.1). As fish can develop a tolerance to MS-222, higher doses may be needed for fish undergoing regular anesthesias (Posner et al. 2013). Lower doses should be considered for young fish in warm, soft water, as the safety margin is narrower (Harms 1999; Roubach et al. 2001).

MS-222 may cause reversible retinal deficits in humans with long-term exposure. Although this is unlikely, staff should limit exposure to the powder in particular, as well as the stock solution and medicated water (Bernstein et al. 1997; Sladky et al. 2001). No changes in retinal structure or function were seen in goldfish (*Carassius auratus*) following repeated exposure to MS-222 (Bailey et al. 2013).

As of 2020, MS-222 is approved by the United States Food and Drug Administration (FDA) for the temporary immobilization of specific teleost families with a 21 day withdrawal period.

Clove Oil, Eugenol, Isoeugenol, and Aqui-S™ Clove oil contains approximately 84% eugenol as well as isoeugenol and methyleugenol. It is also possible to purchase 100% eugenol. Clove oil and eugenol are available over-the-counter and are much less expensive than MS-222. Clove oil and its derivatives (COAD) are incompletely water-soluble, particularly at cold temperatures. Consequently, it is common practice to use 95% ethanol as a solvent with a mixture of one part clove oil to nine parts ethanol (1:9) yielding a 100 mg/mL stock solution. Synthetic isoeugenol products, Aqui-S and Aqui-S 20E, are made in New Zealand with the latter available in the United States. Both products provide a more expensive, water-soluble alternative to natural clove oil compounds (Iverson et al. 2003; Kildea et al. 2004).

Typical induction doses are 20–70 mg/L. Consistent anesthesia and more rapid induction times are observed with natural and synthetic COAD compared to other immersion agents, although longer recoveries are reported (Sladky et al. 2001; Bressler and Ron 2004; Detar and Mattingly 2004; Neiffer and Stamper 2009; Mylniczenko et al. 2014b). Also, compared with MS-222, the degree of excitation during induction in elasmobranchs appears to be less or absent when a COAD product is used (Neiffer and Stamper 2009; Mylniczenko et al. 2014b).

The safety margin in fish varies across taxa. Some studies have claimed increased overall safety (Detar and Mattingly 2004; Neiffer and Stamper 2009; Gladden et al. 2010) while others have reported a narrow safety margin with ventilatory failure and medullary collapse (e.g. pirapitinga, *Piaractus brachypomus*) (Sladky et al. 2001; Silbernagel and Yochem 2016). Possible explanations include direct neurotoxic or hepatotoxic effects and/or the oils coating gill epithelia and interfering with gas exchange. Direct tissue effects are supported by a study that described mild gill necrosis from repeated exposure to eugenol (Afifi et al. 2001). While not experiencing mortality related to COAD, the author has noted gill irritation and increased potency of natural eugenol and Aqui-S, respectively, in southern stingrays (*Hypanus americanus*) compared to other fish.

It is important to note that the United States FDA has provided a Guidance for Industry that states that neither clove oil nor any of its components are subjects of an approved new animal drug application and that they should not be used as an anesthetic in fish (US FDA 2007).

Alfaxalone Alfaxalone is a synthetic steroid that binds to inhibitory gamma-aminobutyric acid (GABA) receptors in the central nervous system to induce muscle relaxation, sedation, and anesthesia. In the United States, the drug is marketed under the trade name Alfaxan®. It is FDA-approved for intravenous use in dogs and cats and is more likely to be found in vet hospitals than other traditional fish anesthetics. Unlike pure alfaxalone which is poorly water-soluble, Alfaxan contains cyclodextrin which results in a water-soluble product with a neutral pH.

Studies have shown that Alfaxan can be used as an immersion anesthetic to achieve surgical anesthesia in several freshwater species including goldfish, koi (*Cyprinus carpio*), and oscars (*Astronotus ocellatus*) (Bauquier et al. 2013; Minter et al. 2014; Bugman et al. 2016; Fernández-Parra et al. 2017). Typical induction and maintenance doses range from 1 to 10 mg/L. No adverse effects were reported in these studies, though dose-dependent depression of opercular rates did occur (Minter et al. 2014).

Alfaxalone combined with alfadalone (Saffan®) was used for immersion anesthesia in fish, but the drug is less available now. Reports included North African catfish (*Clarius gariepinus*), glass catfish (*Kryptopterus bicirrhis*), freshwater elephantfish (*Mormyridae*), and redfin perch (*Perca fluviatilis*) (Bauquier et al. 2013; Minter et al. 2014). Induction, recovery, efficacy, and safety data were similar for all reports of Alfaxan and Saffan, so alfaxalone may be suitable for many freshwater fish species (Bauquier et al. 2013; Minter et al. 2014; Bugman et al. 2016). No literature was identified reporting alfaxalone as an immersion anesthetic in marine species.

Propofol Propofol is an ultra-short-acting anesthetic agent that acts on GABA receptors in the central nervous system. In the United States, propofol is FDA-approved for intravenous use in dogs and cats. It is increasingly used as an immersion anesthetic agent in fish. Studies involving immersion are predominantly in freshwater fish, including European whitefish (*Coregonus lavaretus*), silver catfish (*Rhamdia quelen*), Nile tilapia (*Oreochromis niloticus*), Siberian sturgeon (*Acipenser baerii*), tetra (*Astyanax altiparanae*), rainbow trout, koi, and goldfish (Gholipour Kanani and Ahadizadeh 2013; Gomułka et al. 2014; Oda et al. 2014; Valença-Silva et al. 2014; Gomułka et al. 2015; Ostrensky et al. 2016; Prieto et al. 2017).

Typical dose ranges are 2.5–10 mg/L. Most studies report a wide safety index, although long procedures and high dosages have been associated with prolonged recoveries and mortalities (up to 22% in one study), and the solution may be too opaque for good observation of the fish during anesthesia (Oda et al. 2014). Clinicians should start at low doses for short procedures until more familiar with the drug.

Metomidate Hydrochloride Metomidate hydrochloride is a nonbarbiturate imidazole that is typically used by immersion. It is available in Canada under the trade name Marinil™. It is not approved by the US FDA but is available as an indexed drug that can be used in ornamental fish (Aquacalm®). It is readily water soluble and must be stored in tight, light-protected containers. In addition to immersion, the drug can be given orally (Harvey et al. 1988; Hansen et al. 2003).

Metomidate is a hypnotic agent, inducing sleep rather than general anesthesia. This means that opercular ventilation is maintained for longer than with other immersion anesthetics (Mattson and Riple 1989). Muscle fasciculations and incomplete relaxation may occur at low dosages (Harms 1999). The drug is used for sedation and anesthesia for minor procedures and is particularly useful for sedation during transport to limit transport trauma (Harms 1999; Kilgore et al. 2009). Metomidate should not be used alone for surgical or other noxious procedures (Harms 1999; Hansen et al. 2003).

Metomidate blocks cortisol synthesis (Iversen et al. 2003; Small 2003). One consequence of this is an increase in melanocyte stimulating hormone production, which can cause fish to turn dark in color. Though transient and not of clinical consequence, it is important for the clinician to recognize this drug effect to prevent unnecessary actions (e.g. aborting the procedure) (Harms 1999).

Metomidate is likely contraindicated in gouramis (*Anabantiformes*) and cichlids (*Cichlidae*) in water of pH < 5 (Harms 1999). In Atlantic cod (*Gadus morhua*), recovery times increased with increasing body weight, but not induction time (Zahl et al. 2009). When combined with MS-222, an overall reduction of the MS-222 dose was possible with a marked reduction of both induction and recovery time (Zahl et al. 2009).

Other Immersion Agents Other immersion anesthetic drugs are used to varying degrees in fish. These include benzocaine (the parent compound of MS-222), 2-phenoxyethanol, quinaldine/quinaldine sulfate, and azaperone (Mylniczenko et al. 2014b). Advantages and disadvantages of these compounds are described in the literature. Some are not readily available in the United States.

Inhalant chlorofluorocarbon-based anesthetics (e.g. isoflurane) can be used as immersion agents in fish, but care is indicated (Dunn and Koester 1990; Huang et al. 2010). Poor solubility of these drugs can result in high local concentrations which may result in an anesthetic overdose and makes overall control of anesthetic depth difficult. And drug volatilization and difficulty in scavenging waste gas represent a hazard to both personnel and the environment (Harms 1999; Ross and Ross 2008).

Parenteral Anesthesia

Oral, intracoelomic (ICe), intravenous (IV), and intramuscular (IM) administration of anesthetics are all options for fish. Oral administration is the least reliable in a clinical setting because precise dosing is difficult and the degree and rate of absorption are uncertain, although examples of its application exist (Harms and Bakal 1995; Steers and Sherrill 2001; Hansen et al. 2003; Harms 2003; Raines and Clancy 2009). Both ICe and IV routes require manual and sometimes chemical restraint for administration. The IV route is preferred over ICe administration due to rapid induction and short, predictable duration of effect (Fleming et al. 2003; Hansen et al. 2003). The ICe route, while effective, is associated with a greater risk of visceral damage and inconsistent induction. Intramuscular administration is by far the most common parenteral route used in fish. While manual restraint may be needed for hand injection, use of a pole syringe or darting system may preclude the need to handle larger fish for administration (Harvey et al. 1988; Williams et al. 1988). The preferred site for IM administration is the dorsal epaxial muscles, between the dorsal fin and lateral line on the vertical axis, and the operculum or gill slits and a point approximately 1/3 the distance between the dorsal fin and caudal peduncle on the horizontal axis (Harms and Bakal 1995; Peters et al. 2001). Drug leakage at the injection site should be expected. Induction times may be longer in sedentary species, as movement helps vascular circulation in fish. Large volumes may be required which predisposes the fish to sterile abscess formation at the injection site (Gruber and Keyes 1981; Tytler and Hawkins 1981).

Compared to immersion anesthetic drugs, effects of parenteral anesthesia are less predictable and long recoveries requiring ventilatory support are common (Harms 2003).

Ketamine Hydrochloride Ketamine is a short-acting cyclohexamine dissociative anesthetic. When used alone in fish, periods of apnea and prolonged recoveries with excitement are common, and seizure-like muscle spasms have been seen in elasmobranchs (Oswald 1978; Graham and Iwama 1990; Bruecker and Graham 1993; Stoskopf 1993). Combination protocols are always recommended, e.g. with a reversible α_2-adrenergic agonist such as dexmedetomidine. Ketamine combinations are typically used for capture or initial restraint; other anesthetics such as MS-222 are recommended for maintenance anesthesia. Although IM is the most common route used for administration, IV injections are effective. In these cases, the dosages should be reduced by 1/3 to 1/2 of those considered effective by IM delivery (Oswald 1978; Williams et al. 1988; Bruecker and Graham 1993; Fleming et al. 2003). However, there are a wide range of dose regimens and responses with ketamine combinations, resulting in safe and effective anesthesia in some species, and respiratory depression, bradycardia, and incomplete immobilization in others (Snyder et al. 1998; Fleming et al. 2003; Williams et al. 2004; Di Marco et al. 2011).

Xylazine, Medetomidine, Dexmedetomidine Xylazine, medetomidine, and dexmedetomidine are α_2-adrenergic agonists found in most veterinary clinics. Xylazine was the first α_2-adrenergic agonist used in fish, typically in combination with ketamine. While this combination has provided safe and effective anesthesia in sharks, its use has been associated with apnea, electrocardiogram disturbances, and seizure activity in teleosts, particularly salmonids (Oswald 1978; Andrews and Jones 1990; Stoskopf 1993). Medetomidine with ketamine has not been associated with these side effects in teleosts or elasmobranchs, and medetomidine or dexmedetomidine should be the first choice for clinicians opting to use an α_2-adrenergic agonist (Snyder et al. 1998; Tuttle and Dunn 2003; Williams et al. 2004; Mylniczenko et al. 2014a, b). High-concentration solutions are available from compounding pharmacies to reduce drug volume. As with ketamine, dose regimens and species-specific responses vary enormously. Yohimbine or atipamezole can be given to reverse the effects of xylazine or medetomidine/dexmedetomidine, respectively (Stoskopf 1993; Snyder et al. 1998; Williams et al. 2004).

Midazolam, Diazepam Midazolam and diazepam are benzodiazepine sedatives that are used in other classes to improve muscle relaxation and smooth induction and recovery. Midazolam has been used IM with ketamine and dexmedetomidine to safely sedate black seabass (*Centropristis striata*), but red porgy (*Pagrus pagrus*) showed highly variable responses, including fatal lactic acidosis (Christiansen et al. 2014). Midazolam has been noted to be beneficial for sedation of elasmobranchs, primarily when combined with other drugs (Mylniczenko et al. 2014a). Oral diazepam has been used in fish, but most reports are anecdotal and the few experimental studies show either little to no effect or unpredictable effects (Mylniczenko et al. 2014b).

Propofol Propofol is a short-acting alkylphenol derivative hypnotic with a poorly understood mechanism of action. In the United States and other countries, propofol is labeled for induction and maintenance of anesthesia in dogs and cats. Intravenous propofol has been used for surgical anesthesia in elasmobranchs and sturgeon (*Acipenser* spp.) (Fleming et al. 2003; Miller et al. 2005; Mylniczenko et al. 2014a, b). While safe and effective in most cases, significant respiratory depression has sometimes been noted and prolonged recoveries (>1 hour) have been an issue with some sharks, which makes IV propofol impractical for ram-ventilating species. In addition, the author has observed mortality in African lungfish (*Protopterus annectens*) following IV propofol. While potentially useful for short procedures in sturgeon and non-ram-ventilating elasmobranchs, given other anesthetic options available, the author cannot recommend the use of IV propofol without further studies.

Alfaxalone Several papers describe the use of Saffan (alfaxalone/alfadolone) for IM anesthesia in fish (Oswald 1978; Harvey et al. 1988). Limited information exists for IM use of Alfaxan, an alfaxalone-only product that is available as of 2018. In two marine species, permits (*Trachinotus falcatus*) and schoolmaster snappers (*Lutjanus apodus*), sedation was noted at lower IM doses, but prolonged excitement was noted at higher doses in permits suggesting that this species and possibly other jacks (*Carangidae*) may be more sensitive to Alfaxan (Tuxbury 2017). In freshwater koi, the duration of anesthesia and opercular rate were unpredictable and mortality was as high as 33% at higher dosages (Bailey et al. 2014). Although Alfaxan has been shown to be useful and relatively safe as an immersion agent, use of it as an injectable agent should be approached with caution.

Monitoring, Support, Recovery, and Resuscitation

Anesthetic Depth

Anesthetic depth should be assessed by evaluating a combination of factors, depending on the species, including activity compared to normal, reaction to stimuli, righting reflex, jaw and muscle tone, ventilation (respiratory rate and effort), and heart rate (Oikawa et al. 1994; Stetter 2001; Harms 2003; Myszkowski et al. 2003; Detar and Mattingly 2004). Similar to other vertebrates, broad stages include sedation, loss of equilibrium, and anesthesia (Stetter 2001; Harms 2003). A decrease in caudal fin stroke activity is often the first sign of drug effect followed by a loss of equilibrium and decrease in swimming behavior (for non-sedentary species), respiratory rate, and reaction to stimuli. Some species may go through a short excitement phase on induction, which can result in trauma or jumping from the container, or rapid and repeated flaring of the opercula known as a "coughing" reflex (Harms 1999; Stetter 2001). Onset of surgical anesthesia is marked by a further decrease in respiratory rate and effort and total loss of muscle tone. Non-responsiveness to a firm squeeze at the base of the tail typically indicates general anesthesia is present (Stetter 2001; Harms 2003). It is important to note, however, that depending on the species, drug, and dosage, some stages may not be seen. Also, some signs attributed to drug effect may actually be related to stress. For example, Gulf of Mexico sturgeon (*Acipenser oxyrinchus de soti*) may go into ventrodorsal recumbency when stressed which may be mistakenly interpreted as a loss of righting ability due to anesthesia (Fleming et al. 2003).

In general, with properly dosed immersion drugs, induction should occur within 5–10 minutes, while those administered via other routes can be expected to take longer. Oral drugs, in particular have prolonged, variable, and unpredictable induction times and effects. If fish are kept in immersion anesthesia at induction doses, anesthetic depth will continue to increase; drug level usually needs to be reduced for maintenance anesthesia of longer procedures (e.g. >15–20 minutes).

Cardiopulmonary Activity

Respiratory and heart rates usually decrease as anesthetic dose and duration increase. Gilling is an easily observable behavior in most fish species; however exceptions exist, including species with small opercular cavities, e.g. seahorses and pipefish (*Syngnathidae*), and ram-ventilating species, which show little to no opercular movement, e.g. tuna, pelagic sharks (Harms 1999, 2003). Heart rate is best assessed using ultrasonography, although electrocardiography (ECG) can be used (Harms and Bakal 1995; Harms 1999; Ross and Ross 2008). Doppler or other ultrasound probes can be placed into the opercular slit or directly over the heart (Figure A10.2). For ECG, electrodes can be lightly clamped to the surface of the fins (pectoral and anal fins are often a good combination) or subcutaneous/intramuscular needles can be used which improves signal quality (Harms 1999; Ross and Ross 2008). Pulse oximetry has not been effective for measuring hemoglobin saturation in fish (Harms 1999; Ross and Ross 2008).

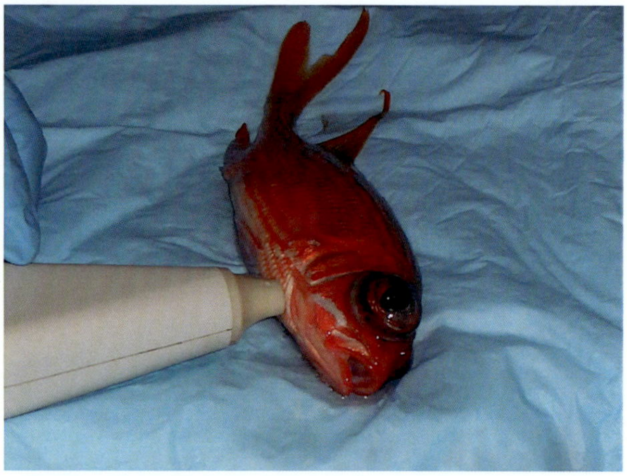

Figure A10.2 Heart rate monitoring using Doppler ultrasound during anesthesia of a longspine squirrelfish (*Holocentrus rufus*). *Source*: Image courtesy of Catherine Hadfield, National Aquarium.

In fish, respiratory arrest typically occurs long before cardiovascular collapse, giving the clinician time to act based on respiratory signs, even if cardiovascular monitoring is not available. That said, even fish that are ventilating well experience anesthesia-induced bradycardia and reduced gill blood flow which may lead to hypoxemia (Tytler and Hawkins 1981). Visual cues of developing hypoxemia include gill and fin pallor (Stetter 2001; Harms 2003). If large enough for blood sampling, respiratory efficiency can be monitored by periodic blood gas sampling to determine pH, oxygen, carbon dioxide, and lactate levels. Arterial blood provides the most information, but venous or mixed samples are more easily obtained in fish and still provide useful information about physiological trends. It is important to note that pH and lactate have often shown higher accuracy than other blood gas results in fish, particularly elasmobranchs, but trends over time in a patient should still be useful (Gallagher et al. 2010; Christiansen et al. 2014; Harter et al. 2015).

Water Quality Monitoring

Monitoring water quality throughout anesthetic procedures should be standard practice in order to reduce anesthetic morbidity and mortality. Temperature, dissolved oxygen, ammonia, and pH are the most useful parameters and should be maintained within appropriate ranges for the individual(s). Temperature tends to change toward ambient during flow-through and recirculating anesthesia. Dissolved oxygen tends to decrease and ammonia increases in any container with fish and during recirculating anesthesia. Problems are particularly common during prolonged procedures or when fish are sequentially anesthetized in the same container. pH can decrease with some immersion agents and tends to decrease over time during recirculating anesthesia. Although a crude assessment, the visual appearance of the water is also useful (e.g. water movement, presence of surface foam due to protein buildup). A solution to most water quality issues consists of exchanging a portion of the water (e.g. 20–50%) in the anesthetic chamber with suitable water. More information on water quality monitoring is available in Chapter A2.

Recovery

With immersion anesthesia, recovery occurs when the fish is placed in anesthetic-free water. For most injectable agents (ketamine, propofol, Alfaxan), recovery depends on the fish metabolizing and excreting the drug. For injectable α_2-agonists, reversal drugs are available which can speed recovery (Snyder et al. 1998; Harms 1999; Horsberg et al. 1999; Williams et al. 2004). Fish should be exposed to suitable, unmedicated water (e.g. in a new container, or after flushing out water used during anesthesia) regardless of anesthesia route, as some drugs and their metabolites can be excreted into the water and reabsorbed through the gills and/or skin. Recovery water should be well-aerated with the fish positioned so its mouth is oriented toward water flow. If additional ventilation is required, anesthetic-free water can be passed over the gills using a syringe, small submersible pump, or inflow line, or the fish may be moved forward through the water with its mouth open until spontaneous ventilation resumes.

Full recovery from immersion anesthetics usually occurs within 5 minutes; recoveries that take more than 10 minutes indicate an excessive anesthetic dose or a compromised animal (Stetter 2001; Ross and Ross 2008). Recovery from oral and parenteral agents is more variable and generally prolonged. Regardless of route of administration, recovery is marked by increasing respiratory rate and effort, return of muscle tone and fin movement, and progressively less ataxia until the fish regains full equilibrium.

It is important to note that an excitement phase may occur during recovery. To limit injury to the fish or staff, nets, lids, foam pads, and other barriers should be used to prevent fish from escaping or traumatizing themselves against the walls of their container (Harms 1999).

Resuscitation

Bradypnea (hypoventilation) can be managed by providing oxygenated water flow over the gills. However, it should be a sign to decrease the anesthetic concentration and potentially increase water flow to prevent subsequent problems (Stetter 2001).

If apnea and bradycardia develop, the anesthetic concentration in the water should be quickly reduced and water flow over the gills should be increased using a suitable syringe or submersible pump. This reduces anesthetic depth and makes use of the buccal flow/heart rate reflex, which causes the heart rate to accelerate in response to an increase in water flow (Ross and Ross 2008).

If the fish does not respond to the steps above, it may require the administration of fluids and/or doxapram. The author has observed a positive response to doxapram at 5 mg/kg IV or ICe in several cases of respiratory arrest. However, doxapram can be a marked stimulant in elasmobranchs, causing them to become excited and dangerous (Stoskopf 1986). Other emergency drugs (e.g. epinephrine, corticosteroids) may be given in the case of physiological collapse or shock.

Analgesia

Despite an increased interest in the use of analgesia in clinical practice, there remains limited information on fish. Without a significant body of definitive studies in the literature to draw from, it remains a challenge for clinicians to discern the difference between a drug providing anesthesia versus immobilization, let alone whether or not the drug provides analgesia.

Fish possess μ and κ opiate receptors within the brain and antinociceptive effects of opioids have been shown in fish. Reports show a reduced response to noxious stimuli using morphine, tramadol, buprenorphine, and dermorphine in rainbow trout, Atlantic cod, koi, goldfish, zebrafish (*Danio rerio*), and winter flounder (*Pseudopleuronectes americanus*) (Harms et al. 2005; Newby et al. 2007; Correia et al. 2011; Jones et al. 2012; Sneddon 2012; Steenbergen and Bardine 2014). Naloxone has been shown to negate or reduce the effectiveness of morphine and buprenorphine, as with other vertebrate taxa (Rose 2002; Correia et al. 2011; Steenbergen and Bardine 2014).

Effects of butorphanol, a mixed opioid agonist–antagonist, have been reported in koi and chain catsharks (*Scyliorhinus retifer*), with opposite outcomes. In koi, butorphanol appeared to provide postsurgical analgesia following exploratory coeliotomy or gonadectomy, while no benefit was noted in dogfish receiving a needle stimulus (Harms et al. 2005; Davis et al. 2006; Baker et al. 2013). It is not clear whether the difference was due to a fundamental difference between elasmobranch and teleost physiology or an insufficient dose or frequency (Davis et al. 2006). It is important to note that in one study involving koi, butorphanol at 10 mg/kg IM led to respiratory depression for several hours following surgery (Baker et al. 2013).

Of the other drugs commonly available to the private veterinarian, lidocaine may prove to be a useful analgesic, at least for intraoperative and postoperative treatments. In a study involving rainbow trout, subcutaneous lidocaine reduced all of the pain indicators associated with injections of acetic acid (Mettam et al. 2011). In zebrafish, injectable lidocaine as an immersion treatment following surgery significantly reduced pain-related behaviors (Schroeder and Sneddon 2017).

Nonsteroidal anti-inflammatory drugs (NSAIDs) have shown variable effects in fish. In a pharmacokinetic study of meloxicam following IV or IM administration in Nile tilapia, researchers demonstrated measurable plasma levels but rapid drug clearance at a dose of 1 mg/kg (Fredholm et al. 2016). While clinical efficacy was not assessed, maximum plasma concentrations were greater than those required for clinical effects in other vertebrate taxa. Two studies showed no obvious analgesic effect of ketoprofen in koi or chain catsharks (Harms et al. 2005; Davis et al. 2006). Carprofen in rainbow trout demonstrated potential analgesia but depressed overall activity, which was considered a deleterious side effect (Mettam et al. 2011). Further details on NSAID use in fish, including toxicity concerns following long-term use, are provided in Chapter A12.

Euthanasia

Euthanasia of fish in clinical practice is usually performed using an overdose of an immersion anesthetic agent. However, immersion alone may be insufficient to ensure death and a two-step euthanasia is preferred, consisting of immersion followed by a secondary method (Harms 1999; Balko et al. 2018; Leary et al. 2020).

The most common immersion drug is buffered tricaine methanesulfonate (MS-222), dosed at more than 5–10 times the anesthetic concentration for a particular species. The container should be dark and quiet to reduce external stimulation and the water quality (including temperature, dissolved oxygen, pH, and salinity) should be appropriate for the individual(s) throughout the euthanasia process. The fish must be maintained in the anesthetic solution for at least 15–30 minutes after cessation of reflexes and opercular movement. Doppler or other ultrasound probes or electrocardiography can be used to identify asystole, but where that equipment is not available, gills should be checked for pallor to ensure the heart has stopped.

Effectiveness of MS-222 for euthanasia varies by species and life stage (Leary et al. 2020). Several studies have shown that common doses of buffered MS-222 do not ensure death and that recovery is possible in some species (Wilson et al. 2009; Collymore et al. 2016; Balko et al. 2018).

Therefore a two-step euthanasia to ensure brain death is recommended. Examples of secondary methods include pithing, decapitation and pithing, macerating, exsanguination, rapid freezing, or pentobarbital (Harms 1999; Balko et al. 2018; Leary et al. 2020). If histologic examination of the brain is required, the best secondary methods may be intravenous pentobarbital or decapitation followed by immediate fixation of the head in formalin.

Pithing can be carried out using large bore needles through the dorsal midline and the back of the orbits toward the brain. Pentobarbital is ideally given intravenously, but can be intracardiac or intracoelomic. The American Veterinary Medical Association (AVMA) Guidelines on Euthanasia recommends 60–100 mg/kg of sodium pentobarbital (0.15–0.25 mL/kg of 390 mg/mL solution), but higher doses are common (e.g. 0.4–1.0 mL/kg of 390 mg/mL solution) (Leary et al. 2020). If pentobarbital is given, the fish should still remain in the anesthetic solution for at least 15–30 minutes after cessation of reflexes and opercular movement.

Other potential options include:

- For large fish, immersion euthanasia may be impractical. In these cases, the recommendation is usually to sedate the fish, then give intravenous pentobarbital (Harms and Bakal 1995).
- For air-breathing species (Box A1.1), sedation followed by intravenous administration of pentobarbital or physical methods of euthanasia are recommended; immersion euthanasia alone should never be relied on.
- For small (<3.8 cm length), tropical or subtropical stenothermic fish, immediate immersion in 2–4°C (36–39°F) water may be considered. The fish must be kept in the water at that temperature for at least 10-20 minutes after cessation of reflexes and opercular movement (Leary et al. 2020).
- Other physical methods as described by the AVMA, providing they are performed with the proper equipment by trained personnel who are regularly monitored for proficiency (Leary et al. 2020)

Unapproved methods include slow chilling or freezing of unanesthetized animals as well as death by anoxia and desiccation.

These are discussed in more detail in the AVMA Guidelines on Euthanasia (Leary et al. 2020). Given the diversity of fish species, practical and legislative factors around anesthetic drug use and disposal, and the different needs following euthanasia, a variety of options are provided. The AVMA Guidelines specify that "euthanasia methods should be tested in one animal or a small group of animals prior to use in a large population for an unfamiliar species" (Leary et al. 2020).

References

Afifi, S., Al-Thobaiti, S., and Rasem, B. (2001). Multiple exposure of Asian sea bass (*Lates calcarifer*, Centropomidae) to clove oil: a histological study. *Journal of Aquaculture in the Tropics* 16: 131–138.

Andrews, J. and Jones, R. (1990). A method for the transport of sharks for captivity. *Journal of Aquariculture and Aquatic Sciences* 5: 70–72.

Bailey, K.M., Hempstead, J.E., Tobias, J.R. et al. (2013). Evaluation of the effects of tricaine methanesulfonate on retinal structure and function in koi carp (*Cyprinus carpio*). *Journal of the American Veterinary Medical Association* 242: 1578–1582.

Bailey, K., Minter, L., Lewbart, G. et al. (2014). Alfaxalone as an intramuscular injectable anesthetic in koi carp (*Cyprinus carpio*). *Journal of Zoo and Wildlife Medicine* 45: 852–858.

Baker, T., Baker, B., Johnson, S., and Sladky, K.K. (2013). Comparative analgesic efficacy of morphine sulfate and butorphanol tartrate in koi (*Cyprinus carpio*) undergoing unilateral gonadectomy. *Journal of the American Veterinary Medical Association* 243: 882–890.

Balko, J.A., Oda, A., and Posner, L.P. (2018). Use of tricaine methanesulfonate or propofol for immersion euthanasia of goldfish (*Carassius auratus*). *Journal of the American Veterinary Medical Association* 12: 1555–1561.

Bassi, M., Klein, W., Fernandes, M. et al. (2005). Pulmonary oxygen diffusing capacity of the South American lungfish, *Lepidosiren paradoxa*: physiological values by the Bohr method. *Physiological and Biochemical Zoology* 78: 560–569.

Bauquier, S., Greenwood, J., and Whittem, T. (2013). Evaluation of the sedative and anaesthetic effects of five different concentrations of alfaxalone in goldfish, *Carassius auratus*. *Aquaculture* 396: 119–123.

Bernstein, P., Digre, K., and Creel, D. (1997). Retinal toxicity associated with occupational exposure to the fish anesthetic MS-222. *American Journal of Ophthalmology* 124: 843–844.

Blank, J., Morrissette, J., Landeira-Fernandez, A. et al. (2004). In situ cardiac performance of Pacific bluefin tuna hearts in response to acute temperature change. *Journal of Experimental Biology* 207: 881–890.

Bond, C. (1996). *Biology of Fishes*, 2e. Philadelphia, PA: Saunders College Publishing.

Braithwaite, V. and Boulcott, P. (2007). Pain perception, aversion, and fear in fish. *Diseases of Aquatic Organisms* 75: 131–138.

Bressler, K. and Ron, B. (2004). Effect of anesthetics on stress and the innate immune system of gilthead bream (*Sparus aurata*). *Israeli Journal of Aquaculture* 56: 5–13.

Bruecker, P. and Graham, M. (1993). The effects of the anesthetic ketamine hydrochloride on oxygen consumption rates and behavior in the fish *Heros (Cichlasoma) citrinellum* (Gunther, 1864). *Comparative Biochemistry and Physiology Part C* 104: 57–59.

Bugman, A., Langer, P., Hadzima, E. et al. (2016). Evaluation of the anesthetic efficacy of alfaxalone in oscar fish (*Astronotus ocellatus*). *American Journal of Veterinary Research* 77: 239–244.

Bushnell, P. and Jones, D. (1994). Cardiovascular and respiratory physiology of tuna: adaptations for support of exceptionally high metabolic rates. *Environmental Biology of Fishes* 40: 303–318.

Christiansen, E., Mitchell, J., Harms, C., and Stoskopf, M. (2014). Sedation of red porgy (*Pagrus pagrus*) and black sea bass (*Centropristis striata*) using ketamine, dexmedetomidine and midazolam delivered via intramuscular injection. *Journal of Zoo and Aquarium Research* 2: 62–68.

Collymore, C., Banks, E.K., and Turner, P.V. (2016). Lidocaine hydrochloride compared with MS222 for the euthanasia of zebrafish (*Danio rerio*). *Journal of the American Association of Laboratory Animal Science* 55: 816–820.

Cooke, S., Suski, C., Ostrand, K. et al. (2004). Behavioral and physiological assessment of low concentrations of clove oil anaesthetic for handling and transporting largemouth bass (*Micropterus salmoides*). *Aquaculture* 239: 509–529.

Correia, A., Cunha, S., Scholze, M., and Stevens, E.D. (2011). A novel behavioral fish model of nociception for testing analgesics. *Pharmaceuticals* 4: 665–680.

Davis, K. and Griffin, B. (2004). Physiological responses of hybrid striped bass under sedation by several anesthetics. *Aquaculture* 233: 531–548.

Davis, M., Mylniczenko, N., Storms, T. et al. (2006). Evaluation of intramuscular ketoprofen and butorphanol as analgesics in chain dogfish (*Scyliorhinus retifer*). *Zoo Biology* 25 (6): 491–500.

Detar, J. and Mattingly, H. (2004). Response of southern redbelly dace to clove oil and MS-222: effects of anesthetic concentration and water temperature. *Proceedings of the Annual Conference of Southeastern Association of Fish and Wildlife Agencies*, Hiltonhead Island, SC.

Di Marco, P., Petochi, T., Longobardi, A. et al. (2011). Efficacy of tricaine methanesulfonate, clove oil, and medetomidine-ketamine and their side effects on the physiology of sturgeon hybrid *Acipenser naccarii* x *Acipenser baerii*. *Journal of Applied Ichthyology* 27: 611–617.

Dunn, R. and Koester, D. (1990). Anesthetics in elasmobranchs: a review with emphasis on halothane-oxygen-nitrous oxide. *Journal of Aquariculture and Aquatic Sciences* 5: 44–52.

Fernández-Parra, R., Donnelly, T., Pignon, C. et al. (2017). Immersion anesthesia with alfaxalone in a goldfish (*Carassius auratus*). *Journal of Exotic Pet Medicine* 26: 276–282.

Ferreira, J., Schoonbee, H., and Smit, G. (1984). The uptake of the anesthetic benzocaine hydrochloride by the gills and the skin of three freshwater fish species. *Journal of Fish Biology* 25: 35–41.

Fleming, G., Heard, D., Floyd, R., and Riggs, A. (2003). Evaluation of propofol and medetomidine-ketamine for short-term immobilization of Gulf of Mexico sturgeon (*Acipenser oxyrinchus desoti*). *Journal of Zoo and Wildlife Medicine* 34: 153–158.

Fredholm, D., Mylniczenko, N., and KuKanich, B. (2016). Pharmacokinetic evaluation of meloxicam after intravenous and intramuscular administration in Nile tilapia (*Oreochromis niloticus*). *Journal of Zoo and Wildlife Medicine* 47: 736–742.

Gallagher, A.J., Frick, L.H., Bushnell, P.G. et al. (2010). Blood gas, oxygen saturation, pH, and lactate values in elasmobranch measured with a commercially available portable clinical analyzer and standard laboratory instruments. *Journal of Aquatic Animal Health* 22: 229–234.

Gelwicks, K. and Zafft, D. (1998). Efficacy of carbonic acid as an anesthetic for rainbow trout. *North American Journal of Fisheries Management* 18: 432–438.

Gholipour Kanani, H. and Ahadizadeh, S. (2013). Use of propofol as an anesthetic and its efficacy on some hematological values of ornamental fish, *Carassius auratus*. *Springerplus* 2 (1): 76.

Gilmour, K., Perry, S., Wood, C. et al. (1998). Nitrogen excretion and the cardiorespiratory physiology of the gulf toadfish, *Opsanus beta*. *Physiological Zoology* 71: 492–505.

Gladden, J.N., Brainard, B.M., Shelton, J.L. et al. (2010). Evaluation of isoeugenol for anesthesia in koi carp (*Cyprinus carpio*). *American Journal of Veterinary Research* 71: 859–866.

Gomes, L., Chippari-Gomes, A., Lopes, N. et al. (2001). Efficacy of benzocaine as an anesthetic in juvenile tambaqui, *Colossoma macropomum*. *Journal of the World Aquaculture Society* 32: 426–431.

Gomułka, P., Wlasow, T., Szczepkowski, M. et al. (2014). The effect of propofol anaesthesia on haematological and biochemical blood profile of European whitefish. *Turkish Journal of Fisheries and Aquatic Sciences* 14: 331–337.

Gomułka, P., Czerniak, E., Dągowski, J. et al. (2015). Effects of propofol and carbon dioxide on acid-base balance in Siberian sturgeon. *Polish Journal of Veterinary Sciences* 18: 267–272.

Graham, J. (1997). *Air-Breathing Fishes: Evolution, Diversity, and Adaptation*. San Diego, CA: Academic Press.

Graham, M. and Iwama, G. (1990). The physiological effects of the anesthetic ketamine hydrochloride on two salmonid species. *Aquaculture* 90: 323–332.

Gruber, S. and Keyes, R. (1981). Keeping sharks for research. In: *Aquarium Systems* (ed. A.D. Hawkins), 373–402. New York: Academic Press.

Hansen, M., Nymoen, U., and Horsberg, T. (2003). Pharmacokinetic and pharmacodynamic properties of metomidate in turbot (*Scophthalmus maximus*) and halibut (*Hippoglossus hippoglossus*). *Journal of Veterinary Pharmacology and Therapeutics* 26: 95–103.

Harms, C. (1999). Anesthesia in fish. In: *Zoo and Wild Animal Medicine, Current Therapy 4* (eds. M.E. Fowler and R.E. Miller), 158–163. Philadelphia, PA: W.B. Saunders Co.

Harms, C. (2003). Fish. In: *Zoo and Wild Animal Medicine 5* (eds. M.E. Fowler and R.E. Miller), 2–20. Philadelphia, PA: W.B. Saunders Co.

Harms, C. and Bakal, R. (1995). Techniques in fish anesthesia. *Journal of Small Exotic Animal Medicine* 3: 19–25.

Harms, C., Lewbart, G., Swanson, C. et al. (2005). Behavioral and clinical pathology changes in koi carp (*Cyprinus carpio*) subjected to anesthesia and surgery with and without intra-operative analgesics. *Comparative Medicine* 55: 221–226.

Harter, T., Morrison, P., Mandelman, J. et al. (2015). Validation of the i-STAT system for the analysis of blood gases and acid-base status in juvenile sandbar shark (*Carcharhinus plumbeus*). *Conservation Physiology* 3: 1–9.

Harvey, B., Denny, C., Kaiser, S., and Young, J. (1988). Remote intramuscular injection of immobilizing drugs into fish using a laser-aimed underwater dart gun. *Veterinary Record* 20: 174–177.

Horsberg, T., Burka, J., and Tasker, R. (1999). Actions and the alpha$_2$ adrenergic agents, medetomidine and atipamezole, in rainbow trout (*Oncorhynchus mykiss*). *Veterinary Anaesthesia and Analgesia* 26: 18–22.

Hseu, J., Yeh, S., Chu, Y., and Ting, Y.Y. (1997). Different anesthetic effects of 2-phenoxyethanol on four species of teleosts. *Journal of the Fisheries Society of Taiwan* 24: 185–191.

Huang, W., Hsieh, Y., Chen, I. et al. (2010). Combined use of MS-222 (tricaine) and isoflurane extends anesthesia time and minimizes cardiac rhythm side effects in adult zebrafish. *Zebrafish* 7: 297–304.

Huntingford, F., Adams, C., Braithwaite, V. et al. (2006). Current issues in fish welfare. *Journal of Fish Biology* 68: 332–372.

Ishimatsu, A. and Itazawa, Y. (1993). Anatomy and physiology of the cardiorespiratory system in air-breathing fish, *Channa argus*. In: *Advances in Fish Research* (ed. B.R. Singh), 55–70. Delhi: Narendra Publishing House.

Iverson, M., Finstad, B., McKinley, R., and Eliassen, R. (2003). The efficacy of metomidate, clove oil, Aqui-S™, and Benzoak® as anaesthetics in Atlantic salmon (*Salmo salar* L.) smolts and their potential stress-reducing capacity. *Aquaculture* 221: 549–566.

Jones, S., Kamunde, C., Lemke, K., and Stevens, E.D. (2012). The dose-response relation for the antinociceptive effect of morphine in a fish, rainbow trout. *Journal of Veterinary Pharmacology and Therapeutics* 35: 563–570.

Kildea, M., Allan, G., and Kearney, R. (2004). Accumulation and clearance of the anaesthetics clove oil and Aqui-S™ from the edible tissue of silver perch (*Bidyanus bidyanus*). *Aquaculture* 232: 265–277.

Kilgore, K., Hill, J., Powell, J. et al. (2009). Investigational use of metomidate hydrochloride as a shipping additive for two ornamental fishes. *Journal of Aquatic Animal Health* 21: 133–139.

Kumlu, M. and Yanar, M. (1999). Effects of the anesthetic quinaldine sulphate and muscle relaxant diazepam on sea bream juveniles (*Sparus aurata*). *Israeli Journal of Aquaculture* 51: 143–147.

Leary, S., Underwood, M., Anthony, R. et al. (2020). AVMA Guidelines for the Euthanasia of Animals: 2020 Edition. https://www.avma.org/sites/default/files/2020-01/2020-Euthanasia-Final-1-17-20.pdf (accessed August 2020).

Mattson, N. and Riple, T. (1989). Metomidate, a better anesthetic for cod (*Gadus morhua*) in comparison with benzocaine, MS-222, chlorobutanol, and phenoxyethanol. *Aquaculture* 83: 89–94.

Mettam, J., Oulton, L., McCrohan, C., and Sneddon, L.U. (2011). The efficacy of three types of analgesic drugs in reducing pain in the rainbow trout, *Oncorhynchus mykiss*. *Applied Animal Behaviour Science* 133: 265–274.

Miller, S., Mitchell, M., Heatley, J. et al. (2005). Clinical and cardiorespiratory effects of propofol in the spotted bamboo shark (*Chiloscyllium plagiosum*). *Journal of Zoo and Wildlife Medicine* 36: 673–676.

Minter, L., Bailey, K., Harms, C. et al. (2014). The efficacy of alfaxalone for immersion anesthesia in koi carp (*Cyprinus carpio*). *Veterinary Anaesthesia and Analgesia* 41: 398–405.

Mylniczenko, N., Clauss, T., and Stamper, M. (2014a). Elasmobranchs and holocephalans. In: *Zoo Animal and Wildlife Immobilization and Anesthesia*, 2e (eds. G. West, D. Heard and N. Caulkett), 261–301. Hoboken, NJ: Wiley.

Mylniczenko, N., Neiffer, D., and Clauss, T. (2014b). Bony fish (lungfish, sturgeon, and teleosts). In: *Zoo Animal and Wildlife Immobilization and Anesthesia*, 2e (eds. G. West, D. Heard and N. Caulkett), 209–260. Hoboken, NJ: Wiley.

Myszkowski, L., Kaminski, R., and Wolnicki, J. (2003). Response of juvenile tench, *Tinca tinca* (L.), to the anaesthetic 2-phenoxyethanol. *Journal of Applied Ichthyology* 19: 142–145.

Neiffer, D. and Stamper, M. (2009). Fish sedation, anesthesia, analgesia, and euthanasia: considerations, methods, and types of drugs. *ILAR Journal* 50: 343–346.

Newby, N.C., Gamperl, A.K., and Stevens, D. (2007). Cardiorespiratory effects and efficacy of morphine sulfate in winter flounder (*Pseudopleuronectes americanus*). *American Journal of Veterinary Research* 68: 592–597.

Oda, A., Bailey, K., Lewbart, G. et al. (2014). Physiologic and biochemical assessments of koi (*Cyprinus carpio*) following immersion in propofol. *Journal of the American Veterinary Medical Association* 245: 1286–1291.

Oikawa, S., Takeda, T., and Itazawa, Y. (1994). Scale effects of MS-222 on a marine teleost, porgy *Pagrus major*. *Aquaculture* 121: 369–379.

Ostrensky, A., Pedrazzani, A., and Vicente, A. (2016). Use of MS-222 (tricaine methanesulfonate) and propofol (2, 6-diisopropylphenol) as anaesthetics for the tetra *Astyanax altiparanae* (Teleostei, Characidae). *Aquaculture Research* 47: 3477–3488.

Oswald, R. (1978). Injection anesthesia for experimental studies in fish. *Comparative Biochemistry and Physiology* 60: 19–26.

Peters, R., Van den Hoek, B., Bretschneider, F., and Struik, M.L. (2001). Saffan®: a review and some examples of its use in fishes (Pisces: Teleostei). *Netherlands Journal of Zoology* 51: 421–437.

Posner, L. (2009). Pain and distress in fish: a review of the evidence. *ILAR Journal* 50: 327–328.

Posner, L.P., Scott, G.N., and Law, J.M. (2013). Repeated exposure of goldfish (*Carassius auratus*) to tricaine methanesulfonate (MS-222). *Journal of Zoo and Wildlife Medicine* 44: 340–347.

Prieto, G., Errecalde, C., Mancini, M. et al. (2017). Anaesthetic effect of propofol on rainbow trout (*Oncorhynchus mykiss*) in two different concentrations. *Iranian Journal of Veterinary Surgery* 12: 18–23.

Raines, J. and Clancy, M. (2009). Sedation by orally administered ketamine in goldfish, *Carassius auratus*; hybrid striped bass, *Morone saxatilis* x *M. chrysops*; and ocellated river stingray, *Potamotrygon motoro*. *Journal of the World Aquaculture Society* 40: 788–794.

Rantin, F., Guerra, C., Kalinin, A., and Glass, M.L. (1998). The influence of aquatic surface respiration (ASR) on cardio-respiratory function of the serrasalmid fish *Piaractus mesopotamicus*. *Comparative Biochemistry and Physiology* 119: 991–997.

Rose, J. (2002). The neurobehavioral nature of fishes and the question of awareness and pain. *Reviews in Fisheries Science* 10: 1–38.

Ross, L. and Ross, B. (2008). *Anaesthetic and Sedative Techniques for Aquatic Animals*. Oxford: Blackwell Science, Ltd.

Rothwell, S., Black, S., Jerrett, A., and Forster, M.E. (2005). Cardiovascular changes and catecholamine release following anaesthesia in Chinook salmon (*Oncorhynchus tshawytscha*) and snapper (*Pagrus auratus*). *Comparative Biochemistry and Physiology Part A* 140: 289–298.

Roubach, R., Gomes, L., and Val, A. (2001). Safest level of tricaine methanesulfonate (MS-222) to induce anesthesia in juveniles of matrinxã, *Brycon cephalus*. *Acta Amazonica* 31: 159–163.

Schroeder, P. and Sneddon, L. (2017). Exploring the efficacy of immersion analgesics in zebrafish using an integrative approach. *Applied Animal Behaviour Science* 187: 93–102.

Silbernagel, C. and Yochem, P. (2016). Effectiveness of the anesthetic Aqui-S® 20 in marine finfish and elasmobranchs. *Journal of Wildlife Diseases* 52: S96–S103.

Sladky, K., Swanson, C., Stoskopf, M. et al. (2001). Comparative efficacy of tricaine methanesulfonate and clove oil for use as anesthetics in red pacu (*Piaractus brachypomus*). *American Journal of Veterinary Research* 62: 337–342.

Small, B. (2003). Anesthetic efficacy of metomidate and comparison of plasma cortisol responses to tricaine methanesulfonate, quinaldine, and clove oil anesthetized channel catfish, *Ictalurus punctatus*. *Aquaculture* 218: 177–185.

Small, B. and Chatakondi, N. (2005). Routine measures of stress are reduced in mature channel catfish during and after Aqui-S anesthesia and recovery. *North American Journal of Aquaculture* 67: 72–78.

Sneddon, L. (2009). Pain perception in fish: indicators and endpoints. *ILAR Journal* 50: 338–342.

Sneddon, L. (2012). Clinical anesthesia and analgesia in fish. *Journal of Exotic Pet Medicine* 21: 32–43.

Snyder, S., Richard, M., Berzins, I. et al. (1998). Immobilization of sandtiger sharks (*Odontaspis taurus*). *Proceedings of the International Association for Aquatic Animal Medicine*, San Diego, CA.

Steenbergen, P.J. and Bardine, N. (2014). Antinociceptive effects of buprenorphine in zebrafish larvae: an alternative for rodent models to study pain and nociception? *Applied Animal Behavior Science* 152: 92–99.

Steers, J. and Sherrill, J. (2001). Use of oral tiletamine-zolazepam for sedation and translocation of captive yellowtail jacks (*Seriola lalandi*). *Proceedings of the International Association for Aquatic Animal Medicine*, Tampa, FL.

Stehly, G. and Gingerich, W. (1999). Evaluation of Aqui-S™ (efficacy and minimum toxic concentration) as a fish anaesthetic/sedative for public aquaculture in the United States. *Aquaculture Research* 30: 365–372.

Stetter, M. (2001). Fish and amphibian anesthesia. *Veterinary Clinics of North America: Exotic Animal Practice* 4: 69–82.

Stoskopf, M. (1986). Preliminary notes on the immobilization and anesthesia of captive sharks. *Erkrankungen Der Zootiere* 28: 145–151.

Stoskopf, M. (ed.) (1993). Shark pharmacology and toxicology. In: *Fish Medicine*, 809–816. Philadelphia, PA: WB Saunders, Inc.

Totland, G., Kryvi, H., Bone, Q., and Flood, P.R. (1981). Vascularization of the lateral muscle of some elasmobranchiomorph fishes. *Journal of Fish Biology* 18: 223–234.

Tuttle, A. and Dunn, J. (2003). Evaluation of intramuscular use of medetomidine (α-2 adrenergic agonist) as an alternative to tricaine methanesulfonate (MS-222, Finquel®) for sedation and anesthesia in teleosts and elasmobranchs. *Proceedings of the International Association of Aquatic Animal Medicine*, Kohala, HI.

Tuxbury, K. (2017). Effects of intramuscular alfaxalone in permit (*Trachinotus falcatus*) and schoolmaster snapper (*Lutjanus apodus*). *Proceedings of the American Association of Zoo Veterinarians*, Dallas, TX.

Tytler, P. and Hawkins, A. (1981). Vivisection, anaesthetics and minor surgery. In: *Aquarium Systems* (ed. A.D. Hawkins), 247–278. New York: Academic Press.

United States Food and Drug Administration (2007). Guidance for Industry: Concerns Related to the Use of Clove Oil as an Anesthetic for Fish. https://www.fda.gov/downloads/AnimalVeterinary/GuidanceComplianceEnforcement/GuidanceforIndustry/ucm052520.pdf (1 November 2018).

Valença-Silva, G., Braz, M., Barreto, R. et al. (2014). Low dose of the anesthetic propofol does not induce genotoxic or mutagenic effects in Nile tilapia. *Transactions of the American Fisheries Society* 143: 414–419.

Walsh, C. and Pease, B. (2002). The use of clove oil as an anaesthetic for the longfinned eel, *Anquilla reinhardtii* (Steindachner). *Aquaculture Research* 33: 627–635.

Williams, T., Christiansen, J., and Nygren, S. (1988). Intramuscular anesthesia of teleosts and elasmobranchs using ketamine hydrochloride. *Proceedings of the American Association of Zoological Parks and Aquariums*, San Diego, CA.

Williams, T., Rollins, M., and Block, B. (2004). Intramuscular anesthesia of bonito and Pacific mackerel with ketamine and medetomidine and reversal of anesthesia with atipamezole. *Journal of the American Veterinary Medical Association* 225: 417–421.

Wilson, J.M., Bunte, R.M., and Carty, A.J. (2009). Evaluation of rapid cooling and tricaine methanesulfonate (MS222) as methods of euthanasia in zebrafish (*Danio rerio*). *Journal of the American Association for Laboratory Animal Science* 48: 785–789.

Zahl, I., Kiessling, A., Samuelsen, O., and Hansen, M.K. (2009). Anaesthesia of Atlantic cod (*Gadus morhua*): effect of preanaesthetic sedation and importance of body weight, temperature, and stress. *Aquaculture* 295: 52–59.

A11

Surgery and Endoscopy

Izidora Sladakovic[1] *and Stephen J. Divers*[2]

[1] *Avian and Exotics Service, Northside Veterinary Specialists, Terrey Hills, New South Wales, Australia*
[2] *College of Veterinary Medicine, University of Georgia, Athens, GA, USA*

Introduction

Surgery and endoscopy have numerous applications in pet fish, aquarium collections, and free-ranging populations. Managed fish often present with disorders requiring surgical intervention. Diagnostic investigations may require endoscopy for internal visualization of organs and lesions and collection of samples. Monitoring and conservation of free-ranging populations may use surgical and endoscopic techniques for research projects. As is the case in domestic animals and increasingly in zoological species, endosurgical procedures are being developed for fish. At this stage, much research still needs to be done in the field of surgery and endoscopy to establish optimal protocols and techniques for fish. However, techniques used in other taxa can be applied to fish, with consideration given to their unique anatomy and physiology. This chapter will provide an overview of general surgery and endoscopy principles, followed by descriptions of specific surgical and endoscopic procedures. Due to the enormous variety of fish anatomy, the procedures described below may need to be modified for different species. Examination of a healthy conspecific can help familiarize the clinician with normal anatomy. Anesthesia and analgesia are covered in Chapter A10 and will not be discussed here.

General Surgical Principles

Preparation of the Patient

Once the patient is anesthetized, it can be removed from the water and placed on a smooth moist surface to prevent damage to the skin. Foam pads with a wedge cut out so the patient can be secured in dorsal or lateral recumbency are commonly used. Fish have a mucus layer covering the epidermis, which has physical, chemical, and biological defense mechanisms that protect fish from environmental pathogens. Aseptic surgical preparation techniques used in terrestrial animals are not applied to fish as they remove the mucus layer and can result in immune compromise. Most commonly, the surgical site is flushed, gently wiped, or dabbed with sterile saline to remove surface debris prior to starting surgery. Gentle application of povidone-iodine may also be used; in a study on rainbow trout (*Oncorhynchus mykiss*), there was no difference in wound healing or histology of the surgical sites when povidone-iodine was applied, compared to the control group (Wagner et al. 1999). Surgical sites may be draped with a transparent plastic drape. The skin should be kept moist throughout surgery. In fish that have large scales, scales may need to be removed along the incision line. The scales can be gently pulled out in the direction of scale growth. Alternatively, a surgical incision can be made through the scales and any incised scales removed at the end of the procedure, prior to skin closure. It is important that all scale material within the incision site is removed as it can incite an inflammatory reaction.

Instrumentation and Visualization

Instrumentation will largely depend on the size of the fish and the surgical procedure. Microsurgical instruments may be required for very small fish or for certain procedures, such as ophthalmic surgery; however, for most medium-sized fish, standard small animal instruments are

Clinical Guide to Fish Medicine, First Edition. Edited by Catherine A. Hadfield and Leigh Ann Clayton.

appropriate. To improve access, retractors such as eyelid retractors or plastic retractors can be used. Plastic self-retaining retractors (Lone Star Retractor, Lone Star Medical Products, Inc., Stafford, TX) are lightweight and can be adjusted to fit patients and incisions of different sizes and shapes (Figure A11.1). Aseptic precautions should be taken. All instrumentation should be autoclaved, gas-sterilized, or cold-sterilized for each patient.

Blood loss needs to be minimized, particularly in small fish. Blood volume varies between species and is generally lower than other vertebrates, ranging from 3 to 8% of body weight (Gamperl and Shiels 2013). Blood loss should be limited to ≤10% of blood volume. Hemostasis can be rapidly provided by radiosurgical devices and vascular clips. Gelatin sponges (Gelfoam, Pfizer distributed by Pharmacia and Upjohn Co., New York, NY) are particularly useful for parenchymal hemorrhage. Handheld electrocautery devices are cheap and readily available, but can cause extensive collateral tissue damage.

In smaller fish, a form of magnification with illumination is essential. Head-mounted operating loupes (e.g. SurgiTel System, General Scientific Corporation, Inc., Ann Arbor, MI) are commonly used, portable, and ergonomic. Operating microscopes can also be used but are costly. A video telescopic operating microscope (VITOM, Karl Storz Veterinary Endoscopy America Inc., Goleta, CA) has been developed to be used with existing endoscopy equipment, and compared to operating loupes, offers the advantage of improved ergonomics and photodocumentation capability (Figure A11.2).

Suture

The skin is the holding layer in fish and is relatively inelastic and tightly adhered to underlying tissue layers. For a novice fish surgeon, practicing on cadavers is recommended to develop appropriate skin closure techniques and familiarize oneself with tissue handling in fish.

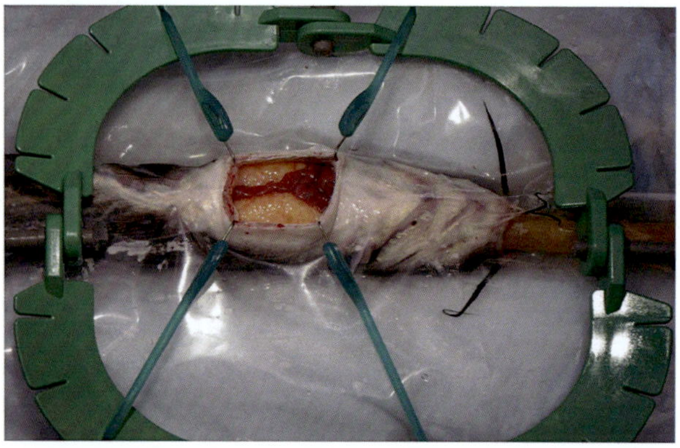

Figure A11.1 A plastic self-retaining retractor in place for an exploratory coeliotomy in a channel catfish (*Ictalurus punctatus*). The retractor can be adjusted for various procedures and sizes of patients which greatly improves visualization and access. *Source:* Courtesy of University of Georgia.

The choice of suture material depends on many factors, including surgery, temperature, and species. In general, absorbable synthetic monofilament suture material is preferred; monofilament suture is less likely to wick pathogens into the incision. The smallest suture size on a reverse-cutting or tapered needle should be used. In koi (*Cyprinus carpio*), five suture materials (silk, monofilament nylon, polyglyconate, polyglactin 910, and chromic gut) were placed in the skin and body wall using a single simple interrupted suture. Monofilament polyglyconate (Maxon) caused the mildest tissue reaction (Hurty et al. 2002). In Siberian sturgeon (*Acipenser baerii*) and juvenile Chinook salmon (*Oncorhynchus tshawytscha*), absorbable monofilament poliglecaprone 25 (Monocryl or Monocryl Plus) was superior to absorbable multifilament and nonabsorbable monofilament suture materials (Deters et al. 2010; Boone et al. 2013). Certain suture materials (e.g. catgut, polydioxanone, polyglactin 910) should be avoided as they can persist for a long time, cause intense inflammation, and predispose to dehiscence and infection. Cyanoacrylate adhesive is not recommended in fish as cutaneous goblet cells produce mucus that removes the adhesive, resulting in dehiscence.

Suture patterns also affect tissue reaction and healing. A tight suture line can lead to necrosis and dehiscence; excessive tension is more problematic in fish than in terrestrial animals. A loose suture line exposes the incision and potentially the coelomic cavity to water. Compared to simple interrupted and interrupted horizontal mattress suture patterns, a subcuticular suture pattern caused the least amount of inflammation and no necrosis in goldfish (*Carassius auratus*) (Nematollahi et al. 2010). This may be related to reduced exposure to the aquatic environment and therefore less risk of infection via the wicking action of the sutures. In juvenile Chinook salmon, a simple interrupted suture pattern caused less ulceration than a horizontal mattress suture pattern (Deters et al. 2012). In general, having less suture material in the fish to incite a foreign body response is preferred. If a subcuticular pattern cannot be performed because of a thin body wall, the authors recommend a simple interrupted or a Ford interlocking suture pattern (Figure A11.3).

Most dermal suture material in fish needs to be removed, although some absorbable suture material may be lost by the time skin healing has occurred. Even if absorbable, dermal suture material should be removed as soon as there is evidence of adequate healing, as suture material can cause ongoing inflammation and impede healing. Skin healing can take two to six weeks depending on the species and water temperature. In koi undergoing exploratory coeliotomy, a

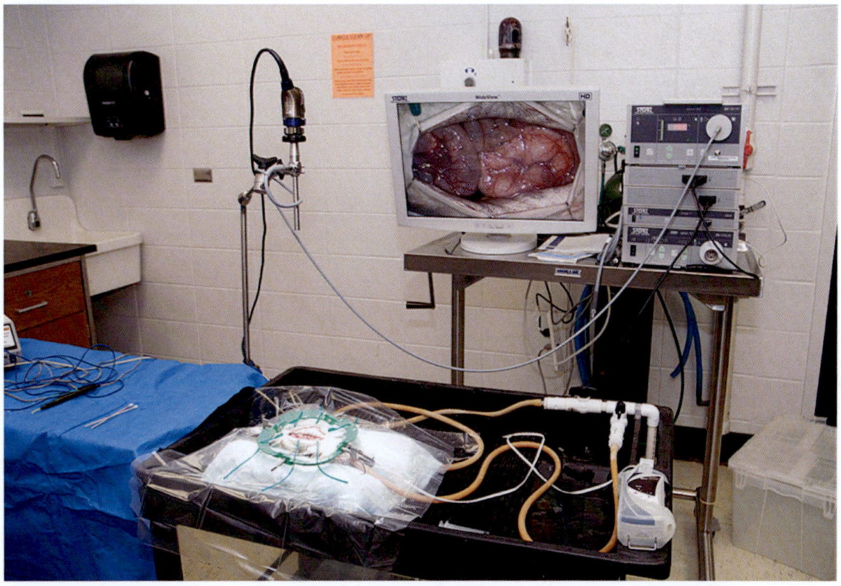

Figure A11.2 The VITOM system (video telescopic operating microscope) positioned for an exploratory coeliotomy. Note the magnification of the surgical site on the monitor. *Source:* Courtesy of University of Georgia.

simple interrupted pattern using polydioxanone resulted in hyperemia, edema, and dehiscence. However, following removal of sutures at day 14, all dehisced wounds healed rapidly by second intention (Christiansen et al. 2015).

Postoperative Management

After surgery, fish are exposed to environmental pathogens that can result in postoperative infections. These are uncommon in fish and there are no studies investigating the use of prophylactic antibiotics to reduce the incidence of infections. Unless the presence of an existing infection is demonstrated, the authors do not recommend prophylactic use of a postoperative antibiotic course, although pre- or intraoperative antibiotics may be considered as per small animal guidelines. For freshwater fish, salt immersion at 1–3 g/L can reduce the risk of postoperative infections by reducing the environmental pathogen load. It also helps with osmoregulation until the integument is healed. Conversely, in marine fish, salinity can be reduced slightly to help with osmoregulation (e.g. from 32 to 28 g/L). Consideration needs to be given to bottom-dwelling fish undergoing ventral surgical approaches; they should be provided with a smooth, clean, nonabrasive and substrate-free surface following surgery. Fish from community tanks may benefit from isolation until healed, as some fish will bite at surgical sites.

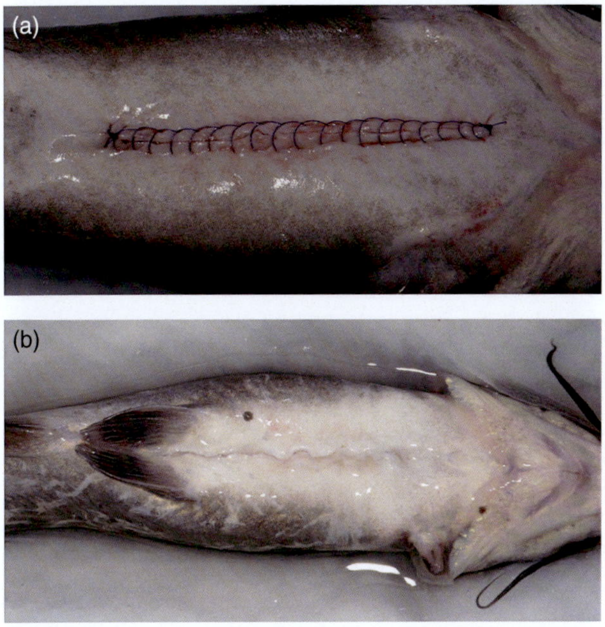

Figure A11.3 Ford interlocking suture pattern (a); subcuticular suture pattern in a channel catfish (*Ictalurus punctatus*) (b). *Source:* Courtesy of University of Georgia.

Surgical Procedures

External Mass Excision/Biopsy

Dermatologic lesions and skin masses are common in fish, including neoplasms, granulomas, abscesses, viral dermatopathies, or exuberant growths (e.g. goldfish wen). External proliferative masses are usually removed by debulking the mass to the level of the skin (Figure A11.4a). Complete excision of masses extending deeper into the tissue layers is often difficult. Radiosurgery, electrocautery, or laser surgery may all be useful for excisions. If present, hemorrhage can be controlled by pressure, gelatin sponges, or radiosurgery. Gelatin sponges or topical pastes often fall off once the fish is placed back in the water. The wound is

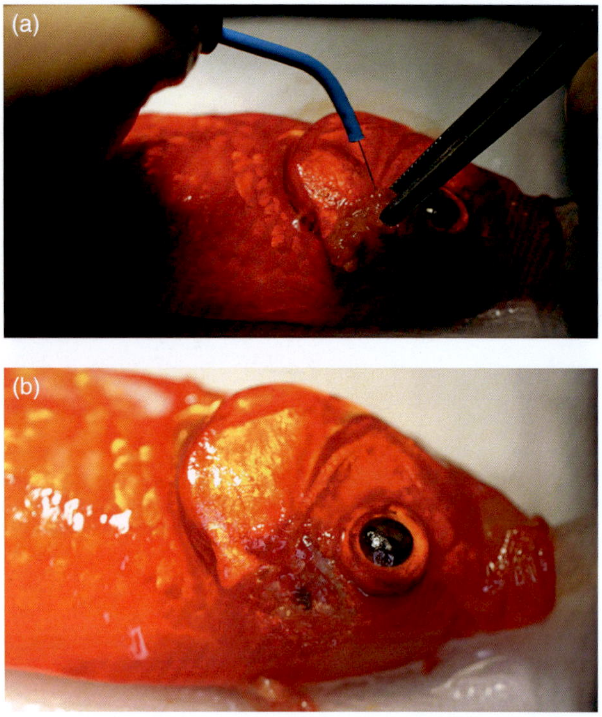

Figure A11.4 Removal of a mass from a goldfish (*Carassius auratus*) (a); postoperative view (b). *Source:* Courtesy of University of Georgia.

usually left open to heal by secondary intention as the relative inelasticity of the skin prevents primary closure (Figure A11.4b). Excised masses may be submitted for culture, cytology, histopathology, or further diagnostics as indicated. Neoplastic or recurrent masses that are unable to be completely excised can be treated with liquid nitrogen cryotherapy or intralesional chemotherapy after debulking, which may result in a curative outcome (Boylan et al. 2015; Vergneau-Grosset et al. 2016). Biopsy techniques used in small animals can be applied to fish. Skin lesions can be biopsied using a punch biopsy and the site allowed to heal by secondary intention. Firm masses can be biopsied using bone or bone marrow biopsy instruments.

Ophthalmic Surgery

Enucleation is indicated with severe ophthalmic disease, particularly in the presence of impaired vision or ocular pain. Common causes include traumatic rupture, infection, cataract with uveitis, or severe exophthalmos or buphthalmos not responsive to other therapies. Fish do not have eyelids. The eye is attached to the orbital rim by the periocular skin. Maxillary and buccal branches of cranial nerve VII and mandibular branch of cranial nerve V pass along the ventrolateral orbital margin. To remove the eye, the periocular skin is transected where it attaches to the globe (Figure A11.5). Periocular muscles are transected close to the globe to minimize hemorrhage. This also reduces the risk of cranial nerve damage. The optic nerve is transected. Hemorrhage can be controlled by pressure, gelatin sponges, a drop of phenylephrine (e.g. phenylephrine hydrochloride 2.5%), or radiosurgery. The socket is left open to heal by secondary intention. The defect typically fills in over days to weeks, but in some cases new skin lines the socket without the space being filled with tissue. Ocular prostheses have been reported in fish but need regular replacement because of tissue remodeling within the socket and should only be used where they benefit the fish, e.g. if euthanasia is the alternative to a prosthesis (Nadelstein et al. 1997).

Cataracts are common in fish and visual impairment may affect quality of life, although some compensation is possible from the lateral line system. In other vertebrates, electroretinograms are routine prior to cataract surgery to ensure the retina is functional. These are possible in fish, but are rarely performed (Bakal et al. 2005). More commonly, cataract removal is carried out when other ocular structures appear healthy on physical examination. Options are phacoemulsification or lens removal (phakectomy). Phacoemulsification has been reported in Gulf sturgeon (*Acipenser oxyrinchus*) with cataracts due to *Diplostomum* spp., with excellent postoperative outcome and return to the wild (Bakal et al. 2005). In aquarium practice, phacoemulsification is typically carried out by veterinary ophthalmologists using standard small animal techniques. Lens removal may be considered as an alternative if phacoemulsification is not available or feasible. It is also commonly used to treat lens luxations. Spectaclectomy and keratectomy were described in three hyperlipidemic moray eels (*Gymnothorax* spp.) for treatment of ocular lipid deposition, which resulted in improved clarity (Clode et al. 2012). Removal of *Philometra* sp. nematodes from the periocular space has been described in redear sunfish (*Lepomis microlophus*) and bluegill (*Lepomis macrochirus*) affected by exophthalmos. The nematodes were removed by making small incisions in the dorsal and ventral conjunctiva, then flushing the periocular space, forcing the parasites through the incision and allowing them to be removed with forceps. Exophthalmos resolved after the removal of the nematodes (Serrano et al. 2011).

Pseudobranch Ablation

Pseudobranch ablation may be considered for management of ocular gas bubble disease in bony fish that is unresponsive to medical management. The pseudobranch is derived from the first gill arch and supplies highly oxygenated blood to the choroid rete and therefore retina, providing a source of gas to the eye. The pseudobranch is accessed

Figure A11.5 Enucleation in a channel catfish (*Ictalurus punctatus*): periocular skin is transected (a); periocular structures are transected to free the globe (b). *Source:* Courtesy of University of Georgia.

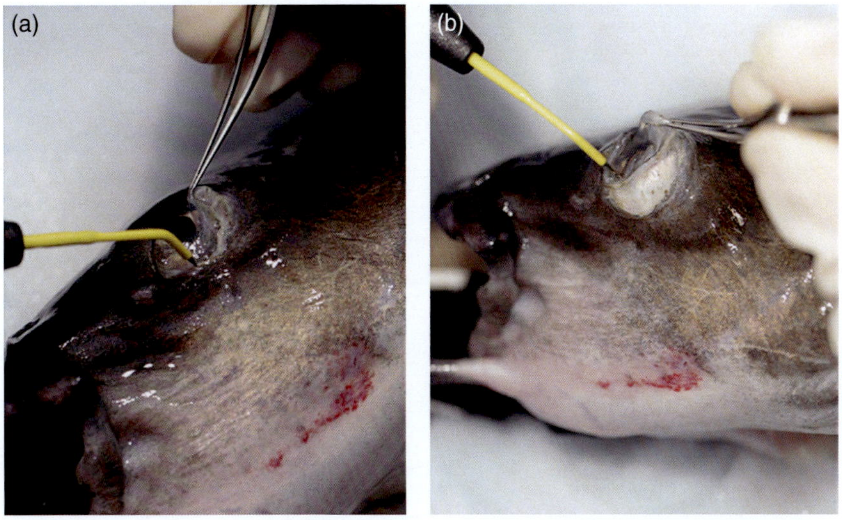

by lifting the operculum and ablated using electrocautery at the base of each primary filament (Figure A11.6) or at the afferent and efferent blood vessels at either end of the gill arch. The pseudobranch is not present or accessible in all fish species, e.g. because of the small opercular slit in filefish (*Monacanthidae*).

Coeliotomy

Indications for exploratory coeliotomy and biopsy collection include the presence of a mass or abnormal tissue architecture on diagnostic imaging, clinicopathologic abnormalities suggestive of organ disease or dysfunction, exploration where other diagnostic investigations have proven inconclusive, or implantation of telemetry devices. In fusiform fish, the fish is typically placed in dorsal recumbency and a ventral midline skin incision is made. The location and extent of the incision are dependent on the procedure and the anatomy of the species. In cases of an exploratory coeliotomy, the incision should extend between the pectoral and pelvic girdles. The skin is the toughest layer and can be difficult to incise in some species. Excess pressure can result in laceration of underlying viscera. The authors recommend creating a skin tent, followed by a stab incision parallel to the body wall using an upward-facing scalpel blade. Alternatively, radiosurgery can facilitate incisions but it is important to minimize collateral damage by using filter-cut settings. The incision can then be extended with scissors or an upward-facing scalpel blade. Once the coeliotomy approach has been made, retractors are placed to aid visualization and access (Figure A11.7). In some cases, the pectoral or pelvic girdles need to be transected for improved exposure; however, this should be avoided if possible to reduce postoperative pain and morbidity. In laterally compressed fish, e.g. surgeonfish (*Acanthuridae*) and flatfish (*Pleuronectiformes*), a lateral incision may be needed, particularly if the dorsal coelomic cavity is the area of interest. Descriptions of exploratory coeliotomy in elasmobranchs are limited. Two case reports in sharks describe a ventral midline approach for foreign body removal (Lécu et al. 2011; Lloyd and Lloyd 2011). A dorsal paramedian coeliotomy approach has been described in subadult southern stingrays (*Hypanus americanus*) for access to the ovary (George et al. 2013). When closing a coeliotomy incision, the skin is the primary holding layer. In small to medium-sized fish (<1–5 kg), a single-layer closure of the skin is usually sufficient. In larger fish, the coelomic membrane and muscle can be closed separately.

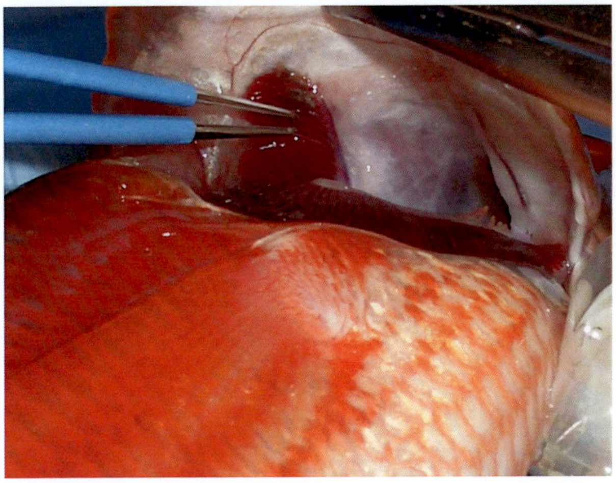

Figure A11.6 Pseudobranch ablation in a squirrelfish (*Holocentrus* sp.). *Source:* Image courtesy of Catherine Hadfield, National Aquarium.

Exploratory Coeliotomy and Biopsy Collection

During exploratory coeliotomy, all internal viscera should be thoroughly evaluated, including the liver, gallbladder,

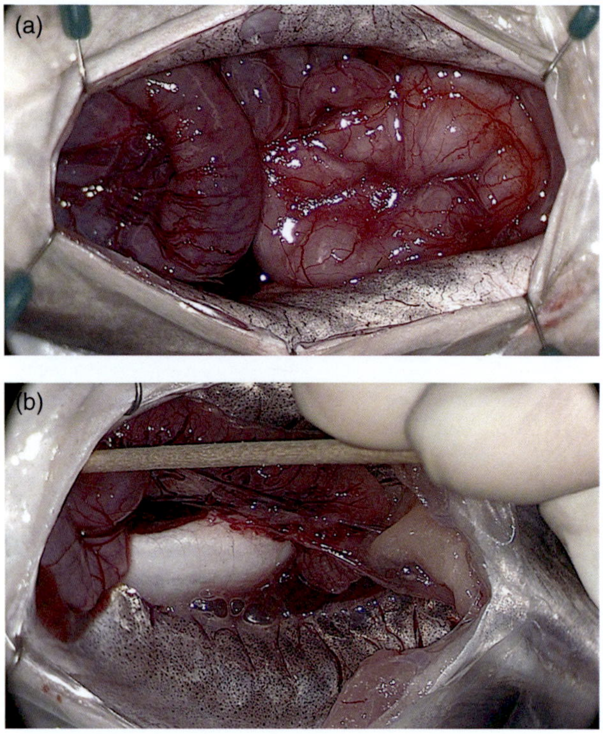

Figure A11.7 Exploratory coeliotomy in a channel catfish (*Ictalurus punctatus*) (a); viscera is gently manipulated using moistened cotton tips (b). *Source:* Courtesy of University of Georgia.

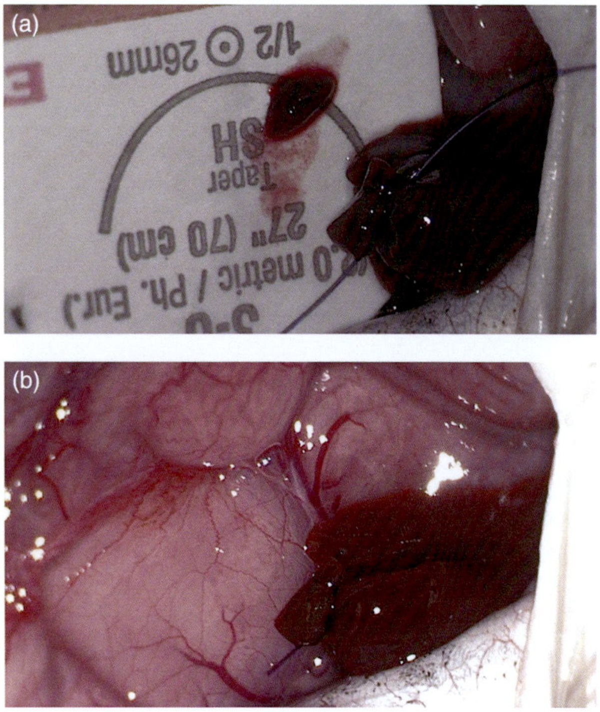

Figure A11.8 Guillotine liver biopsy in a channel catfish (*Ictalurus punctatus*); a suture loop is placed around the edge of the liver and tightened (a), a biopsy is taken distal to the loop, and the suture is cut and the liver lobe released (b). *Source:* Courtesy of University of Georgia.

gastrointestinal tract, reproductive tract, spleen, and swim bladder. Manipulation of the viscera should be gentle, using moistened cotton tips. Some teleost fish have attachments between viscera which may need to be bluntly dissected to aid exploration. Techniques used for biopsy collection are similar to those used in small animals. Liver biopsy can be collected using the guillotine technique with a suture loop (Figure A11.8) (Boone et al. 2008).

Ovariectomy in Teleosts

Indications for ovariectomy include oophoritis, neoplasia, and egg retention. The fish is placed in dorsal recumbency and a coeliotomy approach is made as described above. Ovarian anatomy varies between species. The ovaries may be long and thin, round, or oval, and in some cases may fuse in the midline. In some species, the ovaries may be closely associated with the gastrointestinal tract at the caudal aspect. A long incision is often required. Gentle manipulation is required as the ovary can be friable. The ovary is suspended by the mesovarium and the main blood supply is located at the cranial end. Depending on the size, the blood vessels can be ligated with sutures, vascular clips, or radiosurgery. The mesovarium can be bluntly broken down using hemostats or radiosurgery; this will allow smaller vessels within the ligament to be ligated (Figure A11.9). The coelomic cavity should be flushed and any residual eggs, particularly if the ovary has ruptured during manipulation, should be removed. Ovariectomies have been described in koi and brook trout (*Salvelinus fontinalis*) (Stamper and Norton 2002; Christiansen et al. 2015).

Ovariectomy and Cesarean Section in Elasmobranchs

Literature on elasmobranch reproductive surgery is limited. Significant variations exist between species regarding anatomy and physiology. In many female elasmobranchs, such as cownose rays (*Rhinoptera bonasus*), only the left reproductive tract is functional (Neer and Thompson 2005). Description of batoid ovariectomy is limited to subadult southern stingrays of 50–70 cm disk width. The ray is placed in ventral recumbency. A dorsal approach is made, 2 cm left lateral and parallel to the spinal column. The blood supply is located at the cranial portion of the ovary and is ligated. Caudally, the ovary is attached to the epigonal gland, which is bluntly dissected. The suspensory ligament is bluntly dissected and hemorrhage is controlled if necessary (George et al. 2013). Dystocia is known to occur in elasmobranchs. A cesarean section has been described in a whitetip reef shark (*Triaenodon obesus*). A paramedian approach was made over the caudoventral coelomic wall. Stay sutures were placed in the uterine wall to aid uterine

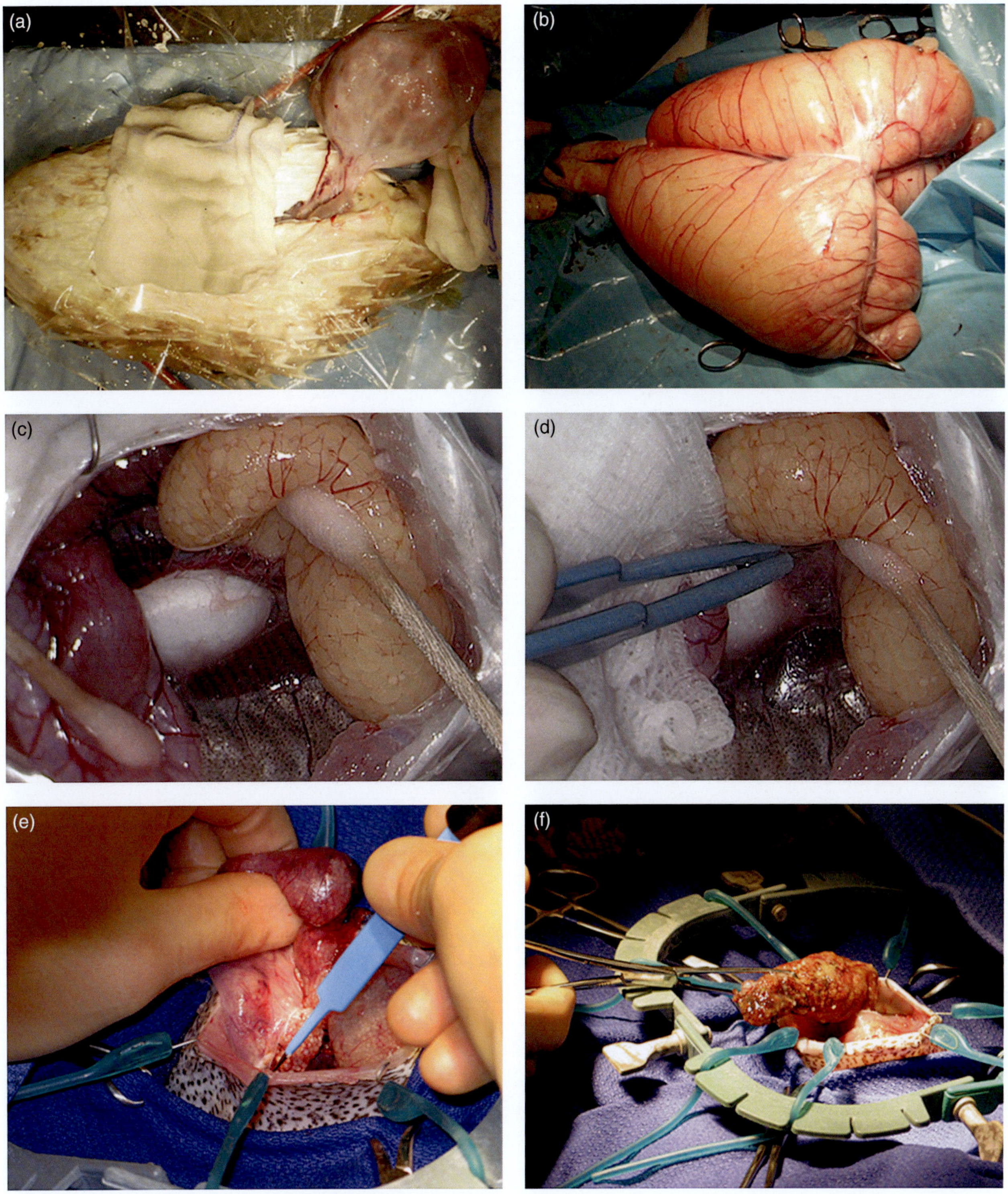

Figure A11.9 Ovariectomy in a spotfin porcupinefish (*Diodon hystrix*) (a); red grouper (*Epinephelus morio*) (b); channel catfish (*Ictalurus punctatus*) (c, d); and red Irish lord (*Hemilepidotus hemilepidotus*) (e, f). *Source:* Images (a-b) courtesy of Catherine Hadfield, National Aquarium. Images (c-f) courtesy of University of Georgia.

manipulation. Pups were removed from the uterine horn, and the fetal membranes and placental attachments removed from the endometrium. The procedure was repeated on the opposite side. The shark recovered well, apart from requiring skin suture replacement due to partial dehiscence (Gearhart et al. 2014). In batoids, a salpingotomy can be performed using the approach described above for a batoid ovariectomy. The uterine material should not

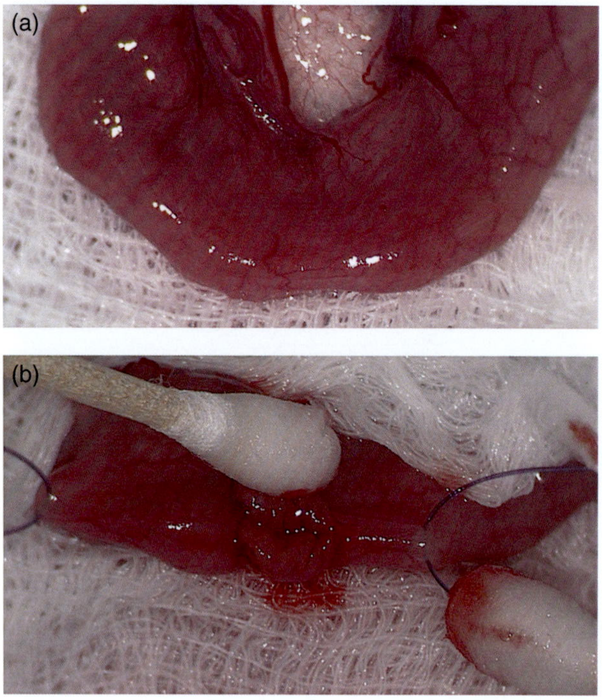

Figure A11.10 Enterotomy in a channel catfish (*Ictalurus punctatus*): a segment of bowel is isolated on a moistened gauze (a); stay sutures are placed at both ends of the incision (b). *Source:* Courtesy of University of Georgia.

be allowed to spill into the coelomic cavity. The uterine incision can be closed as in domestic animals.

Swim Bladder Surgery

Indications for swim bladder surgery include infection, neoplasia, and overinflation. Depending on the anatomy, the swim bladder can be accessed through a ventral midline or lateral incision. A radiograph taken prior to surgery helps in determining the location, anatomy, and pathologic changes associated with the swim bladder. Prior to incising, the region around the swim bladder should be packed with moist gauze or laparotomy sponges to prevent spillage of any pathologic material into the coelomic cavity. A pneumocystoplasty was described in a goldfish with swim bladder overinflation (Britt et al. 2002). Vascular clips were placed transversely across the caudal swim bladder to reduce the volume to an estimated normal volume. The fish died 24 days after surgery. In a goldfish with fungal pneumocystis, a complete pneumocystectomy was performed (Zoller et al. 2017). The goldfish survived for six months following surgery.

Gastrointestinal Surgery

Gastrointestinal surgery is indicated for removal of foreign bodies that cannot be retrieved via endoscopy, repair of perforations and strangulations, and biopsy collection. Foreign body ingestion is common in both teleosts and elasmobranchs (Lécu et al. 2011; Lloyd and Lloyd 2011). Small animal surgical principles apply to piscine gastrointestinal surgery. The area of the tract to be incised is exteriorized and isolated as much as possible. Atraumatic bowel clamps, an assistant's fingers, or stay sutures are placed on either side of the planned incision to prevent leakage (Figure A11.10). At the completion of surgery, the incision is closed in a simple interrupted suture pattern and the incision site tested for leakage. The coelomic cavity should be flushed copiously with sterile saline. In elasmobranchs, sterile fluids with additional sodium chloride and urea may be used for flushing to more closely approximate their plasma osmolality.

Orthopedic Surgery

There have been few reports of orthopedic surgeries in fish. Interfragmentary wire was used to repair mandibular symphyseal fractures in three silver arowana (*Osteoglossum bicirrhosum*) (Lloyd and Sham 2014). Internal stabilization of scoliosis, using cortical bone screws and polymethylmethacrylate, reinforced with Kirschner wire, has been described in two koi. The koi died two to three months postoperatively (Govett et al. 2004).

General Endoscopy Principles

A high standard of care is increasingly expected for fish. This includes minimally invasive diagnostic and surgical procedures, which reduce morbidity and mortality and shorten recovery time. Diagnostic endoscopy has evolved rapidly in zoological medicine and is increasingly applied to fish. Minimally invasive endosurgical techniques are also being developed to replace traditional surgery. Refer to Sections "Introduction" and "General Surgical Principles", which also apply to endoscopic procedures that require a surgical approach.

Rigid Endoscopy Instrumentation

Rigid endoscopy has revolutionized zoological medicine by allowing visualization of internal structures with magnification and collection of samples with precision, from species in which traditional and invasive diagnostic approaches are either risky or almost impossible. Ongoing development and validation of techniques in both diagnostic endoscopy and endosurgery in many non-domestic species have taken the field of zoological medicine to a new level. The application of many of these techniques to fish is an exciting area that will lead to improvement in both diagnostic and therapeutic approaches.

For most fish under 5–10 kg, the 2.7 mm system is suitable and versatile. The 2.7 mm × 18 cm, 30° oblique telescope housed within a 4.8 mm operating sheath allows air or fluid infusion and provides an operating channel for instrument use. A range of 1.7 mm (5-Fr) instruments can be used through the operating channel of a 4.8 mm sheath (Figure A11.11). Biopsy forceps are used for collection of tissue samples for histopathology and microbiology. If sampling a fluid-filled structure, the remote injection/aspiration needle is used. The needle can also be used for intralesional or intracavitary drug delivery. Grasping forceps can be used for debridement of granulomas or retrieval of foreign bodies. Single-action scissors are used to cut through membranes (Divers 2010). The 3.5 mm operating sheath can be used with the telescope for working with multiple 3.5 mm port endosurgery using 3 mm laparoscopy instrumentation. If working with small fish (<250 g), the 1.9 mm integrated telescope, or 1.9 mm telescope within a sheath, may be a more suitable system. The 1.9 mm telescope accommodates 1 mm (3-Fr) instruments, which include the biopsy and grasping forceps. In larger fish (10–200 kg), 5 mm telescopes and instrumentation should be used, while >10 mm may be required for the largest fish.

The light source may be halogen (cheaper and effective for animals <2 kg) or xenon (better quality light and intensity, suitable for larger animals). It is connected to the telescope via a fiber-optic light guide cable for illumination. The telescope eyepiece is connected to an endovideo camera, which is connected to a monitor. The camera allows for image and video documentation. For diagnostic endoscopy, the authors prefer fluid irrigation over gas insufflation. This provides superior visualization of the mucosal and serosal surfaces and avoids postoperative buoyancy issues. Fluid, most often sterile physiologic saline, is used for irrigation. In marine fish, a modified salt solution may be more physiologic, although the benefit of this has not been investigated and the authors have not observed an appreciable difference. A fluid bag is suspended above the operating table and delivered via the ingress port. Flow is controlled by varying the height of the bag above the fish and via the ingress and egress ports of the operating sheath. A list of equipment needs for rigid endoscopy in fish can be found in Box A11.1.

Rigid Endoscope Handling and Use

There are certain principles that should be followed to optimize surgeon ergonomics and improve diagnostic value. The monitor should always be placed in front of the surgeon and the patient should be appropriately positioned for the procedure. Precise control of the telescope is essential when working in small patients or a small space. The telescope is supported using the dominant hand, and the distal sheath is held by thumb and index finger of the inferior hand. This allows the dominant hand to manipulate the telescope, while the inferior hand prevents tremors and unintentional advancing of the telescope, which may result in trauma. For instrument use, the inferior hand grasps the telescope sheath and holds the weight of the entire unit, using the thumb to prevent rotation. The dominant hand is used to pass the instruments down the operating channel (Figure A11.12). The instrument is passed until it appears in the center of the field of view. With the instrument held open, the sheath–telescope unit is moved as a whole to a proposed sampling site. This allows for precision in instrument manipulation, compared to moving the instrument back and forth independently. Once the instrument is closed, it is important not to clamp down on the sample as

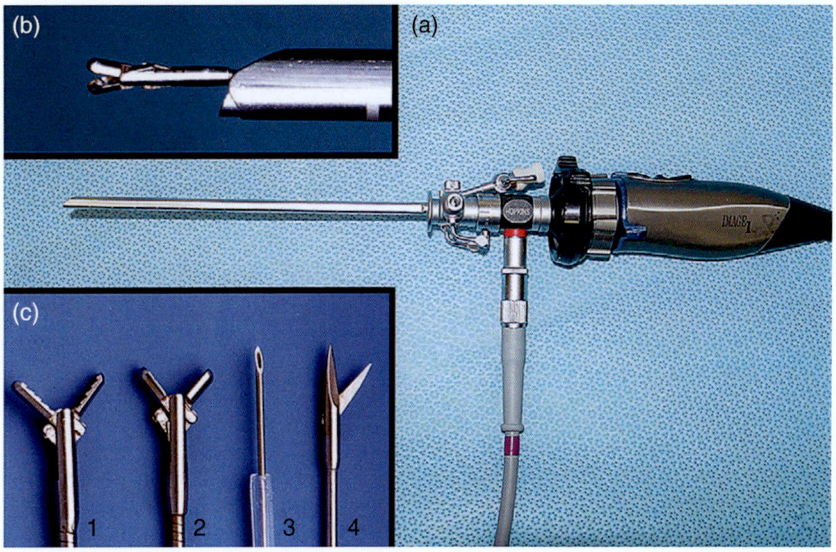

Figure A11.11 A 2.7 mm telescope system: 2.7 mm 30° telescope housed within a 4.8 mm operating sheath, connected to a light cable and an endovideo camera (a); 1.7 mm biopsy forceps inserted down the instrument channel and exiting in front of the telescope (b); 1.7 mm instruments for use through the operating channel (c): retrieval forceps (1), biopsy forceps (2), remote injection/aspiration needle (3), single-action scissors (4). *Source:* Courtesy of University of Georgia.

Box A11.1 Rigid Endoscopy Instrumentation for Fish

Equipment description	Primary indications
Endovideo camera and monitor Xenon light source and light guide cable Digital capture device (e.g. AIDA-Vet)	Required for all endoscopy procedures
1.9 mm × 18.5 cm telescope, 30° oblique, with integrated 3.3 mm operating sheath	Fish <250 g
2.7 mm × 18 cm telescope, 30° oblique 4.8 mm operating sheath	Fish 0.25–10 kg
5 mm × 29 cm telescope, 0°	Fish >10 kg
1 mm biopsy forceps 1 mm grasping forceps	For use with 1.9 mm telescope and integrated sheath
1.7 mm biopsy forceps 1.3 mm single-action scissors 1.7 mm remote injection needle 1.7 mm grasping/retrieval forceps 1.7 mm wire basket retrieval 1.7 mm needle end radiosurgery electrode 1.7 mm polypectomy snare	For use with 2.7 mm telescope and 4.8 mm operating sheath
CO_2 insufflator with silicone tubing	Used for insufflation during coelioscopy
Sterile saline suspended above endoscopy table with intravenous drip line to a port on the operating sheath	Used for irrigation during coelioscopy
Reddick–Olsen dissecting forceps Metzenbaum scissors Babcock forceps Fenestrated grasping forceps Reddick–Olsen dissecting and grasping forceps Short, curved Kelly dissecting and grasping forceps Atraumatic dissecting and grasping forceps Blakesley dissecting and biopsy forceps Scissors with serrated curved double-action jaws Micro hook scissors, single-action jaws Manhes bipolar coagulation forceps Irrigation and suction cannula Palpation probe with cm markings Distensible palpation probe Ultramicro needle holder Knot-tier for extracorporeal suturing Handles (for 2-, 3-, and 5 mm instruments) • Plastic or metal • Manhes-style or haemostat-style racket Cannulae, available in 2.5-, 3.5-, 3.9- (graphite and plastic), and 6 mm (metal)	Rigid instruments, handles and cannulae for multiple-entry coelioscopy
3.8 or 4.0 MHz dual radiofrequency unit with foot pedal Monopolar lead to connect to plastic instrument handles Bipolar lead to connect to 3 mm Manhes bipolar coagulation forceps LigaSure Atlas in 5 and 10 mm	Radiosurgery equipment

this can cause damage and result in increased crush artifact.

Endosurgery

Compared to diagnostic endoscopy, endosurgery requires additional equipment and greater skills for coordinating various instruments through multiple ports. Port cannulae, endosurgical instrumentation, carbon dioxide insufflator, and hemostasis capabilities are required for most endosurgical procedures (Divers 2010).

Flexible Endoscopy

Flexible endoscopy has applications in foreign body removal and gastrointestinal evaluation and biopsy in larger fish where the length of the rigid endoscope is limiting. This has predominantly been applied to elasmobranchs and large teleosts in aquarium collections. There are two main flexible endoscopes available: fiberscopes and video endoscopes. Fiberscopes are available in smaller diameters while video endoscopes provide better image quality. Larger flexible endoscopes have a four-way deflection, instrument channels, air insufflation, and suction

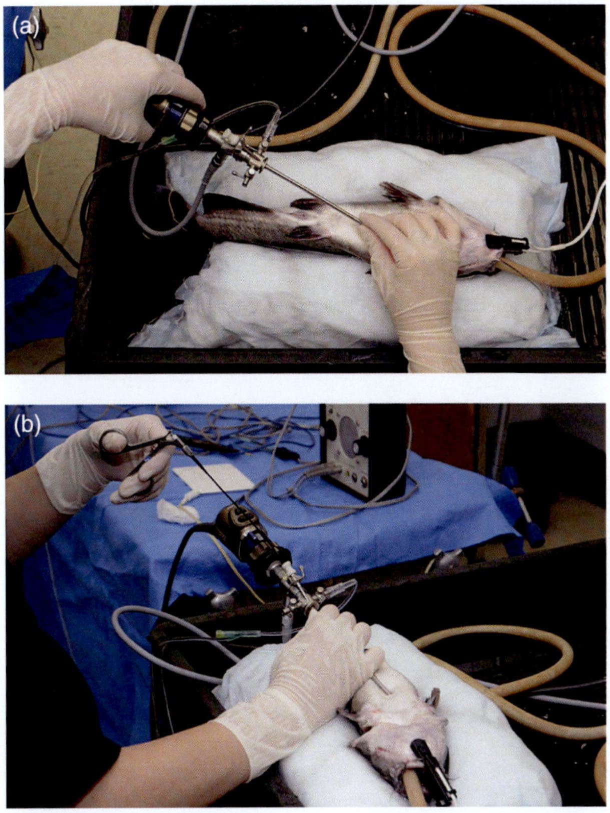

Figure A11.12 Handling of the 2.7 mm telescope housed within a 4.8 mm operating sheath by a left-handed operator: the two-handed technique involves supporting the camera and telescope using the dominant hand, while the thumb and forefinger of the inferior hand stabilize the distal end of the telescope (a); the use of an instrument using the one-handed technique can be facilitated by using the inferior hand to stabilize and take the weight of the telescope unit, while the dominant hand is used to pass the instrument down the operating channel (b). *Source:* Courtesy of University of Georgia.

capabilities. Smaller endoscopes have a one- or two-way deflection, smaller instrument channels, and no insufflation or suction capabilities. The instrument channel can be used for air insufflation; however, this limits its concurrent use with an instrument.

Endoscopic Procedures

Gill Endoscopy and Stomatoscopy

Gill endoscopy is indicated for investigation of gill disease, including parasitic and bacterial infections, and collection of gill samples. Traditional biopsies of the primary filament tips may miss lesions if the disease is focal, at the base of the gill filaments, or hidden from the naked eye. Some teleost fish have small opercula, making visualization of the gills difficult, e.g. frogfish (*Antennariidae*). In elasmobranchs, direct visualization of gills is limited by the anatomy of the gill slits. Endoscopy of the gills provides magnification and improved visualization of the gill filaments and lesions, allowing precise biopsy collection. Gills can be visualized via the operculum or gill slit, or through the oral cavity. The fish is positioned in dorsal recumbency. The pump delivering anesthesia over the gills or keeping the fish partially suspended in water provides irrigation to allow visualization (Figure A11.13).

Stomatoscopy is indicated for investigation of inappetence or dysphagia, sampling of oral lesions, retrieval of foreign bodies, and assessment of dental disease. Some species have a small opening into the oral cavity, further necessitating the use of an endoscope, e.g. parrotfish (*Scarinae*). The fish is positioned in dorsal, ventral, or lateral recumbency, depending on the anatomy. Similar to gill endoscopy, some form of irrigation is often present around the oral cavity, allowing for visualization without additional irrigation (Figure A11.14).

Gastroscopy

Indications for gastroscopy include foreign body retrieval, and investigation of chronic regurgitation/vomiting, weight loss, or inappetence. A gastric disorder may also be suspected based on abnormal diagnostic imaging or clinicopathologic findings. The fish can be placed in dorsal or ventral recumbency. If additional fluid irrigation is needed, a slight reverse Trendelenburg position (head higher than the rest of the body) may be beneficial (Figure A11.15a). As the telescope is advanced past the oral cavity, the ingress port is slightly opened to provide irrigation and aid visualization as the telescope is passed into the stomach (Figure A11.15b, c). In larger fish, if the rigid endoscope is not sufficiently long, a flexible gastroscope is required, using air/saline insufflation to provide a working space. Any identified lesions or foreign bodies can be biopsied or retrieved, respectively. Gastroscopy with a flexible endoscope was used to investigate chronic regurgitation in a green moray eel (*Gymnothorax funebris*) and to manage a reef manta ray (*Manta alfredi*) with substrate retention (Meegan et al. 2012; McDermott et al. 2016).

Cloacoscopy

Indications for cloacoscopy include prolapse, abnormal feces, hematochezia, presence of masses, or reproductive assessment. In elasmobranchs and lungfish, a single external opening (cloaca) is present. In chimaeras and most bony fish, two external openings are visible (an anus and a more cranial opening with urinary and genital pores). The fish is positioned in dorsal recumbency. The telescope is passed through the opening using saline irrigation. The opening is

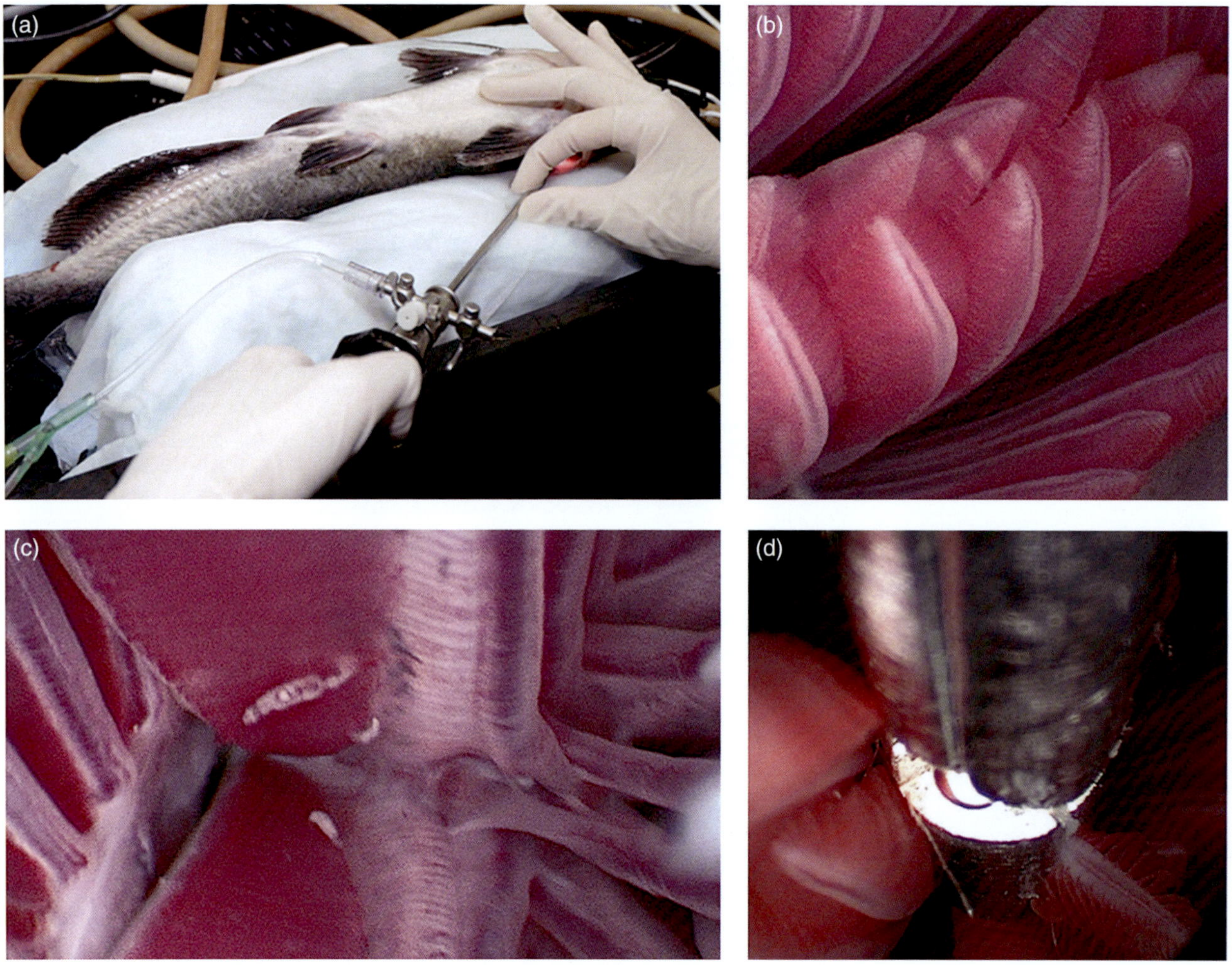

Figure A11.13 Gill endoscopy in a channel catfish (*Ictalurus punctatus*): a 2.7 mm telescope is being used to examine the gills via the operculum (a); endoscopic image of the gill filaments (b); parasites on the proximal gill filaments (c); a gill biopsy taken using 1.7 mm biopsy forceps (d). *Source:* Courtesy of University of Georgia.

pinched at the edge to prevent leakage of infused saline, allowing the lumen to distend for adequate visualization (Figure A11.16). Alternatively, a Trendelenburg position may be used. Fluid irrigation is stopped once adequate visualization is achieved as excessive fluid administration can result in iatrogenic trauma. Any identified lesions can be biopsied, although to avoid perforation the biopsy forceps should be positioned parallel, and not perpendicular, to the intestinal wall.

Coelioscopy

Indications for coelioscopy are similar to those of coeliotomy; it allows for exploration and evaluation of internal viscera as well as biopsy collection. Coelioscopy has also been used for determination of sex and reproductive stages for management and conservation efforts (Divers et al. 2009; Munhofen et al. 2014). Compared to coeliotomy, coelioscopy is less traumatic, provides a more complete and magnified examination of the coelomic cavity, and carries less risk of postsurgical complications, such as wound dehiscence and weight loss (Boone et al. 2008; Macrì et al. 2014).

The coelioscopic approach is dependent on the anatomy of the fish. For dorsoventrally compressed or fusiform fish, a ventral approach is best, with the fish positioned in dorsal recumbency. For laterally compressed fish, a paramedian or lateral approach may be more suitable, with the fish positioned in lateral recumbency. The choice of entrance point also depends on the organ of interest. A small skin incision (~4–5 mm if using a 4.8 mm operating sheath) is made at the entrance point. For a ventral approach, the most common entrance point is approximately 50–70% of the distance from pectoral to pelvic fins. The skin is grasped and elevated. Following incision, small straight hemostats are used to bluntly enter the coelomic cavity through the muscle and coelomic membrane. The hemostats are then

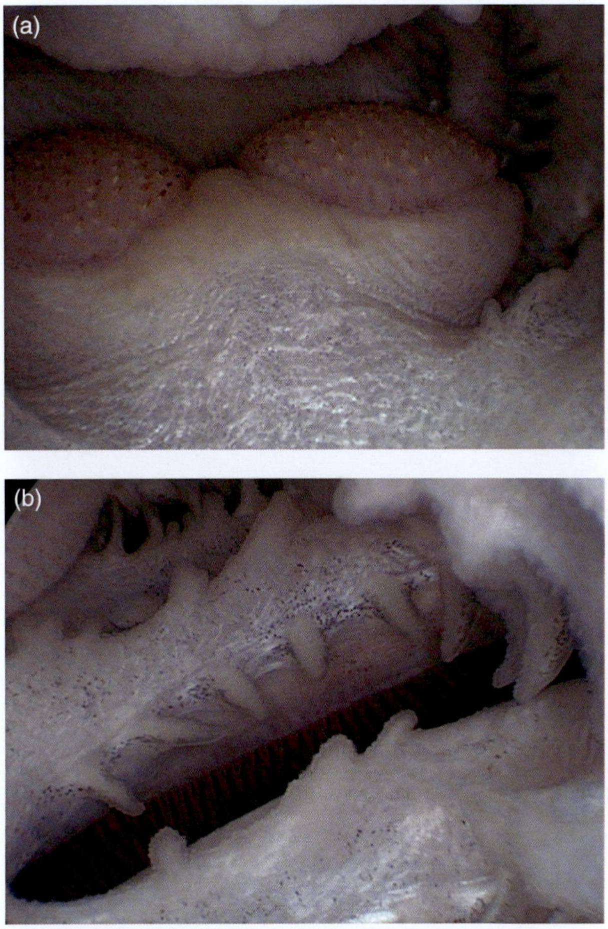

Figure A11.14 Stomatoscopy in a channel catfish (*Ictalurus punctatus*) using a 2.7 mm telescope (a), note the pharyngeal teeth; the gill filaments are visible behind the gill rakers (b). *Source:* Courtesy of University of Georgia.

removed and the telescope-sheath unit is passed through the incision to confirm entrance into the coelomic cavity (Figure A11.17). Alternatively, the operating sheath and obturator can be used (instead of hemostats) and offer the advantage that the coeliotomy hole does not have to be relocated, because once inserted, the obturator is removed and replaced by the telescope. A small skin incision will ensure a snug fit around the sheath, allowing insufflation/irrigation of the coelomic cavity. If the incision is too large and leakage is occurring, a mattress suture can be placed around the telescope to create a seal (Hasson technique).

To create a working space within the coelomic cavity, insufflation with carbon dioxide (CO_2) gas or irrigation with sterile saline is required. Veterinarians have used air pumps for insufflation to deliver room air. The issues with this technique are lack of pressure control, risk of air embolism, drying out of the viscera, and prolonged residual presence of the air. Compared to insufflation, fluid irrigation provides superior detail and allows the organs to "suspend," increasing the access of the telescope between organs, particularly dorsally located structures (Figure A11.18). Fluid irrigation should be stopped once adequate visualization is achieved, as excessive fluid administration in the coelomic cavity may affect cardiac function or cause a prolapse. In fish with substantial lipid in the coelomic cavity or the liver (e.g. elasmobranchs or obese teleosts), the fluid may become cloudy with lipid droplets impeding visualization, particularly if biopsies are taken. For this reason, it is important that biopsies are taken last, after thorough inspection of the coelomic cavity has been performed. CO_2 gas insufflation may be better in these cases, although flushing of the coelomic cavity through the ingress and egress ports may also help. Gas insufflation is required when performing endosurgery or if the integrity of the swim bladder is compromised. If using CO_2, pressures of up to 8 mm Hg provide adequate working space. In some cases, pressures of up to 12 mm Hg may be required. In mammals, pressures over 12 mm Hg are not recommended and can impede ventilation and venous return. Although this is not a problem in fish due to their lack of lungs, excessive pressure may affect cardiac function or cause prolapses (Murray 2010; Stetter 2010). In very small fish, air delivered manually by a syringe through the ingress port can also be used. Organs that can be visualized via coelioscopy include liver, gallbladder, spleen, pancreas (if visible grossly), gastrointestinal tract, reproductive tract, heart (indirectly), kidney, and swim bladder (Figure A11.18). In elasmobranchs, the coelomic cavity can be entered via the abdominal pores lateral to the cloaca, providing a completely nonsurgical approach. Depending on the size of the animal, this approach limits visualization to the caudal coelom and it is not yet known if there are physiological consequences to this approach. At the completion of coelioscopy, any infused air or fluid should be removed to reduce postoperative discomfort. A single suture is used for closure.

Liver Biopsy

To obtain a liver biopsy using the 2.7 mm system, the biopsy forceps are passed through the instrument channel until they appear in the center of the view. Any focal lesion should be biopsied. Otherwise, a liver biopsy is taken from the edge of the liver (Figure A11.19a, b). Using the 1.7 mm biopsy instrument, the liver biopsy specimens obtained are of similar diagnostic quality for histologic evaluation to surgically obtained specimens (Boone et al. 2008). Larger samples may be required for more extensive evaluation. A two-port technique allows sample collection using larger biopsy cups. The use of optical biopsy forceps has been described in free-ranging river sturgeon (*Scaphirhynchus* spp.) to obtain large liver biopsies weighing on average 0.9 g (up to 10% of total liver mass) for toxicologic analysis (Divers et al. 2013).

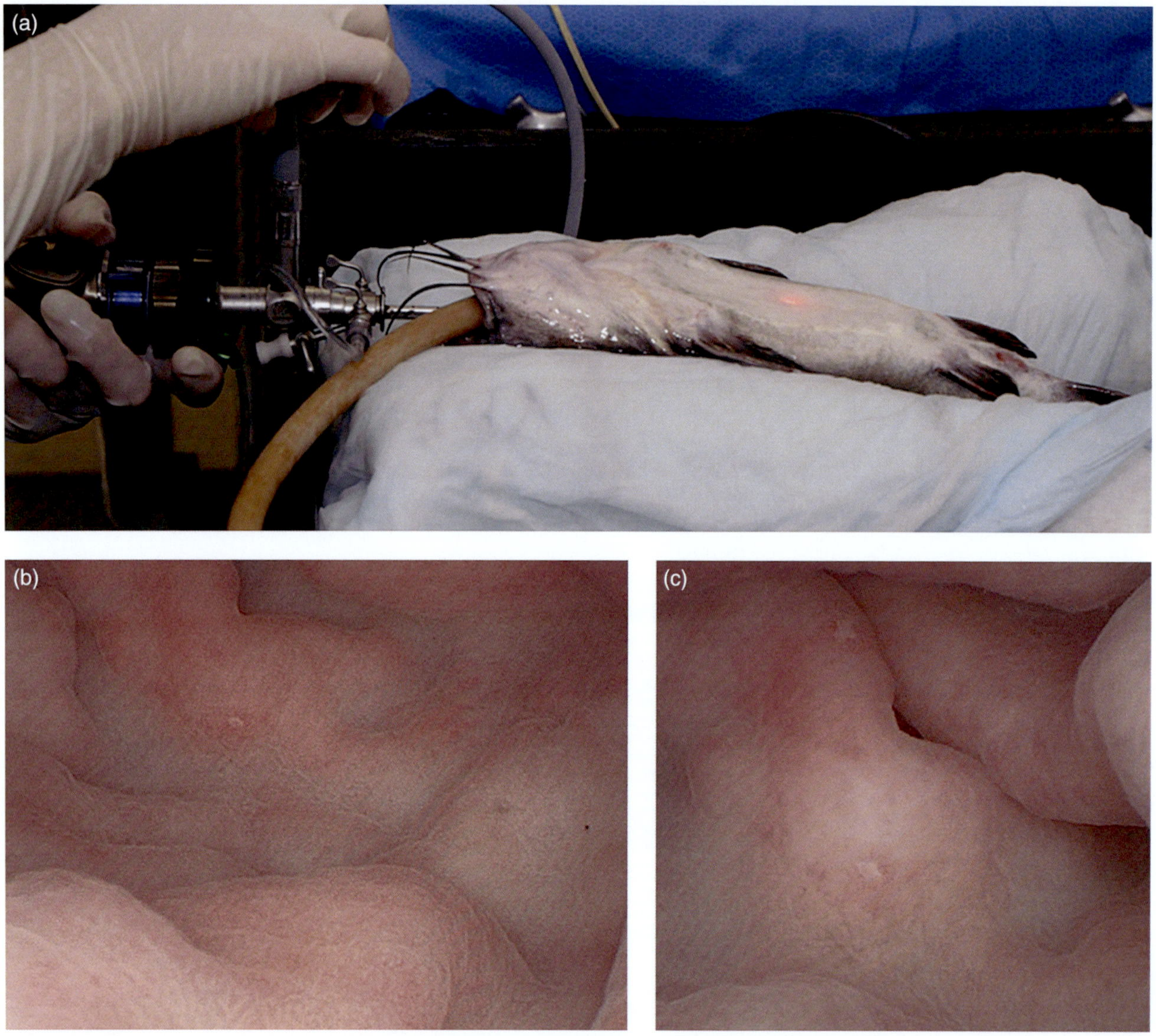

Figure A11.15 Gastroscopy in a channel catfish (*Ictalurus punctatus*) using a 2.7 mm telescope and saline irrigation delivered via the ingress port (a); endoscopic images of the mucosal surface of the stomach (b, c). *Source:* Courtesy of University of Georgia.

Kidney Biopsy

The retrocoelomic position of the kidneys usually necessitates a dorsolateral approach or scissor incision through the dorsal coelomic membrane to access the kidneys for biopsy (Figure A11.19c, d). In some bony fish, ventral or lateral access to the kidney is impeded by the swim bladder, which may need to be collapsed by endoscope-guided needle aspiration. In some bony fish, the cranial kidney can be biopsied through the opercular space using a Tru-cut biopsy tool.

Pneumocystoscopy

Most bony fish have swim bladders and pathology is common. Indications for pneumocystoscopy include buoyancy disorders or swim bladder abnormalities noted on diagnostic imaging. A radiograph taken prior to endoscopy helps in determining the location of the swim bladder and/or location of swim bladder pathology. A mini-coeliotomy (~1 cm) is made over the proposed swim bladder entry site. Once the coelomic cavity is entered, stay sutures can be placed in the swim bladder, which will allow closure after endoscopy, and a small incision is made in the swim bladder. The telescope is then inserted into the swim bladder. Insufflation is not required for pneumocystoscopy as air is already present (Figure A11.20). Fluid should not be instilled into the swim bladder. The authors prefer to close the swim bladder after endoscopy.

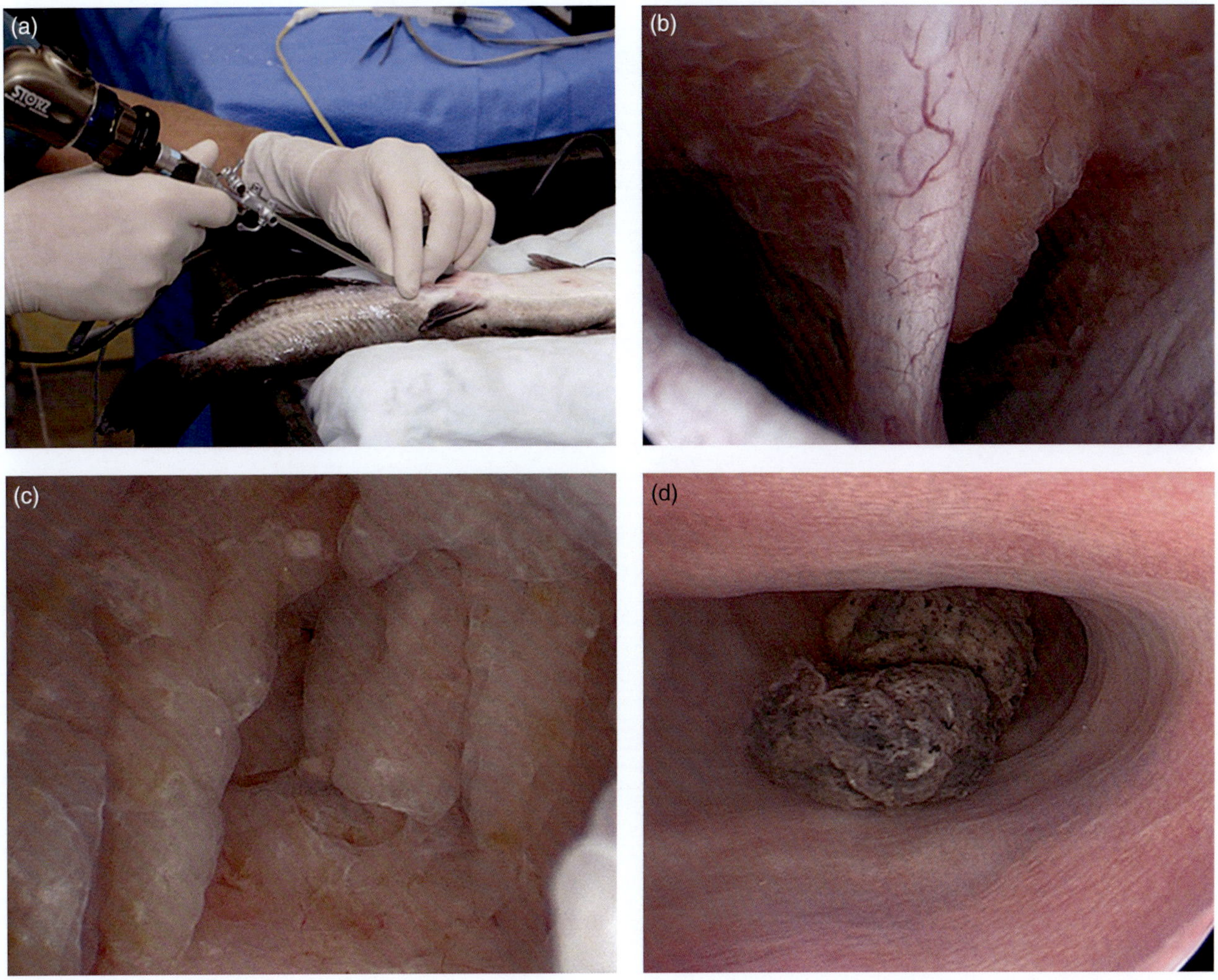

Figure A11.16 Cloacoscopy in a channel catfish (*Ictalurus punctatus*) using a 2.7 mm telescope. The opening is pinched at the edge to prevent infused fluid from escaping, allowing the lumen to distend for visualization (a); endoscopic images of the urogenital opening (b, c); colonoscopy (d). *Source:* Courtesy of University of Georgia.

Biopsy Sample Handling

Samples collected with 1.7 or 1 mm biopsy instruments are small and delicate and need to be handled carefully to prevent damage to the tissue architecture and to avoid artifacts. After collecting a sample, the biopsy cup is placed in a small volume of sterile saline and gently shaken to dislodge the sample. The sample is then decanted onto a sponge and placed in a biopsy cassette before fixation (Figure A11.21). Picking up a sample using a needle or cotton tips can result in sample damage.

Endosurgical Procedures

Endosurgical procedures are in their infancy in fish. In zoological medicine, reproductive tract endosurgery is becoming routine. Reproductive diseases are common in fish, and endosurgery could improve outcomes. This is particularly the case in species in which gonads are elongated, requiring an extensive surgical approach. Endosurgical ovariectomy and orchidectomy, and spermatic and Müllerian duct ligation have been successfully performed in Gulf sturgeon (Figure A11.22). A three-port approach was used. Carbon dioxide insufflation created a working space, while aspiration of the swim bladder further improved access and visualization (Hernandez-Divers et al. 2004).

Endoscopy-assisted surgery allows traditional surgeries to be performed via a smaller incision. A common example is an enterotomy, where a loop of bowel of interest is identified endoscopically and then exteriorized through a minilaparotomy. This facilitates exploration while the actual surgical procedure is carried out through the smallest possible incision.

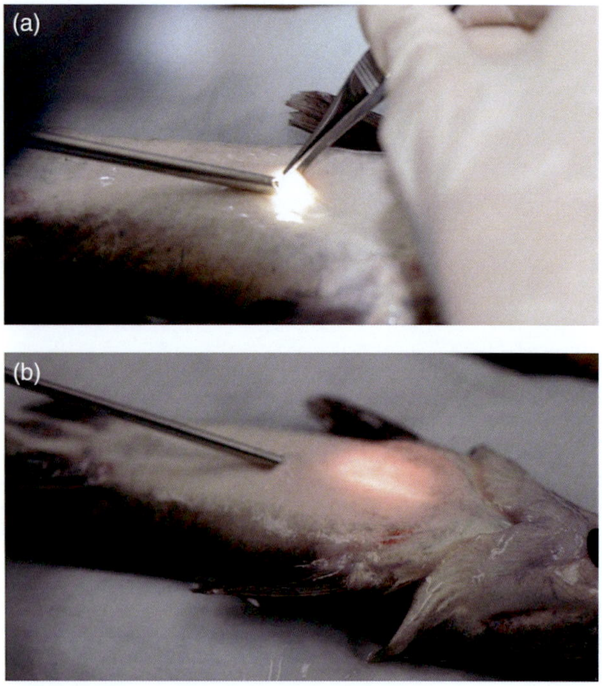

Figure A11.17 A surgical approach is made for a coelioscopy in a channel catfish (*Ictalurus punctatus*) and a 2.7 mm telescope is inserted through the opening (a); the placement of the telescope is confirmed and the coelomic cavity can be insufflated or irrigated (b). *Source:* Courtesy of University of Georgia.

Conclusion

Ongoing development and application of endoscopy and surgery in fish is an exciting and evolving area within zoological medicine. The authors encourage the readers to continue contributing to the literature in the field of fish surgery and endoscopy, including cases with unique anatomy, utilization of novel techniques, and original research.

Acknowledgments

The authors would like to thank Karl Storz Veterinary Endoscopy for their continued support of endoscopy research and development programs. The authors are also thankful to all the technicians, students, interns, residents, and faculty that assist with research and clinical cases at the University of Georgia.

References

Bakal, R.S., Hickson, B.H., Gilger, B.C. et al. (2005). Surgical removal of cataracts due to *Diplostomum* species in Gulf sturgeon (*Acipenser oxyrinchus desotoi*). *Journal of Zoo and Wildlife Medicine* 36: 504–508.

Boone, S.S., Hernandez-Divers, S.J., Radlinsky, M.G. et al. (2008). Comparison between coelioscopy and coeliotomy for liver biopsy in channel catfish. *Journal of the American Veterinary Medical Association* 233: 960–967.

Boone, S.S., Hernandez, S.M., Camus, A.C. et al. (2013). Evaluation of four suture materials for surgical incision closure in siberian sturgeon. *Transactions of the American Fisheries Society* 142: 649–659.

Boylan, S.M., Camus, A., Waltzek, T. et al. (2015). Liquid nitrogen cryotherapy for fibromas in tarpon, *Megalops atlanticus*, Valenciennes 1847, and neoplasia in lined sea horse, *Hippocampus erectus*, Perry 1810. *Journal of Fish Diseases* 38: 681–685.

Britt, T., Weisse, C., Weber, E.S. et al. (2002). Use of pneumocystoplasty for overinflation of the swim bladder in a goldfish. *Journal of the American Veterinary Medical Association* 221: 690–693.

Christiansen, E.F., Cray, C., Lewbart, G.A., and Harms, C.A. (2015). Plasma protein electrophoresis and acute phase proteins in koi carp (*Cyprinus carpio*) following exploratory coeliotomy. *Journal of Exotic Pet Medicine* 24: 76–83.

Clode, A.B., Harms, C., Fatzinger, M.H. et al. (2012). Identification and management of ocular lipid deposition in association with hyperlipidaemia in captive moray eels, *Gymnothorax funebris* Ranzani, *Gymnothorax moringa* (Cuvier) and *Muraena retifera* Goode and Bean. *Journal of Fish Diseases* 35: 683–693.

Deters, K.A., Brown, R.S., Carter, K.M., and Boyd, J.W. (2010). Performance assessment of suture type, water temperature, and surgeon skill in juvenile Chinook salmon surgically implanted with acoustic transmitters. *Transactions of the American Fisheries Society* 139: 888–899.

Deters, K.A., Brown, R.S., Boyd, J.W. et al. (2012). Optimal suturing technique and number of sutures for surgical implantation of acoustic transmitters in juvenile salmonids. *Transactions of the American Fisheries Society* 141: 1–10.

Divers, S.J. (2010). Endoscopy equipment and instrumentation for use in exotic animal medicine. *Veterinary Clinics of North America: Exotic Animal Practice* 13: 171–185.

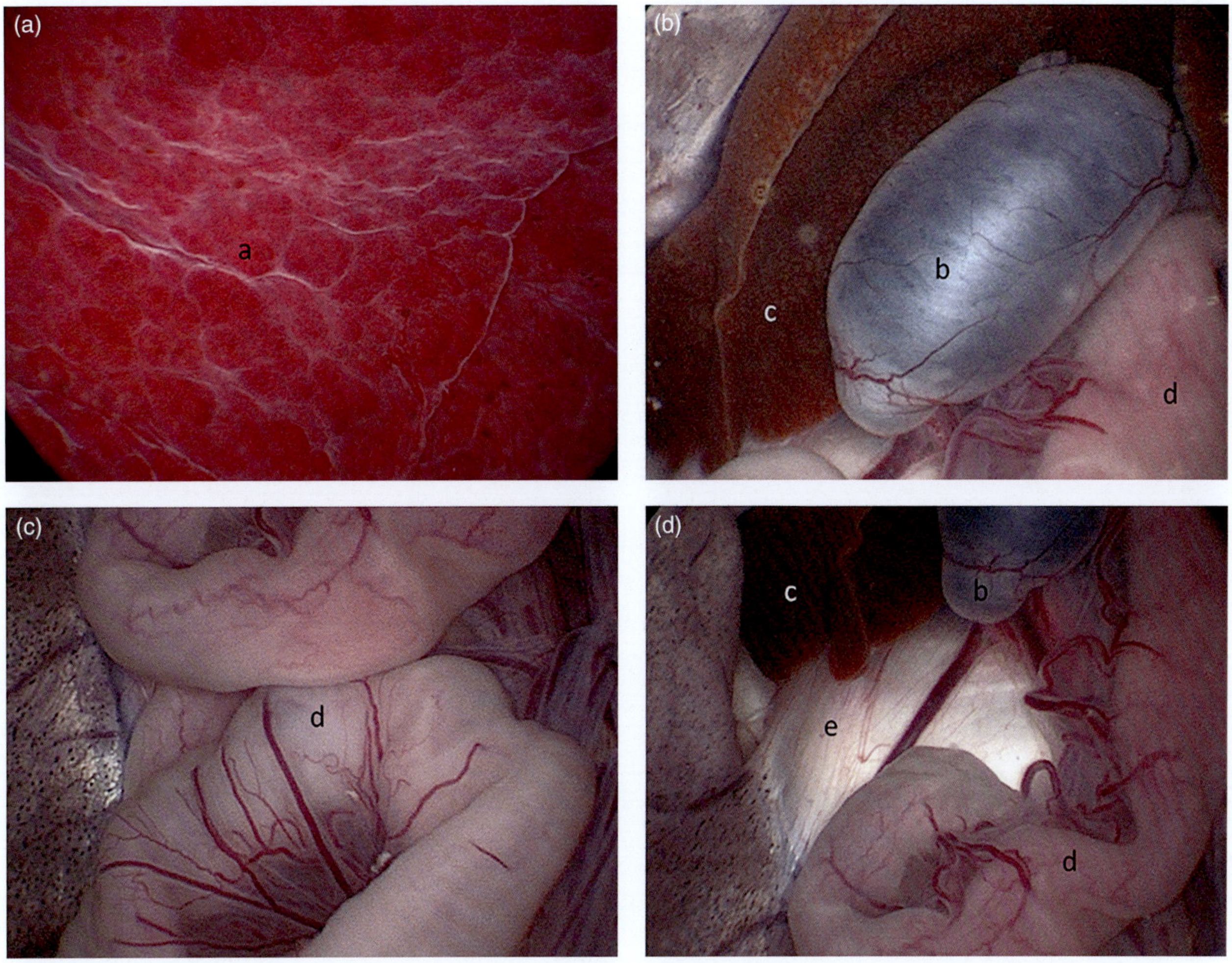

Figure A11.18 Coelioscopy in a channel catfish (*Ictalurus punctatus*) using a 2.7 mm telescope and saline irrigation: spleen (a), gallbladder (b), liver (c), intestinal loop (d), swim bladder (e). *Source:* Courtesy of University of Georgia.

Divers, S.J., Boone, S.S., Hoover, J.J. et al. (2009). Field endoscopy for identifying gender, reproductive stage and gonadal anomalies in free-ranging sturgeon (*Scaphirhynchus*) from the lower Mississippi River. *Journal of Applied Ichthyology* 25: 68–74.

Divers, S.J., Boone, S.S., Berliner, A. et al. (2013). Nonlethal acquisition of large liver samples from free-ranging river sturgeon (*Scaphirhynchus*) using single-entry endoscopic biopsy forceps. *Journal of Wildlife Diseases* 49: 321–331.

Gamperl, A.K. and Shiels, H.A. (2013). Cardiovascular system. In: The Physiology of Fishes, 4e (eds. D.H. Evans, J.B. Claiborne and S. Currie), 36. Boca Raton, FL: CRC Press, Taylor and Francis Group.

Gearhart, S.A., Croft, L.A., and Swider, D.A. (2014). Cesarian section in the whitetip reef shark (*Triaenodon obesus*). *Proceedings of the International Association for Aquatic Animal Medicine Conference*, Gold Coast, Australia.

George, R.H., Steeil, J., and Baine, K. (2013). Ovariectomy of sub-adult southern stingrays (*Dasyatis americana*) to prevent future reproductive problems. *Proceedings of the International Association for Aquatic Animal Medicine Conference*, Sausalito, CA.

Govett, P.D., Olby, N.J., Marcellin-Little, D.J. et al. (2004). Stabilisation of scoliosis in two koi (*Cyprinus carpio*). *Veterinary Record* 155: 115–119.

Hernandez-Divers, S.J., Bakal, R.S., Hickson, B.H. et al. (2004). Endoscopic sex determination and gonadal manipulation in Gulf of Mexico sturgeon (*Acipenser oxyrinchus desotoi*). *Journal of Zoo and Wildlife Medicine* 35: 459–470.

Hurty, C.A., Brazik, D.C., Law, J.M. et al. (2002). Evaluation of the tissue reactions in the skin and body wall of koi (*Cyprinus caprio*) to five suture materials. *Veterinary Record* 151: 324–328.

Lécu, A., Herbert, R., Coulier, L., and Murray, M.J. (2011). Removal of an intracoelomic hook via laparotomy in a sandbar shark (*Carcharhinus plumbeus*). *Journal of Zoo and Wildlife Medicine* 42: 256–262.

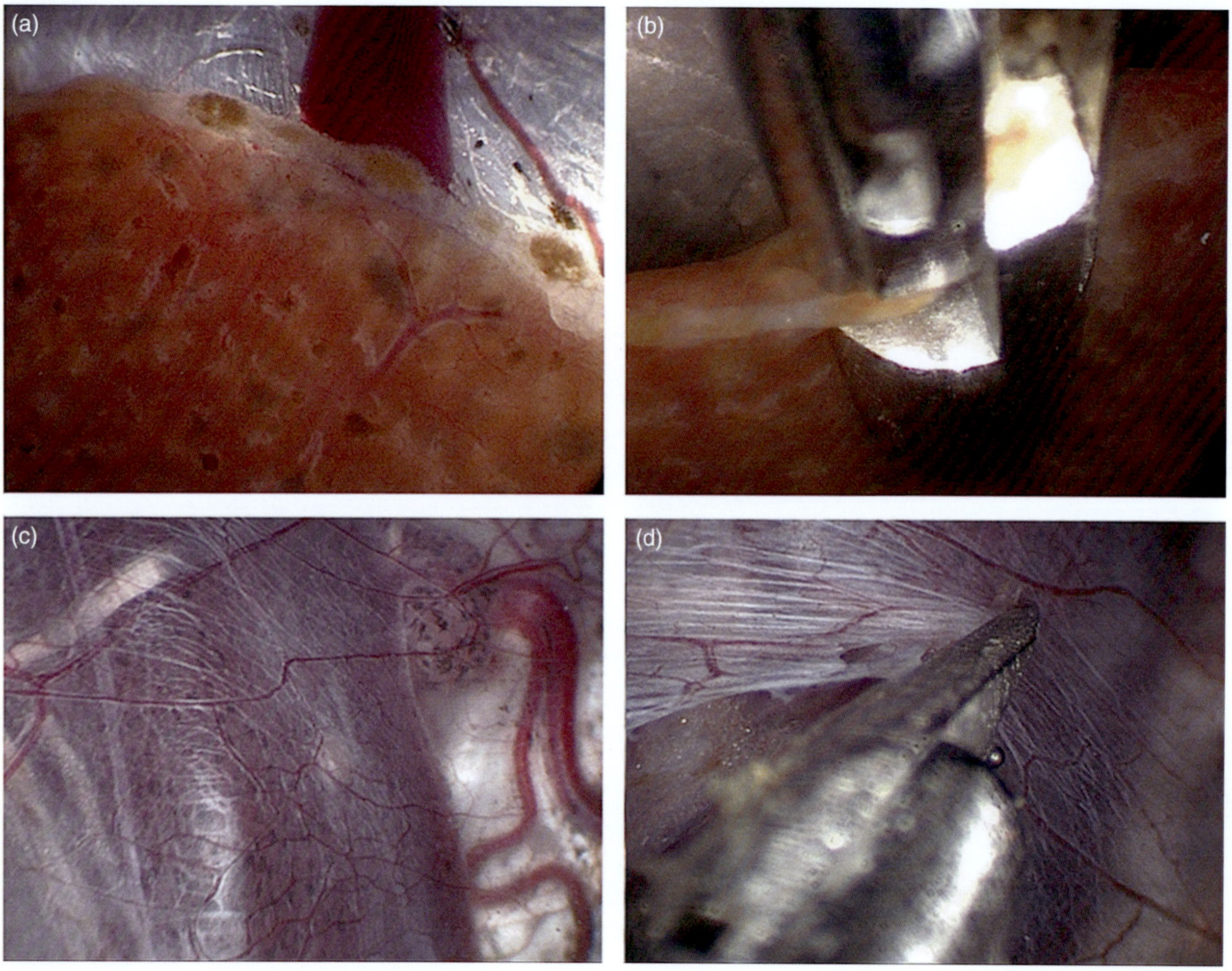

Figure A11.19 Coelioscopy in a channel catfish (*Ictalurus punctatus*) using a 2.7 mm telescope and saline irrigation: endoscopic view of the liver (a), note the detail of the parenchyma and vasculature; liver biopsy using 1.7 mm biopsy forceps (b); endoscopic view of the kidney through the coelomic membrane (c); coelomic membrane incised using 1.7 mm single-action scissors (d). *Source:* Courtesy of University of Georgia.

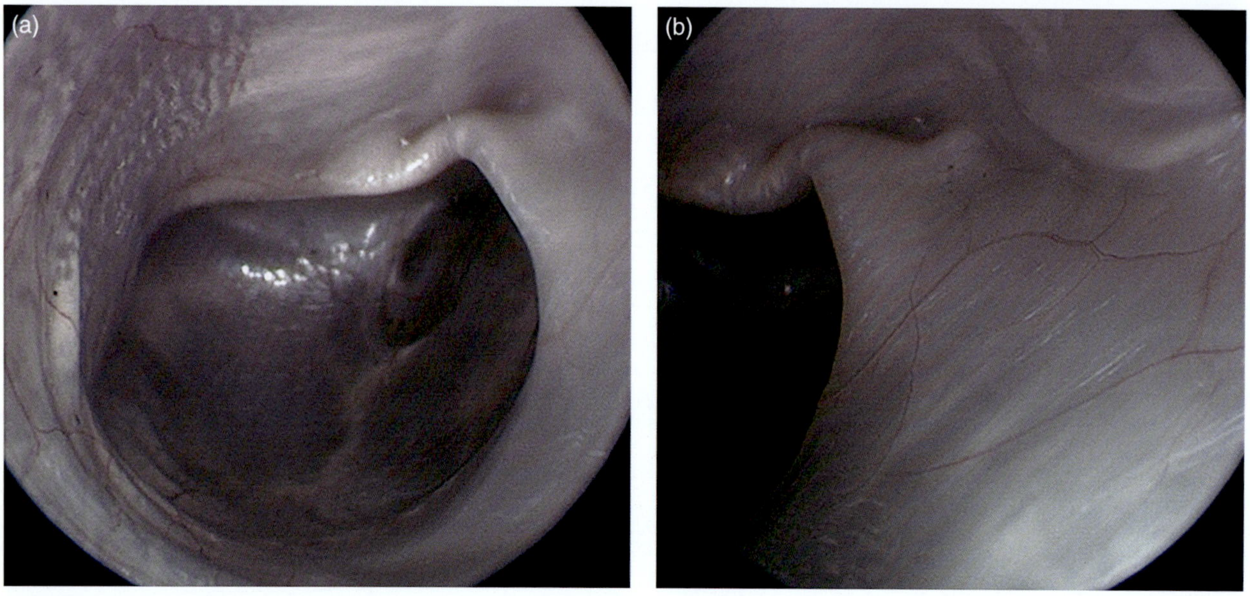

Figure A11.20 Pneumocystoscopy in a channel catfish (*Ictalurus punctatus*) using a 2.7 mm telescope. No insufflation or irrigation is required as the air present in the swim bladder allows visualization. *Source:* Courtesy of University of Georgia.

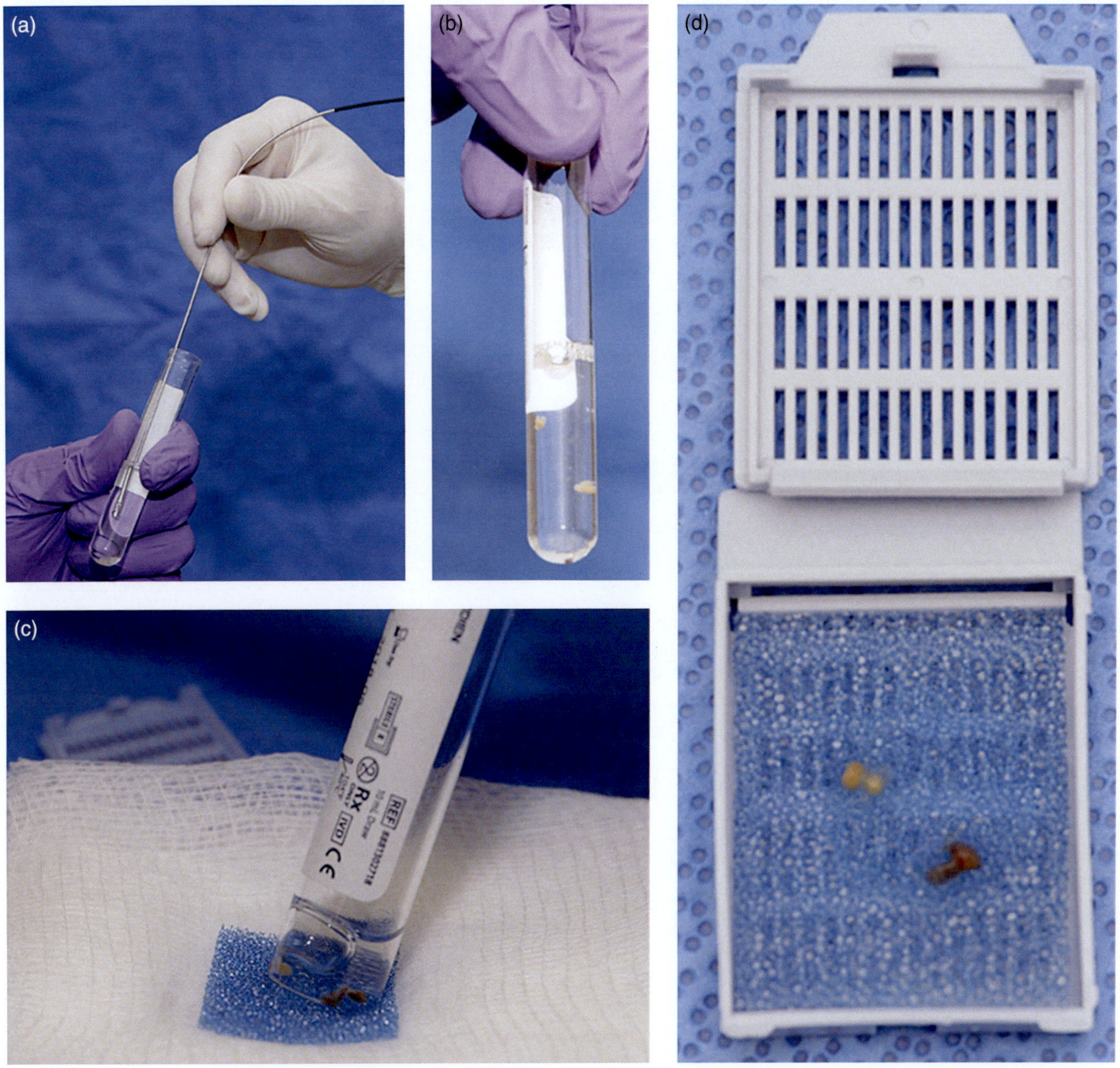

Figure A11.21 Biopsy sample handling: the biopsy cup is placed in a small volume of sterile saline (a) and gently shaken to dislodge the sample (b); the samples are then decanted onto sponges (c) and placed in biopsy cassettes (d). *Source:* Courtesy of University of Georgia.

Lloyd, R. and Lloyd, C. (2011). Surgical removal of a gastric foreign body in a sand tiger shark, *Carcharias taurus* Rafinesque. *Journal of Fish Diseases* 34: 951–953.

Lloyd, R. and Sham, N. (2014). Surgical repair of mandibular symphyseal fractures in three silver arowana (*Osteoglossum bicirrhosum*) using interfragmentary wire. *Journal of Zoo and Wildlife Medicine* 45: 926–930.

Macrì, F., Rapisarda, G., De Stefano, C. et al. (2014). Coelioscopic investigation in European eels (*Anguilla anguilla*). *Journal of Exotic Pet Medicine* 23: 147–151.

McDermott, A.J., Field, C.L., Hoopes, L.A., and Clauss, T.M. (2016). Medical management of coelomic distention, abnormal swimming, substrate retention, and hematologic changes in a reef manta ray (*Manta alfredi*). *Journal of Zoo and Wildlife Medicine* 47: 927–930.

Meegan, J., Sidor, I.F., Field, C. et al. (2012). Endoscopic evaluation and biopsy collection of the gastrointestinal tract in the green moray eel (*Gymnothorax funebris*): application in a case of chronic regurgitation with gastric mucus gland hyperplasia. *Journal of Zoo and Wildlife Medicine* 43: 615–620.

Munhofen, J.L., Jiménez, D.A., Peterson, D.L. et al. (2014). Comparing ultrasonography and endoscopy for early

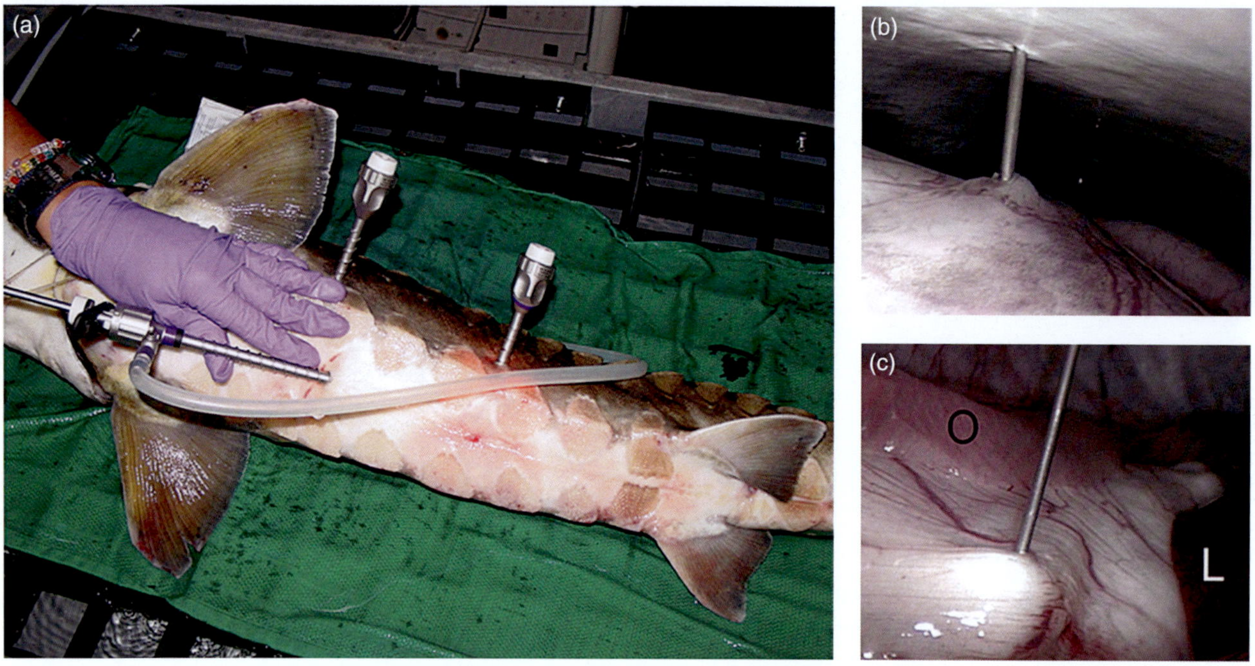

Figure A11.22 Endosurgical ovariectomy in a Gulf sturgeon (*Acipenser oxyrinchus*): a 5 mm telescope is inserted through a ventral cannula and instrument cannulae are inserted laterally (a); endoscopic view of a percutaneous needle inserted into the swim bladder for aspiration (b); a deflated swim bladder improves visualization and access to the ovary (O); liver (L) (c). *Source:* Courtesy of University of Georgia.

gender identification of juvenile siberian sturgeon. *North American Journal of Aquaculture* 76: 14–23.

Murray, M.J. (2010). Endoscopy in sharks. *Veterinary Clinics of North America: Exotic Animal Practice* 13: 301–313.

Nadelstein, B., Bakal, B., and Lewbart, G.A. (1997). Orbital exenteration and placement of a prosthesis in fish. *Journal of the American Veterinary Medical Association* 211: 603–606.

Neer, J.A. and Thompson, B.A. (2005). Life history of the cownose ray, *Rhinoptera bonasus*, in the northern Gulf of Mexico, with comments on geographic variability in life history traits. *Environmental Biology of Fishes* 73: 321–331.

Nematollahi, A., Bigham, A.S., Karimi, I., and Abbasi, F. (2010). Reactions of goldfish (*Carassius auratus*) to three suture patterns following full thickness skin incisions. *Research in Veterinary Science* 89: 451–454.

Serrano, M.E., Mette, J.T., and Dombrowski, D.S. (2011). Mechanical removal of *Philometra* species from the periocular space of redear sunfish (*Lepomis microlophus*) and bluegill (*Lepomis macrochirus*). *Proceedings of the International Association for Aquatic Animal Medicine Conference*, Las Vegas, NV.

Stamper, M.A. and Norton, T. (2002). Ovariectomy in a brook trout (*Salvelinus fontinalis*). *Journal of Zoo and Wildlife Medicine* 33: 172–175.

Stetter, M.D. (2010). Minimally invasive surgical techniques in bony fish (Osteichthyes). *Veterinary Clinics of North America: Exotic Animal Practice* 13: 291–299.

Vergneau-Grosset, C., Summa, N., Rodriguez, C.O. Jr. et al. (2016). Excision and subsequent treatment of a leiomyoma from the periventiduct of a koi (*Cyprinus carpio koi*). *Journal of Exotic Pet Medicine* 25: 194–202.

Wagner, G.N., Stevens, E.D., and Harvey-Clark, C. (1999). Wound healing in rainbow trout following surgical site preparation with a povidone-iodine antiseptic. *Journal of Aquatic Animal Health* 11: 373–382.

Zoller, G., Santamaria-Bouvier, A., De Lasalle, J. et al. (2017). Total pneumocystectomy in a telescope goldfish (*Carassius auratus*) with fungal pneumocystitis. *Journal of Exotic Pet Medicine* 26: 19–28.

A12

Medical Treatment

Claire Vergneau-Grosset and Stéphane Lair

Université de Montréal, Quebec, Canada

Introduction

The diversity of fish species and environmental conditions presents challenges when trying to formulate treatment plans, although some core principles apply. Veterinarians should try to make evidence-based decisions through literature searches, discussions with colleagues, and drug assays. Published pharmacokinetic studies are available, particularly from the aquaculture industry. These can be used as a base, although pharmacokinetics often differ across species, life stages, and environmental conditions. Accurate dosing is essential, and is typically based on fish weight, food weight, or water volume. Whenever treating a group of fish, it is highly recommended to test the medication on a few individuals or a smaller system prior to use on a larger scale (known as a bioassay).

Veterinarians must respect the legal requirements covering the purchase, use, and disposal of medications, and potential environmental residues should always be considered. For medications approved for use in fish, product labels should be considered the definitive source of instructions. Extra-label drug use is possible in nonfood fish under veterinary care, but some readily available drugs are considered a high regulatory priority and should be avoided.

All treatments should be considered within the framework of an integrated management plan. This should include husbandry changes to reduce stressors and transmission, as well as monitoring and prevention to avoid recurrence. These can decrease the need for therapeutics and improve overall success.

This chapter discusses antibiotics, antiparasitics, antifungals, antivirals, anti-inflammatories, hormone treatments, vaccines, and immune stimulants. It is not meant as a formulary. Reviews of drug studies require evaluating the species, life stage, fish size, sample size, water temperature, method of administration, and other husbandry information. Also, more up-to-date information will be available through journals and conferences. Rather, this chapter is meant to help guide clinicians through treatment options that may be available, as well as common routes and dose ranges. Treatments for specific diseases are covered in Section C. Using any of the medications at the doses reported here is at the discretion and responsibility of the attending veterinarian.

Environmental Changes

Medical treatment should be part of an integrated management plan. This will often include environmental changes, especially the reduction or resolution of any stressors. Environmental parameters should be within the optimal ranges for the individuals, including water temperature, dissolved oxygen, salinity, pH, and nitrogenous wastes. Stocking density and nutrition should also be assessed. Without resolving these stressors, the effectiveness of medications will be limited.

In many cases, environmental changes can reduce the need for medications or avoid them altogether. Some important examples include:

- Increasing the frequency of water changes to remove pathogens or toxins.
- Increasing the water temperature above the tolerance range of the pathogen, while still within a suitable range for the fish.
- Reducing the stocking density to reduce transmission rates.
- Removing the source of trauma, e.g. rough décor, inappropriate enclosure size.
- Removing intermediate hosts required for a parasite to complete its life cycle.
- Supplementing the water with missing components, e.g. iodide.

Clinical Guide to Fish Medicine, First Edition. Edited by Catherine A. Hadfield and Leigh Ann Clayton.

Environmental management of specific diseases are discussed in more detail in Section C. However, it is incumbent on veterinarians to consider how environmental changes could be used to reduce the need for medications.

Routes of Administration

Routes of administration depend on the drug pharmacokinetics, number of individuals to be treated, handling considerations, food intake, legislation, and concerns associated with drug residues or adverse effects on nontarget animals. It is possible to reduce the handling stress associated with oral and parenteral drug administration using behavioral conditioning and training, e.g. training zebra sharks (*Stegostoma tigrinum*) for hand injection.

Injectable

Intramuscular (IM) injection is the most common route of parenteral administration. To perform IM injections, the needle should be introduced between dermal scales (if present) into the dorsal musculature. This is usually the epaxial muscles near or just caudal to the dorsal fin(s) (Figure A12.1), but the base of the pectoral fins is often preferred in fancy koi (*Cyprinus carpio koi*) to avoid possible discoloration along the dorsum, and pectoral fins are used in skates and rays. For large animals (e.g. sharks, sawfish), the IM injection can be administered by pole syringe. Portal systems are present in many species, and while their pharmacokinetic effects have not been evaluated in fish, it may be best to administer drugs in the cranial half of the body (Zimmerman et al. 2006). Fish have white and red muscle and these may also affect pharmacokinetic profiles (Bosch et al. 2016). The volume of drug that can be injected into fish muscle without leakage is relatively small compared to mammals and birds of similar sizes. Methods to limit drug leakage include minimizing drug volume, using longer needles, or injecting at an oblique angle (Rigos et al. 2010; Fredholm et al. 2016).

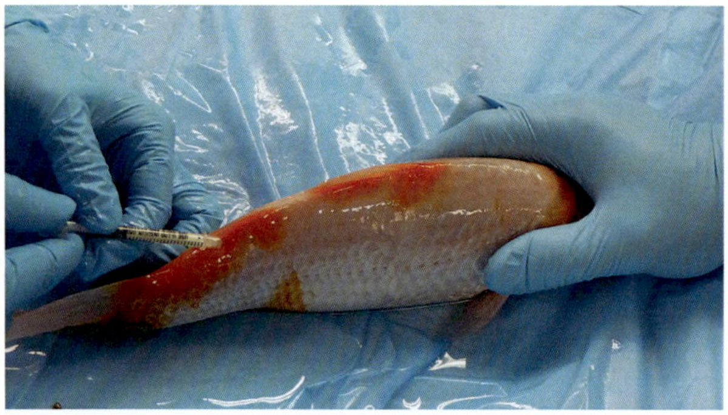

Figure A12.1 Intramuscular injection in the epaxial muscles of a koi (*Cyprinus carpio koi*), caudal to the dorsal fin.

Intracoelomic (ICe) injections are typically performed using a ventral approach, paramedial and cranial to the vent (Figure A12.2). Relatively large volumes of drugs can be administered ICe. Some studies have shown no difference in the pharmacokinetics for certain drugs via IM and ICe routes, while others have shown differences that may be clinically significant (Treves-Brown 2000; Shan et al. 2015). Drugs given intracoelomically may need to be diluted in saline, particularly if drug pH is low (e.g. enrofloxacin). Accidental administration into coelomic organs, such as the gonads, can affect pharmacokinetic parameters (Grosset et al. 2015).

Intravenous administration is less common but is useful for emergency drugs and fluid therapy (Figure A12.3). The most common sites for venipuncture are the ventral tail vein and artery, although it can be hard to know which vessel is accessed and arterial administration is contraindicated with some drugs. More information on venipuncture sites is provided in Chapter A6.

Medications may be administered directly into the swim bladder, for example in cases of pneumocystitis. Where present, most normal swim bladders are located within the coelom, ventral to the lateral line. A lateral approach is usually used. The location may be confirmed using ultrasonography or radiography prior to injection.

The subcutaneous route is rarely recommended in fish, since the skin is poorly elastic in most species and the hypodermis or subcutaneous layer can be difficult to identify.

Oral

For oral administration, drugs may be gavaged directly or added to food. Medicated food avoids the requirement for fish handling if the animals are actively feeding. Tablets or capsules can be introduced into prey items or gel foods.

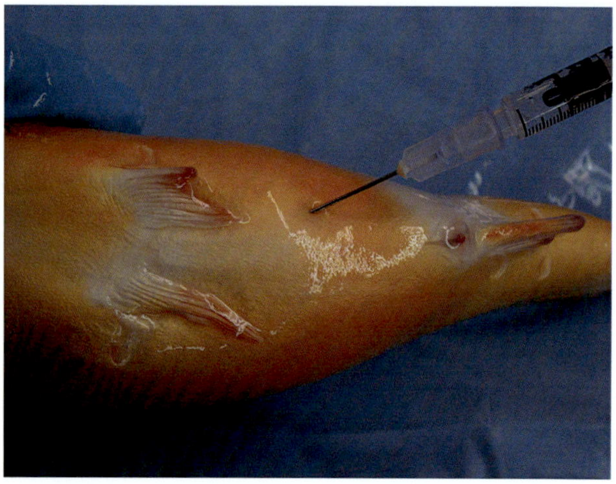

Figure A12.2 Intracoelomic injection in a koi (*Cyprinus carpio koi*).

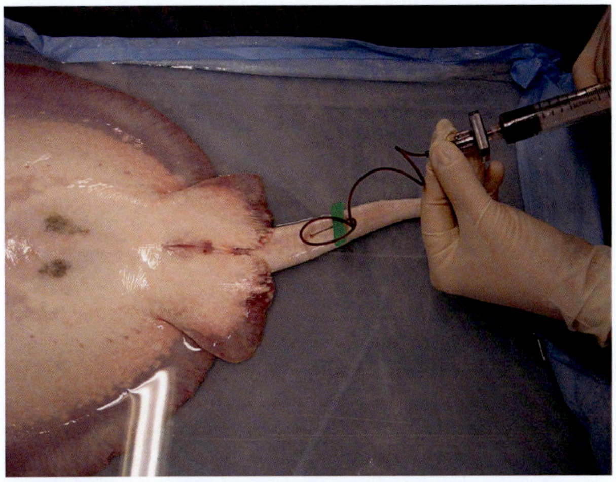

Figure A12.3 Blood transfusion in the ventral tail vein of an Atlantic stingray (*Hypanus sabinus*). *Source*: Image courtesy of Catherine Hadfield, National Aquarium.

Powdered or liquid medications can be put into capsules and fed the same way. Some fish, particularly rays (*Myliobatiformes*), are adept at spitting tablets or capsules in food and intake should be monitored. Powdered or liquid medications can be incorporated into flakes, pellets, or gel foods. Dressing pellets can be improved with the help of vegetable oil (the authors recommend 4 mL of oil per 100 g of pellets). Medicated gel diets can be bought from commercial suppliers or made in-house using medications that are not heat labile (Box A12.1). Thermolabile drugs should not be administered this way, as hot water is needed to prepare the gel and some drugs may be inactivated during the process. The extent of leaching from medicated foods can be hard to predict. Some medicated pelleted diets can be purchased from commercial suppliers; this requires a veterinary feed directive (VFD) in the United States (see below).

For smaller species, bioencapsulation in live prey may be used. This involves the administration of drugs to live invertebrate prey through immersion at a given concentration for a specific duration, prior to feeding the prey to fish. Protocols have been established for the bioencapsulation of metronidazole, enrofloxacin, oxolinic acid, flumequine, erythromycin, oxytetracycline, florfenicol, potentiated sulfonamide, and fenbendazole in brine shrimp (*Artemia* spp.) (Mohney et al. 1990; Chair et al. 1996; Gomez-Gil et al. 2001; Cook and Rust 2002; Roiha et al. 2010; Touraki et al. 2010; Allender et al. 2011; Allender et al. 2012; Touraki et al. 2012).

Oral medications can also be provided directly by tube feeding (gavage). This is the most reliable way to provide

Box A12.1 Preparing Medicated Gel Foods

1) Calculations:
   a) Use the planned dose and the feeding rate (e.g. 2%) to calculate the concentration of medication in the medicated gel:

      Concentration of medication in feed (g/kg feed)
      = dose (mg/kg) / [feed rate (%BW/d) × 10]

   b) Use the weight of fish, feeding rate, and number of treatments to calculate the total amount of medicated feed needed:

      Total medicated feed needed (kg)
      = weight of fish (kg) × feed rate (%BW/d)
      × 0.01 × number of treatment days

   c) Use those results to calculate the amount of medication to add to the gel:

      Total medication to be added to medicated feed (g)
      = total medicated feed needed (kg)
      × target concentration (g/kg of feed)

   d) Confirm the amount of medicated gel to be fed per day:

      Medicated feed per day (kg)
      = weight of fish (kg) × feed rate (%BW/d) × 0.01

2) Make the gel following the label instructions, except withhold an equivalent weight of powder to match the drug that will be added. After adding the near-boiling water, mix thoroughly for two minutes (to allow the mix to cool), then add the medication. Homogenize for two more minutes.
3) Pour into a lidded container of the desired size/shape. Place the medicated gel in the refrigerator or freezer (if medication is stable when frozen) and handle like seafood.

For example: To feed metronidazole gel at a dose of 20 mg/kg for 10 days, a feeding rate of 2%, to 30 fish weighing 0.5 kg each:

Concentration of medication in feed = 20/(2 × 10)
= 1 g/kg

Total medicated feed needed = 30 × 0.5 × 2 × 0.01 × 10
= 3 kg

Total medication to be added = 3 × 1 = 3 g

Medicated feed per day = 30 × 0.5 × 2 × 0.01 = 0.3 kg

When making up the gel food, withhold 3 g of the food powder to replace it with medication.

oral medications but requires handling and is rarely practical for groups of fish. It could also affect pharmacokinetics if the medication is not administered in food. Tube feeding of fish is described in Chapter A4.

Immersion

Immersion treatments vary from a dip of a few seconds to a prolonged immersion (or bath) over several weeks. Immersion treatments are practical for groups of fish and inappetent animals and may not require fish handling. Human exposure and disposal of medicated water must be considered prior to use. Water volumes should be calculated accurately to determine the drug needs; this volume should exclude the space occupied by substrate and décor and include sump(s) and the life support system. Some volume calculations are listed in Box A12.2.

Immersion treatments may be carried out in isolated containers or in the primary enclosure. Isolated containers limit the effects of the medication to the target animals and reduce overall drug needs. The water should be from the original system, and dissolved oxygen, temperature, pH, and ammonia must remain within target ranges throughout treatment. Isolated containers may be as simple as a 5 gallon bucket or a 100 gallon Rubbermaid® container. Alternatively, a tank may be taken off-line for treatment (i.e. isolated from all life support equipment), as long as water quality parameters can be maintained. The same principles can be applied to net pens by enclosing them in a barrier.

Immersion treatments in the primary enclosure carry much higher potential risks and should only be considered when other options are not available. Medications can have unexpected and serious effects on the water quality, life support system, and nontarget animals. Drug needs are often higher, with more concerns about how to dispose of medicated water. Ozone, ultraviolet, and carbon filters, as well as foam fractionators must be off-line during immersion treatments in systems, as they are likely to degrade or adsorb medications. Many immersion medications can affect bacterial populations and damage the biological filtration. The effects can be unpredictable and increased monitoring of dissolved oxygen, ammonia, and nitrite is warranted during and following immersion treatments. Some medications that can be used by immersion are light-sensitive, including tetracycline, oxytetracycline, and chloroquine. Immersion treatments of systems are covered in more detail in Chapter A13.

Topical

Direct topical application in fish is primarily used for the treatment of skin and eye lesions. They can be applied under manual or chemical restraint. The most commonly reported topical medication is the recombinant platelet-derived growth factor becaplermin (Regranex®, 0.01% gel, Ortho-McNeil Pharmaceutical Inc., Raritan, NJ, USA). Becaplermin can improve healing of lateral line depigmentation when the underlying stressors are removed (Fleming et al. 2008). Other commercial products have been described including a paste for gingival wounds containing pectin, gelatin, and methylcellulose (Orabase®, ConvaTec, Bridgewater Township, NJ, USA) (Harms and Wildgoose 2001). The use of a compounded gel containing 0.0024% misoprostol, 2% phenytoin, and a gelling agent has also been advocated for wound treatment (Clarke 2016). However, in an experimental trial to evaluate healing of superficial wounds in brook trout (*Salvelinus fontinalis*) using a more concentrated formulation of this gel, there was no improvement compared to the controls (Coutant et al. 2019). A list of topical medications used in elasmobranchs, and their manufacturers, is available in Mylniczenko and Clauss (2017). Topical administration of medications on the gills may allow systemic absorption of some emergency drugs (e.g. doxapram).

Box A12.2 Calculating Water Volumes

Volume of a rectangular container

- Volume (L) = length (cm) × width (cm) × depth (cm)/1000
- Volume (L) = length (m) × depth (m) × average depth (m) × 1000
- Volume (US gallons) = length (ft) × width (ft) × depth (ft) × 7.48
- Volume (US gallons) = length (in.) × width (in.) × depth (in.)/231
- Volume (acre-ft) = surface area (acres) × average depth (ft)

Volume of a cylindrical container

- Volume (L) = 3.14 × radius^2 (cm) × depth (cm)/1000
- Volume (US gallons) = 3.14 × radius^2 (ft) × depth (ft) × 7.48
- Volume (US gallons) = 3.14 × radius^2 (in.) × depth (in.)/231

For ponds, if average depth is unknown, maximum depth × 0.4 can be used as an estimate.

Alternatively, a container of known volume or water with a known flow rate can be used to empty or fill the container.

Other Routes

Other routes are possible but under-reported in fish. These include per cloaca/per rectum, intrauterine, subconjunctival, intraocular, and intrathecal routes.

Commonly Used Medical Treatments

Using any of the medications at the doses reported here is at the discretion and responsibility of the attending veterinarian. Medication use must follow all legislation regarding use and disposal. The drugs discussed in this section apply largely to ornamental fish under veterinary care. Most are not approved for use in food fish. Legislation in North America and Europe is covered in more detail at the end of this chapter.

Antibiotics

Antibiotics should only be used to treat specific pathogens based on culture and sensitivity results or other ancillary testing. Indiscriminate use of antibiotics can damage target and nontarget animals and contribute to antibiotic-resistant bacteria (Seepersadsingh and Adesiyun 2003; Blackburn et al. 2010; Mohammed and Arias 2015).

Only a few antibiotics are approved by the United States Food and Drug Administration (FDA) for use in fish: florfenicol, sulfadimethoxine–ormetoprim, sulfamerazine, and oxytetracycline, and they are approved for specific products, taxa, and indications (US FDA 2019a). All antibiotic use in ornamental fish is considered extra-label in the United States.

Amikacin

Amikacin is a concentration-dependent bactericidal aminoglycoside antibiotic. It is effective against many Gram-negative bacteria and has shown some in vitro effect against piscine mycobacteriosis (Chang and Whipps 2015). There have been no pharmacokinetic studies or reports of toxicity in fish. It must be administered parenterally. Doses are empirical with 2.5–5 mg/kg IM q72h commonly used. It is also used intravenously at similar doses.

Cefovecin

Cefovecin is a time-dependent bactericidal third-generation cephalosporin. It is effective against Gram-negative bacteria. It must be administered parenterally. In common stingrays (*Dasyatis pastinaca*), cefovecin at 8 mg/kg IM did not remain above potential therapeutic concentration for more than 24 hours, whereas in white-spotted bamboo sharks (*Chiloscyllium plagiosum*), the same dose subcutaneously was detected for four days (Garcia-Parraga et al. 2010; Steeil et al. 2014). A higher dose of 16 mg/kg SC in copper rockfish (*Sebastes caurinus*) maintained therapeutic plasma concentration for seven days, but with significant interindividual variation (Seeley et al. 2016). These differences may be due to differences in protein binding between species, therefore extrapolating between fish species should be done with caution.

Ceftazidime

Ceftazidime is a time-dependent bactericidal third-generation cephalosporin. It is effective against Gram-negative bacteria, with particularly good activity against *Pseudomonas* spp. Of note, it is prohibited from veterinary use in some European countries. Ceftazidime is available as a powder. Following reconstitution, aliquots can be frozen to increase the life span and thawed prior to administration. Ceftazidime must be administered parenterally. It is commonly used in teleost fish at 20 mg/kg IM q72h, supported by a pharmacokinetic study in koi (Govett et al. 2009). A pharmacokinetic study in cownose rays (*Rhinoptera bonasus*) recommended 20 mg/kg IM q48h based on minimum inhibitory concentrations (MIC) extrapolated from mammals and reptiles (Myers et al. 2014). It is also used intravenously at similar doses. Higher doses would likely be required for ICe administration, based on lower peak plasma concentrations observed in koi (Govett et al. 2009).

Ceftiofur

Ceftiofur is a time-dependent bactericidal third-generation cephalosporin. It is most effective against Gram-negative bacteria but has some action against Gram-positive ß-lactamase producing bacteria. It must be administered parenterally. There have been few studies in fish. Pharmacokinetics of short-acting ceftiofur sodium (Naxcel®, Pfizer Animal Health, New York, NY, USA) has been studied in Nile tilapia (*Oreochromis niloticus*) with a dose recommendation of 5 mg/kg IM q3–6h (Khalil et al. 2016). Pharmacokinetics of an extended release formulation, ceftiofur crystalline-free acid (CCFA, Excede®, Pfizer Animal Health), have been studied in koi with a dose recommendation of 60 mg/kg IM q14d (Grosset et al. 2015). However, there was high individual variability in pharmacokinetics (Grosset et al. 2015). Minor adverse effects included avascular necrosis at the site of IM injection; these lesions resolved spontaneously (Grosset et al. 2015). In smooth dogfish (*Mustelus canis*), a single dose of 6.6 mg/kg IM maintained pooled plasma levels at more than double the reported MIC for *Aeromonas* spp. for more than seven days (Fayette et al. 2019).

Enrofloxacin

Enrofloxacin is a bactericidal concentration-dependent second-generation fluoroquinolone. It is effective against

Gram-negative and Gram-positive bacteria, particularly *Aeromonas*, *Vibrio*, *Yersinia*, and *Streptococcus* spp. It is used commonly in exotic pet species in the United States but is prohibited in certain countries within the European Union. Pharmacokinetics of enrofloxacin have been studied in a wide variety of fish, including pirapitinga (*Piaractus brachypomus*), snakehead fish (*Channa argus*), Amur catfish (*Silurus asotus*), Atlantic salmon (*Salmo salar*), rainbow trout (*Oncorhynchus mykiss*), goldfish (*Carassius auratus*), and koi (Bowser et al. 1992; Lewbart et al. 1997; Stoffregen et al. 1997; Lewbart et al. 2005a; Kim et al. 2006; Udomkusonsri et al. 2007; Kyuchukova et al. 2015; Fang et al. 2016). Conversion of enrofloxacin into the active metabolite ciprofloxacin has been investigated in a wide variety of teleosts and the results vary across species (Lewbart et al. 1997; della Rocca et al. 2004; Danyi et al. 2011; Fang et al. 2011; Kyuchukova et al. 2015; Fang et al. 2016; Fan et al. 2017). Where the conversion is seen, the level of ciprofloxacin is usually low (Lewbart et al. 1997; Danyi et al. 2011; Kyuchukova et al. 2015; Fang et al. 2016).

Possible routes of administration include immersion, oral, and injectable (IM, ICe, slow IV). Oral administration results in lower peak plasma concentrations than parenteral administration, but a longer half-life, possibly due to an entero-hepatic cycle (Bowser et al. 1992; Lewbart et al. 1997). Therefore, less frequent administrations of higher doses are recommended for oral administration compared to parenteral administration. Compared to other fluoroquinolones such as oxolinic acid, enrofloxacin has a higher oral bioavailability and a longer half-life (Martinsen and Horsberg 1995). Recommended parenteral doses range from 5 to 10 mg/kg IV or IM q24–48h, and 10 mg/kg ICe q96h. Common oral doses are 10–20 mg/kg PO q24–48h.

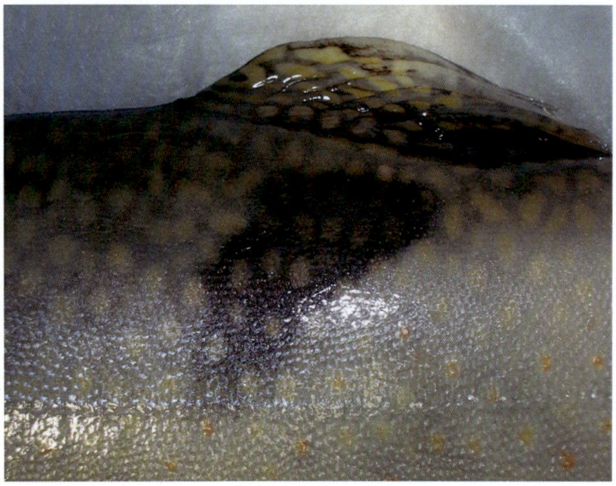

Figure A12.4 Local skin hyperpigmentation in a brook trout (*Salvelinus fontinalis*) following intramuscular injection of enrofloxacin.

Intramuscular administration of enrofloxacin (22.7 mg/mL) can be associated with local skin discoloration (Figure A12.4), muscle hemorrhage, inflammation, and necrosis (Scott et al. 2020). Intracoelomic administration does not seem to be associated with significant tissue reaction, but it is common practice to dilute the enrofloxacin 50:50 with sterile saline due to the low pH. As with other vertebrates, enrofloxacin should be used with caution in juvenile fish. Spinal deformities have been reported in juvenile Siberian sturgeons (*Acipenser baerii*) treated with high oral doses of enrofloxacin (Wang et al. 2016). The high-concentration enrofloxacin (100 mg/mL) should not be used by injection as muscle necrosis is common.

Immersion treatment requires higher doses in seawater than freshwater as fluoroquinolones complex with divalent cations (Phillips et al. 2016). Enrofloxacin immersion doses range from 2.5–10 mg/L for at least five hours q24–48h (Lewbart et al. 1997). Immersion treatment can damage ammonia-oxidizing bacteria in biological filtration; a dose-dependent effect has been observed at 5–40 mg/L (Nimenya et al. 1999). Appropriate disposal of the medicated water must be considered.

Ciprofloxacin

Ciprofloxacin is a bactericidal concentration-dependent second-generation fluoroquinolone. It has the same target range as enrofloxacin (Gram-negative and Gram-positive bacteria) and is a metabolite of enrofloxacin in some species. It is usually administered orally but can be given parenterally or by immersion. Oral doses are often 10–20 mg/kg PO q24–48h (Guo et al. 2005). Required doses may be higher than for enrofloxacin because of lower bioavailability (Papich 2017). A dose of 15 mg/kg IM q2–5d has been suggested in rainbow trout, common carp (*Cyprinus carpio*), and North African catfish (*Clarias gariepinus*) (Nouws et al. 1988). Immersion treatment at 10 mg/L q24h has been recommended (Guo et al. 2005).

Oxolinic Acid

Oxolinic acid (also reported as oxalinic acid) is a bactericidal concentration-dependent quinolone antibiotic. It is most effective against Gram-negative bacteria. Oxolinic acid is approved for use in aquaculture fish in Europe. Oral, injectable, and immersion administrations are described, with immersion being most common in practice. Immersion treatments have been described at 20 mg/L for two hours to 200 mg/L for 72 hours (Samuelsen 1997; Touraki et al. 2012). Veterinarians often use 10–20 mg/L as a leave-in immersion. Oxolinic acid is better absorbed in soft water and at low pH, because divalent cations chelate quinolones. Doses at the high end of the range are recommended in hard water (Noga 2010a). Oral doses range from

10 to 25 mg/kg q24h (Martinsen and Horsberg 1995; Noga 2010a). Bioencapsulation in brine shrimp nauplii is performed by placing nauplii in a 12 mg/mL emulsion in the dark for 24 hours (Touraki et al. 2012). Parenteral doses include 20–25 mg/kg IV and 50 mg/kg ICe (Hustvedt et al. 1991; Martinsen and Horsberg 1995; Samuelsen et al. 2003). Oxolinic acid elimination half-life is lower than that of enrofloxacin and frequent dosing may be required (Martinsen and Horsberg 1995).

Azithromycin

Azithromycin is a bactericidal concentration-dependent macrolide antibiotic. It is effective against some Gram-negative bacteria and some Gram-positive bacteria. It does have some activity against *Chlamydiales*. It is typically administered at 30–40 mg/kg PO q24h (Fairgrieve et al. 2005; Fairgrieve et al. 2006). Following ICe dosing in salmonids, azithromycin has shown a longer half-life than erythromycin (Fairgrieve et al. 2006). However, due to lower cost and fewer resistance concerns, erythromycin is used more commonly in fish.

Erythromycin

Erythromycin is a bacteriostatic time-dependent macrolide antibiotic. It is most effective against Gram-positive bacteria and is typically used to treat *Renibacterium* and *Streptococcus* spp. In other classes, it is also used as a prokinetic for the upper gastrointestinal tract. It can be administered orally, parenterally, or by immersion but oral treatment at 50–200 mg/kg q24h is preferred. Several forms are available including erythromycin phosphate, erythromycin stearate, erythromycin estolate, erythromycin hydrate, and crystalline erythromycin (Cook and Rust 2002). Erythromycin phosphate is available in a water-soluble solution and may be used for immersion, oral, or injectable treatments (Fairgrieve et al. 2005; Fairgrieve et al. 2006). Erythromycin estolate is the best absorbed through the oral route in mammals but this has not been evaluated in fish (Plumb 2015). Erythromycin hydrate is water-soluble but can lead to water turbidity (Cook and Rust 2002). Erythromycin stearate is not water-soluble and should not be used for immersion (Cook and Rust 2002). Phosphate and stearate forms appear to be the most appropriate for bioencapsulation in brine shrimp (Cook and Rust 2002). Erythromycin immersion can damage biological filtration (Noga 2010a).

Florfenicol

Florfenicol is a primarily bacteriostatic time-dependent antibiotic. It is effective against a variety of Gram-negative bacteria. It is also effective against some Gram-positive bacteria, such as *Streptococcus* spp. As of 2019, florfenicol is approved in the United States for *Edwardsiella ictaluri*, *Flavobacterium columnare*, *Flavobacterium psychrophilum*, *Aeromonas salmonicida*, and *Streptococcus iniae* in catfish and freshwater-reared finfish with a 15-day withdrawal (Aquaflor®, Merck Animal Health) (US FDA 2019a). It must be used under a veterinary feed directive (VFD). It is closely related to chloramphenicol but lacks the para-nitro group that is responsible for aplastic anemia in humans.

Pharmacokinetics have been published in pirapitinga, koi, olive flounder (*Paralichthys olivaceus*), channel catfish (*Ictalurus punctatus*), three-spot gourami (*Trichogaster trichopterus*), and Asian swamp eels (*Monopterus albus*) (Lewbart et al. 2005b; Yanong et al. 2005; Lim et al. 2011; Gaunt et al. 2012; Gaunt et al. 2013; Xie et al. 2013). Elasmobranchs are under-represented, but pharmacokinetics have been published for white-spotted bamboo sharks (Zimmerman et al. 2006). Florfenicol is used via oral and parenteral routes. Immersion administration was ineffective in koi (Yanong et al. 2005). The approved dose is 10–15 mg/kg body weight PO for 10 days and most pharmacokinetic studies support this dose regimen. A higher dose of 20 mg/kg PO for 10 days has been recommended for *F. psychrophilum* (Meinertz et al. 2014). An IM dose of 20–40 mg/kg has been recommended, with intervals ranging from 24 hours in pirapitinga to five days in olive flounder and bamboo sharks (Lewbart et al. 2005b; Zimmerman et al. 2006; Lim et al. 2011). Florfenicol has a high therapeutic margin with doses up to 100 mg/kg PO q24h for 10 days reported as safe in Atlantic salmon (Inglis et al. 1991). Immersion treatment with any medication can affect biological filtration, although studies have shown variable effects with the closely related antibiotic chloramphenicol (Collins et al. 1976; Nimenya et al. 1999; Meinertz et al. 2014).

Oxytetracycline

Oxytetracycline is a bacteriostatic concentration-dependent antibiotic in the tetracycline class. It is effective against Gram-positive and Gram-negative bacteria, although resistance is commonly reported. It has some activity against *Chlamydiales*. As of 2019, oxytetracycline dihydrate is approved in the United States for specific bacterial diseases in catfish and salmonids with a 21-day withdrawal (Terramycin 200 for Fish®) (US FDA 2019a).

Oxytetracycline can be administered via oral, injectable, or immersion routes. Typical oral doses are 55–85 mg/kg body weight q24h for 10 days, based on studies in salmonids and channel catfish (Miller et al. 2012). Oral bioavailability is low in common carp and European bass (*Dicentrarchus labrax*) with resulting high fecal residues (Treves-Brown 2000).

Intramuscular doses usually range from 3 to 5 mg/kg q24–48h, although 7 mg/kg q24h IM has been recommended in pirapitinga (Doi et al. 1998). Extended-release oxytetracycline pharmacokinetics have been described at 50 mg/kg IM in grouper with high plasma concentrations maintained for more than 48 hours (Rigos 2010). Intracoelomic administration at 25–50 mg/kg may be a more appropriate route with better absorption than the IM route (Treves-Brown 2000). A dose of 10 mg/kg ICe has shown an immune stimulant effect in rainbow trout (Siwicki et al. 1989).

Typical doses for immersion range from 10 to 100 mg/L q12–24h for three to four days (Goodwin et al. 2005). Divalent cations chelate oxytetracycline; little of the administered drug dose is active in seawater (Lunestad and Goksoyr 1990). In seawater and hard freshwater, alternative treatments should be considered. If oxytetracycline is indicated, higher doses may be required and/or divalent cations in the water should be kept low (e.g. calcium < 10 mg/L or hardness < 20 mg/L). At a calcium concentration of 5.1 mg/L, an immersion dose of 400 mg/L reached target plasma concentrations in giant danios (*Devario aequipinnatus*), but buffer was required to counteract the low pH of oxytetracycline at that dose (Vorbach et al. 2019).

Therapeutic index is high at low water temperature. For example, no mortalities were reported in yellow perch (*Perca flavescens*) fingerlings up to 748 mg/L for 12 hours at 12°C (54°F) (Unkenholz et al. 1997). However, mortality rate increased with temperatures over 20°C (68°F) at 500 mg/L (Brooks et al. 1994). The drug is light-sensitive and darkens on exposure, so light should be kept to a minimum during treatment (Pouliquen et al. 2007). Ultraviolet and ozone disinfection must be disconnected. Gloves should be worn when working with medicated water, as degradation products may be toxic to humans (Montoliu et al. 1981). Immersion treatment may affect biological filtration, with inhibition reported at 12.5–75.0 mg/L in some studies, while another reported no effect at 50 mg/L (Collins et al. 1976; Klaver and Matthews 1994).

Nitrofurans

Nitrofuran antibiotics, including nitrofurazone and furazolidone, are still found in some products sold over-the-counter. These products are carcinogenic and have been placed under high regulatory priority by the US FDA. Their use should be avoided in fish.

Sulfamerazine

Sulfamerazine is a bacteriostatic sulfonamide. It was approved by the FDA in the 1960s for use in food fish but is no longer available in the United States. Sulfamerazine is available elsewhere in the world and formulations for other species are on the market in North America. Oral dose includes 220 mg/kg q24h for 14 days (Noga 2010a).

Sulfadimethoxine–Ormetoprim

Sulfadimethoxine–ormetoprim is a bacteriostatic potentiated sulfonamide. It is effective against many Gram-negative and Gram-positive bacteria, although resistance is reported commonly. It also has some anticoccidial effects. As of 2019, this combination is FDA-approved in the United States for *Edwardsiella ictaluri* and *Aeromonas salmonicida* in catfish and salmonids (Romet-30® and Romet-TC®, Pharmaq-AS, Overhalla, Norway) with a 3–42-day withdrawal (US FDA 2019a). The optimal ratio of sulfadimethoxine to ormetoprim is debated, with Romet having a 5:1 ratio.

Administration is usually oral, and it can be provided by bioencapsulation into live prey (Mohney et al. 1990). Pharmacokinetics have been described in striped bass (*Morone* spp.) and Atlantic salmon (Samuelsen et al. 1995; Horsberg et al. 1997; Bakal et al. 2004). Reported oral doses are 29–50 mg/kg body weight, based on pharmacokinetics in salmonids and catfish (Bakal et al. 2004). Rectal prolapses have been reported in cownose rays with coccidia infections that were treated with sulfadimethoxine at 50 mg/kg PO (McDermott et al. 2016). Folate-deficiency anemia secondary to prolonged treatment with potentiated sulfonamides has not been reported in fish. Absorption of sulfonamides via immersion varies widely depending on temperature, pH, and salinity and is very low for sulfadimethoxine (Samuelsen et al. 1997).

Trimethoprim–Sulfamethoxazole

Trimethoprim–sulfamethoxazole (TMP–SMX) is a bacteriostatic potentiated sulfonamide. It is effective against Gram-negative and Gram-positive bacteria, except enterococci. It is typically given orally or via immersion, although immersion pharmacokinetics in Atlantic halibut (*Hippoglossus hippoglossus*) showed that sulfamethoxazole is poorly absorbed compared to other sulfonamides (Samuelsen et al. 1997). Common immersion doses are 20–30 mg/L for 6–10 hours immersion repeated q24h. Higher doses may be needed in freshwater compared to salt water (Samuelsen et al. 1997). Efficacy of bioencapsulation into *Artemia* sp. has been shown in turbot (*Scophthalmus maximus*) and European seabass larvae, with therapeutic concentrations maintained for more than 24 hours after a single feeding (Chair et al. 1996). Pellets may be also coated with trimethoprim–sulfamethoxazole with a concentration 1.5 g/kg of food, as described in goldfish (Liu et al. 2012).

Trimethoprim–Sulfadiazine

Trimethoprim–sulfadiazine is a bacteriostatic potentiated sulfonamide. It is effective against Gram-negative and Gram-positive bacteria. As of 2019, it is approved for salmonids in Canada and Europe (Tribrissen 40% Powder®, Merck Animal Health) (Health Canada 2010). The optimal ratio of trimethoprim and sulfadiazine in fish is debated, with Tribrissen having a 1:5 ratio. More sulfadiazine may be beneficial based on pharmacokinetic and MIC data and these products may be available from compounding pharmacies (Horsberg et al. 1997). Pharmacokinetics have been described in Atlantic salmon and mandarin fish (*Siniperca chuatsi*) (Horsberg et al. 1997; Wang et al. 2015). Administration can be oral, intracoelomic, or by immersion. Doses range from 30–120 mg/kg body weight PO q24h, 30–125 mg/kg ICe, and 20 mg/L immersion for five hours q24h (Noga 2010a; Wang et al. 2015). Elimination half-life is much higher with multiple-dose administration than with a single administration; therefore, dosing intervals may need to be extended over time (Wang et al. 2015).

Antiparasitics

Chitin Synthase Inhibitors

Diflubenzuron Diflubenzuron is a chitin synthase inhibitor that is used to treat crustacean parasites such as branchiurans and copepods. It is a white powder. Administration can be oral or via immersion. Diflubenzuron is active during parasite ecdysis; therefore, frequency of administration should be adapted to the life cycle under the current temperature and environmental conditions (e.g. potentially every 5–14 days). Immersion doses range from 0.03 to 0.05 mg/L for 8–24 hours q5–14d (Noga 2010a). Oral doses include 75 mg/kg q24h for 14 days (Horsberg and Hoy 1991; Noga 2010a).

Immersion treatment with diflubenzuron can affect nontarget crustaceans and other invertebrates containing chitin. No adverse effects have been reported in jellyfish or algae (Crossley et al. 2009; Langford et al. 2014). Diflubenzuron is persistent in the environment with a half-life of nine days in freshwater at 36°C (97°F), although organic matter contributes to the degradation (Fischer and Hall 1992). An Environmental Protection Agency (EPA) permit is required to purchase and use diflubenzuron in the United States and label instructions must be followed. Alternative crustacean treatments include emamectin and trichlorfon.

Lufenuron Lufenuron is a chitin synthase inhibitor that is used to treat crustacean parasites such as branchiurans and copepods in ornamental fish. It also has some antifungal activity. Treatment is usually by immersion. Typical doses include 0.1 mg/L q7d for three to five weeks (Mayer et al. 2013). Lufenuron persists in the environment, although light can increase the rate of degradation (FAO 2008). Light should be minimized and UV filtration removed during immersion treatment. Immersion treatment can affect nontarget invertebrates containing chitin, and anecdotal observations suggest toxicity to echinoderms. Exposure of nontarget invertebrates should be avoided.

Oxidants

Copper Copper can be used to treat ectoparasites (particularly *Cryptocaryon* spp.) and oomycetes (water mold). Copper may also be used to kill algae and snails. It is commonly used in quarantine of marine teleosts (Hadfield and Clayton 2011). Two types of copper can be used: ionic copper sulfate pentahydrate (also known as bluestone), or chelated copper such as copper citrate, EDTA, or ethanolamine (e.g. Coppersafe™, Mardel, Fritz Aquatics, Mesquite, TX, USA). The copper sulfate form has a lower applied dose, since more ionic copper is available, but requires even greater care and attention to detail to minimize toxicity. A sudden increase in copper ions is harmful, so the medication should be fully dissolved prior to use and doses should be administered slowly and uniformly. A common method is to dilute the copper and administer the dose over several hours via a drip system. Copper ions readily form salts (e.g. copper chloride, copper carbonate) that are inactive. A reduction in pH will rapidly release toxic copper ions from the salts. Since copper becomes bound in systems (particularly within substrate, rocks, and porous walls), its release can happen long after treatment was terminated. Acute copper toxicity is negatively correlated with alkalinity and hardness, i.e. if alkalinity or hardness decrease, copper toxicity increases (Chakoumakos 1979). Therefore, copper is contraindicated in poorly buffered water, often listed as alkalinity <50 mg/L (Noga 2010a).

When using copper sulfate in salt water, the target free copper ion concentration is often 0.15–0.22 mg/L redosed as needed to maintain therapeutic levels for 14–30 days. Dose calculations are based on copper sulfate having 25.5% active copper ions (Box A12.3). Conservative dosing is recommended to avoid sudden increases in copper ion concentration; it is often recommended to use five to seven days to reach therapeutic concentration. Copper ion concentration should be measured q12–24h throughout and following treatment. Assays for copper ions are readily available, but colorimetric assays from local aquarium stores are less accurate than the results from a benchtop colorimeter or spectrophotometer. Copper sulfate can be removed with water changes and activated carbon filtration.

When using chelated copper in salt water, the target concentration is higher, often 0.4–0.5 mg/L on assays that measure total copper concentration. Removal of chelated copper usually relies primarily on water changes as it does not adsorb well to carbon (Noga 2010a).

Copper treatment is much less common in freshwater, but can be a useful alternative to formalin, particularly in aquaculture pond systems. Alkalinity should be >50 mg/L. Copper should not be used in ponds with heavy algal growth, as the algicidal activity of copper could precipitate a drop in dissolved oxygen. This can be assessed objectively using turbidity, e.g. a Secchi disk reading of >50 cm (18 in.). Where treatment is essential despite algal growth, the total dose may be split into four and each quadrant of the pond dosed at separate times while dissolved oxygen is monitored closely. In freshwater, the active component is considered the copper sulfate molecule, so dose calculations are based around the product being 100% active. The copper sulfate reacts with carbonates in the water to form inactive copper carbonate, so the target concentration is based on the alkalinity, usually 1% of alkalinity, although lower doses may be effective (Box A12.3). In freshwater, it is typically redosed based on the parasite life cycle, e.g. q48h for 4 doses for *Ichthyophthirius* sp.

Copper is toxic to most elasmobranchs, some teleosts, and most invertebrates (Table A12.1) (Hadfield and Clayton 2011; LaDouceur et al. 2016). Signs of direct copper toxicity in fish may include acute mortality without clinical signs, or a brief period (e.g. 24 hours) of reduced feeding, change in coloration, or increased hiding prior to acute mortality. It is important to immediately stop copper therapy if potential premonitory signs are seen. Copper may also lead to mortality through immune suppression and treatment may need to be stopped if other diseases that are not susceptible to copper are seen (e.g. *Brooklynella* spp., viral infections). Copper is also toxic to vascular plants, algae, and phytoplankton. The potential toxicity of copper to so many species creates problems when copper is needed to treat teleosts in complex, multispecies systems. There are two solutions that can still allow the use of copper.

- For *Cryptocaryon* spp. in coral systems, the best option is often to remove the susceptible teleosts and treat them in an isolated system.
- For *Cryptocaryon* spp. in systems with teleosts and elasmobranchs, the best option may be to remove the elasmobranchs while the system is treated.

Copper immersion treatment can damage biological filtration, depending on the oxidizing bacteria present and prior exposure, although this is rare (Collins et al. 1975; Mohan and Aiken 2004). However, as with any immersion treatment, water quality should be monitored closely.

Copper is not routinely given orally. However, anecdotal reports of using an insoluble oral formulation of copper wire particles to treat *Eimeria southwelli* in cownose rays have shown promise (Clarke et al. 2015).

Box A12.3 Calculation of Copper Sulfate Doses

Freshwater

Alkalinity should be >50 mg/L
Secchi reading must be >50 cm (18 in.)
Copper sulfate dose (mg/L) = alkalinity (mg/L)/100
To a maximum concentration of 2.5 mg/L copper sulfate
Copper sulfate dose (g) = volume (L) × dose (mg/L)/1000
Copper sulfate dose (g) = volume (gallons) × dose (mg/L) × 0.0038
Copper sulfate dose (lb) = volume (acre/ft) × dose (mg/L) × 2.72

Salt water

Target copper sulfate dose is usually 0.15–0.22 mg/L, but individual doses are usually incremental, e.g. 0.03 mg/L
Copper sulfate dose (g) = volume (gallons) × dose (mg/L) × 0.015
Copper sulfate dose (g) = volume (L) × dose (mg/L) × 0.004
Apply slowly, e.g. dilute and apply using a drip system over 12 hours

Chloramine-T Chloramine-T is a chlorinated and deprotonated sulfonamide that is typically used as a nonselective disinfectant. It is also used to treat external bacteria and protozoa in fish. It is a white powder. As of 2019, it is approved in the United States for treatment of *Flavobacterium* spp. in freshwater-reared salmonids, walleye (*Sander vitreus*), and warm-water finfish with a 0-day withdrawal (Halamid Aqua, Syndel USA (previously Western Chemical, Inc.), Ferndale, WA, USA) (US FDA 2019a). It is considered 100% active. It is used as an immersion treatment. When dissolved in water, chloramine-T forms hypochlorous acid (HOCl), a strong disinfectant, and hypochlorite ion (OCl^-), a weak disinfectant. So, chloramine-T is more active at low pH. Doses range from 2.5 to 20 mg/L depending on pH and hardness (Noga 2010a).

Chloramine-T is considered safer than chlorine because it does not form trihalomethanes with organic matter (Noga 2010a). The doses reported above are considered generally safe in warm-water fish, but toxicity has been reported. Clinical signs include dyspnea and tachypnea (Powell et al. 1995). At high doses, it can also inhibit normal swim bladder inflation in freshwater angelfish fry (*Pterophyllum scalare*) (Sanabria et al. 2009).

Formalin Formalin is a common immersion treatment for various ectoparasites and oomycetes in bony fish. In a survey of fish quarantine in zoos and aquariums, 64% used formalin (Hadfield and Clayton 2011). As of 2019, formalin

Table A12.1 Marine fish and invertebrate groups that may show increased sensitivity to copper treatment.

Fish group	High risk of adverse effects; alternative treatments or conservative dosing recommended	Lower risk of adverse effects
Bony fish	Seahorses and pipefish (*Syngnathidae*); juvenile butterflyfish (*Chaetodontidae*) and marine angelfish (*Pomacanthidae*); juvenile pufferfish (*Tetraodontidae*); needlefish (*Belonidae*); some wrasses (*Labridae*); light-emitting fish; fry	Adult marine tropical teleosts
Elasmobranchs	Most elasmobranchs, particularly pelagic and reef sharks	Cownose rays (*Rhinoptera bonasus*)
Invertebrates	Most invertebrates, including corals	Potentially horseshoe crabs (*Limulus* spp.)

is approved in the United States to treat specific external protozoa and monogeneans in finfish and oomycetes in freshwater-reared finfish and their eggs (Parasite-S® by Syndel USA, Formalin-F® by Natchez Animal Supply Co., and Formacide-B® by B.L. Mitchell, Inc.) with a 0-day withdrawal (US FDA 2019a). In the United States, it is available over-the-counter without prescription. Formalin use in fish is banned in the European Union because it is a potential carcinogen. Personal protective equipment should include goggles and gloves when handling the medication or medicated water and additional ventilation may be needed in enclosed spaces (Wooster et al. 2005).

Formalin typically contains 37% formaldehyde, 10–15% methanol, and water. It is considered 100% active (i.e. 1000 mg/mL). Doses are usually given in mg/L of formalin. Prolonged immersion doses range from 12.5 to 25 mg/L (equivalent to 0.013–0.025 mL/L). Higher doses are used for shorter duration, e.g. 100–250 mg/L (0.10–0.25 mL/L) for 60 minutes, but mortalities and histopathologic gill lesions have been reported within this dose range (Chmelova et al. 2016).

Formalin immersion decreases dissolved oxygen concentration, so additional aeration or oxygenation should always be provided during treatment, and dissolved oxygen should be monitored during and following treatment. Formalin is toxic to some fish, particularly scaleless fish and fry, and mortality increases with formalin dose (Intorre et al. 2007; Dolezelova et al. 2009). Formalin is more toxic in acidic soft water and at high water temperature; it should be used with caution in water temperatures >27°C (81°F). Toxicity may present with dyspnea, tachypnea, lethargy, erratic swimming, and acute mortalities up to 48 hours following treatment (Intorre et al. 2007). Gill lesions may be seen (Buchmann et al. 2004; Chmelova et al. 2016). Formalin is not used in elasmobranchs. Formalin is toxic to algae, vascular plants, and most invertebrates. Great care should be used prior to using formalin in a pond or other system that has significant algal growth, as the algal die-off can cause a catastrophic drop in dissolved oxygen. If it must be used, it is recommended to split the dose into four and apply to each quadrant over a period of several days.

Formalin can be rapidly aerosolized or degraded by microbial flora. Important factors included prior exposure, water temperature, dose, and total surface area (Pedersen et al. 2010; Knight et al. 2016). Fish density did not affect the rate of formalin degradation (Knight et al. 2016). This degradation means that repeated formalin treatments will often fall below therapeutic level, unless assays are used to monitor the in-water concentration and guide dosing (e.g. Formaldehyde Test Kit, Model FM-1, Hach, Loveland, CO, USA).

Formalin can affect the biological filtration, particularly at the higher end of the dose range (Collins et al. 1975; Pedersen et al. 2010). Of note, formalin immersion will artifactually increase ammonia concentration measured using the Nessler method (Heinen et al. 1995). Formalin should never be mixed with potassium permanganate since this could result in fire or explosion. Formalin should be stored above 4°C (39°F) in the dark to prevent paraformaldehyde precipitation, which is toxic to fish. The methanol in commercial formalin preparations reduces this risk, but formalin should always be inspected and discarded if white particulate is found.

Hydrogen Peroxide Hydrogen peroxide (H_2O_2) is an oxidizing agent used to treat external Gram-negative bacteria, fungi, protozoa, and metazoa. It is a colorless liquid. It is also used as a nonselective disinfectant. As of 2019, hydrogen peroxide is approved in the United States for *Flavobacterium branchiophilum*, *Flavobacterium columnare*, oomycetes, and gyrodactylids in a variety of freshwater-reared finfish and eggs with 0-day withdrawal (35% Perox-Aid, Syndel USA) (US FDA 2019a). The 35% preparation is equivalent to 350 mg/mL and is used by immersion. Medical-grade 3% hydrogen peroxide is available over-the-counter. Doses range from 3–100 mg/L for 30–60 minutes to 500–1000 mg/L for 15–20 minutes (Montgomery-Brock 2001; Vera and Migaud 2016), with lower doses used for columnaris and protozoal ectoparasites and higher doses for egg treatments. Certain strains of sealice have recently developed resistance to hydrogen peroxide (Helgesen et al. 2015). Peracetic acid and sodium percarbonate (sometimes referred to as sodium carbonate peroxyhydrate) can be used instead, as these generate hydrogen peroxide. Doses of peracetic acid are typically 0.1–2.0 mg/L q24h for three days. Doses of sodium percarbonate are often similar to hydrogen peroxide, e.g. 10–120 mg/L for one to six hours.

Toxicity has been reported with mortalities at routine doses in three spot gourami, walleye, pallid sturgeon (*Scaphirhynchus albus*), sixfinger threadfin (*Polydactylus sexfilis*), suckermouth catfish (*Hypostomus plecostomus*), paddlefish (*Polyodon spathula*), and northern pike (*Esox lucius*) (Rach et al. 1997; Montgomery-Brock 2001; Russo et al. 2007). Toxicity increases with increasing water temperature (Rach et al. 1997). Fry are usually more sensitive than adult fish. Typical signs are dyspnea and tachypnea and acute mortalities. Hydrogen peroxide is degraded to water and oxygen so there are no residue concerns. It is a strong oxidizer and suitable personal protective equipment should be worn.

Malachite Green Malachite green is a triarylmethane dye that was often used in conjunction with formalin due to synergistic effects on oomycetes and ectoparasitic protozoa. However, it is carcinogenic and genotoxic. Its use is prohibited in food animal species in the United States, European Union, United Kingdom, and Canada, and it has been placed under high regulatory priority by the FDA (European Food Safety Authority 2016; Canada Food Inspection Agency 2017; US FDA 2019a). The use of malachite green in pet fish should be discouraged.

Potassium Permanganate Potassium permanganate ($KMnO_4$) is a strong oxidizing agent used to treat external bacterial, fungal, protozoal, and monogenean infections in freshwater and brackish-water fish. It is available in crystal or powder form and must be dissolved in water prior to use. It is used by immersion and should be dosed based on permanganate demand, which is affected by organic load. A simple assay can be done using four small containers of system water. Potassium permanganate should be added at 2, 4, 6, and 8 mg/L. The therapeutic concentration is the lowest dose that maintains a faint pink color for 15 minutes. This dose should be increased by 2 mg/L to produce the dose required to maintain 2 mg/L in the pond. For example, if 2 mg/L maintained a faint pink color, the dose should be 4 mg/L. If >8 mg/L is indicated by the bioassay, organic material should be removed and another bioassay should be performed. A more accurate assay can be done using ORP (redox potential), with a target ORP of 450–500 mV. If an immersion dose of 2 mg/L produces an ORP < 450 mV, more potassium permanganate should be added. If ORP reaches >600 mV, 0.04 mL/L of 3% hydrogen peroxide (30 mg H_2O_2/mL) should be added to inactivate the potassium permanganate. An effective dose should maintain a faint pink color in the system for >8 hours; if the water turns brown, the dose was too low, if the water stays dark purple, the dose was too high. To reduce the risk of toxicity, wait at least four days before considering redosing.

Potassium permanganate is contraindicated in marine fish. Adverse effects have also been reported in some freshwater fish, including lethargy, erratic swimming, dyspnea, tachypnea, dysbiosis, and mortalities (Intorre et al. 2007; Mohammed and Arias 2015). Potassium permanganate can be toxic to algae and its use may deplete oxygen in the system. Supplemental aeration or oxygenation is mandatory during treatment. Ultraviolet filters should be shut down during treatment. Immersion treatment does not usually affect biological filtration (Collins et al. 1975). Potassium permanganate must never be used with formalin as it could result in fire or explosion. It is a strong oxidizer and suitable personal protective equipment should be worn.

Imidazoles

Fenbendazole Fenbendazole is a benzimidazole used to treat nematodes; it may have some effect against monogeneans, flagellates, and microsporidia. Pharmacokinetics have been studied in several species, including channel catfish and rainbow trout (Kitzman et al. 1990; Soukupova-Markova et al. 2015). It can be administered orally or by immersion. Oral treatments may show greater efficacy than immersion treatment, even for external parasites, and reduce disposal concerns (Forwood et al. 2013). Immersion treatments range from 2 to 25 mg/L. Oral treatments range from 10 to 75 mg/kg of body weight q24–48h for a few treatments (Noga 2010a). Bioencapsulation into *Artemia* spp. has been described (60 minutes at 2 g/L in freshwater, resulting in a fenbendazole concentration of ~4.5 mg/g of shrimp) (Allender et al. 2012).

Elasmobranchs and temperate demersal freshwater species have been reported as susceptible to fenbendazole toxicity at routine doses, but all fish may be susceptible, particularly following gavage dosing (Myers et al. 2007; Reed et al. 2012). Signs of toxicity have included neurologic signs and acute mortalities (Myers et al. 2007; Reed et al. 2012). Histology in rays has shown digestive and epigonal organ lesions (Garner 2013). Leukopenia and anemia have been documented in elasmobranchs, so blood transfusions might be an option in case of toxicity (Myers et al. 2007). Of note, most adverse effects occurred after four to six days of treatment (Reed et al. 2012). This medication should be used with caution and bioassays are essential prior to dosing groups of fish.

Metronidazole Metronidazole is a bactericidal antibiotic in the nitroimidazole class. It is active against protozoa and some bacteria, particularly anaerobes. It is used to treat gastrointestinal flagellates (e.g. *Spironucleus/Hexamita* spp.) and ectoparasitic protozoa. It is relatively insoluble in water but not at typical therapeutic doses (Noga 2010a). Various doses have been described for prolonged immersion treatments, ranging from 5 to 25 mg/L q24–48h for 3–40 days (Noga 2010a; Hadfield and Clayton 2011; Webb et al. 2013). A practical spectrophotometric assay method is reported in Webb et al. (2013) and its use is recommended to better understand drug levels in the water. Oral doses include 25–50 mg/kg body weight q24h for 10 days to 125 mg/kg once (Tojo and Santamarina 1998b). Bioencapsulation in *Artemia* spp. has been described (15 minutes at 10 g/L in freshwater, resulting in a metronidazole concentration of ~2 mg/g of shrimp) (Allender et al. 2011). Anecdotal cases of neurologic signs and death have been suspected in fish, especially pipefish, after oral overdose but the drug seems relatively safe at low doses. It seems to be relatively safe for invertebrates (Kołodziejska et al. 2013).

Other Antiparasitics

Emamectin Emamectin is an avermectin, a family of lactone macrocyclic antibiotics. Emamectin is active against crustaceans, nematodes, and potentially monogeneans. It is also used as an insecticide. As of 2019, emamectin benzoate (Slice®, Merck Animal Health) is approved in several countries, including Canada, United Kingdom, Norway, and Chile, as an in-feed treatment of fish lice in salmonids (Health Canada 2010). The dose is equivalent to 0.05 mg/kg body weight q24h for seven days, and it likely remains efficacious for more than a week after the end of an oral treatment (Olsvik et al. 2008). This dose has also been effective against swim bladder and intracoelomic nematodes (Larrat et al. 2012; Collymore et al. 2014; Béland et al. 2020). Emamectin is toxic to some aquatic invertebrates and exposure of nontarget invertebrates should be avoided (Langford et al. 2014).

Chloroquine Chloroquine is an aminoquinoline drug that can be used to treat external protozoa such as *Cryptocaryon irritans*, *Amyloodinium ocellatum*, trichodinids, and scuticociliates. It is available in several forms but immersion with chloroquine diphosphate, also known as chloroquine phosphate, is the most common form in fish (Verbeeck et al. 2005). Based on clinical experience, the authors recommend 10–15 mg/L for 1–21 days to control external protozoa in marine fish. Higher doses are described, up to 40 mg/L (Picón-Camacho et al. 2011). Recurrence of *Cryptocaryon irritans* has been reported anecdotally, even after long courses. Oral administration of chloroquine at 40 g/kg feed for 10 days was ineffective against *Ichthyobodo* and *Gyrodactylus* sp. in rainbow trout but actual intake of medicated feed was unknown (Tojo and Santamarina 1998a, b). No pharmacokinetic study of chloroquine in fish is available, to the authors' knowledge.

Chloroquine is damaged by exposure to UV, so UV filters should be shut down during immersion treatments (Owoyale 1989). It may be worth providing shade for medicated systems exposed to sunlight, but it does not appear to be necessary to reduce light levels for indoor systems. Unlike formalin and praziquantel, chloroquine often persists in water, and a single dose may maintain therapeutic levels for days to weeks. Assays are recommended to avoid overdosing the system. High doses of chloroquine or rapid increases in chloroquine can damage biological filtration, although concentrations of 10–15 mg/L rarely do. It may be useful to monitor phosphate levels if chloroquine diphosphate is used in aquaria containing invertebrates. Caution is advised if ozone is used to remove chloroquine, as unknown and potentially toxic by-products may be produced.

Toxic effects on echinoderms and corals have been reported anecdotally (Noga 2010a). The medication may be safe in other invertebrates, e.g. some shrimp and crabs (*Decapoda*). Bioassays are still recommended prior to treatment.

Levamisole Levamisole is a synthetic imidazothiazole that is used in fish to treat nematodes and as an immune stimulant. It is a white powder. Administration may be oral, by immersion or, more rarely, parenteral. Oral and intramuscular doses range from 2.5 to 10 mg/kg body weight q24h (Blanc et al. 1992; Noga 2010a). Immersion doses range from 1 mg/L for 24 hours to 50 mg/L for two hours (Taraschewski et al. 1988; Harms 1996). Toxicity has been reported at higher doses, e.g. 100 mg/L for 25 minutes was associated with mortalities in adult three-spined sticklebacks (*Gasterosteus aculeatus*) (Schmahl and Taraschewski 1987). Levamisole can improve the specific and nonspecific immune response in fish and it has been used as a vaccine adjuvant in fish (Siwicki et al. 1989; Lie et al. 2006).

Residue concerns prevent licensed use, as the drug can cause leukopenia and vasculitis in humans (Poon et al. 2011). A dose-dependent inhibition of the biological filtration has been noted with immersion at 4–32 mg/L (Nimenya et al. 1999).

Niclosamide Niclosamide is a salicylanilide derivative used to treat protozoa, nematodes, snails, and lampreys. It is particularly effective against *Tetrahymena* spp. in vitro. Niclosamide (Bayluscide®, Bayer, Leverkusen, Germany) is considered a pesticide and is regulated by the EPA in the United States and by Health Canada in Canada. It may be administered by oral or immersion routes. Oral doses of 200 mg/kg PO q24h for 14 days have been reported (Leibowitz et al. 2010). Immersion doses include 0.03–0.06 mg/L for 24 hours (Hubert et al. 2005). It has been used in open systems such as rivers, often in combination with 3-trifluoromethyl-4-nitrophenol (Dawson 2003).

Niclosamide has a low safety index in fish (Schmahl and Taraschewski 1987). Juvenile lake sturgeons (*Acipenser fulvescens*) are particularly sensitive (Boogaard et al. 2003). Niclosamide is photosensitive, so light should be minimized during immersion treatment and UV disinfection should be disconnected (Dawson 2003).

Phytotherapy Phytotherapeutic agents are products with medicinal properties obtained from plants. They can act directly on pathogens or modulate the immune system of the host (Bulfon et al. 2015; Valladão et al. 2015). Most studies involve treatment of monogeneans. Crude extracts of a variety of plants provided by immersion have been shown to reduce the load of *Dactylogyrus* spp. in goldfish (Liu et al. 2010; Ji et al. 2012; Hu et al. 2014). Oral crushed garlic and immersion with garlic oil can reduce monogenean load in guppies (*Poecilia reticulata*) (Fridman et al. 2014; Schelkle et al. 2015). Tea tree oil immersion reduced *Gyrodactylus* sp. load in three-spined stickleback (Steverding et al. 2005). Plant extracts have also shown good effects against protozoa such as *Ichthyophthirius* and *Trichodina* spp., bacteria such as *Aeromonas hydrophila*, and oomycetes (Ekanem et al. 2004; Chitmanat et al. 2005; Harikrishnan et al. 2010; Fu et al. 2014). A good review of phytotherapy studies can be found in Valladão et al. (2015).

Many products are available over-the-counter. However, quality controls are rare and composition is not guaranteed. While toxic effects of herbal products in fish have not been reported often, adverse effects associated with herbal products have been reported in human medicine (Schoepfer et al. 2007).

Praziquantel Praziquantel is a quinoline anthelminthic that is active against monogeneans, digenes, and cestodes. It is most effective on adults and larvae; eggs and cysts are rarely affected, so repeated treatments based on the prepatent period are required for egg-laying parasites. It is available in various formulations for use as an oral, injectable, or immersion treatment.

Pharmacokinetic studies have been conducted in several fish species (Kim et al. 2001; Tubbs and Tingle 2006a, b; Xie et al. 2015; Xu et al. 2016). Effective oral doses are often higher than in other classes, e.g. 50–330 mg/kg q1–4d (Szekely and Molnar 1991; Kim and Cho 2000; Tubbs and Tingle 2006b; Williams et al. 2007). Doses at the higher end of that range are consistently more effective, but poor palatability and regurgitation are common, particularly with surface-coated pellets (Hirazawa et al. 2004; Williams et al. 2007; Forwood et al. 2013). Microencapsulation of praziquantel has been attempted to improve palatability in yellowtail amberjack (*Seriola lalandi*) but effective doses remained unpalatable (Partridge et al. 2014). Lower doses for longer courses are a commonly reported compromise (Williams et al. 2007). In Korean rockfish (*Sebastes schlegelii*), concomitant administration of oral cimetidine at 200 mg/kg allowed for a higher praziquantel plasma concentration at a lower applied dose (Kim and Kim 2002).

Immersion treatment with praziquantel is common. The drug is poorly soluble in water. Manual dissolution through a mesh is effective and common, but usually does not result in full dissolution. Initial dissolution in ethanol can be used (e.g. 1 mL/g to produce a thick paste), but the ethanol can act as a carbon source in aquatic systems and the subsequent bacterial growth can deplete dissolved oxygen, so this method is less common. Typical immersion doses are 2–20 mg/L, with shorter durations often reported for the higher doses (e.g. 10 mg/L for 90 minutes). Praziquantel is degraded by bacteria in the system. In salt water, degradation time was much faster with repeated treatments (Thomas et al. 2016). Higher applied doses may be needed to attain therapeutic levels during repeated treatments. Assays are the best way to assess the applied dose and typically rely on high-performance liquid chromatography (HPLC) (Gilde and Herzig 2016). Praziquantel usually has no effect on the biological filter.

Injectable treatments are less commonly reported. Typical injectable doses include 5–25 mg/kg IM repeated after an interval of days to weeks. This treatment was reported more efficacious than copper to treat turbellarians in bluespine unicornfish (*Naso unicornis*) (Justine et al. 2009)

Salinity Changes Salinity changes can be useful when pathogens have a different tolerance range than the fish hosts, especially for some ectoparasitic protozoa and monogeneans (Noga 2010a). Increased salinity may also be used in freshwater to treat oomycetes, carp edema virus, nitrite toxicity, and to reduce osmotic stress (Miyazaki et al. 2005; Noga 2010a).

For large changes in salinity, three to five minutes duration dips are typically used (e.g. freshwater dip of marine teleosts, or saltwater dip of freshwater teleosts). The water must be the same pH and temperature as the system water and have suitable oxygen levels (typically 95–100%

saturation). Fish commonly show tachypnea, lethargy, and recumbency during the dip but recover immediately when returned to system water. While most species of teleost can tolerate these dips, the fish should be closely monitored and removed if there are concerns.

Smaller changes in salinity are usually done progressively and maintained for prolonged periods. Typical salinities for prolonged hyposalinity treatments of marine fish are 18–28 g/L. Sensitive fish (e.g. reef sharks) may not be able to handle the lower end of the range (Cavin et al. 2015a). Prolonged exposure to <18 g/L is not recommended for marine, stenohaline species. Typical doses for freshwater fish are 1–5 g/L. Some fish (e.g. channel catfish) are routinely maintained at 1–3 g/L. Most freshwater fish will tolerate this range, but there are exceptions, e.g. elephantfish (*Mormyridae*). Prolonged exposure to higher doses should be used with caution, for example 10 g/L was the mean lethal concentration (LC50) in zebrafish (*Danio rerio*) (Dolezelova et al. 2009). Signs of inappropriate salinity may include lethargy, dyspnea, tachypnea, inappetence, and mortalities (Burgdorf-Moisuk et al. 2011). Gradual changes in salinity do not usually affect the biological filtration (Collins et al. 1975).

Pure uniodized sodium chloride or a seawater mix should be used for hypersalinity baths. Table salt may be used in small aquariums. This should not be confused with Himalayan salt or Epsom salt which contain various amount of magnesium and sulfur. Some salts contain anti-caking agents (e.g. sodium ferrocyanide) and these must be avoided as they can be highly toxic to fish (Noga 2010a). Calculating the quantity of salt or freshwater to add to a tank is described in Boxes A12.4 and A12.5.

Toltrazuril Toltrazuril is a triazine that may be used to treat coccidia. An oral dose of 10 mg/kg q24h for five days may have suppressed *Eimeria southwelli* in some cownose rays (Stamper et al. 1998). Immersion treatment at 2 μg/L for 6–24 hours every other day has been described as a treatment for microsporidiosis (Schmahl et al. 1990).

Trichlorfon or Metrifonate Trichlorfon or metrifonate are the nonproprietary names of an organophosphate whose active form is *O,O*-dimethyl 2,2,2-trichloro-1-hydroxyethyl phosphonate. The most common formulation used in the United States is Dylox® (Bayer). It is a white powder. It can be used as an immersion treatment for branchiurans, copepods, and monogeneans. Typical effective doses are 0.25–0.50 mg/L of active compound for 3–24 hours q7–10d for two to three treatments (Noga 2010a). The label should be read carefully to determine the level of active compound, e.g. Dylox®420SL has 37.3% active ingredient but an active concentration of 420 mg/mL because the carrier solution is heavier than water.

Human contact with this drug or medicated water must be avoided as it is toxic and can be absorbed transdermally. Suitable personal protective equipment is essential. Trichlorfon is regulated by the EPA in the United States. Regulations on the use and disposal must be followed.

The safety margin of trichlorfon, and its degradation product dichlorvos, is low, especially in elasmobranchs. Adverse effects include leukopenia, anemia, and sudden death. Atropine may be administered prior to treatment to mitigate toxicity from the cholinesterase inhibition. This is likely most effective by intramuscular administration (e.g. 0.05–0.10 mg/kg IM), but oral administration is reported anecdotally. Concomitant administration of the immune stimulant propolis has been shown to mitigate adverse effects in koi (Yonar et al. 2015).

Antifungals

Fungal diseases and fungal-like oomycetes (water molds, e.g. *Saprolegnia* spp.) in fish are often treated with copper sulfate, formalin, hydrogen peroxide, albendazole, or salinity changes, but typical antifungals have been used. They are often divided into:

- Triazoles, e.g. fluconazole, itraconazole, posaconazole, and voriconazole.
- Imidazoles, e.g. clotrimazole.
- Echinocandins, e.g. caspofungin.
- Polyene antifungals, e.g. nystatin, bronopol, and fumagillin.

Reports of triazoles in fish are primarily limited to systemic fungal diseases in ornamental fish. Prognosis is usually poor, but the following doses have been reported without adverse effects: itraconazole 20 mg/kg PO q48h for two to eight weeks and voriconazole 10–50 mg/kg PO (Pereira

Box A12.4 Calculation of Salt to be Added to Increase Salinity

$$\text{Salt quantity}(\text{g})\text{ to add} = \text{volume}(\text{L}) \times \left(\text{final salinity}\left[\text{g}/\text{L}\right] - \text{initial salinity}\left[\text{g}/\text{L}\right]\right)$$

$$\text{Salt water}(\text{L})\text{ to add} = \text{volume}(\text{L}) \times \left(\text{final salinity}\left[\text{g}/\text{L}\right] - \text{initial salinity}\left[\text{g}/\text{L}\right]\right) / \text{salinity of added water}(\text{g}/\text{L})$$

Box A12.5 Calculation of Freshwater to be Added to Decrease Salinity

$$\text{Freshwater}(\text{L})\text{ to add} = \text{volume}(\text{L}) \times (\text{initial salinity}[\text{g/L}] - \text{final salinity}[\text{g/L}]) / \text{initial salinity}(\text{g/L})$$

et al. 2002; Cavin and Brodt 2014). No pharmacokinetic data are available.

Fumagillin has been reported as a potential option for microsporidiosis. It can decrease the number of xenomas and the proportion of fish with xenomas. However, severe adverse effects are common (Lauren et al. 1989). Fumagillin has been shown to cause reversible thrombocytopenia in humans. Alternative treatments for microsporidiosis include benzimidazoles, toltrazuril, and monensin, although success has been variable (Sanders et al. 2012).

Antivirals

Few studies have investigated the use of antivirals in fish. In vitro effects have been documented for acyclovir (9-[2-hydroxyethoxymethyl] guanine) against channel catfish virus and salmon herpesvirus (Kimura et al. 1983; Buck and Loh 1985). Other antiviral agents have been less efficient in vitro, including adenine-β-D-arabinofuranoside, phosphonoacetic acid, phosphonoformic acid, and 5-iodo-2′-deoxyuridine (Buck and Loh 1985). Overall, management of viral infections in fish relies on minimizing stressors, good biosecurity, and vaccination.

Anti-inflammatories

Nonsteroidal Anti-inflammatories

Among nonsteroidal anti-inflammatory drugs (NSAIDs), meloxicam, ketoprofen, carprofen, robenacoxib, and indomethacin have been evaluated in fish (Harms et al. 2005; Davis et al. 2006; Lovy et al. 2007; Mettam et al. 2011; Ward et al. 2012; Larouche et al. 2018; Fredholm et al. 2016; Raulic et al. 2020). They are used to reduce inflammation and for analgesia. NSAIDs can be absorbed injectably (IM, ICe, IV), orally, or via immersion.

Meloxicam pharmacokinetics have been studied at 1 mg/kg IM or IV in Nile tilapia (Fredholm et al. 2016). Significant leakage of the drug was seen following IM injection. Elimination was rapid but injections were performed in the caudal third of the body and the portal systems may have had some effect. Ketoprofen at 0.5–2.0 mg/kg IM in goldfish reduced the MAC (minimum anesthetic concentration) of MS-222 but this was not seen at 4.0 mg/kg IM in chain catsharks (*Scyliorhinus retifer*) (Davis et al. 2006; Ward et al. 2012). Ketoprofen at 2 mg/kg IM once was found to decrease postoperative creatine kinase in koi (Harms et al. 2005). Carprofen at 2.5–5.0 mg/kg IM once following acetic acid injection in rainbow trout reduced the time taken for fish to resume feeding compared to controls (Mettam et al. 2011).

Adverse effects associated with some NSAIDs have been reported in fish. Degenerative and necrotic renal and branchial lesions have been associated with diclofenac in rainbow trout (Schwaiger et al. 2004). Perforations of the proximal intestine associated with severe coelomitis and mortalities were noted in trout administered indomethacin at 5–15 mg/kg PO q24h for 30 days (Lovy et al. 2007). Ibuprofen and diclofenac can act as endocrine disruptors in fish (Ji et al. 2013; Guiloski et al. 2015). No histopathologic lesions attributed to the meloxicam were seen in goldfish after a single injection at 5 mg/kg IM (Larouche et al. 2018). No histopathologic lesions were seen in rainbow trout after a single injection of robenacoxib at 2 mg/kg IM (Raulic et al. 2020).

Steroidal Anti-inflammatories

Indications for steroid use in fish are extrapolated from mammals. These include adjunctive treatment of shock, trauma, inflammation, and palliative treatment of tumors (Petervary et al. 1992). Steroids may be administered injectably (IM, ICe, IV), orally, or via immersion. Empirical doses of 1–2 mg/kg dexamethasone sodium phosphate IM PRN or q12h have been suggested.

Very high doses of 50–100 mg/kg dexamethasone IM induced apoptosis in lymphoid organs of elasmobranchs (Walsh et al. 2002). Dexamethasone has shown dose-dependent immune suppressive effects in fish at doses as low as 0.03 μg/kg ICe (Ribas et al. 2016). Prednisolone at 1.4 mg/kg ICe has been used to induce immune suppression in experimental studies (Samuelsen et al. 2003). Immersion in dexamethasone at 20 mg/L has been shown to slow wound healing and ~1 g/L led to osteopenia (Wei et al. 2013; Ochandio et al. 2015).

Hormones

Human Chorionic Gonadotropin

Human chorionic gonadotropin (hCG) is a hormone used to induce spawning in male and female bony fish. As of 2019, it is approved in the United States for use in finfish (Chorulon®, Merck Animal Health) with 0-day withdrawal (US FDA 2019a). It is administered by IM injection or by inoculation through the genital pore. Doses vary greatly (e.g. 30–1000 IU/kg) and may be repeated. In a study on goldfish, a single injection of hCG led to ovulation in 100% of individuals compared to 13% of control females (Targonska and Kucharczyk 2011). Survival to the eyed-egg stage was also highest in the group receiving hCG (Targonska and Kucharczyk 2011).

Gonadotropin-Releasing Hormone Agonists

Gonadotropin-releasing hormone (GnRH) agonists produce an initial increase followed by downregulation of follicle stimulating hormone, luteinizing hormone, testosterone, progesterone, and estradiol. GnRH agonists can be used to induce ovulation in bony fish. Some commonly used formulations contain a synthetic analog of salmon GnRH and a dopamine antagonist such as domperidone or metoclopramide (e.g. Ovaprim®, Syndel USA; Ovopel, Unic-trade, Budapest, Hungary). Doses are typically 0.5–1.0 mL/kg IM or ICe. Studies have shown high fecundity and spawning rates, but efficacy varies across species (Hill et al. 2009). Some species, such as Philippine catfish (*Clarias batrachus*), have shown particularly low spawning rates (Ngamvongchon et al. 1988; Chowdhury et al. 2010). Some studies have reported mortalities of up to 35% (Hill et al. 2009). More blinded studies are needed.

A depot formulation of deslorelin (Suprelorin®, Virbac Laboratories, Carros, France) has been tested in female yellow-spotted river stingrays (*Potamotrygon* sp.) to try to prevent breeding (Hanna 2015). Both 17ß-estradiol and progesterone concentrations increased over four months, compared to the control animals. However, hormonal concentrations have been shown to be unreliable indicators of deslorelin effects in other species and more studies are needed to investigate the effect of this product in fish (Petritz et al. 2013). A depot formulation of leuprolide acetate (Lupron, Abbvie, St. Laurent, QC, Canada) has been used anecdotally at 0.15 mg/kg IM in a pelagic stingray (*Pteroplatytrygon violacea*). No definitive effect was observed on mating behavior nor testosterone levels (Stremme et al. 2007).

Progestins

Progestins are synthetic progestogens used for contraception and treatment of certain reproductive disorders. Medroxyprogesterone acetate has been used at 20 mg/kg IM once a month in stingrays to treat polycystic ovaries in all-female groups of stingrays (*Myliobatiformes*) (Cavin et al. 2015b). Medroxyprogesterone had no contraceptive effect on southern stingrays (*Hypanus americanus*) in a preliminary report (George et al. 2009). A dose of 1 mg/kg ICe has been associated with immunosuppression in common carp (Pietsch et al. 2011).

Vaccines

Vaccines are used in fish to prevent or reduce severity of disease caused by specific bacteria and viruses. Experimental vaccines are also available for some parasitic diseases. Vaccines may be killed (also known as inactivated), modified-live (also known as attenuated), subunit, toxoid, or recombinant. As with other classes, killed vaccines are often safer but less immunogenic. They can be administered by IM or ICe injection, orally, or by immersion. Oral vaccines typically show low efficacy in fish. Some pathogens are particularly suitable for vaccine prophylaxis due to strong immunogenic responses, including *Vibrio* spp., *Yersinia ruckeri*, and infectious hematopoietic necrosis virus.

As of 2019, licensed vaccines in the United States are commercially available for salmonids against infectious salmon anemia (ISA), infectious pancreatic necrosis (IPN), *Aeromonas salmonicida*, *Vibrio anguillarum*, *Vibrio ordalii*, *Aliivibrio salmonicida*, *Edwardsiella ictaluri*, *Yersinia ruckeri*, *Flavobacterium columnare*, and *Renibacterium salmoninarum*. Of these, ISA and IPN are usually killed vaccines while the others are modified live vaccines. A modified live vaccine against cyprinid herpesvirus 3 (Cavoy, Novartis Animal Health, Charlottetown, Canada) was briefly licensed for koi in the United States, but adverse effects were noted in certain facilities and the product was removed from the US market (O'Connor et al. 2014; Weber et al. 2014).

Many more vaccines are reported in the literature and these may be available experimentally. Alternatively, customized vaccines can be produced to a specific pathogen isolated at a specific facility. These are usually known as autogenous vaccines. The term autologous vaccine may be used, although this technically applies to vaccines derived from the same individual. Autogenous vaccines can be produced for bacterial pathogens that can be cultured readily, e.g. *Aeromonas*, *Vibrio*, *Photobacterium*, *Flavobacterium*, *Yersinia*, and *Streptococcus* spp. Autogenous vaccines may be useful for pathogens where strain variation means that a generic vaccine is unlikely to be effective (e.g. *Aeromonas hydrophila*). Commercial vaccines are a better choice for pathogens with low antigenic diversity (e.g. *Aeromonas salmonicida salmonicida*) (Gudmundsdottir et al. 2003). Autogenous vaccines contain adjuvants to amplify the immune response, e.g. aqueous aluminum phosphate, aluminum hydroxide, or oil-based Freund's adjuvant (Gudmundsdottir et al. 2003). Oil-based adjuvants typically result in greater antibody titers and longer protection but may be associated with more injection site reactions (Gudmundsdottir et al. 2003; Fukushima et al. 2017).

In the United States, the oversight of a veterinarian or other qualified fish health specialist is required, and the vaccine must be produced by a USDA-licensed vaccine production facility. Pure cultures should be submitted as soon as possible after isolation and the number of subcultures should be kept to a minimum as they may affect surface antigens. The vaccine should be kept refrigerated and used in less than one to two weeks. Immune stimulants may be given for two weeks before and after vaccination to improve success. Vaccines are most effective when given prior to exposure or clinical signs.

Immune Stimulants

Immune stimulants are naturally occurring compounds that can increase resistance to disease. They may reduce or avoid the need for chemotherapeutics, particularly for *Aeromonas*, *Vibrio*, *Yersinia*, *Edwardsiella*, and *Streptococcus* infections. They can have some effect against ciliates and monogeneans, although the effect is much stronger in vitro than in vivo. They show little to no effect against intracellular organisms (e.g. viruses, *Mycobacterium* spp.) and large parasites (e.g. nematodes, copepods) (Sakai 1999). Immune stimulants can also be used as vaccine adjuvants. Readily available immune stimulants include beta-glucans, garlic (allicin), propolis, and vitamin C.

Beta-glucans

Beta-glucans are nondigestible glucose polysaccharides found within cell walls of bacteria, plants, and fungi (e.g. brewer's yeast, *Saccharomyces* spp.). Beta-glucans, particularly ß-1,3- and ß-1,6-glucans, are used extensively as immune-stimulants in aquaculture (Meena et al. 2013). Beta-glucans are best administered orally or by ICe injection. Most studies have shown improved survival in teleosts when beta-glucans are given at suitable doses prior to challenge with *Aeromonas*, *Vibrio*, *Edwardsiella*, and *Streptococcus* spp. (Meena et al. 2013; Petit and Wiegertjes 2016). Studies have shown reduced parasite load or reduced lesion severity if given prior to challenge with *Ichthyophthirius multifiliis*, *Dactylogyrus* sp., and *Loma salmonae*, although the in vivo effects are mild (Guselle et al. 2010; Lauridsen and Buchmann 2010; del Rio-Zaragoza et al. 2011). Some studies have shown improved wound healing time (Przybylska-Diaz et al. 2013). Typical doses vary by product but for the most commonly reported product (Macrogard, Biorigin, Brazil), effective doses are often 10–50 mg/kg ICe q48h for 3 doses or 0.5–2.0 g/kg diet for one to two weeks.

Longer courses (>4 weeks) typically show no additional benefits, although short courses may have some prolonged effects on immunity (Yoshida et al. 1995; Petit and Wiegertjes 2016). Higher doses can lead to immune suppression and reduced survival compared to lower doses (Meena et al. 2013). The main indication for beta-glucan supplementation is for short courses at suitable doses prior to a stressor such as transport, or during an unavoidable stressor (Barros et al. 2014).

Garlic (Allicin)

Crushed garlic (*Allium sativum*) contains allicin (diallyl thiosulfinate) and other sulfur-allyl compounds. These have immune-stimulant, antioxidant, hypolipidemic, antimicrobial, and antihypertensive properties (Lee and Gao 2012). Whole garlic is not effective. Crushed garlic works well and various commercial solutions are available (e.g. Allyl products by Millipore Sigma, Saint-Louis, MO, USA). The actual dose of active compounds is usually unknown. Many studies have shown improved survival when administered prior to challenge with external bacteria, with some effect against protozoa and monogeneans (Aly and Mohamed 2010; Lee and Gao 2012; Fridman et al. 2014; Schelkle et al. 2015). These products are best administered orally with recommended doses typically 5–10 g/kg of feed for two to four weeks (Shahsavani et al. 2011). Higher doses and longer courses should be avoided as oxidative tissue damage and acute mortalities have been reported (Breyer et al. 2015).

Propolis

Propolis is produced by honeybees using plant resins and beeswax. The ethanol-extracted form is typically more effective than crude propolis. Several active compounds have been identified, including flavonoid aglycones, terpenoids, and cinnamic acid derivatives (Sforcin 2007). Studies usually show increased resistance to certain infectious diseases, such as *Aeromonas hydrophila*, and some effect on monogeneans (Sforcin 2007; El-Asely et al. 2014; Dotta et al. 2015). Propolis also has a protective effect against the toxic effects of certain pesticides, e.g. trichlorfon, malathion, and cypermethrin (Kandiel et al. 2014; Yonar et al. 2015). It is most effective orally or by injection. Typical oral doses are often 5–10 g/kg of feed for up to four weeks (El-Asely et al. 2014; Dotta et al. 2015). No adverse effects have been reported in fish.

Vitamin C

Vitamin C, or ascorbic acid, is an essential vitamin in teleosts. Elasmobranchs, sturgeon, gar, lungfish, and jawless fish seem able to synthesize some vitamin C (Moreau and Dabrowski 1996). Minimum vitamin C requirements for survival are often ~50 mg/kg, but requirements are higher in juvenile fish and may increase 3- to 10-fold when fish are under stress (Kim and Kang 2015). These higher levels appear to have a strong immune-stimulant effect. Vitamin C can be administered orally or by IM injection. Since the vitamin is heat labile and light-sensitive, stabilized oral forms (e.g. L-ascorbyl-2-polyphosphate) should be used and appropriate storage and preparation of products are essential. Oral doses that have resulted in improved fish survival following challenges are typically 500–1500 mg/kg of feed (Kumari and Sahoo 2005; Azad et al. 2007; Ibrahem et al. 2010; Barros et al. 2014; Kim and Kang 2015). No adverse effects have been noted and no ceiling effect has been seen, so maintaining high dietary levels long-term may be a safe way to improve immune function in fish. The requirement for vitamin C is affected by the level of vitamin E in the diet, with recommended vitamin E doses ranging from 50 to 250 mg/kg of feed (Azad et al. 2007; Garcia et al. 2007; Lim et al. 2010). For more information, the reader can refer to Oliva-Teles (2012) and Chapter A4.

Critical Care

Critical care of individual fish is based primarily on clinical experience and anecdotal information, with limited information available in the literature.

Resuscitation of a Nonresponsive Fish

Resuscitation of fish is extrapolated from the sequence reported in other vertebrates (following the acronym ABCD: Airway, Breathing, Circulation, Drugs).

1) Note the time and call for help if needed.
2) Airway: Suitable water must be provided for ventilation. It should have sufficient dissolved oxygen (95–120%) and no anesthetic agents. Any obvious obstruction affecting water flow over the gills should be addressed (e.g. oral foreign body).
3) Breathing: Ventilation can be provided using hand movements, a syringe, a mechanical pump, or by manually swimming the fish through the water to push water through the mouth and over the gills.
4) Circulation: Cardiac compression and management of rhythm abnormalities have not been reported in fish. Of note, cardiac muscle contraction typically continues long after cessation of opercular movement in fish, so a focus on improving ventilation may be more clinically helpful.
5) Emergency drugs: These are given based on doses and responses reported in other vertebrate classes (Table A12.2). Intravenous fluid therapy may be indicated to improve blood pressure (see below).
6) Correction of the primary issue, if known, e.g. control of severe hemorrhage, intravenous atropine following organophosphate toxicity, intravenous antibiotics for acute bacterial septicemia.
7) Cardiovascular support may include gently swimming the fish to improve venous return.
8) Monitoring of heart rate, respiratory rate, blood gases, lactate, water quality (including temperature, dissolved oxygen, nitrogenous wastes, and pH) may be indicated.

Fluid Therapy

Marine teleosts are hyposmotic to their environment and dehydration is a common consequence of disease; fluid

Table A12.2 Proposed doses for emergency drugs in fish.

Drug	Dose	Indication
Atropine sulfate	0.01–0.03 mg/kg IV or IM	Bradycardia; higher doses are used for organophosphate toxicity
Dexamethasone sodium phosphate	1–3 mg/kg IV or IM	Shock, more potent than prednisolone
Dobutamine	0.0005–0.02 mg/kg SLOW IV	Theoretical treatment for acidemia
Doxapram	1–2 mg/kg IV, IM, or topically on the gills	Apnea; hyperactivity and sudden arousal has been reported in elasmobranchs (Stamper 2004)
Epinephrine	0.01–0.2 mg/kg IV	Cardiovascular collapse
Parenteral fluids (0.9% saline, lactated Ringer's, Normosol, Plasmalyte, elasmobranch Ringer's)	5 mL/kg IV bolus Up to 30 mL/kg ICe or SLOW IV	Cardiovascular support, acidemia
Prednisolone sodium succinate (Solu-delta)	1–10 mg/kg IV or IM	Shock
Methylprednisolone sodium succinate (Solu-medrol)	1–20 mg/kg SLOW IV or IM	Shock
Sodium acetate or sodium bicarbonate	1 mEq/kg SLOW IV, best in fluids	Acidemia not responsive to fluid therapy; blood pH should be monitored closely

therapy should always be considered for a sick marine teleost. It is likely that any sick fish could benefit from fluid therapy to improve cardiovascular or renal function and reduce lactic acidosis. Fluids may be administered orally by gavage, intravenously, or intracoelomically. Oral fluid administration can often be done under manual restraint. Dechlorinated freshwater or common isotonic fluids (e.g. lactated Ringer's) may be used. Parenteral fluid administration often requires chemical restraint. Intravenous is the most effective route, although intracoelomic administration is reported. Various common isotonic fluids have been used in fish, including lactated Ringer's, 0.9% normal saline, and various Normosol and Plasmalyte combinations. The authors are not aware of any comparison of fluid type in fish. These fluids typically have an osmolarity of 270–310 mOsm/L. Marine elasmobranchs have a much higher plasma osmolarity (900–1500 mOsm/L) due to high urea, sodium, trimethylamine *N*-oxide (TMAO), chloride, and calcium. It may be best to provide marine elasmobranchs with fluids that have additional salts to more closely approximate their osmolarity. A possible elasmobranch Ringer's solution has been described, consisting of lactated Ringer's with additional sodium chloride (10 g/L), urea (26 g/L), and sodium bicarbonate (0.1 g/L) to reach an osmolarity of ~960 mOsm/L and pH of 7.3 (Andrews and Jones 1990). Four other recipes for elasmobranch-adapted fluids are provided in Mylniczenko and Clauss (2017). Solutions should be passed through a 22 μm filter before being administered parenterally.

Colloids may be administered intravenously to improve fluid volume (e.g. Hemaccel, Hetastarch, or plasma). Transfusions may be used in cases of acute, severe anemia or hemorrhage (Delaune et al. 2017). Cross-matching is recommended, ideally both major and minor. However, in a study involving seven species of elasmobranchs, cross-matches were negative among all conspecifics (Hadfield et al. 2010).

Legislation

This section is intended to give a general overview of the legislation that may apply to medication use in fish. It is not meant as legal advice. Legal advice should only be sought from the relevant regulatory authority, legislation, or a qualified attorney, lawyer, solicitor, or legal advisor with suitable experience of the field and the region.

International Legislation

Some international regulations apply to fish, such as the Convention on International Trade in Endangered Species of Wild Flora and Fauna, the International Air Transport Association (IATA) Live Animal Regulation transport guidelines, and the Aquatic Animal Health Code from the World Organisation for Animal Health (OIE). However, fish medical treatments are not regulated internationally and there is great variability between countries and over time. For example, a drug may be available over-the-counter in one country and prohibited in another.

Legislation in the United States

In the United States, several groups regulate fish therapeutics.

- Drugs are regulated by the Food and Drug Administration's (FDA) Center for Veterinary Medicine (CVM).
- Animal vaccines are regulated by the Animal Plant Health Inspection Service (APHIS) in the Department of Agriculture (USDA).
- Pesticides (e.g. diflubenzuron, lufenuron, trichlorfon) and water discharge are regulated by the Environmental Protection Agency (EPA).
- Water discharge may also be regulated by a local National Pollutant Discharge Elimination System (NPDES) in the state in which the drug use is occurring.

The FDA approves drugs for use in fish, under the authority of the Federal Food, Drug, and Cosmetic Act (FFDCA) and its amendments. The FFDCA defines a "drug" by its intended use. For example, oxygen and sodium chloride are drugs when they are used to mitigate or treat disease.

Drug products are approved for specific species, dosages, and indications, and must be manufactured by specific companies (US FDA 2019a). They must be used according to the approved label instructions. When a product is approved, a withdrawal time is included on the label. The withdrawal period must be followed prior to harvest. Only a few drugs are FDA-approved for use in aquaculture. As of 2019, these are florfenicol (Aquaflor), sulfadimethoxine–ormetoprim (Romet-30 and Romet-TC), sulfamerazine (no longer on the US market), oxytetracycline dihydrate (Terramycin 200 for Fish), oxytetracycline hydrochloride (for vertebral marking; various trade names), hydrogen peroxide (35% Perox-aid), formalin (various trade names), chorionic gonadotropin (Chorulon), chloramine-T (Halamid Aqua), and tricaine methanesulfonate (Tricaine-S®). Of note, tricaine methanesulfonate is approved for temporary immobilization of fish with a 21-day withdrawal. It is not approved for euthanasia. Drug products can also be conditionally approved by the FDA (pending additional data), but none are currently listed for fish. References that provide complete lists of approved drugs in aquaculture include FDA CVM's Aquaculture page (https://www.fda.gov/

AnimalVeterinary/DevelopmentApprovalProcess/Aquaculture/ucm132954.htm) and the US Fish and Wildlife Service (USFWS) guidelines (https://www.fws.gov/fisheries/aadap/aquaculture.html). Additional assistance can be requested at askCVM@fda.hhs.gov.

Off-label or extra-label drug use (ELDU) is defined as the actual or intended use of an approved drug in an animal in a manner that is not in accordance with the approved labeling (e.g. different species, dosage, or indication). ELDU is permitted by veterinarians under the Animal Medicinal Drug Use Clarification Act (AMDUCA; 21 CFR 530). Specific criteria must be met:

- There must be oversight by a licensed veterinarian with a valid veterinarian–client–patient relationship.
- The veterinarian must take appropriate measures to guarantee an adequate withdrawal period is followed, or that the animal and its food products will not enter the human food supply.
- It must be used to treat a disease, where morbidity or mortality would result from failure to treat.

ELDU is not allowed in feed according to the FFDCA and AMDUCA. However, the FDA recognized a significant need for ELDU of medicated feed and published compliance policy guide (CPG) 615.115; this describes the conditions when FDA would not take enforcement action against a veterinarian prescribing extra-label use of a medicated feed. Since January 2017, there are three marketed medicated feed products in aquaculture that are Veterinary Feed Directives (Terramycin 200 for Fish, Romet 30/TC, and Aquaflor). These products can be used in an ELDU manner for minor species provided the veterinarian follows the conditions prescribed in the CPG, including the following:

- The medicated feed is already approved for use in aquatic species.
- There is state-licensed veterinary oversight within a valid veterinarian–client–patient relationship, following a recent examination of the fish. The veterinarian provides the completed VFD form to the client and registered feed distributor/producer.
- Doses and withdrawal periods must be followed.
- The owner must meet specific record requirements (e.g. instructions, invoices, and treatment dates are kept for at least two years), be able to identify treated animals, and meet appropriate withdrawals where applicable.
- Refills are not allowed.

Some drugs are prohibited in food-fish in the US. Prohibited drugs include chloramphenicol, fluoroquinolones, vancomycin, dimetridazole, metronidazole, nitrofurans, malachite green, and steroid hormones (21 CFR 530.41). It is best to also avoid these in ornamental fish if possible, because of safety concerns and to reduce the risk of resistance to antibiotics that are considered critical in human medicine.

Some drugs are listed as low regulatory priority, meaning that they are not formally approved but the FDA is unlikely to object to their use as a treatment within sound management practices. These include sodium chloride, calcium chloride, carbon dioxide, garlic, and povidone iodine (CVM Program Policy and Procedures Manual 1243.4200). Two drugs commonly used in fish are not considered low regulatory priority but regulatory action is being deferred pending further study: copper sulfate and potassium permanganate.

Full drug approval through the FDA is costly and time consuming. For ornamental fish, an alternative is drug indexing, regulated by the Minor Use/Minor Species (MUMS) Act (US FDA 2014). Indexed drugs are evaluated for safety and effectiveness through an alternative FDA review process for use in nonfood animals. Similar to approved drugs, these are for specific species, dosages, and indications, and must be manufactured by specific companies. They cannot be used in food fish and cannot be used in an ELDU manner. As of 2019, metomidate hydrochloride (Aquacalm®, Syndel USA) and the GnRH agonist Ovaprim are indexed drugs for fish. The FDA routinely publishes a list of indexed drugs and veterinarians should regularly check these lists (https://www.fda.gov/AnimalVeterinary/DevelopmentApprovalProcess/MinorUseMinorSpecies/ucm125452.htm).

A drug may also be administered under the Investigational New Animal Drug regulations (INAD; 21 CFR 511). This allows sponsors to use a drug for clinical investigations. The process is monitored through the FDA and can be used in support of a new drug approval. For example, 10% eugenol (Aqui-S 20E®, Aqui-S New Zealand Ltd., New Zealand) and erythromycin (Erymicin 200®, Syndel USA) are being evaluated as INADs under USFWS Aquatic Animal Drug Approval Partnership Program (AADAP; https://www.fws.gov/fisheries/aadap/home.htm).

Compounding refers to altering the ingredients or formulation of a drug (e.g. creating a liquid from tablets). Current US law permits compounding of animal drugs by veterinarians or pharmacists when the source of the active ingredient is an FDA-approved drug, provided the conditions for legal extra-label drug use are followed. The law does not permit compounding from bulk drug substances, but the FDA recognizes that there are circumstances where there are no suitable commercial drugs. A draft guidance was published on the FDA website in November 2019 (GFI #256; US FDA 2019b). It states that the FDA does not intend to take enforcement action for products that meet the following criteria:

- There is no medically appropriate drug that is FDA-approved, conditionally approved, or indexed.
- There is oversight by a licensed veterinarian with a valid veterinarian–client–patient relationship.
- The drug is intended for use in nonfood-producing species (e.g. aquarium and ornamental fish) (exceptions to this are described in the draft guidance under "antidotes for food-producing animals").
- The drug is compounded by or under the direct supervision of a veterinarian or a pharmacist in a state-licensed pharmacy or federal facility using a patient-specific prescription (exceptions to this are described in the draft guidance for "office stock").
- The drug is compounded in accordance with the current US Pharmacopeia and National Formulary.
- The drug is not a copy of an FDA-approved, conditionally approved, or indexed drug; a copy consists of the same active ingredient, at a similar concentration, given by the same route. More detail on this topic is available within the draft guidance.
- The medical rationale should be noted in the patient's medical record.
- The prescription label includes (in addition to normal label requirements): "This is a compounded drug" and "Caution: Federal law restricts this drug to use by or on the order of a licensed veterinarian."
- Any adverse effects are reported to the FDA (form FDA 1932a).

The guidance does not apply to INADs. The guidance specifically excludes controlled drugs.

All pesticides used in the United States must be registered with the EPA according to the Federal Insecticide, Fungicide, and Rodenticide Act (FIFRA). The EPA has the authority to register, restrict, or prohibit the use of pesticides. Pesticide registration decisions balance the risks with the benefits. Veterinarians must get certified to purchase and use restricted use pesticides such as diflubenzuron, lufenuron, and trichlorfon (EPA 2016). Pesticide use must follow label instructions.

Water discharge is also regulated by the EPA under the Clean Water Act (or Federal Water Pollution Control Act) which sets minimum water quality standards. This includes the discharge of copper sulfate and chelated copper compounds. The discharge of pesticides from aquaculture facilities is regulated through the National Pollutant Discharge Elimination System permit (NPDES).

State or local legislation may be more stringent than national legislation. It is essential that veterinarians are familiar with the legislation that applies to their situation.

There are many medications available in pet stores, agricultural cooperatives, and online. If a product is making drug claims and has not been approved, conditionally approved, or indexed, then it is considered an unapproved drug and marketing of it may be illegal. The FDA would not have reviewed these products to ensure they are effective, safe, and properly labeled and manufactured. These products may have misinformation on the label and may not contain the ingredients they say they do. Caution should be exercised if using these products.

Legislation in Europe

In the European Union (EU), legislation regarding fish treatments is made by the European Commission and translated into legislation in each member state (country), which can be more restrictive. *Salmonidae* are considered major food-producing species in the EU, while other fish are classified as minor food-producing species (EMEA 2002). In some EU states, several ornamental fish species are considered domestic animals, e.g. common carp, goldfish, zebrafish, guppies, and bettas (*Betta splendens*) in France (Ministère de l'Ecologie 2006).

Currently approved drugs include bronopol, diflubenzuron, emamectin, florfenicol, flumequine (a first-generation fluoroquinolone), gentamicin, oxolinic acid, oxytetracycline, and trimethoprim–sulfadiazine. Withdrawal times are based on the maximal residue levels (MRLs) defined by the European Food Safety Authority (EFSA).

Prohibited drugs for foodstuff of animal origin are listed in Annex IV of the European regulations and include chloramphenicol, chlorpromazine, colchicine, dimetridazole, metronidazole, nitrofurans, and ronidazole (European Union CEE 2377/1990). Some EU countries further prohibit the use of certain antibiotics in all animal species, which may include vancomycin, certain fluoroquinolones, third- and fourth-generation cephalosporins such as ceftazidime, and antibiotics used against mycobacteriosis. In addition, certain antibiotics can only be used if a bacterial culture has determined that they are the only available treatment (Ministère de l'Agricuture 2016).

Similar to the ELDU in the United States, extra-label drug use is possible for veterinarians treating minor species, using an algorithm known as the cascade (EMEA 2002).

1) Veterinarians must use a drug authorized for that species and indication, if it exists.
2) If none exists, veterinarians can use a drug that is authorized for the same species for a different indication or authorized in the member state for another species.
3) If there is no such product, the options are:

- A drug authorized in the member state for human use can be used if not specifically prohibited from veterinary use. Antibiotics may be specifically excluded.
- Special manufacture of a drug prepared for this occasion by a pharmacy holding an appropriate authorization and under veterinary prescription for a specific case.
- A drug authorized in another EU member state in accordance with the Special Import Authorization Scheme; if used in food fish, it must be authorized for food-producing species.
- In exceptional circumstances, medicines may be imported from countries outside of the EU by the Special Import Authorization Scheme, which takes many months.

A minimum withdrawal period of 500 degree days is required (number of days = 500/water temperature (°C)). Storage and disposal of these drugs and their remnants are under the strict responsibility of the veterinarian who must follow specific regulations.

Conclusion

Despite knowledge gained from aquaculture, ornamental fish therapeutics remains in its infancy and more experimental studies are needed to refine treatment administration.

References

Allender, M.C., Kastura, M., George, R. et al. (2011). Bioencapsulation of metronidazole in adult brine shrimp (*Artemia* sp.). *Journal of Zoo and Wildlife Medicine* 42: 241–246.

Allender, M.C., Kastura, M., George, R. et al. (2012). Bioencapsulation of fenbendazole in adult *Artemia*. *Journal of Exotic Pet Medicine* 21: 207–212.

Aly, S.M. and Mohamed, M.F. (2010). *Echinacea purpurea* and *Allium sativum* as immunostimulants in fish culture using Nile tilapia (*Oreochromis niloticus*). *Journal of Animal Physiology and Animal Nutrition* 94: e31–e39.

Andrews, A.J.C. and Jones, R.T. (1990). A method for the transport of sharks for captivity. *Journal of Aquariculture and Aquatic Sciences* 5: 70–72.

Azad, I.S., Dayal, J.S., Poornima, M., and Ali, S.A. (2007). Supra dietary levels of vitamins C and E enhance antibody production and immune memory in juvenile milkfish, *Chanos chanos* (Forsskal) to formalin-killed *Vibrio vulnificus*. *Fish & Shellfish Immunology* 23: 154–163.

Bakal, R.S., Bai, S.A., and Stoskopf, M.K. (2004). Pharmacokinetics of sulfadimethoxine and ormetoprim in a 5:1 ratio following intraperitoneal and oral administration, in the hybrid striped bass (*Morone chrysops* x *Morone saxitalis*). *Journal of Veterinary Pharmacology and Therapeutics* 27: 1–6.

Barros, M.M., Falcon, D.R., Orsi Rde, O. et al. (2014). Non-specific immune parameters and physiological response of Nile tilapia fed beta-glucan and vitamin C for different periods and submitted to stress and bacterial challenge. *Fish & Shellfish Immunology* 39: 188–195.

Béland, K., Séguin, G., and Lair, S. (2020). Emamectin benzoate as a safe and effective anthelmintic to treat the coelomic nematode *Philometra rubra* in striped bass *Morone saxatilis*. *Diseases of Aquatic Organisms* 142: 47–53.

Blackburn, J.K., Mitchell, M.A., Blackburn, M.C. et al. (2010). Evidence of antibiotic resistance in free-swimming, top-level marine predatory fishes. *Journal of Zoo and Wildlife Medicine* 41: 7–16.

Blanc, G., Loussouarn, S., and Pinault, L. (1992). Biodisponibilité immédiate du lévamisole chez l'anguille Européenne (*Anguilla anguilla* L.) hôte définitif des nématodes *Anguillicola* Yamaguti, 1974. In: *Chemotherapy in Aquaculture: From Theory to Reality* (eds. C. Michel and D.J. Alderman), 468–486. Paris: Office International des Epizooties.

Boogaard, M.A., Bills, T.D., and Johnson, D.A. (2003). Acute toxicity of TFM and a TFM/niclosamide mixture to selected species of fish, including lake sturgeon (*Acipenser fulvescens*) and mudpuppies (*Necturus maculosus*), in laboratory and field exposures. *Journal of Great Lakes Research* 29: 529–541.

Bosch, A.C., O'Neil, B., Sigge, G.O. et al. (2016). Mercury accumulation in yellowfin tuna (*Thunnus albacares*) with regards to muscle type, muscle position and fish size. *Food Chemistry* 190: 351–356.

Bowser, P.R., Wooster, G.A., St Leger, J., and Babish, J.G. (1992). Pharmacokinetics of enrofloxacin in fingerling rainbow trout (*Oncorhynchus mykiss*). *Journal of Veterinary Pharmacology and Therapeutics* 15: 62–71.

Breyer, K.E., Getchell, R.G., Cornwell, E.R. et al. (2015). Efficacy of an extract from garlic, *Allium sativum*, against infection with the furunculosis bacterium, *Aeromonas salmonicida*, in rainbow trout, *Oncorhynchus mykiss*. *Journal of the World Aquaculture Society* 46: 273–282.

Brooks, C.R., Heidinger, R.C., and Kohler, C.C. (1994). Mass-marking otoliths of larval and juvenile walleyes by immersion in oxytetracycline, calcein, or calcein blue.

North American Journal of Fisheries Management 14: 143–150.

Buchmann, K., Bresciani, J., and Jappe, C. (2004). Effects of formalin treatment on epithelial structure and mucous cell densities in rainbow trout, *Oncorhynchus mykiss* (Walbaum), skin. *Journal of Fish Diseases* 27: 99–104.

Buck, C.C. and Loh, P.C. (1985). In vitro effect of acyclovir and other antiherpetic compounds on the replication of channel catfish virus. *Antiviral Research* 5: 269–280.

Bulfon, C., Volpatti, D., and Galeotti, M. (2015). Review article: current research on the use of plant-derived products in farmed fish. *Aquaculture Research* 46: 513–551.

Burgdorf-Moisuk, A., Mitchell, M., and Watson, M. (2011). Clinical and physiologic effects of sodium chloride baths in goldfish (*Carassius auratus*). *Journal of Zoo and Wildlife Medicine* 42: 586–592.

Canada Food Inspection Agency (2017). CFIA aquaculture therapeutant residue monitoring list [online]. http://www.inspection.gc.ca/food/fish-and-seafood/manuals/standards-and-methods/eng/1348608971859/1348609209602?chap=7 (accessed 1 December 2016).

Cavin, J.M. and Brodt, J.F. (2014). Medical management of acute positive buyancy in a leafy sea dragon (*Phycodurus eques*). *Proceedings of the International Association for Aquatic Animal Medicine Conference*, Gold Coast, Australia.

Cavin, J.M., Innis, C.J., Tuxbury, K.A. et al. (2015a). Elasmobranch reproductive physiology, disorders, and treatment. *Proceedings of the International Association for Aquatic Animal Medicine Conference*, Chicago, IL.

Cavin, J.M., Innis, C.J., Tuxbury, K.A. et al. (2015b). The trials (and errors) of learning about a new species: veterinary management of blacknose sharks (*Carcharhinus acronotus*). *Proceedings of the International Association for Aquatic Animal Medicine Conference*, Chicago, IL.

Chair, M., Nelis, H.J., Leger, P. et al. (1996). Accumulation of trimethoprim, sulfamethoxazole, and N-acetylsulfamethoxazole in fish and shrimp fed medicated *Artemia franciscana*. *Antimicrobial Agents and Chemotherapy* 40: 1649–1652.

Chakoumakos, C. (1979). Toxicity of copper to cutthroat trout (*Salmo clarki*) under different conditions of alkalinity, pH, and hardness. *Environmental Science and Technology* 13: 213–219.

Chang, C.T. and Whipps, C.M. (2015). Activity of antibiotics against *Mycobacterium* species commonly found in laboratory zebrafish. *Journal of Aquatic Animal Health* 27: 88–95.

Chitmanat, C., Tongdonmuan, K., and Nunsong, W. (2005). The use of crude extracts from traditional medicinal plants to eliminate *Trichodina* sp. in tilapia (*Oreochromis niloticus*) fingerlings. *Songklanakarin Journal of Science and Technology* 27: 359–364.

Chmelova, L., Sehonova, P., Doubkova, V. et al. (2016). Effects of therapeutic formalin bath on selected indices in fish. *Neuro Endocrinology Letters* 37: 67–77.

Chowdhury, M., Chatterjee, A., Mondal, A., and Chatterji, U. (2010). Ovaprim abrogates expression of GnRH receptor-II in the Indian catfish. *International Journal of Biology* 2: 189–198.

Clarke, E.O.I. (2016). Topical application of misoprostol and phenytoin gel for treatment of dermal ulceration in teleosts. *Proceedings of the International Association for Aquatic Animal Medicine Conference*, Virginia Beach, VA.

Clarke, E.O.I., Grzenda, K., Murphy, D. et al. (2015). Successful treatment of *Eimeria southwelli* in a cownose ray (*Rhinoptera bonasus*) using oral copper wire particles. *Proceedings of the International Association for Aquatic Animal Medicine Conference*, New Orleans, LA.

Collins, M., Gratzek, J., Daw, D. et al. (1975). Effects of parasiticides agents on nitrification. *Journal of the Fisheries Research Board of Canada* 32: 2033–2037.

Collins, M., Gratzek, J., Shotts, F., and Al, E. (1976). Effects of antibacterial agents on nitrification in an aquatic recirculating system. *Journal of the Fisheries Research Board of Canada* 33: 215–218.

Collymore, C., Watral, V., White, J.R. et al. (2014). Tolerance and efficacy of emamectin benzoate and ivermectin for the treatment of *Pseudocapillaria tomentosa* in laboratory zebrafish (*Danio rerio*). *Zebrafish* 11: 490–497.

Cook, M.A. and Rust, M.B. (2002). Bioencapsulation of five forms of erythromycin by adult *Artemia salina* (L.). Bioencapsulation of five forms of erythromycin by adult *Artemia salina*. *Journal of Fish Diseases* 25: 165–170.

Coutant, T., Vergneau-Grosset, C., and Lair, S. (2019). Effect of a misoprostol/phenytoin gel on experimentally induced wounds in brook trout (*Salvelinus frontinalis*) – a randomized study. *Journal of Aquatic Animal Health* 31: 214–221.

Crossley, S.M., George, A.L., and Keller, C.J. (2009). A method for eradicating amphipod parasites (hyperiidae) from host jellyfish, *Chrysaora fuscescens* (Brandt, 1835), in a closed recirculating system. *Journal of Zoo and Wildlife Medicine* 40: 174–180.

Danyi, S., Widart, J., Douny, C. et al. (2011). Determination and kinetics of enrofloxacin and ciprofloxacin in Tra catfish (*Pangasianodon hypophthalmus*) and giant freshwater prawn (*Macrobrachium rosenbergii*) using a liquid chromatography/mass spectrometry method. *Journal of Veterinary Pharmacology and Therapeutics* 34: 142–152.

Davis, M.R., Mylniczenko, N., Storms, T. et al. (2006). Evaluation of intramuscular ketoprofen and butorphanol as analgesics in chain dogfish (*Scyliorhinus retifer*). *Zoo Biology* 25: 491–500.

Dawson, V.K. (2003). Environmental fate and effects of the lampricide bayluscide: a review. *Journal of Great Lakes Research* 29: 475–492.

Del Rio-Zaragoza, O.B., Fajer-Ávila, E.J., and Almazán-Reuda, P. (2011). Influence of ß-glucan on innate immunity and resistance of *Lutjanus guttatus* to an experimental infection of dactylogyrid monogeneans. *Parasite Immunology* 33: 483–494.

Delaune, A.J.M., Field, C.L., and Clauss, T.M. (2017). Whole blood transfusions to treat severe anemia in seven cownose rays (*Rhinoptera bonasus*) and one short-tail stingray (*Dasyatis brevicaudata*). *Journal of Zoo and Wildlife Medicine* 48: 1172–1180.

Della Rocca, G., Di Salvo, A., Malvisi, J., and Sello, M. (2004). The disposition of enrofloxacin in seabream (*Sparus aurata* L.) after single intravenous injection or from medicated feed administration. *Aquaculture* 232: 53–62.

Doi, A.M., Stoskopf, M.K., and Lewbart, G.A. (1998). Pharmacokinetics of oxytetracycline in the red pacu (*Colossoma brachypomum*) following different routes of administration. *Journal of Veterinary Pharmacology and Therapeutics* 21: 364–368.

Dolezelova, P., Macova, S., Plhalova, L. et al. (2009). Comparison of the sensitivity of different fish species to medical substances. *Neuroendocrinology Letters* 30 (Suppl. 1): 248–252.

Dotta, G., Brum, A., Jeronimo, G.T. et al. (2015). Effect of dietary supplementation with propolis and *Aloe barbadensis* extracts on hematological parameters and parasitism in Nile tilapia. *Revista Brasileira de Parasitologia Veterinária* 24: 66–71.

Ekanem, A.P., Obiekezie, A., Kloas, W., and Knopf, K. (2004). Effects of crude extracts of *Mucuna pruriens* (Fabaceae) and *Carica papaya* (Caricaceae) against the protozoan fish parasite *Ichthyophthirius multifiliis*. *Parasitology Research* 92: 361–366.

El-Asely, A.M., Abbass, A.A., and Austin, B. (2014). Honey bee pollen improves growth, immunity and protection of Nile tilapia (*Oreochromis niloticus*) against infection with *Aeromonas hydrophila*. *Fish & Shellfish Immunology* 40: 500–506.

Environmental Protection Agency (EPA) (2016). How to get certified as a pesticide applicator [online]. https://www.epa.gov/pesticide-worker-safety/how-get-certified-pesticide-applicator (accessed 2 December 2016).

European Agency for the Evaluation of Medicinal Products (EMEA) (2002). Points to consider regarding efficacy requirements for minor species and minor indications. *Veterinary Medicines and Inspections* [online]. http://www.ema.europa.eu/docs/en_GB/document_library/Scientific_guideline/2009/10/WC500004682.pdf (accessed 7 December 2016).

European Food Safety Authority (EFSA) (2016). Malachite green in food. EFSA panel on contaminants in the food chain. *EFSA Journal* 14: 4530.

Fairgrieve, W., Masada, C., Mcauley, W. et al. (2005). Accumulation and clearance of orally administered erythromycin and its derivative, azithromycin, in juvenile fall chinook salmon *Oncorhynchus tshawytscha*. *Diseases of Aquatic Organisms* 64: 99–106.

Fairgrieve, W., Masada, C., Peterson, M. et al. (2006). Concentrations of erythromycin and azithromycin in mature Chinook salmon *Oncorhynchus tshawytscha* after intraperitoneal injection, and in their progeny. *Diseases of Aquatic Organisms* 68: 227–234.

Fan, J., Shan, Q., Wang, J. et al. (2017). Comparative pharmacokinetics of enrofloxacin in healthy and *Aeromonas hydrophila*-infected crucian carp (*Carassius auratus gibelio*). *Journal of Veterinary Pharmacology and Therapeutics* 40: 580–582.

Fang, X., Liu, X., Liu, W., and Lu, C. (2011). Pharmacokinetics of enrofloxacin in allogynogenetic silver crucian carp, *Carassius auratus gibelio*. *Journal of Veterinary Pharmacology and Therapeutics* 35: 397–401.

Fang, X., Zhou, J., and Liu, X. (2016). Pharmacokinetics of enrofloxacin in snakehead fish, *Channa argus*. *Journal of Veterinary Pharmacology and Therapeutics* 39: 209–212.

Fayette, M.A., Rose, J.B., Hunter, R.P. et al. (2019). Naïve-pooled pharmacokinetics of ceftiofur crystalline free acid after single intramuscular administration in smooth dogfish (*Mustelus canis*). *Journal of Zoo and Wildlife Medicine* 50: 466–469.

Fischer, S.A. and Hall, L.W. (1992). Environmental concentrations and aquatic toxicity data on diflubenzuron (Dimilin). *Critical Reviews in Toxicology* 22: 45–79.

Fleming, G.J., Corwin, A., McCoy, A.J., and Stamper, M.A. (2008). Treatment factors influencing the use of recombinant platelet-derived growth factor (Regranex) for head and lateral line erosion syndrome in ocean surgeonfish (*Acanthurus bahianus*). *Journal of Zoo and Wildlife Medicine* 39: 155–160.

Food and Agriculture Organization of the United Nations (2008). Lufenuron. FAO specifications and evaluations for agricultural pesticides [online]. http://www.fao.org/agriculture/crops/thematic-sitemap/theme/pests/jmps/ps-new/en/ (accessed 2 December 2016).

Forwood, J.M., Harris, J.O., and Deveney, M.R. (2013). Efficacy of bath and orally administered praziquantel and fenbendazole against *Lepidotrema bidyana* Murray, a monogenean parasite of silver perch, *Bidyanus bidyanus* (Mitchell). *Journal of Fish Diseases* 36: 939–947.

Fredholm, D.V., Mylniczenko, N.D., and Kukanich, B. (2016). Pharmacokinetic evaluation of meloxicam after intravenous and intramuscular administration in Nile tilapia (*Oreochromis niloticus*). *Journal of Zoo and Wildlife Medicine* 47: 736–742.

Fridman, S., Sinai, T., and Zilberg, D. (2014). Efficacy of garlic-based treatments against monogenean parasites infecting the guppy (*Poecilia reticulata* (Peters)). *Veterinary Parasitology* 203: 51–58.

Fu, Y., Zhang, Q., Xu, D.H. et al. (2014). Parasiticidal effects of *Morus alba* root bark extracts against *Ichthyophthirius multifiliis* infecting grass carp. *Diseases of Aquatic Organisms* 108: 129–136.

Fukushima, H.C., Leal, C.A., Cavalcante, R.B. et al. (2017). *Lactococcus garvieae* outbreaks in Brazilian farms lactococcosis in *Pseudoplatystoma* sp. – development of an autogenous vaccine as a control strategy. *Journal of Fish Diseases* 40: 263–272.

Garcia, F., Pilarski, F., Onaka, E.M. et al. (2007). Hematology of *Piaractus mesopotamicus* fed diets supplemented with vitamins C and E, challenged by *Aeromonas hydrophila*. *Aquaculture* 271: 39–46.

Garcia-Parraga, D., Rodriguez J.M., Alvaro, T. et al. (2010). Preliminary study of cefovecin (Convenia©) pharmacokinetics in several aquatic species. *Proceedings of the European Association of Aquatic Mammals Conference*, Lisbon, Portugal.

Garner, M.M. (2013). A retrospective study of disease in elasmobranchs. *Veterinary Pathology* 50: 377–389.

Gaunt, P.S., Langston, C., Wrzesinski, C. et al. (2012). Single intravenous and oral dose pharmacokinetics of florfenicol in the channel catfish (*Ictalurus punctatus*). *Journal of Veterinary Pharmacology and Therapeutics* 35: 503–507.

Gaunt, P.S., Langston, C., Wrzesinski, C. et al. (2013). Multidose pharmacokinetics of orally administered florfenicol in the channel catfish (*Ictalurus punctatus*). *Journal of Veterinary Pharmacology and Therapeutics* 39: 502–506.

George, R.H., Allender, M.C., and Irvin, L. (2009). Ultrasonography as a tool in defining and managing the reproductive cycle of *Dasyatis americana* and *Aetobatus narinari* in captivity. *Proceedings of the International Association of Aquatic Animal Medicine Conference*, San Antonio, TX.

Gilde, K. and Herzig, B. (2016). Praziquantel determination in aquarium water by direct injection on a monolithic silica column. *Proceedings of the Marine Aquaculture Conference of North America*, San Diego, CA.

Gomez-Gil, B., Cabanillas-Ramos, J., Paez-Brambila, S., and Roque, A. (2001). Standardization of the bioencapsulation of enrofloxacin and oxytetracyclin in *Artemia franciscana* Kellogs, 1906. *Aquaculture* 196: 1–12.

Goodwin, A.E., Park, E., and Nowak, B.F. (2005). Short communication: successful treatment of largemouth bass, *Micropterus salmoides* (L.), with epitheliocystis hyperinfection. *Journal of Fish Diseases* 28: 623–625.

Govett, P.D., Buur, J., Krein, A. et al. (2009). Pharmacokinetics of ceftazidime in koi (*Cyprinus carpio*) after single dose intramuscular or intracoelomic administration. *Proceedings of the International Association of Aquatic Animal Health Conference*, San Antonio, TX.

Grosset, C., Weber, E.S., Gehring, R. et al. (2015). Evaluation of an extended-release formulation of ceftiofur crystalline-free acid in koi (*Cyprinus carpio*). *Journal of Veterinary Pharmacology and Therapeutics* 38: 606–615.

Gudmundsdottir, S., Lange, S., Magnadottir, B., and Gudmundsdottir, B.K. (2003). Protection against atypical furunculosis in Atlantic halibut, *Hippoglossus hippoglossus* (L.); comparison of a commercial furunculosis vaccine and an autogenous vaccine. *Journal of Fish Diseases* 26: 331–338.

Guiloski, I.C., Ribas, J.L., Pereira Lda, S. et al. (2015). Effects of trophic exposure to dexamethasone and diclofenac in freshwater fish. *Ecotoxicology and Environmental Safety* 114: 204–211.

Guo, L., Xie, Z., Lin, X. et al. (2005). Pharmacokinetics of ciprofloxacin in eels by high-performance liquid chromatography with fluorescence detection. *Analytical Biochemistry* 341: 275–279.

Guselle, N.J., Speare, D.J., and Markham, R.J.F. (2010). Efficacy of intraperitoneally and orally administered ProVale, a yeast ß-(1,3)-d-glcan product, in inhibitoring xenoma formation by the microsporidian *Loma salmonae* on rainbow trout gills. *North American Journal of Aquaculture* 72: 65–72.

Hadfield, C.A. and Clayton, L.A. (2011). Fish quarantine: current practices in public zoos and aquaria. *Journal of Zoo and Wildlife Medicine* 42: 641–650.

Hadfield, C.A., Haines, A.N., Clayton, L.A., and Whitaker, B.R. (2010). Cross matching of blood in carcharhiniform, lamniform, and orectolobiform sharks. *Journal of Zoo and Wildlife Medicine* 41: 480–486.

Hanna, J. (2015). The effects of deslorelin implantation on the reproductive steroid hormones of female freshwater stingrays. *Proceedings of the Regional Aquatic Workshop*, Monterey, CA.

Harikrishnan, R., Balasundaram, C., and Heo, M.S. (2010). Potential use of probiotic- and triherbal extract-enriched diets to control *Aeromonas hydrophila* infection in carp. *Diseases of Aquatic Organisms* 92: 41–49.

Harms, C.A. (1996). Treatments for parasitic diseases of aquarium and ornamental fish. *Seminars of Avian and Exotic Pet Medicine* 5: 54–63.

Harms, C.A. and Wildgoose, W. (2001). Surgery. In: *BSAVA Manual of Ornamental Fish*, 2e (ed. W. Wildgoose), 159–266. Quedgeley: British Small Animal Veterinary Association.

Harms, C.A., Lewbart, G.A., Swanson, C.R. et al. (2005). Behavioral and clinical pathology changes in koi carp (*Cyprinus carpio*) subjected to anesthesia and surgery with and without intra-operative analgesics. *Comparative Medicine* 55: 221–226.

Health Canada (2010). List of veterinary drugs that are authorized for sale by Health Canada for use in food-producing aquatic animals. *Drug and Health Products* [online]. http://www.hc-sc.gc.ca/dhp-mps/vet/legislation/pol/aquaculture_anim-eng.php (accessed 12 November 2016).

Heinen, J.M., Weber, A.L., Noble, A.C., and Morton, J.D. (1995). Tolerance to formalin by a fluidized-bed biofilter and rainbow trout *Oncorhynchus mykiss* in a recirculating culture system. *Journal of the World Aquaculture Society* 26: 65–71.

Helgesen, K.O., Romstad, H., Aaen, S.M., and Horsberg, T.E. (2015). First report of reduced sensitivity towards hydrogen peroxide found in the salmon louse *Lepeophtheirus salmonis* in Norway. *Aquaculture Reports* 1: 37–42.

Hill, J.E., Kilgore, K.H., and Pouder, D.B. (2009). Survey of Ovaprim use as a spawning aid in ornamental fishes in the United States as administered through the University of Florida Tropical Aquaculture Laboratory. *North Amercian Journal of Aquaculture* 71: 206–209.

Hirazawa, N., Mitsuboshi, T., Hirata, T., and Shirasu, K. (2004). Susceptibility of spotted halibut *Verasper variegatus* (Pleuronectidae) to infection by the monogenean *Neobenedenia girellae* (Capsalidae) and oral therapy trials. *Aquaculture* 238: 83–95.

Horsberg, T.E. and Hoy, T. (1991). Tissue distribution of 14C-diflubenzuron in Atlantic salmon (*Salmo salar*). *Acta Veterinaria Scandinavica* 32: 527–533.

Horsberg, T.E., Martinsen, B., Sandersen, K., and Zernichow, L. (1997). Potentiated sulfonamides: in vitro inhibitory effect and pharmacokinetic properties in Atlantic salmon in seawater. *Journal of Aquatic Animal Health* 9: 203–210.

Hu, Y., Ji, J., Ling, F. et al. (2014). Screening medicinal plants for use against *Dactylogyrus intermedius* (Monogenea) infection in goldfish. *Journal of Aquatic Animal Health* 26: 127–136.

Hubert, T.D., Bernardy, J.A., Vue, C. et al. (2005). Residues of the lampricides 3-trifluoromethyl-4-nitrophenol and niclosamide in muscle tissue of rainbow trout. *Journal of Agricultural and Food Chemistry* 53: 5342–5346.

Hustvedt, S.O., Salte, R., and Vassvik, V. (1991). Absorption, distribution and elimination of oxolinic acid in Atlantic salmon (*Salmo salar* L.) after various routes of administration. *Aquaculture* 95: 193–197.

Ibrahem, M.D., Fathi, M., Mesalhy, S., and Abd El-Aty, A.M. (2010). Effect of dietary supplementation of inulin and vitamin C on the growth, hematology, innate immunity, and resistance of Nile tilapia (*Oreochromis niloticus*). *Fish & Shellfish Immunology* 29: 241–246.

Inglis, V., Richards, R.H., Varma, K.J. et al. (1991). Florfenicol in Atlantic salmon, *Salmo salar L.*, parr: tolerance and assessment of efficacy against furunculosis. *Journal of Fish Diseases* 14: 343–351.

Intorre, L., Meucci, V., Di Bello, D. et al. (2007). Tolerance of benzalkonium chloride, formalin, malachite green, and potassium permanganate in goldfish and zebrafish. *Journal of the American Veterinary Medical Association* 231: 590–595.

Ji, J., Lu, C., Kang, Y. et al. (2012). Screening of 42 medicinal plants for in vivo anthelmintic activity against *Dactylogyrus intermedius* (Monogenea) in goldfish (*Carassius auratus*). *Parasitology Research* 111: 97–104.

Ji, K., Liu, X., Lee, S. et al. (2013). Effects of non-steroidal anti-inflammatory drugs on hormones and genes of the hypothalamic-pituitary-gonad axis, and reproduction of zebrafish. *Journal of Hazardous Materials* 254–255: 242–251.

Justine, J.-L., Leblanc, P., Keller, F., and Lester, R.J.G. (2009). Turbellarian black spot disease in bluespine unicornfish *Naso unicornis* in New Caledonia, caused by the parasitic turbellariam *Piscinquilinus* sp. *Diseases of Aquatic Organisms* 85: 245–249.

Kandiel, M.M., El-Asely, A.M., Radwan, H.A., and Abbass, A.A. (2014). Modulation of genotoxicity and endocrine disruptive effects of malathion by dietary honeybee pollen and propolis in Nile tilapia (*Oreochromis niloticus*). *Journal of Advanced Research* 5: 671–684.

Khalil, W.F., Shaheen, H.M., and Abdou, R.H. (2016). Ceftiofur pharmacokinetics in Nile tilapia *Oreochromis niloticus* after intracardiac and intramuscular administrations. *Diseases of Aquatic Organisms* 121: 29–35.

Kim, K.H. and Cho, J.B. (2000). Treatment of *Microcotyle sebastis* (Monogenea: Polyopisthocotylea) infestation with praziquantel in an experimental cage simulating commercial rockfish *Sebastes schlegeli* culture conditions. *Diseases of Aquatic Organisms* 40: 229–231.

Kim, J.-H. and Kang, J.-C. (2015). Influence of dietary ascorbic acid on the immune responses of juvenile korean rockfish *Sebastes schlegelii*. *Journal of Aquatic Animal Health* 27: 178–184.

Kim, K.H. and Kim, C.S. (2002). Cimetidine enhances the plasma praziquantel concentation and treatment efficacy against *Microcotyle sebastis* in cultured rockfish *Sebastes schlegeli*. *Diseases of Aquatic Organisms* 49: 45–49.

Kim, K.H., Kim, C.S., and Kim, J.-W. (2001). Depletion of praziquantel in plasma and muscle tissue of cultured rockfish *Sebastes schlegeli* after oral and bath treatment. *Diseases of Aquatic Organisms* 45: 203–207.

Kim, M.-S., Lim, J.-H., Park, B.-K. et al. (2006). Pharmacokinetics of enrofloxacin in Korean catfish (*Silurus asotus*). *Journal of Veterinary Pharmacology and Therapeutics* 29: 397–402.

Kimura, T., Suzuki, S., and Yoshimizu, M. (1983). In vitro antiviral effect of 9-(2-hydroxyethoxymethyl) guanine on the fish herpesvirus, *Oncorhynchus masou* virus (OMV). *Antiviral Research* 3: 93–101.

Kitzman, J.V., Holley, J.H., Huber, W.G. et al. (1990). Pharmacokinetics and metabolism of fenbendazole in channel catfish. *Veterinary Research Communications* 14: 217–226.

Klaver, A.L. and Matthews, R.A. (1994). Effects of oxytetracycline on nitrification in a model aquatic system. *Aquaculture* 123: 237–247.

Knight, S.J., Boles, L., and Stamper, M.A. (2016). Response of recirculating saltwater aquariums to long-term formalin treatment. *Journal of Zoo and Aquarium Research* 4: 77–84.

Kołodziejska, M., Maszkowska, J., Białk-Bielińska, A. et al. (2013). Aquatic toxicity of four veterinary drugs commonly applied in fish farming and animal husbandry. *Chemosphere* 92: 1253–1259.

Kumari, J. and Sahoo, P.K. (2005). High dietary vitamin C affects growth, non-specific immune response and disease resistance in Asian catfish (*Clarias batrachus*). *Molecular and Cellular Biochemistry* 280: 25–33.

Kyuchukova, R., Milanova, A., Pavlov, A., and Lashev, L. (2015). Comparison of plasma and tissue disposition of enrofloxacin in rainbow trout (*Oncorhynchus mykiss*) and common carp (*Cyprinus carpio*) after a single oral administration. *Food Additive and Contaminants Part A: Chemistry, Analysis, Control, Exposure and Risk Assessment* 32: 35–39.

Ladouceur, E.E., Wynne, J., Garner, M.M. et al. (2016). Lesions of copper toxicosis in captive marine invertebrates with comparisons to normal histology. *Veterinary Pathology* 53: 648–658.

Langford, K.H., Oxnevad, S., Schoyen, M., and Thomas, K.V. (2014). Do antiparasitic medicines used in aquaculture pose a risk to the Norwegian aquatic environment? *Environmental Science and Technology* 48: 7774–7780.

Larouche, C.B., Limoges, M.J., and Lair, S. (2018). Absence of acute toxicity of a single intramuscular injection of meloxicam in goldfish (*Carassius auratus auratus*): A randomized controlled trial. *Journal of Zoo and Wildlife Medicine* 49: 617–622.

Larrat, S., Marvin, J., and Lair, S. (2012). Safety and efficacy of emamectin benzoate to treat *Anguillicoloides crassus* (Kuwahara, Niimi and Itagaki) infections in American eels (*Anguilla rostrata*, Lesueur). *Journal of Fish Diseases* 35: 467–470.

Lauren, D.J., Wishkovsky, A., Groff, J.M. et al. (1989). Toxicity and pharmacokinetics of the antibiotic fumagillin in yearling rainbow trout (*Salmo gairdneri*). *Toxicology and Applied Pharmacology* 98: 444–453.

Lauridsen, J.H. and Buchmann, K. (2010). Effects of short- and long-term glucan feeding of rainbow trout (Salmonidae) on the susceptibility to *Ichthyophthirius multifiliis* infections. *Acta Ichthyologica et Piscatoria* 40: 61–66.

Lee, J.-Y. and Gao, Y. (2012). Review of the application of garlic, *Allium sativum*, in aquaculture. *Journal of the World Aquaculture Society* 43: 447–458.

Leibowitz, M.P., Chettri, J.K., Ofir, R., and Zilberg, D. (2010). Treatment development for systemic *Tetrahymena* sp. infection in guppies, *Poecilia reticulata* Peters. *Journal of Fish Diseases* 33: 473–480.

Lewbart, G.A., Vaden, S., Deen, J. et al. (1997). Pharmacokinetics of enrofloxacin in the red pacu (*Colossoma brachypomum*) after intramuscular, oral and bath administration. *Jounal of Veterinary Pharmacology and Therapeutics* 20: 124–128.

Lewbart, G.A., Butkus, D.A., Papich, M.G. et al. (2005a). Evaluation of a method of intracoelomic catheterization in koi. *Journal of the American Veterinary Medical Association* 226: 784–788.

Lewbart, G.A., Papich, M.G., and Whitt-Smith, D. (2005b). Pharmacokinetics of florfenicol in the red pacu (*Piaractus *brachypomus*) after single dose intramuscular administration. *Journal of Veterinary Pharmacology and Therapeutics* 28: 317–319.

Lie, G., Guo, Y., Zhao, D. et al. (2006). Effects of levamisole on the immune response and disease resistance of *Clarias fuscus*. *Aquaculture* 253: 212–217.

Lim, C., Yildirim-Aksoy, M., Welker, T., and Klesius, P.H. (2010). Growth performance, immune response, and resistance to *Streptococcus iniae* of Nile tilapia, *Oreochromis niloticus*, fed diets containing various levels of vitamins C and E. *Journal of the World Aquaculture Society* 41: 35–48.

Lim, J.-H., Kim, M.-S., Hwang, Y.-H. et al. (2011). Pharmacokinetics of florfenicol following intramuscular and intravenous administration in olive flounder (*Paralichthys olivaceus*). *Journal of Veterinary Pharmacology and Therapeutics* 34: 206–208.

Liu, Y.T., Wang, F., Wang, G.X. et al. (2010). In vivo anthelmintic activity of crude extracts of *Radix angelicae pubescentis, Fructus bruceae, Caulis spatholobi, Semen aesculi,* and *Semen pharbitidis* against *Dactylogyrus intermedius* (Monogenea) in goldfish (*Carassius auratus*). *Parasitology Research* 106: 1233–1239.

Liu, Y., Zhou, Z., Wu, N. et al. (2012). Gibel carp *Carassius auratus* gut microbiota after oral administration of trimethoprim/sulfamethoxazole. *Diseases of Aquatic Organisms* 99: 207–213.

Lovy, J., Speare, D.J., and Wright, G.M. (2007). Pathological effects caused by chronic treatment of rainbow trout with indomethacin. *Journal of Aquatic Animal Health* 19: 94–98.

Lunestad, B.T. and Goksoyr, J. (1990). Reduction in the antibacterial effect of oxytetracycline in seawater by complex formation with magnesium and calcium. *Diseases of Aquatic Organisms* 9: 67–72.

Martinsen, B. and Horsberg, T.E. (1995). Comparative single-dose pharmacokinetics of four quinolones, oxolinic acid, flumequine, sarafloxacin, and enrofloxacin, in Atlantic salmon (*Salmo salar*) held in seawater at 10 degrees C. *Antimicrobial Agents and Chemotherapy* 39: 1059–1064.

Mayer, J., Hensel, P., Mejia-Fava, J. et al. (2013). The use of lufenuron to treat fish lice (*Argulus* sp.) in koi (*Cyprinus carpio*). *Journal of Exotic Pet Medicine* 22: 65–69.

Mcdermott, A.J., Field, C.L., Hoopes, L.A., and Clauss, T.M. (2016). Medical management of coelomic distention, abnormal swimming, substrate retention, and hematologic changes in a reef manta ray (*Manta alfredi*). *Journal of Zoo and Wildlife Medicine* 47: 927–930.

Meena, D.K., Das, P., Kumar, S. et al. (2013). Beta-glucan: an ideal immunostimulant in aquaculture (a review). *Fish Physiology and Biochemistry* 39: 431–457.

Meinertz, J.R., Hess, K.R., Bernardy, J.A. et al. (2014). Florfenicol residues in rainbow trout after oral dosing in recirculating and flow-through culture systems. *Journal of Aquatic Animal Health* 26: 243–250.

Mettam, J., Oulton, L., Mccrohan, C., and Sneddon, L. (2011). The efficacy of three types of analgesic drugs in reducing pain in the rainbow trout, *Oncorhynchus mykiss*. *Applied Animal Behaviour Science* 133: 265–274.

Miller, R.A., Pelsor, F.R., Kane, A.S., and Reimschuessel, R. (2012). Oxytetracycline pharmacokinetics in rainbow trout during and after an orally administered medicated feed regimen. *Jounal of Aquatic Animal Health* 24: 121–128.

Ministère de l'Agriculture de l'Agroalimentaire et de la Forêt (2016). Arrêté du 18 mars 2016 fixant la liste des substances antibiotiques d'importance critique prévue à l'article L. 5144-1-1 du code de la santé publique et fixant la liste des méthodes de réalisation du test de détermination de la sensibilité des souches bactériennes prévue à l'article R. 5141-117-2. *Journal Officiel de la République Française* [online]. https://www.legifrance.gouv.fr/jo_pdf.do?id=JORFTEXT000032291325 (accessed 7 December 2016).

Ministère de l'Ecologie et du Développement Durable (2006). Arrêté du 11 août 2006 fixant la liste des espèces, races ou variétés d'animaux domestiques. *Journal Officiel de la République Française* [online]. https://www.legifrance.gouv.fr/affichTexte.do?cidTexte=JORFTEXT000000789087anddateTexte=andcategorieLien=id (accessed 17 March 2017).

Miyazaki, T., Isshiki, T., and Katsuyuki, H. (2005). Histopathological and electron microscopy studies on sleepy disease of koi *Cyprinus carpio* koi in Japan. *Diseases of Aquatic Organisms* 65: 197–207.

Mohammed, H.H. and Arias, C.R. (2015). Potassium permanganate elicits a shift of the external fish microbiome and increases host susceptibility to columnaris disease. *Veterinary Research* 46: 82.

Mohan, P.J. and Aiken, A. (2004). Water quality and life support system. In: *The Elasmobranch Husbandry Manual: Captive Care of Sharks, Rays and their Relatives* (eds. M. Smith, D. Warmolts, D. Thoney and R. Hueter), 69–88. Columbus: Ohio Biological Survey.

Mohney, L.L., Lightner, D.V., Williams, R.R., and Bauerlein, M. (1990). Bioencapsulation of therapeutic quantities of the antibacterial Romet-30 in nauplii of the brine shrimp *Artemia* and in the nematode *Panagrellus redivivus*. *Journal of the World Aquaculture Society* 21: 186–191.

Montgomery-Brock, D. (2001). The application of hydrogen peroxide as a treatment for the ectoparasite *Amyloodinium ocellatum* (Brown 1931) on the Pacific threadfin *Polydactylus sexfilis*. *Journal of the World Aquaculture Society* 32: 250–254.

Montoliu, J., Carrera, M., Darnell, A., and Revert, L. (1981). Lactic acidosis and Fanconi's syndrome due to degraded tetracycline. *British Medical Journal* 283: 1576–1577.

Moreau, R. and Dabrowski, K. (1996). The primary localization of ascorbate and its synthesis in the kidneys of acipenserid (*Chondrostei*) and teleost (*Teleostei*) fishes. *Journal of Comparative Physiology B* 166: 178–183.

Myers, G.E., Garner, M.M., Barrie, M.T. et al. (2007). Fenbendazole toxicity in sharks. Paper presented at the *American Association of Zoo Veterinarians*, Knoxville, TN.

Myers, D.A., Galvenek, E.A., and Coetzee, J.F. (2014). Pharmacologic evaluation of ceftazidime in cownose rays (*Rhinoptera bonasus*). *Proceedings of the International Association of Aquatic Animal Health Conference*, Gold Coast, Australia.

Mylniczenko, N.D., and Clauss, T. (2017) Pharmacology of elasmobranchs: updates and techniques. In: *The Elasmobranch Husbandry Manual II: Recent Advances in the Care of Sharks, Rays and their Relatives* (eds M. Smith, D. Warmolts, D. Thoney, R. Hueter, M. Murray, and J. Ezcurra), pp. 289–302. Ohio Biological Survey, Columbus.

Ngamvongchon, S., Pawaputanon, O., Leelapatra, W., and Johnson, W.E. (1988). Effectiveness of LHRH analogue for the induced spawning of carp and catfish in Northeast Thailand. *Aquaculture* 74: 35–40.

Nimenya, H., Delaunois, A., La Duong, D. et al. (1999). Short-term toxicity of various pharmacological agents on the in vitro nitrification process in a simple closed aquatic system. *Alternatives to Laboratory Animals* 27: 121–135.

Noga, E.J. (2010a). Pharmacopoeia. In: *Fish Disease: Diagnosis and Treatment*, 2e (ed. E.J. Noga), 375–420. Ames, IO: Wiley.

Nouws, J.F.M., Grondel, J.L., Schutte, A.R., and Laurensen, J. (1988). Pharmacokinetics of ciprofloxacin in carp, African catfish and rainbow trout. *The Veterinary Quarterly* 10: 211–216.

Ochandio, B., Bechara, I., and Parise-Maltempi, P. (2015). Dexamethasone action on caudal fin regeneration of carp *Cyprinus carpio* (Linnaeus, 1758). *Brazilian Journal of Biology* 75: 442–450.

O'Connor, M.R., Farver, T.B., Malm, K.V. et al. (2014). Protective immunity of a modified-live cyprinid herpesvirus 3 vaccine in koi (*Cyprinus carpio koi*) 13 months after vaccination. *American Journal of Veterinary Research* 75: 905–911.

Oliva-Teles, A. (2012). Nutrition and health of aquaculture fish. *Journal of Fish Diseases* 35: 83–108.

Olsvik, P.A., Lie, K.K., Mykkeltvedt, E. et al. (2008). Pharmacokinetics and transcriptional effects of the anti-salmon lice drug emamectin benzoate in Atlantic salmon (*Salmo salar* L.). *BMC Pharmacology* 8: 16.

Owoyale, J.A. (1989). Decomposition profile of ultraviolet-irradiated chloroquine. *International Journal of Pharmaceutics* 52: 179–181.

Papich, M.G. (2017). Ciprofloxacin pharmacokinetics in clinical canine patients. *Journal of Veterinary Internal Medicine* 31: 1508–1513.

Partridge, G.J., Michael, R.J., and Thuillier, L. (2014). Praziquantel form, dietary application method and dietary inclusion level affect palatability and efficacy against monogenean parasites in yellowtail kingfish. *Diseases of Aquatic Organisms* 109: 155–163.

Pedersen, L.-F., Pedersen, P.B., Nielsen, J.L., and Nielsen, P.H. (2010). Long term/low dose formalin exposure to small-scale recirculation aquaculture systems. *Aquacultural Engineering* 42: 1–7.

Pereira, N.P., Nunes, G.D., Baylina, N. et al. (2002). *Fusarium solani* infection of the eye, brain, otic capsule and endolymphatic tubes in captive Port Jackson sharks (*Heterodontus portusjacksoni*). *Proceedings of the International Association of Aquatic Animal Health Conference*, Albufeira, Portugal.

Petervary, N., Gillette, D., and Lewbart, G.A. (1992). Pathology of a renal tumor in a red oscar, *Astronotus ocellatus*, and occurrence of renal tumors in various tropical fish species. *Proceedings of the International Association of Aquatic Animal Health Conference*, Hong Kong.

Petit, J. and Wiegertjes, G.F. (2016). Long-lived effect of administering ß-glucans: indications for trained immunity in fish. *Developmental and Comparative Immunology* 64: 93–102.

Petritz, O.A., Sanchez-Migallon Guzman, D., Paul-Murphy, J. et al. (2013). Evaluation of the efficacy and safety of single administration of 4.7-mg deslorelin acetate implants on egg production and plasma sex hormones in Japanese quail (*Coturnix coturnix japonica*). *American Journal of Veterinary Research* 74: 316–323.

Phillips, B.E., Harms, C.A., Lewbart, G.A. et al. (2016). Population pharmacokinetics of enrofloxacin and its metabolite ciprofloxacin in the green sea urchin (*Strongylocentrotus droebachiensis*) following intracoelomic and immersion administration. *Journal of Zoo and Wildlife Medicine* 47: 175–186.

Picón-Camacho, S.M., Ruiz De Ybanez, M.R., Holzer, A.S. et al. (2011). In vitro treatments for the theront stage of the ciliate protozoan *Cryptocaryon irritans*. *Diseases of Aquatic Organisms* 94: 167–172.

Pietsch, C., Neumann, N., Preuer, T., and Kloas, W. (2011). In vivo treatment with progestogens causes immunosuppression of carp *Cyprinus carpio* leucocytes by affecting nitric oxide production and arginase activity. *Journal of Fish Biology* 79: 53–69.

Plumb, D.C. (2015). Plumb's Veterinary Drug Handbook, 8e. Ames, IO: Wiley.

Poon, S.H., Baliog, C.R., Sams, R.N. et al. (2011). Syndrome of cocaine-levamisole-induced cutaneous vasculitis and immune-mediated leukopenia. *Seminars in Arthritis and Rheumatism* 41: 434–444.

Pouliquen, H., Delépée, R., Larhantec-Verdier, M. et al. (2007). Comparative hydrolysis and photolysis of four antibacterial agents (oxytetracycline, oxolinic acid, flumequine and florfenicol) in deionised water, freshwater and seawater under abiotic conditions. *Aquaculture* 262: 23–28.

Powell, M., Speare, D., and Wright, G. (1995). Morphological changes in rainbow trout (*Oncorhynchus mykiss*) gill epithelia following repeated intermittent exposure to chloramine-T. *Canadian Journal of Zoology* 73: 154–165.

Przybylska-Diaz, D.A., Schmidt, J.G., Vera-Jimenez, N.I. et al. (2013). Beta-glucan enriched bath directly stimulates the wound healing process in common carp (*Cyprinus carpio* L.). *Fish & Shellfish Immunology* 35: 998–1006.

Rach, J.J., Schreier, T.M., Howe, G.E., and Redman, S.D. (1997). Effect of species, life stage, and water temperature on the toxicity of hydrogen peroxide to fish. *The Progressive Fish-Culturist* 59: 41–46.

Raulic, J., Beaudry, F., Beauchamp, G. et al. (2020). Pharmacokinetic, pharmacodynamic and toxicology study of robenacoxib in rainbow trout (*Oncorhynchus mykiss*). *Proceedings of the International Association of Aquatic Animal Health Conference*, Tampa, FL.

Reed, A.N., Clayton, L.A., and Hadfield, C.A. (2012). Morbidity and mortality associated with fenbendazole use in teleost fish at the National Aquarium, Baltimore. *Proceedings of the International Association for Aquatic Animal Medicine Conference*, Atlanta, GA.

Ribas, J.L., Zampronio, A.R., and Silva De Assis, H.C. (2016). Effects of trophic exposure to diclofenac and dexamethasone on hematological parameters and immune response in freshwater fish. *Environmental Toxicology and Chemistry* 35: 975–982.

Rigos, G., Katharios, P., and Papandroulakis, N. (2010). Single intramuscular administration of long-acting oxytetracycline in grouper (*Epinephelus marginatus*). *Turkish Journal of Veterinary and Animal Sciences* 34: 441–445.

Roiha, I.S., Otterlei, E., Litlabo, A., and Samuelsen, O.B. (2010). Uptake and elimination of florfenicol in Atlantic cod (*Gadus morhua*) larvae delivered orally through bioencapsulation in the brine shrimp *Artemia franciscana*. *Aquaculture* 310: 27–31.

Russo, R., Curtis, E.W., and Yanong, R.P.E. (2007). Preliminary investigations of hydrogen peroxide treatment of selected ornamental fishes and efficacy against external bacteria and parasites in green swordtails. *Journal of Aquatic Animal Health* 19: 121–127.

Sakai, M. (1999). Current research status of fish immunostimulants. *Aquaculture* 172: 63–92.

Samuelsen, O.B. (1997). Efficacy of bath-administered flumequine and oxolinic acid in the treatment of vibriosis in Atlantic halibut. *Jounal of Aquaric Animal Health* 9: 127–131.

Samuelsen, O.B., Ervik, A., and Wennevik, V. (1995). Absorption, tissue distribution, metabolism and excretion of ormetoprim and sulphadimethoxine in Atlantic salmon (*Salmo salar*) after intravenous and oral administration of Romet. *Xenobiotica* 25: 1169–1180.

Samuelsen, O.B., Lunestad, B.T., and Jelmert, A. (1997). Pharmacokinetic and efficacy studies on bath-administering potentiated sulphonamides in Atlantic halibut, *Hippoglossus hippoglossus* L. *Journal of Fish Diseases* 20: 287–296.

Samuelsen, O.B., Kvenseth, P.G., Andreassen, J.H. et al. (2003). The efficacy of a single intraperitoneal injection of oxolinic acid in the treatment of bacterial infections in goldsinny wrasse (*Ctenolabrus rupestris*) and corkwing wrasse (*Symphodus melops*) studied under field and laboratory conditions. *Journal of Veterinary Pharmacology and Therapeutics* 26: 181–186.

Sanabria, C., Diamant, A., and Zilberg, D. (2009). Effects of commonly used disinfectants and temperature on swim bladder non-inflation in freshwater angelfish, *Pterophyllum scalare* (Lichtenstein). *Aquaculture* 292: 158–165.

Sanders, J.L., Watral, V., and Kent, M.L. (2012). Microsporidiosis in zebrafish research facilities. *ILAR Journal* 53: 106–113.

Schelkle, B., Snellgrove, D., Jones, L.L., and Cable, J. (2015). Efficacy of commercially available products against *Gyrodactylus turnbulli* infections on guppies *Poecilia reticulata*. *Diseases of Aquatic Organisms* 115: 129–137.

Schmahl, G. and Taraschewski, H. (1987). Treatment of fish parasites. 2. Effects of praziquantel, niclosamide, levamisole-HCl, and metrifonate on monogenea (*Gyrodactylus aculeati*, *Diplozoon paradoxum*). *Parasitology Research* 73: 341–351.

Schmahl, G., El Toukhy, A., and Ghaffar, F. (1990). Transmission electron microscopic studies on the effects of toltrazuril on *Glugea anomala*, Moniez, 1887 (Microsporidia) infecting the three-spined stickleback

Gasterosteus aculeatus. *Parasitology Research* 76: 700–706.

Schoepfer, A.M., Engel, A., Fattinger, K. et al. (2007). Herbal does not mean innocuous: ten cases of severe hepatotoxicity associated with dietary supplements from Herbalife® products. *Journal of Hepatology* 47: 521–526.

Schwaiger, J., Ferling, H., Mallow, U. et al. (2004). Toxic effects of the non-steroidal anti-inflammatory drug diclofenac. Part I: histopathological alterations and bioaccumulation in rainbow trout. *Aquatic Toxicology* 68: 141–150.

Scott, G., Law, M., Christiansen, E.F. et al. (2020). Evaluation of localized inflammatory reactions secondary to intramuscular injections of enrolofloxacin in striped bass (*Morone saxatilis*). *Journal of Zoo and Wildlife Medicine* 51: 46–52.

Seeley, K.E., Wolf, K.N., Bishop, M.A. et al. (2016). Pharmacokinetcs of long-acting cefovecin in copper rockfish (*Sebastes caurinus*). *American Journal of Veterinary Research* 77: 260–264.

Seepersadsingh, N. and Adesiyun, A.A. (2003). Prevalence and antimicrobial resistance of *Salmonella* spp. in pet mammals, reptiles, fish aquarium water, and birds in Trinidad. *Journal Veterinary Medecine B Infectious Diseases and Veterinary Public Health* 50: 488–493.

Sforcin, J.M. (2007). Propolis and the immune system: a review. *Journal of Ethnopharmacology* 113: 1–14.

Shahsavani, D., Baghshani, H., and Alishahi, E. (2011). Efficacy of allicin in decreasing lead (Pb) accumulation in selected tissues of lead-exposed common carp (*Cyprinus carpio*). *Biological Trace Element Research* 142: 572–580.

Shan, Q., Zhu, X., Liu, S. et al. (2015). Pharmacokinetics of cefquinome in tilapia (*Oreochromis niloticus*) after a single intramuscular or intraperitoneal administration. *Journal of Veterinary Pharmacology and Therapeutics* 38: 601–605.

Siwicki, A.K., Anderson, D.P., and Dixon, O.W. (1989). Comparisons of nonspecific and specific immunomodulation by oxolinic acid, oxytetracycline and levamisole in salmonids. *Veterinary Immunology and Immunopathology* 23: 195–200.

Soukupova-Markova, Z., Doubkova, V., Marsalek, P. et al. (2015). Degradation rate of praziquantel and fenbendazole in rainbow trout following oral administration. *Neuro Endocrinology Letters* 36 (Suppl. 1): 64–67.

Stamper, M.A. (2004). Immobilization of elasmobranchs. In: *The Elasmobranch Husbandry Manual: Captive Care of Sharks, Rays and their Relatives* (eds. M. Smith, D. Warmolts, D. Thoney and R. Hueter), 281–295. Columbus: Ohio Biological Survey.

Stamper, M.A., Lewbart, G.A., Barrington, P.R. et al. (1998). *Eimeria southwelli* infection associated with high mortality of cownose rays. *Jounal of Aquaric Animal Health* 10: 264–270.

Steeil, J.C., Schumacher, J., George, R.H. et al. (2014). Pharmacokinetics of cefovecin (Convenia) in white bamboo sharks (*Chiloscyllium plagiosum*) and Atlantic horseshoe crabs (*Limulus polyphemus*). *Journal of Zoo and Wildlife Medicine* 45: 389–392.

Steverding, D., Morgan, E., Tkaczynski, P. et al. (2005). Effect of Australian tea tree oil on *Gyrodactylus* spp. infection of the three-spined stickleback *Gasterosteus aculeatus*. *Diseases of Aquatic Organisms* 66: 29–32.

Stoffregen, D.A., Wooster, G.A., Bustos, P.S. et al. (1997). Multiple route and dose pharmacokinetics of enrofloxacin in juvenile Atlantic salmon. *Jounal of Veterinary Pharmacology and Therapeutics* 20: 111–123.

Stremme, D.W., Grandinetti, N., and Kind, M. (2007). Testosterone levels in a male pelagic stingray (*Pteroplatytrygon violacea*) after an injection of Lupron (leuprolide acetate) depot given to control aggressive mating behavior. *Proceedings of the International Association of Aquatic Animal Health Conference*, Orlando, FL.

Szekely, C. and Molnar, K. (1991). Praziquantel (Droncit) is effective against diplostomosis of grasscarp *Ctenopharyngodon idella* and silver carp *Hypophthalmichthys molitrix*. *Diseases of Aquatic Organisms* 11: 147–150.

Taraschewski, H., Renner, C., and Mehlhorn, H. (1988). Treatment of fish parasites: effects of levamisole HCl, metrifonate, fenbendazole, mebendazole, and ivermectin on *Anguillicola crassus* (nematodes) pathogenic in the air bladder of eels. *Parasitology Research* 74: 281–289.

Targonska, K. and Kucharczyk, D. (2011). The application of hCG, CPH and Ovopel in successful artificial reproduction of goldfish (*Carassius auratus auratus*) under controlled conditions. *Reproduction in Domestic Animals* 46: 651–655.

Thomas, A., Dawson, M.R., Ellis, H., and Stamper, M.A. (2016). Praziquantel degradation in marine aquarium water. *PeerJ* 4: e1857.

Tojo, J.L. and Santamarina, M.T. (1998a). Oral pharmacological treatments for parasitic diseases of rainbow trout *Oncorhynchus mykiss*. II. *Gyrodactylus* sp. *Diseases of Aquatic Organisms* 33: 187–193.

Tojo, J.L. and Santamarina, M.T. (1998b). Oral pharmacological treatments for parasitic diseases of rainbow trout *Oncorhynchus mykiss*. III. *Ichthyobodo necator*. *Diseases of Aquatic Organisms* 33: 195–199.

Touraki, M., Ladoukakis, M., and Karagiannis, V. (2010). Efficacy of flumequine administered by bath or through medicated nauplii of *Artemia franciscana* (L.) in the treatment of vibriosis in sea bass larvae. *Aquaculture* 306: 146–152.

Touraki, M., Niopas, I., and Karagiannis, V. (2012). Treatment of vibriosis in European sea bass larvae, *Dicentrarchus labrax* L., with oxolinic acid administered by bath or through medicated nauplii of *Artemia franciscana* (Kellogg): efficacy and residual kinetics. *Journal of Fish Diseases* 35: 513–522.

Treves-Brown, K.M. (2000). *Applied Fish Pharmacology*. Boston, MA: Kluwer Academic Publishers.

Tubbs, L.A. and Tingle, M.D. (2006a). Bioavailability and pharmacokinetics of a praziquantel bolus in kingfish *Seriola lalandi*. *Diseases of Aquatic Organisms* 69: 233–238.

Tubbs, L.A. and Tingle, M.D. (2006b). Effect of dose escalation on multiple dose pharmacokinetics of orally administered praziquantel in kingfish *Seriola lalandi*. *Aquaculture* 261: 1168–1174.

Udomkusonsri, P., Arthitvong, S., Klangkaew, N., and Kusucharit, N. (2007). Pharmacokinetics of enrofloxacin in koi carp (*Cyprinus carpio*) after various routes of administration. *Kasetsart Journal (Natural Science)* 41: 62–68.

Unkenholz, E.G., Brown, M.L., and Pope, K.L. (1997). Oxytetracycline marking efficacy for yellow perch fingerlings and temporal assays of tissue residues. *The Progressive Fish-Culturist* 59: 280–284.

US Food and Drug Administration (2014). Drug indexing [online]. http://www.fda.gov/AnimalVeterinary/DevelopmentApprovalProcess/MinorUseMinorSpecies/ucm070206.htm (accessed 2 December 2016).

US Food and Drug Administration (2019a). Aquaculture [online]. https://www.fda.gov/animal-veterinary/development-approval-process/aquaculture (accessed 23 November 2019).

US Food and Drug Administration (2019b). Compounding drugs from bulk drug substances [online]. https://www.fda.gov/media/132567/download (accessed 24 November 2019).

Valladão, G.M., Gallani, S.U., and Pilarski, F. (2015). Phytotherapy as an alternative for treating fish disease. *Jounal of Veterinary Pharmacology and Therapeutics* 38: 417–428.

Vera, L.M. and Migaud, H. (2016). Hydrogen peroxide treatment in Atlantic salmon induces stress and detoxification response in a daily manner. *Chronobiology International* 33: 530–542.

Verbeeck, R.K., Junginger, H.E., Midha, K.K. et al. (2005). Biowaiver monographs for immediate release solid oral dosage forms based on biopharmaceutics classification system (BCS) literature data: chloroquine phosphate, chloroquine sulfate, and chloroquine hydrochloride. *Journal of Pharmaceutical Sciences* 94: 1389–1395.

Vorbach, B.S., Chandasana, H., Derendorf, H., and Yanong, R.P.E. (2019). Pharmacokinetics of oxytetracycline in the giant danio (*Devario aequipinnatus*) following bath immersion. *Aquaculture* 498: 12–16.

Walsh, C.J., Wyffels, J.T., Bodine, A.B., and Luer, C.A. (2002). Dexamethasone-induced apoptosis in immune cells from peripheral circulation and lymphomyeloid tissues of juvenile clearnose skates, *Raja eglanteria*. *Developmental and Comparative Immunology* 26: 623–633.

Wang, W., Luo, L., Xiao, H. et al. (2015). A pharmacokinetic and residual study of sulfadiazine/trimethoprim in mandarin fish (*Siniperca chuatsi*) with single- and multiple-dose oral administrations. *Jounal of Veterinary Pharmacology and Therapeutics* 39: 309–314.

Wang, D., Li, S., and Lu, T. (2016). Rule of accumulation of enrofloxacin in *Acipenser baerii* and drug-induced damage to the tissues. *Experimental Biology and Medicine (Maywood)* 241: 1977–1984.

Ward, J.L., Mccartney, S.P., Chinnadurai, S.K., and Posner, L.P. (2012). Development of a minimum-anesthetic-concentration depression model to study the effects of various analgesics in goldfish (*Carassius auratus*). *Journal of Zoo and Wildlife Medicine* 43: 214–222.

Webb, D.H., Marrero, C., Ellis, H. et al. (2013). A simple reagent-free spectrophotometric assay for monitoring metronidazole therapy in aquarium water. *Journal of Aquatic Animal Health* 25: 165–170.

Weber, E.P., Malm, K.V., Yun, S.C. et al. (2014). Efficacy and safety of a modified-live cyprinid herpesvirus 3 vaccine in koi (*Cyprinus carpio koi*) for prevention of koi herpesvirus disease. *American Journal of Veterinary Research* 75: 899–904.

Wei, Y.J., Wang, C.M., Cai, X.T. et al. (2013). Establishment of zebrafish osteopenia model induced by dexamethasone. *Yao Xue Xue Bao* 48: 255–260.

Williams, R.E., Ernst, I., Chambers, C.B., and Whittington, I.D. (2007). Efficacy of orally administered praziquantel against *Zeuxapta seriolae* and *Benedenia seriolae* (Monogenea) in yellowtail kingfish *Seriola lalandi*. *Diseases of Aquatic Organisms* 77: 199–205.

Wooster, G.A., Martinez, C.M., and Bowser, P.R. (2005). Human health risks associated with formalin treatments used in aquaculture: initial study. *North American Journal of Aquaculture* 67: 111–113.

Xie, L.-L., Wu, Z.-X., Chen, X.-X. et al. (2013). Pharmacokinetics of florfenicol and its metabolite, florfenicol amine, in rice field eel (*Monopterus albus*) after a single-dose intramuscular or oral administration. *Jounal of Veterinary Pharmacology and Therapeutics* 36: 229–235.

Xie, X., Zhao, Y., Yang, X., and Hu, K. (2015). Comparison of praziquantel pharmacokinetics and tissue distribution in fresh and brackish water cultured grass carp (*Ctenopharyngodon idellus*) after oral administration of single bolus. *BMC Veterinary Research* 11: 84.

Xu, N., Dong, J., Yang, Y., and Ai, X. (2016). Pharmacokinetics and residue depletion of praziquantel in rice field eels *Monopterus albus*. *Diseases of Aquatic Organisms* 119: 67–74.

Yanong, R.P.E., Curtis, E.W., Simmons, R. et al. (2005). Pharmacokinetic studies of florfenicol in koi carp and threespot gourami *Trichogaster trichopterus* after oral and intramuscular treatment. *Journal of Aquatic Animal Health* 17: 129–137.

Yonar, M.E., Yonar, S.M., Pala, A. et al. (2015). Trichlorfon-induced haematological and biochemical changes in *Cyprinus carpio*: ameliorative effect of propolis. *Diseases of Aquatic Organisms* 114: 209–216.

Yoshida, T., Kruger, R., and Inglis, V. (1995). Short communication: augmentation of non-specific protection in African catfish, *Clarias gariepinus* (Burchell), by the long-term oral administration of immunostimulants. *Journal of Fish Diseases* 18: 195–198.

Zimmerman, D.M., Armstrong, D.L., Curro, T.G. et al. (2006). Pharmacokinetics of florfenicol after a single intramuscular dose in white-spotted bamboo sharks (*Chiloscyllium plagiosum*). *Journal of Zoo and Wildlife Medicine* 37: 165–173.

A13

Environmental Considerations of Immersion Medications

M. Andrew Stamper[1], Kent J. Semmen[1] and Michael J. Murray[2]

[1] *Disney's Animals, Science and Environment, Lake Buena Vista, FL, USA*
[2] *Monterey Bay Aquarium, Monterey, CA, USA*

Introduction

Immersion medications are often used on fish and invertebrates to treat parasites, bacteria, and oomycetes. They may be more effective and practical than oral or parenteral medications, particularly when dealing with a group of fish. They can be applied in different ways, but a major distinction should be made between the following:

- Treatment within a temporary isolation system; a smaller body of water with little organic material and no filtration.
- Treatment within an established system with organic material, biological filtration, and potentially mechanical and chemical filtration.
- Treatment of a flow-through system.

Immersion treatment with little organic material and no filtration is almost always the best option because of more predictable effects, lower drug costs, and smaller volumes of medicated water for disposal. However, there are times when treatment of established systems is required, e.g. because a pathogen has an environmental reservoir, or because it is impossible to remove all susceptible fish for treatment. Immersion treatment of established systems is quite common for pathogens such as *Cryptocaryon*, *Neobenedenia*, and *Lepeophtheirus* spp. Avoiding these situations is a principal benefit of good quarantine and biosecurity practices.

Immersion treatments in established systems have potentially significant and unpredictable effects on the biological filtration, the animals, and the medication. This is because of differences in biotic factors (such as the microbiome, animal, and plant populations) and abiotic factors (such as the drug composition, pH, salinity, oxidation-reduction, and life support systems). This makes it extremely challenging to extrapolate the actual impact of medications between systems or even on the same system at different points in time. So it is particularly important to consider potential impacts and appropriately monitor for water quality and animal side effects when using immersion treatments in established systems.

Immersion treatment in a flow-through raceway-type system is typically done by adding the treatment solution to the inflow of the system and allowing it to flush through once, or by metering in a constant flow of the treatment solution to maintain a calculated concentration for the duration of the treatment. Flush treatments usually result in uneven distribution of the product throughout the water column and are therefore not appropriate for regulated products. Constant dosing of a flow-through system can be costly and raises discharge issues.

The following categories and examples can help guide clinical decisions surrounding immersion medications:

- Impacts of water chemistry on immersion medications
  - How will factors such as pH, temperature, and salinity impact the medication?
  - Has the system already been exposed to the medication?
  - How will the biological load affect the rate of drug metabolism?

Clinical Guide to Fish Medicine, First Edition. Edited by Catherine A. Hadfield and Leigh Ann Clayton.

- Effects of water clarification and disinfection on immersion medications
  - Are activated carbon, ultraviolet, or ozone present and can they be removed to prevent drug degradation?
- Effects of immersion medications on the biological filtration and microbiome
  - Will the medication adversely affect the biological filtration?
  - Will the medication cause a bacterial bloom? Could this increase turbidity or decrease dissolved oxygen?
- Effects on target and nontarget species
  - Are there animals present that tend to show adverse reactions at lower drug levels?
  - Could the medication negatively impact plants in the system?
- Medication assays
  - How can the level of the medication and potential byproducts be measured?
  - If not possible, are there indirect measurements, e.g. water clarity, oxygen levels?
- Human exposure to medicated water
  - Is snorkeling or diving needed during or following treatment?
- Disposal of medicated water
  - What regulations and recommendations exist for disposal of medicated water?

Reviews of these topics are followed by a detailed discussion of some common immersion medications: formalin, trichlorfon, praziquantel, copper, and chloroquine.

Impacts of Water Chemistry on Immersion Medications

Physical aspects of the water, such as temperature, pH, salinity, hardness, and total organic load, can have many effects on drugs. They can impact the dissolution of medications, the forms that are available (known as chemical speciation), and the rate of degradation.

The dissolution of a medication depends on its lipophilic or hydrophilic properties as well as the application method. These also impact the ability of a medication to be absorbed through the animals' gills, skin, or gastrointestinal tract, or to be bound by microbes, algae, or substrate. An example of a commonly used immersion medication that is poorly soluble in water is praziquantel, and specific application methods are used to improve dissolution (discussed below).

Temperature affects the rate of drug degradation. Typically, higher water temperatures lead to faster drug degradation, as seen with the organophosphate trichlorfon. Temperature also affects the physiology of the animals and microbes, changing their enzyme activity and their ability to bind and/or transform drugs.

Water pH has huge impacts on the form that chemicals take (speciation). One example is trichlorfon, which is easily converted to the more toxic dichlorvos at higher pH. When the drug is used in the lower pH of freshwater, it is relatively less toxic than when the same dose is used in salt water.

Salinity can also affect the chemical form of medications. For instance, as salinity increases, copper binding (adsorption) to surfaces decreases, which increases the concentration of copper ions in the water and can increase the risk of toxicity. Salinity can also have a physiological impact on medication levels in the fish, for example, rising salinity increased the renal elimination rate of praziquantel in grass carp (*Ctenopharyngodon idella*) (Xie et al. 2015).

Water hardness can also influence the effectiveness of medications. For example, the high levels of magnesium and calcium ions in salt water bind and neutralize tetracyclines. These same cations in the water and substrate (e.g. calcium carbonate in crushed coral) bind copper, reducing the levels of copper ions in the water. This is why it can be difficult to get copper to therapeutic levels in naïve systems; if they have not previously been exposed to copper, more of the calcium carbonate binding sites are available. Leaching of copper from these binding sites explains why copper levels can persist after a treatment has been discontinued.

Total organic carbon (TOC, the amount of carbon in a system) can also affect medications. Organic compounds are known to bind to metals such as copper, making them less available and less toxic. This is why chelated or organically bound copper (e.g. Cupramine™) has a higher therapeutic dose than ionic copper sulfate.

Effects of Water Clarification and Disinfection on Immersion Medications

Water clarity is often improved for aesthetic reasons using activated carbon filtration, ozone, and ultraviolet (UV) light. Disinfection in fish systems commonly involves UV and/or ozone. These techniques can have dramatic effects on medications and usually need to be discontinued during immersion treatments.

Activated carbon, often referred to as GAC (granular activated carbon), is a highly porous, crystalline filtration material with a tremendous surface area-to-volume ratio. There are a finite number of exposed binding sites, so activated carbon is often described by its surface area and porosity. It is most effective against carbon-based molecules (e.g. organics, formalin, praziquantel). It can adsorb heavy metals, although not as efficiently and dependent largely on the speciation of the metals (e.g. organically bound versus ionic) (Bhatnagar et al. 2013). It also removes oxidants like ozone and chlorine by oxidation of its outer surfaces – not within its pore structure. GAC should be used immediately after mechanical filtration to remove particulate matter that could occlude it. It can be effectively used in in-line canister-type filters or larger sand filter vessels. It may be used continuously, but short-term use is more common due to concerns that critical organics/nutrients may be depleted by overuse. Binding sites become exhausted over time through binding or occlusion by microbial growth and the media must be changed periodically. The GAC manufacturer's representative can be consulted for sizing and replacement rate based on use.

In-line UV disinfection can degrade many medications including praziquantel, chloroquine, tetracycline, and oxytetracycline. Natural sunlight can also cause deterioration of these chemotherapeutics and some systems may need to be protected from direct sunlight during treatment. The rate of this degradation increases with increasing pH and alkalinity, and it is important to bear in mind that potentially toxic by-products may result from light degradation of some drugs such as chloroquine and tetracycline (Nord et al. 1991; Karim et al. 1994; López-Peñalver et al. 2010; Havlíková et al. 2016; Čizmić et al. 2017).

Ozone or other oxidation techniques can also degrade many medications. It may be possible to predict sensitivity to oxidants based on the presence and number of oxidation-prone carbon-carbon double bonds; however, it is likely best to simply stop ozone disinfection during immersion treatment.

In practical terms, these mean that activated carbon, UV, and ozone should all be removed from a system during immersion treatment. This can have adverse effects on water clarity and pathogen load that should be discussed prior to starting treatment. It also means that activated carbon, ultraviolet, and ozone may be used to try to help with management of medicated water after treatment.

Effects of Immersion Medications on the Biological Filtration

The impact of immersion medications on the biological filtration is one of the most important considerations when adding therapeutic agents to water. Any chemical addition to a system could damage or destroy the bacteria that are critical to the biological filtration. There are several papers on the effects of chemicals on biofilters (Tables A13.1 and A13.2) (Collins et al. 1975, 1976; Klaver and Matthews 1994; Nimenya et al. 1999; Schwartz et al. 2000; Pedersen et al. 2010; Knight et al. 2016). In spite of this, the exact impact is hard to predict, as it depends on the in-water drug concentration and the sensitivity of the ammonia-oxidizing bacteria (AOB) and nitrite-oxidizing bacteria (NOB) in that particular system. Other factors that might alter the impact are duration of treatment, thickness of the biofilm, water hardness, and binding agents such as organic carbon. In addition, it is not an all-or-nothing effect. By destroying some of the AOB or NOB, medication can select for other bacteria. For this reason, it is important not to rely too heavily on information from other systems and to be prepared for unexpected effects on the biological filtration any time an immersion medication is used.

To reduce the risk of adverse effects on the animals, measures should be in place prior to treatment to monitor drug, ammonia, and nitrite levels regularly; often daily for a medication that is new to that system. It is also important to be prepared to respond to an increase in ammonia or nitrite. This may mean making more water available for potential water changes or acquiring ammonia-binding compounds prior to starting treatment. It is helpful to maintain a biofarm (nitrifying bacteria cultured in a similar isolated system) to allow for rapid recolonization of AOB and NOB. These may be fed using ammonium chloride or ammonium sulfate titrated to effect, or kept with fish considered of low infectious disease risk. Alkalinity, phosphate, and oxygenation may need to be monitored and adjusted to help a struggling biofilter or to reestablish a biofilter.

Effects of The Microbiome

The microbiome consists of all the microbes in a given environment, including viruses, bacteria, archaea, protists, fungi, and phytoplankton. In an aquarium system, the microbes exist throughout the water and within the biofilm across all the surfaces, not just within the biofilters. A healthy, diverse microbiome is likely important to fish and invertebrate health. These microbes can have dramatic impacts on immersion medications.

The high standards for water clarity and clean surfaces within aquarium exhibit systems essentially starve these microbes into inactivity. When the microbes are provided with a nutrient that was previously limited (e.g. carbon, phosphate), they can show rapid blooms. This is a common response when carbon-based nutrients are added to water in a form that one or more of the species in the microbiome can break down. Many of the common immersion medications in fish are carbon-based and can trigger this bacterial bloom, including formalin and praziquantel, as well as

Table A13.1 Chemicals where impact on biological filtration has been shown, both for ammonia-oxidizing bacteria (AOB) and nitrite-oxidizing bacteria (NOB).

Chemical	Dose	Comments
Ampicillin	Dose-dependent 34–136 mg/L	AOB and NOB impacted[a]
Chloramine T	Dose-dependent 5–40 mg/L	AOB and NOB impacted[a]
Chloramphenicol	10–80 mg/L	Impacts varied across papers[a,c]
Enrofloxacin	Dose-dependent 5–40 mg/L	Only NOB impacted[a]
Erythromycin	Dose-dependent 10–80 mg/L	AOB and NOB impacted[a]
Levamisole	Dose-dependent 4–32 mg/L	AOB and NOB impacted[a]
Methylene blue	Dose-dependent 1–8 mg/L	AOB and NOB impacted[a,b]
Nifurpirinol	50 mg/L	AOB and NOB impacted[c]
Oxytetracyline	50 mg/L; 12.5–75.0 mg/L (>50 mg/L completely inhibited)	Impacts varied across papers[c,d]
Polymyxin B	Dose-dependent 1–8 mg/L	AOB and NOB impacted[a]
Sulfamerazine	50 mg/L	AOB and NOB impacted[c]

[a] Nimeyna et al. 1999
[b] Collins et al. 1975
[c] Collins et al. 1976
[d] Klaver and Matthews 1994

Table A13.2 Chemicals where reports have suggested no impact on biological filtration.

Chemical	Dose
Copper II sulfate	1–16 mg/L[a,b]
Formalin	25 mg/L every other day[b,c]
Formalin + malachite green	25 mg/L + 0.1 mg/L every other day[b]
Kanamycin disulfate	10–80 mg/L[a]
Malachite green	2–16 mg/L[a,b]
Neomycin sulfate	10–80 mg/L[a]
Potassium penicillin G	20–160 mg/L[a]
Potassium permanganate	4 mg/L[b]
Sodium chloride	5000 mg/L[b]
Tetracycline	10–80 mg/L[a]
Trimethoprim sulfadoxine	40–160 mg/L[a]

[a] Nimeyna et al. 1999
[b] Collins et al. 1975
[c] Pedersen et al. 2008

ethanol that may be used as a solvent. Ethanol can have a particularly profound effect as it is a short-chained carbon molecule that can be used by almost any microbe. This process can be responsible for three effects:

- A rapid drop in dissolved oxygen used by the microbes.
- Turbidity caused by microbial blooms (often transient).
- Degradation of the medication.

The exponential decay of formalin and praziquantel levels in a treated body of water is consistent with this microbial digestion (Figures A13.1 and A13.2) (Knight et al. 2016; Thomas et al. 2016). On the other hand, chloroquine was very stable in the water column in at least one experiment (Figure A13.3).

The extent of these effects will vary with the different microbial communities in each system. Therefore, it is important to invest in the procedures needed to monitor chemical concentrations and dissolved oxygen in water during and after treatments. This monitoring is very important for effective and safe immersion treatments.

There may be a temptation to add an antibiotic to the water to eliminate any bacteria that might digest the medication. While this is an interesting idea, the antibiotic would not kill all the bacteria in the microbiome and the void left by the antibiotic treatment would be rapidly filled by other bacterial species.

The environmental biota can have other impacts on medications. Copper is known to bind to microbial surfaces and this process is regulated by, and directly proportional to, copper concentration. About four times as much copper is bound at 50 ppb as at 5 ppb (Millero 1996). Bacteria and algae are also known to release extracellular ligands that can form complexes with copper, reducing the level of active, ionic copper in the water (Gledhill et al. 1999; Croot et al. 2000). Even vascular plants such as the wetland grasses (*Phragmites* spp.) can impact medication concentrations, such as by concentrating praziquantel

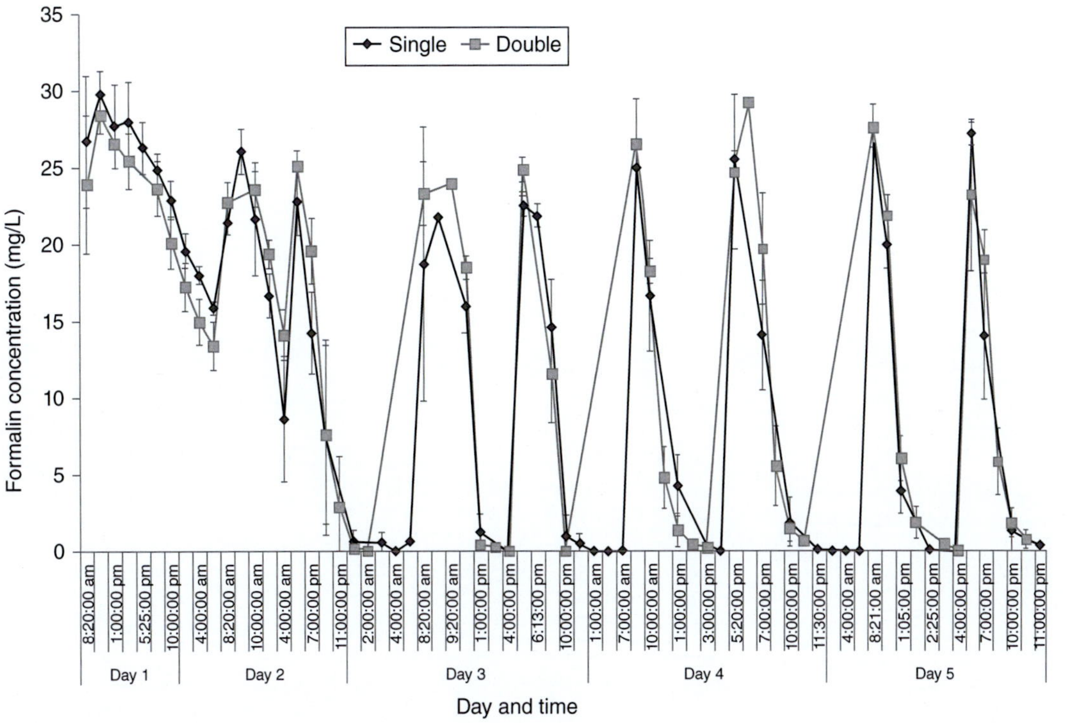

Figure A13.1 Formalin degradation rates in saltwater aquariums following sequential additions of formalin. Formalin added at 08:00 and 17:00. Rate of formalin degradation increased with subsequent formalin additions. The pattern was consistent across systems and across single-fish density (SD) and double-fish density (DD) treatments. The increased degradation is suggestive of microbe populations adapting to using formalin as a food source (Knight et al. 2016).

in their tissues and lowering the amount in the water (Marsik et al. 2017).

Effects on Target and Nontarget Species

One of the problems with immersion medications in established systems is that both target and nontarget species are exposed to the medication and its by-products. Morbidity and mortality may be seen in either group because of potential sensitivity to the medications and the unpredictable effects discussed above. And deaths of small invertebrates and microbes in the system (e.g. within large undergravel filters) can release a large amount of nutrients into the system, affecting ammonia and dissolved oxygen.

It is important to try to determine the root cause (i.e. physiology or environmental dynamics). If adverse effects are seen, they should be carefully documented and reported in the literature and to the associated regulatory group, e.g. to the US Food and Drug Administration (FDA) for FDA-approved drugs.

Novel treatment regimens should always be bioassayed prior to use on a large scale, where negative impacts could be severe and/or challenging to correct. This usually means testing the drug on a few individuals to identify possible fish/invertebrate sensitivities to the drug itself. However, this disregards the system effects described above. If possible, a bioassay that tests the drug on a smaller, similar system can help identify other adverse effects. Even though each system will have its own dynamics, it will give more information on likely effects. Because quality control can be an issue with unregulated drugs, bioassays should also be considered when a new lot of medication has been acquired. Bioassays are most effective with the following steps:

- The medication should be from the same lot that will be used for the larger treatment.
- The medication should be tested on a few individuals of the same species and life stages, ideally a cohort taken from the treatment group. All exposed species should be considered, including nontarget species.
- Monitoring should continue after the treatment has been discontinued, in case of delayed effects on the animals, plants, microbes, or filtration.

Bioassays are an invaluable tool in trying to mitigate the unpredictable effects of immersion medications.

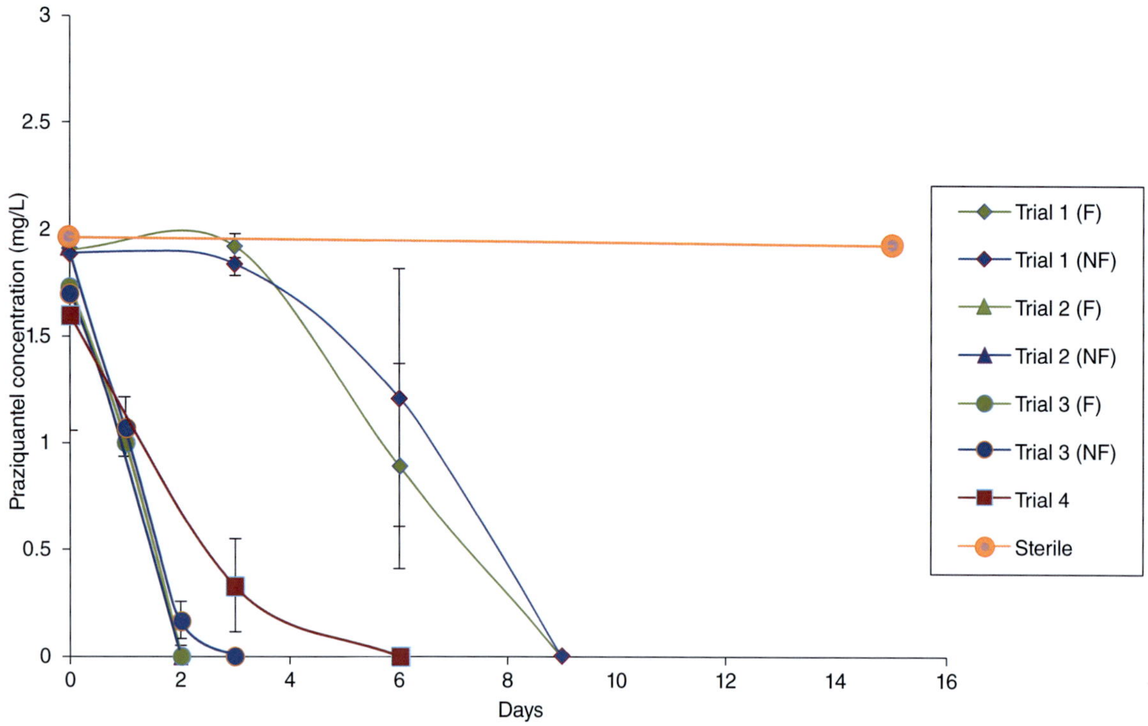

Figure A13.2 Praziquantel degradation rates in saltwater aquariums following the addition of praziquantel. Rate of degradation increased with subsequent praziquantel additions. The degradation pattern was consistent across systems and across systems with fish (F) and without fish (NF). In the sterile trial, using sterilized water, the drug concentration remained statistically unchanged for 15 days, suggesting that it is stable under these conditions (Thomas et al. 2016).

Medication Assays

Especially with bulk immersion medications, the clinician should question the composition, purity, and/or expiration of pharmaceuticals. Any manufacturer of these products should be able to provide its certificate of analysis (COA), which is a good place to start, but may still leave doubts and unanswered questions about the product's integrity. When this occurs, and the cost of the chemical or potential negative effects warrants it, the product should be submitted to a pharmaceutical lab for analysis, following the United States Pharmacopeia standards in the United States.

Talking to colleagues can provide anecdotal information on how drug levels change over time; however, because of dynamic variables between systems, the information may not be applicable. It is much better to repeatedly assess drug concentrations in the water to ensure appropriate levels are present throughout and following treatment. Colorimetric analysis methods available from local aquarium stores, e.g. for copper levels, are too inaccurate and should not be relied upon. An in-house colorimeter or spectrophotometer can be used to measure free ionic copper levels accurately. In-house benchtop water quality analyzers can often be used to measure chloroquine and formalin. More sophisticated chemical analyzers such as high-performance liquid chromatography (HPLC) systems or mass spectrophotometers are required for other chemicals, such as praziquantel. Investment in these units is advised for institutions with large systems. For more sensitive analytical techniques, such as inductively coupled plasma mass spectrometry (ICP-MS) or atomic absorption (AA), a local environmental laboratory is often needed.

Diving or Swimming in Medicated Water

The management of large aquatic systems often involves divers using surface or self-contained air. For the purposes of this discussion, the term diver will be used to describe humans who may be breathing compressed gases from SCUBA, breathing surface-supplied air, snorkeling, or swimming. When medications are put into these systems, potential known and unknown human health and safety hazards must be considered before divers are allowed to enter the water. This evaluation must include not only the primary compound, but also potential breakdown chemicals. Unfortunately, many of these breakdown compounds are unknown.

Historically, diver safety into medicated water was a simple matter of arithmetic. The normal human dose of the drug was compared to the concentration of the same drug in

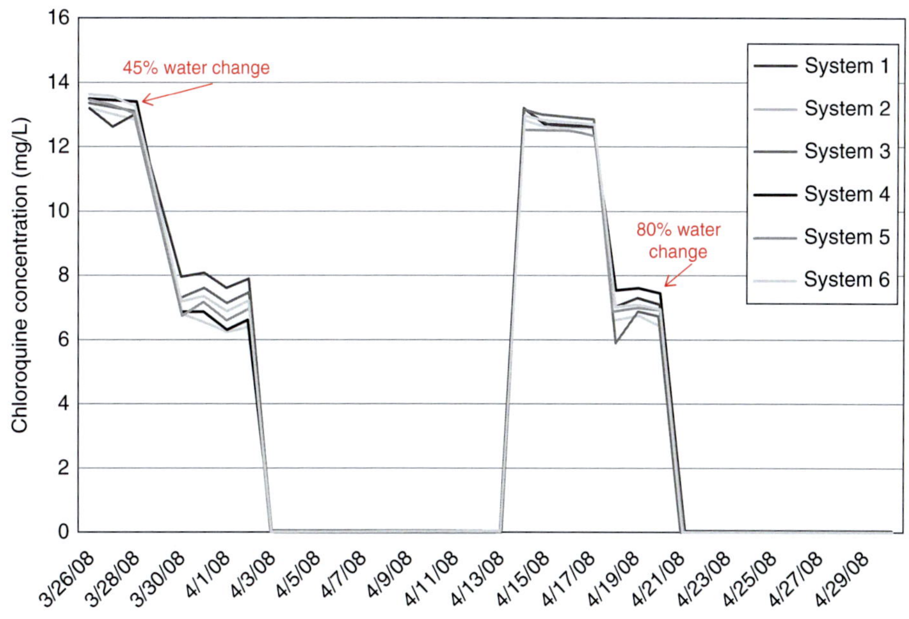

Figure A13.3 Chloroquine degradation rates in saltwater aquariums following sequential additions of chloroquine. Rate of chloroquine degradation was stable with each addition (unpublished data).

aquatic solution. Arithmetic calculations then determined how much water the diver would need to drink to meet or exceed the published dose. The resulting volume was typically measured in at least tens of liters, and so toxic effects were considered unlikely. However, this approach does not take into account route of exposure, such as cutaneous, conjunctival, intranasal, or regulator-generated aerosol; routes that are generally not evaluated during drug trials.

While limited, there are some resources available to better understand the risks. All chemicals used in immersion-based medications have source-provided Safety Data Sheets (SDS), formerly known as Material Safety Data Sheets (MSDS). These outline hazards associated with the specific chemical compound. Included on the SDS are hazard identification, exposure control and personal protective equipment (PPE) requirements, physical and chemical properties, stability and reactivity, and toxicologic information.

Further information may be garnered by working with dive control boards, dive physicians, pharmacists, and water quality chemists. Literature reviews may also provide insight. Unfortunately, there is no single source for the answer to the question: "Is diving in the water safe?"

In most areas, national and regional regulators have roles to play in the evaluation and mitigation of hazardous employment activities. Discussions presented within this venue are based on information from the US Occupational Safety and Health Administration (OSHA) and/or the US Environmental Protection Agency (EPA). Readers from outside of the US are encouraged to investigate or contact analogous national, regional, or local agencies in their areas.

Medicated water is generally considered to be "polluted water". The EPA defines polluted water as water that could make a diver sick (now or later), increase a diver's risk of developing cancer, or cause any undesirable outcome for the diver, tender, or other persons that may have contact. Even if the water is considered safe, unexplained symptoms in a diver may open up the question of whether the water caused it, whether it did or not. As such, all diving in medicated water must be considered "polluted water diving", and it is incumbent on the institution to ensure that steps are taken to protect individuals exposed from the affected water.

OSHA has not produced specific regulations for the chemicals that are encountered as immersion therapeutics. There is, however, regulatory oversight through their General Duty clause (OSHA section 5), the mandate to provide a place of employment free from recognized hazards. Since in most cases there is little known about the danger associated with the parent or by-product chemicals used in immersion therapy, it is prudent to consider diving in those waters hazardous and plan accordingly.

The US federal General Industry Standards Hazardous Waste Operations and Emergency Response (29 CFR 1910.120) requires the development of written health and safety programs which provide standard operating procedures and site-specific health and safety plans. In other words, any time there is a plan to allow human contact with medicated water, especially diving, there must be a plan in place to mitigate hazards. The plan should be unique to each circumstance, location, and drug.

Avoidance is the simplest option and diving in medicated water should be avoided wherever possible. Guest and volunteer dive programs should always be discontinued, and staff dives should be canceled or rescheduled if possible. Institutions that may require immersion therapy of large systems that rely on dive operations should develop contingency plans to be implemented when operations need to be canceled.

If diving in medicated water cannot be avoided, there must be a thorough and specific plan for diver health and safety. The first aspect is who would dive; only suitably trained staff should be considered. The hazardous diving plan should also include assessment of the hazards associated with the chemotherapeutic agent, personal protective equipment (PPE), a specific and detailed work plan, diver decontamination plan, and methods to determine when normal operations are safe to resume.

The US EPA has a great deal of experience diving in polluted water. As a result, they have developed a set of recommendations for PPE when diving in polluted water (Figure A13.4). The primary routes of exposure for the diver are inhalation, ingestion, and skin contact. Inhalation and ingestion are prevented by utilizing full face masks or helmets with positive pressure and a redundant breathing system. Mouth piece regulators must be avoided. The use of a vulcanized rubber hazmat dry suit with attached boots mitigates skin contact. Dry gloves and protective gauntlets further reduce opportunities for direct water to skin contact. Neoprene wetsuits should be avoided.

When divers exit the water, there needs to be a rinse station to remove and discharge the medicated water. In most cases, a hose with potable water which is either discharged to municipal sewer or via the institution's normal discharge route is appropriate.

The decision on when to resume normal dive operations depends on various factors, such as the medication, method for management of the medicated water, the type of system treated, and the specific treatment protocol. Ideally, assays of the parent compound in the water should be used as objective data to guide the decision. Even then, there needs to be some degree of thought put into the nature of the by-products of chemical breakdown. Systems with substrate, especially carbonate-bearing substrate (e.g. crushed coral), artificial rockwork, and/or other tank furnishings, can accumulate chemicals within these materials. Over time, these chemicals may leach back into the water, posing a potentially hazardous situation for divers.

Disposal of Medicated Water

A significant aspect of the decision-making process when contemplating an immersion therapy must be the disposal of the medicated water. Practically speaking, there are five basic methods for disposal:

- Discharge to municipal sanitary sewer.
- Discharge to a natural body of water.
- Return to the institution's water system.
- Biotic or abiotic removal or destruction of the compound.
- Transfer to an evaporation pond with subsequent removal of the resulting sludge.

Each method has advantages and disadvantages. The most common in aquarium medicine is probably discharge to municipal sanitary sewer, in part because the volumes used are relatively small. However, potential environmental impacts and disposal regulations must be considered prior to initiation of therapy. Best practices should include making sure the relevant national, regional and/or local regulatory agency discharge regulations are determined in regard to the medication(s), dose, volume, and frequency used. Disposal is just as important a consideration as dose and duration.

Discharge to Municipal Sanitary Sewer

Discharging medicated water to the municipal sanitary sewer is generally relatively straightforward and simple. It is not necessarily an environmentally sound practice or inexpensive. Some communities in areas with little annual rainfall are reluctant to accept seawater, either natural or artificial, into their wastewater system. This is especially true in areas in which efforts are being made to replenish ground water supplies with treated water from municipal wastewater plants. It is not unusual for water treatment districts to employ metering systems to measure the amount of water, either fresh or salt water, being discharged and to charge the user accordingly.

Discharge via sanitary sewer does avoid direct contamination of natural bodies of water. Additionally, routine wastewater treatment increases the opportunity for biotic or abiotic breakdown of some chemotherapeutics. However, some medications are not removed by routine wastewater treatment facilities, e.g. fenbendazole, estrogens (Kaczala and Blum 2016). Some wastewater facilities employ more robust wastewater treatment methods to better remove pollutants, but even then, not all are effective (Jones et al. 2007). Eventually, the effluent will be discharged from the treatment facility into the environment. For those chemotherapeutics that remain, their fate is quite similar to that of chemotherapeutics discharged directly into natural bodies of surface or underground water. Discharge to the municipal sanitary sewer is not ideal.

Discharge to a Natural Body of Water

This may arguably be the easiest and cheapest method available. These advantages are outweighed by the numerous environmental, public health, and ethical problems

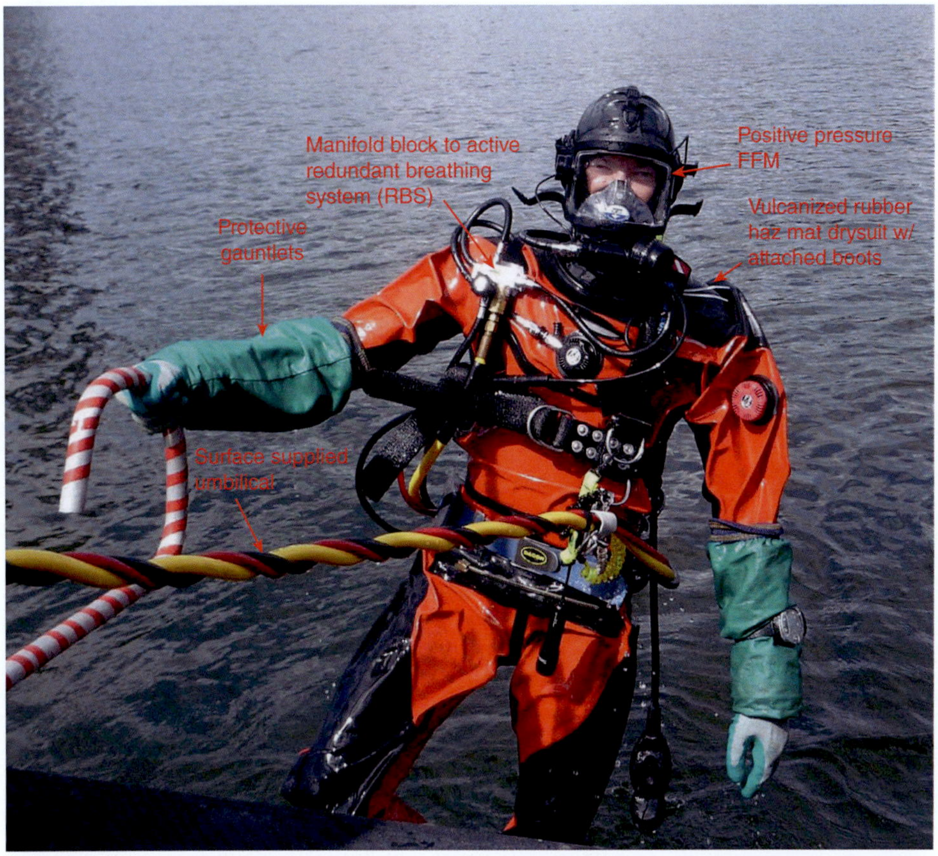

Figure A13.4 This diver is wearing appropriate personal protective equipment (PPE) for immersion in medicated water. Exposure via inhalation, ingestion, and skin contact is avoided with a vulcanized rubber hazmat dry suit with attached boots, positive pressure full face mask, redundant breathing systems, and protective gauntlets. *Source*: Image courtesy of Sean Sheldrake, US Environmental Protection Agency.

associated with open discharge. While some might argue that the "solution to pollution is dilution", the cavalier dumping of medicated water into natural bodies of water is an antiquated, irresponsible method of disposal. While dilution may mitigate some of the acute and lethal impacts on animals, plants, and ecosystems, it does not prevent the chronic, sublethal impacts that these chemotherapeutics may have (Prichard and Granek 2016). Compounds may become concentrated (bioaccumulate) in animals, plants, and sediments, which may release the pollutant when disturbed. Impacts not only occur locally, but move with the water to affect downstream surface water and potentially ground water, which could contaminate drinking water (Helperin et al. 2001). And discharge of medicated salt water from large systems into freshwater bodies (e.g. lakes, rivers) can have significant ecological impacts, including decreased biodiversity, changes in the natural character of aquatic ecosystems, and lower productivity (Williams 2001).

There is evidence of increasing antibiotic resistance in aquatic environments, both freshwater and marine, including offshore predatory marine fish (Kummerer 2009b; Blackburn et al. 2010; Marsik et al. 2017). Discharge of medicated water must be prevented to avoid contributing to this problem (Bártíková et al. 2016).

Discharge of medicated water is regulated at multiple levels in most locations. Failure to comply may not only result in significant financial penalties but will likely result in unwanted and damaging publicity. In addition, the increased scrutiny by both FDA and USDA in the United States may eventually threaten to make many of the immersion medications unavailable in the future.

Return to the Institution's Water System

Returning medicated water to the main water system is also inexpensive and easily accomplished. While the environmental, public health, and ethical concerns are not as great as those described above, there are aspects of this method that warrant consideration.

Since the medicated water is placed back into general circulation, there may be widespread impacts on animals and plants within the institution as well as the critical biological filtration. For the reasons described above, these effects can be unpredictable. Dilution and microbial degradation of some drugs can mitigate some of the direct, acute effects; however, long-term, chronic exposure may be significant. The problem of bioaccumulation in living organisms remains the same as mentioned above. Medications may also bind to filter media, substrate, real or artificial rockwork, and other tank décor. They may then leach back out into the water column with significant impacts. For example, copper is known to bind with carbonates, which are components of crushed coral and other marine substrates. A decrease in pH or increase in salinity may result in the release of copper back into the water, potentially intoxicating susceptible species like invertebrates or elasmobranchs (Keith 1981; Cardeilhac and Whitaker 1988).

In most cases, returning medicated water to the main water system is not recommended, unless there is a process in place to remove the agent first. A more complete discussion of methods of removal or destruction is given below.

Biotic or Abiotic Removal or Destruction of the Medication

A fourth option for medications is to use natural (biotic) or physical (abiotic) methods to remove the drugs from the water. These methods are most effective when the water levels of the particular agent can be measured. It is important to bear in mind that some of the methods may result in the breakdown of the parent compound into different chemicals, and their form and behavior may not be well-understood.

These methods are typically less convenient and more expensive than immediate discharge. When evaluating the cost, it is important to include the costs associated with disposal of the waste generated when absorptive methods are used, such as activated carbon.

Biotic elimination is a process of biodegradation by microbes, including bacteria, protists, algae, or fungi. These organisms may be part of the system's natural microbiome, or they may be organisms that have been compound-adapted to specifically aid in the degradation of the drug. These biotic processes have not been well-studied. The dramatic decrease in the half-life of praziquantel due to plant and microbial degradation suggests that this may be an effective strategy to remove praziquantel from water (Knight et al. 2016; Thomas et al. 2016; Marsik et al. 2017). Most antibiotics tested have not been subject to biodegradation (Kummerer 2009a).

Common abiotic methods include adsorption, photolysis, oxidation, and reduction (Kummerer 2009a). Nanofiltration and ultrafiltration methods show promise.

Adsorption is typically accomplished using activated carbon, making use of the high surface area and abundant binding sites. It can be used in both freshwater and saltwater systems. Some products are marketed specifically for aquarium and pond applications, e.g. Norit® Aquarium Carbon 3-6. As mentioned above (see Section "Effects of Water Clarification and Disinfection on Immersion Medications"), activated carbon is effective at removing many organic compounds including formalin, trichlorfon, chloroquine, and praziquantel. However, important chemotherapeutic agents, such as inorganic copper, are poorly adsorbed unless bound to organics, and many compounds have yet to be evaluated. There is some evidence to suggest that the water solubility of compounds also influences affinity to carbon; hydrophilic compounds break through (escape) carbon more readily than hydrophobic ones (Snyder et al. 2007). Activated carbon can be expensive and messy to work with. Carbon needs to be backwashed frequently and replaced before the bindings sites are used up or overgrown by microbes (Snyder et al. 2007). Replacement frequency can be determined by drug assays or based on the manufacturer's recommendation. An important consideration of carbon is that the adsorption process mechanically binds the compound and does not alter or eliminate it; it is simply moved from the water column onto the carbon particle, which must be discarded through appropriate hazardous waste disposal (Singh et al. 1996; Jiuhui 2008).

Other composite adsorbents, such as zeolite, may prove effective in removing immersion drugs from the water. However, they tend to be selective, may alter the parent compound into one or more unknown chemicals, and are likely to be expensive (Jiuhui 2008).

Light-based destruction of chemotherapeutics may occur due to UV or traditional lighting. Drugs that are known to be degraded by UV light include praziquantel, chloroquine, tetracycline, and oxytetracycline. Reports of visible light sensitivity are often anecdotal and supporting data may be scant. Degradation through UV may result in toxic by-products, so potential breakdown products should be assessed before using this technique. The best source of information concerning the light sensitivity of a chemotherapeutic is the pharmaceutical literature and drug inserts.

Oxidative processes, such as ozonation, are fairly common in aquatic systems containing fish and invertebrates. While effective at degrading organic compounds, ozone and other potent oxidizers can react with compounds to create toxic by-products, about which little is known (Kim et al. 2002). Their use in the degradation of medications requires further investigation and should only be used under close monitoring.

Nanofiltration and ultrafiltration using membrane technology have been used for the management of potable drinking water and may have applications in the removal of chemotherapeutics from water. Molecular size and water solubility influence the ability of nanofiltration and ultrafiltration membranes to remove dissolved compounds from water (Yoon et al. 2006, 2007). It is anticipated that the cost of these membrane technologies will decrease over time, increasing the opportunity for use in fish health programs.

Unfortunately, there is no single biotic and abiotic method that is effective for all drugs in all cases. Veterinarians, husbandry staff, life support staff, and water quality staff should develop methods that are best suited to each circumstance.

Transfer to an Evaporation Pond

There are rare circumstances in which none of the previously described options for discharge are feasible due to environmental, infrastructure, and/or regulatory considerations. Such cases may mandate the use of evaporation ponds. These are shallow, artificial ponds with a large surface area that enhances water evaporation by sunlight and high temperatures. This results in the pollutants accumulating in either a crystalline or concentrated sludge form. The sludge then requires proper handling, treatment, and disposal. This is usually a complete service provided by some hazardous waste disposal companies.

This approach allows the same on-site management of medicated water regardless of the compound being used, therefore fewer protocols are needed. Evaporation ponds are either lined or unlined. Lined ponds use synthetic liners to contain the liquid and an alarm system to detect leaks, so there is no impact on groundwater. Unlined ponds may be more problematic from an environmental perspective. Substrate materials should be compacted and consist of soil, such as clay, which has very low permeability, protecting groundwater. There should be adequate geological and hydrological information and ongoing monitoring for contamination of the water table. Evaporation ponds must include fencing and nets to avoid wildlife and humans accessing the water. Even with those safeguards, the potential for untoward environmental impacts cannot be guaranteed (Helperin et al. 2001). The institution needs to thoroughly investigate and understand the process at their hazardous waste facility, to ensure it is done in an environmentally appropriate manner.

Environmental considerations aside, evaporation ponds tend to be expensive. This includes the cost of the transport of medicated water to the treatment facility, the use of the pond, and the final disposal of the chemical sludge.

Record-Keeping

The use and subsequent disposal of immersion mediations must be carefully recorded. These compounds are either therapeutic or prophylactic and so are considered drugs by overseeing agencies. Best practices, as well as regulatory and accreditation standards, require proper documentation of all drug prescriptions, including immersion medications, within the veterinarian–client–patient relationship. Reporting requirements associated with the disposal of medicated water may also include documentation of pre-use approval.

Specific Drug Examples

Some of the most common immersion fish medications (formalin, trichlorfon, praziquantel, copper, and chloroquine) can be used as representative models for other therapeutics. Below is a comprehensive look at each of the chemicals.

Formalin

Full chemical name or formula: Formalin is a generic term that refers to a solution of 37% formaldehyde gas (CH_2O) dissolved in water, with 10–15% methanol. Prescribed treatment doses must specify formalin or formaldehyde concentration to avoid confusion between the prescriber and those performing the application.

Trade names: Formacide-B®, Formalin-F®, Paracide-F®, Parasite-S®.

Typical uses: Formalin is used commonly to treat ectoparasites and oomycetes. Doses are usually given in mg/L of formalin. Prolonged immersion doses range from 12.5 to 25 mg/L. Higher doses are used for shorter duration, e.g. 100–250 mg/L for 60 minutes (Noga 2011).

Unpredictability: Formalin can cause a rapid decrease in dissolved oxygen. This effect is most pronounced in systems with algae and limited gas exchange. Formalin can combine with organic matter in the system, reducing its treatment efficacy. Formalin can become more toxic at higher water temperature and should not be used in water >27°C (80°F) (Alderman 1992; Francis-Floyd 1996). It is also more toxic in soft, low-pH water (Noga 2011). Formalin can be rapidly degraded by bacteria within the microbiome (Figure A13.1) (Knight et al. 2016). Paraformaldehyde is a highly toxic by-product that can develop, particularly following exposure to temperature extremes. Formalin should never be used if a white precipitate or cloudiness is observed in the bottle, as that may indicate the presence of paraformaldehyde (Francis-Floyd 1996).

Effects on water quality: Formalin in an aquatic system quickly consumes oxygen, both directly and indirectly. It reacts directly with dissolved oxygen at a ratio of 5:1 – each 5 mg/L of formalin applied can remove 1 mg/L dissolved oxygen (Noga 2011). Formalin indirectly decreases oxygen by rapidly killing algae and phytoplankton (Francis-Floyd 1996; Bowker et al. 2011). Increased aeration should be provided during treatment and dissolved oxygen should always be monitored. Increased ammonia may be seen. Use of Nessler's reagent to test for ammonia in formalin-treated systems may give falsely elevated results. The ammonium salicylate method should be used instead.

Bioassay: Bioassays are strongly recommended prior to treatment of a new species or high concentration baths, e.g. >100 mg/L at >21°C (70°F), to evaluate potential adverse effects.

Measuring drug levels: Samples must be analyzed immediately. The preferred method to assay concentrations of 3–500 µg/L formaldehyde (CH_2O) is a colorimetric method using a reagent known as MBTH (3-methyl-2-benzothiazoline hydrazone). CH_2O reacts with MBTH and a developing solution to produce a blue color that can be measured with a standard spectrophotometer. The measurement wavelength is 630 nm. The color intensity is proportional to the formaldehyde concentration.

Effects on target and nontarget species: There are many reports of formalin toxicity in fish, although environmental conditions must be considered. Particularly susceptible groups include some scaleless fish and elasmobranchs (Francis-Floyd 1996; Noga 2011). Signs of toxicity may include dyspnea, tachypnea, pallor, excess mucous, erratic swimming, inappetence, and death, often within 24–48 hours (Wedemeyer 1971; Noga 2011). Formalin is also toxic to many invertebrates, algae, and vascular plants. Toxicity increases with increasing water temperature and decreasing pH.

Effects on biofiltration and microbiome: At ≤25 mg/L, formalin generally has limited deleterious effect on nitrifying bacteria; however, higher doses can damage the biological filtration. Some microbes can use formalin as a food source, and the resultant bacterial bloom can cause turbidity and metabolize oxygen (Figure A13.1).

Human exposure: All SDS safety precautions should be followed. Formalin should be stored in the dark in a cabinet designed for flammables and should be protected from temperature extremes to inhibit the formation of paraformaldehyde.

Disposal: Formaldehyde is hazardous waste and national, regional, or local permissible municipal sewer disposal concentrations should be determined. Fortunately, formaldehyde shows rapid degradation in water where it reacts with oxygen to form formic acid: $2CH_2O + O_2 \rightarrow 2CH_2O_2$. Formic acid then undergoes metabolic oxidation by micro-organisms to form carbon dioxide and water: $2CH_2O_2 + O_2 \rightarrow 2CO_2 + 2H_2O$. Aeration has also been shown to increase formalin degradation in aquaria (Chinabut et al. 1988). And formaldehyde can be destroyed by ozone according to the following reaction: $CH_2O + 2O_3 \rightarrow CO_2 + H_2O + 2O_2$. Medicated water can also be treated with granular activated carbon or UV prior to disposal. Activated carbon should then be disposed of as hazardous waste.

Trichlorfon or Metrifonate

Full chemical name or formula: O,O-dimethyl 2,2,2-trichloro-1-hydroxyethyl phosphonate (DTHP).

Trade names: D50®, Dipterex®, Dylox®, Foschlor®, Masoten®, Neguvon®, Trichlorophene®.

Typical uses: Trichlorfon may be used to treat copepods, branchiurans, leeches, and monogeneans. Typical doses are reported as 0.25–0.50 mg/L, although reports do not always clarify if this is based on weight of drug or active compound.

Unpredictability: The concentration and effectiveness of trichlorfon can depend on its source, carrier, age, and exposure. It is important to know the source's active concentration for dosing calculations: most are 50 or 80%. Mixing with other therapeutics must be avoided as it could result in dangerous by-products. It is well-established that this chemical is very susceptible to microbial digestion. Microbial digestion and/or possible parasite resistance can increase over time in a system, so it should not be used routinely as a prophylactic. Dichlorvos (2,2-dichlorovinyl dimethyl phosphate) is the major transformation product of trichlorfon (Hofer 1981). This is rapidly formed by hydrolysis in water but can also be formed by photolysis. Dichlorvos is at least 100 times more toxic than trichlorfon. The rate of trichlorfon transformation to dichlorvos increases with increasing alkalinity and increasing temperature (Deer and Beard 2001).

Effects on target and nontarget species: The primary mode of action is inhibition of the enzyme cholinesterase (ChE) that breaks down acetylcholine. It leads to an accumulation of the neurotransmitter acetylcholine, causing disruptions in the central nervous system. It is toxic to a wide range of taxa because acetylcholine is an important and ubiquitous neurotransmitter. It is moderately toxic to most fish, particularly elasmobranchs, and highly toxic to invertebrates and waterfowl. Symptoms of toxicity include hyperactivity, tremors, seizures, and death (Jensen and Gaufin 1964; IPCS 1986). Leukopenia and anemia have also been reported. Atropine may be administered prior to treatment to mitigate toxicity from the cholinesterase inhibition. Concomitant administration of the immune stimulant propolis has been shown to mitigate adverse effects in koi (*Cyprinus carpio koi*) (Yonar et al. 2015). The potential for bioaccumulation is low because of low persistence in water and its hydrophilic properties; it tends to remain in water and not in sediment or suspended solids (HSDB 1999).

Effects on biofiltration and microbiome: Trichlorfon does not typically interfere with biological filtration. Degradation of the medication is much faster in nonsterile soils than in sterile substrates, so microbial digestion seems likely (Rosenberg and Alexander 1979). It can cause microbial blooms.

Effects on water quality: It is readily water-soluble and will not discolor the water, although the carrier or contaminants may. Due to the toxic effects and subsequent mortality of invertebrates, as well as possible microbial blooms in the system, a decrease in oxygen or increase in ammonia could occur.

Bioassay: Bioassays are essential because of the toxicity of trichlorfon and its unpredictable transformation to the exponentially more toxic by-product, dichlorvos. Close observation during the bioassay is essential.

Measuring drug levels: There is no simple or inexpensive methodology for measuring trichlorfon concentration in water. It can be measured using gas chromatography and recent methods have been developed to analyze trichlorfon through liquid chromatography-mass spectroscopy (LC-MS) (Zhu et al. 2007).

Human exposure: Trichlorfon is particularly hazardous as it can be absorbed transdermally in humans, with the same anticholinesterase effects. Suitable personal protective equipment (e.g. chemical gloves and face mask during dosing) are essential. All SDS safety precautions must be followed. It should be stored in a hazardous chemical cabinet.

Disposal: Trichlorfon is considered hazardous waste. National, regional, or local permissible municipal sewer disposal concentrations should be determined. Levels should be reduced using granular activated carbon treatment or ozone prior to disposal. The activated carbon should then be disposed of as hazardous waste.

Praziquantel

Full chemical name or formula: 2-cyclohexyl-carbonyl-4-oxo-1,2,3,6,7,11*b*-hexahydro, 4*H*-pyrazino[2,1-*a*]isoquinoline.

Trade names: Droncit®, Drontal®.

Typical uses: Praziquantel immersion is often used for the treatment of monogeneans and it has activity against digenes, cestodes, and acanthocephalans. Typical immersion doses are 2–20 mg/L (Noga 2011).

Unpredictability: Praziquantel is lipophilic and dissolves poorly in water. Two methods are commonly used to improve dissolution, but the effective dose can be hard to estimate due to this solubility issue. Praziquantel can be manually dissolved into aquarium water by squeezing through a very fine mesh net or filter material. Alternatively, it can be dissolved in just enough 95% ethyl alcohol to form a thick paste (~1 mL/g praziquantel) prior to dosing. This carries the risk of providing a good carbon source for bacterial blooms. If praziquantel is not dissolved properly it can be irritating to fish gills and may result in potentially fatal gill damage (Reed et al. 2009). The major degradation product of praziquantel has been elucidated and the rate of decomposition is affected by temperature and light exposure (Saeed and Hamid 2004). Praziquantel is also subject to rapid degradation by the microbial community of the aquatic system (Figure A13.2) (Thomas et al. 2016).

Effects on target and nontarget species: Praziquantel has a wide safety index for fish and plants when used properly. It has a no observable effect level (NOEL) when given orally to vertebrates at 20 g/kg/d (Hempel et al. 2006). It can act on monogeneans and other parasites through exposure within the water column and through absorption by the fish (Kim and Cho 2000). The effect on monogeneans is reduced for parasites that reside deep within the gill lamellae, are protected by gill inflammation, or are encapsulated as ova (Chisholm and Whittington 2002; Reed et al. 2009).

Effects on biofiltration and microbiome: Praziquantel does not typically interfere with biological filtration. Some microbes can use praziquantel as a food source and bloom, metabolizing oxygen (Figure A13.2). A bacterial bloom can also be induced if praziquantel is administered in ethyl alcohol.

Effects on water quality: Praziquantel typically has no effect on dissolved oxygen, alkalinity, pH, turbidity, or color. However, a bacterial bloom can occur, particularly when the praziquantel is dissolved in ethanol; this can cause turbidity, low dissolved oxygen, and increased ammonia.

Bioassay: Praziquantel has a wide safety index, but a bioassay testing a small cohort of individuals is advised with new species.

Measuring drug levels: Modern HPLC methods allow rapid analysis of praziquantel and show good recovery of the drug in plasma, tissue, freshwater, and salt water (Kim et al. 2001; Tubs and Tingle 2006; Horvat et al. 2012; Xie et al. 2015; Thomas et al. 2016). The assays can be used to determine if target concentrations are reached and for what duration. They can also show possible by-product formation.

Human exposure: All SDS safety precautions should be followed. Praziquantel does not typically have any specific storage requirements.

Disposal: National, regional, or local permissible municipal sewer disposal concentrations should be determined. Levels can be reduced using granular activated carbon treatment, ozone, or UV, but the drug is also likely rapidly degraded by bacteria. Praziquantel has not previously been detected in environmental water samples.

Copper Sulfate, Chelated Copper

Full chemical name or formula: Copper sulfate ($CuSO_4$) is also known as bluestone. Organic copper salts include chelated copper and copper citrate ($C_6H_8Cu_2O_7^{4+}$). Copper citrate stock solution can be prepared in-house by adding 2.23 g of copper sulfate pentahydrate and 1.5 g of citric acid to 1 L of distilled water to make 0.56 mg of copper/mL (Noga 2011).

Trade names: Cupramine™ (amine-bound copper complex), CopperSafe™ (unknown copper chelation).

Typical uses: Copper immersion is often used to treat ectoparasites (particularly *Cryptocaryon* spp.) and oomycetes. Copper may also be used as an algaecide and to eradicate snails. The therapeutic range depends on the salinity, alkalinity, product, and parasite (see Chapter A12).

Unpredictability: High temperatures, low alkalinity, and low pH increase the risk of toxicity by increasing the proportion of ionic copper and the uptake of copper by fish (Cardeilhac and Whitaker 1988). Therefore, treatment regimens are different in salt water compared to freshwater (see Chapter A12). Copper more readily precipitates out at higher alkalinities and also binds to calcareous materials (e.g. dolomite, crushed coral, oyster shell) affecting the level of copper in solution. This is especially true when the non-chelated, more reactive bluestone form of copper is used. Copper can also be absorbed by living organisms, including bacteria and algae. Bacteria will exponentially increase uptake rate during the course of treatment and are instrumental in the eventual reduction of copper back to trace levels. These reasons make it challenging to maintain therapeutic levels during treatment and to remove copper from a system post-treatment. These dynamics may also explain some of the apparent variability in copper sensitivities between fish species.

Effects on target and nontarget species: Copper may be acutely toxic to some species of finfish, most elasmobranchs, and most invertebrates (see Chapter A12). As well as species sensitivities, age can have an effect: some papers report increased toxicity in older fish, others report increased toxicity in juveniles (Howarth and Sprague 1978; Bunton et al. 1987; Pickering and Lazorchak 1995; Furuta et al. 2008). Copper can be directly toxic to a variety of tissues and damage to the immune system can increase the risk of secondary disease. Signs of toxicity may include inappetence, changes in coloration, lethargy, and acute mortalities. A slow increase to reach the therapeutic concentration is recommended. A common problem is a sudden increase in ionic copper sulfate following rapid dosing, or if dosing continues at the same rate after the binding sites are exhausted. Knowledge of how a specific system handles copper additions is invaluable – it helps to judge required doses and when dosing should be reduced as saturation of the surface binding sites is reached. Copper can also be toxic to algae and vascular plants.

Effects on biofiltration and microbiome: Copper can have an inhibitory effect on biological filtration, particularly following rapid dosing. Water quality must be monitored regularly throughout and after treatment. Common ammonia-binding compounds like Amquel® cannot be used with copper since they will increase copper toxicity by reducing Cu^{2+} to Cu^{+}.

Effects on water quality: Copper does not cause turbidity or discoloration of the water. It can cause an increase in ammonia and nitrite due to the inhibition of nitrifying bacteria. It can also lead to increased ammonia and decreased dissolved oxygen due to the death and decay of invertebrates, algae, and vascular plants.

Bioassay: A bioassay on a small cohort of individuals and conservative dosing are advised with new species or life stages.

Measuring drug levels: A colorimeter or spectrophotometer using the colorimetric porphyrin method is typically used to measure free copper ion levels in-house. Less-expensive colorimetric analysis methods available from local aquarium stores are too inaccurate and should not be relied upon. Also, some only measure total copper, and not the biologically active free copper ion. More sensitive analytical techniques such as ICP-MS can also be used. Methods of analysis for the therapeutic free copper ion are the same regardless of the copper formulation used. A total copper method in addition to the free copper method should be used according to manufacturer recommendations when chelated copper is used.

Human exposure: All SDS safety precautions should be followed. Copper does not typically have any specific storage requirements.

Disposal: Activated carbon and water changes are typically used to remove copper, but copper concentration may need to be checked regularly for several weeks after cessation of treatment, as it may leach back into the system from adsorbent surfaces. In the United States as of 2020, copper is considered low regulatory priority by the FDA. However, it is best practice to contact your local state or county for permissible municipal sewer disposal concentrations.

Chloroquine

Full chemical name or formula: Chloroquine diphosphate – sometimes referred to as chloroquine phosphate ($C_{18}H_{26}ClN_3\cdot 2H_3PO_4$), chloroquine hydrochloride ($C_{18}H_{26}ClN_3\cdot 2HCl$), chloroquine sulfate ($C_{18}H_{26}ClN_3\cdot H_2O_4S$). The most common form used in fish medicine is chloroquine diphosphate.

Trade names: Aralen®, Aralen HCl®, Plaquenil™.

Typical uses: Chloroquine immersion is typically used to treat external protozoa such as *Cryptocaryon irritans*, *Amyloodinium ocellatum*, trichodinids, and scuticociliates. A common therapeutic dose for prolonged bath treatment is 10 mg/L, based on drug weight (Noga 2011). It is important to note that this is equivalent to a chloroquine (base salt) dose of 6.2 mg/L, since the phosphate makes up the other 3.8 mg of the weight.

Unpredictability: Increased toxicity is seen with increasing pH. Unlike formalin and praziquantel, chloroquine is usually stable in aquatic systems (Figure A13.3). It is, however, readily degraded by UV light. Chloroquine does reduce the bioavailability of praziquantel in rats and humans, so the two medications may interact in an aquarium system and should not be used together.

Effects on target and nontarget species: Chloroquine can be toxic to some invertebrates and algae. There are anecdotal reports of toxicity in some teleost species, particularly at higher doses (>30 mg/L drug weight).

Effects on biofiltration and microbiome: Chloroquine may have an inhibitory effect on biological filtration, either directly or indirectly, particularly at high doses. Water quality must be monitored regularly throughout and following treatment.

Effects on water quality: Chloroquine can cause an increase in ammonia and nitrite due to inhibition of nitrifying bacteria. It can also lead to increased ammonia and decreased dissolved oxygen due to the death and decay of invertebrates and algae. Repeated treatments of chloroquine diphosphate with limited water turnover may increase phosphate level in the water, but it is unlikely to be clinically significant in fish systems.

Bioassay: A bioassay by testing a small cohort of individuals is always advised with new species.

Measuring drug levels: Measuring chloroquine levels is essential because of its prolonged survival in water (Figure A13.3). Routine redosing without measuring drug levels can lead to toxicity in the fish and damage to the biological filtration. Levels can be measured using the UV absorbance method on a UV spectrophotometer at 329 nm. Customized standard curves must be run using the water of the system to be tested. This accounts for any organic interferences within the water column.

Human exposure: All SDS safety precautions should be followed. Chloroquine should be protected from direct light.

Disposal: National, regional, or local permissible municipal sewer disposal concentrations should be determined. It is preferable to treat medicated water with activated carbon, ozone, or UV prior to disposal.

References

Alderman, D. (1992). Chemotherapy in aquaculture today. In: *Chemotherapy in Aquaculture. From Theory to Reality*. Office International des Epizootics, University of California, CA.

Bártíková, H., Podlipná, R., and Skálová, L. (2016). Veterinary drugs in the environment and their toxicity to plants. *Chemosphere* 144: 2290–2301.

Bhatnagar, A., Hogland, W., Marques, M., and Sillanpää, M. (2013). An overview of the modification methods of activated carbon for its water treatment applications. *Chemical Engineering Journal* 219: 499–511.

Blackburn, J.K., Mitchell, M.A., Blackburn, M.-C.H. et al. (2010). Evidence of antibiotic resistance in free-swimming, top-level marine predatory fishes. *Journal of Zoo and Wildlife Medicine* 41: 7–16.

Bowker, J., Trushenski, J., Tuttle-Lau, M. et al. (2011). Guide to Using Drugs, Biologics, and Other Chemicals in Aquaculture. Bethesda, MD: American Fisheries Society, Fish Culture Section.

Bunton, T.E., Baksi, S.M., George, S.G., and Frazier, J.M. (1987). Abnormal hepatic copper storage in a teleost fish (*Morone americana*). *Veterinary Pathology* 24: 515–524.

Cardeilhac, P.T. and Whitaker, B.R. (1988). Tropical fish medicine. Copper treatments. Uses and precautions. *Veterinary Clinics of North America: Small Animal Practice* 18: 435–448.

Chinabut, S., Limsuwan, C., and Sangjan, M. (1988). Formalin: its toxicity to *Aeromonas hydrophila*, plankton and degradation. *Network of Aquaculture Centers in Asia-Pacific* WP/88/72.

Chisholm, L.A. and Whittington, I.D. (2002). Efficacy of praziquantel bath treatments for monogenean infections of the *Rhinobatos typus*. *Journal of Aquatic Animal Health* 14: 30–234.

Čizmić, M., Ljubas, D., Ćurković, L. et al. (2017). Kinetics and degradation pathways of photolytic and photocatalytic oxidation of the anthelmintic drug praziquantel. *Journal of Hazardous Materials* 323: 500–512.

Collins, M.T., Gratzek, J.B., Dawe, D.L., and Nemetz, T.G. (1975). Effects of parasiticides on nitrification. *Journal of the Fisheries Research Board of Canada* 32: 2033–2037.

Collins, M.T., Gratzek, J.B., Dawe, D.L., and Nemetz, T.G. (1976). Effects of antibacterial agents on nitrification in an aquatic recirculating system. *Journal of the Fisheries Research Board of Canada* 33: 215–218.

Croot, P.L., Moffett, J.W., and Brand, L.E. (2000). Production of extracellular Cu complexing ligands by eucaryotic phytoplankton in response to Cu stress. *Limnology and Oceanography* 45: 619–627.

Deer, H.M. and Beard, R. (2001). Effect of water pH on the chemical stability of pesticides. *AG/Pesticides* 14: 1–3.

Francis-Floyd, R. (1996). Use of formalin to control fish parasites. *University of Florida IFAS Extension* Electronic Data Information Source #VM-77. https://edis.ifas.ufl.edu/pdffiles/VM/VM06100.pdf (accessed 1 December 2018).

Furuta, T., Iwata, N., and Kikuchi, K. (2008). Effects of fish size and water temperature on the acute toxicity of copper for Japanese flounder, *Paralichthys olivaceus*, and red sea bream, *Pagrus major*. *Journal of the World Aquaculture Society* 39: 766–773.

Gledhill, M., Nimmo, M., Hill, S.J., and Brown, M.T. (1999). The release of copper-complexing ligands by the brown alga *Fucus vesiculosus* (Phaeophyceae) in response to increasing total copper levels. *Journal of Phycology* 35: 501–509.

Havlíková, L., Šatínsky, D., and Solich, P. (2016). Aspects of decontamination of ivermectin and praziquantel from environmental waters using advanced oxidation technology. *Chemosphere* 144: 21–28.

Hazardous Substances Database (1999). National Library of Medicine Bethesda, Maryland, available at https://toxnet.nlm.nih.gov/cgi-bin/sis/htmlgen?HSDB. (accessed December 2018)

Helperin, A.N., Beckman, D.S., Inwood, D. et al. (2001). California's contaminated groundwater. *Natural Resources Defense Council* 4: 3–18.

Hempel, H., Scheffczyk, A., Schallnaß, H.J., and Lumaret, J.P. (2006). Toxicity of four veterinary parasiticides on larvae of the dung beetle *Aphodius constans* in the laboratory. *Environmental Toxicology and Chemistry* 25: 3155–3163.

Hofer, W. (1981). Chemistry of metrifonate and dichlorvos. *Basic and Clinical Pharmacology and Toxicology* 49: 7–14.

Horvat, A.J., Babić, S., Pavlović, D.M. et al. (2012). Analysis, occurrence and fate of anthelmintics and their transformation products in the environment. *Trends in Analytical Chemistry* 31: 61–84.

Howarth, R.S. and Sprague, J.B. (1978). Copper lethality to rainbow trout in waters of various hardness and pH. *Water Research* 12: 455–462.

International Program on Chemical Safety (1986). Environmental Health Criteria for Organophosphorus Insecticides – A General Introduction 63. World Health Organization.

Jensen, L.D. and Gaufin, A.R. (1964). Effects of ten organic insecticides on two species of stonefly naiads. *Transactions of the American Fisheries Society* 93: 27–34.

Jiuhui, Q.U. (2008). Research progress of novel adsorption processes in water purification: a review. *Journal of Environmental Sciences (China)* 20: 1–13.

Jones, O.A.H., Green, P.G., Voulvoulis, N., and Lester, J.N. (2007). Questioning the excessive use of advanced treatment to remove organic micropollutants from wastewater. *Environmental Science and Technology* 41: 5085–5089.

Kaczala, F. and Blum, S. (2016). The occurrence of veterinary pharmaceuticals in the environment: a review. *Current Analytical Chemistry* 12: 169–182.

Karim, E.I., Ibrahim, K., Abdelrahman, A., and Fell, A. (1994). Photodegradation studies on chloroquine phosphate by high-performance liquid chromatography. *Journal of Pharmaceutical and Biomedical Analysis* 12: 667–674.

Keith, R.E. (1981). Loss of therapeutic copper in closed marine systems. *Aquaculture* 24: 355–362.

Kim, K.H. and Cho, J.B. (2000). Treatment of *Microcotyle sebastis* (*Monogenea: Polyopisthocotylea*) infestation with praziquantel in an experimental cage simulating commercial rockfish *Sebastes schlegeli* culture conditions. *Diseases of Aquatic Organisms* 40: 229–231.

Kim, K.H., Kim, C.S., and Kim, J.W. (2001). Depletion of praziquantel in plasma and muscle tissue of cultured rockfish *Sebastes schlegeli* after oral and bath treatment. *Diseases of Aquatic Organisms* 45: 203–207.

Kim, B.S., Fujita, H., Sakai, Y. et al. (2002). Catalytic ozonation of an organophosphorus pesticide using microporous silicate and its effect on total toxicity reduction. *Water Science and Technology* 46: 35–41.

Klaver, A.L. and Matthews, R.A. (1994). Effects of oxytetracycline on nitrification in a model aquatic system. *Aquaculture* 123: 237–247.

Knight, S.J., Boles, L., and Stamper, M.A. (2016). Response of recirculating saltwater aquariums to long-term formalin treatment. *Journal of Zoo and Aquarium Research* 4: 77–84.

Kummerer, K. (2009a). Antibiotics in the aquatic environment-a review-part I. *Chemosphere* 75: 417–434.

Kummerer, K. (2009b). Antibiotics in the aquatic environment-a review-part II. *Chemosphere* 75: 435–441.

López-Peñalver, J.J., Sánchez-Polo, M., Gómez-Pacheco, C.V., and Rivera-Utrilla, J. (2010). Photodegradation of tetracyclines in aqueous solution by using UV and UV/ H_2O_2 oxidation processes. *Journal of Chemical Technology and Biotechnology* 85: 1325–1333.

Marsik, P., Podlipna, R., and Vanek, T. (2017). Study of praziquantel phytoremediation and transformation and its removal in constructed wetland. *Journal of Hazardous Materials* 323: 394–399.

Millero, F.J. (1996). Chemical Oceanography, 2e. New York: CRC press.

Nimenya, H., Delaunois, A., La Duong, D. et al. (1999). Short-term toxicity of various pharmacological agents on the in vitro nitrification process in a simple closed aquatic system. *Alternatives to Laboratory Animals* 27: 121–135.

Noga, E.J. (2011). *Fish Disease: Diagnosis and Treatment*, 2e. Ames, IA: Wiley.

Nord, K., Karlsen, J., and Tønnesen, H.H. (1991). Photochemical stability of biologically active compounds. IV. Photochemical degradation of chloroquine. *International Journal of Pharmaceutics* 72: 11–18.

Pedersen, L.F., Pedersen, P.B., Nielsen, J.L. et al. (2008). Formaldehyde induced variation in biofilter performance and microbial composition. Paper presented at *International Conference on Recirculating Aquaculture*, Roanoke, VA.

Pedersen, L.F., Pedersen, P.B., Nielsen, J.L., and Nielsen, P.H. (2010). Long term/low dose formalin exposure to small-scale recirculation aquaculture systems. *Aquacultural Engineering* 42: 1–7.

Pickering, Q.H. and Lazorchak, J.M. (1995). Evaluation of the robustness of the fathead minnow, *Pimephales promelas*, larval survival and growth test, US EPA method 1000.0. *Environmental Toxicology and Chemistry* 14: 653–659.

Prichard, E. and Granek, E.F. (2016). Effects of pharmaceuticals and personal care products on marine organisms: from single-species studies to an ecosystem-based approach. *Environmental Science and Pollution Research* 23: 22365–22384.

Reed, P., Francis-Floyd, R., and Klinger, R. (2009). Monogenean parasites of fish. *University of Florida IFAS Extension* Electronic Data Information Source #FA-28/FA033. https://edis.ifas.ufl.edu/pdffiles/FA/FA03300.pdf (accessed 1 December 2018).

Rosenberg, A. and Alexander, M. (1979). Microbial cleavage of various organophosphorus insecticides. *Applied and Environmental Microbiology* 37: 886–891.

Saeed, A.E. and Hamid, A.E. (2004). Photo-thermal stability of praziquantel. *Saudi Pharmaceutical Journal* 12: 157–162.

Schwartz, M.F., Bullock, G.L., Hankins, J.A. et al. (2000). Effects of selected chemotherapeutants on nitrification in fluidized-sand biofilters for coldwater fish production. *International Journal of Recirculating Aquaculture* 1: 61–81.

Singh, B., Madhusudhanan, S., Dubey, V. et al. (1996). Active carbon for removal of toxic chemicals from contaminated water. *Carbon* 34: 327–330.

Snyder, S.A., Adham, S., Redding, A.M. et al. (2007). Role of membranes and activated carbon in the removal of endocrine disruptors and pharmaceuticals. *Desalination* 202: 156–181.

Thomas, A., Dawson, M., Ellis, H., and Stamper, M.A. (2016). Praziquantel degradation in marine aquarium water. *PeerJ* 4:e1857.

Tubbs, L.A. and Tingle, M.D. (2006). Bioavailability and pharmacokinetics of a praziquantel bolus in kingfish *Seriola lalandi*. *Diseases of Aquatic Organisms* 69: 233–238.

Wedemeyer, G. (1971). The stress of formalin treatments in rainbow trout (*Salmo gairdneri*) and coho salmon (*Oncorhynchus kisutch*). *Journal of the Fisheries Board of Canada* 28: 1899–1904.

Williams, W.D. (2001). Anthropogenic salinisation of inland waters. In: *Saline Lakes* (eds. J.M. Melack, R. Jellison and D.B. Herbst), 329–337. Dordrecht: Springer.

Xie, X., Zhao, Y., Yang, X., and Hu, K. (2015). Comparison of praziquantel pharmacokinetics and tissue distribution in fresh and brackish water cultured grass carp (*Ctenopharyngodon idellus*) after oral administration of single bolus. *BMC Veterinary Research* 11: 84.

Yonar, M.E., Yonar, S.M., Pala, A. et al. (2015). Trichlorfon-induced haematological and biochemical changes in *Cyprinus carpio*: ameliorative effect of propolis. *Diseases of Aquatic Organisms* 114: 209–216.

Yoon, Y., Westerhoff, P., Snyder, S.A., and Wert, E.C. (2006). Nanofiltration and ultrafiltration of endocrine disrupting compounds, pharmaceuticals and personal care products. *Journal of Membrane Science* 270: 88–100.

Yoon, Y., Westerhoff, P., Snyder, S.A. et al. (2007). Removal of endocrine disrupting compounds and pharmaceuticals by nanofiltration and ultrafiltration membranes. *Desalination* 202: 16–23.

Zhu, H.Z., Cui, Y.M., Zheng, X.W. et al. (2007). Determination of trace trichlorfon by high performance liquid chromatography with UV detection based on its catalytic effect on sodium perborate oxidizing benzidine. *Analytica Chimica Acta* 584: 166–171.

A14

Acquisition and Transport

Jamie M. Torres[1], *Andrew B. Pulver*[2] *and Leigh A. Clayton*[3]

[1] *Audubon Nature Institute, New Orleans, LA, USA*
[2] *National Aquarium, Baltimore, MD, USA*
[3] *New England Aquarium, Boston, MA, USA*

Introduction

Fish acquisition and transport cover an enormous range of circumstances. Examples of this diversity include a pet fish that needs to be removed from a small aquarium and transported by car to a new home; the transport of several hundred teleosts from a vendor to a zoological facility; and the transport of large elasmobranchs by air across international borders. Despite this variability, core principles apply to all: maintain appropriate dissolved oxygen, pH, and temperature; reduce ammonia buildup; avoid abrupt changes in water chemistry; and reduce the risk of trauma. Focusing on these principles will help ensure fish arrive at their destination healthy. Suboptimal water quality, temperature changes, trauma, or other adverse transport events can lead to physiologic complications (e.g. ammonia toxicity, hypoxia, acidosis, ionic imbalance, hyperlactemia) that may precipitate morbidity and mortality.

There are four main steps related to fish acquisition and transport; pre-transport planning (e.g. goal-setting, sourcing, and logistics), the transport itself, acclimation on arrival, and a post-transport review. Goal-setting and post-transport reviews are often skipped, but are critical, particularly for large and complex shipments. Goal-setting helps guide the level of planning and allows consensus on expectations (e.g. $x\%$ of fish look healthy on arrival or $x\%$ clear quarantine). Following each transport, it should be routine to critically review the process and the results to identify possible improvements.

Source and Sustainability

The twenty-first century has rightly brought higher expectations for animal welfare; these apply to fish as much as mammals. Hobbyists and professionals working with fish are invested in having healthy fish, though the details of what this actually means can vary. Increasingly, hobbyists and aquarium professionals see it as their responsibility to ensure they can provide excellent care throughout the animal's life span.

Prior to acquisition planning, the natural history of the species should be thoroughly reviewed to ensure that the needs can be met for the whole life of the animal (e.g. water parameters, habitat preferences, nutritional requirements, social needs, reproductive cycles, maximum life span and size). The habitat and care available should dictate if an acquisition is suitable. For example, there are species routinely available in the hobbyist trade that often outgrow their aquariums within a few years of acquisition. It is important to review available data regarding the species longevity under professional care, as well as any previous quarantine records.

Sources must be evaluated in detail to ensure that fish are collected or cultured sustainably, that only healthy fish are transported, and that transport conditions are optimal. Many freshwater teleosts and some marine teleosts are available from captive-bred populations, and the number of captive-bred species available continues to increase (Box A14.1). A large proportion of ornamental

Clinical Guide to Fish Medicine, First Edition. Edited by Catherine A. Hadfield and Leigh Ann Clayton.

Box A14.1 Examples of Ornamental Fish Species That Are Commonly Bred under Human Care

Freshwater
- Oscars (*Astronotus ocellatus*)
- Barbs (*Barbus, Capoeta, Puntius* spp.)
- Catfish and plecos (*Callichthys, Corydoras, Hypostomus* spp.)
- Goldfish (*Carassius auratus*)
- Gouramis (*Helostoma, Trichogaster* spp.)
- Common carp and koi (*Cyprinus carpio*)
- Zebrafish and other minnows (*Danio* spp.)
- Freshwater sharks (*Epalzeorhynchos, Labeo* spp.)
- Various tetras (*Gymnocorymbus, Hemigrammus, Hyphessobrycon, Paracheirodon* spp.)
- Guppies and mollies (*Poecilia* spp.)
- Freshwater angelfish (*Pterophyllum scalare*)
- Rasbora (*Rasbora* spp.)
- Discus (*Symphysodon* spp.)
- Swordtails and platies (*Xiphophorus* spp.)

Marine
- Clownfish (*Amphiprion* spp.)
- Some seahorses (*Hippocampus* spp.)
- Some cardinalfish (*Pterapogon, Sphaeramia* spp).

fish are wild-caught. Currently, it is estimated that over 11 million marine fish are imported into the United States annually, representing over 150 families from nearly 40 different countries (Rhyne et al. 2012). Some of these animals are collected using sustainable means, but not all. Collection methods should be evaluated to ensure they do not negatively impact wild populations. In reality, it can be challenging to clearly identify sources and collection methods. Consumer focus on this can help support vendors who are transparent about their business model and methods.

For institutions that acquire large numbers of fish, it is incumbent on them to routinely assess sources, as well as transport and quarantine success rates. Each shipment should be assessed on arrival to evaluate the impact of transportation on fish health. This knowledge guides immediate management choices and helps direct future acquisition choices. If vendors routinely ship fish that are in poor condition or arrive with excessive transport-related morbidity and mortality, a new source should be sought. Overall fish welfare can be improved by only acquiring fish that consistently do well with transport and quarantine, or where modifications are possible to improve success rates. Choosing species that have a high likelihood of thriving also reduces overall financial costs.

Cultured or Previously Wild-Caught Fish

Fish that have been bred under human care or have been under human care for a period of time after being wild-caught often adjust well to new managed habitats. They may be available from a variety of sources, including reputable vendors, aquaculture facilities, government hatcheries, research facilities, private collections, zoos, or aquariums. The source often has a significant impact on the health of the incoming fish; useful traits include open communication, known medical history, stable populations, and a history of well-managed transports.

Recently Wild-Caught Fish

Wild-caught fish may be available from vendors or wildlife collectors or may be collected by the institution. Permits are generally needed to remove animals from the wild and this may fall under federal, state, and local regulations. Public zoos and aquariums typically have additional requirements, such as Scientific Collecting Permits. Permits for transport may also be required. Obtaining permits can be time-consuming, taking as little as 24 hours or as long as 12 months, depending on the jurisdiction. Collection methods vary and can directly impact the health of the animals being obtained. Potential impacts on wild populations must be considered with all wild-caught fish.

Wild-caught fish may be more likely to carry a variety of pathogens and it can take longer for the animals to adjust to managed care. Common issues include difficulty switching to managed diets, trauma, and immunosuppression secondary to catch and transport stressors.

General Principles of Acquisition and Transport

Some common features are important to consider across all events, although details will vary. Catching fish can present a risk of trauma and exertional myopathy, particularly for large, fast-swimming species and ram-ventilating sharks. There are also a variety of common water quality concerns. Fish use oxygen and excrete ammonia and carbon dioxide. In a closed transport container, the available oxygen can be used up, the ammonia buildup is directly toxic, and the carbon dioxide lowers water pH. The reduced pH provides some protection from the ammonia toxicity, as it shifts a higher percentage of ammonia to the less toxic, ionized form. However, when the closed container is opened at the end of transport and the carbon dioxide is released, the pH can increase rapidly. This increases the proportion of ammonia that is in the more toxic unionized form and clinical signs from ammonia toxicity may develop. Other common problems during transport and on arrival include temperature and water chemistry fluctuations. Fish physiology is adapted to match their temperature and water chemistry and sudden changes are detrimental. Even if the changes are within a range that the species can normally tolerate, the cumulative effect of all the stressors can lead to morbidity and mortality.

To try to minimize these consequences, there are some general principles that apply to every fish acquisition and transport:

1) Reduce the risk of trauma to the fish, e.g. soft knotless nets, short catch and handling time, smooth transport containers, short transport time, quiet recovery time after transport, net or stretcher training, avoiding high-risk species.
2) Maintain appropriate dissolved oxygen throughout the transport, e.g. closed system with added oxygen, or the provision of air or oxygen during transport.
3) Reduce ammonia buildup, e.g. pre-transport fasting, short transport time, low stocking density, largest practical water volume, ammonia-locking compounds.
4) Maintain appropriate pH and manage the buildup of carbon dioxide, e.g. adequate buffer, off-gassing during long transports.
5) Reduce or avoid temperature fluctuations, e.g. careful timing, insulation, climate control, heat or cooling packs, short transport time, effective acclimation.
6) Minimize water chemistry changes, e.g. review and match the source and destination water chemistry, effective acclimation.

Preparation

Risk Assessment

Responsible animal acquisition and transport begins with a risk assessment from origin to destination. Fish present greater challenges than most other animals because of the need to transport in water and their sensitivity to environmental changes. The following factors affect the level of risk associated with catch and transport.

Physical factors

- Distance and transport time: Longer transports are more susceptible to water quality and environmental problems, e.g. oxygen depletion, ammonia buildup, temperature fluctuations. The risk of morbidity and mortality increases with transport time.
- Complexity of transport and number of parties involved: It is possible for there to be several different couriers involved in a large shipment or long-distance transport and good coordination is required. Minimizing the number of parties involved reduces the risk of complications or delays.
- Differences in the source and destination: Differences in water temperature, water chemistry, or habitat can have profound impacts on fish. It is important to take the time to evaluate these differences prior to transport. For high-risk or high-profile individuals, it may help to have a written comparison of the source and destination in order to allow a thorough risk assessment.
- Volume of transport water: A larger water volume typically represents a lower risk but a higher transport cost. Pelagic species are particularly difficult as they usually need sufficient water and a suitable enclosure shape to allow normal swimming throughout transport.
- Water quality management: Normal respiration and excretion degrade water quality over time in a closed transport container. Water changes, buffers, ammonia-locking compounds, or full life support systems may be needed for longer transports. Water quality testing should be performed upon arrival at the receiving facility.
- Experience: If the owner does not have experience with the species or the catch and transport conditions, they should seek out experienced people for advice or to manage the acquisition.
- Holidays: Transporting animals close to major holidays should be avoided as this reduces the personnel available for catch, transport, and acclimation, and increases transport delays, particularly with air travel.
- Weather: Extreme temperatures, winter storms, and other adverse weather can have significant effects on transports and should be avoided, where forecast.

Animal factors

- Species and life stages: There are significant differences in resilience among fish. As a rule of thumb, fine-scaled fish, fast-swimming or pelagic fish, ram-ventilating elasmobranchs, and small fry carry the highest risks (Young et al. 2002; Correia et al. 2011; Silva et al. 2015). Even within these groups, resilience varies (Mandelman and Skomal 2009; Hyatt et al. 2011). Intertidal species, more sessile species, and small pond fish often present lower risks (Silva et al. 2015).
- Animal size: In general, larger specimens are more tolerant of some of the environmental changes that can occur but are more prone to trauma and need larger transport containers.

- Oxygenation requirements: Fish consume more oxygen during transport than under normal conditions. Some fish species and life stages are more sensitive to low dissolved oxygen than others. Ram-ventilating elasmobranchs and pelagic fish often have high oxygen needs. Benthic species, species that live in cool or deep water, and species that live in warm, shallow water are often more tolerant of low oxygen levels.
- Health state of the specific individuals prior to transport: Recent morbidity or mortality should prohibit transport, except in an emergency. Animals that are in thin body condition or that have not been eating reliably are also poor candidates for transport.
- Physiologic state of the specific individuals prior to transport: If fish have recently experienced significant stressors, e.g. chasing to catch from an exhibit or several hours on a hook and line, they present much higher transport risks. These animals may benefit from a rest period prior to shipment.

The risk assessment helps to identify which transports require more planning and preparation and what other resources may be required. There is some information in the published literature comparing methods or outcomes (Colburn et al. 2008; Kilgore et al. 2009; Hyatt et al. 2011; Silva et al. 2015). However, specialists with extensive fish transport experience are often the best resource for more complex shipments. If the risks to the fish are deemed too high, canceling the acquisition should be considered.

Pre-Shipment Conditioning

The risks associated with a catch and transport can be reduced by conditioning the fish; this means preparing the fish to better tolerate the transport and any differences in environmental conditions at the receiving institution (e.g. water parameters or diet).

Housing fish in a suitable, isolated system prior to transport can allow for conditioning and close monitoring prior to transport. This helps ensure that there is no morbidity or mortality prior to shipping. It allows for any pre-shipment examinations that may be required. It also allows for pre-shipment fasting that may not be possible in large multispecies habitats.

If the target destination has different water temperatures, water chemistry, habitats, or anticipated diets, it can be very helpful to approximate those changes prior to transport. Common areas to focus on include matching water temperature, matching cation and other water chemistry levels, and converting to the new diet prior to transport. This level of focus is currently reserved for high-risk or high-profile animals.

If significant stress or trauma occurred during the initial catch, housing fish in a suitable holding system allows them to recover prior to shipping. This is particularly relevant if the catch from the holding system can be easily accomplished. Recovery can take several weeks to months depending on the impact of the initial catch.

For large elasmobranchs, conditioning them to the smaller glide paths they will experience during transport may make a difference, particularly if they have been in large open exhibits for several years. This can be accomplished by using barriers to restrict their available swim space for increasing periods of time.

Mock Transports

For particularly large or high-risk fish, many zoos and aquariums do mock transports (run-throughs) without the animal to assess the logistics and timing of the catch, transport, and release plans. This can be an excellent way to identify potential failures points (e.g. availability of a suitable forklift or limited access to a loading dock) and improve practices.

Mock transports using animals are common in aquaculture to assess whether a group of fish is ready for transport, before putting the entire group at risk. This typically involves transferring a subset of the fish into a transport container and monitoring how they do for a period equal to the duration of the planned transport; the fish can be returned to their habitats if there are any signs of morbidity. This is a valuable tool in assessing if a population is in good enough condition to ship. It is important that the fish are given sufficient recovery time before transport; this may take several weeks.

Mock transports using animals are less common in the zoo and aquarium field, but have proven valuable in the authors' experience, particularly for large, high-risk individuals such as ram-ventilating sharks. For example, the planned transport container can be set up next to the holding system and the fish transferred to the transport container for predetermined periods of time. If the fish begins to do poorly, it can be moved back immediately, without this dilemma unfolding for the first time on the road.

Feeding and Fasting

Fasting fish prior to transport reduces ammonia excretion during transport. Ammonia can build up surprisingly quickly in small volumes of water. However, fasting too long prior to a transport can deplete glycogen stores, particularly in under-conditioned, small, or fast-moving fish, causing them to be hypoglycemic upon arrival. Guidelines are hard to provide, as gastrointestinal transit times vary

Box A14.2 Possible Fasting Times for Fish Prior to Transport

Fish <5 g – typically 0–24 hours
Bony fish 10–300 g – often fasted 12–48 hours; longer for herbivorous or cold-water fish
Bony fish >300 g – often fasted for several days; longer for herbivorous or cold-water fish
Elasmobranchs that usually eat daily – minimal fasting, <8 hours
Elasmobranchs that usually fast between feeds – typically fasted 48–72 hours

across fish species, diet, and water temperature, and the condition of the fish must be considered; however, general suggestions are provided (Box A14.2) and some specific references are available (Lim et al. 2003).

There is increasing interest in using immune stimulants prior to transport fasting to reduce the risk of secondary disease after transport. While most research has focused on disease challenges in static populations, some have shown reduced mortality rates following transport. For example, vitamin C at 2000 mg/kg orally once daily for 10 days reduced cumulative mortality of guppies (*Poecilia reticulata*) following shipment (Lim et al. 2003).

Catch and Handling Recommendations

It is essential to minimize stress and trauma during the catch in order to reduce the risk of morbidity and mortality during or after transport.

Aquarium or Pond Bony Fish

Most aquarium and pond fish can be caught with a net. Individual experience plays a large role in successful, low-stress catches. It is important to avoid chasing and to stop attempts if the catch attempt is prolonged. Removing décor, isolating fish into smaller areas of the habitat, and/or draining some water can improve net proficiency and decrease catch times. The least stressful net catch makes use of positive reinforcement training to teach the fish to swim into a net or other restraint (e.g. stretcher or tube) on cue. Clear nets and plastic bags that are slowly advanced around the animal are another method that can cause minimal stress.

There are many nets available. Professional aquarists rely largely on rubber mesh nets and clear vinyl bag nets with vinyl coated fine mesh bottoms (Figure A14.1).

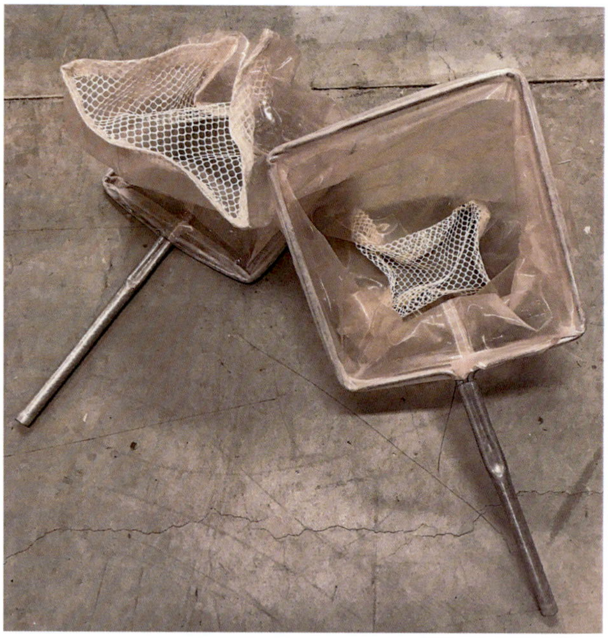

Figure A14.1 Vinyl nets used for catching fish.

Knotted nets and knotless nylon should be avoided as they are more likely to cause scale damage or even adhere to fish scales. The size of the fish should dictate the mesh opening; mesh size needs to prevent escapes or entrapment by the operculum or spines.

Some teleosts have extremely delicate skin and do not typically do well when caught with a net, e.g. harvestfish (*Peprilus paru*) and Atlantic silversides (*Menidia menidia*). They do best when caught and moved in a bucket or vinyl bag.

Aquarium Cartilaginous Fish

Small cartilaginous fish (<3–4 kg) are often caught using nets as above. For large sharks, vinyl stretchers or tunnels are commonly used to provide support for the whole body (Figure A14.2a). For large rays and skates, a flat stretcher with reinforced beams helps reduce the risk of trauma (Figure A14.2b). To facilitate restraint in the stretcher, most large elasmobranchs are confined to a smaller pool and then guided into the stretcher or tunnel by divers. In large systems, vinyl corral systems may be deployed to funnel the fish into a smaller space where a catch is possible (Figure A14.2c). These may be deployed days before the catch to give the animals time to make the new space part of their regular swimming pattern.

Free-Ranging Bony Fish

Catching fish with rod and reel can be effective. The least traumatic, barbless, zero-offset, circle hooks are

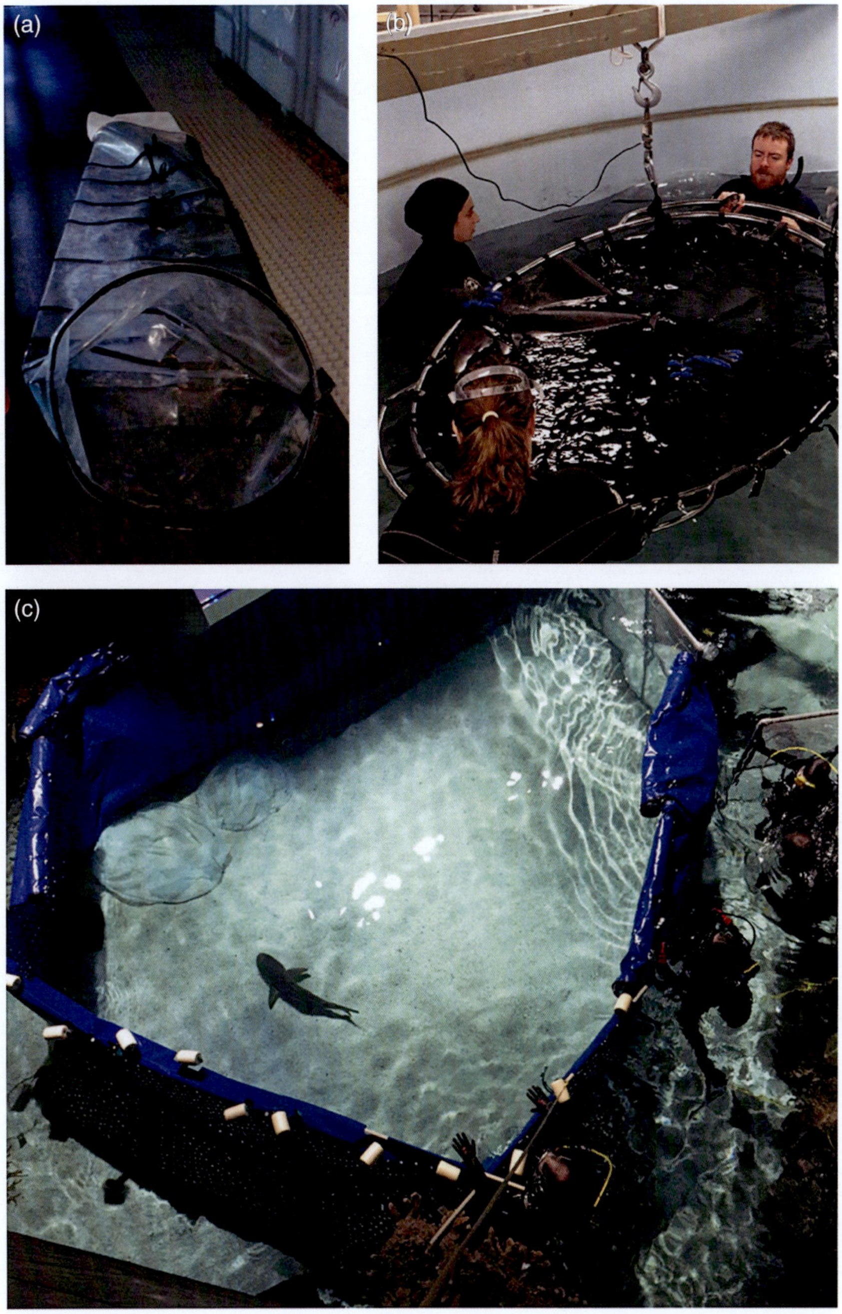

Figure A14.2 Clear tunnel that can be used to catch and transfer a large shark (a) and vinyl stretcher that can be used for a large ray (b). Vinyl corral system used to lead a large fish into a catch area (c). *Source:* Image (a) courtesy of Jack Jewel, Shark Reef Aquarium and (b–c) courtesy of Catherine Hadfield, National Aquarium.

recommended. Minimizing the depth of water at which bony fish are hooked at, ideally to <5 m (15 ft), can significantly reduce the risk of barotrauma.

Commercially available fish traps or pots can be used to target specific species. These traps should be assessed for hole size and any sharp edges that could injure fish. Some states require the addition of turtle excluder devices on traps and inclusion of trap descriptions on permit applications. Traps should be monitored regularly to minimize the time that animals may spend in them.

Seine nets may be used in shallow areas. These are used to encircle an area and collect all the animals within, so this method has a much higher potential for by-catch. Seine material should be knot-free. Mesh size should be chosen carefully: it should be slightly less than the smallest target fish size, allowing smaller fish to swim out. The goal is for fish to be trapped inside of the net, not through the holes as with a gill net. The length and size of the seine are also important, as using a large seine will increase the by-catch and the time required to assess and release any entrapped animals. Legal seine dimensions are often dictated by state permit offices; these should be checked and the seine dimensions should be included on the permit request.

Gill nets or other types of set nets may be used in deeper water. Traditionally, these nets are set and then patrolled for a specific amount of time. Some size selectivity can occur based on the gauge of netting used. In gill nets, fish can become entangled by getting their body, gill opercula, or fins and spines entangled in the mesh. These are rarely used because of higher associated mortality (Hubert et al. 2012).

Divers can also be used to catch fish by hand-net. This allows divers to target specific species and individuals to minimize by-catch. This is often labor-intensive and requires experienced divers. With a proficient team, a barrier net (not a seine or gill net) can be used to encircle a school of fish, then a diver can hand-net individual fish within the confined space. Any fish that are caught at deeper water depths should be transferred to a recompression chamber or brought to the surface slowly, in stages, in order to reduce the risk of barotrauma.

Barotrauma of bony fish becomes increasingly common as catch depth increases. In general, atmospheric pressure increases by 1 atmosphere (atm) or 15 pounds per square inch (psi) for every 10 m (33 ft) of water depth. In one study, fish started showing signs of barotrauma when caught at depths >6 m (18 ft) (Schreer et al. 2009). Barotrauma can present as positive buoyancy, distension of the swim bladder, rupture of the swim bladder, buphthalmos or exophthalmos, or prolapse of the stomach. Management options include slow or staged ascents using decompression barrels, recompression chambers, or needle decompression.

- Barrels can be used to hold fish at designated depths over several hours to allow them to be brought to the surface without barotrauma. The barrel can be equipped with closed circuit TV to observe the fish throughout the process.
- Recompression chambers at the surface can be used after ascent to repressurize the fish to a pressure that resolves any visible barotrauma (Figure A14.3). Recompression chambers have also been used underwater to keep fish at their catch depth pressure during the ascent to a boat, and once aboard, the fish can be slowly depressurized in the chamber under constant observation.
- Needle decompression involves inserting a needle into the swim bladder to allow gas to escape. Though this can be successful, there is risk of improper placement of the venting needle and infection that could result in morbidity or mortality; recompression treatment in a chamber is preferred.

Releasing fish suffering from barotrauma overboard is likely to result in mortality (Curtis et al. 2015). If a fish showing signs must be released, it should be returned by a diver to catch depth at the original collection site as soon as possible, instead of releasing at the surface.

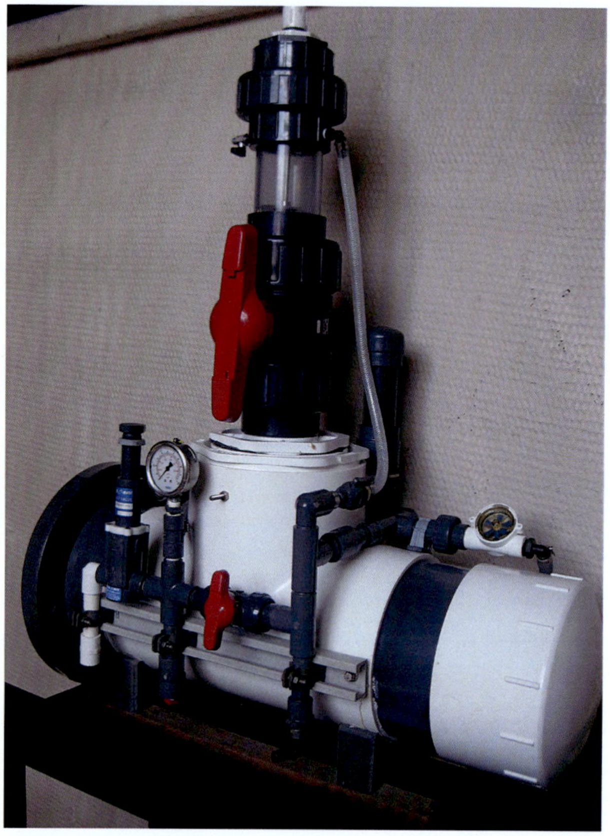

Figure A14.3 A boat-based recompression chamber. *Source:* Image courtesy of Joe Welsh, Monterey Bay Aquarium.

When catching free-ranging fish, suitable temporary enclosures are required, often on a boat or truck. Making use of a local facility to observe the animals over a few days following the catch and prior to transport can be invaluable. It is essential that these staging locations provide suitable space and water parameters for the animals; if not, they will compound existing physiologic problems. Some jurisdictions allow release back to the wild for a short period of time after capture, if that is deemed the best option for the fish. Commercial vendors that are collecting and selling free-ranging fish typically hold them for a few weeks prior to shipping.

There are still some fish collectors that use methods to temporarily stun the fish in order to make them easier to catch. Electrofishing uses an electrical current through the water to stun all fish in the surrounding area. The shock causes muscle tremors and contractions which can result in spinal fractures. Another method is sodium cyanide, which is sprayed into the habitat to temporarily stun fish making them easier to catch. This chemical is harmful to the environment and damages the aquatic community. Up to 70% of fish that are caught with cyanide will die within 48 hours of exposure (Rubec et al. 2001). Both methods must be discouraged and avoided.

Free-Ranging Cartilaginous Fish

Public aquariums or commercial collectors often catch specific elasmobranchs using long-lines (Figure A14.4). These consist of main lines with baited hooks tied off at intervals using gangions. Vinyl airline tubing over the steel gangions can help protect the eyes and skin of the fish. PVC rigs on the hooks should be used to reduce the risk of the animal swallowing the hook (Figure A14.5). The time fish spend on the line, known as the soak time, should be limited to a maximum of 60 minutes to prevent morbidity and mortality, particularly for ram-ventilating sharks.

Sharks can also be caught using rod and reel methods. There is some evidence to suggest that using circle hooks causes less trauma than more traditional hooks, but other studies show no significant difference. Rod and reel methods lessen the amount of time animals spend on a line.

Finally, some sharks, skates, and rays are caught in gill or seine nets. This method typically has the highest rate of post-catch mortality for ram-ventilating sharks as the net can prevent normal respiration and should be avoided.

Transport Containers

Shipping Bags

Sealed shipping bags in insulated containers are the most common way to transport fish. Each represents a fully closed system, with no air or water exchange. Polyethylene bags that are 3–10 mil are recommended for durability (bag thickness of 0.08–0.25 mm). Square-bottomed gusseted bags allow bags to sit upright. Determining the correct bag size and stocking density comes with experience but some references have specific recommendations in cm/L, g/L, or g/m^3 (Table A14.1; Lim et al. 2003; Colburn et al. 2008; Silva et al. 2015). These recommendations are typically aimed at cost-effective commercial transports; stocking

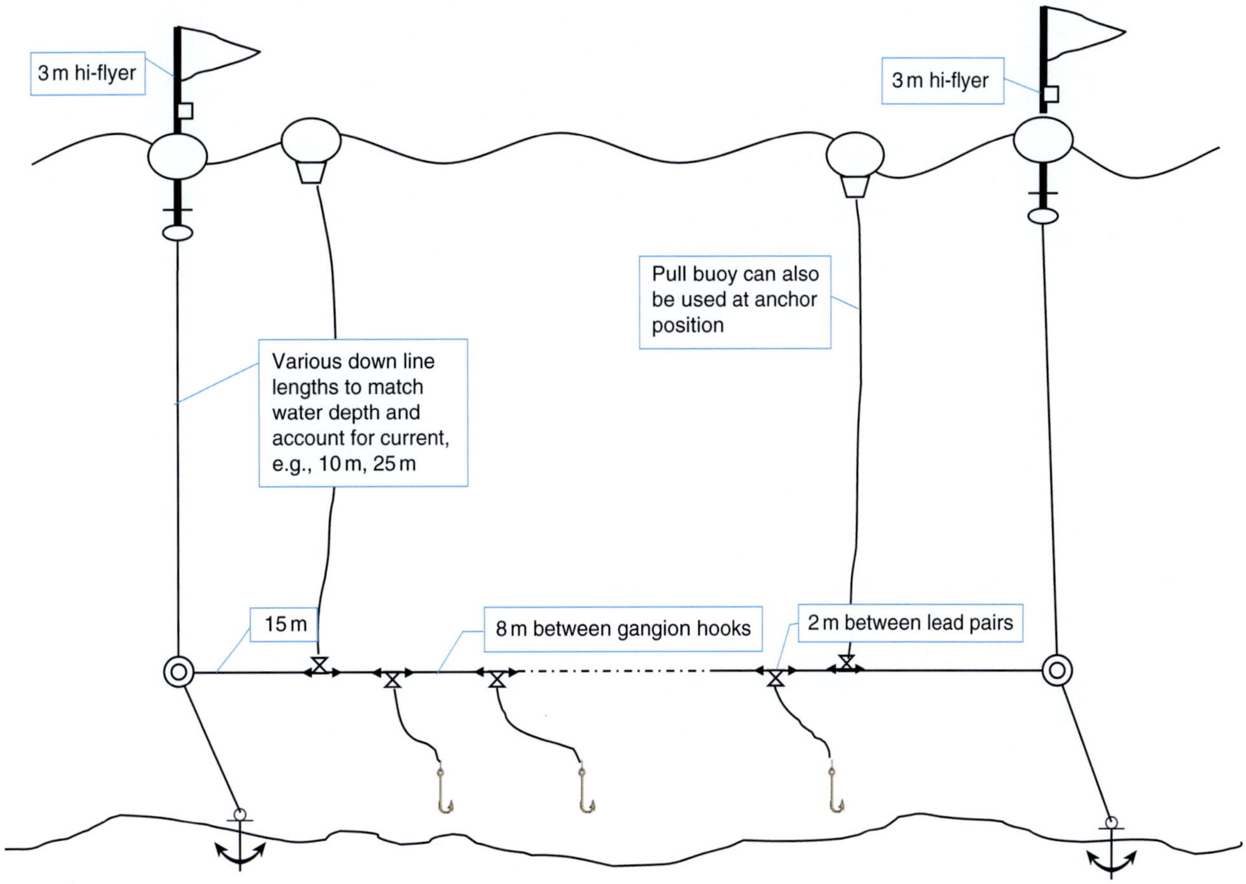

Figure A14.4 Sketch of a 400 m long, bottom set long-line system. *Source:* Image courtesy of Andy Dehart, National Aquarium.

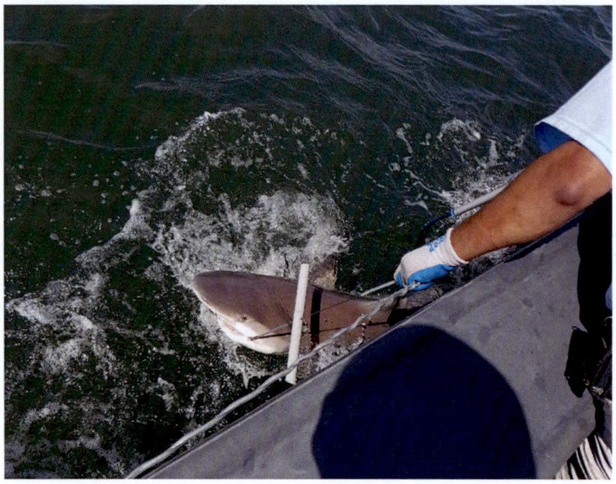

Figure A14.5 PVC pipe used to reduce the risk of a hook being swallowed.

Table A14.1 Recommended bag sizes for individual fish.

Size	Dimension (cm)	Volume (L)	Fish length (cm)
Eighth bag	14.4×11.9×45.0	3	2.5–7.5
Quarter bag	18.8×18.8×50.0	5	7.5–12.5
Half bag	18.8×37.5×55.0	8–10	12.5–20.0
Full bag	37.5×37.5×55.0	15–20	20–30

density should be kept lower where possible. The bag should always contain water from the fish's current system to reduce changes in the water chemistry. The recommended ratio is 1/3 water to 2/3 air or oxygen. While air can be used, oxygen is the better option, and pet stores may provide this service to hobbyists. To fill the bags with oxygen after transferring the fish, the free end of the bag is twisted down on itself with the rigid oxygen airline in the middle of the twist (Figure A14.6a, b). The bag should be twisted down to the water level to expel any ambient air. The oxygen flow is turned on to fill the space with pure oxygen. Once full, the rigid tubing can be pulled out and the bag end twisted further upon itself. The twist should be clamped down using a durable rubber band (e.g. number 64), castrating band tool, or metal c-ring (Figure A14.6c). The corners of the bags may be taped to prevent animals from becoming wedged. It is best to double bag, particularly for longer transports, with newspaper in between and on the outside; this allows greater protection and also makes it obvious if the inside bag leaks. Fish species known to puncture bags with their fin spines or bite through bags should be contained within the bags using a perforated, hard-plastic container; a soldering iron can be used to ensure that the perforations are smooth (Figure A14.6d).

This packing method with oxygen typically results in a dissolved oxygen of 250% at the start of transport, above 150% after 24 hours and ~100% after 48 hours, which should be the maximum duration for bagged transport (Lim et al. 2003).

These bags can be put into a polystyrene (Styrofoam™) box within a cardboard box or into a cooler to help maintain temperature. The practice of inverting the bags in the packing box is not recommended as there is a higher risk of a catastrophic leak. All empty spaces between bags should be filled with cushioning material (e.g. newspaper). The packing area should be dry to avoid damaging any cardboard. All box seams should be taped to provide additional strength to the box. If the boxes are being transported by a shipping company or airline, the boxes must be labeled with "LIVE ANIMALS" and any specific care instructions for the species. Writing the contents of the box on the outside helps, particularly if there are multiple boxes. The name of the receiving institution, address, and point of contact with a telephone number should be written in at least one place on the outside of each box. Most commercial carriers now require the shipping party to obtain an International Safe Transit Association (ISTA) certification before becoming approved to ship fish through them.

Rigid Transport Containers

Rigid transport containers should be used for fish that are likely to damage bags, e.g. scorpionfish (*Scorpaenidae*). They should also be used for large specimens, particularly large elasmobranchs, as they allow the addition of filtration systems and pumps to ensure continuous water flow and encourage free swimming.

Open-topped rigid transport containers are useful in some situations, e.g. a deep transport well in a boat to transport recently caught fish back to shore. It is important that fish cannot jump out of the containers and that water can be added as needed should spilling occur. There are some advantages to open transport containers, such as off-gassing of accumulating carbon dioxide and the ability to visually monitor the fish.

Lidded rigid transport containers help prevent water spillage and fish jumping. Examples include a five gallon bucket with a lid, a large cooler, or a large, round or oval polyethylene or fiberglass tank. Aeration can be provided via air pumps or compressed oxygen with air stones, or water pumps with spray bars. On a small scale, pumps can be powered using a power converter in the cigarette lighter of a car. Holes can be drilled in lids to allow passage of airlines, cables, or pump tubing while the lid is closed. Viewing windows at the top or sides of lidded transport containers allow monitoring of the animals. Lidded transports may be sealed shut to become true

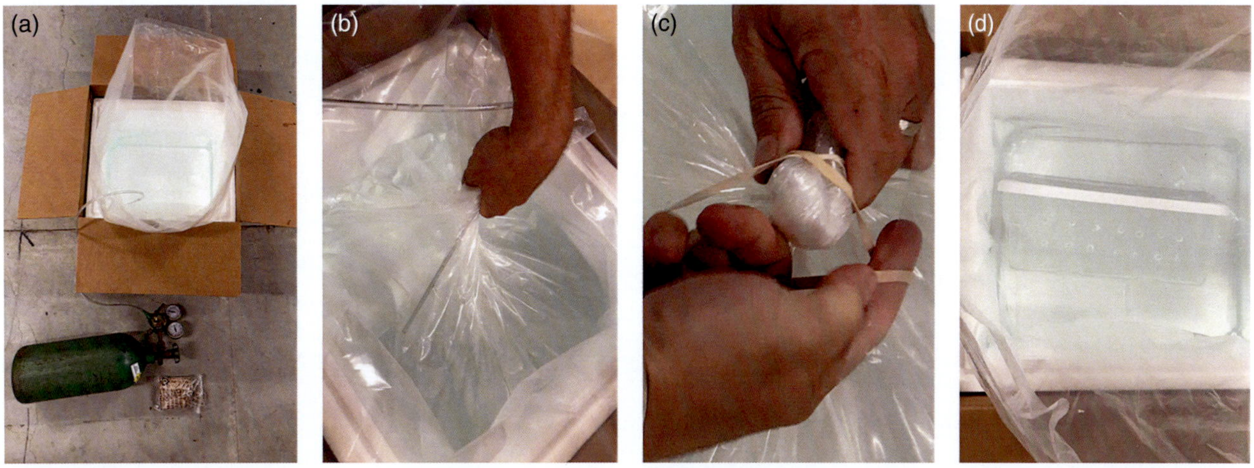

Figure A14.6 To fill a fish transport bag with oxygen, the rigid line should be in place when the bag is twisted (a, b) and removed after filling and prior to clamping (c). Fish that may perforate a plastic bag should be contained within a perforated, hard-plastic container (d).

closed systems. For longer transports, these usually require filtration systems to manage ammonia, oxygen, and carbon dioxide.

Additives

Various additives may be used during fish transports to maintain water chemistry and reduce the risk of secondary disease.

Water pH usually drops over the course of a shipment. Buffers such as sodium bicarbonate ($NaHCO_3$, baking soda), sodium carbonate (Na_2CO_3, soda ash), or tris-hydrooxymethyl aminomethane (tris) can be used to help stabilize the pH (Smith et al. 2004). They should be added to the water as needed during shipping to keep the pH stable (Correia et al. 2011). This can be particularly important during the transport of large sharks.

Ammonia-locking compounds, such as Amquel® added directly to the transport water, are commonly used in large-scale transports (Correia et al. 2011). For freshwater transports, ion-exchange resins such as zeolite can be added to the transport water or wrapped in a net bag to adsorb ammonia. The direct addition of a commercial nitrifying bacteria consortia to the transport water may be useful. In one study, one of two consortia tested reduced ammonia buildup during a simulated transport (Dhanasiri et al. 2011). These should all be considered adjunct control methods. Suitable fasting and low stocking densities in shipping containers are essential.

A low level of salt is often used in freshwater fish transports, especially for hatcheries transporting baitfish or salmonids. This can help reduce osmotic stress and may reduce the impact of any nitrite buildup (Carneiro and Urbinati 2001). The dose is often 0.5–3.0 g/L (Lim et al. 2003). It is important to use sodium chloride or a commercial aquarium saltwater mix.

Anesthetics such as metomidate hydrochloride, tricaine methanesulfonate (MS-222), 2-phenoxyethanol, and isoeugenol products have been used to reduce the activity level, metabolic rate, and stress response of fish during transport (Kilgore et al. 2009). Doses are much lower than used for examinations and diagnostic sampling. Excessive anesthetic depth and hypoventilation are risks, particularly where observation and intervention options are limited. When using anesthetics, it is particularly important to run mock transports well in advance of the anticipated shipment to evaluate species response. Medication use must follow all legislation regarding use and disposal. Physical restraint of fish during transports should be avoided.

There are several over-the-counter products sold in pet stores that are marketed to help protect fish during transports. These products' ingredients are often proprietary, but they usually claim to help protect the skin from wounds and to bind ammonia. Few studies have evaluated the efficacy of these products.

Temperature Control

Controlling ambient temperature to match the target water temperature throughout transport is the best way to minimize temperature stressors, but this is often impractical. Transport timing is also important, for example, transporting tropical teleosts during cold, winter temperatures should be avoided. As well as season, anticipated weather conditions along the route should be considered, and transports avoided if there is a high risk of adverse weather or severe storms.

Good insulation of bags or rigid transport containers is important to slow temperature changes, but supplemental heat or cooling may be needed. If heat or ice packs are necessary, great care should be used to ensure they do not heat or cool the water too much; mock transports can help with this calculation.

Filtration and Monitoring Systems

Long transports (>24 hours) of any fish and short transports of large fish usually require additional water monitoring, filtration, and/or water changes.

Dissolved oxygen meters and compressed oxygen are common with longer transports. Target dissolved oxygen is often 120–160%, but wider ranges are used (e.g. 100–300%).

Filtration can be used to reduce the buildup of nitrogenous waste, particularly where water changes during the transport are impractical. Filter size and type are dependent on the size of the transport system. It could be as simple as a filter pad (e.g. Poly-Filter®) or a canister filter with mechanical and mature biological filtration. More complex filtration systems may include foam fractionation, carbon filtration, and degassing options. Any filtration system requires power. Batteries are often the most practical option, but generators or power inverters may be needed. For biological filters, it is wise to start seeding the filter with system bacteria for at least two weeks prior to transport. This can be done by adding the filter to an already cycled system or using biomedia from an already cycled system in the new filter. This will help ensure that the filter is able to process the bioload during transport.

Long transports may be staged, stopping at designated locations to allow partial water changes. This allows greater monitoring and helps to stabilize water quality during transport. Possible locations to stop and manage any issues should also be considered as part of the contingency planning.

The level of monitoring that is possible can directly impact overall success. Where monitoring of the fish during transport is available, important features include swimming pattern and speed, respiration, and skin color. Of particular concern are pelagic species that are resting on the substrate, lateral recumbency, ataxia, dyspnea or bradypnea, blotchy skin, or visible trauma.

Water quality monitoring at the end of or during transport should always be considered. For closed, unaccompanied transports, dissolved oxygen, temperature, salinity, pH, ammonia, and nitrite should be assessed on arrival to determine the transport stress and the duration of acclimation needed. For accompanied transports, particularly for long transports, these values should be monitored throughout. Low dissolved oxygen can be improved using additional air or oxygen. Temperature issues can be hard to resolve during transport, but air conditioning/heating, cold/heat packs, and water changes may be used. pH can be used to assess the level of dissolved carbon dioxide and the need for off-gassing, buffer, or water changes. Elevated ammonia can be improved using ammonia-locking compounds, additional filtration, or water changes.

Staffing and Medical Intervention

The number of people required for a fish transport depends on the type and length of transport and the species. For small fish that are traveling a short distance by car or truck, a single person is usually adequate. Longer overland transports may require several people so that drivers can be rotated. Large elasmobranchs may require a person to be physically present to visually monitor the animals, in addition to drivers. One person should have overall control and be the liaison for the various groups involved in a transport. When transports are planned, the personnel available should be part of that plan.

Various medications have been used during transport of large fish, particularly elasmobranchs. These include glucose, antibiotics, steroids, sodium bicarbonate, and vitamin E. Pre-transport treatment with some of these medications may disrupt animal physiology and should be avoided. A better approach is to optimize health and diet prior to transport and to be able to provide supportive care if needed during or following transport.

Transport Options

By Road

This is often the most straightforward option, as temperature control is easier to guarantee and there are typically fewer major delays. Trucks can be designed to carry large rigid transport containers, along with suitable monitoring, aeration, filtration, and power.

By Air

While this is usually faster than road transport, it is also the most likely to suffer delays. Direct flights are recommended or the fewest connections and shortest total travel time. Choosing flight paths and times that are followed by several more flights the same day is recommended, so that transport boxes can get on a following flight if the first is missed. Air cargo carriers typically offer Next Flight Guaranteed (NFG) status, giving the owner assurance that the transport will go through. Holidays and labor union strikes are two scenarios that should preclude air transport, as they significantly increase the risk of the transport being delayed or boxes getting lost. Weather also needs to be considered. Storms can delay flights for hours to days. It is best to check the weather along the flight path before delivering the animals to the airport to try to minimize the risk of delays.

Additional considerations include temperature control throughout the flight and while at the airports, and if the fish can be accompanied and checked in flight. It is also essential to check that any equipment going on the flight has been cleared for use; regulations may exist for compressed oxygen cylinders and power sources.

By Boat

This route often allows for excellent water quality during transport. Fish shipped in the live-well of a boat can receive frequent water changes, so long as water parameters match. However, this method is impractical for large shipments or for transports across landmasses or oceans.

By Parcel Carrier

To ship using parcel carriers (e.g. FedEx®, UPS®), the sender must be pre-approved as a live fish shipper; this often includes trial transports to evaluate packaging standards. Once approved, this can be the most convenient method to ship low numbers of boxes on a regular basis. Door-to-door service is usually available. Caution should be exercised when using this method toward the end of a working week as Friday delivery dates can be delayed and weekend availability varies. Holidays are high-volume periods which put the fish at risk; transports over holidays should be avoided. Weather also needs to be considered as parcel vehicles are rarely climate-controlled and fish can be exposed to both warm and cold temperature extremes.

Acclimation on Arrival

Acclimation refers to using gradual water changes to help fish adapt to the water chemistry and temperature of the destination habitat. Proper acclimation improves short- and long-term survival of all fish. Water chemistry is complex, and even if temperature, salinity, and pH of the transport and destination water match, there may be other components that could be physiological stressors if changed suddenly. Acclimation is almost always recommended.

The major exceptions to providing a gradual acclimation is if a bag drained in transport, or if fish arrive in obviously fouled water or are showing significant morbidity; those fish should be moved immediately to better water as their prognosis worsens the longer they are in those conditions. There are some situations when acclimation may not be considered essential, e.g. transporting fish from a flow-through system to another flow-through system with the same source water, or a short transport to the veterinarian prior to returning the fish to the original system. However, even in those cases, there may be a change in water temperature that necessitates an acclimation period.

The main tenets of acclimation are slow and steady, with minimal external stressors. There are two basic methods.

1) The simplest is to float the transport bag in the destination system and slowly add the new water using a small container over 20–60 minutes (Figure A14.7a) until the water in the bag is mostly new water. Equivalent amounts of shipping water may need to be removed. Temperature equalization occurs gradually through the bag's immersion. Other water parameters slowly change to match the new water chemistry. When most of the water volume has been changed, the water and fish can be gently poured into the new water. This method can be difficult with large shipments as the bags may not all fit across the surface of the destination system and this is obviously unsuitable for large, hard-sided shipment containers.
2) Drip acclimation is used by large wholesalers and many zoos and aquariums. These make use of airline tubing from the destination system to drip the new water into the transport containers. A knot in the airline tubing after starting a siphon usually creates an ideal drip rate for acclimation (Figure A14.7b). Commercial wholesalers use a distribution line from the destination system to process large numbers of incoming containers.

Fish should be continuously monitored during acclimation. It may help to keep lighting low during acclimation, particularly for fish that have been in the dark for >10 hours, to let them adjust slowly. It is helpful to keep noise and other stressors to a minimum, including handling. If treatments are planned for when fish arrive (e.g. formalin dips), these should be applied after acclimation and before moving the fish to their new enclosures.

The systems that the fish are being released into may require changes to improve post-release survival. This may include additional natural or artificial hides or adjusting the water flow or lighting. It is also important to consider the impacts of animals already in the system. Introducing new fish to an established population can increase aggression and displacement and can limit feeding opportunities. Established aggressive or active fish may need to

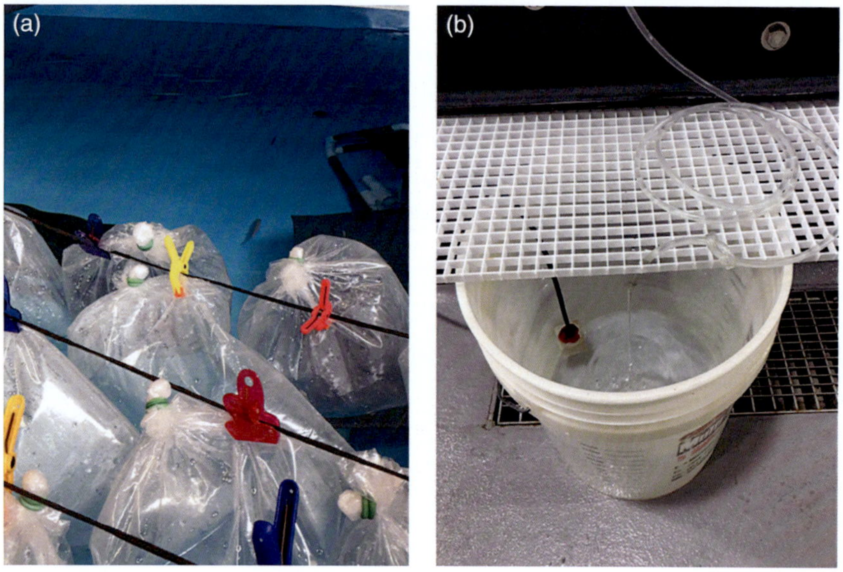

Figure A14.7 Acclimating fish in floating bags; the bags will be opened and water gradually introduced in aliquots (a). Acclimating fish using a drip system (b).

be temporarily removed to allow new fish to adjust. If fish must be added to an established population, providing a heavy feed before releasing the new fish and releasing into areas of the enclosure that are open territory can be helpful. "Howdy cages" are often used in public aquarium exhibits to house new fish for 12–48 hours while they adjust to a new system safely away from other animals. After that, the door of the howdy cages can be opened to allow the fish to leave when they choose.

Legislation

Animal acquisitions and transports must follow all federal, state, and local legislation. For fish, legislation typically applies to collecting wild animals, protected species, transport across state lines or international borders, and transport for release. This is a brief orientation of some of the relevant legislation, with a focus on US legislation. This is not meant as legal advice. Legal advice should only be sought from the relevant regulatory authority, legislation, or a qualified attorney, lawyer, solicitor, or legal advisor with suitable experience of the field and the region.

- The Convention on International Trade in Endangered Species of Wild Fauna and Flora (CITES) regulates international trade in listed species. Fish that are protected by CITES include arowana (*Scleropages* spp.), arapaima (*Arapaima gigas*), sturgeon (*Acipenseridae*), seahorses (*Hippocampus* spp.), humphead wrasse (*Cheilinus undulatus*), totoaba (*Totoaba macdonaldi*), and some elasmobranchs. The Endangered Species Act (ESA) is the legislation within the United States that carries out the provisions outlined by CITES. The US Fish and Wildlife Service (USFWS) administers the ESA and oversees all international import/export permits.
- The International Air Transport Association (IATA) Live Animal Regulations (LAR) apply to any live animals that are shipped on a commercial flight. They include details of shipping containers.
- The Magnuson-Stevens Act governs marine fisheries management in US federal waters and includes transport restrictions.
- The US Department of Agriculture (USDA) registers veterinarians that are able to complete Veterinary Certificates of Inspection (health certificates) for transport across state lines and internationally. It is important to note that health certificate regulations for each state or country that animals will be traveling through must be followed.
- The US Department of Transportation (DOT) has regulations that impact the shipment of live animals, along with several other federal, state, and local government agencies. Agencies may interpret those regulations uniquely within their jurisdiction.

Conclusion

Every acquisition should be considered for suitability and sustainability. A well-planned transport is vital to ensuring that healthy animals arrive at their destination.

Careful attention to detail and mock transports can help ensure that fish are exposed to as few stressors as possible. While some stressors are unavoidable, minimizing others is vital to the overall health and welfare of the animals being shipped. An appropriate acclimation is important to help fish adjust to changes in their water parameters on arrival. Following these basic principles will go a long way to ensuring that animals' needs are met to the best of our ability during acquisition and transport.

References

Carneiro, P.C.F. and Urbinati, E.C. (2001). Salt as a stress response mitigator of matrinxã, *Brycon cephalus* (Günuther), during transport. *Aquaculture Research* 32: 297–304.

Colburn, H.R., Walker, A.B., and Berlinsky, D.L. (2008). Factors affecting survival of cobia, *Rachycentron canadum*, during simulated transport. *Journal of the World Aquaculture Society* 39: 678–683.

Correia, J.P.S., Graça, J.T.C., Hirofumi, M., and Kube, N. (2011). Long-term transportation, by road and air, of chub mackerel (*Scomber japonicus*) and Atlantic bonito (*Sarda sarda*). *Zoo Biology* 30: 459–472.

Curtis, J.M., Johnson, M.W., Diamond, S.L., and Stunz, G.W. (2015). Quantifying delayed mortality from barotrauma impairment in discarded red snapper using acoustic telemetry. *Marine and Coastal Fisheries* 7: 434–449.

Dhanasiri, A.K.S., Kiron, V., Fernandes, J.M.O. et al. (2011). Novel application of nitrifying bacterial consortia to ease ammonia toxicity in ornamental fish transport units: trials with zebrafish. *Journal of Applied Microbiology* 111: 278–292.

Hubert, W.A., Pope, K.L., and Dettmers, J.M. (2012). Passive capture techniques. In: Fisheries Techniques, 3e (eds. A.V. Zale, D.L. Parrish and T.M. Sutton), 223–265. Bethesda, MD: American Fisheries Society.

Hyatt, M.W., Anderson, P.A., O'Donnell, P.M., and Berzins, I.K. (2011). Assessment of acid-base derangements among bonnethead sharks (*Sphyrna tiburo*), bull (*Carcharhinus leucas*), and lemon (*Negaprion brevirostris*) sharks from gillnet and longline capture and handling methods. *Comparative Biochemistry and Physiology Part A* 162: 113–120.

Kilgore, K.H., Hill, J.E., Powell, J.F.F. et al. (2009). Investigational use of metomidate hydrochloride as a shipping additive for two ornamental fishes. *Journal of Aquatic Animal Health* 21: 133–139.

Lim, L.C., Dhert, P., and Sorgeloos, P. (2003). Recent developments and improvements in ornamental fish packaging systems for air transport. *Aquaculture Research* 34: 923–935.

Mandelman, J.W. and Skomal, G.B. (2009). Differential sensitivity to capture stress assessed by blood acid-base status in five carcharhinid sharks. *Journal of Comparative Physiology Part B* 179: 267–277.

Rhyne, A.L., Tlusty, M.F., Schofield, P.J. et al. (2012). Revealing the appetite of the marine aquarium fish trade: the volume and biodiversity of fish imported into the United States. *PLoS One* 7 (5): e35808.

Rubec, P.J., Cruz, F., Pratt, V. et al. (2001). Cyanide-free net-caught fish for the marine aquarium trade. *Aquarium Sciences and Conservation* 3: 37–51.

Schreer, J.F., Gokey, J., and DeGhett, V.J. (2009). The incidence and consequences of barotrauma in fish in the St. Lawrence River. *North American Journal of Fisheries Management* 29: 1707–1713.

Silva, R.E., Morais, H.A., Rodrigues, N.V. et al. (2015). Optimising sealed transports of small ornamental fish. *Journal of Zoo and Aquarium Research* 3: 141–150.

Smith, M.F.L., Marshall, A., Correia, J.P., and Rupp, J. (2004). Elasmobranch transport technique and equipment. In: Elasmobranch Husbandry Manual (eds. M. Smith, D. Warmolts, D. Thoney and R. Hueter), 105–131. Columbus: Ohio Biological Survey, Inc.

Young, F.A., Kajiura, S.M., Visser, G.J. et al. (2002). Notes on the long-term transport of the scalloped hammerhead shark (*Sphyrna lewini*). *Zoo Biology* 21: 243–251.

A15

Fish Quarantine

Catherine A. Hadfield

Seattle Aquarium, Seattle, WA, USA

Introduction

The primary goal of fish quarantine is to reduce the risk of introducing significant pathogens into an established collection. There is ample evidence that lack of quarantine can put collections at risk of sustained morbidity and mortality (Poynton et al. 1997; Dove and Clauss 2008; Kik et al. 2011). Fish are susceptible to a wide range of opportunistic pathogens that are common in the environment and on other animals. These infectious diseases often show clinically following stressors such as transport and environmental changes. Keeping fish isolated after transport allows these diseases to be identified and treated. Quarantine also allows fish to recover from transport and adapt to new environments and diets. Some fish need additional support during this period and close monitoring can improve the overall outcome. Additionally, the quarantine period can provide training opportunities that will help the fish in the long term.

There are six core concepts with all fish quarantine: acquisition planning, appropriate isolation, ideal environmental conditions, monitoring, reactive diagnostics and treatments, and accurate records. These apply in every quarantine situation, whether the quarantine is for a hobbyist acquiring a few goldfish (*Carassius auratus*), a large aquarium acquiring a variety of ornamental species, or a research facility acquiring a large group of zebrafish (*Danio rerio*). However, no single quarantine plan is applicable to every situation; plans are most effective when designed for the systems, species, common diseases, and available resources.

The value of quarantine is best exemplified in isolated collections, such as facilities with recirculating systems that use municipal freshwater and/or artificial seawater. If these systems have limited organics and foods are usually commercial or frozen, the primary infectious disease risk comes from the acquisition of new animals. A well-managed quarantine can significantly reduce the risk of a serious disease outbreak and the loss of established animals. However, high welfare standards need to be maintained at all times. If conditions in quarantine systems are suboptimal, increased morbidity and mortality during quarantine are likely. If suitable quarantine systems are not available on-site, isolated off-site options should be considered.

For systems where there are multiple potential sources of infectious diseases, quarantine plans need to be considered within this larger framework. Some additional sources of infectious diseases include:

- Open or semi-open systems with regular inflow of untreated surface water;
- Exposure to wild fish;
- Diets that include fresh or live fish and invertebrates;
- Systems that are rich in organic material.

However, even with these additional exposures to infectious diseases, a well-managed quarantine can still help fish recover and adapt to new environments and reduce the risk of introducing novel pathogens. For example, even if a *Cryptocaryon* sp. is already present in a large system, quarantine can reduce the risk of introducing a novel or virulent strain of *Cryptocaryon* and allows the incoming fish to overcome transport stressors before they are exposed to the resident strain.

It is important to have measurable quarantine goals. One goal may be no new infectious disease outbreaks in the

Clinical Guide to Fish Medicine, First Edition. Edited by Catherine A. Hadfield and Leigh Ann Clayton.

collection. Another goal may be to successfully quarantine a species that has been problematic in the past. A common goal with public aquariums is for animals to be in an exhibit by a specified date. This is one of the more problematic goals, and it is important early on to discuss possible contingencies to avoid rushing animals into habitats. A useful quantitative assessment of overall quarantine success is the percentage of healthy fish that clear quarantine, compared to the number that came in. High mortalities should never be considered an inherent part of fish quarantine. With good planning, appropriate isolation, ideal environmental conditions, close monitoring, and appropriate diagnostics and treatments, quarantine success of >90% should be readily possible. By making fish quarantine success a specific goal at the National Aquarium, it was increased to and maintained at >95%.

Critical Components

Acquisition Planning

If a fish species is new to a collection, the natural history and recommended husbandry care should be reviewed. Useful sources include the literature, hobbyist boards, and colleagues. If the fish species has been acquired before, records should be reviewed to evaluate prior sources, quarantine history (husbandry, morbidity, mortality, and treatments), time in the collection, and subsequent causes of morbidity and mortality.

Sourcing of the animals should be considered before collection plans are put together and prior to each acquisition. Every effort should be made to acquire fish only from reliable institutions or sustainable wild sources. Good transport planning is also important, since transport is a significant stressor. The onus is on the shipper and receiver to minimize the stress of catch and transport and to minimize the environmental changes the animals are exposed to. Sourcing, transport, and acclimation are covered in more detail in Chapter A14.

Acquisition planning must consider the available quarantine space. This includes keeping bony fish, cartilaginous fish, and invertebrates in separate systems for quarantine. This is primarily because these groups show different tolerances to common medications. Animals should only be added to systems that have established biological filters. The nitrifying bacteria in systems without fish or invertebrates can be fed using ammonium chloride, urea, or seafood additions. Three weeks is usually the minimum time required to cycle a new system or a system that has had a major environmental change. However, more time may be needed, particularly at low temperatures. Systems should be cycled at the preferred environmental parameters (e.g. temperature, salinity, pH) for the incoming species or the pre-transport parameters if these are different. For example, if striped bass (*Morone saxatilis*) are held at a salinity of 5 g/L pre-transport but are destined to be held at 25 g/L, the quarantine system should be cycled at 5 g/L, then the salinity gradually increased after the fish have been introduced. While temperature, salinity, and pH are core parameters, matching of more parameters, such as alkalinity and cations, can be helpful for high-risk transports (e.g. pelagic sharks).

Fish acquisitions should be avoided prior to major holidays and other closures, as reduced personnel availability may impact monitoring during the critical early stages of quarantine. Ideally, fish should arrive early in the day to allow for monitoring throughout the day, and in small enough groups that acclimation can be done smoothly.

All-in-all-out practices are an excellent way to minimize disease transmission; in these, a quarantine system is used for a single group, then remains empty until the next group arrives. Cleaning and disinfection may be used between groups. Incoming fish should not be added to established fish populations. This can lead to aggression and reduced feeding opportunities, and puts the resident fish at risk from novel infectious diseases. These can result in higher morbidity and mortality in both the resident fish and the new fish. Continuing to add new fish to quarantine systems over several weeks until they are considered at full capacity also increases morbidity and mortality. Quarantine success was improved at the National Aquarium by only allowing quarantine systems to receive additional new fish for a maximum of seven days after the initial additions. After those seven days, the system was closed and new fish, even from the same supplier, were placed in a different quarantine system.

Acquisition plans should include any diet items that may be needed. It is also helpful to discuss likely medications, routes, and discharge plans for any medicated water. It is helpful to be clear on roles and responsibilities prior to fish acquisitions, for example how medications would be accessed after hours in the event of an emergency.

Contingency plans should be considered in case of a life support failure, water quality problems, or a significant disease event that may require a longer quarantine or alternative housing. For example, sufficient suitable water should be available to allow several large water changes in the quarantine systems.

Isolation

Isolation is a core component of good biosecurity (Box A15.1). At best, isolation means independent quarantine

Box A15.1 Important Biosecurity Factors in Fish Quarantine

- Geographically separated from systems with collection animals or free-ranging animals.
- Dedicated systems, sufficiently far apart to not allow water to splash between.
- Managed as all-in-all-out quarantine systems.
- Dedicated staff.
- Limited/no movement of nonessential staff (e.g. visitors).
- Dedicated nets, hoses, brushes, scrapers, feeding poles, buckets, and décor for each system.
- Décor that can be cleaned and disinfected (e.g. PVC pipes and frames, felt strips, plastic plants).
- As little organic material and substrate as possible, unless needed by the species.
- Clear signage that indicates quarantine status.
- Low-pathogen incoming water source (e.g. municipal water or mechanical filtration then ozone and/or ultraviolet disinfection of incoming surface water).
- Ultraviolet disinfection of recirculating water and discharge water.
- Suitable food sources and food inspection and preparation protocols.
- Routine use of gloves (hand and full-sleeve) and hand-washing stations with soap, warm water, and clean towels.
- If ground contamination may be a source of disease transmission, suitable foot cleaning stations and disinfection baths may help, although dedicated boots are better.
- Appropriate heating, ventilation, and air-conditioning (HVAC) system.
- Good integrated pest management program.
- Good cleaning and disinfection protocols.
- Outdoor systems may benefit from a roof and bird deterrents.
- System breakdown and disinfection protocols in case of serious infectious disease outbreak.

systems that are in a different location from the systems that house the collection. They should be in a quiet area without through-traffic. Where possible, staff should be dedicated to managing quarantine systems only, or at least should manage quarantine systems after finishing work with the collection.

Each quarantine system should be isolated from any other quarantine system in case of a disease outbreak in one. This requires separate equipment for each system, suitable personal protective equipment (e.g. gloves) and hand-washing areas, and adequate space between the systems (Box A15.1). Figures A15.1 and A15.2 demonstrate potential quarantine systems for aquarium fish. Other references provide additional information for aquaculture systems (e.g. Maes and Carmichael 2002). Within a quarantine system, it is often useful to have more than one tank, e.g. two 45 gallon (170 L) tanks on the same system, or one 1800 gallon (6800 L) system with an 80 gallon (300 L) saddle tank (Figure A15.3). This allows fish to be separated from the group if needed while being kept in the same water and on the same treatments.

The Association of Zoos and Aquariums (AZA) recommends at least 30 days of isolation. Shorter periods provide less protection and should be avoided (Whittington and Chong 2007). Since many diseases take longer to present, the minimum duration of quarantine could be extended for groups at high risk of infectious disease outbreaks (e.g. confiscations by customs officers, pond-reared fish). Also, some treatments take time. For example, quarantine of tropical marine teleosts treated with copper sulfate immersion is often at least 40–45 days.

Mechanical filtration and disinfection of incoming water is recommended where surface water is used or where water is coming from other systems holding animals. Disinfection of the recirculating water should also be considered for fish quarantine systems. Water disinfection using ultraviolet (UV) filtration can help reduce pathogen load, particularly viruses and bacteria. It is less effective against larger parasites at typical doses. UV disinfection is simple and safe, but the filters do require regular maintenance including bulb replacements and cleaning of the bulb sleeves. Ozone disinfection is also effective but can be hard to manage in quarantine systems because of the variation in the bioload. Disinfection of water discharged from fish quarantine systems is also recommended to reduce the risk of transferring pathogens.

Environmental Conditions

Ideal environmental conditions are essential. It can be tempting to be less fastidious about conditions because quarantine is temporary, but doing so can significantly increase morbidity and mortality.

Stocking density has been a major factor in quarantine success at National Aquarium. Stocking densities of >1.0 cm/L (or >1.5 in./gallon), based on estimated total lengths, led to higher mortality. Consistently starting quarantine with stocking densities of <1.0 cm/L significantly improved quarantine success.

Enclosure shape and size should be appropriate for the species, numbers, and life stages. Large quarantine systems can accommodate larger animals and larger groups, are

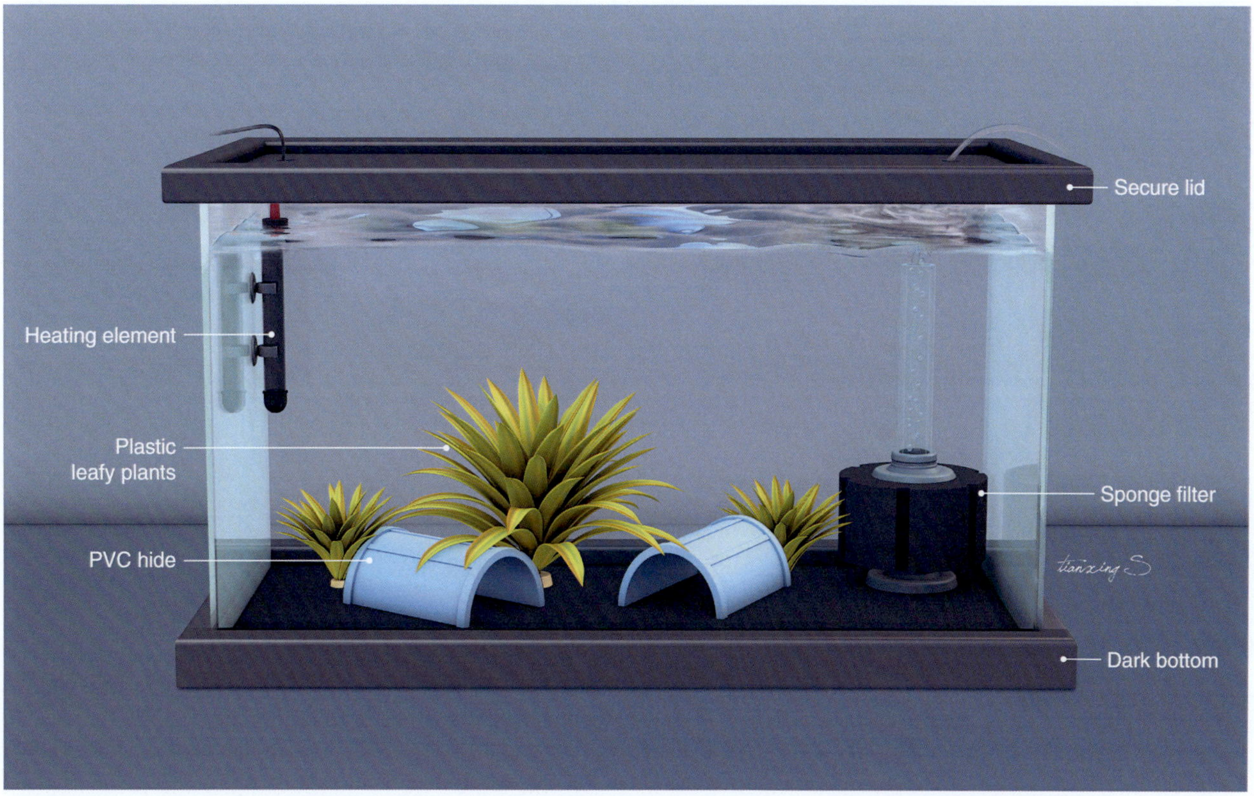

Figure A15.1 Example of a quarantine system that would be suitable for a small group of teleosts, such as neon tetras (*Paracheirodon innesi*). *Source*: Image courtesy of Tianxing Shi; copyright reserved.

generally more stable, and provide more space for individuals to choose their niche. However, large quarantine systems are also harder to manage in the event of an infectious disease outbreak as it may be more challenging to access animals or carry out large water changes, and the medication cost is higher.

Water temperature needs to be stable and appropriate for all the animals. Contingency plans should be available for systems that are relying on heat exchangers (e.g. a cold-water system housed in a warm room, or where the temperature of the incoming water may change). All water quality parameters should be ideal, including dissolved oxygen, salinity, pH, hardness, and alkalinity. There should be no nitrogenous wastes. This can be challenging in quarantine systems as bioload tends to vary significantly; cycling of biological filtration on quarantine systems should be targeted for the maximum anticipated bioload. Suitable water for water changes should always be available. Ammonia-locking compounds such as Amquel® (Kordon LLC, Hayward, CA) should also be available in case elevated ammonia cannot be managed with water turnover or husbandry changes.

The social needs of the animals must be considered during quarantine. Social incompatibility is a common source of trauma and stress. Even with good planning, fish may need to be separated if there is any sign of displacement or aggression. Suitable substrate should be provided if it is needed for the species and life stages. Enrichment should be included to allow expression of natural behaviors (e.g. hiding, burying, foraging, egg-laying). There is sometimes a balance between ideal environmental conditions and ease of cleaning and monitoring, but the goal should always be to provide the best conditions. This may mean adding a sand substrate that is regularly siphoned and is discarded after quarantine, or judicious placement of PVC pipes so that fish within them are still visible from observation windows.

Fish in quarantine are often transitioning onto new diets. This is particularly challenging with some wild-caught fish, e.g. scorpionfish (*Scorpaenidae*) and seahorses (*Syngnathidae*). A wide variety of food items should be available in order to help transition the fish. This may include live foods such as brine shrimp, rotifers, copepods, bloodworms, glass shrimp, minnows, or mollies. Acquiring these for immediate use is not ideal; it is much safer to use live foods that are from a stable, healthy population, which typically means acquiring live foods well before starting fish quarantine and maintaining them under ideal environmental conditions. A variety of options for herbivorous fish is also important and may

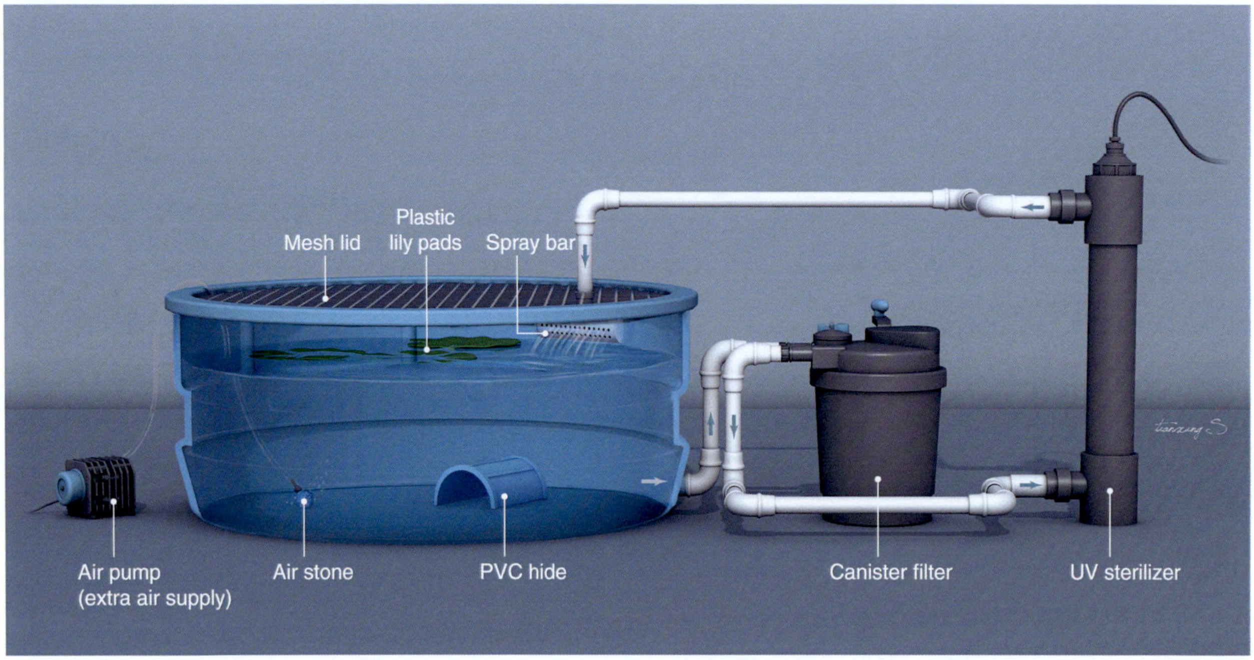

Figure A15.2 Example of a quarantine system that would be suitable for koi (*Cyprinus carpio koi*) or similar fish. *Source*: Image courtesy of Tianxing Shi; copyright reserved.

include pellets, flake foods, gel foods, algae, leafy greens, and vegetables.

Close Monitoring

Close monitoring is key to quarantine success. Infectious diseases are likely, and if caught early, both morbidity and mortality can be significantly reduced. For example, prognosis is much worse if *Ichthyophthirius multifiliis* is identified when there are obvious white spots and mortalities rather than earlier when fish show subtle behavioral changes. Social issues, such as displacement or competition for food, also need to be caught early to reduce morbidity and mortality.

Water quality monitoring is essential, particularly temperature, dissolved oxygen, salinity, pH, ammonia, and nitrite. Chlorines are important to assay in freshwater. Ideally other parameters, such as total gas pressure, nitrate, hardness, and alkalinity, should also be measured. The frequency of testing should be higher than in well-established systems, often once a day for the first few weeks in recirculating systems.

Regular visual examinations with adequate lighting are essential and should be done at least twice a day and during feeding. Monitoring is improved by having side windows in fiberglass tanks (Figure A15.4). Glass or acrylic tanks allow for easy monitoring, but provide limited opportunities for cover and do not make ideal quarantine tanks; they can be improved by covering two or three sides in black material. Habitat lighting should be sufficient to allow monitoring while being suitable for the species present. Flashlights are particularly useful to catch early signs, such as subtle changes on the fins.

Clinical signs during fish quarantine that warrant further investigation include:

- Dyspnea, tachypnea, e.g. increased opercular flaring, piping at the surface, gathering at areas of turbulence;
- Pruritus, e.g. flashing, agitated swimming, clamped fins;

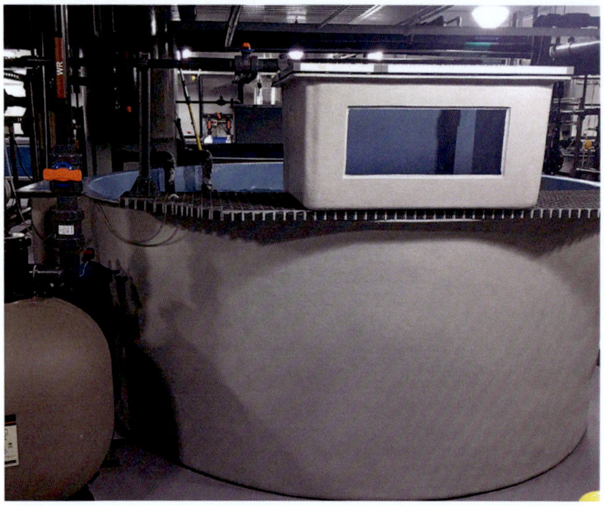

Figure A15.3 Example of a saddle tank that allows fish within a quarantine group to be separated if needed. The same water is circulated through both tanks.

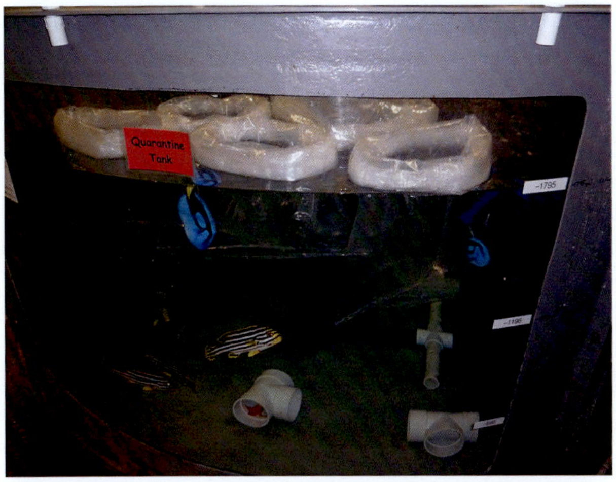

Figure A15.4 Large window in the side of a fiberglass tank used for fish quarantine. The quarantine status is clearly labeled and a variety of hides are available. The fish are part-way through acclimation.

- Skin changes, particularly hyperemia, pallor, darkening, ulceration, white spots, black spots, visible parasites, or trauma;
- Poor food intake, decreased food intake, poor body condition;
- Abnormal posture or position, e.g. increased hiding, isolated schooling fish, recumbency of mid-water fish;
- Abnormal swimming, e.g. fast swimming, whirling;
- Mortalities.

The time needed for feeding and monitoring fish during quarantine is typically much higher than for established animals. Communication about quarantine also needs to be more frequent and detailed than for collection animals. In order to minimize morbidity and mortality, staff with extensive fish husbandry experience should be responsible for quarantine.

Diagnostics and Treatments

With close monitoring, morbidity can be identified early allowing for additional diagnostics and treatments as indicated. Some of the common categories of problems during quarantine are:

- Trauma, often from catch, transport, décor, or cohorts;
- Ammonia toxicity, often due to naïve or damaged biological filtration;
- Poor feeding response;
- Protozoal ectoparasites, particularly the ciliates *Cryptocaryon irritans* in salt water and *Ichthyophthirius multifiliis* in freshwater;
- Monogenean ectoparasites, particularly *Capsalidae* and *Gyrodactylidae*;
- Opportunistic bacteria, such as *Vibrio* and *Aeromonas* spp., particularly soon after transport;
- Viral infections, e.g. nervous necrosis virus, herpesvirus, lymphocystivirus;
- Oomycetes, often secondary to skin damage;
- Metazoan endoparasites, e.g. digenes, nematodes;
- Crustaceans and other large ectoparasites, e.g. copepods, leeches, branchiurans.

While a few of the problems above can affect individual fish, they more commonly affect some or all of a group. Even if clinical signs are only visible in one fish, it is important to always consider that the problem may be more widespread.

If the cause of morbidity is not obvious based on the history, visual examination, and water quality, additional diagnostics should be considered as soon as possible. One exception to this may be morbidity immediately after transport; this often resolves over 24–48 hours if fish are given good environmental conditions and quiet recovery time. Useful diagnostics in the event of morbidity during quarantine include:

- Physical examination and assessment of body condition;
- Skin scrape, fin clip, and gill biopsy for direct examination under bright-field microscopy;
- Physical removal of any visible parasites for direct examination;
- Fecal sample for direct examination;
- Aspirates or scrapes of any lesions for direct examination and stained cytologies and cultures;
- Blood sample or aspirate of an effusion for bacterial culture;
- PCR testing for common viral diseases, e.g. gill swab for koi herpes virus.

Where hands-on diagnostics are indicated, it is worth considering what supportive care can be provided during the handling. For example, if an inappetent fish is being sedated for a gill biopsy, gavage feeding should be considered. Environmental tests for infectious diseases may also be useful, e.g. sock filters to collect monogenean eggs or membrane filters to collect mycobacteria (Crim et al. 2017). If a diagnosis has not been reached based on these tests, particularly if a group is affected, euthanasia of a sick or moribund fish may be the most effective way to reach a diagnosis.

Necropsies should always be carried out on mortalities during quarantine. These are most useful on fresh specimens, but even autolyzed specimens can provide useful information. The priorities for necropsies of fish in quarantine are often different from animals in established collections. The main areas of focus for a quarantine necropsy are:

- Physical examination for signs of external trauma, skin lesions, parasites, and to assess body condition.
- Skin scrape, fin clip, and gill biopsy to identify pathogens, signs of irritation, or gas emboli.
- Examination of the gastrointestinal contents to assess recent food intake and examination of the coelomic fat stores to assess long-term feeding history.
- Evidence of systemic inflammation, for example generalized hyperemia, skin ulceration, congestion, widespread granulomas, and organomegaly.

Ancillary testing such as cultures, histology, and other tissue analyses can be frustratingly slow with an emerging group issue in quarantine but can be invaluable in understanding the process, even in retrospect. If fish are due to be introduced to a particularly valuable established collection, it is likely worth holding the fish in quarantine pending these slower results.

Reactive treatments can be targeted to the known diagnosis or the most likely diagnosis (Hadfield and Clayton 2011). Common treatments reported in quarantine include:

- Supportive care;
- Antibiotic therapy;
- Praziquantel immersion and/or orally;
- Formalin immersion for freshwater and marine teleosts;
- Copper sulfate or chelated copper immersion for marine teleosts;
- Chloroquine immersion for marine teleosts.

More information on treatments is available in Chapters A12 and A13 and Section C, but a brief overview as it relates to quarantine is provided here.

Sensitivity to medications depends on a wide variety of factors, including species, life stages, overall health, temperature, water chemistry, microbiome, drug source, dosing regimen, and other stressors. For example, morbidity from copper sulfate immersion treatment during quarantine is often lower if started 10–14 days after arrival than when started soon after arrival (Zec et al. 2017). To minimize risks, information should be sought from the literature and colleagues, as well as reviewing in-house historical records. Some general guidelines can be used.

- Juvenile fish often show a greater sensitivity to immersion medications than adults or subadults.
- Elasmobranchs often show a greater sensitivity to immersion medications, particularly copper sulfate and formalin. Pelagic elasmobranchs show a low tolerance to salinity changes compared to other groups.
- Some teleost groups often show a greater sensitivity to immersion medications and handling, including seahorses, pipefish, and seadragons (*Syngnathidae*).
- Scaleless and fine-scaled teleosts may show a greater sensitivity to immersion medications than other groups, e.g. knifefish (*Gymnotiformes*).
- Fish with skin lesions, e.g. abrasions or ulcerations, are likely to show a greater sensitivity to immersion medications.
- Some fish have adaptations that may be affected by treatments, e.g. the bacteria in bioluminescent fish such as lantern fish (*Myctophidae*) and flashlight fish (*Anomalopidae*) may be affected by any treatment that also has antibacterial activity, such as copper sulfate or chloroquine.

Bioassays (testing the drug on a subset of the population) can be invaluable in identifying any unexpected consequences of treatment. It is particularly helpful to carry out bioassays under similar environmental conditions as the target group.

Biological filtration can be damaged by a number of immersion medications and environmental changes; more details are covered in Chapters A12 and A13. The effect varies enormously depending on the microbiota present, the environmental conditions, and the exposure history. Common quarantine immersion medications that may damage biological filtration include copper sulfate, formalin, chloroquine, oxolinic acid, and other antibiotics. Whenever immersion medications are used, environmental parameters should be monitored closely and contingency plans should be available in the event of filter damage, dissolved oxygen concerns, or a potential drug reaction in the fish.

Life support systems can alter immersion medications. In general, ultraviolet and ozone disinfection, activated carbon filtration, and foam fractionation should be discontinued or taken off-line for the duration of an immersion treatment. The addition of ozone filtration after an immersion treatment can result in the production of unknown and potentially toxic by-products and it may be better to rely on mechanical removal of medications through water changes and activated carbon filtration. This carbon may need to be disposed of as hazardous waste, which is why likely medications and their disposal should be discussed as part of the acquisition planning process.

For animals that shipped and acclimated well, a treatment dip (e.g. formalin, freshwater for marine fish) prior to transfer to the quarantine enclosure can reduce the risk of introducing pathogens into the quarantine system. An added layer of safety can be achieved by using similar dips after animals leave quarantine and before they go into their next habitat. These are essentially dose-and-move strategies and they can be extremely helpful in reducing reinfection by environmental stages.

Accurate Records

Accurate records are essential in evaluating how a quarantine group is fairing. Important information to record includes:

- Source;
- Date of arrival;
- Transport conditions;
- Species, numbers, and estimated sizes on arrival;
- Water quality results and subsequent actions;
- Feeding;
- Behavior notes;
- Morbidity (species, sizes, dates, clinical signs, progression, diagnostic tests, final diagnoses);
- Mortality (species, sizes, dates, condition, diagnostic tests, final diagnoses);
- Treatments including sources, lot numbers, doses, durations, assays, complications;
- Date of clearing quarantine and duration of quarantine;
- Species, numbers, and estimated sizes on clearing quarantine.

These records are the most reliable way to evaluate quarantine practices and allow improvement over time.

Risk Assessment Approach

The six core principals of planning, appropriate isolation, ideal environmental conditions, monitoring, reactive diagnostics and treatments, and accurate records can be used to build a good quarantine plan. However, a more tailored plan provides additional benefits. This is because the likelihood of specific diseases and the possible treatments depend on a variety of factors, including:

- Water source;
- Fish source;
- Species and life stages;
- Transport time and conditions;
- Time of year;
- Diets available;
- Facilities available;
- Medications available and user familiarity;
- History of the collection;
- History of the geographic area (if outdoors or using surface or ground water);
- Quarantine goals and collection goals.

It is possible to use a risk assessment approach to anticipate likely problems and plan for specific diagnostics and preventative or reactive treatments (Pye et al. 2018). The risk assessment may also indicate where an acquisition is inappropriate, e.g. if the quarantine system size or shape presents a high risk of skin trauma to a pelagic shark, or if appropriate diets cannot be provided. This risk assessment approach is being increasingly advocated for determining quarantine needs in zoological collections and movement of live fish through international trade (Whittington and Chong 2007; Rimmer et al. 2015; Pye et al. 2018).

Risk assessments are best done on a group-by-group basis. A rigid quarantine protocol, particularly if applied across different species, systems, or institutions, may actually increase morbidity and mortality. For example, using high concentrations of formalin on all incoming fish, regardless of species or life stage, may lead to morbidity and mortality in larval and juvenile fish. This risk assessment should be considered fluid. For example, a group of juvenile French grunts (*Haemulon flavolineatum*) from an AZA institution may be considered low risk, but if the transport goes poorly, their risk of disease issues increases. This approach can be time-consuming initially, but rapidly becomes second nature and can reduce costs and improve quarantine efficiency in the long run. Examples are provided below to illustrate this approach.

Once potential problems have been identified, they can be categorized based on their cost and probability.

- Cost (or impact) can be financial (including cost of treatment in quarantine or in the collection and cost of replacement fish) and ethical (including animal welfare, sustainability, and staff morale). As an example, *Neobenedenia* spp. of monogenean often have a high cost in a large display exhibit as the parasites tend to cause chronic morbidity and mortality and may require regular treatment to control clinical signs.
- Probability will depend on the species and life stages being acquired, the time of year, and the sources; for example, salmon smolts are at higher risk of infectious disease than adult stages, and cardinal tetras (*Paracheirodon axelrodi*) from a local pet store have a higher probability of *Ichthyophthirius multifiliis* than ones from a small private collection.

To guide discussion and planning, potential risks can be divided into four broad categories:

- High cost and common, where preventative measures should be considered;
- High cost and uncommon, where screening should be considered;

- Low cost and common, where screening should be considered;
- Low cost and uncommon, where routine monitoring should be sufficient.

Some diseases will always fall in the same category, e.g. *Cryptocaryon irritans* is likely to be considered high cost and common in all wild-caught or commercially acquired tropical marine teleosts. However, in most cases, the categories are not inherent. For example, the monogenean *Benedeniella posterocolpa* may be considered a high cost for a colony of cownose rays (*Rhinoptera bonasus*) that is known to be clear of the parasites, but a lower cost if the parasites are already present in the colony.

This process allows quarantine plans to be tailored to the needs of the animals and the specifics of the situation, which improves welfare, minimizes morbidity and mortality, and guides organizational resource allocation both in quarantine and in the collection.

Example 1: Quarantine of Koi for an Established Koi Pond

A lot is known about diseases of koi (*Cyprinus carpio koi*) and some of these diseases present a significant threat to an existing collection, particularly koi herpes virus (KHV) and carp edema virus (CEV). Koi can have significant financial and emotional value and routine veterinary care is more common than for other pet fish. Source is a particularly important consideration for koi, because specific infectious disease screening exists.

Table A15.1 is an example of a risk assessment for the quarantine of koi for an established pond. Based on the table, a tentative quarantine plan may consist of the following.

1) *Acquisition planning*: Evaluate the source and their infectious disease testing, particularly for KHV, CEV, and spring viremia of carp. Avoid acquiring koi when the water temperature is <15°C (<59°F), as KHV is dormant at this temperature and would not show clinically.
2) *Isolation*: All-in-all-out management. Provide a suitable habitat isolated from other fish, or at least other cyprinids, for a minimum of 30 days (e.g. Figure A15.2).
3) *Ideal environmental conditions*: During quarantine, provide water temperature of >18°C (>64°F) to increase the likelihood of clinical signs in fish with latent KHV; if previous water temperature was different, slowly approximate to the target temperature. Dechlorinate source water. Consider increasing salinity to 5 g/L during quarantine to reduce the risk of CEV.
4) *Close monitoring*: Visual checks twice daily and during feeding; watch closely for visible ectoparasites, signs of skin or gill irritation, or behavioral changes. Check ammonia, pH, chlorine, and water temperature at least daily.
5) *Reactive diagnostics and treatments*: Sedated examinations in the event of any morbidity and full necropsies, histology, and PCR testing for KHV with any mortality. Develop a plan for treatment of *Ichthyophthirius multifiliis* and crustaceans that can be applied if needed. Consider sedated physical examination of all fish, or a subset of fish, for skin scrapes, gill biopsies, and PCR testing for KHV +/− CEV prior to clearing quarantine.
6) *Accurate records*: Record quarantine events in an electronic file or on a log sheet that can be scanned and saved.

Example 2: Quarantine of Neon Tetras for a New Home Aquarium

Neon tetras (*Paracheirodon innesi*) are one of many characids that are common in home aquariums and routinely available at local pet stores. A reputable source will help reduce the risk of infectious diseases and in-breeding. The owner should be aware that these fish are prone to a number of common pathogens.

Table A15.2 is an example of a risk assessment for this quarantine group or similar species. Based on the table, a tentative quarantine plan may consist of the following.

1) *Acquisition planning*: Evaluate several local pet stores to identify healthy looking populations. Purchase the fish

Table A15.1 An example of a risk assessment for koi going into an established koi pond.

High cost and common	High cost and uncommon	Low cost and common
Ichthyophthirius multifiliis ciliates	Koi herpes virus	Trauma
Argulus spp. branchiurans	Carp edema virus	Lymphocystis
Lernaea spp. anchor worms	Spring viremia of carp	Carp pox
		Trichodinid ciliates
		Dactylogyrid and gyrodactylid monogeneans
		Chlorines in tap water

Table A15.2 An example of a risk assessment for neon tetras going into a new home aquarium.

High cost and common	High cost and uncommon	Low cost and common
Ichthyophthirius multifiliis ciliates	Temperature failure	Neutral water pH
Mycobacteriosis		Chlorines in tap water
Microsporidiosis		
Ammonia toxicity		
Oomycetes		

when ambient temperatures are similar to the water temperature.

2) *Isolation*: Since the fish are going into a new home aquarium, an isolated quarantine can be done in that aquarium. However, if other species are acquired at the same time, particularly from another source, there is some benefit to having a separate, suitable enclosure for the other group in case of disease and because some fish (e.g. *Pangio* spp. loaches) may be less tolerant of immersion treatments than characids.
3) *Ideal environmental conditions*: Start with a very low stocking density to reduce the risk of ammonia toxicity. Provide an appropriate temperature and pH; neon tetras can tolerate low temperatures and neutral pH, but do best at 24–27°C (75–81°F) and a pH of ~6.5. Aerate tap water for 24 hours prior to use to off-gas chlorines.
4) *Close monitoring*: Visual checks twice daily and during feeding, watch closely for behavioral or skin changes, particularly white spots, nodules, pallor, or white cotton-like growths. Check ammonia, pH, chlorine, and water temperature at least daily.
5) *Reactive diagnostics and treatments*: Identify what treatments for *Ichthyophthirius multifiliis* are available at local pet stores and suitable for the species. Consider purchasing the treatment in advance, as these ciliates can build up quickly. Determine what diagnostic and treatment options are available at a local vet practice in the event of morbidity or mortality.
6) *Accurate records*: Record quarantine events in an electronic file or on a log sheet that can be scanned and saved.

Example 3: Quarantine of a Group of Tropical Marine Teleosts for a Display Aquarium

Infectious diseases introduced into a large display aquarium can carry high potential costs, as the size and complexity of these systems often limit diagnostic and treatment options. The primary quarantine goal is typically to avoid introducing significant pathogens. These may be known pathogens (e.g. *Neobenedenia* spp.) or unknown (e.g. a suspected viral disease). Since most large display aquaria have veterinarians on-site and the fish are cared for by animal care professionals, routine diagnostics are common, more treatment options are available, and preventative treatments are more likely. Since incoming fish may be sourced from far afield, both source and transport plans can have an enormous impact on overall success.

Table A15.3 is an example of a risk assessment for Indo-Pacific tropical teleosts. Based on the table, a tentative quarantine plan may consist of the following.

1) *Acquisition planning*: Identify the best source. Cycle all possible systems prior to fish arrival and develop plans in case of damage to the biological filtration. Minimize transport time and other transport stressors. Acquire the fish for one system within one week, when experienced staff are available. Carefully consider compatibility of species, sexes, and life stages. Have a variety of foods, including live foods, available and ready to use. Consider likely treatments and possible drug sensitivities. Have likely medications in sufficient

Table A15.3 An example of a risk assessment for marine Indo-Pacific tropical teleosts going into a large display aquarium.

High cost and common	High cost and uncommon	Low cost and common
Cryptocaryon irritans ciliates	*Cryptosporidium* spp.	Trauma
Neobenedenia spp. monogeneans	Novel virulent virus	Scuticociliates
Brooklynella spp. ciliates		Myxozoans
Poor appetite		Digenes
Conspecific aggression		
Post-shipping bacterial infection in small fish		
Biological filtration damage from immersion treatments		

quantity, particularly formalin, praziquantel, copper, chloroquine, and suitable antibiotics.

2) *Isolation*: All-in-all-out management. Isolate for a minimum of 45 days to provide enough time for treatments. A longer quarantine may be needed if problems are seen.
3) *Ideal environmental conditions*: Provide suitable conditions for each species and individual; consider social situation carefully (e.g. Moorish idols (*Zanclus cornutus*) and anthias (*Anthiadinae*) may do best if kept only with a school of conspecifics). Keep fish that have more specific dietary or environmental requirements in smaller systems or smaller tanks on the same system.
4) *Close monitoring*: Check the water quality in the transport bags on arrival. Visual checks at least twice daily and during feeding (identifying every individual wherever possible). Move décor carefully if needed to look for sick or dead fish in larger systems. Routine water quality testing (including dissolved oxygen) daily after arrival and both during and after immersion treatments; the interval can be extended when the system is stable.
5) *A – Reactive diagnostics and treatments*: Investigate any morbidity immediately, e.g. physical examinations with skin scrapes, gill biopsies, and other testing as indicated. Perform a necropsy and ancillary testing as soon as a mortality is found.

   B – Preventative treatments:
   - If fish have shipped and acclimated well, provide a formalin (37%) dip at 50 mg/L for two hours prior to transfer to the quarantine enclosure to reduce the risk of introducing ectoparasites.
   - If fish shipped poorly or seem particularly susceptible to transport trauma (e.g. anthias) consider a short course of antibiotics post-transport.
   - Copper sulfate immersion or hyposalinity treatment in species and life stages that can tolerate the treatment to reduce the risk of *Cryptocaryon* spp. For copper sulfate immersion, target dose may be 0.17–0.20 mg/L ionic copper for 21 days, starting 7–10 days after acquisition with a slow increase to therapy over seven days. Assay ionic copper daily until levels have returned to baseline. For hyposalinity treatment, consider a slow decrease to 18 g/L, maintained for >3 weeks.
   - Praziquantel immersion to reduce the risk of monogeneans. Suggested regimen for *Neobenedenia* spp. may be 4 mg/L repeated every four days for eight treatments as a pulse therapy. Assay drug levels if possible to determine actual dose and duration of treatment.
   - Praziquantel medicated feed to reduce the risk of internal digenes and external monogeneans. Suggested dose may be 250 mg/100 g food weight orally once daily for three days (equivalent to 50 mg/kg of body weight if eating 2% of body weight).
   - Freshwater dips, matched to pH and temperature, during the transfer to the exhibit.
6) *Accurate records*: Record quarantine events including source, water quality, feeding, morbidity, mortality, diagnostics, and treatments on the medical records system. Regularly review the records.

Example 4: Quarantine of Pelagic, Ram-ventilating Sharks for a Display Aquarium

Elasmobranch quarantine is usually straightforward as long as the animals are kept in ideal conditions and transport has gone well. However, particularly in suboptimal conditions, traumatic lesions and secondary infectious diseases are seen. Wild-caught elasmobranchs may be difficult to transition onto a diet of frozen-thawed seafood, and it is helpful to discuss potential nutritional support options early on. Wild-caught adult females may be gravid and plans should include that possibility.

Table A15.4 is an example of a risk assessment for a bonnethead shark (*Sphyrna tiburo*). Based on the table, a tentative quarantine plan may consist of the following.

1) *Acquisition planning*: Identify the best source and review the prior husbandry conditions and any known medical history for that individual or cohorts from that source. Decide whether a male or female is more appropriate for the collection. Plan the transport to minimize the risk of trauma, poor water quality, and capture myopathy. Plan to quarantine alone in a suitable, cycled system; this reduces disease risks and allows individual management for problems such as inappetence. The system should have viewing windows on the sides. Have likely medications in sufficient quantity, particularly praziquantel and suitable antibiotics. Medications such as organophosphates and chitin inhibitors may be needed.

Table A15.4 An example of a risk assessment for bonnethead sharks (*Sphyrna tiburo*) going into a large display aquarium.

High cost and common	High cost and uncommon	Low cost and common
Poor appetite	*Fusarium* spp. fungi	Gravid female
Aggression	Meningitis	
Trauma, particularly to rostrum, fins, eyes	Poor water quality	
Erpocotyle spp. monogeneans	Environmental toxins	
Trauma from hook catches		

2) *Isolation*: Isolate for a minimum of 90 days to provide time for potential subclinical diseases to show and to train the animal to feed at a specific target.
3) *Ideal environmental conditions*: Large oval tank with additional markings on enclosure walls (e.g. vertical stripes or bubble nets) to reduce the risk of abrasions. Use tight, knot-less netting or high walls to ensure the enclosure is escape-proof. Maintain water temperature at 25–26°C (77–79°F). Have redundant heat exchangers. Have a wide variety of potential food items available.
4) *Close monitoring*: Monitor the water quality within the transport container, ideally before, during, and at the end of the shipment. Visual checks at least twice daily and during feeding. Continuous in-line monitoring of temperature and dissolved oxygen. Automated water level sensors. Routine water quality testing (including dissolved oxygen) daily after arrival and both during and after immersion treatments; the interval can be extended when the system is stable. Check water for heavy metals. Routine physical examination including ultrasound, fecal examination, endoscopic examination (oral/gill cavities), and bloodwork (e.g. hematology, biochemistry, vitamins, and heavy metal levels).
5) *A – Reactive diagnostics and treatments*: Investigate any morbidity immediately. Dewormers should be used with extreme caution in elasmobranchs.

   B – Preventative treatments: Praziquantel immersion to reduce the risk of monogeneans. Suggested regimen may be 5 mg/L repeated every seven days for four treatments as a pulse therapy. Assay drug levels if possible to determine actual dose and duration of treatment.
6) *Accurate records*: Record quarantine events including source, water quality, feeding, morbidity, mortality, diagnostics, and treatments on the medical records system. Regularly review the records.

Example 5: Quarantine of Tilapia for an Established Tilapia Culture Facility

An important consideration is whether the fish might enter the human food chain, as associated policies must be followed (e.g. Food and Drug Administration regulations in the United States). This has a significant impact on available medications and dosages. Most culture facilities are familiar with the diseases that are common in their species and region. Biosecurity measures should already be in place but are worth reviewing.

Table A15.5 is an example of a risk assessment for tilapia in aquaculture. Based on the table, a tentative quarantine plan may consist of the following.

1) *Acquisition planning*: Look for specific pathogen-free populations and review the infectious disease testing of the source fish. Select a suitable time to acquire the fish and the target size/age of fish.
2) *Isolation*: All-in-all-out management and other biosecurity measures. Isolate for a minimum of 30 days; the fish may stay in that system after quarantine.
3) *Ideal environmental conditions*: Stocking density is often high, which represents a stressor. Keep other stressors to a minimum. Follow feeding recommendations.
4) *Close monitoring*: Visual checks at least twice daily and during feeding. Check dissolved oxygen, ammonia, nitrite, nitrate, pH, alkalinity, hardness, turbidity, and water temperature; the frequency depends on fish density and risk assessments.
5) *Reactive diagnostics and treatments*: Rapidly investigate morbidity or mortality above target levels using necropsy, cultures, and PCR testing. In the case of a large group, consider sacrificing a few apparently healthy fish for diagnostics early in quarantine. If diseases are identified, treatments must follow legislative guidelines for food fish.
6) *Accurate records*: Record quarantine events on the records system. Maintain records according to the associated regulations (usually at least two years).

Training and Enrichment

Animals learn with every interaction, including during feeding, cleaning, and water changes. It is enormously helpful to consider if any behavioral management in

Table A15.5 An example of a risk assessment for Nile tilapia in a culture facility.

High cost and common	High cost and uncommon	Low cost and common
Flavobacterium columnare	Betanodavirus	Poor water quality
Francisella spp.		Trichodinids
Motile aeromonad septicemia		*Dactylogyrus* spp. monogeneans
Streptococcus iniae, *S. agalactiae*		*Argulus* spp. branchiurans
Ichthyophthirius multifiliis		Copepods

quarantine will help fish adjust to their new environment, new social situation, or new diet (e.g. using a visual cue for feeding). Many fish have additional learning needs. These may include feeding at a station or desensitization to divers or touch. Operant conditioning during quarantine can also reduce stress and risk of trauma associated with husbandry behaviors (e.g. likely catch methods and diagnostic or treatment procedures). Additional details are available in Chapter A5 and in Pierce and Cheney (2008) and Kazdin (1994).

"Failing" Quarantine

Some groups may present too high a risk to clear quarantine and join an established collection. The most likely situation is a pathogen that is causing high morbidity and mortality, cannot be eliminated, and has not been seen in conspecifics in the collection. If the disease cannot be managed in quarantine, then depopulation, cleaning, and disinfection may be indicated. If only one species in a group is affected, others may be held in a prolonged quarantine for additional monitoring and testing. If the disease can be managed in quarantine, but the animals are likely to be carriers, options such as prolonged quarantine and additional testing should be discussed in detail. Accurate epidemiological information is not available for most fish diseases (e.g. likely host range), so caution is usually indicated with a valuable established collection.

One other situation is a group that presents with multiple issues or where there is chronic morbidity and mortality with varying or nonspecific findings. If their current environmental parameters are good and the group does not stabilize, they risk ongoing chronic morbidity and mortality and present an unknown risk to an established collection. These fish should typically go through a prolonged quarantine with additional testing and may still not clear quarantine if the risk to the collection is deemed too high.

Clearing Quarantine

Criteria to allow fish to clear quarantine should include the following:

- Visual examination to ensure that the fish look healthy and show no visible signs of disease.
- Review of the quarantine records.
- A set period of time from any morbidity or mortality (e.g. seven days) to reduce the risk that it represented the start of an outbreak.
- A set period of time free from medications (e.g. 7–14 days) in case of adverse reaction to the medication or in case the medications were suppressing but not clearing an infectious disease of concern.
- Diagnostic testing results, if indicated based on the risk assessment.

It is not possible to eliminate the risks of introducing infectious diseases, but through good quarantine practices and excellent husbandry and welfare standards, the risks can be reduced significantly.

Reviewing Quarantine Results

It is the responsibility of veterinarians and husbandry personnel to ensure suitable standards in quarantine and to promote responsible and sustainable quarantine practices. A part of this process is regularly reviewing quarantine goals, procedures, morbidity and mortality, and overall success rate. It is always possible to identify areas of improvement and build on quarantine success over time.

References

Crim, M.J., Lawrence, C., Livingston, R.S. et al. (2017). Comparison of antemortem and environmental samples for zebrafish health monitoring and quarantine. *Journal for the American Association of Laboratory Animal Science* 56: 412–424.

Dove, A.D.M. and Clauss, T.M. (2008). Infestations of demersal elasmobranchs in a large aquarium by the leech *Branchellion torpedinis*. *Proceedings of the Eastern Fish Health Workshop*, Atlantic Beach, NC.

Hadfield, C.A. and Clayton, L.A. (2011). Fish quarantine: current practices in public zoos and aquaria. *Journal of Zoo and Wildlife Medicine* 42: 641–650.

Kazdin, A. (1994). *Behavior Modification in Applied Settings*, 5e. Pacific Grove, CA: Brooks/Cole Publishing Company.

Kik, M.J.L., Janse, M., and Benz, G.W. (2011). The sea louse *Lepeophtheirus acutus* (Caligidae, Siphonostomatoida, Copepoda) as a pathogen of aquarium-held elasmobranchs. *Journal of Fish Diseases* 34: 793–799.

Maes, R.A. and Carmichael, G. (2002). A small-scale quarantine facility for existing fish hatcheries. *American Journal of Aquaculture* 64: 136–143.

Pierce, W. and Cheney, C. (2008). *Behavior Analysis and Learning*, 4e. New York: Psychology Press.

Poynton, S.L., Campbell, T.W., and Palm, H.W. (1997). Skin lesions in captive lemon sharks *Negaprion brevirostris* (Carcharhinidae) associated with the monogenean *Neodermophthirius harkemai* Price, 1963 (Microbothriidae). *Diseases of Aquatic Organisms* 31: 29–33.

Pye, G., Adkesson, M.J., Guthrie, A. et al. (2018). Risk analysis: changing the quarantine paradigm? *Journal of Zoo and Wildlife Medicine* 49: 513–519.

Rimmer, A.E., Becker, J.A., Tweedie, A. et al. (2015). Detection of dwarf gourami iridovirus (infectious spleen and kidney necrosis virus) in populations of ornamental fish prior to and after importation into Australia, with the first evidence of infection in domestically farmed platy (*Xiphophorus maculatus*). *Preventative Veterinary Medicine* 122: 181–194.

Whittington, R.J. and Chong, R. (2007). Global trade in ornamental fish from an Australian perspective: the case for revised import risk analysis and management strategies. *Preventative Veterinary Medicine* 81: 92–116.

Zec, S., Hadfield, C., and Hungerford, L. (2017). Retrospective review of copper sulfate immersion treatment of marine teleosts during quarantine at the National Aquarium from 2004-2016. *Proceedings of the International Association of Aquatic Animal Medicine*, Cancun, Mexico.

Section B

Presenting Problems

Introduction

Section B provides a quick reference to common clinical presentations. This is intended to help guide initial responses and point out areas for further investigation. It is arranged in chapters: acute mortalities, respiratory or cardiovascular signs, cutaneous signs, gastrointestinal or coelomic signs, musculoskeletal signs, and ocular signs. For each presentation, there is an overview of possible etiologies and diagnostic and management approaches. The most likely etiologies are mentioned first, followed by a list of differentials categorized using a DAMNVITAL acronym; the L stands for "life support system/ environmental". The diagnostic and management approaches are not meant as scripts; that is impossible with the enormous variety in the field of fish medicine. The goal is to provide some guidance and ideas.

B1

Acute Mortalities in a Group

Catherine A. Hadfield

Seattle Aquarium, Seattle, WA, USA

Overview

- Acute mortalities in a group of fish often indicate an environmental or infectious process.
- The most common differentials are low dissolved oxygen, ammonia toxicity, bacterial infections, *Ichthyophthirius multifiliis* (in freshwater), or *Cryptocaryon irritans* (in salt water).
- There are often several factors that contribute to an event. The primary etiology may be evident, but it is important to identify and resolve any contributory factors.

Signalment

- Any fish can be affected.
- Fish under severe or chronic stressors or multiple stressors are more susceptible.
- Juveniles are more susceptible.

Clinical Findings

- There may be no signs other than peracute death.
- Where signs are seen, skin or gill changes and flared operculi are common.

Etiologies

- Some etiologies are particularly common in specific scenarios.
    - Following recent fish additions: ammonia toxicity, bacterial infections, *Ichthyophthirius multifiliis*, and *Cryptocaryon irritans*.
    - During catch and transport: trauma, barotrauma, ammonia toxicity, low dissolved oxygen, and metabolic derangements (e.g. acidosis, exertional myopathy).
- Metabolic
    - Nephroliths.
- Infectious/inflammatory
    - Viruses, particularly rhabdoviruses (e.g. IHNV, VHSV, SVCV), infectious pancreatic necrosis, and some herpesviruses (e.g. KHV), ranaviruses, megalocytiviruses.
    - Bacteria, particularly vibriosis, *Aeromonas*, *Citrobacter*, *Pseudomonas*, *Edwardsiella*, *Flavobacterium*, *Yersinia*, *Streptococcus*, *Francisella* spp.
    - Fungi or fungal-like organisms, specifically atypical oomycetes.
    - Protozoa, particularly *Cryptocaryon*, *Brooklynella* spp. (SW); *Ichthyophthirius*, *Heteropolaria* spp. (FW).
    - Metazoa, particularly monogeneans (e.g. gyrodactylids, *Neobenedenia* spp.).
- Toxic
    - Ammonia, nitrites.
    - Chlorines, chloramines.
    - Heavy metals (e.g. copper).
    - Drug toxicity (e.g. inappropriate drug, inaccurate dose, contamination, idiosyncratic reaction).
    - Pesticides, herbicides, fertilizers.
    - Paint fumes.
    - Nicotine.
    - Detergents.
    - Hydrogen sulfide.
    - Cyanide.
    - Harmful algal blooms.
- Trauma
    - Cnidarian nematocysts.
- Life support system/environmental
    - Low dissolved oxygen.
    - Gas supersaturation.
    - Rapid change in water temperature, pH, salinity.
    - Electrical trauma.

Clinical Guide to Fish Medicine, First Edition. Edited by Catherine A. Hadfield and Leigh Ann Clayton.

- Severe weather (e.g. lightning, heavy rain).
- Loss of water.

Diagnostic Approach

- Visually assess the animals.
  - Identify the species, size classes, and percentage of population impacted.
  - Identify clinical signs, particularly changes to the skin or fins, respiratory rate and effort, or behavior.
- Visually assess the habitat.
  - Stagnant or turbid water may suggest low dissolved oxygen or ammonia toxicity, particularly with abundant organic material.
  - Microbubbles in the system and ocular or skin gas bubbles in the fish suggest gas supersaturation.
  - Look for sources of possible contaminants above or around the system (e.g. drips falling into the water, recent painting, fertilizer use near a pond).
- Check the life support system (e.g. pumps that are not running, loose airlines, water pooling on the ground). If possible, assess the system for stray voltage over 24–48 hours.
- Check the water quality, particularly temperature, dissolved oxygen, ammonia, salinity, pH, copper, and chlorine. Compare results to target ranges and any previous records.
- Freeze 1 L of water in a clean plastic bottle for later analysis if needed (e.g. for pesticides, cations, drugs). In the United States, state fish diagnostic laboratories can often help identify water testing options.
- Consider freezing a sample of the top layer of sediment or substrate for later analysis (e.g. for pesticides). Water bottles or sturdy bags can be used.
- Review the recent history, in particular:
  - When animals were first added to the system.
  - Recent animal additions and the history of those animals.
  - Quarantine and other biosecurity protocols.
  - When animals were last fed and the feeding response.
  - Water source and any additives used (e.g. salts, conditioners).
  - Volume and timing of recent water changes.
  - When the mortalities started and which species were affected.
  - Known causes of prior morbidity and mortality.
  - Recent medications, including applied doses and method of dosing.
  - Recent life support system changes.
  - Recent weather for outdoor systems (e.g. lightning, heavy rain).
- Examine the mortalities. The best diagnostic samples are collected from sick fish that were recently euthanized. However, earlier mortalities can still be helpful. Start with the freshest fish (i.e. reddest gills) as soon as possible. Collect skin scrapes, gill biopsies, and fin biopsies to examine under direct microscopy. Most ectoparasites on the differential list can be identified with these diagnostics. If no cause is identified from those samples, carry out a full necropsy with additional testing as indicated, e.g.:
  - Photographs.
  - Cultures, particularly bacterial (e.g. blood, liver, kidney).
  - Wet mounts and impression smears (e.g. liver, spleen, kidney, gastrointestinal tract, any lesions).
  - Histology.
  - Further diagnostics (e.g. swabs or tissues for PCR testing for IHNV, VHSV, SVCV, KHV, *Yersinia ruckeri*).
  - Archive samples (e.g. gill, muscle, liver, spleen, kidney, brain, frozen at −20°C (−4°F) or ideally −80°C (−112°F) and fixed in 95% ethanol and electron microscopy fixative).
  - Label all samples fully.
- Limit diagnostics on surviving fish to situations where the cause has not been identified from the other sources of information, to minimize further stress on those fish.
- If unexpected mortalities occurred after a drug exposure, confirm the identity of the drug, record lot numbers and acquisition dates, and save a sample; some pharmaceutical companies may be able to assess content or purity.

Management Approach

- Remove dead fish as soon as possible, place in labeled bags, and refrigerate or put on ice for necropsy.
- If there are no obvious signs of gas supersaturation (e.g. microbubbles in the water or ocular and skin gas bubbles), increase aeration and water flow; target dissolved oxygen may be 95–100%.
- If the source water is considered appropriate (i.e. similar temperature, salinity and pH, with no risk of contamination), carry out a 20–50% water change.
- Remove any decomposing plants and organic debris.
- Treat or manage any known problems (e.g. restore power, discontinue medication, add activated carbon filtration, treat with suitable antiparasitic or antibacterial).
- If a known problem cannot be corrected (e.g. contamination of a pond) or the cause is unknown and a suitable system exists, consider moving the fish. Minimize stress on the fish through a short, atraumatic catch and transport and provide an acclimation (gradually introducing

the new water). A move is usually contraindicated if fish are showing severe dyspnea. If in doubt, move one to two fish and assess their response.

- In freshwater systems, consider supplementation with salt (sodium chloride or a commercial salt mix) at 2–3 g/L to reduce osmotic stress.
- Reduce feeding in the short term unless fish are very small or emaciated.
- Reduce lighting and visual stressors; this may include covering tank windows.
- Consider short courses of corticosteroids to reduce the inflammatory response that is commonly seen in sick fish (e.g. dexamethasone SP 0.5–1.0 mg/kg IM for 2–3 doses).
- If mortalities were high (e.g. 90%) due to an infectious or toxic cause, consider euthanasia of the remaining fish, as prognosis for the whole group is usually poor.
- Continue to monitor the fish and the system closely in case of secondary disease.

Abbreviations/Acronyms

- FW: Freshwater
- IHNV: Infectious hematopoietic necrosis virus
- KHV: Koi herpesvirus
- PCR: Polymerase chain reaction
- SVCV: Spring viremia of carp virus
- SW: Salt water
- VHSV: Viral hemorrhagic septicemia virus

B2

Respiratory or Cardiovascular Signs

Catherine A. Hadfield

Seattle Aquarium, Seattle, WA, USA

Dyspnea and Tachypnea

Overview

- Dyspnea and tachypnea are common presentations in fish.
- These clinical signs represent a true emergency and can affect a single fish or an entire system. Associated mortality can be high.
- Dyspnea and tachypnea in a group of fish are typically due to an environmental problem or an acute ectoparasitic or bacterial disease causing gill damage or anemia.
- There are often several factors that contribute to an event. The primary etiology may be evident, but it is important to identify and resolve any contributory factors.

Signalment

- Any fish can be affected.
- Fish under severe or chronic stressors or multiple stressors are more susceptible.
- Air-breathing fish are less susceptible (see Table A1.1).

Clinical Findings

- One or more fish may be affected.
- Dyspnea is often easier to appreciate than tachypnea. In general, opercular or gill slit movement in fish is subtle. Dyspnea may be represented by increased flaring of the operculi or gill slits, gaping of the mouth, and head or body movements associated with ventilation.
- Tachypnea can be assessed by measuring respiratory rate against prior values or normal conspecifics.
- Fish may gather near areas of highest oxygen, i.e. at the surface, near inflowing water, or near areas of turbulence. Gasping at the surface may be seen (piping).
- Rigid body posture or reduced responsiveness to food or other stimuli may be seen.
- Oral or gill pathology may be grossly visible.
- Mortalities may show obvious opercular flaring and mouth gaping (Figure B2.1).

Etiologies

- The most common differentials are low dissolved oxygen, ammonia toxicity, contaminated water, columnaris, ciliates, and monogeneans.
- Neoplasia/hyperplasia
  - Goiter.
  - Oral, pharyngeal, branchial.
- Vascular
  - Anemia.
  - Cardiovascular disease.
- Infectious/inflammatory (branchial or systemic)
  - Viruses, particularly KHV, herpesviral hematopoietic necrosis, carp edema virus, infectious salmon anemia, Atlantic salmon paramyxovirus.
  - Bacteria, particularly *Flavobacterium* spp.
  - Fungi or fungal-like organisms, particularly *Branchiomyces* spp., oomycetes, some *Microsporidia*.
  - Protozoa, particularly *Cryptocaryon*, *Brooklynella*, *Ichthyobodo*, *Amyloodinium* spp., scuticociliates, amoebic gill disease (SW); *Ichthyophthirius*, *Chilodonella*, *Cryptobia*, *Ichthyobodo*, *Piscinoodinium* spp., trichodinids, scuticociliates, sessile ciliates (e.g. *Heteropolaria*, *Capriniana* spp.) (FW).
  - Metazoa, particularly capsalids, dactylogyrids, gyrodactylids, polyopisthocotyles, blood flukes (aporocotylids/sanguinicolids), leeches, copepods, isopods.
  - Myxozoa, particularly *Henneguya* spp., *Myxobolus koi*.

Clinical Guide to Fish Medicine, First Edition. Edited by Catherine A. Hadfield and Leigh Ann Clayton.

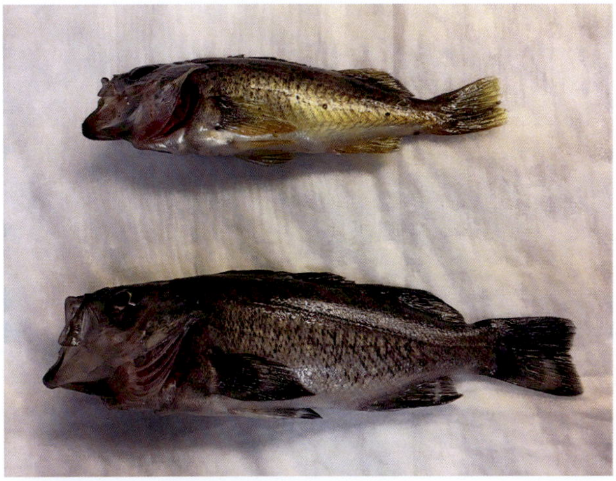

Figure B2.1 Flared operculi and gaping mouths in two rockfish (*Sebastes* spp.) presented for necropsy.

- Toxic
  - Ammonia, nitrites, nitrates.
  - Chlorines, chloramines.
  - Heavy metals (e.g. copper, lead, iron).
  - Drug toxicity (e.g. inappropriate drug, inaccurate dose, contamination, idiosyncratic reaction).
  - Hydrogen sulfide.
  - Cyanide.
  - Harmful algal blooms.
- Trauma
  - Cohort, décor, or catch trauma.
  - Barotrauma.
  - Aggression, displacement, chasing.
  - Cnidarian nematocysts.
- Life support system/environmental
  - Low dissolved oxygen.
  - Gas supersaturation.
  - High water temperature.
  - Excessive turbidity.
  - Rapid change in pH.

Diagnostic Approach

- Visually assess the animals.
  - Identify the species, size classes, and percentage of population impacted.
  - Identify any other clinical signs, particularly to try to differentiate between acute disease (e.g. erythema, flashing) or chronic or acute-on-chronic disease (e.g. weight loss, poor coloration).
- Visually assess the habitat.
  - Stagnant or turbid water may suggest low dissolved oxygen or ammonia toxicity, particularly with abundant organic material.
  - Microbubbles in the system and ocular or skin gas bubbles in the fish suggest gas supersaturation.
- Check the life support system (e.g. pumps that are not running, loose airlines).
- Check the water quality, particularly temperature, dissolved oxygen, ammonia, pH, and chlorine. Compare results to target ranges and any previous records.
- Review the recent history, in particular:
  - When animals were first added to the system.
  - Recent animal additions and the history of those animals.
  - Quarantine and other biosecurity protocols.
  - When animals were last fed and the feeding response.
  - Water source and any additives used (e.g. salts, conditioners).
  - Volume and timing of recent water changes.
  - Any recent mortalities.
  - Known causes of prior morbidity and mortality.
  - Recent medications, including applied doses and method of dosing.
  - Recent life support system changes.
  - Recent weather for outdoor systems (e.g. lightning, heavy rain).
- Examine any mortalities, if available. The best diagnostic samples are collected from sick fish that were recently euthanized. Start with the freshest fish (i.e. reddest gills) as soon as possible. Examine the oral cavity and gills. Collect skin scrapes and gill biopsies to examine under direct microscopy (Figure B2.2). If no cause is identified from those samples, carry out a full necropsy with additional testing as indicated, e.g.:
  - Wet mounts and impression smears (e.g. liver, spleen, kidney, any lesions).
  - Histology.
  - Further diagnostics (e.g. swabs or tissues for PCR testing for KHV).
  - Archive samples (e.g. gill, liver, kidney, frozen at −20°C (−4°F) or ideally −80°C (−112°F) and fixed in 95% ethanol and electron microscopy fixative).
- If the cause is still unknown, handling of live fish is often required. Fish that are dyspneic or tachypneic can decompensate with handling: minimize the number of fish examined, provide a short and atraumatic catch and restraint, and provide high levels of dissolved oxygen. Be prepared to ventilate the fish manually.
  - Examine the oral cavity for any mass effect or other changes.
  - Examine the gills for color, structure, and obvious ectoparasites or masses.
  - Examine skin scrapes and gill biopsies under direct microscopy.
  - Consider blood samples to assess PCV, TS, blood gases, lactate, and additional hematology.

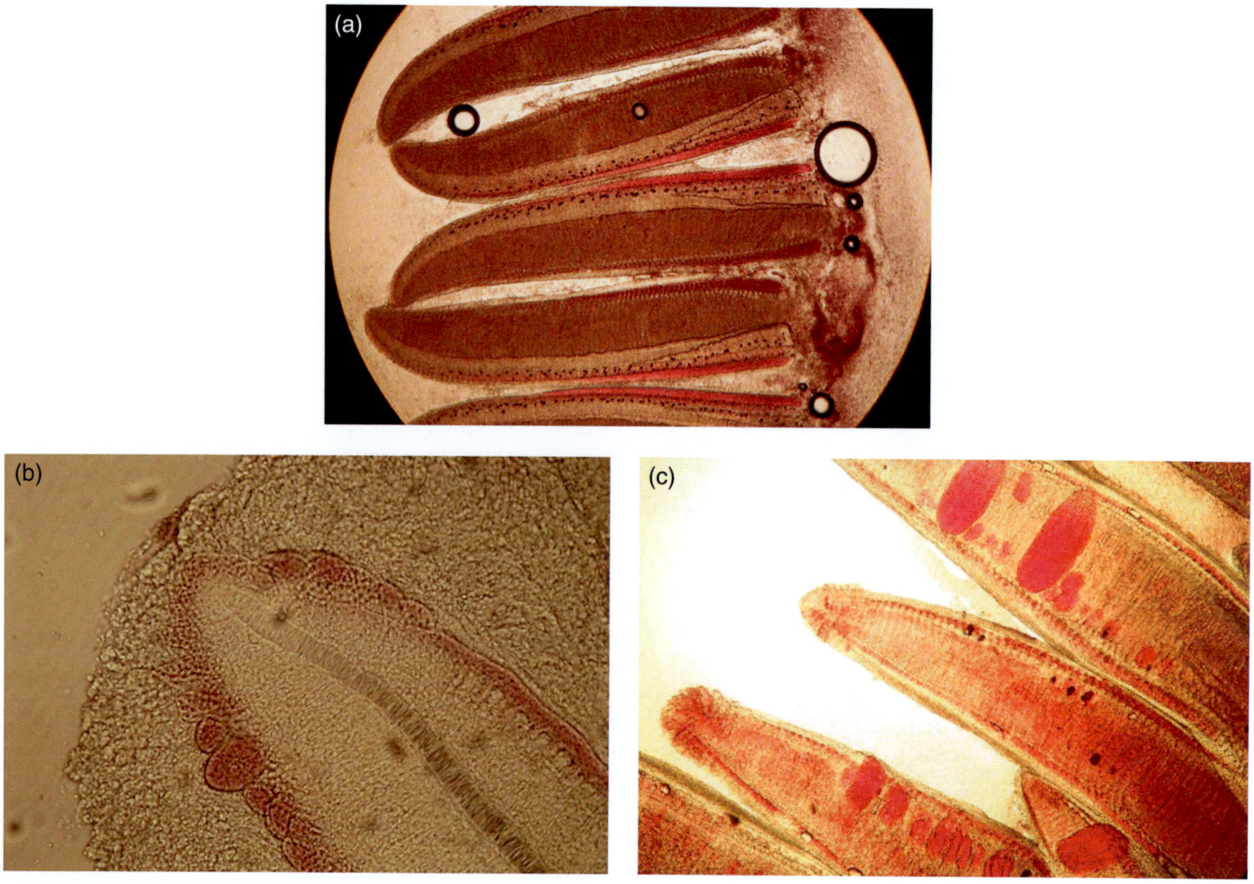

Figure B2.2 Gill wet mounts under direct microscopy: normal gills (a), increased mucus (b), and telangiectasia (c).

Management Approach

- Remove dead fish as soon as possible, place in labeled bags, and refrigerate or put on ice for necropsy.
- If there are no obvious signs of gas supersaturation (e.g. microbubbles in the water or ocular and skin gas bubbles), increase aeration and water flow; target dissolved oxygen may be 95–100%.
- If the source water is considered appropriate (i.e. similar temperature, salinity and pH, with no risk of contamination), carry out a 20–50% water change.
- Remove any decomposing plants and organic debris.
- Treat or manage any known problems (e.g. restore power, discontinue medications, add activated carbon filtration, treat with suitable antiparasitic or antibacterial).
- In freshwater systems, consider supplementation with salt (sodium chloride or a commercial salt mix) at 2–3 g/L to reduce osmotic stress.
- Reduce feeding in the short term unless fish are very small or emaciated.
- Reduce lighting and visual stressors; this may include covering tank windows.
- Consider short courses of corticosteroids to reduce the inflammatory response that is commonly seen in sick fish (e.g. dexamethasone SP 0.5–1.0 mg/kg IM for 2–3 doses).
- Continue to monitor the fish and the system closely in case of secondary disease.

Abbreviations/Acronyms

- FW: Freshwater
- KHV: Koi herpesvirus
- PCR: Polymerase chain reaction
- PCV: Packed cell volume
- SW: Salt water
- TS: Total solids

Gill Pallor

Overview

- Gill pallor in living fish is typically due to anemia and may be associated with lethargy, dyspnea, or tachypnea.
- Anemia in a group of fish may indicate an infectious disease, nutritional deficiency, or toxin.
- Following death, gills become pale then tan-colored due to autolysis. This should not be overinterpreted as pathology.

Signalment

- Any fish can be affected.

Clinical Findings

- One or more fish may be affected.
- Normal gill color in living fish is dark red (Figure B2.3a).
- Abnormal gills may be pale red, pink, brown, gray, yellow, or white (Figure B2.3b–c). Lesions may be focal, multifocal, or generalized.
- Parasites or other pathology may be seen on the skin or gills.
- Lethargy, dyspnea, or tachypnea may be seen.

Etiologies

- The most common differentials are infectious and toxic.
- Artifact
  - Postmortem.
  - Autolysis.
- Nutritional
  - Deficiency of vitamin C, E, K, several Bs (e.g. folate, niacin, pantothenic acid, pyridoxine), iron.
  - Suboptimal fatty acid or carbohydrate composition of diet.
- Neoplasia
  - Particularly hematopoietic, kidney, spleen.

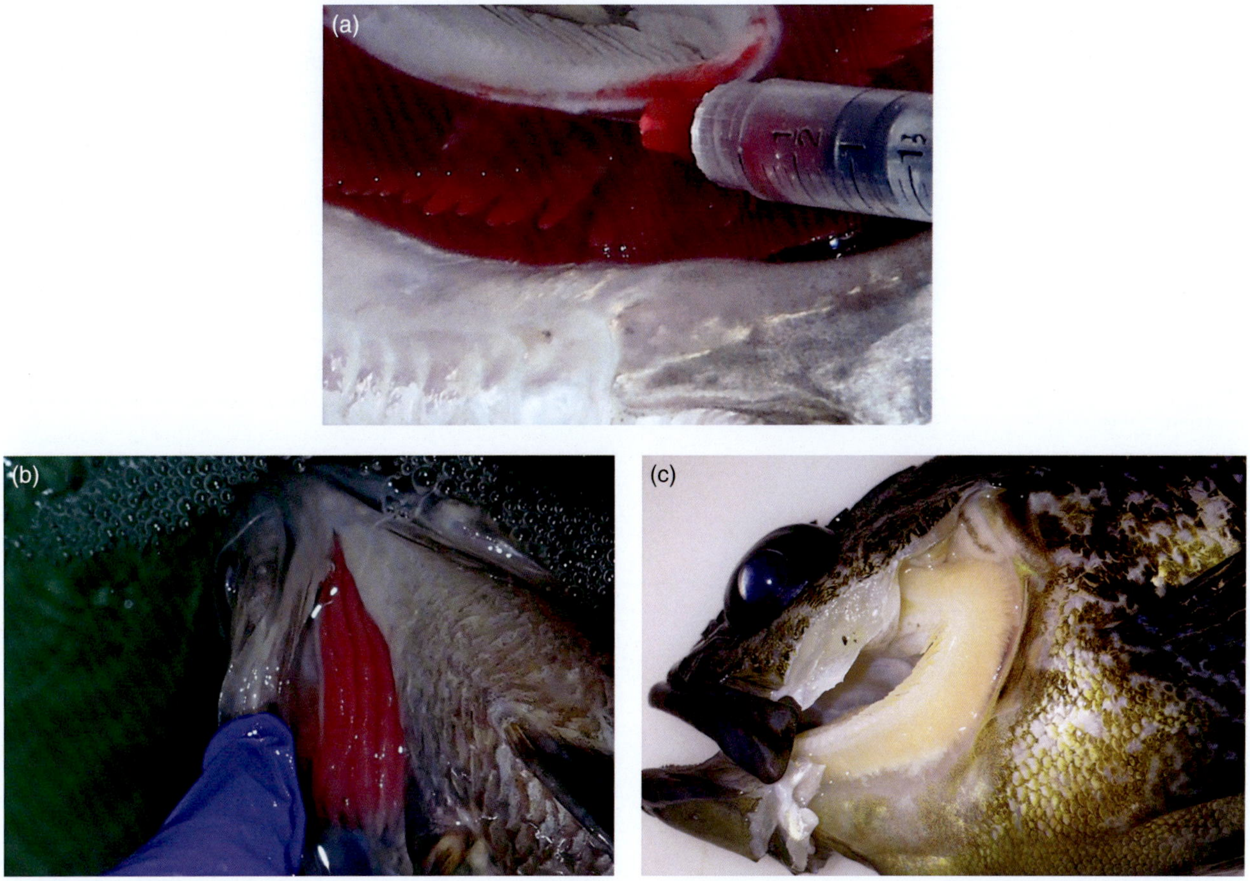

Figure B2.3 Normal dark red gills (seen during venipuncture) (a), moderate gill pallor (b), and severe gill pallor (c) in bony fish.

- Infectious (through hemorrhage, hemolysis, or chronic disease)
  - Most viruses, particularly rhabdoviruses (e.g. IHNV, VHSV, SVCV), some herpesviruses (e.g. KHV), carp edema virus, red seabream iridovirus, infectious salmon anemia, viral erythrocytic necrosis, erythrocytic inclusion body syndrome.
  - Most bacteria, such as vibriosis, *Aeromonas*, *Yersinia*, *Edwardsiella*, *Mycobacterium*, *Flavobacterium*, *Francisella*, piscirickettsial-like spp.
  - Chronic fungal infections.
  - Protozoa, particularly *Ichthyobodo*, *Cryptobia* spp., scuticociliates, trypanosomes.
  - Metazoa, particularly gill monogeneans, polyopisthocotyles, blood flukes (aporocotylids/sanguinicolids), leeches, anguillicolid nematodes, copepods.
  - Chronic myxozoan infections.
  - Apicomplexa, particularly gregarines, piroplasms.
- Inflammatory
  - Vasculitis.
  - Transfusion reaction.
- Idiopathic
  - Chronic liver disease.
  - Chronic kidney disease.
- Toxic
  - Nitrites, nitrates.
  - Chlorines.
  - Heavy metals (e.g. copper, lead, zinc).
  - Hydrogen sulfide.
  - Anticoagulants.
  - Mycotoxins.
- Trauma
  - Cohort, décor, or catch trauma.

Diagnostic Approach

- Review the history, in particular:
  - Recent animal additions and the history of those animals.
  - Food eaten, including storage and preparation.
  - Known causes of prior morbidity and mortality.
  - Chronicity of clinical signs.
- Visually assess the animals, in particular check for:
  - Dyspnea or tachypnea.
  - Erythema, hyperemia, or ulcers that may suggest systemic inflammation.
  - Obvious signs of external trauma.
  - Bloody discharges.
  - Large parasites such as leeches.
- Check the water quality, particularly nitrite, copper, chlorine, and zinc if possible. Compare results to target ranges and any previous records.
- Necropsy any mortalities, if available. The best diagnostic samples are collected from sick fish that were recently euthanized. There is likely to be generalized pallor of the gills, heart, spleen, kidney, and intestinal tract. Splenomegaly, hepatomegaly, or renomegaly may be seen if the anemia is hemolytic or has an infectious etiology. Include additional testing as indicated, e.g.:
  - Peripheral blood smears and hematology, if fresh enough.
  - Cultures, often bacterial, mycobacterial, and fungal (e.g. blood, kidney).
  - Wet mounts and impression smears (e.g. gill, skin, liver, spleen, kidney, gastrointestinal tract, any lesions).
  - Histology.
  - Further diagnostics (e.g. swabs or tissues for PCR testing for KHV or infectious salmon anemia virus).
  - Archive samples (e.g. gill, liver, spleen, kidney, frozen at −20°C (−4°F) or ideally −80°C (−112°F) and fixed in 95% ethanol and electron microscopy fixative).
- Examine fecal samples under direct microscopy and floatation to look for intestinal parasites.
- If the cause is still unknown, handling of live fish is often required. Fish that are dyspneic or tachypneic can decompensate with handling: minimize the number of fish examined, provide a short and atraumatic catch and restraint, and provide high levels of dissolved oxygen. Be prepared to ventilate the fish manually.
  - Examine the skin, eyes, gills, oral cavity, and cloaca/anus for gross abnormalities or parasites.
  - Examine skin scrapes and gill biopsies under direct microscopy (unless the gills are white).
  - Collect a blood sample for culture, hematology, biochemistry, and heavy metal levels. Samples from the ventral tail vein/artery typically provide the most reliable results. A reduced PCV and total solids or total proteins is required to show anemia. The type of anemia and chronicity is often hard to determine in fish, but if a fish is asymptomatic with a PCV of <8%, it is likely to be chronic. Note that sampling effects can falsely indicate anemia, e.g. small needle size, excessive negative pressure, or rapid temperature change.
  - Consider radiography and ultrasonography to look for coelomic masses, effusions, or ingested foreign bodies.
  - Collect an aspirate of any coelomic effusion for cultures, cytology, and fluid analysis.
  - Consider an aspirate or biopsy of the cranial kidney in bony fish to look for changes in hematopoiesis; the sample should be sent to a clinical pathologist with experience in fish histology.

Management Approach

- Increase aeration and water flow; target dissolved oxygen may be 95–100%.
- Treat or manage any known problems (e.g. treat polyopisthocotyles, separate aggressive fish).
- If a toxin is suspected and suitable water exists, carry out a 20–50% water change once daily for several days or consider moving the fish.
- Improve the diet or food handling, if indicated.
- Provide supportive care of individual fish (e.g. fluid therapy, blood transfusion, erythropoietin or darbepoetin treatment, nutritional support, analgesia).

Abbreviations/Acronyms

- IHNV: Infectious hematopoietic necrosis virus
- KHV: Koi herpesvirus
- PCR: Polymerase chain reaction
- PCV: Packed cell volume
- SVCV: Spring viremia of carp virus
- VHSV: Viral hemorrhagic septicemia virus

B3

Cutaneous Signs

Catherine A. Hadfield

Seattle Aquarium, Seattle, WA, USA

Red/Erosive Skin Lesions

Overview

- Erythema, hyperemia, skin ulcers, and fin erosions are common in fish.
- A single lesion without other signs is most commonly due to trauma or focal inflammation.
- Diffuse or multifocal lesions are usually an indication of systemic inflammation, which may have a bacterial, parasitic, viral, fungal, or toxic etiology.

Signalment

- Any fish can be affected.

Clinical Findings

- Focal ulcers or erosions with hyperemia and edema are often inflammatory.
- Focal ulcers without inflammation look like an area of scale loss or exposure of fascia, muscle, or bone with no hyperemia or edema.
- Diffuse erythema or hyperemia and multifocal ulcers or erosions are often indicators of systemic inflammation (Figure B3.1). They may be associated with lethargy, reduced appetite, dyspnea, tachypnea, or mortalities.

Etiologies

- Neoplasia
  - Cutaneous, e.g. papillomatosis, dermal sarcoma.
- Infectious/inflammatory
  - Viruses particularly rhabdoviruses (e.g. IHNV, VHSV, SVCV), infectious pancreatic necrosis virus, carp edema virus, and some herpesviruses (e.g. KHV), ranaviruses, megalocytiviruses.
  - Most bacteria, particularly vibriosis, *Aeromonas*, *Citrobacter*, *Pseudomonas*, *Edwardsiella*, *Flavobacterium*, *Tenacibaculum*, *Yersinia*, *Streptococcus*, *Erysipelothrix*, *Francisella*, *Mycobacterium*, *Nocardia*, piscirickettsial-like spp.
  - Fungi or fungal-like organisms, particularly atypical oomycetes, *Fusarium* spp.
  - Protozoa, particularly scuticociliates, *Chilodonella*, *Heteropolaria*, *Spironucleus*, *Ichthyobodo* spp.
  - Metazoa, particularly monogeneans, copepods, leeches.
- Toxic
  - Ammonia.
  - Polycyclic aromatic hydrocarbons, organochlorines.
  - Drug toxicity (e.g. inappropriate drug, contamination, idiosyncratic reaction).
  - Detergents.
- Trauma
  - Conspecific or interspecific aggression.
  - Abrasions from inappropriate enclosure size, shape, substrate, walls, or décor, or due to startling stimuli.
  - Catch or handling trauma.
  - Fish spine perforation.
  - Positive buoyancy and exposure to air.
  - Negative buoyancy and damage from the substrate.
- Life support system/environmental
  - Sunburn or excess UV light exposure.

Clinical Guide to Fish Medicine, First Edition. Edited by Catherine A. Hadfield and Leigh Ann Clayton.

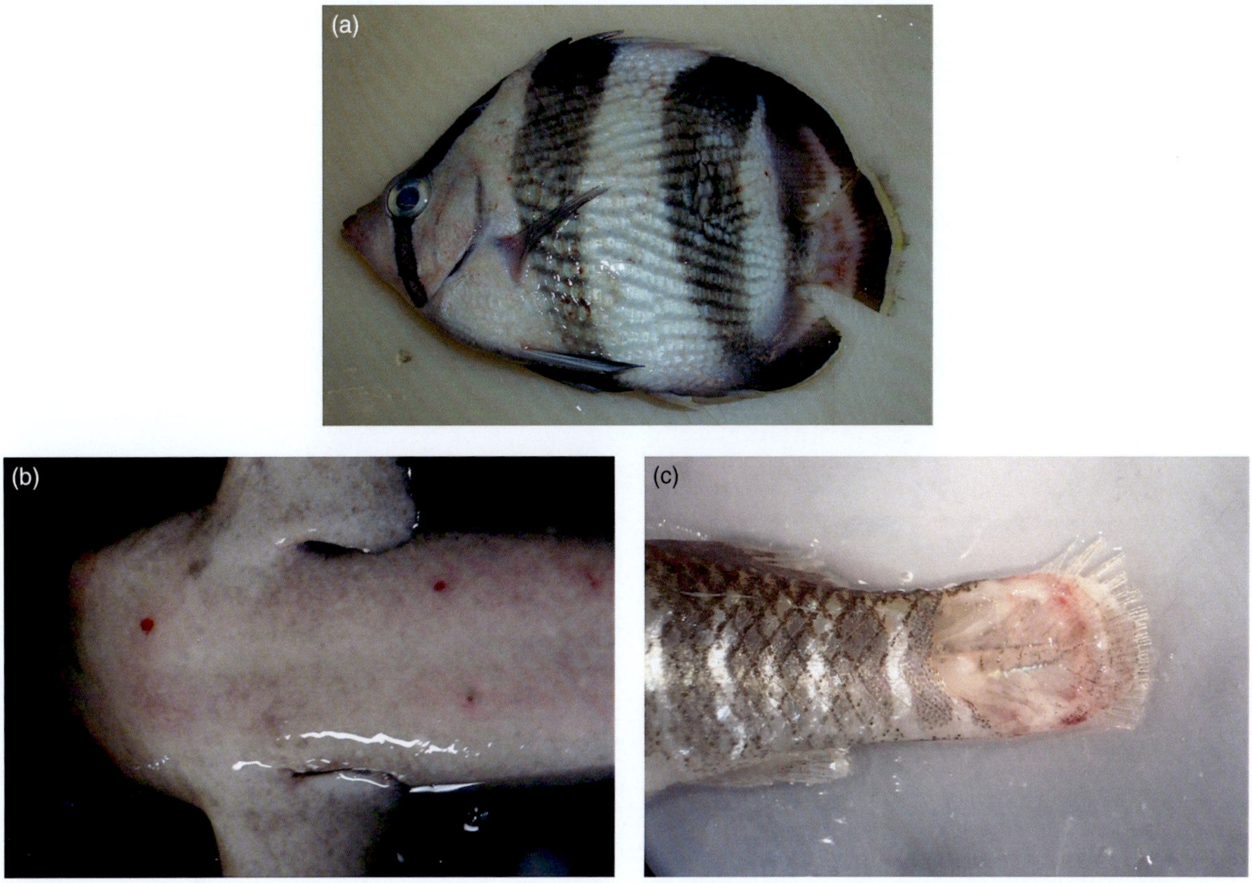

Figure B3.1 Signs of systemic inflammation including generalized hyperemia in a banded butterflyfish (*Chaetodon striatus*) (a), cutaneous ulcers in a whitetip reef shark (*Triaenodon obesus*) (b), and fin and peduncle erosions in a killifish (*Fundulus* sp.) (c).

  - Residual oxidants.
  - Inappropriate pH.
  - Rapid change in water temperature or high water temperature.

Diagnostic Approach

- Review the history, in particular:
  - Recent animal additions and the history of those animals.
  - Quarantine and other biosecurity protocols.
  - Water source and any additives used (e.g. salts, conditioners).
  - Any recent mortalities.
  - Known causes of prior morbidity and mortality.
  - Recent handling or transport.
  - Chronicity and progression of clinical signs.
- Check the water quality. Compare results to target ranges and any previous records.
- Visually assess the animals.
  - Identify the species, size classes, and percentage of population impacted.
  - Assess the severity and location of lesions.
  - Observe the social dynamics in the system for signs of aggression or displacement.
- Visually assess the habitat.
  - Look for possible sources of trauma (e.g. rough fiberglass, lack of appropriate resting space, right-angled corners or tight turning circles for pelagic species).
- Necropsy any mortalities, if available. The best diagnostic samples are collected from sick fish that were recently euthanized. Include additional testing as indicated, e.g.:
  - Cultures, often bacterial, mycobacterial, and fungal (e.g. blood, liver, kidney).
  - Wet mounts and impression smears (e.g. gill, skin, liver, spleen, kidney, gastrointestinal tract, any lesions).

- Histology.
- Further diagnostics (e.g. swabs or tissues for PCR testing for IHNV, VHSV, SVCV, KHV, *Yersinia ruckeri*).
- Archive samples (e.g. gill, muscle, liver, spleen, kidney, frozen at −20°C (−4°F) or ideally −80°C (−112°F) and fixed in 95% ethanol and electron microscopy fixative).

- If the cause is still unknown, handling of live fish is often required; anesthesia should be used to facilitate restraint.
  - Perform a full clinical examination.
  - Examine skin scrapes of the affected areas under direct microscopy and impression smears (e.g. Dif-Quik, Gram, and acid-fast stains).
  - Examine gill biopsies under direct microscopy and potentially histology.
  - Consider biopsies of the edges of skin lesions for histology.
  - Consider blood cultures and cultures from under the edges of skin lesions.
  - Consider endoscopic coeliotomy for biopsies and cultures of the liver or spleen.
- Consider diagnostic freshwater or salt water dips (matched to pH and temperature) to look for ectoparasites.

Management Approach

- Reduce or remove any possible sources of trauma, e.g. adjust the social structure, add soft barriers such as bubbles or kelp strips to keep pelagic animals off the walls, remove abrasive décor.
- Treat any identified bacterial pathogens, ideally based on cytology, culture, and sensitivity results. However, empirical antibiotic therapy may be used based on most likely pathogens.
- Treat any identified parasites or other etiologies.
- Reduce or resolve stressors.
- Consider slightly increasing the salinity with freshwater fish or slightly decreasing the salinity with salt water teleosts to reduce the osmotic stress.
- Consider analgesia and anti-inflammatory medications, e.g. short courses of corticosteroids.
- If the lesions are severe and fish do not show a rapid improvement with management, prognosis is guarded.

Abbreviations/Acronyms

- IHNV: Infectious hematopoietic necrosis virus
- KHV: Koi herpesvirus
- SVCV: Spring viremia of carp virus
- UV: Ultraviolet
- VHSV: Viral hemorrhagic septicemia virus

Light Skin Lesions

Overview

- Light-colored skin lesions are common in fish, particularly white spots, but plaques and filamentous lesions are also seen.
- If white spots are seen on teleosts, it is important to rapidly identify or rule out *Cryptocaryon irritans* (in salt water) and *Ichthyophthirius multifiliis* (in freshwater). These can be highly pathogenic and a rapid response is critical.
- If these parasites are ruled out, a number of other differentials should be considered for white spots. Diagnosis can usually be based on skin scrapes and gill biopsies examined under direct microscopy.
- Pale plaques are more typically viral in origin, but these can look like spots early in the disease process.

Signalment

- Any fish can be affected, particularly bony fish.

Clinical Findings

- One or more fish may be affected.
- Multifocal light-colored lesions typically cluster into the following categories.
  - Small white spots, often associated with other signs such as increased hiding, dark coloration, dyspnea, tachypnea, pruritus, or mortalities.
  - Large, cream-colored foci or plaques, particularly on the fins, usually with no other signs.
  - White cotton-like lesions, often associated with underlying skin erosions. The material may become gray, brown, or green over time.
  - Fine, round or linear bubbles that catch the light, which may be associated with other signs such as lethargy.

Etiologies

- The most common differentials can be tentatively based on appearance.
  - Small spots are often due to *Cryptocaryon* (Figure B3.2), *Ichthyophthirius*, sessile ciliates, monogeneans, or *Flavobacterium* spp.
  - Plaques are often viral.

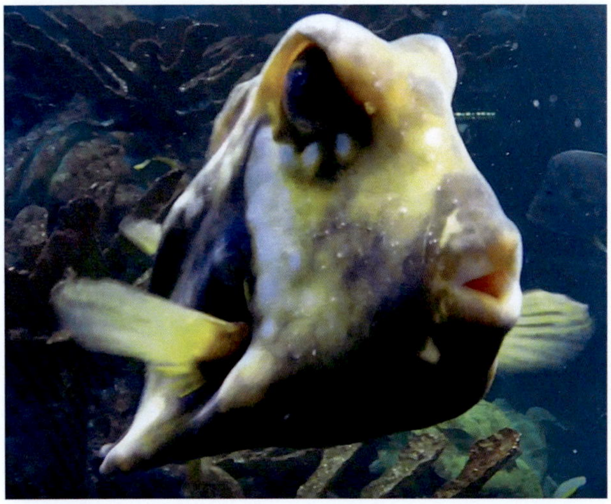

Figure B3.2 White spots due to *Cryptocaryon irritans* in a smooth trunkfish (*Lactophrys triqueter*). *Source*: Image courtesy of New England Aquarium.

  - Cotton-like lesions are often due to oomycetes or sessile ciliates.
  - Bubbles are often due to gas supersaturation.
- Metabolic
  - Calcinosis cutis or calcinosis circumscripta.
- Neoplasia
  - Cutaneous, e.g. papillomatosis, dermal sarcoma.
- Normal anatomy
  - Nuptial tubercles of male cyprinids during the breeding season.
- Infectious/inflammatory
  - Viruses, particularly lymphocystis, carp pox, adenoviruses.
  - Bacteria, particularly *Mycobacterium*, *Nocardia*, *Edwardsiella*, *Streptococcus*, *Flavobacterium*, *Tenacibaculum* spp., *Renibacterium salmoninarum*, epitheliocystis or other CLOs.
  - Fungi or fungal-like organisms, particularly oomycetes, microsporidian xenomas (e.g. *Glugea* spp.), *Mesomycetozoea*.
  - Protozoa, particularly *Cryptocaryon* spp., scuticociliates, *Amyloodinium* spp., amoebic gill disease (SW); *Ichthyophthirius* spp., scuticociliates, sessile ciliates (e.g. *Heteropolaria* spp.) (FW).
  - Metazoa, particularly monopisthocotyle monogeneans, digenean metacercariae, turbellaria, leeches, copepods, branchiurans, mussel glochidia.
  - Myxozoa, particularly *Henneguya* spp.
- Trauma
  - Venomous fin ray (e.g. lionfish) or barb (e.g. stingray).
  - Foreign bodies (e.g. fiberglass, gravel).
  - Abrasions from inappropriate enclosure size, shape, substrate, walls, or décor.
- Life support system/environmental
  - Gas supersaturation.

Diagnostic Approach

- Review the history, in particular:
  - Recent animal additions and the history of those animals.
  - Quarantine and other biosecurity protocols.
  - Water source.
  - Any recent mortalities.
  - Known causes of prior morbidity and mortality.
  - Recent life support system changes.
  - Chronicity and progression of clinical signs.
- Visually assess the animals.
  - Identify the species, size classes, and percentage of population impacted.
  - Identify any other clinical signs, particularly increased hiding, pruritus, dyspnea, or tachypnea.
- Check the water quality. Compare results to target ranges and any previous records.
- Necropsy any mortalities, if available. The best diagnostic samples are collected from sick fish that were recently euthanized. Examine the skin and gills. Collect skin scrapes, gill biopsies, and fin biopsies to examine under direct microscopy. Most differentials can be identified with these diagnostics. Consider additional testing as indicated, e.g.:
  - Histology of skin and gill samples.
  - Cultures, often bacterial (e.g. from within or under lesions).
  - Archive samples (e.g. skin and gill frozen at −20°C (−4°F) or ideally −80°C (−112°F) and fixed in 95% ethanol and electron microscopy fixative).
- If the cause is still unknown, handling of live fish is recommended; anesthesia should be used to facilitate restraint, but since immersion anesthesia can affect parasite loads, samples should be taken as soon as the fish are sufficiently sedated.
  - Perform a full clinical examination.
  - Examine skin scrapes, gill biopsies, and fin biopsies on several affected fish.
  - Consider biopsy of lesions for histology and culture if no ectoparasites were found.
- Consider diagnostic freshwater or salt water dips (matched to pH and temperature) to look for ectoparasites.

Management Approach

- If there are no obvious signs of gas supersaturation (e.g. microbubbles in the water or ocular and skin gas bubbles), increase aeration and water flow; target dissolved oxygen may be 95–100%.
- Reduce or resolve stressors.
- Further management depends on the cause (see Section C).

Abbreviations/Acronyms

- CLO: Chlamydia-like organisms
- FW: Freshwater
- SW: Salt water

Dark Skin Lesions

Overview

- Dark spots or plaques on the skin are less common in fish than light-colored spots.
- The most common cause is encysted digenes.
- In general, morbidity and mortality from these lesions are low and investigation is not as urgent as with white spots, although *Amyloodinium* can cause more severe signs.

Signalment

- Any fish can be affected, particularly bony fish.

Clinical Findings

- One or more fish may be affected.
- Dark foci or plaques are often chronic.
- Fish typically show no other clinical signs.
- If lesions are associated with clinical signs, particularly dyspnea, tachypnea, or pruritus, diagnostics are more urgent.

Etiologies

- The most common differential is encysted digenes.
- Neoplasia/hyperplasia.
  - Cutaneous.
- Normal
  - Nuptial tubercles on male cyprinids during the breeding season.
  - Anal fin spots on some male African cichlids during the breeding season.
- Infectious/inflammatory
  - Bacteria, particularly *Flavobacterium*, *Tenacibaculum* spp.
  - Fungi or fungal-like organisms, particularly oomycetes.
  - Protozoa, particularly *Amyloodinium* spp.
  - Metazoa, particularly digenes (e.g. *Clinostomum* spp.), capsalid and monocotylid monogeneans, turbellaria, leeches, nematodes (e.g. *Huffmanela* spp.), copepods, branchiurans.
- Trauma
  - Venomous fin ray (e.g. lionfish) or barb (e.g. stingray).
  - Foreign bodies.
  - Abrasions from inappropriate enclosure size, shape, substrate, walls, or décor.

Diagnostic Approach

- Review the history, in particular:
  - Recent animal additions and the history of those animals.
  - Quarantine and other biosecurity protocols.
  - Access to snail hosts (currently or in the past).
  - Chronicity and progression of clinical signs.
- Visually assess the animals.
  - Identify the species, size classes, and percentage of population impacted.
  - Identify any other clinical signs.
- Check the water quality. Compare results to target ranges and any previous records.
- Handling of live fish is usually required for diagnosis; anesthesia should be used to facilitate restraint.
  - Perform a full clinical examination.
  - Examine skin scrapes, gill biopsies, and fin biopsies on several affected fish, targeting the lesions.
  - Consider biopsy of lesions for histology.

Management Approach

- Reduce or resolve stressors.
- Further management depends on the cause (see Section C); no management changes may be indicated for encysted digenes.

Pruritus

Overview

- Pruritus may be shown by flashing, clamped fins, erratic or agitated swimming, increased jumping, dyspnea, or tachypnea.
- Flashing describes the fast rub on substrate or décor that many fish show in response to skin or gill irritation.
- Pruritus is a common presenting sign in fish and is often due to ectoparasites or chemical or particulate irritants.

Signalment

- Any fish can be affected.

Clinical Findings

- Healthy fish flash occasionally and flashing may be seen as part of a social display.
- An increase in frequency or duration, or flashing of multiple fish in succession is usually an indicator of pruritus.
- Pruritus may also be associated with increased activity, dyspnea, or tachypnea. Fins may be in an abnormal position.
- Parasites, discoloration (e.g. white spots, hyperemia, dull coloration), ulcers, or other pathology may be visible on the skin.
- Parasites, discoloration (e.g. white spots, gray foci, pallor, hyperemia, congestion), edema, or other pathology may be visible on the gills.
- Fish scales may be seen in the water column or on the substrate.

Etiologies

- The most common differentials are ectoparasites on the skin or gills, particularly protozoa, and environmental irritants.
- Infectious
  - Bacteria, particularly *Flavobacterium*, *Tenacibaculum* spp.
  - Protozoa, particularly *Cryptocaryon*, *Ichthyobodo*, *Amyloodinium* spp., scuticociliates, amoebic gill disease (SW); *Ichthyophthirius*, *Ichthyobodo*, *Piscinoodinium* spp., scuticociliates, sessile ciliates (e.g. *Heteropolaria* spp.) (FW).
  - Metazoa, particularly monogeneans, leeches, gastrointestinal nematodes.
- Inflammatory
  - Branchitis, dermatitis.
  - Enteritis, cloacitis.
- Toxic
  - Ammonia.
  - Chlorines.
  - Drug toxicity (e.g. inappropriate drug, contamination, idiosyncratic reaction).
  - Inappropriate pH.
  - Detergents.
  - Harmful algal blooms.
- Trauma
  - Cnidarian nematocysts.

Diagnostic Approach

- Review the recent history, particularly:
  - Recent animal additions and the history of those animals.
  - Quarantine and other biosecurity protocols.
  - Water source and any additives used (e.g. salts, conditioners).
  - Any recent mortalities.
  - Known causes of prior morbidity and mortality.
  - Recent medications, including applied doses and method of dosing.
- Check the water quality, particularly ammonia, salinity, pH, and chlorine. Compare results to target ranges and any previous records.
- Visually assess the animals.
  - Identify the species, size classes, and percentage of population impacted.
  - Identify any other clinical signs, particularly changes to the skin or fins, respiratory rate and effort, or behavior.
- Necropsy any mortalities, if available. The best diagnostic samples are collected from sick fish that were recently euthanized. Collect skin scrapes, gill biopsies, fin biopsies, and intestinal scrapes to examine under direct microscopy. If no cause is identified from those samples, carry out a full necropsy with additional testing as indicated, e.g.:
  - Histology.
  - Archive samples (e.g. gill, muscle, liver, spleen, kidney, frozen at −20°C (−4°F) or ideally −80°C (−112°F) and fixed in 95% ethanol and electron microscopy fixative).
- Examine fecal samples under direct microscopy and floatation to look for intestinal parasites.
- If the cause is still unknown, handling of live fish is recommended; anesthesia should be used to facilitate restraint, but since immersion anesthesia can affect parasite loads, samples should be taken as soon as the fish are sufficiently sedated.
  - Perform a full clinical examination.
  - Examine skin scrapes, gill biopsies, fin biopsies, and fecal samples under direct microscopy.
- Consider diagnostic freshwater or salt water dips (matched to pH and temperature) to look for ectoparasites.
- If the cause is still unknown, freeze 1 L of water in a clean plastic bottle for later analysis if needed (e.g. for pesticides, drugs).

Management Approach

- Increase aeration and water flow; target dissolved oxygen may be 95–100%.
- If the source water is considered appropriate (i.e. similar temperature, salinity and pH, with no risk of contamination), carry out a 20–50% water change.
- Reduce or resolve stressors.

- Consider short courses of corticosteroids to reduce the inflammatory response (e.g. dexamethasone SP 0.5–1.0 mg/kg IM for 2–3 doses).
- Further management depends on the cause (see Section C).

Abbreviations/Acronyms

- FW: Freshwater
- SW: Salt water

B4

Gastrointestinal or Coelomic Signs

Catherine A. Hadfield

Seattle Aquarium, Seattle, WA, USA

Inappetence, Weight Loss

Overview

- Inappetence and weight loss are common presenting signs in fish.
- They can be secondary to almost any disease. They may also be seen due to unsuitable environmental parameters, particularly water temperature, diet, and social situation.
- It is helpful to determine if the problem is a lack of response to food, an inability to prehend or ingest food, or weight loss despite a normal appetite, as these alter the differentials.
- It is also helpful to determine if the problem is acute or chronic. Chronic weight loss usually carries a guarded prognosis unless there is an obvious environmental cause.
- It can sometimes be hard to determine when a reduced appetite is a concern and when supplemental feeding is indicated. These decisions depend on the species, life stage, history, and experience. Species that normally feed frequently are more likely to benefit from early nutritional support than species that feed intermittently.

Signalment

- Any fish can be affected.

Clinical Findings

- One or more fish may be affected.
- Lethargy may be seen.
- Visible abnormalities around the mouth may be seen.
- Fecal output is reduced with inappetence.
- Body condition may be reduced.
  - Signs of poor body condition include reduced muscle mass (particularly visible within the epaxial muscle) and a flat to concave (or "pinched") coelomic cavity (Figure B4.1).
  - Eyes may look sunken.
  - Muscle tone is usually poor.
  - Negative buoyancy may be seen in elasmobranchs due to loss of lipid in the liver. This may be seen as longer resting periods, increased swimming effort, or tail-down swimming.
- A small liver, empty gastrointestinal (GI) tract, and enlarged gallbladder (if present) may be seen on diagnostic imaging, at surgery, or at necropsy. Bony fish also show a lack of coelomic fat.

Etiologies (Reduced Feeding Response)

- Metabolic
  - Nephrolithiasis.
- Nutritional
  - Inappropriate feed items, timing, or method of presentation.
  - Rancid food.
  - New diets.
  - Competition for food.
  - Dental disease.
  - Gastrointestinal foreign bodies (e.g. hook, décor, sealant).
- Infectious
  - Viruses, particularly some herpesviruses, rhabdoviruses, ranaviruses, megalocytiviruses, betanodaviruses, alphaviruses.

Clinical Guide to Fish Medicine, First Edition. Edited by Catherine A. Hadfield and Leigh Ann Clayton.

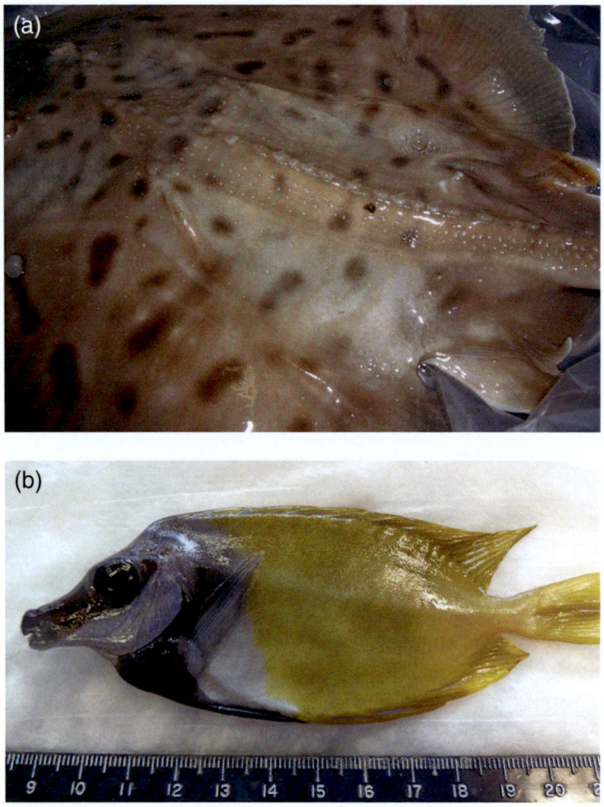

Figure B4.1 Emaciation in a clearnose skate (*Raja eglanteria*) (a) and foxface rabbitfish (*Siganus vulpinus*) (b).

  - Most bacteria, particularly vibriosis, *Aeromonas*, *Citrobacter*, *Pseudomonas*, *Edwardsiella*, *Flavobacterium*, *Yersinia*, *Streptococcus*, *Renibacterium*, *Francisella*, *Mycobacterium*, *Nocardia*, piscirickettsial-like spp.
  - Fungi or fungal-like organisms, particularly atypical oomycetes, *Exophiala*, *Fusarium*, *Paecilomyces* spp., *Microsporidia*, *Mesomycetozoea*.
  - Protozoa, particularly *Cryptocaryon, Brooklynella*, *Ichthyobodo*, *Amyloodinium* spp., scuticociliates, amoebic gill disease (SW); *Ichthyophthirius*, *Chilodonella*, *Cryptobia*, *Ichthyobodo*, *Piscinoodinium*, *Hexamita*, *Spironucleus* spp., trichodinids, scuticociliates, or sessile ciliates (e.g. *Heteropolaria* spp.) (FW).
  - Metazoa, particularly monogeneans, digenes, cestodes, leeches, nematodes, branchiurans.
  - Myxozoa, particularly *Ceratonova*, *Enteromyxum*, *Henneguya*, *Myxobolus* spp.
  - Apicomplexa, particularly *Cryptosporidium*, *Eimeria* spp.
- Inflammatory
  - Any inflammatory condition (e.g. oophoritis, hepatitis, enteritis, ocular or neurologic inflammation).
- Idiopathic
  - Egg retention or binding.
- Toxic
  - Ammonia, nitrites.
  - Chlorines, chloramines.
  - Heavy metals (e.g. lead, zinc, copper).
  - Drug toxicity (e.g. inappropriate drug, contamination, idiosyncratic reaction).
  - Hydrogen sulfide.
  - Pesticides.
  - Melamine.
- Trauma
  - Cohort, décor, or catch trauma.
  - Cnidarian nematocysts.
- Life support system/environmental
  - Inappropriate water temperature, particularly if low.
  - Inappropriate lighting (e.g. flashing, lights staying on at night).
  - Inappropriate social structure.
  - Breeding season.
  - Noise or vibration (e.g. nearby construction or pumps).
  - Stray voltage.
  - Low dissolved oxygen, high carbon dioxide, gas supersaturation.

Etiologies (Normal Feed Response, Inability to Prehend or Ingest Food)

- Neoplasia/hyperplasia
  - Goiter.
  - Oral, pharyngeal.
- Nutritional
  - Inappropriate feed items (e.g. pellets that are too large).
  - Oropharyngeal foreign bodies (e.g. hook, fish spine).
  - Dental overgrowth or malalignment.
  - Myopathy (particularly seahorses, *Syngnathidae*).
- Infectious/inflammatory
  - Any neurologic or musculoskeletal disease (e.g. betanodavirus, vibriosis, osteoarthritis).
- Trauma
  - Spinal or jaw fracture.
  - Oral hematoma.

Etiologies (Weight Loss in Spite of Normal Food Intake)

- Neoplasia
  - Any neoplasia.
  - Primary gastrointestinal neoplasia in fish is rare but has been reported (e.g. gastric carcinoma).
- Nutritional
  - Inappropriate feed items.
  - Deficiency of macro- or micronutrients.

- Infectious/inflammatory
  - Granulomatous disease, particularly *Mycobacterium*, *Nocardia*, *Francisella*, *Streptococcus*, *Renibacterium*, piscirickettsial-like spp.
  - Metazoa, particularly digenes, cestodes, nematodes.
  - Myxozoa, particularly *Ceratonova*, *Enteromyxum* spp.
  - Apicomplexa, particularly *Cryptosporidium*, *Eimeria* spp.

Diagnostic Approach

- Review the history, in particular:
  - Recent animal additions and the history of those animals.
  - Food offered, including storage, preparation, and presentation.
  - Feeding response.
  - Food eaten.
  - Any recent mortalities.
  - Known causes of prior morbidity and mortality.
  - Chronicity of clinical signs.
- Check the water quality. Compare results to target ranges and any previous records.
- Visually assess the animals.
  - Check the body condition of all the animals in the system.
  - Look for signs of displacement or inappropriate social groups.
  - Observe feeding to try to determine if there are problems with feeding method, response, or prehension.
- Visually assess the habitat.
  - Check the suitability for the species.
  - Look for access to potential foreign bodies.
- Examine fecal samples under direct microscopy, floatation, Dif-Quik, Gram, and acid-fast stains.
- Necropsy any mortalities, if available. The best diagnostic samples are collected from sick fish that were recently euthanized. Include additional testing as indicated, e.g.:
  - Radiographs.
  - Cultures, often bacterial, mycobacterial, and fungal (e.g. blood, liver, kidney, gonad, brain).
  - Wet mounts and impression smears (e.g. gill, skin, liver, spleen, kidney, gonad, gastrointestinal tract, any lesions).
  - Histology.
  - Further diagnostics (e.g. swabs or tissues for PCR testing for *Mycobacterium* spp.).
  - Archive samples (e.g. gill, muscle, liver, spleen, kidney, gonad, brain, frozen at −20°C (−4°F) or ideally −80°C (−112°F) and fixed in 95% ethanol and electron microscopy fixative).
- If the cause is still unknown, handling of live fish is recommended for diagnostics, fluid therapy, and nutritional support. Anesthesia should be used to facilitate restraint.
  - Perform a full clinical examination.
  - Check body weights and lengths and compare to any previous records.
  - Consider if an internal or external identifier (e.g. PIT tag, fin clip) would help with tracking changes in individuals.
  - Examine skin scrapes and gill biopsies under direct microscopy.
  - Consider cloacal or rectal washes to collect fecal material if no free-catch samples are available.
  - Consider plain and contrast radiography to examine the skull, coelom, and skeletal system and to look for foreign bodies.
  - Consider ultrasonography to evaluate liver size and echogenicity and any coelomic abnormalities.
  - Consider upper gastrointestinal endoscopy.
  - Consider coelomic endoscopy or exploratory coeliotomy to examine and biopsy liver, spleen, gonad, and kidney.
  - Consider hematology and biochemistry to look for signs of infectious or other systemic disease. It is relatively common to see low glucose, protein, urea, and PCV with hyponutrition and chronic disease.
- Consider diagnostic freshwater or saltwater dips (matched to pH and temperature) to look for ectoparasites.
- The underlying etiology is often not determined, but supportive care may still resolve clinical signs.

Management Approach

- Treat any obvious primary cause (e.g. endoscopic retrieval of foreign bodies, jaw fracture repair).
- Encourage free feeding:
  - Ensure that food is of excellent quality; rancidity is easily detected by fish.
  - Provide appropriate feed items, timing, and feeding cues.
  - Increase variety and availability of food items.
  - Change delivery method and/or location (e.g. from hand feeding to broadcast feeding). For carnivorous and omnivorous fish, blood in the water and movement of the food can help.
  - Temporarily relax any prior behavioral criteria (e.g. feeding at a specific station).
  - Consider isolating affected animals, as long as this is not an additional stressor.
  - Monitor closely for subtle improvements (e.g. orienting towards food, picking at food overnight).
- Provide supportive care if environmental changes do not resolve the issue or while waiting to see a response to environmental changes. This is particularly helpful

when supporting fish after a transport while they adjust to new environments.
  - Provide fluid support for inappetent or thin marine fish as they will be dehydrated. Oral is the most common route, but intravenous and intracoelomic fluids can be used.
  - Gavage (tube) feed or force feed using a slurry of wild-type diet and/or commercial feeds. The interval depends on the species, life stage, and handling considerations and may vary from twice daily (e.g. juvenile *Raja* spp. skates) to monthly (e.g. adult *Sebastes* spp. rockfish).
  - Gradually increase the volume to allow the GI tract to respond and prevent a potential refeeding syndrome, although this has not been reported in fish.
  - Continue supportive care until the animal is able to satisfy its caloric requirements through free feeding, unless the handling stress is considered a greater risk. Many animals will free feed while being intermittently gavage fed.
- Consider short courses of corticosteroids to reduce the inflammatory response that is commonly seen in sick fish (e.g. dexamethasone SP 0.5–1.0 mg/kg IM for 2–3 doses).
- Monitor behavior, weights, and body condition scores (see Chapter A4).

Abbreviations/Acronyms
- FW: Freshwater
- SW: Salt water

Coelomic Distension

Overview
- Coelomic distension is a common presenting sign in fish.
- It is usually due to fluid or increased soft tissue, or a combination of both. The most common causes are obesity, hepatomegaly, eggs, or systemic infection.
- Coelomic distension is occasionally due to gas; this is associated with signs of positive buoyancy and is covered in Chapter B5: *Positive Buoyancy*.
- Coelomic distension is colloquially known as dropsy or pine cone disease due to the raised scales seen in some species.
- This is usually an individual animal problem. Where multiple fish are affected, infectious diseases should be higher on the differential list.

Signalment
- Any fish can be affected.

Clinical Findings
- One or more fish may be affected.
- Coelomic distension may be the only presenting sign. It may be generalized and symmetric (e.g. effusion, fat; Figure B4.2a) or focal and asymmetric (e.g. neoplasia, renomegaly).
- Lethargy, reduced feeding response, or cloacal/anal protrusion or prolapse may be seen.
- If skin erythema, hyperemia, or ulceration is visible, an infectious or inflammatory process is more likely, although ulcers can form due to pressure effects.

Etiologies
- The most common differentials are obesity, hepatomegaly, large ovaries, and systemic inflammation or infection.

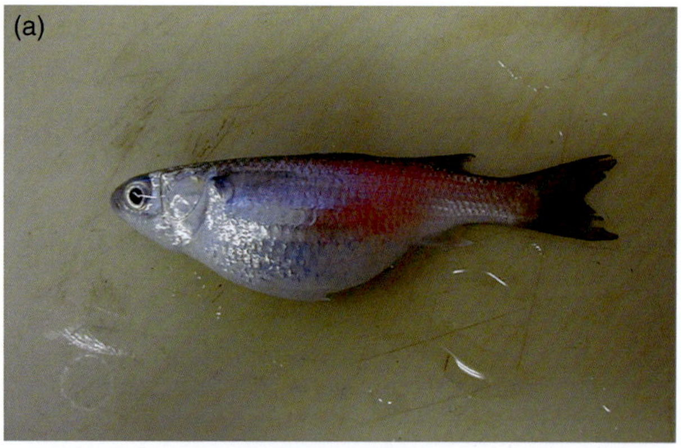

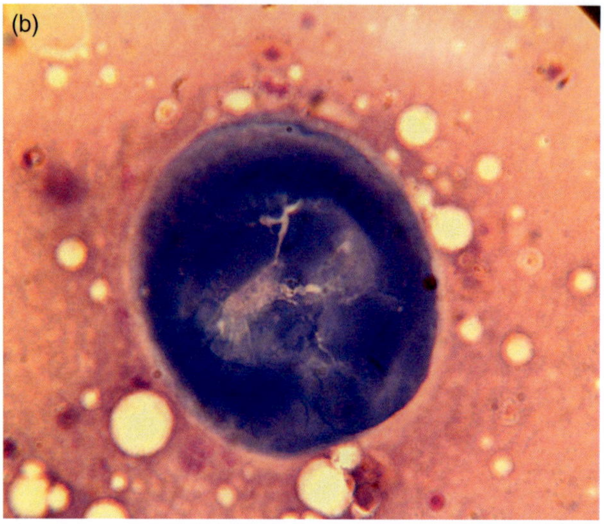

Figure B4.2 Coelomic distension in a mullet (*Mugil* sp.) (a) and Dif-Quik stain of the coelomic aspirate showing an ovum at x1000 (b).

- Developmental
  - Genetic predisposition to polycystic kidneys in goldfish (*Carassius auratus*), common carp (*Cyprinus carpio*), and white sturgeon (*Acipenser transmontanus*).
- Metabolic
  - Nephrolithiasis and urolithiasis.
- Neoplasia
  - Any coelomic neoplasia due to the mass or associated effusion or hemorrhage; gonadal and hepatic neoplasias are the most common.
- Nutritional/gastrointestinal
  - Obesity.
  - Hepatomegaly or hepatic lipidosis.
  - Intestinal torsion or perforation.
  - Gastrointestinal foreign bodies (e.g. substrate, décor, sealant).
  - Hypoproteinemia.
  - Deficiency of some micronutrients (e.g. vitamin A, C, or E) causing effusion or edema.
- Normal anatomy
  - Normal ovarian or testicular development.
  - Late gestation.
- Infectious
  - Most viruses, particularly rhabdoviruses (e.g. IHNV, VHSV, SVCV), infectious pancreatic necrosis, carp edema virus, and some herpesviruses (e.g. KHV), ranaviruses, megalocytiviruses, retroviral-associated neoplasia.
  - Most bacteria, particularly vibriosis, *Aeromonas*, *Citrobacter*, *Pseudomonas*, *Edwardsiella*, *Flavobacterium*, *Yersinia*, *Streptococcus*, *Renibacterium*, *Francisella*, *Mycobacterium*, *Nocardia*, piscirickettsial-like spp.
  - Fungi or fungal-like organisms, particularly *Exophiala* spp. and *Microsporidia*.
  - Protozoa, particularly scuticociliates, *Cryptobia*, *Hexamita/Spironucleus* spp.
  - Metazoa, particularly cestodes, large nematodes, pentastomids, acanthocephalans.
  - Myxozoa, particularly *Ceratonova*, *Enteromyxum*, *Hoferellus*, *Tetracapsuloides* spp.
  - Apicomplexa, particularly *Eimeria* spp.
- Inflammatory
  - Vasculitis.
  - Disseminated intravascular coagulopathy.
  - Hepatitis, steatitis, oophoritis, nephritis, enterocolitis, coelomitis (including vaccine-induced coelomitis).
- Idiopathic
  - Congestive heart failure.
  - Egg retention or binding.
  - Dystocia.
  - Uterine mucometra and ovarian cysts in female rays.
  - Chronic liver disease or polycystic liver.
  - Chronic kidney disease or polycystic kidney.
  - Protein-losing enteropathy.
- Toxic
  - Indomethacin.
  - Heavy metals.
- Trauma
  - Coelomic hemorrhage.
  - Hematomas.
- Life support system/environmental
  - High pH.

Diagnostic Approach

- Review the history, in particular:
  - Food eaten, including storage and preparation.
  - Fecal output.
  - Reproductive history.
  - Known causes of prior morbidity and mortality.
  - Chronicity of clinical signs; acute presentations are often due to fluid rather than soft tissue.
- Check the water quality, particularly pH. Compare results to target ranges and any previous records.
- Visually assess the animals.
  - Identify the sexes (if possible) (Table A1.3).
  - Identify any other clinical signs such as skin lesions, abnormal buoyancy, or cloacal/anal distension, prolapse, or discharge.
  - Look for access to potential foreign bodies.
  - Try to assess fecal output.
- Necropsy any mortalities, if available. The best diagnostic samples are collected from sick fish that were recently euthanized. Include additional testing as indicated, e.g.:
  - Cultures, often bacterial and mycobacterial (e.g. blood, coelomic mass or effusion).
  - Wet mounts and impression smears (e.g. gill, skin, liver, spleen, kidney, gonad, gastrointestinal tract, any lesions).
  - Histology.
  - Further diagnostics (e.g. swabs or tissues for PCR testing for IHNV, VHSV, SVCV).
  - Archive samples (e.g. gill, muscle, liver, kidney, gonad, frozen at −20°C (−4°F) or ideally −80°C (−112°F) and fixed in 95% ethanol and electron microscopy fixative).
- If the cause is still unknown, handling of live fish is usually required; anesthesia should be used to facilitate restraint, although palpation and ultrasound can be done in some species without restraint.
  - Palpate the coelom to try to assess if the distension is soft tissue, fluid, or gas, or if foreign bodies can be palpated.
  - Examine the cloaca, anus, and urogenital openings for any abnormalities or discharges. If large enough, do a

digital examination of the cloaca to palpate any abnormalities, check the status of the cervix (if present), and identify any gonadal or fetal tissue.
  - In elasmobranchs, check the abdominal pores lateral to the cloaca and apply gentle pressure to the coelom to see if there is any discharge from the pores or cloaca. In female elasmobranchs with uterine effusion, consider aspiration of the fluid using a red rubber tube passed through the cervix.
  - Use ultrasonography to differentiate between soft tissue and fluid in the coelom and to evaluate the size and echogenicity of the liver, gonads, gastrointestinal tract, heart, and any cysts or masses. In viviparous species, check if the fish is gravid.
  - Consider radiography or computed tomography to evaluate the coelom; positive contrast agents are often required.
  - Collect aspirates of any coelomic effusion or abnormal viscera, under ultrasound guidance if possible. Check under direct microscopy, Dif-Quik, Gram, and acid-fast stains. Ovaries, testes, liver, spleen, and fat tend to exfoliate recognizable cells (Figure B4.2b). If fluid is collected, evaluate specific gravity and protein. Samples with high specific gravity (>1.020), high protein (>30 g/L), high cellularity (abundant cells on smear, e.g. >5000/μL), numerous leukocytes or necrotic cells are suggestive of inflammation. Infectious agents may be seen (e.g. bacteria, fungi, myxozoans). Consider aerobic and mycobacterial cultures. Serosanguinous fluid is often due to contamination; a true hemorrhagic effusion is uncommon in fish.
  - Consider tru-cut biopsies, coelomic endoscopy, or exploratory coeliotomy if enlarged organs or masses are present.

Management Approach

- Further management depends on the cause (Figure B4.3) (see Section C for egg retention, obesity, gastrointestinal foreign bodies, dystocia, and specific infectious diseases).
- Provide appropriate fluid and nutritional support if affected fish are not showing adequate food intake.
- Consider analgesia and anti-inflammatory medications.
- For distension due to coelomic effusion, treat the underlying cause (e.g. systemic antibiotics if bacterial). Coeliocentesis may help reduce pressure effects, but does not help support respiration, unlike in other vertebrate classes. Consider diuretics, although they have not been reported commonly in fish.
- If hepatic disease is suspected, consider hepatoprotective medication (e.g. silymarin, *S*-adenosyl-methionine (SAMe), or milk thistle).

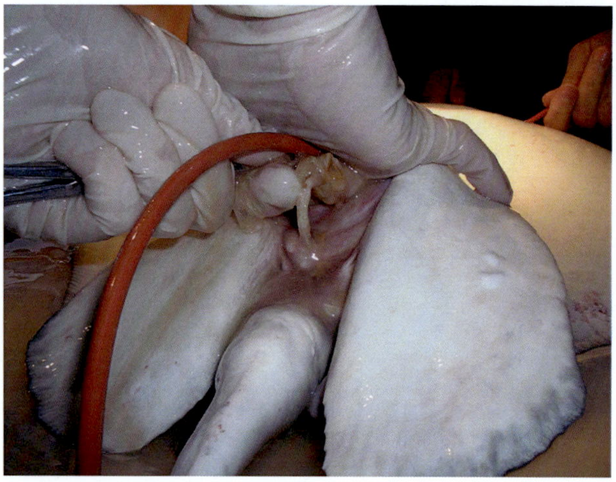

Figure B4.3 Per cloaca removal of a necrotic fetus in a cownose ray (*Rhinoptera bonasus*). The red rubber catheter is used to insert sterile lubricant.

- If a coelomic mass or visceral pathology is identified, surgical or endosurgical management may be possible.
  - Abnormal gonads can be excised relatively easily in most bony fish; the surgery is more complicated in elasmobranchs.
  - Removal of hepatic masses is possible, but diffuse hepatic disease is more common in fish.
  - Removal of renal and gastrointestinal masses is often difficult in fish.
- Monitor fish based on clinical signs, weights, ultrasonography, and coeleocentesis.

Bibliography

Lovy, J., Speare, D.J., and Wright, G.M. (2007). Pathological effects caused by chronic treatment of rainbow trout with indomethacin. *Journal of Aquatic Animal Health* 19: 94–98.

Marselas, G.A., Stoskopf, M.K., Brown, M.J. et al. (1998). Abdominal ascites in electric eels (*Electrophorus electricus*) associated with hepatic hemosiderosis and elevated water pH. *Journal of Zoo and Wildlife Medicine* 29: 413–418.

Abbreviations/Acronyms

- IHNV: Infectious hematopoietic necrosis virus
- KHV: Koi herpesvirus
- SVCV: Spring viremia of carp virus
- VHSV: Viral hemorrhagic septicemia virus

Dental Disease

Overview

- Dental overgrowth is typically a husbandry-related problem seen in fish that evolved to feed or graze on hard items (e.g. bivalves, crustaceans, corals, rocks). These fish have beaks or dental plates that often overgrow when fed softer food items.
- Other dental pathology may include tooth loss, accretions on teeth, and gingivitis.
- Affected fish often present with a reduced feeding response or weight loss.
- This is usually an individual animal problem, unless conspecifics have been in the collection for a similar amount of time.
- Management often includes long-term changes to the diet.

Signalment

- Dental overgrowth is common in parrotfish (*Scaridae*), pufferfish (*Tetraodontidae*), and some rays, particularly eagle rays (*Myliobatidae*).
- Gingivitis is common in some sharks such as sand tigers (*Carcharias taurus*).

Clinical Findings

- One or more fish of the same species may be affected.
- Overgrown teeth or dental plates may be visible or the mouth may not be able to close normally (Figure B4.4).
- Missing teeth or gingival hyperemia and erosions may be seen.
- Inappetence, reduced feeding, poor body condition, or poor growth may be seen. Fish may drop food, particularly hard foods.

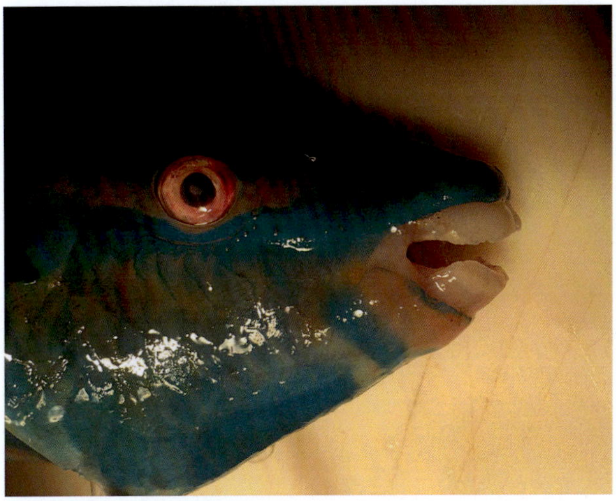

Figure B4.4 Mild beak overgrowth in a parrotfish (*Scaridae*).

Etiologies

- The most likely differential is an inappropriate diet.
- Developmental
  - Abnormal bone or cartilage development.
- Nutritional
  - Soft diets (e.g. lack of rock for grazers; lack of whole bivalves, crustaceans, and echinoderms for benthic feeders).
  - Inappropriate composition of plaster of Paris used to make diet blocks for parrotfish.
  - Deficiency of micronutrients.
- Neoplasia
  - Oral, pharyngeal (e.g. squamous cell carcinoma, melanoma, osteoma).
- Infectious/inflammatory
  - Particularly osteomyelitis or osteoarthritis.
- Trauma
  - Particularly to skull bones or dental plates.

Diagnostic Approach

- Review the history, in particular:
  - Food offered, including storage and preparation.
  - Food eaten.
  - Previous diets.
  - Chronicity of clinical signs.
- Visually assess the animals.
  - Observe normal feeding to check feed response and prehension.
  - Check all conspecifics.
- Handling of live fish is usually required for diagnosis and treatment; anesthesia should be used to facilitate restraint.
  - Examine the oropharyngeal cavity in detail.
  - Check the range of motion of the jaws.
  - Consider radiography and computed tomography of the skull.
  - If a mass is identified, consider aspirates or incisional or excisional biopsies.
  - If erosive lesions are identified, consider cultures, cytology, and histology.

Management Approach

- Provide appropriate fluid and nutritional support if the affected fish is not showing adequate food intake.
- For dental overgrowth:
  - Trim overgrown dental plates. The tissue is firm and high-speed dental burs or low-speed drills (e.g. Dremel®) are often needed.

- Increase hard items in the diet if needed to reflect wild-type diets (e.g. clams or mussels in shells, hard-shelled crabs, whole shrimp or crayfish, live rocks, or put feed items into suitable plaster molds to allow grazing). If using plaster molds, use a product with a high setting strength of ≥6500 psi to try to prevent concretions on pharyngeal teeth.
- Even with diet correction, chronic management of the dental plates is often required after an overgrowth event.

- For oral masses, consider excision or local treatment.
- If the animal is unlikely to be able to eat again, consider euthanasia.

Cloacal/Anal Distension or Prolapse

Overview

- Elasmobranchs, lungfish, and coelacanths have a true cloaca where urogenital and gastrointestinal tracts merge into a single collection chamber. Most teleosts have separate anus, urinary, and genital pores, although the urinary and genital pores are often closely associated.
- Cloacal/anal distension or prolapse in fish is often associated with coelomic distension and reproductive or intestinal disease.
- It is often impossible to reduce the prolapse or distension in fish without fixing the underlying problem.

Signalment

- Any fish can be affected; signs may be more likely in females.

Clinical Findings

- One or more fish of the same species may be affected, but this is more commonly an individual fish problem.
- Coelomic distension is often seen with cloacal/anal distension or prolapse.
- Lethargy, reduced feeding response, or abnormal swimming may be seen.
- Hyperemia and skin ulcers may be seen, particularly around the cloaca/anus.
- Discharge from the cloaca, anus, urogenital openings, or from the abdominal pores in elasmobranchs may be seen.
- Mucosal changes may be seen (Figure B4.5); normal mucosa should be pale, flat, with no petechiae.
- Prolapsed tissue may be gonad, gonaduct, rectum, or intestine. Prolapse of a urinary bladder is rare.

Etiologies

- The most common differentials are large ovaries, oophoritis, cloacitis, enterocolitis, and systemic inflammation.
- The full list also includes any differential that can cause coelomic distension (see above).
- Normal anatomy that may be mistaken for pathology includes gonopodia and urogenital papillae.

Diagnostic Approach

- Review the history, in particular:
  - Food eaten, including storage and preparation.
  - Fecal output.
  - Reproductive history.
- Visually assess the animals.
  - Identify the sexes (if possible) (Table A1.3).
  - Identify any other clinical signs such as coelomic distension, skin lesions, or abnormal buoyancy.
  - Look for access to potential foreign bodies.
  - Try to assess fecal output.
- Necropsy any mortalities, if available. The best diagnostic samples are collected from sick fish that were recently euthanized. Include additional testing as indicated, e.g.:

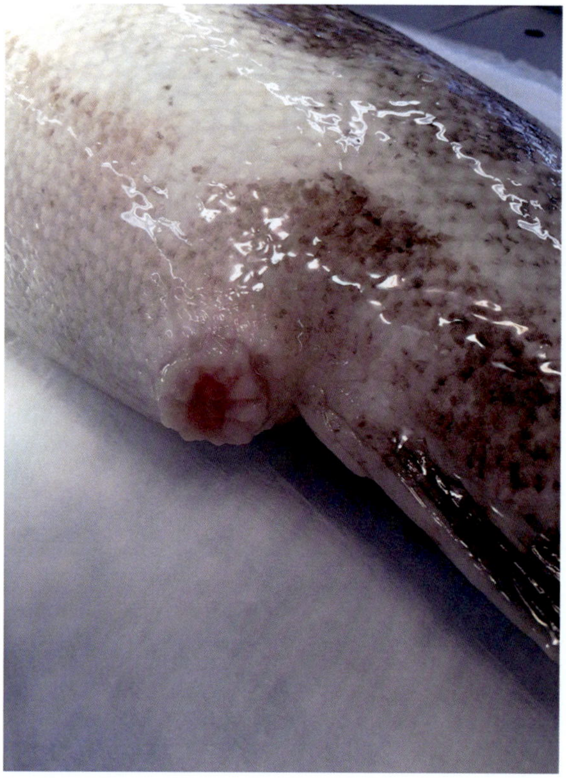

Figure B4.5 Anal distension in a seabass (*Centropristis* sp.).

  - Cultures, often bacterial and mycobacterial (e.g. blood, coelomic effusion, ovaries).
  - Wet mounts and impression smears (e.g. gill, skin, liver, spleen, kidney, gonad, gastrointestinal tract, cloaca/anus, any lesions).
  - Histology.
  - Further diagnostics (e.g. swabs or tissues for PCR testing).
  - Archive samples (e.g. liver, spleen, kidney, gonad, frozen at −20°C (−4°F) or ideally −80°C (−112°F) and fixed in 95% ethanol and electron microscopy fixative).
- If the cause is still unknown, handling of live fish is usually required; anesthesia should be used to facilitate restraint.
  - Palpate the coelom and cloaca, anus, and urogenital openings, if size allows.
  - Check impression smears of the distended tissue on direct cytology, Dif-Quik, Gram, and acid-fast stains.
  - Use ultrasonography to identify any coelomic effusion and to evaluate the size and echogenicity of the liver, gonads, gastrointestinal tract, heart, and any cysts or masses.
  - Consider plain and contrast radiography to evaluate the coelom and look for foreign bodies.
  - Consider endoscopy of the cloaca, distal intestines, and reproductive tract to assess the mucosa, identify and potentially remove foreign bodies, or identify and biopsy any masses.

Management Approach

- Distension and prolapses are best managed by resolving the underlying issue (e.g. ovariectomy, mass removal).
- Minor prolapses may not need additional treatment.
- Manual replacement is often difficult and recurrence is common if the underlying problem is not resolved, even with purse string sutures or -pexy surgeries.
- Consider analgesia and anti-inflammatory medications.
- Provide supportive care as indicated (e.g. fluid and nutritional support).

B5

Musculoskeletal or Neurologic Signs

Catherine A. Hadfield

Seattle Aquarium, Seattle, WA, USA

Spinal Deformity

Overview

- Spinal deformities may include a lateral curvature (scoliosis), dorsal/convex curvature (kyphosis), or ventral/concave curvature (lordosis). These may be combined (e.g. kyphoscoliosis).
- Swimming and buoyancy may be affected.
- Diagnostic imaging and histology are the most useful diagnostics.
- The etiology is often hard to determine.
- Treatment is usually unrewarding and prevention is essential.

Signalment

- Any fish can be affected, but reports are common in:
  - Larval bony fish in aquaculture.
  - Sand tigers (*Carcharias taurus*) under human care, typically starting at three to eight years old.

Clinical Findings

- One or more fish may be affected, usually of the same species.
- Fish may present with obvious curves in the spine.
- Reduced appetites or growth rates are common.
- Abnormal swimming is common; abnormal buoyancy may be seen.
- Paresis, muscle wasting, or changes in skin coloration caudal to a lesion may be seen.
- Other deformities may be seen (e.g. short or curved jaw, short opercula). In sand tigers, gingival hyperplasia, curled pectoral fins, and transient luxation of the lower jaw ("drop jaw") have been associated with spinal deformities.

Etiologies

- Spinal deformities are likely to be multifactorial with etiologies varying by species and life stages. The insult may have happened long before clinical signs are appreciated, so determining the etiology can be challenging.
- Degenerative
  - Osteoarthritis.
- Developmental
  - Genetic abnormality.
  - Triploidy.
  - High water temperature, high water flow, or low dissolved oxygen during development.
  - Inappropriate light schedules during development, particularly long photoperiods.
  - Failure of swim bladder inflation.
  - Selective breeding for characteristic deformities (e.g. fancy goldfish (*Carassius auratus*), balloon kissing gourami (*Helostoma temminckii*), balloon molly (*Poecilia sphenops*)).
- Neoplasia
- Nutritional
  - Deficiency of vitamin A, B1, C, E, tryptophan, phosphorus, potassium, zinc.
  - Excess vitamin A or E.
  - Overfeeding and rapid growth rates.
  - Suboptimal fatty acid composition of diet.
- Infectious/inflammatory
  - Bacteria, particularly *Mycobacterium*, *Streptococcus* spp., *Flavobacterium psychrophilum* survivors.
  - Fungi or fungal-like organisms, particularly *Microsporidia* (e.g. *Pseudoloma* spp.), *Mesomycetozoea.*

Clinical Guide to Fish Medicine, First Edition. Edited by Catherine A. Hadfield and Leigh Ann Clayton.

- Metazoa, particularly digenes.
- Myxozoa, particularly *Myxobolus* spp.

- Iatrogenic
  - Intraperitoneal vaccination using oil adjuvants.
  - Local injection site reactions.
- Toxic
  - Selenium.
  - Pesticides, herbicides.
  - Heavy metals (e.g. arsenic, cadmium, copper, lead, mercury, zinc).
  - Mycotoxins.
- Trauma
  - Cohort, décor, or catch trauma, particularly when animals are young.
  - Electrical stunning.
- Life support system/environmental
  - Inappropriate enclosure size or design; short glide distances and reduced time gliding correlate with spinal deformities in sand tigers.
  - High carbon dioxide.
  - Stray voltage and poor electrical grounding.
  - Lightning strike.

Diagnostic Approach

- Review the history, in particular:
  - Food eaten, including storage and preparation.
  - Previous diets.
  - Environmental conditions during development.
  - Recent weather if outdoors, particularly lightning storms.
  - Chronicity of clinical signs; acute presentations are often traumatic.
- Check the water quality, particularly heavy metals and carbon dioxide. Compare results to target ranges and any previous records.
- Visually assess the animals.
  - Identify the species, size classes, and percentage of population impacted.
  - Look for obvious spinal deformity and check for abnormal head or tail position, swimming patterns, fin movements, or buoyancy.
  - Identify any other clinical signs, such as skin discoloration or muscle atrophy caudal to a possible lesion.
- Visually assess the habitat.
  - Check the suitability for the species.
- Check the life support system for possible sources of stray voltage (e.g. frayed electrical leads). A voltmeter should be used to assess for any stray voltage in the system, ideally over 24–48 hours since changes may be transient.
- Necropsy any mortalities, if available. Include additional testing as indicated, e.g.:
  - Radiographs (with orthogonal views) or computed tomography.
  - Cultures, often bacterial, mycobacterial, and fungal (e.g. blood, vertebral).
  - Wet mounts and impression smears (e.g. liver, kidney, vertebrae, adjacent musculature).
  - Histology; this may show acute or chronic inflammatory infiltrate, degeneration, fibrosis, proliferation, necrosis, hemorrhage, neoplasia, or parasites.
  - Archive samples (e.g. serum, liver, vertebrae, and muscle, frozen at −20°C (−4°F) or ideally −80°C (−112°F) for possible assessment of vitamins A, C, E, and zinc).
- If the cause is still unknown, handling of live fish may be required; anesthesia should be used to facilitate restraint and reduce the risk of trauma.
  - Palpate the spine.
  - Use radiography (with orthogonal views), computed tomography, or MRI to determine the extent of the spinal pathology (Figure B5.1). Common changes include fractures, luxations, subluxations, compression, fusion, changes in bone density, and obvious lysis or proliferation. Witten et al. (2009) provides a good nomenclature system for describing bony pathology.
  - Consider hematology and biochemistry to look for an inflammatory leukogram and changes in alkaline phosphatase, calcium, or phosphorus and to assess serum levels of vitamins A, C, E, and zinc.
  - Consider aspirate and/or biopsy of bony lesions and adjacent musculature for cytology, histology, and cultures (Figure B5.2).

Management Approach

- Treat the primary cause where known, e.g. antibiotics based on culture and sensitivity for bacterial osteomyelitis.
- Ground the system in case of stray voltage.
- Consider supplementing the diet with additional vitamins C and E and potassium; these usually have a wide safety index. Consider supplementing with vitamin A, phosphorous, or zinc if there is a known deficiency.
- Individual mild cases may be managed with supportive care, analgesia, muscle relaxants, and low-light laser therapy.
- Lesions often progress. In cases of severe changes or where there is no response to supportive care, consider euthanasia for welfare reasons.
- A detailed investigation of the system and population is warranted to prevent further cases.

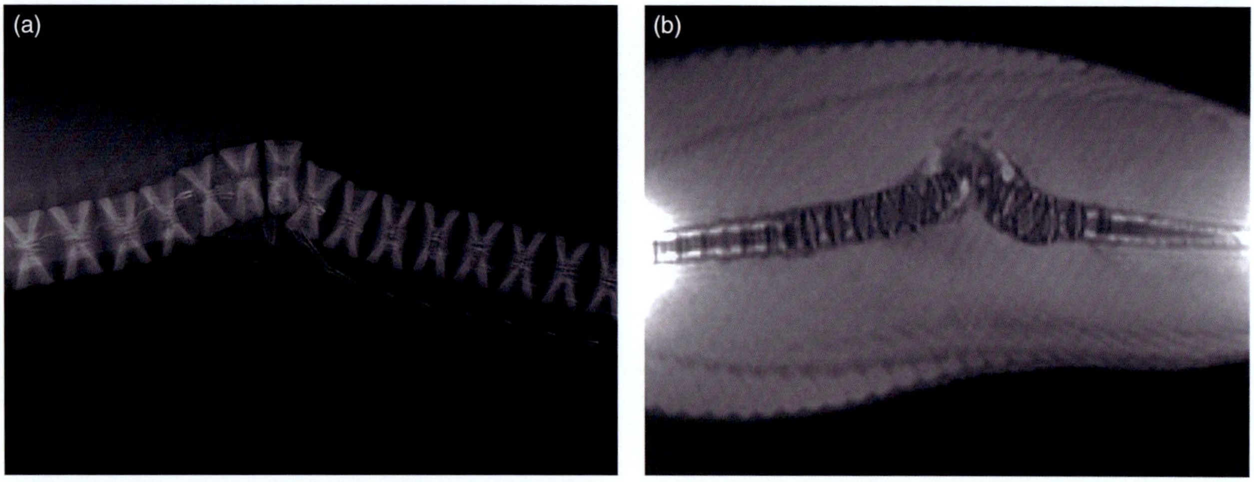

Figure B5.1 Scoliosis and kyphosis in a sand tiger shark (*Carcharias taurus*) seen on a lateral radiograph (a) and MRI (b); the radiograph also shows the gas-filled stomach. *Source*: Images courtesy of New England Aquarium.

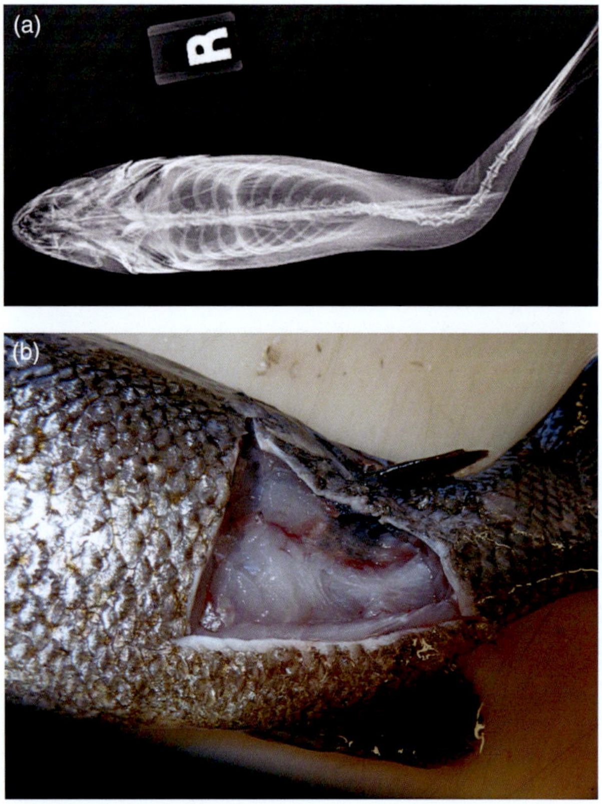

Figure B5.2 Radiograph showing lordoscoliosis in a spangled perch (*Leiopotherapon unicolor*) (a) and myositis seen at necropsy (b).

Bibliography

Anderson, P.A., Huber, D.R., and Berzins, I.K. (2012). Correlations of capture, transport, and nutrition with spinal deformities in sand tiger sharks, *Carcharias Taurus*, in public aquaria. *Journal of Zoo and Wildlife Medicine* 43: 750–758.

Berg, B.A., Yurtzeva, A., Hansen, T. et al. (2012). Vaccinated farmed Atlantic salmon are susceptible to spinal and skull deformities. *Journal of Applied Ichthyology* 28: 446–452.

Boglione, C., Gavaia, P., Koumoundouros, G. et al. (2013a). Skeletal anomalies in reared European fish larvae and juveniles. Part 1: normal and anomalous skeletogenic processes. *Reviews in Aquaculture* 5: S99–S120.

Boglione, C., Gisbert, E., Gavaia, P. et al. (2013b). Skeletal anomalies in reared European fish larvae and juveniles. Part 2: main typologies, occurrences and factors. *Reviews in Aquaculture* 5: S121–S167.

Martens, L.G., Lock, E.J., Fjelldal, P.G. et al. (2010). Dietary fatty acids and inflammation in the vertebral column of Atlantic salmon, *Salmo salar* L., smolts: a possible link to spinal deformities. *Journal of Fish Diseases* 33: 957–972.

Nordgreen, A.H., Slinde, E., Møller, D., and Roth, B. (2008). Effects of various electric field strengths and current durations on stunning and spinal injuries of Atlantic herring. *Journal of Aquatic Animal Health* 20: 110–115.

Tate, E.E., Anderson, P.A., Huber, D.R., and Berzins, I.K. (2013). Correlations of swimming patterns with spinal deformities in the sand tiger shark, *Carcharias Taurus*. *International Journal of Comparative Psychology* 26: 75–82.

Witten, P.E., Gil-Martens, L., Huysseune, A. et al. (2009). Towards a classification and an understanding of developmental relationships of vertebral body malformations in Atlantic salmon (*Salmo salar* L.). *Aquaculture* 295: 6–15.

Abbreviations/Acronyms

- MRI: Magnetic resonance imaging

External Masses

Overview

- Masses on the skin, especially around the mouth and the fins, are common in fish.
- Single masses are often neoplastic, although focal abscesses are seen. Multifocal masses have a greater range of differentials.
- Cytology and histology are usually required for definitive diagnosis.
- The masses can often be removed. Recurrence is common but systemic spread is less common.
- Masses in the oral or gular area are most commonly goiters; these are covered in Chapter C2.

Signalment

- Any fish can be affected.
- These are particularly common in bony fish.

Clinical Findings

- One or more fish of the same species may be affected, but this is more commonly an individual fish problem.
- Masses vary in size and may be ulcerated.
- Single masses are more common than multifocal lesions.
- Mass effects may be seen, e.g. opercular flaring, dyspnea, or tachypnea with oral masses.
- Fish can have large masses with no other appreciable clinical signs and no apparent impact on quality of life.

Etiologies

- The most common differentials for a single skin mass are neoplastic, particularly spindle cell tumors.
- Metabolic
  - Calcinosis cutis or calcinosis circumscripta.
- Neoplasia
  - Spindle cell tumors (e.g. fibromas, neurofibromas, fibrosarcomas).
  - Pigmented tumors (e.g. melanomas, chromatophoromas, chromatoblastomas).
  - Lymphomas and lymphosarcomas.
  - Lipomas.
  - Xanthomas.
  - Papillomatosis.
- Normal anatomy (e.g. nuptial tubercles, cloacal protuberances, goldfish wen)
- Infectious (cysts, abscesses, or granulomas)
  - Viruses, particularly lymphocystis, carp pox, adenoviruses.
  - Bacteria, particularly *Edwardsiella*, *Mycobacterium*, *Nocardia* spp.
  - Fungi or fungal-like organisms, particularly microsporidial xenomas.
  - Metazoa, particularly pentastomids.
  - Myxozoa, particularly myxozoan pseudocysts.
  - Algal granulomas.
- Inflammatory
  - Panniculitis, dermatitis, steatitis.
- Trauma
  - Venomous fin ray (e.g. lionfish) or barb (e.g. stingray).
  - Foreign bodies (e.g. fiberglass, gravel).
  - Abrasions and hyperplasia from inappropriate enclosure size, shape, or décor.
  - Hematomas.

Diagnostic Approach

- Review the history, in particular:
  - Age.
  - Known causes of prior morbidity and mortality.
  - When a mass was first seen and the progression.
- Visually assess the animals.
  - Identify any other clinical signs, including behavioral changes.
- Handling of live fish is usually required; anesthesia should be used to facilitate restraint.
  - Perform a full clinical examination.
  - Examine the masses and any possible effects (e.g. compression of adjacent tissues, ulceration).
  - Consider radiography, ultrasonography, computed tomography, or other diagnostic imaging to look for signs of local invasion or obvious systemic spread.
  - Collect scrapes, aspirates, and impression smears of the mass. Examine samples under direct microscopy and Dif-Quik, Gram, acid-fast, and potentially other special stains. Consider cultures (e.g. aerobic, mycobacterial, fungal). Consider incisional or excisional biopsies. Skin preparation is not indicated, although large scales may need to be removed over the site. Bone cutters may be needed for firm masses. Fix samples in formalin for histology. If enough tissue is available, place some into sterile cryovials for freezing and fixing in 95% ethanol or other fixatives. Biopsy sites are typically left to heal by second intention.
  - Consider endoscopic or exploratory coeliotomy to look for systemic lesions.

Management Approach

- Consider surgical removal under general or local anesthesia and analgesia. Closure is usually by second intention unless there has been coelomic exposure or the tissue is under tension.
- Provide supportive care (e.g. analgesia, fluid and nutritional support), if needed.
- Further management of neoplastic diseases is described in Chapter C2.

Circling or Spiraling

Overview

- Central neurologic system (CNS) problems may present with circling or spiral (corkscrew) swimming (sometimes referred to as whirling), or changes in posture or behavior.
- The most common differentials are toxic and infectious, with some viruses, bacteria, and parasites preferring the CNS.
- Peripheral neurologic signs are harder to identify in fish but may be seen, such as loss of fin movement on one side.
- Pruritus can often look neurologic, so parasites and irritants should be considered.

Signalment

- Any fish can be affected.

Clinical Findings

- One or more fish may be affected.
- Circling and spiraling are usually obvious, although they may be intermittent.
- More subtle signs such as changes in posture (e.g. listing, head-down, tail-down), behavior (e.g. spy-hopping), or feeding (e.g. missing food strikes) may be seen.
- Paralysis or paresis may be seen. This may be unilateral or caudal.
- Seizures have not been specifically reported in fish.
- Spinal deformity, skin color changes, or muscle atrophy may be seen secondary to a spinal lesion.
- Reduced feeding, inappetence, regurgitation, or weight loss may be seen.
- Blindness may be seen. Vision can be hard to evaluate in fish because of their sensitivity to water movement and vibration, but most fish should show a startle response to a sudden movement above the water.

Etiologies

- The most common differentials include *Vibrio* or *Streptococcus* spp. and myxozoan infections in the CNS.
- Developmental
- Metabolic
  - Acid–base, glucose, or electrolyte changes.
- Neoplasia
  - Nervous system.
  - Musculoskeletal.
- Nutritional
  - Deficiency of vitamin E, several vitamin Bs (e.g. thiamine, riboflavin, niacin, folate, pyridoxine, cyanocobalamin), selenium, calcium, or phosphorus can cause neurologic signs in other classes.
- Vascular
  - Ischemic or vascular event.
- Infectious/inflammatory (septicemia, meningitis, encephalitis, myositis)
  - Viruses, particularly betanodaviruses, rhabdoviruses, herpesviruses, birnaviruses, ranaviruses.
  - Bacteria, particularly vibriosis, *Edwardsiella*, *Carnobacterium*, *Serratia*, *Streptococcus*, *Francisella* spp., *Flavobacterium psychrophilum*.
  - Fungi or fungal-like organisms, particularly *Exophiala* spp. and *Microsporidia* (e.g. *Pleistophora*).
  - Protozoa, particularly scuticociliates.
  - Metazoa, particularly philometrid nematodes, digenes.
  - Myxozoa, particularly *Myxobolus cerebralis*.
- Idiopathic
  - Chronic liver disease.
  - Chronic kidney disease.
- Toxic
  - Ammonia.
  - Chlorines.
  - Heavy metals (e.g. copper, lead, zinc).
  - Drug toxicity (e.g. trichlorfon, contamination, idiosyncratic reaction).
  - Pesticides, herbicides.
  - Paint fumes.
  - Cyanide.
- Trauma
  - Physical trauma, particularly to the spine or head.
  - Electrical stunning.
- Life support system/environmental
  - Stereotypies.
  - Inappropriate enclosure shape.
  - Stray voltage and poor electrical grounding.
  - Lightning strike.

Diagnostic Approach

- Review the history, in particular:
  - Recent animal additions and the history of those animals.
  - Quarantine and other biosecurity protocols.
  - Water source.
  - Food eaten, including storage and preparation.
  - Any recent mortalities.
  - Known causes of prior morbidity and mortality.
  - Recent medications, including applied doses and method of dosing.
  - Chronicity and progression of clinical signs.
- Check the water quality, particularly ammonia, copper, and chlorine. Compare results to target ranges and any previous records.

- Visually observe the animals.
  - Try to confirm that the signs look neurologic, rather than pruritic or associated with musculoskeletal or swim bladder pathology.
  - With CNS disease, fish often show no effort to correct posture, buoyancy is usually unaffected, and signs are often continuous or triggered by a visual or tactile stimulus.
- Visually assess the habitat.
  - Look for sources of possible contaminants above or around the system.
- Consider freezing 1 L of water in a clean plastic bottle for later analysis if needed.
- Necropsy any mortalities, if available. The best diagnostic samples are collected from sick fish that were recently euthanized. Include additional testing as indicated, e.g.:
  - Radiographs.
  - Cultures, often bacterial (e.g. blood, liver, kidney, brain, CSF).
  - Wet mounts and impression smears (e.g. liver, kidney, brain, CSF).
  - Histology.
  - Further diagnostics (e.g. CSF analysis, tissues for virus isolation).
  - Archive samples (e.g. liver, kidney, brain, frozen at −20°C (−4°F) or ideally −80°C (−112°F) and fixed in 95% ethanol and electron microscopy fixative).
- If the cause is still unknown, handling of live fish may be required; anesthesia should be used to facilitate restraint and reduce the risk of trauma.
  - Perform a full clinical examination.
  - Use radiography or computed tomography to look for possible skull or spinal pathology.
  - Consider hematology, biochemistry, and blood gases to look for inflammation, anemia, acidosis, hypoglycemia, and electrolytes changes, and consider testing for lead (whole blood) or zinc (plasma).
  - Consider sampling the CSF in elasmobranchs to look for inflammation or infectious agents on cytology and culture.

Management Approach

- Treat the underlying cause, if identified.
- Modify the environment to prevent additional trauma (e.g. minimal substrate and décor, reduce lighting and cover windows to reduce startle responses).
- Ground the system in case of stray voltage.
- Provide supportive care (e.g. fluid and nutritional support, intravenous vitamin B complex), if needed.
- Consider anti-inflammatory or shock doses of corticosteroids (e.g. dexamethasone SP, methylprednisolone).
- In cases of severe spinal trauma, or where there is no response to supportive care, consider euthanasia.
- If a group is affected and no infectious diseases are identified, consider moving the animals to a new system in case of unknown contaminants.

Abbreviations/Acronyms

- CNS: Central neurologic system
- CSF: Cerebrospinal fluid

Positive Buoyancy

Overview

- Positive buoyancy typically presents as a bony fish that is unable to swim down through the water column or that requires more effort than normal to swim down or stay low in the water. It may be in a normal or abnormal orientation (e.g. lateral).
- It is important to differentiate this presentation from a neurologic or respiratory disorder or displacement.
- Positive buoyancy is usually due to abnormal gas accumulation in the swim bladder, gastrointestinal tract, coelom, subcutis, or pouch.
- Common causes of positive buoyancy are swim bladder disease and barotrauma.
- Abnormal gas accumulations can be removed by centesis. While this can resolve signs, recurrence is common.

Signalment

- Any bony fish can be affected, but some species are over-represented:
  - Fancy goldfish (*Carassius auratus*) such as orandas, moors, lionheads, bubble-eyes, ryukins, and ranchus.
  - Seahorses (*Syngnathidae*) due to swim bladder or pouch inflation or subcutaneous gas emboli.
  - Deep-water species such as red-banded rockfish (*Sebastes babcocki*).

Clinical Findings

- One or more fish may be affected, but this is more commonly an individual fish problem.
- Fish are often at the surface and may be in a lateral, ventrodorsal, dorsoventral, or vertical position.
- Fish may be unable to swim down or may be able to swim down but only with vigorous swimming. In chronic cases, this may be associated with secondary skin damage.
- Fish may swim normally but float up to the surface when at rest.
- Exophthalmos or buphthalmos may be seen.

- Dyspnea or tachypnea may be seen but are not common.

Etiologies

- The most common differentials are swim bladder disease and barotrauma.
- Developmental
  - Selective breeding for characteristic deformities (e.g. fancy goldfish).
- Anomalous
  - Swallowing of air when out of the water (e.g. during restraint or transfer).
  - Lack of access to breeding females in male seahorses with gas in the pouch.
- Metabolic
  - Acidosis (theoretically).
- Neoplasia
  - Swim bladder.
  - Kidney or other tissue near the swim bladder or pneumatic duct.
  - Nervous system.
- Nutritional
  - Floating foods allowing swallowing of air.
  - Dry foods that can expand in the gastrointestinal tract.
  - Foreign body obstruction of the pneumatic duct.
- Normal behavior
  - Several species perch in vertical or ventrodorsal orientations that can look like positive buoyancy (e.g. rockfish, upsidedown catfish (*Synodontis nigriventris*)).
- Infectious/inflammatory – any systemic, swim bladder, renal, gastrointestinal, or neurologic inflammation, and pouch inflammation in seahorses
  - Viruses, particularly spring viremia of carp and largemouth bass virus.
  - Bacteria, particularly vibriosis, *Aeromonas*, *Streptococcus*, *Mycobacterium* spp.
  - Fungi or fungal-like organisms, particularly *Exophiala*, *Phoma* spp.
  - Metazoa, particularly anguillicolid nematodes, encysted pentastomids.
  - Myxozoa, particularly *Hoferellus*, *Sphaerospora* spp.
  - Apicomplexa, particularly *Goussia* spp.
- Trauma
  - Barotrauma (e.g. recent catch from depth).
  - Physical trauma, particularly to the spine, swim bladder, or pneumatic duct.
  - Electrical stunning.
- Life support system/environmental
  - Gas supersaturation.
  - Low pH (theoretically).
  - Stray voltage and poor electrical grounding.
  - Lightning strike.

Diagnostic Approach

- Visually assess the animals.
  - Try to confirm if this is a true buoyancy disorder, rather than due to a neurologic or respiratory disorder or displacement.
  - With positive buoyancy, gas emboli may be grossly visible (e.g. in or around the eyes or under the skin). If you gently push the fish down, it is likely to float back to the surface; this can help identify which part of the body is positively buoyant. The fish may try to vigorously swim down.
  - With neurologic issues, fish often show no effort to correct an abnormal posture or position and may show abnormal swimming, including circling or spiraling.
  - With respiratory issues, fish may gather at the surface, but commonly show dyspnea and tachypnea.
  - Fish may be displaced into abnormal locations in the water column, such as at the surface. The behavioral interactions are often seen if the fish are monitored closely and may resolve if the social group is changed.
- Review the history, in particular:
  - Food eaten, including presentation.
  - Recent life support system changes.
  - Recent husbandry changes.
  - Recent handling or transport.
  - Chronicity of clinical signs.
- Check water quality, including gas pressures over 24–48 hours. If a total gas pressure meter is not available, a dissolved oxygen meter can be used to see if oxygen is supersaturated, although this is less useful. Compare results to target ranges and any previous records.
- Check the life support system for visible cracks and check the water for microbubbles, which can be suggestive of supersaturation.
- Necropsy any mortalities, if available. The best diagnostic samples are collected from sick fish that were recently euthanized. A normal swim bladder wall is usually thin and translucent or thick, white, and opaque, although there may be pigmented areas. Abnormal findings include serosanguinous fluid, purulent exudate, soft tissue, petechiae or ecchymoses, adhesions, or tears. Include additional testing as indicated, e.g.:
  - Cultures, often bacterial, mycobacterial, and fungal (e.g. abnormal fluid or tissue near the swim bladder).
  - Wet mounts and impression smears (e.g. gill, skin, liver, kidney, gastrointestinal tract, swim bladder).
  - Histology.
  - Further diagnostics (e.g. swabs or tissues for PCR testing for spring viremia of carp or largemouth bass virus).

- Archive samples (e.g. gill, liver, kidney, swim bladder, frozen at −20°C (−4°F) or ideally −80°C (−112°F) and fixed in 95% ethanol and electron microscopy fixative).
- If the cause is still unknown, handling of live fish is usually required for diagnosis and treatment; anesthesia should be used to facilitate restraint.
  - Perform a full clinical examination.
  - Examine gill and fin biopsies under direct microscopy to look for gas emboli.
  - Use radiography, ultrasonography, or computed tomography to identify the site and volume of abnormal gas. For radiography, include both resting (vertical beam) and standing (horizontal beam) lateral views. Swim bladder volume is often reported as 4–7% of body volume, with freshwater species at the higher end of the range. However, this is a rough guideline and clinically normal fish can have larger swim bladders. It is helpful to compare to radiographs of a normal conspecific.
  - Consider rigid endoscopy of the coelom or swim bladder for diagnosis and treatment.

Management Approach

- Ensure that any exposed skin or fins remain wet (e.g. high local humidity, correction of the positive buoyancy).
- Recompression is usually the preferred treatment for excess gas accumulation. This may involve weighted crates that can be sunk to specific depths, or chambers that can be pressurized. Chambers are not available commercially but can be built. One system is described in Smiley and Drawbridge (2007).
- Remove swim bladder gas (pneumocentesis) or free gas to provide temporary relief, using a suitable-sized needle on a syringe or short extension set and a lateral approach. This can be done under radiographic or ultrasound guidance. Recurrence over several days is common.
- Remove subcutaneous or pouch gas in seahorses by percutaneous aspiration or by catheter, respectively.
- Treat any primary cause, if identified (e.g. antibiotics, gastroprotectants).
- Consider acetazolamide, a carbonic anhydrase inhibitor that can reduce the concentration of carbon dioxide in the eyes and plasma and may reduce oxygen secretion. Typical doses are 2.5–5.0 mg/kg IM every three to seven days for up to three treatments. High doses can be associated with negative buoyancy, neurologic signs, and mortalities.
- Consider surgical correction of swim bladder pathology (e.g. pneumocystoplasty, pneumocystectomy).
- Provide supportive care (e.g. fluid or nutritional support), if needed.
- In marine fish, consider reducing the salinity slightly to help the fish maintain buoyancy.
- It is possible to inject fluid (e.g. hetastarch) into the swim bladder to try to reduce buoyancy and gas secretion.
- For idiopathic cases in fancy goldfish, there are anecdotal reports of improvements with feeding fresh, crushed, or cooked peas; fasting for two to three days; using magnesium sulfate to reduce constipation; and managing buoyancy using small weights attached to the fish.

Bibliography

Britt, T., Weisse, C., Weber, E.S. et al. (2002). Use of pneumocystoplasty for overinflation of the swim bladder in a goldfish. *Journal of the American Veterinary Medical Association* 221: 690–693.

Holzer, A.S., Hartigan, A., Patra, S. et al. (2014). Molecular fingerprinting of the myxozoan community in common carp suffering swim bladder inflammation (SBI) identifies multiple etiological agents. *Parasites & Vectors* 7: 398–407.

Lewbart, G.A., Stone, E.A., and Love, N.E. (1995). Pneumocystectomy in a Midas cichlid. *Journal of the American Veterinary Medical Association* 207: 319–321.

Pees, M., Pees, K., and Kiefer, I. (2010). The use of computed tomography for assessment of the swim bladder in koi carp (*Cyprinus carpio*). *Veterinary Radiology & Ultrasound* 51: 291–298.

Perlberg, S.T., Diamant, A., Ofir, R., and Zilberg, D. (2008). Characterization of swim bladder non-inflation (SBN) in angelfish, *Pteropyllum scalare* (Schultz), and the effect of exposure to methylene blue. *Journal of Fish Diseases.*

Smiley, J.E. and Drawbridge, M.A. (2007). Techniques for live capture of deepwater fishes with special emphasis on the design and application of a low-cost hyperbaric chamber. *Journal of Fish Biology* 70: 867–878.

Abbreviations/Acronyms

- CT: Computed tomography
- IM: Intramuscular

Negative Buoyancy

Overview

- Fish maintain neutral buoyancy using a variety of methods, including a gas-filled swim bladder, fat deposition in the liver, and body shape and movement.
- Negative buoyancy typically presents as a fish that is on the substrate, lower in the water column than normal, or swimming with a tail-down posture.
- Negative buoyancy may be due to neurologic, musculoskeletal, gastrointestinal, or swim bladder pathology, or loss of body condition.
- Prognosis is usually guarded for fish with negative buoyancy.

Signalment

- Any fish can be affected.
- Larval bony fish in aquaculture are particularly susceptible.

Clinical Findings

- One or more fish may be affected, but this is more commonly an individual fish problem.
- Fish may be seen on the substrate, upright or recumbent, or may be low in the water column. Affected fish may swim with a tail-down posture.
- Lethargy is often seen.
- Respiratory rate and effort are often normal.
- Edematous or ulcerative skin or eye lesions may develop in dependent areas (e.g. leading edge of the anal fin).

Etiologies

- The most common differentials are swim bladder disease in bony fish with swim bladders, and loss of fat reserves in cartilaginous fish.
- Developmental
    - Failure to inflate the swim bladder as fry.
    - Selective breeding for characteristic deformities (e.g. fancy goldfish (*Carassius auratus*)).
    - Genetic abnormalities.
    - Methylene blue exposure during development.
- Neoplasia
    - Swim bladder (e.g. swim bladder sarcoma virus).
    - Kidney or other tissue near the swim bladder or pneumatic duct.
    - Nervous system.
- Nutritional
    - Loss of fat reserves, particularly in the liver.
    - Inability to swallow air.
    - Foreign body obstruction of the pneumatic duct.
    - Myopathy (particularly seahorses, *Syngnathidae*).
- Infectious/inflammatory
    - Viruses, particularly spring viremia of carp, Atlantic salmon swim bladder sarcoma.
    - Bacteria, particularly vibriosis, *Aeromonas*, *Mycobacterium* spp.
    - Fungi or fungal-like organisms, particularly *Exophiala*, *Phoma* spp.
    - Metazoa, particularly anguillicolid nematodes, encysted pentastomids, encysted digenes.
    - Myxozoa, particularly *Hoferellus*, *Sphaerospora* spp.
    - Apicomplexa, particularly *Goussia* spp.
- Toxic
    - Drug toxicity (e.g. acetazolamide, idiosyncratic reaction).
- Trauma
    - Physical trauma, particularly to the spine, swim bladder, or pneumatic duct

Diagnostic Approach

- Visually assess the animals.
    - Try to confirm if this is a true buoyancy disorder, rather than due to a neurologic disorder or displacement.
    - With negative buoyancy, if you move the fish higher in the water column, it is likely to drift back down. The fish may try to vigorously swim up.
    - With neurologic issues, fish often show no effort to correct an abnormal posture or position and may show abnormal swimming, including circling or spiraling.
    - Fish may be displaced into abnormal locations in the water column, such as towards the substrate. The behavioral interactions are often seen if the fish are monitored closely and may resolve if the social group is changed.
- Review the history, in particular:
    - Food eaten, including storage and preparation.
    - Age.
    - Recent handling or transport.
    - History of positive buoyancy.
    - Chronicity of clinical signs.
- Necropsy any mortalities, if available. The best diagnostic samples are collected from sick fish that were recently euthanized. Include additional testing as indicated, e.g.:
    - Cultures, often bacterial, mycobacterial, and fungal (e.g. abnormal fluid or tissue near the swim bladder).
    - Wet mounts and impression smears (e.g. gill, skin, liver, kidney, gastrointestinal tract, swim bladder).
    - Histology.
    - Archive samples (e.g. gill, muscle, liver, kidney, swim bladder, frozen at −20°C (−4°F) or ideally −80°C (−112°F) and fixed in 95% ethanol and electron microscopy fixative).

- If the cause is still unknown, handling of live fish is usually required; anesthesia should be used to facilitate restraint.
  - Perform a full clinical examination.
  - Use radiography or computed tomography to identify any swim bladder or skeletal abnormalities. For radiography, include both resting (vertical beam) and standing (horizontal beam) lateral views. Swim bladder volume is often reported as 4–7% of body volume, with freshwater species at the higher end of the range. However, this is a rough guideline. It is helpful to compare to radiographs of a normal conspecific.
  - If fluid or soft tissue abnormalities are seen, collect aspirates for aerobic, mycobacterial, and fungal cultures and cytology (e.g. Dif-Quik, Gram, and acid-fast stains).
  - Consider ultrasonography to evaluate liver size and echogenicity and any coelomic abnormalities.
  - Consider rigid endoscopy of the coelom or swim bladder.

Management Approach

- Provide supportive care. Nutritional support is particularly important for elasmobranchs showing negative buoyancy to restore fat reserves in the liver.
- Provide a substrate that is smooth and clean (e.g. round gravel or smooth fiberglass).
- Treat any primary cause, if identified.
- Consider increasing the salinity slightly to help the fish maintain buoyancy, if tolerated.
- Consider injecting air into small swim bladders. Sterile air should be used; this can be taken from inside a fluid bag. Recurrence is common.
- For idiopathic cases in fancy goldfish, there are anecdotal reports of managing buoyancy temporarily with floats attached to the fish.

B6

Ocular Signs

Catherine A. Hadfield

Seattle Aquarium, Seattle, WA, USA

Exophthalmos or Buphthalmos

Overview

- Exophthalmos means protrusion of the globe. This is typically due to retrobulbar gas or soft tissue. In rare cases, it may be due to retrobulbar fluid.
- Buphthalmos means enlargement of the globe. This can be due to increased intraocular gas, soft tissue, or fluid.
- Both are referred to colloquially as popeye.
- It is important to differentiate the cause of the distension (gas, soft tissue, or fluid) and the location (intraocular, retrobulbar) as this will affect the differential list, prognosis, and management plans. However, in many cases, fish will present with a combination of ocular signs.

Signalment

- Any bony fish can be affected, but some are particularly susceptible:
  - Groupers (*Epinephelus* spp.).
  - Dhufish (*Glaucosoma hebraicum*).
  - Rockfish (*Sebastes* spp.).
  - Squirrelfish and soldierfish (*Holocentridae*).
- This is rare in elasmobranchs.

Clinical Findings

- One or more fish may be affected.
- One or both eyes may be affected.
- An enlarged eye is readily visible, but it can be hard to differentiate between exophthalmos and buphthalmos. In general, a hands-on examination is required.
- Ocular opacities, ulceration, perforation, or hemorrhage may be seen.
- Affected fish often show no other clinical signs, although positive buoyancy, reduced appetite, lethargy, or skin changes may be seen.

Etiologies (Gas)

- The most common differentials are gas supersaturation and low hydrostatic pressure; inflammation is often secondary.
- Metabolic
  - Pseudobranch pathology.
  - Renal disease (theoretically).
  - Acidosis (theoretically).
- Trauma
  - Cohort, décor, or catch trauma.
  - Startling stimuli.
  - Barotrauma (e.g. catch from depth within several days).
- Life support system/environmental
  - Gas supersaturation.
  - Shallow systems for deep-water fish.
  - High or increasing water temperature.

Etiologies (Soft Tissue or Fluid, Including Blood)

- If only one eye is affected, trauma and neoplasia are the most common differentials. If both eyes are affected, nutritional or infectious causes are more likely.
- Neoplasia
  - Retrobulbar.
  - Intraocular.
- Nutritional
  - Excess fat behind the eye.
  - Deficiency of micronutrients (e.g. vitamin A, C, E, folate, pyridoxine).

Clinical Guide to Fish Medicine, First Edition. Edited by Catherine A. Hadfield and Leigh Ann Clayton.

- Infectious/inflammatory
  - Viruses, particularly rhabdoviruses, herpesviruses, infectious pancreatic necrosis virus, infectious salmon anemia, cardiomyopathy syndrome.
  - Bacteria, particularly vibriosis, *Aeromonas*, *Citrobacter*, *Pseudomonas*, *Edwardsiella*, *Flavobacterium*, *Yersinia*, *Streptococcus*, *Mycobacterium*, *Francisella* spp.
  - Fungi or fungal-like organisms, particularly *Fusarium* spp., *Mesomycetozoea*.
  - Protozoa, particularly scuticociliates.
  - Metazoa, particularly philometrid nematodes.
  - Myxozoa, particularly *Tetracapsuloides bryosalmonae*.
- Toxic
  - Ammonia.
- Trauma
  - Cohort, décor, or catch trauma.
  - Startling stimuli.
- Life support system/environmental
  - Stray voltage and poor electrical grounding.

Diagnostic Approach

- Review the history, in particular:
  - Recent animal additions and the history of those animals.
  - Quarantine and other biosecurity protocols.
  - Habitat dimensions, particularly depth.
  - Recent life support system changes.
  - Recent catch, handling, or transport.
  - External events, such as sudden lighting changes.
  - Chronicity and progression of clinical signs.
- Check the water quality, particularly dissolved oxygen and total gas pressures. Compare results to target ranges and any previous records.
- Visually assess the animals.
  - Identify the species, size classes, and percentage of population impacted.
  - Identify if lesions are unilateral or bilateral.
  - Try to differentiate between gas or soft tissue/fluid (Figure B6.1) (gas can produce small bubbles in the anterior chamber).
  - Evaluate vision (e.g. assess the response to a sudden movement above the water).
  - Identify any other clinical signs (e.g. skin hyperemia or ulceration, behavioral changes).
- Handling of live fish is usually required; anesthesia should be used to facilitate restraint and reduce the risk of trauma.
  - Examine the eyes, oral cavity, and gills. A slit lamp and direct or indirect ophthalmoscope are helpful.
  - Measure intraocular pressure. Reported values for teleosts have typically been 10–20 mmHg. Comparison with a normal conspecific helps with interpretation.
  - Collect a fine-needle aspirate from the affected space for gas or fluid removal and cytology, fluid analysis, or cultures as indicated.
  - Examine gill and fin biopsies under direct microscopy to check for gas emboli.
  - Consider ultrasonography, radiography, or computed tomography to identify pathology within and around the eyes.

Management Approach

- Prevent further ocular trauma by removing complex décor, reducing the lighting, and partially covering any windows to reduce startle responses.
- Treat any infection with systemic, topical, conjunctival, or intraocular medications.
- Consider analgesia and anti-inflammatory medications.
- If gas supersaturation is suspected, identify and remove the source. Agitate the water gently to help with off-gassing. If the problem cannot be resolved, consider moving affected fish to a different system.
- For intraocular or retrobulbar gas, consider recompression treatment. Recompression chambers for fish can be built; one system is described in Smiley and Drawbridge (2007). For intransient intraocular gas, consider pseudobranch ablation.
- Prognosis for retrobulbar gas is usually good. In some cases, clinical signs may remain or recur but systemic signs and mortality are rare.
- Prognosis for intraocular gas is worse due to lens and retina damage. Return to normal function is possible, although uncommon with chronic cases. The eye may progress to phthisis bulbi. Enucleation may improve overall prognosis.
- Prognosis with severe inflammatory lesions is guarded. Enucleation may improve overall prognosis if the disease is not systemic.

Bibliography

Smiley, J.E. and Drawbridge, M.A. (2007). Techniques for live capture of deepwater fishes with special emphasis on the design and application of a low-cost hyperbaric chamber. *Journal of Fish Biology* 70: 867–878.

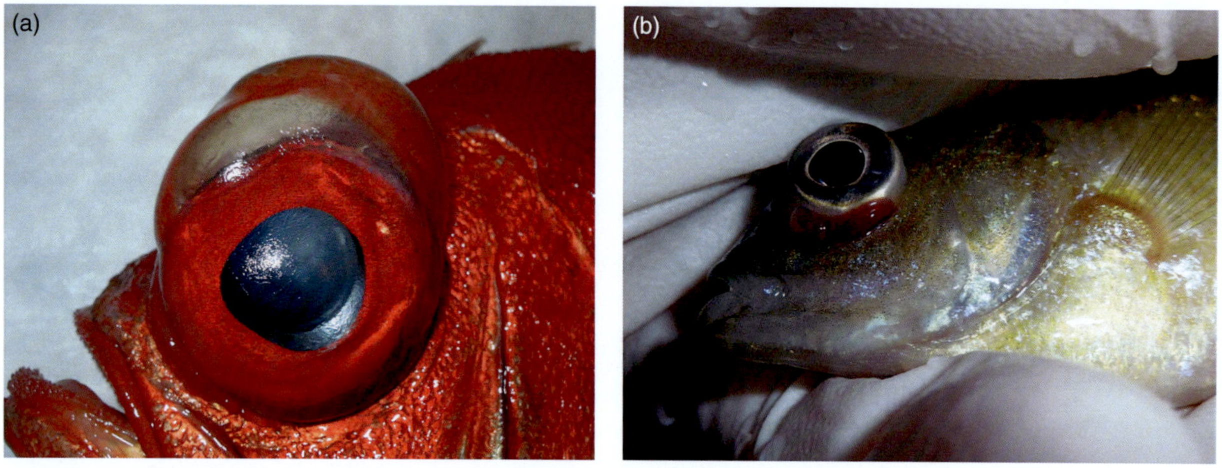

Figure B6.1 Exophthalmos in a short bigeye (*Pristigenys alta*) due to gas (a) and in a bluegill (*Lepomis macrochirus*) due to philometrid nematodes (b).

Ocular Opacity

Overview

- Ocular opacities can be due to changes in the conjunctiva, cornea, anterior chamber, or lens.
- Diffuse ocular opacities are common and often due to keratitis and uveitis. Lesions are frequently traumatic or infectious in origin. Bilateral lesions can suggest systemic infection.
- Lenticular opacities (cataracts) are also common.
- Lipid keratopathy can cause white plaques within the cornea and conjunctiva not associated with inflammation.

Signalment

- Any fish can be affected, but species with protruding eyes are particularly susceptible.

Clinical Findings

- One or more fish may be affected.
- One or both eyes may be affected.
- If only the lens is affected, the globe, cornea, iris, and anterior chamber look normal (Figure B6.2).
- If the cornea or anterior chamber is involved, the affected eye usually looks diffusely white, although lesions can be red, gray, black, or erosive.
- Affected eyes may be exophthalmic or buphthalmic.
- Reduced appetite, inappetence, weight loss, lethargy, or skin changes may be seen and are more likely to be associated with systemic disease.

Etiologies

- If only one eye is affected, trauma is more likely. If both eyes are affected, infectious or environmental causes are more likely.
- Nutritional
  - Abnormal lipid deposition.
  - Deficiency of micronutrients.
- Infectious/inflammatory (uveitis, keratitis)
  - Bacteria, particularly vibriosis, *Aeromonas*, *Citrobacter*, *Pseudomonas*, *Edwardsiella*, *Flavobacterium*, *Yersinia*, *Streptococcus*, *Francisella* spp.
  - Fungi or fungal-like organisms, particularly atypical oomycetes.
  - Protozoa, particularly *Cryptocaryon*, scuticociliates (SW); *Ichthyophthirius*, scuticociliates (FW).
  - Metazoa, particularly capsalids (e.g. *Neobenedenia* spp.), digenes (e.g. *Diplostomum* spp.), turbellarians, copepods.
- Toxic
  - Ammonia, nitrites.
  - Polycyclic aromatic hydrocarbons.
- Trauma
  - Cohort, décor, or catch trauma.
  - Startling stimuli.
  - Barotrauma.
  - Lens luxation.
- Life support system/environmental
  - Rapid change in pH or salinity.
  - High, low, or fluctuating water temperature.
  - High carbon dioxide.
  - Insufficient or excessive UV from overhead lighting.
  - Sudden lighting changes.
  - Residual oxidants.

Diagnostic Approach

- Review the history, in particular:
  - Recent animal additions and the history of those animals.
  - Quarantine and other biosecurity protocols.
  - Environmental conditions.

- Recent catch, handling, or transport.
- Chronicity and progression of clinical signs.
- Check the water quality, particularly pH, carbon dioxide, oxidants, and ORPs (with ozone). Compare results to target ranges and any previous records.
- Visually assess the animals.
  - Identify the species, size classes, and percentage of population impacted.
  - Identify if lesions are unilateral or bilateral.
  - Try to differentiate between opaque corneas or lenses.
  - Evaluate vision (e.g. assess the response to a sudden movement above the water).
  - Identify any other clinical signs (e.g. buphthalmos, skin hyperemia or ulceration, behavioral changes).
- Handling of live fish is usually required; anesthesia should be used to facilitate restraint and reduce the risk of trauma.
  - Examine the eyes, oral cavity, and gills. A slit lamp and direct or indirect ophthalmoscope are helpful.
  - Consider corneal cultures, particularly if lesions are not healing as expected.
  - Examine an impression smear of the corneal surface to identify bacteria, parasites (e.g. *Neobenedenia* spp.), and cell type and morphology.
  - Measure intraocular pressure. Comparison with a normal conspecific under the same husbandry conditions helps with interpretation.
  - Use topical fluorescein stain to assess for ulcerative keratitis.
  - Consider ultrasonography to evaluate the posterior chamber and retrobulbar space.
  - If there is concomitant exophthalmos or buphthalmos, consider aspiration of the retrobulbar or intraocular space.
- Histology of the eye and retrobulbar tissues following enucleation or at necropsy is often required for diagnosis, although the underlying etiology may remain unknown.

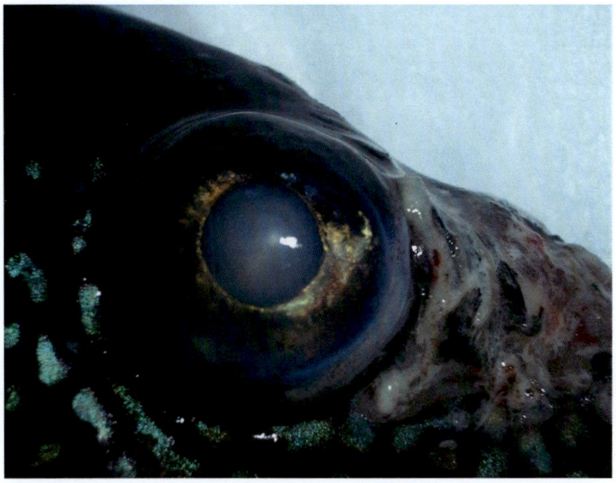

Figure B6.2 Cataract and cutaneous ulceration.

Management Approach

- Prevent further ocular trauma by removing complex décor, reducing the lighting, and partially covering any windows to reduce startle responses.
- Treat any infection with systemic, topical, conjunctival, or intraocular medications.
- Consider analgesia and anti-inflammatory medications.
- For lens luxations or cataracts, consider surgical management.
- For ulcerative keratitis, consider a grid keratotomy with a 25 ga needle or cotton-tipped applicator.
- Fish can often heal ocular lesions unless the inflammation is severe or there are ongoing insults. Enucleation may improve overall prognosis if the disease is not systemic.

Abbreviations/Acronyms

- FW: Freshwater
- ORP: Oxidation–reduction potential
- SW: Salt water
- UV: Ultraviolet

Section C

Diseases of Fish

Introduction

Section C covers common diseases seen in practice, with clinically-relevant information in a bullet-point format. Chapters are divided into noninfectious diseases, viruses, bacteria, fungi and fungal-like organisms, protozoa, metazoa, and myxozoa and coccidia. For each disease, the initial overview highlights important points. This is followed by information on etiology; please bear in mind that for infectious diseases, taxonomic names and groups are updated frequently as new information emerges and some disagreement may exist as to how to name or classify organisms. For infectious diseases, etiology is followed by information on life cycle and transmission. Signalment and risk factors are reviewed, followed by typical signs and clinical findings, differential diagnoses, and possible diagnostics. Management options are divided up into husbandry (e.g. increased mechanical cleaning) and medical (e.g. drug treatment). Prevention is also discussed, as is the zoonotic risk for infectious diseases. These details are as up-to-date as we could reasonably achieve, but we are all constantly learning and the reader should review recent literature for additional information.

C1

Noninfectious Diseases (Environmental)

Catherine A. Hadfield

Seattle Aquarium, Seattle, WA, USA

Introduction

This first chapter on noninfectious diseases focuses on environmental problems related to water quality. These include low dissolved oxygen, gas supersaturation, barotrauma, temperature stress, pH stress, and toxicity from ammonia, nitrites, nitrates, chlorines, heavy metals, hydrogen sulfide, and pesticides. Where available, information is provided on etiology, signalment, clinical signs, diagnosis, husbandry and medical management, and prevention.

Low Dissolved Oxygen

Overview

- Low dissolved oxygen (DO) is the most common environmental problem of fish. It can lead to high mortality in wild and managed fish.
- Target DO for most fish systems is >90% saturation, equivalent to 6–15 mg/L depending on the salinity and water temperature.
- Husbandry changes should be instigated rapidly to resolve low dissolved oxygen.

Etiology

- Almost all fish rely on oxygen (O_2) that is dissolved in water for respiration.
- A few fish are obligate air-breathers and use oxygen in air (Table A1.1). They are not susceptible to low dissolved oxygen in water but require access to air.
- DO comes from atmospheric diffusion and photosynthesis by aquatic plants (when sunlight is available). Water movement increases the oxygen content.
- Low DO can be due to a wide variety of factors:
  - Low aeration or water flow (e.g. aerator or pump failure, blocked lines, lack of wind or rainfall).
  - High water temperature.
  - High salinity.
  - High organic load, high stocking density, or heavy feeding.
  - Small water volume or surface area (e.g. during transport or restraint).
  - Some immersion treatments (e.g. formalin).
  - Granular activated carbon filtration.
  - Reduced photosynthesis (e.g. at dawn, after an algal die-off, in the fall and winter); low DO is particularly common in ponds on cloudy days in the fall.
  - Ice cover over shallow ponds, particularly if decaying matter is present.
  - Groundwater (e.g. deep wells).
  - Low barometric pressure or high altitude.
  - Reversal of a thermocline (warm surface water and cold deep water) during the summer in lakes or ponds following wind, rain, or thunderstorms.

Signalment

- Species sensitivity varies.
- Most species are sensitive to low DO, particularly:
  - Salmon and trout (*Salmonidae*).
  - Tropical marine teleosts.
  - Most elasmobranchs.
- Some species are more tolerant of low DO; these are typically slow-moving, freshwater species that have evolved in environments where DO can be low, e.g.:
  - Tilapia (*Oreochromis* and *Tilapia* spp.).

Clinical Guide to Fish Medicine, First Edition. Edited by Catherine A. Hadfield and Leigh Ann Clayton.

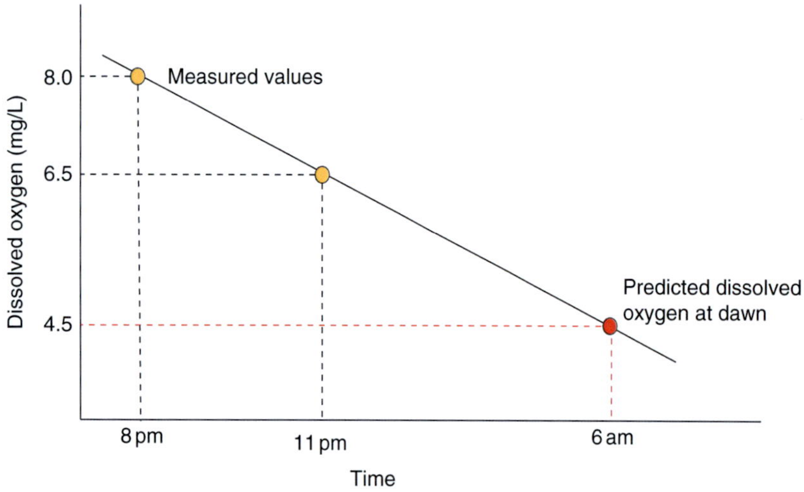

Figure C1.1 Predicting early morning dissolved oxygen levels in a pond using measured values at dusk and two to three hours after dusk.

- Crucian carp (*Carassius carassius*), goldfish (*Carassius auratus*).
- Epaulette sharks (*Hemiscyllium ocellatum*).
- Facultative and obligate air-breathing fish (Table A1.1).

- Larger individuals are often more sensitive to low DO than smaller individuals.

Signs/Clinical Findings

- Multiple fish from one or more species are usually affected.
- Lethargy is common.
- Acute inappetence is common.
- Dyspnea or tachypnea is common (e.g. flared opercula or gill slits, piping or gasping at the surface, gathering near the surface or in areas of high flow or turbulence).
- Blotchy skin may be seen in sharks.
- The water may show a change in color if there has been an algal die-off.
- The water may look stagnant and there may be a smell of decomposition.
- Acute mortality can reach 100%.

Differential Diagnoses

- Acute mortalities with dyspnea or tachypnea are typically due to an environmental failure (e.g. low DO, ammonia toxicity, contaminated water) or an acute ectoparasitic or bacterial disease (e.g. *Cryptocaryon irritans*, columnaris).

Diagnosis

- DO must be measured where the fish are found. It cannot be reliably measured from a water sample or from another location in the system (e.g. in the sump).
- DO should be measured with a DO meter. Calibration is required each time a meter is turned on. DO is reported as saturation percentage, with normal being 90–100% in most systems. DO is also measured in mg/L, but absolute values vary based on salinity and water temperature, with less oxygen dissolved at higher temperature and higher salinity (see Chapter A2).
- Where a DO meter is not available, environmental cues and clinical signs can be suggestive.

Husbandry Management

- Increase aeration immediately; target DO is often 95–100% in the face of morbidity or mortality.
  - Emergency aeration can be provided by air stones placed low in the water column, but they are relatively inefficient. Fine-pore stones that produce very small bubbles are more efficient than ones that produce large bubbles.
  - Direct oxygenation is often needed and can be provided from oxygen cylinders, liquid oxygen, or oxygen generators. It may be theoretically possible to cause problems by over-supplementing with oxygen, so pure oxygen is best used where DO meters are available.
  - Packed column aerators, aeration cones, and Venturi oxygen injectors should be considered where long-term solutions are needed.
- Check the life support system to ensure it is running normally. If filters or pumps are not working, their outflow should be diverted before they are turned back on to ensure that any anoxic products (such as hydrogen sulfide) are discarded. These products must be flushed out prior to connecting to the system.
- Minimize stressors; handling should be avoided if possible as fish may decompensate acutely.
- Remove any unnecessary organic material.
- Reduce feeding temporarily to reduce oxygen consumption.
- Monitor biological filtration closely (e.g. daily ammonia and nitrite testing) as it can be damaged by low DO.

Medical Management

- Management typically relies on husbandry changes.

Prevention

- DO should be measured on a routine basis.
- Low DO in outdoor ponds can be prevented by monitoring because it drops in a predictable manner overnight. Measure DO at dusk and two to three hours later, extrapolating the decrease until dawn (Figure C1.1). If DO is predicted to fall too low, aeration can be increased.
- Aerators can be put on electrical timers to routinely provide additional aeration during the late evening or overnight, or connected to sensors and turned on when DO is approaching the lower acceptable limit.
- In the event of a sustained power outage:
  - Battery-powered or generator-powered air pumps can be used.
  - Temperature, DO, and ammonia should be monitored.
  - Feed should be withheld.
  - Suitable water should be available for water changes.
- The concentration of algae (including phytoplankton) in surface waters should be monitored routinely (e.g. with Secchi disks) to identity changes that may impact DO.

Bibliography

Pollock, M.S., Clarke, L.M.J., and Dubé, M.G. (2007). The effects of hypoxia on fishes: from ecological relevance to physiological effects. *Environmental Reviews* 15: 1–14.

Abbreviations/Acronyms

- DO: Dissolved oxygen

Gas Supersaturation

Overview

- Gas supersaturation occurs when the sum of the gas pressures in the water is higher than atmospheric pressure (also known as barometric pressure).
- Gas supersaturation is common in aquarium fish, particularly following gas entrainment into a pump, and in cold-water aquaculture where gas pressures are kept high.
- Gas supersaturation is one of the causes of gas bubble disease (GBD).
- Clinical signs may be seen with only transient increases in gas pressure.
- Prognosis is usually good if the supersaturation can be resolved.

Etiology

- The typical composition of atmospheric air is 78% nitrogen, 20.9% oxygen, 0.03% carbon dioxide, and 0.93% argon.
- The partial pressures of these gases when dissolved in water depend on atmospheric pressure, water temperature, salinity, pH, biological activity, and gas exchange.
- Supersaturation is due to increased partial pressures of dissolved gases and can cause GBD.
  - High partial pressure of nitrogen is the most common cause of GBD, since that gas is more soluble and abundant.
  - High partial pressure of carbon dioxide can sometimes cause GBD.
  - Supersaturation with oxygen rarely causes GBD and may be more likely to cause oxygen toxicity or gill damage.
- There are several potential causes of supersaturation:
  - Entrainment of air into a pump or valve due to a crack or leak upstream.
  - Rapid increase in water pressure or temperature.
  - Excessive supplementation of gases.
  - Turbulent water flow or entrainment of air across large pressure differentials (e.g. aquarium and life support equipment on different floors, waterfalls, spillways of hydroelectric dams).
  - Water sourced from springs, deep wells, or the bottom of dams or spillways.
  - Unusually high levels of photosynthesis (e.g. phytoplankton blooms).

Signalment

- All fish species are susceptible, although sensitivity varies.
- Larger and more active bony fish are often the most susceptible.

Signs/Clinical Findings

- Multiple fish from one or more species are usually affected.
- Exophthalmos, buphthalmos, corneal edema, or intraocular and periocular gas or hemorrhage are common.

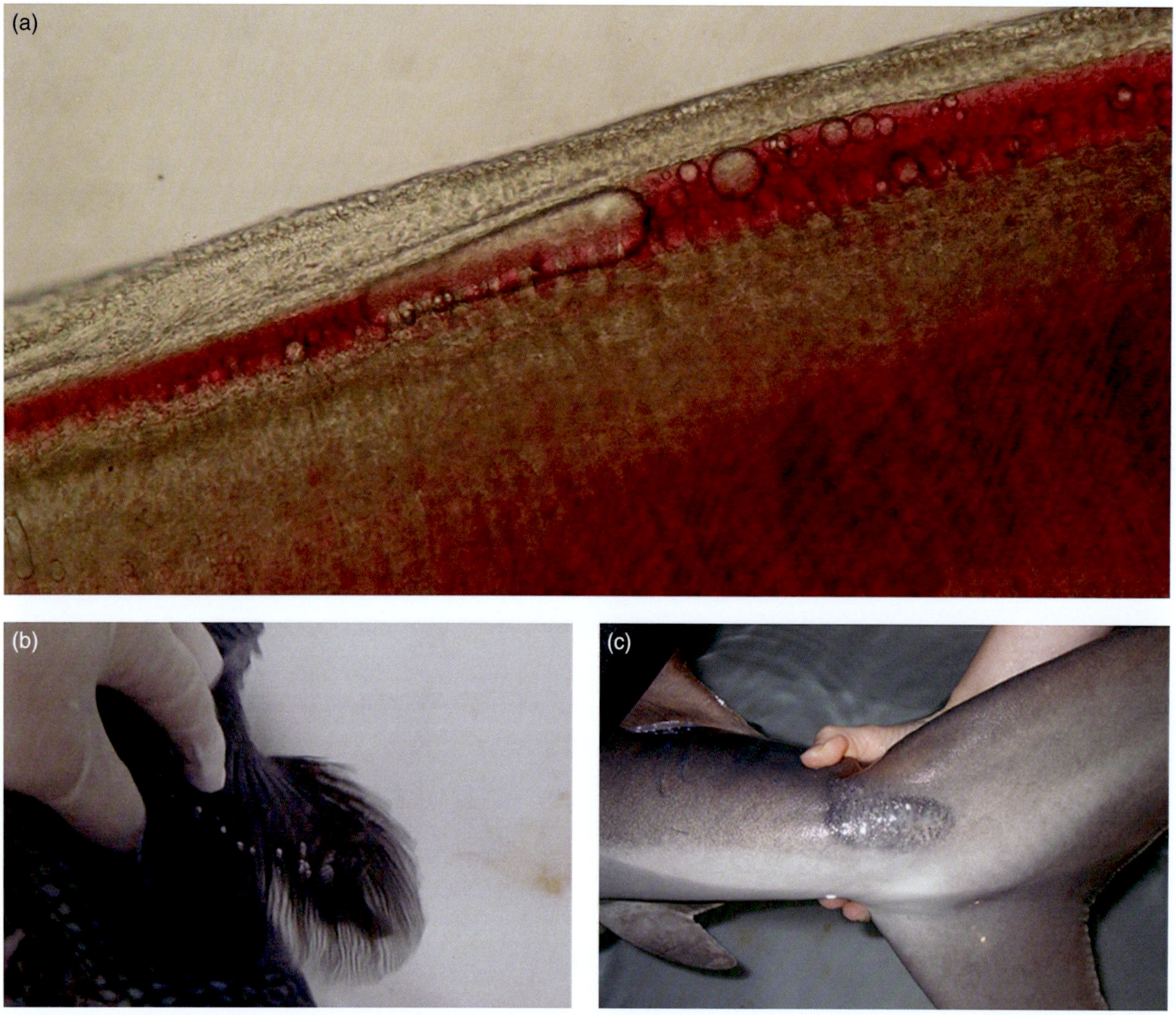

Figure C1.2 Gas emboli on a gill wet mount under direct microscopy (a), on the pectoral fins of a black grouper (*Mycteroperca bonaci*) (b), and on the skin of a sandbar shark (*Carcharhinus plumbeus*).

Gas may displace the lens and lead to cataracts and inflammation.

- Skin darkening may be seen. Focal pallor may be seen in sharks.
- Gas emboli may be visible in the skin or fins as small white or gray spots or larger blisters. Male seahorses (*Syngnathidae*) may show gas within the brood pouch.
- Dyspnea or tachypnea is common. Flared opercula and "coughing" or "yawning" may be seen.
- Lethargy or increased activity (e.g. jumping, swimming into walls) may be seen.
- Fish may avoid areas of gas supersaturation (e.g. gathering in unusual positions).
- Positive or negative buoyancy is possible due to swim bladder enlargement or rupture.
- Reduced appetite or poor growth rates may be seen.
- Mortality can reach 100%.
- If the source is removed, air bubbles under the skin resolve within hours to days.
- Intraocular gas is slower to resolve and intraocular structures may be permanently damaged. Common sequelae include cataracts and ophthalmitis. The eye may progress to phthisis bulbi.

Differential Diagnoses

- Gas emboli on gill biopsies may also be due to barotrauma (e.g. fish recently brought up from depth) or may accumulate in the perimortem period (e.g. moribund fish on a skimmer or in turbulent water). Lesions may develop postmortem from the gill cut, in which case the

emboli are only near the cut edge and not within the capillaries of the secondary lamellae.
- Intraocular or periocular gas may be due to infectious or inflammatory processes in the eye, barotrauma, or physical trauma.

Diagnosis
- Diagnosis is usually based on gas emboli in the fish; these may be grossly visible on physical examination or seen on gill or fin biopsies on microscopy (Figure C1.2). Gas emboli glisten, are round or elongated with rounded ends, and typically follow blood vessels.
- Necropsy often shows emphysema (e.g. corneal, orbital, cutaneous). Gills may show edema, gas emboli, or epithelial degeneration. Gas emboli or hemorrhage may be seen in any tissues.
- To confirm the diagnosis, total gas pressure (TGP) should be measured using a TGP meter, also known as a saturometer.
  - TGP must be measured where the fish are found.
  - While single values are useful, it is important to determine baseline levels and monitor trends over time.
  - Results are reported as a percentage relative to atmospheric pressure of air at the water surface and mg/L.
  - >103% is suspicious.
  - >110% is likely to cause acute lesions.
- Specific reports of morbidity and mortality due to increased TGP include:
  - 115% led to clinical signs in seven days in rainbow trout (*Oncorhynchus mykiss*).
  - 120% for 40–120 hours led to 20% mortality in Chinook salmon juveniles (*Oncorhynchus tshawytscha*).
  - 122% for 56–96 hours led to acute mortalities in white seabass juveniles (*Atractoscion nobilis*).
  - 130% for 10 minutes led to clinical signs and 130% for two to three hours led to 4% mortality in rock carp juveniles (*Procypris rabaudi*).
- If a TGP meter is not available, dissolved oxygen (DO) can be used. Gas supersaturation may be suspected if DO is >100%, but this is a crude assessment.
- It is important to note that if DO is >100% due to oxygen supplementation, rather than air supplementation, supersaturation seems rare.

Husbandry Management
- Check the life support system to look for problems along the lines, such as visible cracks or salt deposits. Problematic components may need to be taken off-line.
- Minimize stressors; handling should be avoided if possible as fish may decompensate acutely.
- Agitate the surface water to improve off-gassing.
- Reduce feeding temporarily to reduce activity levels.
- Consider increasing the water depth to help reduce gas pressures.
- Consider slowly reducing the water temperature, if tolerated by the animals.
- Consider recompression treatment of individual fish to >1 atmosphere for 6–24 hours followed by gradual decompression over several hours or days. One chamber design is described in Smiley and Drawbridge (2007).
- If incoming water is supersaturated, or the problem cannot be fixed, well-designed degassing towers are likely required.

Medical Management
- Common treatments (see Chapters A12 and A13 for more details):
  - Aspiration of free gas in the eye, coelom, or pouch can resolve signs temporarily. For the eye, the smallest possible needle gauge should be used (22–27 ga in most fish). For the pouch, an IV catheter or small red rubber tube works well. However, recurrence is common if the source is not resolved.
  - Acetazolamide may be used for GBD. This is a carbonic anhydrase inhibitor that can reduce the concentration of carbon dioxide in the eyes and plasma and may reduce oxygen secretion. Typical doses are 2.5–5.0 mg/kg IM every three to seven days for up to three treatments. High doses can be associated with negative buoyancy, neurologic signs, and mortalities.
  - Systemic antibiotic coverage may be considered, particularly in seahorses where bacterial dermatitis is commonly associated with GBD.
- Other reported treatments (see Chapters A12 and A13 for more details):
  - Dorzolamide, a topical carbonic anhydrase inhibitor.
  - Systemic anti-inflammatories.
- All legislation regarding medication use and disposal must be followed.

Prevention
- Routine TGP measurements are helpful to establish baselines.
- Good life support system design, maintenance, and monitoring are important. Degassing towers should be used with all large or intensive systems.
- Providing large habitats with variable depths may reduce the risk.

Bibliography

Gültepe, N., Ateş, O., Hisar, O., and Beydemir, S. (2011). Carbonic anhydrase activities from the rainbow trout lens correspond to the development of acute gas bubble disease. *Journal of Aquatic Animal Health* 23:134–139.

LePage, V., Young, J., Dutton, C.J. et al. (2015). Diseases of captive yellow seahorse *Hippocampus kuda* Bleeker, pot-bellied seahorse *Hippocampus abdominalis* Lesson and weedy seadragon *Phyllopteryx taeniolatus* Lacépède. *Journal of Fish Diseases* 38: 439–450.

Llizo, S. (2004). Medical management of syngnathids with buoyancy disorders. *Proceedings of the International Association for Aquatic Animal Medicine Conference*, Galvastan, TX.

Smiley, J.E. and Drawbridge, M.A. (2007). Techniques for live capture of deep-water fishes with special emphasis on the design and application of a low-cost hyperbaric chamber. *Journal of Fish Biology* 70: 867–878.

Smiley, J.E., Drawbridge, M.A., Okihiro, M.S., and Kaufmann, R.S. (2010). Acute effects of gas supersaturation on juvenile cultured white seabass. *Transactions of the American Fisheries Society* 140: 1269–1276.

Smiley, J.E., Okihiro, M.S., Drawbridge, M.A., and Kaufmann, R.S. (2012). Pathology of ocular lesions associated with gas supersaturation in white seabass. *Journal of Aquatic Animal Health* 24: 1–10.

Wang, Y., Liang, R., Tuo, Y., and Li, K. (2015). Tolerance and avoidance behaviour towards gas supersaturation in rock carp *Procypris rabaudi* with a history of previous exposure. *North American Journal of Aquaculture* 77: 478–484.

Abbreviations/Acronyms

- DO: Dissolved oxygen
- GBD: Gas bubble disease
- IM: Intramuscular
- TGP: Total gas pressure

Barotrauma

Overview

- Barotrauma refers to physical tissue damage caused by a change in air or water pressure. It is typically seen when fish are brought up from depth.
- Barotrauma can lead to swim bladder hyperinflation and rupture, exophthalmos, buphthalmos, organ compression, and esophageal, gastric, cloacal, or anal prolapse.
- It is one of the reasons for high by-catch mortality in bony fish.
- Recompression can improve short-term and long-term survival.

Etiology

- The most common cause of barotrauma in bony fish is rapid ascent from depth during commercial or recreational fishing without adequate decompression.
  - Surface atmospheric pressure is 1 atmosphere (1 ATA). Pressure increases with water depth (Pascal's law). At a water depth of 10 m (33 ft), total pressure is 2 ATA; at 20 m (66 ft), total pressure is 3 ATA; at 30 m (98 ft), total pressure is 4 ATA, etc.
  - As pressure decreases (e.g. when fish are brought up through the water column), gas expands (Boyle's law).
  - The greatest pressure differential happens between 10 m and the surface.
- Barotrauma can also be seen in fish passing up through hydroelectric turbines or transported by airplane or helicopter.

Signalment

- Physoclistous teleosts are more susceptible than physostomous fish, as the swim bladder is a closed space.
- A few physoclistous fish such as the Samson fish (*Seriola hippos*) and silver trevally (*Pseudocaranx georgianus*) have a specialized anatomical structure that lets them vent the swim bladder during ascent. These species should be less susceptible to barotrauma.
- Fish without swim bladders (e.g. elasmobranchs, adult flatfish) should be less susceptible to barotrauma.

Signs/Clinical Findings

- Signs are often immediately obvious.
- Positive buoyancy (e.g. recumbent at the surface) immediately post-catch is the most common sign.
- Dyspnea or tachypnea is common.
- Ataxia or hyperactivity may be seen.
- Exophthalmos is common; buphthalmos or hemorrhage may be seen.
- Prolapse of the esophagus and potentially the stomach may be seen in the mouth.
- Prolapse of the cloaca or anus may be seen.
- Gas emboli may be seen in the skin and fins.
- Exophthalmos can develop days after decompression (seven to nine days in two studies) and progress over several weeks.
- Mortality may be immediate or delayed and can reach 100%.

Differential Diagnoses

- Positive buoyancy immediately after an ascent is almost always barotrauma.

Diagnosis

- Diagnosis is based on the history and clinical signs.
- Gill and fin biopsies may show gas emboli.
- Radiography and computed tomography can be helpful to assess the swim bladder and other gas-filled spaces.
- Necropsy may show distension or rupture of the swim bladder, free gas in the coelom, emphysema, gas emboli, hemorrhage, and gastrointestinal prolapse.

Husbandry Management

- Recompression treatment can resolve signs even after severe barotrauma. Where signs resolve, long-term prognosis can be good. Retinal function is often unaffected by the exophthalmos, although it can be damaged by sunlight exposure at the surface.
  - Start recompression immediately; a delay of even 15 minutes increases morbidity and mortality.
  - Recompress to water pressures equivalent to where the fish were collected (e.g. 2.5 ATA at 15 m (50 ft) depth) for ~6–24 hours then gradually decompress over several hours or days.
  - Fish may become negatively buoyant because of the swim bladder damage; this usually resolves over days to weeks.
  - Recompression chambers may consist of weighted crates that can be sunk to specific depths, or PVC or acrylic chambers that can be pressurized. They are not available commercially but can be built easily. One system is described in Smiley and Drawbridge (2007).

Medical Management

- Common treatments:
  - Percutaneous aspiration of gas from the swim bladder is common. Aspiration is done with a sterile needle from a lateral approach at the point of greatest distension. This can help individual cases, but studies often show this has no significant effect on mortality compared to untreated fish, particularly deep-water fish. Recompression is recommended wherever possible.

Prevention

- The risk can be reduced by only catching fish at shallow depths (<6 m).
- For deep-water catches, either a slow ascent with decompression stops spread over hours or days, a staging area (e.g. 10-m deep pens), or immediate recompression and slow decompression at the surface should be part of the catch process.
- Increased use of recompression chambers may reduce by-catch mortality in recreational fisheries.

Bibliography

Brill, R., Magel, C., Davis, M. et al. (2008). Effects of rapid decompression and exposure to bright light on visual function in black rockfish (*Sebastes melanops*) and Pacific halibut (*Hippoglossus stenolepis*). *Fisheries Bulletin* 106: 427–437.

Hall, K.C., Broadhurst, M.K., and Butcher, P.A. (2014). Clinical signs of barotrauma in golden perch, *Macquaria ambigua* (Richardson), and associated effects on post-release mortality and healthy. *Journal of Fish Diseases* 37: 251–264.

Hughes, J.M., Rowland, A.J., Stewart, J., and Gill, H.S. (2016). Discovery of a specialized anatomical structure in some physoclistous carangid fishes which permits rapid ascent without barotrauma. *Marine Biology* 163: 169.

Humborstad, O.-B., Ferter, K., Kryvi, H., and Fjelldal, P.G. (2017). Exophthalmia in wild-caught cod (*Gadus morhua* L.): development of a secondary barotrauma effect in captivity. *Journal of Fish Diseases* 40: 41–49.

Munday, E.S., Tissot, B.N., Heildel, J.R., and Miller-Morgan, T. (2015). The effects of venting and decompression on yellow tang (*Zebrasoma flavescens*) in the marine ornamental aquarium fish trade. *Peer J* 3: e756.

Pribyl, A.L., Schreck, C.B., Kent, M.L. et al. (2012). Recovery potential of black rockfish, *Sebastes melanops* Girard, recompressed following barotrauma. *Journal of Fish Diseases* 35: 275–286.

Smiley, J.E. and Drawbridge, M.A. (2007). Techniques for live capture of deepwater fishes with special emphasis on the design and application of a low-cost hyperbaric chamber. *Journal of Fish Biology* 70: 867–878.

Wild, G.R. (2009). Does venting promote survival of released fish? *Fisheries* 23: 20–28.

Abbreviations/Acronyms

- ATA: Atmosphere

Temperature Stress

Overview

- Almost all fish are poikilothermic and many are sensitive to even small changes in water temperature.
- Changes in water temperature affect activity and appetite and can expose animals to new pathogens, suppress the immune system, and alter drug pharmacokinetics. High water temperature also reduces dissolved oxygen and increases evaporation, salinity, bacterial and algal populations, and ammonia toxicity.
- Fast temperature changes are more hazardous than slow.
- In general, rapid changes of >3°C (5°F) should be avoided.
- Water temperature can be corrected slowly using heat exchangers, new water, or adjusting the external temperature.

Etiology

- There are several possible causes of an acute water temperature change:
  - Heater/chiller/heat exchanger malfunction (e.g. power outage, switch failure).
  - Changes in ambient temperature.
  - Addition of water (e.g. cold incoming lines or rainfall).
  - Inadequate temperature control or insulation during transport or restraint.
  - Lack of acclimation prior to moving fish to a new system.
  - Reversal of a normal thermocline (warm surface water and cold deep water) during the summer in lakes or ponds due to wind, rain, or thunderstorms.

Signalment

- All fish are susceptible, although sensitivity depends on the species, life stage, and individual history. Tropical fish and cold-water fish are typically more susceptible than temperate fish.
- Systems that rely on heat exchangers to maintain a water temperature that is different from ambient are at highest risk.
- Temperate fish acclimated to life in outdoor ponds are often able to tolerate changes in water temperature well.

Signs/Clinical Findings

- Multiple fish from one or more species are usually affected.
- High water temperature:
  - Increased or decreased activity may be seen.
  - Dyspnea or tachypnea may be seen.
  - Erythema or skin ulcers may be seen.
  - Mortalities may be seen.
- Low water temperature:
  - Decreased feeding and growth rates are common.
  - Decreased activity is common.
  - Bradypnea may be seen.
  - Mortalities may be seen.

Differential Diagnoses

- The clinical signs are variable and nonspecific. Section B reviews differentials in more detail.

Diagnosis

- Water temperature must be measured on-site.
- A variety of thermometers are available and accuracy and precision can vary. Meters should be certified (e.g. by the National Institute of Standards and Technology in the United States), checked routinely against known temperatures, and the same meters should be used for serial measurements.
- Rate of change and historical water temperatures are important variables to consider (e.g. fish housed under stable conditions are less tolerant of changes than ones habituated to diurnal or seasonal fluctuations).
- Monitoring of specific diseases may need to increase, e.g. oomycetes and *Flavobacterium psychrophilum* in freshwater salmonids at low water temperature.

Husbandry Management

- High water temperature:
  - Slowly decrease water temperature if possible (e.g. adjust or add heat exchangers, change water if suitable water exists, add fans, decrease ambient temperature).
  - Increase aeration; target dissolved oxygen may be 95–100%.
  - Decrease feeding temporarily.
- Low water temperature:
  - Slowly increase water temperature if possible.
  - Increase insulation of the system (e.g. lids).
  - Decrease feeding temporarily.

Medical Management

- Management typically relies on husbandry changes.

Prevention

- Heat exchangers should be chosen based on target water temperature and volume, ambient temperature range, and heat generated by the life support system.
- Systems that differ significantly from ambient temperature should be avoided or have insulation and redundant heat exchangers or power sources.
- Water temperature changes must be minimized during transport and restraint.
- Slow acclimation is essential when fish are moved into new water, i.e. exposure to new water should always be gradual (see Chapter A14).

pH Stress

Overview

- Each species of fish has an optimal environmental pH range. Values outside this range or any rapid fluctuations can contribute to morbidity and mortality.
- The typical range for most marine fish is 7.5–8.5. The range for freshwater or estuarine fish can be much wider.
- Low pH is more common. It affects physiology and increases dissolution and uptake of heavy metals. High pH increases the proportion of toxic ammonia.
- pH can be corrected slowly using water or other additives; pH should not be changed by more than 0.5 units/d.

Etiology

- pH is affected by weak acids (e.g. carbon dioxide (CO_2), tannic, humic, fulvic acids), strong acids (e.g. hydrochloric or sulfuric acid), and bases or buffers (e.g. carbonates, bicarbonates, phosphates, hydroxides).
- The concentration of buffers in the water is known as alkalinity.
- Low pH can be associated with:
  - Low alkalinity.
  - Addition of reverse osmosis or deionized water.
  - Acidic rainfall.
  - High stocking density and poor off-gassing of CO_2.
  - Closed transport containers.
  - Decreased photosynthesis (e.g. in early morning).
- High pH can be associated with:
  - High alkalinity.
  - Addition of strong buffers.
  - Opening of closed transport containers, releasing built-up CO_2.
  - Increased photosynthesis.
  - Leaching from inadequately cured concrete.

Signalment

- All fish are susceptible, although sensitivity depends on the species, life stage, and individual history.

Signs/Clinical Findings

- Multiple fish from one or more species may be affected.
- Low pH:
  - Increased activity or tremors may be seen.
  - Dyspnea or tachypnea may be seen.
  - Increased mucus production may be seen.
- High pH:
  - Dyspnea or tachypnea may be seen.
  - Skin pallor may be seen.
  - Corneal opacities may be seen.
  - Coelomic effusion may be seen.

Differential Diagnoses

- The clinical signs are variable and nonspecific. Section B reviews differentials in more detail.

Diagnosis

- pH can be measured using portable pH meters or colorimetric tests. Meters must be calibrated prior to each use.
- Alkalinity can be measured using commercial test kits and spectrophotometry.
- Carbon dioxide can be measured using commercial test kits.
- Results should be compared to any previous values to assess rate of change and trends.

Husbandry Management

- pH should be corrected slowly; not more than 0.5 units/d. pH should be monitored closely during changes.
- Low pH:
  - Increase aeration; target dissolved oxygen may be 95–100%.
  - Do not correct pH if ammonia levels are high; correct the ammonia issue first.
  - Change 20–30% of the water if suitable water is available.
  - Slowly add buffer if alkalinity is low. Monitor closely.
  - Slowly add calcium hydroxide (limewater) or sodium hydroxide solution to convert CO_2 or carbonic acid into carbonates. Monitor closely.
  - Consider reducing stocking density.
  - Consider adding a CO_2 scrubber or packed-column aerator for long-term correction.
- High pH:
  - Change 20–30% of the water with lower pH water (e.g. reverse osmosis or deionized water).
  - Add driftwood, almond leaves, or peat.
  - Remove excess plants.
  - Consider CO_2 injectors or reactors for long-term correction.

Medical Management

- Management typically relies on husbandry changes.

Prevention

- pH and alkalinity should be monitored routinely and systems should be maintained between predetermined target ranges.
- pH should be checked in closed containers after transport.
- In closed systems, routine partial water changes with suitable water helps to maintain alkalinity and pH.

Bibliography

Boyd, C.E., Tucker, C.S., and Somridhivej, B. (2016). Alkalinity and hardness: critical but elusive concepts in aquaculture. *Journal of the World Aquaculture Society* 47: 6–14.

Holland, A., Duivenvoorden, L.J., and Kinnear, S.H.W. (2014). The double-edged sword of humic substances: contrasting their effect on respiratory stress in eastern rainbow fish exposed to low pH. *Environmental Science and Pollution Research* 21: 1701–1707.

Ammonia Toxicity

Overview

- Ammonia is a nitrogenous waste product that is excreted by most fish.
- It can build up in closed systems unless it is oxidized by nitrifying bacteria or removed through water changes.
- Ammonia exists in an ionized and unionized form; the unionized form is more toxic to fish. The proportion of unionized ammonia is highest in warm freshwater.
- Ammonia toxicity is a common problem in aquarium fish, often due to immature or damaged biological filters. It is common in aquaculture due to high stocking densities.
- Husbandry changes should be instigated rapidly to resolve the problem.

Etiology

- There are multiple possible sources of ammonia in fish systems:
  - Protein waste products, bacterial fermentation, and organic decomposition.
  - Municipal or groundwater.
  - Leaching of fertilizers, industrial emissions, and volcanic activity.
- In most open systems, ammonia is diluted and removed by water flow.
- In closed systems, ammonia builds up rapidly. Closed systems may be recirculating (e.g. most aquariums or recirculating fish anesthesia systems) or static (e.g. transport bags). Nitrifying bacteria or water changes are required to remove ammonia. Ammonia-locking compounds can be used to make ammonia unavailable.
- Nitrifying bacteria use ammonia, dissolved oxygen (DO), and bicarbonate ions to convert ammonia to nitrite, then nitrate. They are known as ammonia-oxidizing and nitrite-oxidizing bacteria. They grow on every surface, including within biological filters. They require sufficient DO and alkalinity.
- There are many examples of how ammonia can build up due to damaged or insufficient nitrifying bacteria:
  - Newly established systems with immature biological filtration (known as new tank syndrome).
  - Recent animal additions.
  - High stocking densities.
  - High organic load and high feed volumes.
  - Reduced water changes.
  - Acute environmental changes (e.g. rapid temperature, pH, or salinity changes).
  - Reduced water flow through the system or filter media (e.g. power failure, channeling of water).
  - Low dissolved oxygen.
  - Low alkalinity.
  - High water pH, particularly >8.0.
  - High water temperature.
  - High ammonia, which can actually inhibit nitrification.
  - Recent algal bloom and die-off.
  - Some antibiotics (e.g. enrofloxacin, erythromycin).
  - Some antiparasitics (e.g. formalin, chloroquine, levamisole), especially in a naïve system where the bacteria have not previously been exposed to the medication.
- Ammonia exists as ionized ammonium (NH_4^+) and unionized ammonia (NH_3, known as UIA). Combined, these make up total ammonia nitrogen (TAN). The unionized form (UIA) is much more toxic to fish as it can diffuse across the gills. More of the ammonia is in the toxic form (UIA) at high pH, high water temperature, and low salinity (e.g. a freshwater pond after a hot day).
- Closed transport containers (e.g. sealed shipping bags) present a specific risk. Ammonia from the fish builds up over time. When these closed transport containers are opened, built-up carbon dioxide escapes, the pH increases, and the proportion of toxic ammonia increases rapidly. For this reason, acclimation should be started as soon as containers are opened.

Signalment

- Some species are particularly sensitive to elevated ammonia, such as tetras (*Characidae*) and salmonids (*Salmonidae*).
- Air-breathing species are typically more tolerant of ammonia (Table A1.1).

Signs/Clinical Findings

- Multiple fish from one or more species are usually affected.
- Acute toxicity is most commonly reported.
  - Lethargy is common.
  - Inappetence or reduced feeding is common.
  - Dyspnea or tachypnea is common.
  - Erythema, dark coloration, or increased mucus production is common.
  - Neurologic signs may be seen (e.g. circling, erratic swimming).
- Chronic toxicity is likely under-reported.
  - Reduced feeding, weight loss, or poor growth rates may be seen.
  - Dyspnea or tachypnea may be seen.
  - Increased skin mucus may be seen.
  - Neurologic signs may be seen (e.g. erratic swimming).
  - Secondary infections may be the primary presenting sign.
- Mortality depends on the UIA level and rate of increase, fish species and life stages, and the presence of other stressors. With rapid increases in ammonia, the mortality rate can reach 100%.
- Secondary infections are common and systems should be closely monitored for several weeks after an ammonia increase.
- A subsequent increase in nitrite is common.

Differential Diagnoses

- Acute mortalities with dyspnea or tachypnea are typically due to an environmental failure (e.g. low dissolved oxygen, ammonia toxicity, contaminated water) or an acute ectoparasitic or bacterial disease (e.g. *Cryptocaryon irritans*, columnaris).

Diagnosis

- Diagnosis is based on water testing and consistent clinical signs.
- Ammonia is colorless and odorless at these levels; high levels cannot be diagnosed by observation.
- Ammonia can be measured using a variety of commercial test kits and ion-specific electrodes (see Chapter A2). Most commercial tests report TAN. Since UIA is the toxic form, UIA should be calculated from TAN based on pH and temperature. Tables are available (Table A2.3, on test kits, and online).
- UIA should be <0.02 mg/L. Typical toxic values are 0.5–1.0 mg/L, but species sensitivities vary. Some median lethal doses are listed below, from most to least sensitive, reported as UIA 96 hours LC_{50}. Most studies were under optimal environmental conditions.
  - Cardinal tetra (*Paracheirodon axelrodi*) 0.32 mg/L.
  - Marbled hatchetfish (*Carnegiella strigata*) 0.37 mg/L.
  - Winter flounder (*Pseudopleuronectes americanus*) 0.52 mg/L.
  - Lesser bleeding-heart tetra (*Hyphessobrycon socolofi*) 0.61 mg/L.
  - Rummy-nose tetra (*Hemigrammus rhodostomus*) 0.66 mg/L.
  - Pirarucu (*Arapaima gigas*) 0.70 mg/L.
  - Rainbow trout (*Oncorhynchus mykiss*) 0.82 mg/L.
  - Matrinchã (*Brycon amazonicus*) 0.83 mg/L.
  - Agassiz's dwarf cichlid (*Apistogramma agassizii*) 0.85 mg/L.
  - Tambaqui (*Colossoma macropomum*) 1.09 mg/L.
  - Green neon tetra (*Paracheirodon simulans*) 1.14 mg/L.
  - Corydora (*Corydoras schwartzi*) 1.16 mg/L.
  - Gilthead seabream (*Sparus aurata*) 1.27–2.5 mg/L.
  - European bass (*Dicentrarchus labrax*) 1.7 mg/L.
  - Oscar (*Astronotus ocellatus*) 1.75 mg/L.
  - Marbled spinefoot rabbitfish (*Siganus rivulatus*) 1.86 mg/L.
  - Turbot (*Scophthalmus maximus*) 2.6 mg/L.
  - Three-spined stickleback (*Gasterosteus aculeatus*) 2.93 mg/L.
  - Channel catfish (*Ictalurus punctatus*) 3.1 mg/L.
- Clinical pathology abnormalities may include dermal hyperplasia or gill hyperplasia, hypertrophy, and fusion. Secondary infections may be identified.
- Plasma and tissue ammonia levels are rarely used as sample handling requirements are restrictive, requiring immediate analysis or rapid freezing to −80°C (−112°F).

Husbandry Management

- Increase aeration; target DO may be 95–100%.
- Change 30–50% of the water daily, if suitable water exists (i.e. similar temperature, pH, and salt composition). Reduce this when ammonia is starting to decrease to allow the nitrifying bacteria to mature.
- Remove any unnecessary organic material (e.g. uneaten food, dead leaves).
- Reduce or stop feeding or spread out feeds temporarily. Fasted fish do still continue to excrete some ammonia.
- Check the life support system and adjust if needed. Common solutions include unclogging a filter or mixing filter media to improve water flow. However, if a filter has been off for several hours, flush it well to remove any anoxic by-products prior to connecting it to the system.
- Consider adding a new source of organic carbon (e.g. chopped hay) as carbon can be a limiting nutrient for the nitrifying bacteria.

- Consider adding mature gravel or filter media from another system to provide more nitrifying bacteria. The source system should be evaluated to determine the risk of transferring pathogens.
- In freshwater, consider adding zeolite to adsorb ammonia. Once used, this can be reactivated with an overnight soaking in 50 g/L (5%) salt solution followed by thorough rinsing.
- Consider moving some or all the fish if the ammonia cannot be removed.
- Once the ammonia has been reduced, increase alkalinity if needed to support nitrification (e.g. with sodium bicarbonate). Buffer must not be added while ammonia levels are high as this may increase the proportion of toxic ammonia.
- Ammonia is not removed by activated carbon.
- Review long-terms plans for the system if the life support is insufficient for the target stocking density.

Medical Management

- Common treatments (see Chapters A12 and A13 for more details):
  - Some commercial products that bind ammonia are available. They are typically proprietary mixes, e.g. AmQuel® and AmQuel Plus™ (Kordon LLC, Hayward, CA) and AMMO-LOCK® (API, Mars Fishcare, Chalfont, PA). Because these do not remove or break down the ammonia, ammonia test results remain high.
  - In freshwater, 1–3 g/L of salt can reduce physiologic stress.
- All legislation regarding medication use and disposal must be followed.

Prevention

- Ammonia should be tested every one to two weeks in most systems and more frequently with an immature filter or after the addition of animals or immersion medications. Any ammonia should trigger a response.
- Dissolved oxygen and alkalinity should be maintained within appropriate ranges.
- Biological filtration should be planned around the maximum bioload.
- With new systems, biological filters can be matured with ammonium chloride or urea over three to eight weeks. If that is not possible, filters can be seeded with media from a suitable system; the risk of transferring pathogens should be assessed.
- If no cycling is possible prior to adding fish, the initial stocking density should be very low (e.g. total length of all fish in the system <0.3 cm/L or <0.4 in./gallon) and consist of fish that are relatively tolerant of ammonia. Ammonia should be monitored daily for two to four weeks and no further fish should be added until after the ammonia level decreases.
- Any environmental changes (e.g. salinity or temperature) should be slow.
- For redundancy, filter media can be maintained under similar environmental conditions without fish and fed with ammonium chloride or urea. These biofarms provide an excellent and safe source of nitrifying bacteria.
- Ponds should be covered to reduce leaf debris and if fertilizer must be used in the area, it should contain only phosphate with no nitrogenous compounds.
- Fish should be fasted prior to shipping and transported at the lowest possible stocking density and as quickly as possible.

Bibliography

Barbierie, E. and Bondioli, A.C.V. (2015). Acute toxicity of ammonia in pacu fish (*Piaractus mesopotamicus*, Holmberg, 1887) at different temperature levels. *Aquaculture Research* 46: 565–571.

Person-Le Ruyet, J., Chartois, H., and Quemener, L. (1995). Comparative acute ammonia toxicity in marine fish and plasma ammonia response. *Aquaculture* 136: 181–194.

Roumieh, R., Barakat, A., Abdelmeguid, N.E. et al. (2013). Acute and chronic effects of aqueous ammonia on marbled spinefoot rabbitfish, *Siganus rivulatus* (Forsskål 1775). *Aquaculture Research* 44: 1777–1790.

Souza-Bastos, L.R. and Val, A.L. (2015). Are Amazonian fish more sensitive to ammonia? Toxicity of ammonia to eleven native species. *Hydrobiologia* 789: 143–155.

Abbreviations/Acronyms

- DO: Dissolved oxygen
- LC_{50}: Median lethal concentration, synonymous with the median tolerance limit (TLm)
- TAN: Total ammonia nitrogen
- UIA: Unionized ammonia

Nitrite Toxicity

Overview

- Nitrite is a by-product of ammonia oxidation and can build up in closed systems. While toxic, it is less toxic than ammonia on a mg/L basis.
- Toxicity is most commonly seen in freshwater systems; chloride ions in salt water inhibit uptake of nitrite by fish.
- Exposure to nitrite can cause methemoglobinemia, giving it the common name of brown blood disease.
- Signs are similar to those of low dissolved oxygen, as nitrite blocks oxygen transport.
- The most common treatments are water changes, aeration, and sodium chloride additions.

Etiology

- Ammonia is converted to nitrite by ammonia-oxidizing bacteria (AOB). Nitrite is converted to nitrate by nitrite-oxidizing bacteria (NOB).
- Increased ammonia is typically followed by an increase in nitrite, because if AOB are damaged or insufficient, the same is likely true of the NOB.

Signalment

- Freshwater fish in recirculating systems are the most susceptible.
- Salmonids (*Salmonidae*), cichlids (*Cichlidae*), cyprinids (*Cyprinidae*), and channel catfish and related species (*Ictalurus* spp.) are particularly susceptible.
- Perch (*Percidae*), pike (*Esocidae*), bass and bluegill (*Centrarchidae*) are usually more resistant.
- Marine fish are typically resistant, although nitrite may act as a stressor.

Signs/Clinical Findings

- Multiple fish from one or more species are usually affected.
- Dyspnea or tachypnea is common.
- Gills may be red, pink, tan, or brown.
- Poor growth rates may be seen with chronic exposure.
- Morbidity and mortality are typically low.

Differential Diagnoses

- Dyspnea or tachypnea in freshwater fish is typically due to an environmental failure (e.g. low dissolved oxygen, ammonia toxicity, contaminated water) or a ciliate or monogenean infection (e.g. *Ichthyophthirius multifiliis*).
- Tan or brown gills in freshwater fish may be due to nitrite, nitrate, or chloramine toxicity, or autolysis.

Diagnosis

- Diagnosis is based on water testing and consistent clinical signs in freshwater fish.
- Commercial test kits are typically colorimetric assays that report nitrite–nitrogen (NO_2–N). To convert to total nitrite levels, the NO_2–N test result should be multiplied by 3.3, i.e. 1 mg/L NO_2–N = 3.3 mg/L NO_2.
- Nitrite in water should be <0.1 mg/L. Signs may be seen at 0.5–1.0 mg/L. Some median lethal levels of nitrite are listed below, from most to least sensitive, reported as NO_2–N 96 hours LC_{50}.
  - Rainbow trout (*Oncorhynchus mykiss*) 0.2–11 mg/L.
  - Channel catfish (*Ictalurus punctatus*) 7 mg/L.
  - Nile tilapia (*Oreochromis niloticus*) 8–81 mg/L for large to small fish.
  - Blue tilapia (*Oreochromis aureus*) 16 mg/L.
  - Fathead minnow (*Pimephales promelas*) 45–70 mg/L.
  - Largemouth bass (*Micropterus salmoides*) 140 mg/L.

Husbandry Management

- Husbandry changes are similar to those for ammonia toxicity.
- Increase aeration; target dissolved oxygen may be 95–100%.
- Change 30–50% of the water daily, if suitable water exists. Reduce this when nitrite is <0.5 mg/L to allow the nitrifying bacteria to mature.
- Remove unnecessary organic material.
- Reduce or stop feeding temporarily.
- Check the life support system and adjust if needed.
- If alkalinity and ammonia levels are low, increase alkalinity slowly (e.g. with sodium bicarbonate).
- Nitrite is not removed by activated carbon.
- Review long-terms plans for the system if the life support is insufficient for the target stocking density.

Medical Management

- Common treatments (see Chapters A12 and A13 for more details):
  - The most common treatment is sodium chloride at 3–10 mg/L of chloride for each 1 mg/L of NO_2–N. This is usually done with sea salt or aquarium salt.
  - Calcium chloride can be more effective than sodium chloride. Typical doses are 1.5 mg/L of chloride for each 1 mg/L of NO_2–N.
- All legislation regarding medication use and disposal must be followed.

Prevention

- Prevention methods are similar to those for ammonia toxicity.
- Some fish, particularly channel catfish, may be maintained at low salinity to avoid nitrite toxicity.

Bibliography

Atwood, H.L., Fontenot, Q.C., Tomasso, J.R., and Isely, J.J. (2001). Toxicity of nitrite to Nile tilapia: effect of fish size and environmental chloride. *North American Journal of Aquaculture* 63: 49–51.

Lewis, W.M. and Morris, D.P. (1986). Toxicity of nitrite to fish: a review. *Transactions of the American Fisheries Society* 115: 183–195.

Abbreviations/Acronyms

- AOB: Ammonia-oxidizing bacteria
- NOB: Nitrite-oxidizing bacteria
- LC_{50}: Median lethal concentration, synonymous with the median tolerance limit (TLm)

Nitrate Toxicity

Overview

- Nitrates build up in closed systems due to oxidization of nitrogenous compounds by nitrifying bacteria.
- They are chronic stressors and endocrine disruptors.
- Nitrates are less toxic than ammonia or nitrite on a mg/L basis, but they often reach high levels in long-established, large recirculating systems.
- Nitrates can be removed through water changes, plants, or anaerobic bacteria in denitrification systems.

Etiology

- Most nitrates in aquarium systems are the end result of oxidation of ammonia from fish and other organic material. Nitrates can also come from urban, agricultural, industrial, or sewage runoff.
- Risk factors for nitrate toxicity include:
  - Long-established, large recirculating systems.
  - Limited water changes.
  - No denitrification.
  - Contamination of ponds (e.g. with pesticide or fertilizer).
  - No or few live plants.

Signalment

- Freshwater fish and marine elasmobranchs in recirculating systems are most susceptible.
- Eggs, fry, and small fish are more sensitive than older or larger fish in most studies.

Signs/Clinical Findings

- Several fish are typically affected.
- Signs are usually chronic.
- Lethargy may be seen.
- Inappetence, reduced appetite, or reduced growth rates may be seen.
- Dyspnea or tachypnea may be seen.
- Gills may be pale or tan-colored.
- Erythema may be seen.
- Muscle rigidity may be seen.
- Goiters may be visible as ventral throat swelling in elasmobranchs or unilateral or bilateral opercular distension in bony fish.
- Feminization of male fish may be seen.
- Mortality is typically low but chronic mortalities may be seen.

Differential Diagnoses

- The clinical signs are variable and nonspecific. Section B reviews differentials in more detail.

Diagnosis

- Diagnosis is based on water testing, consistent clinical signs, and response to management changes.
- Commercial test kits are typically colorimetric assays that report nitrate–nitrogen (NO_3–N). To convert to total nitrate levels, the NO_3–N test result should be multiplied by 4.4, i.e. 1 mg/L NO_3–N = 4.4 mg/L NO_3.
  - Total nitrate should be <50 mg/L for most fish, <15 mg/L for fish systems with invertebrates, and <2 mg/L for particularly sensitive freshwater species.
  - In large recirculating fish systems without denitrification, levels are often much higher (e.g. total nitrate 200–500 mg/L).
  - Total nitrate of 44 mg/L (10 mg/L nitrate–nitrogen) is the EPA maximum for drinking water.

- Some median lethal levels of nitrate in freshwater fish are listed below, from most to least sensitive, reported as NO_3–N 96 hours LC_{50}.
  - Guppy fry (*Poecilia reticulata*) 191 mg/L.
  - Siberian sturgeon (*Acipenser baerii*) 397–1028 mg/L for large to small fish.
  - Fathead minnow larvae (*Pimephales promelas*) 1010–1607 mg/L.
  - Guadalupe bass fingerlings (*Micropterus treculii*) 1261 mg/L.
  - Chinook salmon fingerlings (*Oncorhynchus tshawytscha*) 1310 mg/L.
  - Rainbow trout fingerlings (*Oncorhynchus mykiss*) 1355 mg/L.
  - Channel catfish fingerlings (*Ictalurus punctatus*) 1355–1423 mg/L.
  - Bluegill fingerlings (*Lepomis macrochirus*) 2110 mg/L.
- Reported lethal levels for most marine teleosts are usually higher, but a few have low NO_3–N 96 hours LC_{50} values.
  - Planehead filefish fingerlings (*Monacanthus hispidus*) 573 mg/L.
  - Florida pompano fingerlings (*Trachinotus carolinus*) 1000 mg/L.
- Morbidity and mortality are seen in marine elasmobranchs at lower levels than most marine teleosts.
  - Clearnose skate fingerlings (*Raja eglanteria*) NO_3–N 96 hours LC_{50} >960 mg/L.
  - Whitespotted bamboo shark juveniles (*Chiloscyllium plagiosum*) showed diffuse hyperplastic goiter at NO_3–N 70 mg/L for 29 days, in spite of adequate iodide in the diet and water.

Husbandry Management

- Management typically relies on long-term husbandry changes.
- Increase water changes using suitable water.
- Remove unnecessary organic material.
- Consider reducing the stocking density.
- Consider adding live plants; these also provide environmental enrichment and alternative food sources for the animals.
- Consider adding denitrification filtration for long-term correction (see Chapter A3).

Medical Management

- Common treatments (see Chapters A12 and A13 for more details):
  - Supportive care may be indicated.
  - Iodide supplementation may be considered for goiters (e.g. potassium iodide in water or food).
- All legislation regarding medication use and disposal must be followed.

Prevention

- High water exchange rates physically remove nitrates, but water availability and discharge restrictions may limit this option.
- Denitrification filters are usually required to manage nitrates in large recirculating systems.
- The risk is lower in systems with abundant live plants.

Bibliography

Camargo, J.A., Alonso, A., and Salamanca, A. (2005). Nitrate toxicity to aquatic animals: a review with new data for freshwater invertebrates. *Chemosphere* 58: 1255–1267.

Crow, G.L., Atkinson, M.J., Ron, B. et al. (1998). Relationship of water chemistry to serum thyroid hormones in captive sharks with goiters. *Aquatic Geochemistry* 4: 469–480.

Hamlin, H.J. (2003). Nitrate toxicity in Siberian sturgeon (*Acipenser baeri*). *Aquaculture* 253: 688–693.

Morris, A.L., Hamlin, H.J., Francis-Floyd, R. et al. (2011). Nitrate-induced goiter in captive whitespotted bamboo sharks *Chiloscyllium plagiosum*. *Journal of Aquatic Animal Health* 23: 92–99.

Abbreviations/Acronyms

- EPA: Environmental Protection Agency
- LC_{50}: Median lethal concentration, synonymous with the median tolerance limit (TLm)

Chlorine and Chloramine Toxicity

Overview

- Chlorine and chloramine toxicity are common in fish, typically through exposure to untreated municipal water.
- Treatment and prevention involve removing the compounds using sodium thiosulfate, aeration, or activated carbon filtration.

Etiology

- Chlorines (Cl_2, OCl^-, and HOCl) and chloramines (chlorine bound to ammonia) are found in municipal water for disinfection and to reduce the production of trihalomethanes. They are often present at levels that may be toxic to fish (e.g. 0.5–3.0 mg/L). Untreated municipal water is a common cause of chlorine exposure.
- Another source of chlorine is bleach contamination (e.g. from equipment disinfection).
- Chlorines and chloramines can be created through ozone disinfection, although bromines are more common. These should be confined to the ozone contact chamber and not released into the fish habitat.
- Chloramine-T is sometimes used as an immersion treatment for fish.
- Chlorines are also common in industrial effluents.
- Risk factors include high water temperature, low organic load, and low hardness and pH (<7.5).

Signalment

- Freshwater fish are more susceptible.
- Smaller fish are more susceptible.

Signs/Clinical Findings

- Multiple fish from one or more species are usually affected.
- Lethargy, abnormal swimming, and hiding are common and may progress to increased jumping, tetany, and other erratic movements.
- Tachypnea or dyspnea is common.
- Inappetence or reduced feeding may be seen.
- Pallor, darkened skin, or increased mucus may be seen.
- Gills may be pale or tan-colored due to hemolytic anemia or methemoglobin formation.
- Mortalities are possible and can occur within hours.

Differential Diagnoses

- Signs are nonspecific.
- Tan gill discoloration in freshwater fish may be due to nitrite, nitrate, or chloramine toxicity, or autolysis.

Diagnosis

- This is typically diagnosed based on level of free and total chlorine in the water and clinical signs.
  - Free chlorine includes Cl_2, OCl^-, and HOCl.
  - Total chlorine includes free chlorine and combined chlorine such as chloramines.
- Levels can be measured by colorimetry, potentiometry, or handheld meters.
- Total chlorine should be <0.03 mg/L for most fish and <0.01 mg/L for sensitive species.
- It may be possible to smell the gas if total chlorine is >0.2 mg/L.
- Cytology or histology may show gill hyperplasia.
- Chlorines can damage biological filtration; ammonia should be monitored closely after an event.

Husbandry Management

- Change 30–50% of the water daily, if suitable water exists.
- Vigorously aerate the system water using air or oxygen for several days.
- Vigorously aerate new water for ~24 hours prior to use to remove chlorines and some chloramines.
- Add an activated carbon filter to adsorb chlorines and chloramines; note that removal of chloramine is much slower than chlorine and therefore the water requires a longer contact time. Monitor dissolved oxygen as well as chlorine levels.
- Consider reducing the water temperature slightly.
- Consider moving the fish if chlorines or chloramines cannot be removed.

Medical Management

- Common treatments (see Chapters A12 and A13 for more details):
  - Sodium thiosulfate immersion neutralizes chlorines and chloramines. A common dose is 7.4 mg/L for each 1 mg/L of chlorine, but needs can vary with the water pH. This process releases ammonia from chloramines, but in amounts that can usually be handled by active biological filtration.
  - Several commercial products bind chlorines and chloramines, e.g. AmQuel® and AmQuel Plus™ (Kordon LLC) and AMMO-LOCK® (API). These are liquids that are added to the system water. Label instructions should be followed.
- All legislation regarding medication use and disposal must be followed.

Prevention

- Water with chlorines or chloramines should always be treated prior to use with fish using sodium thiosulfate, activated carbon filtration, or aeration. Ionized and total chlorine should be checked prior to use.

Bibliography

Mahjoor, A.A. and Loh, R. (2008). Some histopathologic aspects of chlorine toxicity in rainbow trout (*Oncorhynchus mykiss*). *Asian Journal of Animal and Veterinary Advances* 3: 303–306.

Zillich, J.A. (1972). Toxicity of combined chlorine residuals to freshwater fish. *Water Pollution Control Federation* 44: 212–220.

Heavy Metal Toxicity

Overview

- Sources of heavy metals in fish systems include contamination of water from plumbing, décor, therapeutic agents, runoff, groundwater, or food contamination.
- Copper toxicity is the most common heavy metal toxicity in fish. Other heavy metals that can cause toxicity in fish include zinc and lead.
- Heavy metals are usually more toxic at low pH, hardness, and alkalinity and at high water temperatures.
- Treatment typically involves removing the source. Activated carbon filters can adsorb heavy metals.

Etiology

- Many heavy metals are essential at trace concentrations (e.g. copper, zinc, iron, chromium, manganese) but can result in toxicity at higher levels. Others are not considered essential (e.g. lead, mercury, cadmium, cesium). Exposure may be from immersion or ingestion.
- Copper:
  - Immersion appears to be the primary route of exposure, usually from copper sulfate treatment or copper or brass plumbing. Antifouling paints used for watercraft also contain copper.
  - Toxicity from ingestion does not appear common because of low oral bioavailability in most species.
- Zinc:
  - Ingestion appears to be the primary route of exposure in fish.
  - Exposure may be from coins containing zinc (e.g. US one-cent coins since 1983), galvanized steel tanks or plumbing, or sacrificial zinc anodes. High levels may also be found in effluent from galvanizing, paint, or textile plants.
- Lead:
  - Sources include lead plumbing, lead-based paints, and metal strips used to anchor live plants.
- Iron:
  - The most common source is contaminated well water.
- There are many risk factors beyond exposure.
  - Low pH, hardness, and alkalinity increase heavy metal dissolution and uptake at the gills. A sudden drop in pH can release metal ions that were previously in a nontoxic chelated form.
  - High water temperature increases absorption.
  - Low dissolved organic carbon increases their availability.
  - Heavy metal levels can interact, e.g. zinc can decrease absorption of copper ions.

Signalment

- Sensitivity varies by species and life stage.
- Some groups are often considered to have a low tolerance for copper ions:
  - Most elasmobranchs, with exceptions such as cownose rays (*Rhinoptera bonasus*).
  - Most invertebrates, with potential exceptions such as horseshoe crabs (*Limulus polyphemus*).
  - Teleosts housed in soft, acidic freshwater.
  - Larval and juvenile teleosts.
  - Seahorses, seadragons, and pipefish (*Syngnathidae*).

Signs/Clinical Findings

- Multiple fish from one or more species may be affected.
- Signs are variable and often nonspecific.
- Lethargy, erratic swimming, or loss of equilibrium may be seen.
- Inappetence, reduced feeding, or poor growth rates may be seen.
- Skin darkening may be seen.
- Tachypnea or dyspnea may be seen, particularly with copper, lead, or iron toxicity.
- Gill pallor from non-regenerative anemia may be seen. Gill hyperplasia, edema, and curling of the distal tips of the primary lamellae have been described with copper toxicity in teleosts.
- Coelomic distension due to gastric distension and ileus may be seen.
- Abnormal growth or development may be seen.
- Secondary disease due to immune suppression may be seen; in these cases, the disease typically continues after the heavy metals have been removed.
- Acute or chronic mortalities are possible.

Differential Diagnoses

- The clinical signs are variable and nonspecific.

Diagnosis

- The concentration of heavy metals in water can be measured. Ionic forms are more toxic and tests that measure ionic forms are more useful diagnostically. Commercial tests are available for ionic and total copper and iron. Atomic absorption spectrophotometry is usually used for broader assays.
- If levels cannot be measured immediately, 1 L of water can be frozen for later analysis.
- Interpretation of results can be challenging, and trends over time or comparisons with unaffected systems can be useful. Rapid increases are more problematic than slow increases.

- Literature reports of toxic levels can be used as guides, but not absolute limits. Effects vary by species, life stage, rate of change, water chemistry, water temperature, and the presence of other stressors.
- Some median lethal levels of copper are listed below, from most to least sensitive, reported as 96 hours LC_{50} for the copper salt, not the ionic form.
  - Mummichog (*Fundulus heteroclitus*) 0.3 mg/L.
  - Spiny dogfish (*Squalus acanthias*) ~0.8–1.0 mg/L.
  - Sheepshead (*Archosargus probatocephalus*) 1.1 mg/L.
  - Carp (*Capoeta fusca*) 1.1–7.5 mg/L in soft to hard water.
  - Hardhead catfish (*Arius felis*) 2.4 mg/L.
  - Pinfish (*Lagodon rhomboides*) 2.8 mg/L.
  - Atlantic croaker (*Micropogonias undulatus*) 5.6 mg/L.
  - Gulf toadfish (*Opsanus beta*) 21.6–36.1 mg/L.
- Morbidity and mortality in fish from zinc toxicity has been reported at 0.02–100 mg/L of zinc sulfate.
- Morbidity and mortality in fish from lead toxicity has been reported at 0.05–30 mg/L.
- There are often no gross changes on necropsy, although foreign body ingestion may be seen (e.g. coins, lead strips).
- Lesions may be seen on histology but are usually nonspecific.
  - Hyperplasia, sloughing, or necrosis of epithelial surfaces is the most common, particularly gill and renal tubular epithelium. Inclusions may be seen.
  - Liver and kidney parenchymal necrosis may be seen.
- Heavy metal concentrations in serum may be useful. Some reference levels exist for comparison, e.g. smooth dogfish (*Mustelus canis*).
- Heavy metal levels in tissues are likely to be more reliable than from serum.
  - Gill, kidney, and liver are often the sites of greatest accumulation, although muscle, skin, and intestines may also be useful.
  - For accurate results, acid-cleaned instruments or whole fish should be used for analysis to avoid contamination from necropsy instruments.
  - Tissues can be frozen in plastic for later analysis if needed.
  - Some reference levels exist, e.g. Greenland sharks (*Somniosus microcephalus*), tiger sharks (*Galeocerdo cuvier*).
- Biochemical changes seen in mammals and birds (e.g. changes in aminolevulinic acid or protoporphyrins due to exposure to lead) have not been assessed in fish.

Husbandry Management

- Remove the source of contamination as soon as possible.
- Change 30–50% of the water once daily, if suitable water exists.
- Add activated carbon filters.
- Consider adding zeolite or other ion-exchange resin filters to freshwater systems.
- Consider water conditioners designed to bind heavy metals (e.g. Rid-Metals™ (Kordon)).
- For iron toxicity, add vigorous aeration followed by mechanical filtration to oxidize and remove the iron.

Medical Management

- Common treatments (see Chapters A12 and A13 for more details):
  - Chelating agents such as ethylenediaminetetraacetate (EDTA) and dimercaptosuccinic acid (DMSA) may be useful but are poorly described in fish. Calcium disodium EDTA at 28 mg/kg IM every 72 hours for 5 doses followed by DMSA at 35 mg/kg PO every three to four days for three weeks were associated with improved signs and lower blood lead values in an electric eel (*Electrophorus electricus*). DMSA immersion at 1.5 mg/L for two weeks improved signs in rainbow trout (*Oncorhynchus mykiss*).
  - Fluid therapy and other supportive care may be indicated.
- All legislation regarding medication use and disposal must be followed.

Prevention

- Copper sulfate immersion treatment of fish should only be used where alkalinity is >50 mg/L of $CaCO_3$, increases should be slow, and levels should be measured at least once daily. Rapid changes in pH during treatment must be avoided. If the fish may be sensitive to ionic copper, a chelated copper compound or alternative treatment should be considered (e.g. hyposalinity).
- Only aquarium-safe products should be added to aquariums. Lead strips used to anchor aquatic plants should be removed before plants are added. Aluminum- or magnesium-based anodes should be used in preference to zinc.
- Coins and other foreign material dropped into fish systems should be removed as soon as possible.
- Ponds should be situated out of reach of possible contaminants.
- Ground freshwater that is high in heavy metals should be run through activated carbon, zeolite, or other ion-exchange filter prior to use.

Bibliography

Blanchard, J. and Grosell, M. (2006). Copper toxicity across salinities from freshwater to seawater in the euryhaline fish *Fundulus heteroclitus*: is copper an ionoregulatory toxicant in high salinities? *Aquatic Toxicology* 80: 131–139.

De Boeck, G., Hattink, J., Franklin, N.M. et al. (2007). Copper toxicity in the spiny dogfish (*Squalus acanthus*): urea loss contributes to the osmoregulatory disturbance. *Aquatic Toxicology* 84: 133–141.

Ebrahimpour, M., Alipour, H., and Rakhshah, S. (2010). Influence of water hardness on acute toxicity of copper and zinc on fish. *Toxicology and Industrial Health* 26: 361–365.

Endo, T., Hisamichi, Y., Haraguchi, K. et al. (2008). Hg, Zn and Cu levels in the muscle and liver of tiger sharks (*Galeocerdo cuvier*) from the coast of Ishigaki Island, Japan: relationship between metal concentrations and body length. *Marine Pollution Bulletin* 56: 1774–1780.

Firat, O., Cogun, H.Y., Yüzereroglu, T.A. et al. (2011). A comparative study on the effects of a pesticide (cypermethrin) and two metals (copper, lead) to serum biochemistry of Nile tilapia, *Oreochromis niloticus*. *Fish Physiology and Biochemistry* 37: 657–666.

Grosell, M., McDonald, M.D., Wood, C.M., and Walsh, P.J. (2004). Effects of prolonged copper exposure in the marine gulf toadfish (*Opsanus beta*) I. Hydromineral balance and plasma nitrogenous waste products. *Aquatic Toxicology* 68: 249–262.

Mathews, T. and Fisher, N.S. (2009). Dominance of dietary intake of metals in marine elasmobranch and teleost fish. *Science of the Total Environment* 407: 5156–5161.

McMeans, B.C., Borga, K., Bechtol, W.R. et al. (2007). Essential and non-essential element concentrations in two sleeper shark species collected in arctic waters. *Environmental Pollution* 148: 281–290.

Mebane, C.A., Dillon, F.S., and Hennessy, D.P. (2012). Acute toxicity of cadmium, lead, zinc, and their mixtures to stream-resident fish and invertebrates. *Environmental Toxicology and Chemistry* 31: 1334–1348.

Park, K. and Heo, G.-J. (2008). Acute and subacute toxicity of copper sulfate pentahydrate ($CuSO_4 \cdot 5H_2O$) in the guppy (*Poecilia reticulata*). *Journal of the Veterinary Medical Science* 71: 333–336.

Persky, M.E., Williams, J.J., Burks, R.E. et al. (2012). Hematologic, plasma biochemistry, and select nutrient values in captive smooth dogfish (*Mustelus canis*). *Journal of Zoo and Wildlife Medicine* 43: 842–851.

Wenger, S., Pendl, H., Tahas, S. et al. (2018). Clinical signs, diagnosis, and treatment of lead intoxication in an electric eel (*Electrophorus electricus*). *Journal of Zoo and Wildlife Medicine* 49: 1029–1031.

Abbreviations/Acronyms

- IM: Intramuscular
- LC_{50}: Median lethal concentration, synonymous with the median tolerance limit (TLm)
- PO: Orally

Hydrogen Sulfide Toxicity

Overview

- Hydrogen sulfide (H_2S) is a gas produced under anoxic conditions, which may be seen in deep sediment or filters with poor water flow. Levels can also be high in groundwater.
- It is acutely toxic to most fish and exposure can lead to rapid mortalities.
- Prognosis is typically poor unless fish can be moved to an uncontaminated system.

Etiology

- Hydrogen sulfide is a toxic, soluble, flammable gas that is produced from sulfates by anaerobic bacteria (particularly *Desulfovibrio* spp.) in anoxic conditions.
- Any long-standing sediment can become anoxic if there is poor water flow or aeration (e.g. pond sediment, deep sand in an aquarium, filter media after >two hours without water flow). The hydrogen sulfide can be released into the system (e.g. in ponds after high winds or thunderstorms, reconnecting a filter that had become anoxic, stirring a deep sand bed in an aquarium).
- Hydrogen sulfide can be high in groundwater and hot springs and may be present in wastewater from paper mills and chemical plants.
- Some poorly managed denitrification systems can also produce hydrogen sulfide.
- The effects are worse at low pH and high water temperature.
- The gas creates sulfhemoglobin, which directly damages gills and blocks oxygen transport using a similar mechanism to methemoglobin.

Signalment

- Almost all fish species are susceptible.
- Toxicity is more likely in saltwater and brackish water fish, as more sulfates are available.
- Fry are particularly susceptible.

Signs/Clinical Findings

- Most, if not all, fish in the system are usually affected.
- Lethargy is common.
- Inappetence or reduced feeding is common.
- Dyspnea or tachypnea is common, often progressing to bradypnea.
- Gill pallor may be seen.
- Acute mortalities are common and mortality can reach 100%.

Differential Diagnoses

- Acute mortalities with dyspnea or tachypnea are typically due to an environmental failure (e.g. low dissolved oxygen, ammonia toxicity, contaminated water) or an acute ectoparasitic or bacterial disease.

Diagnosis

- There may be a distinctive sulfide smell, similar to rotten eggs, at >0.3 µg/L H_2S.
- In some cases, black material may be seen on substrate or in the water due to the formation of metal sulfides.
- Water levels can be measured with commercial test kits. For accurate results, the water must be kept anoxic prior to sampling. Any H_2S is detrimental (i.e. >0.1 µg/L); 0.5–10 µg/L can cause acute mortalities. It is important to check the diagnostic range of tests kits as some have a lowest detectable limit that is higher than the toxic limit for most fish and some can only be used in freshwater.
- Gill biopsies may show clubbing and hyperplasia of lamellae.

Husbandry Management

- Aerate vigorously, ideally with oxygen, to support gas exchange and convert sulfides to sulfates.
- Move fish as soon as possible to an uncontaminated system. If that is not possible, change 80–100% of the water rapidly.
- Reduce water temperature slightly, if possible.
- Consider increasing pH slightly.

Medical Management

- Management typically relies on husbandry changes.
- Individual animal supportive care may be indicated.
- All legislation regarding medication use and disposal must be followed.

Prevention

- Groundwater should be degassed and aerated prior to use.
- Substrate that is >10 cm deep should be avoided, well-aerated, or regularly stirred.
- Excess organic material should be removed from systems.
- Filter media should be monitored closely for signs of channeling or poor water flow.
- Filters that have held stagnant water for >two hours should be taken off-line to run water through, or drained and cleaned before use.

Bibliography

Affonso, E.G., Polez, V.L.P., Corrêa, C.F. et al. (2004). Physiological responses to sulphide toxicity by the air-breathing catfish, *Hoplosternum littorale* (Siluriformes, Callichthyidae). *Comparative Biochemistry and Physiology, Part C* 139: 251–257.

Torrans, E.L. and Clemens, H.P. (1982). Physiological and biochemical effects of acute exposure of fish to hydrogen sulfide. *Comparative Biochemistry and Physiology, Part C* 71: 183–190.

Organophosphate and Carbamate Toxicity

Overview

- Organophosphates and carbamates are common pesticides; exposure is often from runoff into ponds. Some organophosphates are also used for immersion treatment of ectoparasites in fish.
- These are toxic to all animals, including humans, and can be absorbed transdermally.
- Treatment relies on removing the source and providing supportive care.

Etiology

- Organophosphates and carbamates inhibit acetylcholinesterase, leading to increased potentiation of neurotransmitter effects.

- Exposure is typically from leaching into surface water or immersion treatment of fish.
- Trichlorfon (Dylox) is the most common organophosphate used on fish, often to treat copepods or leeches.
- Organochlorines (e.g. DDT and aldrin) are used less commonly now and will not be discussed in this section.

Signalment

- Many elasmobranch species are considered particularly sensitive to organophosphates.
- *Serrasalmidae* (e.g. red hooks and pacu) may be particularly sensitive to organophosphates.
- Ponds near agricultural land are most likely to be affected by accidental exposure.

Signs/Clinical Findings

- Multiple fish from one or more species may be affected.
- Signs are usually acute.
- Reduced feeding or inappetence is common.
- Neurologic signs including erratic swimming, seizures, or vertebral fractures are common. Pectoral fins may be held cranially. Lethargy or paralysis may be seen.
- Dyspnea or tachypnea may be seen.
- Acute mortalities are likely.

Differential Diagnoses

- Differentials for acute neurologic signs in a group of fish include toxin exposure, nutritional deficiencies, and bacterial, viral, or parasitic infections affecting the central nervous system.

Diagnosis

- Diagnosis is typically based on a history of known exposure.
- Organophosphate concentration in water can be measured at specialist laboratories using gas chromatography and liquid chromatography-mass spectroscopy.
- Decreased acetylcholinesterase activity in blood or tissues (e.g. brain) may be found.
- There are no specific necropsy or histology findings.

Husbandry Management

- If exposure is suspected, suitable human personal protective equipment is required to prevent human exposure.
- Consider moving fish to an uncontaminated system.
- Change 50–80% of the water daily. Treatment and discharge of the contaminated water must follow all relevant legislation.
- Add activated carbon filters.
- Consider adding zeolite or other ion-exchange resin filters to freshwater systems.

Medical Management

- Reported treatments (see Chapters A12 and A13 for more details):
  - Supportive care is indicated.
  - Atropine 0.1–0.5 mg/kg IM or IV is used commonly.
- All legislation regarding medication use and disposal must be followed.

Prevention

- The main prevention is avoidance. Outdoor systems should be situated in such a way that they cannot be exposed to contaminated runoff.
- When immersion treatment with an organophosphate is required, a bioassay is essential and the minimum effective dose should be used. Pretreatment of the animals with intramuscular atropine may reduce the risk of toxicity.

Bibliography

Ozxan, O.E., Uner, N., Sevgiler, Y. et al. (2006). Sublethal effects of organophosphate diazinon on the brain of *Cyprinus carpio*. *Drug and Chemical Toxicology* 29: 57–67.

Thangnipon, W., Thangnipon, W., Luangpaiboon, P., and Chinabut, S. (1995). Effects of the organophosphate insecticide, monocrotophos, on acetylcholinesterase activity in the Nile tilapia fish (*Oreochromis niloticus*) brain. *Neurochemical Research* 20: 587–591.

Abbreviations/Acronyms

- DDT: Dichlorodiphenyltrichloroethane
- IM: Intramuscular
- IV: Intravenous

C2

Noninfectious Diseases (Other)

Catherine A. Hadfield

Seattle Aquarium, Seattle, WA, USA

Introduction

This chapter focuses on other noninfectious diseases of fish, including trauma, exertional myopathy, lateral line depigmentation, thyroid hyperplasia, mucometra and ovarian cysts, egg retention or binding, dystocia, cataracts, lipid keratopathy, micronutrient deficiency, gastrointestinal foreign bodies, and neoplasia. Where available, information is provided on etiology, signalment, clinical signs, diagnosis, husbandry and medical management, and prevention.

Physical Trauma

Overview

- Trauma is a common cause of morbidity and mortality in fish.
- Typical sources are catch and transport, cohorts, or inappropriate enclosure design.
- A history and examination of the environment and wounds often help determine the cause.
- Traumatic lesions in fish often heal readily when provided with good environmental conditions. Fish can often heal lesions that might carry a poor prognosis in other vertebrate classes.

Etiology

- Physical trauma may be due to:
  - Inappropriate enclosure size or shape (e.g. inadequate rest areas, narrow turns for pelagic species).
  - Inappropriate décor (e.g. abrasive surfaces in tubes used by moray eels (*Muraenidae*), damaged fiberglass surfaces).
  - Inappropriate cohorts resulting in bite wounds or chasing (Figure C2.1) (e.g. ambush predators such as pike (*Esocidae*), frogfish (*Antennariidae*), scorpionfish (*Scorpaenidae*), and wobbegongs (*Orectolobidae*); territorial fish such as damselfish (*Pomacentridae*), triggerfish (*Balistidae*), and bettas (*Betta splendens*)).
  - Mating behaviors in elasmobranchs (Figure C2.1).
  - Predators at outdoor systems (e.g. herons, racoons).
  - Jumping.
  - Sudden stimuli such as lights turning on.
  - Inappropriate catch techniques.
  - Rough handling.
  - Inappropriate transport containers.
- The probability of physical trauma increases if the affected fish is sick or already has an external abnormality (e.g. ulcer, mass), or during particular behaviors (e.g. extrusion of the valvular intestine in requiem sharks (*Carcharhinidae*) and sawfish (*Pristidae*)).
- Thermal trauma from contact with heaters is particularly common in species such as seahorses (*Syngnathidae*), as they may perch around heaters.
- Electrical trauma is covered in a later section.

Signalment

- All fish species are susceptible.
- Pelagic fish are particularly prone to trauma from the enclosure (e.g. blue sharks (*Prionace glauca*), tuna (*Thunnus* spp.)).
- Fish with fine scales or no scales may be more susceptible to skin trauma (e.g. butterfish (*Peprilus triacanthus*)).
- Fish with dermal plates are less sensitive to trauma at those sites (e.g. sturgeon (*Acipenseridae*)).

Clinical Guide to Fish Medicine, First Edition. Edited by Catherine A. Hadfield and Leigh Ann Clayton.

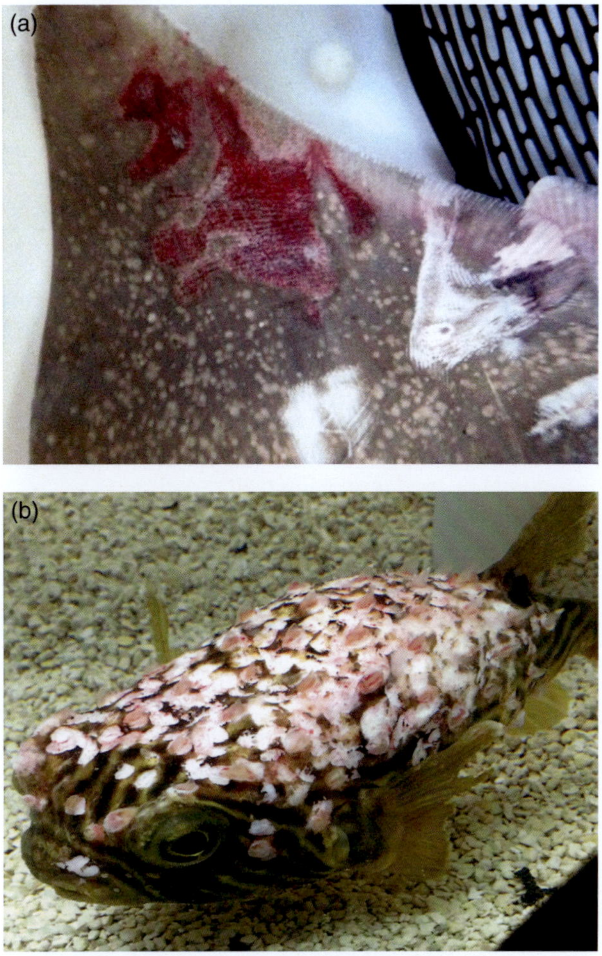

Figure C2.1 Bite wounds to the pectoral fin of a female bullnose ray (*Myliobatis freminvillii*) from a male during mating (a) and to a striped burrfish (*Chilomycterus schoepfii*) from a tankmate (b).

Signs/Clinical Findings

- External wounds are usually obvious and tend to reflect the source of the trauma (e.g. rostral abrasions are often associated with habitat problems and bite or crush wounds can be used to try to identify the aggressor).
- Bloody discharge may be visible from the gill cavity, cloaca, anus, or urogenital openings.
- Severe hemorrhage is rare but may be seen if a large vessel is torn (e.g. gill arch fracture) or secondary to a coagulopathy.
- Lethargy and gill pallor may be seen, particularly with internal trauma (e.g. liver or cloacal laceration).
- Abnormal swimming or buoyancy may be seen (e.g. with spinal or swim bladder trauma). Darkening of the caudal skin, often with a clear delineation from normal skin, is suggestive of a spinal lesion at that location.
- Dyspnea or tachypnea may be seen due to increased activity, pain, or anemia.
- Acute collapse or mortalities with no other clinical signs may occur due to severe internal or head trauma.
- White, brown, or green cotton-like growth on the wounds of freshwater fish may be seen due to secondary oomycete or columnaris infection.

Differential Diagnoses

- There may be no need for differentials (e.g. if teeth marks are visible, or there was a recent hook catch). However, an underlying inflammatory cause should be considered with any nonspecific external lesion. This may be viral, bacterial, fungal, parasitic, or neoplastic.
- Blood from the oral or pharyngeal cavity may be from the oropharyngeal mucosa, gills, thyroid tissue, or more rarely the upper gastrointestinal tract. Differentials include inflammation, infection, neoplasia, and trauma.
- Blood from the cloaca may be from the caudal gastrointestinal, reproductive, or urinary tract. Differentials include inflammation, infection, neoplasia, and trauma.

Diagnosis

- The wounds and environment should be assessed visually to determine the etiology and if hands-on examination, diagnostics, or treatments are required.
- Physical examination is indicated if hemorrhage cannot be controlled, lesions look unusual, etiology is unknown, or healing is not progressing normally. A neurologic examination may help; spinal fractures may result in loss of response to noxious stimuli caudal to the fracture.
- Clinical pathology:
  - Direct and stained cytology of lesion scrapes should be done to rule out pathogens such as scuticociliates, oomycetes, columnaris, and myxozoans.
  - PCV and TS can help assess the degree of hemorrhage.
  - Hematology and blood culture can be useful in case of systemic inflammation or infection.
- Radiology and computed tomography can help identify skeletal lesions and internal fish hooks.
- Ultrasound can be used to look for internal trauma (e.g. liver or intestinal laceration, hemocoelom).
- Metal detectors have been used in large sharks to detect fish hooks.

Husbandry Management

- Remove the source of the trauma where possible (e.g. move or separate animals; remove, move, or block décor to prevent access or disrupt territories; add suitable lids).
- Fish can heal severe injuries when provided with good environmental conditions. They are capable of

regenerating retinal and neural tissue due to progenitor cells found at all life stages. If a lesion is going to heal, it typically shows improvement in a few days. Large defects should heal fully over weeks.

- If hemorrhage is severe, increase dissolved oxygen to 95–100% to support gas exchange.

Medical Management

- Common treatments (see Chapters A12 and A13 for more details):
  - If hemorrhage is severe, hemostasis can be encouraged with direct pressure, ligation, hemostatic sponges (e.g. VetSpon® by Elanco Animal Health, Greenfield, IN; Gelfoam® by Pfizer, New York, NY; or Celox™ by Medtrade, UK), hemostatic agents (e.g. Yunnan Baiyou; QuikClot® by Z-Medica, Wallingford, CT), electrocautery, or local infiltration of epinephrine or phenylephrine.
  - In rare cases, fluid therapy and whole blood transfusion may be indicated (e.g. PCV < 10%). This can include oral administration of dechlorinated freshwater or isotonic saline, particularly for marine fish. Intravenous options include isotonic fluids, colloids, or whole blood from a healthy conspecific after cross-matching. Intracoelomic routes can be used where intravenous access is not possible, but absorption is highly variable.
  - Hemoglobin-based oxygen carriers (e.g. Oxyglobin) may improve blood oxygenation. Reported doses in fish have been 2.5–7.7 mL/kg IV with no sustained deleterious effects; transient lethargy and tissue discoloration were seen in rainbow trout (*Oncorhynchus mykiss*).
  - Erythropoietin has been used in fish and does stimulate erythropoiesis in goldfish (*Carassius auratus*).
  - Analgesia is indicated, but the risk of exacerbating traumatic lesions should be considered. For example, if a net capture is needed for flighty fish with ocular trauma, the risk of further trauma may outweigh the benefits of injectable analgesia, and oral or immersion routes should be considered.
  - Antibiotics may be indicated if wounds are extensive, although fish appear less susceptible to secondary bacterial infection than other vertebrate classes. Where antibiotics are used, they should be based on culture and sensitivity results, but it is common to use an antibiotic with broad Gram-negative aerobic coverage and a wide dosing interval (e.g. ceftazidime, enrofloxacin, florfenicol, amikacin).
  - Topical treatments are rarely indicated but can help in some cases.
    - Flushing of fish wounds with sterile saline is rarely indicated unless contamination is severe.
    - Becaplermin 0.01% gel (Regranex®, Smith & Nephew, Andover, MA) is a platelet-derived growth factor that can accelerate re-epithelialization. It is best applied topically to an open tissue bed after gentle debridement of the edges. Suitable PPE should be used to avoid human exposure.
    - Naltrexone 0.03% cream has shown similar wound closure rates to becaplermin in mammalian models and is more readily available.
    - Misoprostol 0.0024% and phenytoin 2% powder can be compounded with a gelling agent and applied topically to try to accelerate healing. Suitable PPE should be used to avoid human exposure.
    - Collagen products (e.g. Collasate®, PRN Pharmacal, Pensacola, FL) may accelerate healing.
    - Topical antiseptics (e.g. povidone iodine) may damage tissues and are not indicated.
  - Surgical repair is rarely indicated for skin and muscle injuries, as the lack of tissue elasticity limits primary closure and most wounds heal best by second intention. Surgical repair may be indicated with signs of necrosis or infection, to improve tissue apposition (e.g. a body wall flap, fractured mandible), for gastrointestinal trauma (e.g. laceration of the valvular intestine), or to restore critical anastomoses. During debridement, tissue appearance and texture are more useful in assessing viability than vascularity. Tail fractures on skates and rays may be reduced at surgery but heal better by second intention than primary repair. Xenografts can help provide an extracellular matrix to accelerate healing of large skin defects. Of these, BioSIST (SurgiVet, Dublin, OH) use has been reported in fish on the skin and cornea, although multiple sutures are required to reduce disintegration in water.
  - If a hook is identified, endoscopic or surgical removal should be attempted to avoid sequelae such as esophageal or gastric perforation, hepatic laceration, pericarditis, coelomitis, and bacterial septicemia.
  - Nutritional support may be indicated.
  - Euthanasia may be warranted if trauma is severe, particularly with spinal lesions or severe underlying disease, but if fish are otherwise healthy, welfare is adequate, and environmental conditions are good, medical management is often rewarding.
- All legislation regarding medication use and disposal must be followed.

Prevention

- The size and shape of all habitats (including quarantine and holding) should dictate the species and individuals that can be housed.
- Careful attention to stocking density and compatibility is essential.
- Appropriate jump barriers or lids should be in place on every system (Figure C2.2).
- Overhead lighting should come on gradually, mimicking dawn and dusk wherever possible.
- For fish such as seahorses, in-tank heaters should have a guard around them.
- Manual or chemical restraint and transports should be planned carefully. Behavioral conditioning should be used wherever possible to reduce the need for catch and restraint.
- With outdoor systems, nets or other defenses may be needed to reduce predation by nuisance animals.

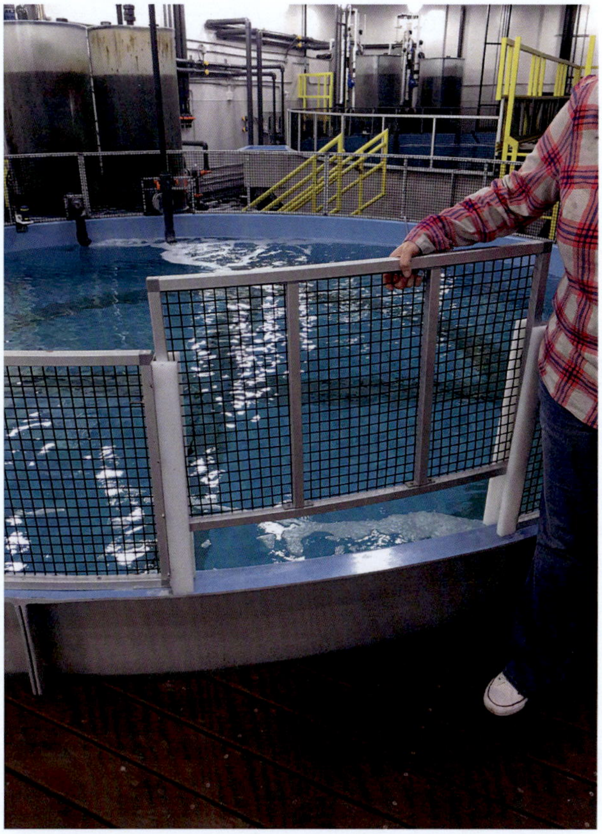

Figure C2.2 Barrier to prevent fish from jumping out of the system. The panels are easy to remove for access.

Bibliography

Borucinksa, J., Kohler, N., Natanson, L., and Skomal, G. (2002). Pathology associated with retained fishing hooks in blue sharks, *Prionace glauca* (L.), with implications for their conservation. *Journal of Fish Diseases* 25: 515–521.

Lécu, A., Herbert, R., Coulier, L., and Murray, M.J. (2011). Removal of an intracoelomic hook via laparotomy in a sandbar shark (*Carcharhinus plumbeus*). *Journal of Zoo and Wildlife Medicine* 42: 256–262.

McLaughlin, P.J., Cain, J.D., Titunick, M.B. et al. (2017). Topical naltrexone is a safe and effective alternative to standard treatment of diabetic wounds. *Advances in Wound Care* 6: 279–288.

Mylniczenko, N.D., Clayton, L.A., Greenwell, M.G. et al. (2002). Effects of oxyglobin administration in rainbow trout (*Oncorhycnhus mykiss*). *Proceedings of the America Association of Zoo Veterinarians Conference*, Milwaukee, WI.

Mylniczenko, N.D. and Travis, E.K. (2004). Techniques using vet BioSIST in aquatic animals. *Proceedings of the American Association of Zoo Veterinarians Conference*, San Diego, CA.

Nordgreen, A.H., Slinde, E., Møller, D., and Roth, B. (2008). Effect of various electric field strengths and current durations on stunning and spinal injuries of Atlantic herring. *Journal of Aquatic Animal Health* 20: 110–115.

Tagliatela, R. and Corte, F.D. (1997). Human and recombinant erythropoietin stimulate erythropoiesis in the goldfish *Carassius auratus*. *European Journal of Histochemistry* 41: 301–304.

Abbreviations/Acronyms

- IV: Intravenous
- PCV: Packed cell volume
- PPE: Personal protective equipment
- TS: Total solids

Electrical Trauma

Overview

- Fish can receive electrical trauma from lightning storms, stray voltage, power surges, or electrical stunning.
- Typical findings include spinal fractures and abnormal swimming.
- Electrical trauma can also act as a chronic stressor with non-specific clinical signs.
- Prognosis is poor if signs are obvious.

Etiology

- Fish can be exposed to electrical trauma from a variety of sources:
  - Lightning around outdoor pens and ponds.
  - Stray voltage from ungrounded life support equipment.
  - Power surges (changes in the flow of electricity) through life support equipment.
  - Electrical stunning, also known as electrofishing; this is used to render fish unconscious for commercial catch or slaughter.

Signs/Clinical Findings

- Fish may be asymptomatic with low-level exposure.
- If signs are seen, several fish are usually affected.
- Abnormal swimming is common.
- Spinal abnormalities are common, including kyphosis, scoliosis, or lordosis.
- Skin discoloration may be visible caudal to a spinal lesion.
- Acute mortalities may be seen and the rate can be high.

Differential Diagnoses

- Differentials for acute spinal lesions in a group of fish are primarily electrical or physical trauma.

Diagnosis

- The cause may be obvious in the history (e.g. storms, electrical stunning).
- Stray voltage can be measured using a voltmeter, but increases are often transient and trends over time should be checked.
- Radiology or computed tomography may show kyphosis, scoliosis, lordosis, or spinal fractures or luxations.
- Necropsy or coeliotomy may show spinal lesions and hematomas or necrosis.

Husbandry Management

- Avoid further exposure (e.g. replace suspect pumps or heat exchangers).

Medical Management

- Common treatments (see Chapters A12 and A13 for more details):
  - Supportive care, including analgesia, may be indicated.
  - Euthanasia may be indicated with severe clinical signs.
- All legislation regarding medication use and disposal must be followed.

Prevention

- Recommendations are available for electrical stunning of fish based on fish species and water volume.
- Pumps and heat exchangers should be routinely grounded and on a regular preventative maintenance schedule.
- Surge protectors should be considered for all pumps and heat exchangers.

Bibliography

Nordgreen, A.H., Slinde, E., Møller, D., and Roth, B. (2008). Effect of various electric field strengths and current durations on stunning and spinal injuries of Atlantic herring. *Journal of Aquatic Animal Health* 20: 110–115.

Exertional Myopathy

Overview

- Exertional myopathy is an under-reported cause of morbidity and mortality in fish.
- Some species are particularly susceptible (e.g. ram-ventilating elasmobranchs).
- It is seen following exertion (e.g. catch, transport, manual restraint) and exacerbated by hypoxia or hypoventilation (e.g. prolonged anesthesia, air exposure) and lack of recovery time.
- Typical signs include changes in swimming behavior or respiration, elevated lactate, and acidosis.

- Once clinical signs are seen, prognosis is guarded.

Etiology

- Strenuous exertion in fish requires some energy to be produced anaerobically. This leads to an increase in lactic acid and carbon dioxide. If the fish is not able to recover aerobically or buffer the blood appropriately, blood pH starts to decrease (acidemia). The resulting acidosis may be respiratory, metabolic, or mixed.
- Greater effort and longer duration of exertion increase the risk (e.g. prolonged soak time on long lines, repeated catch attempts, or long transport time). Other factors that increase the risk include:
  - Low dissolved oxygen or hypoventilation.
  - Low alkalinity.
  - High water temperature.
  - Lack of sufficient recovery time.

Signalment

- Ram-ventilating sharks are particularly vulnerable, but susceptibility varies within this group, e.g. blacktip (*Carcharhinus limbatus*), blacktip reef (*Carcharhinus melanopterus*), dusky (*Carcharhinus obscurus*), Atlantic sharpnose (*Rhizoprionodon terraenovae*), and bonnethead sharks (*Sphyrna tiburo*) are more susceptible than sandbar (*Carcharhinus plumbeus*), tiger (*Galeocerdo cuvier*), and lemon sharks (*Negaprion brevirostris*).
- Bony fish are also susceptible, particularly active species (e.g. tuna (*Thunnus* spp.)).
- The effect of size varies across studies, however larger individuals are often more susceptible during transport and restraint.

Signs/Clinical Findings

- Signs may be seen at the time of exertion or several hours afterwards.
- Reduced swimming activity and tachypnea or dyspnea are typical early signs.
- Muscle rigidity and immobility usually develop over several hours.
- Acute mortalities are common. Mortality of around 80% from exertional myopathy and lactic acidosis is reported for recreational fisheries and by-catch of susceptible species.

Differential Diagnoses

- Acute morbidity or mortality following exertion may also be due to low dissolved oxygen, other environmental stressors, trauma, or acute infectious disease, but the primary differential should be exertional myopathy.

Diagnosis

- Exertional myopathy is typically diagnosed based on clinical signs, clinical pathology, histology, and ruling out differentials.
- Blood gases and lactate can be measured on an i-STAT® (Abbott, Princeton, NJ) or Heska E-POC™ (Heska Corporation, Loveland, CO). These units provide temperature correction based on human blood characteristics. Alternative equations are available (e.g. Gallagher et al. 2010).
- Lactate can be measured reliably from venous, arterial, or mixed samples. Blood gases are normally only reliable on arterial samples (e.g. ventral tail artery), and accuracy of results in fish is questioned.
- Reference values for blood gases and lactate in fish are available, although method of sampling should be considered as handling will affect results. Commonly reported normal ranges for fish include:
  - pH 7.2–7.5
  - pCO_2 5–10 mmHg
  - HCO_3^- 3–7 mmol/L
  - Lactate < 2.0 mmol/L
- Lactate values of >5 mmol/L are a concern; reports of recovery with lactate >20 mmol/L are extremely rare.
- Increases in glucose, potassium, sodium, lactate dehydrogenase, and creatine kinase may be seen.
- Necropsy or coeliotomy results are typically normal. Histologic lesions may include multifocal skeletal and cardiac muscle necrosis consistent with rhabdomyolysis.

Husbandry Management

- Increase dissolved oxygen (e.g. 110–130%) and increase water flow to assist ventilation.
- Provide excellent water quality and appropriate water temperature.

Medical Management

- Common treatments (see Chapters A12 and A13 for more details):
  - Treatment may involve ventilation, hyperoxygenation, fluid therapy, sodium bicarbonate or acetate, and vitamin E/selenium. It can be hard to balance the diagnostic and treatment needs with minimizing activity and stress on the animal.
  - Ventilation may involve water pumps or syringes or walking the animal through the water to ensure well-oxygenated water flows readily over all the gills.
  - Fluid therapy should be used to correct acidosis and hypovolemia. In marine elasmobranchs, it may help to

modify electrolyte solutions to match their high osmolality, but if unavailable, isotonic solutions such as lactated Ringer's can be used. Doses may include 5 mL/kg IV boluses, up to 30 mL/kg slow ICe.
  - The fluid volume required in large fish is usually a limiting factor, so sodium bicarbonate or sodium acetate are often used (e.g. at 1 mEq/kg or 1 mg/kg IV PRN respectively). Intramuscular routes are not typically recommended. Blood pH should be monitored to prevent overcorrection.
  - Analgesics should be considered to reduce muscle pain.
- Other reported treatments (see Chapters A12 and A13 for more details):
  - Intravenous calcium supplementation is sometimes advocated.
  - Injectable corticosteroids are sometimes advocated.
  - Intravenous dobutamine may improve microvascular perfusion.
  - Muscle relaxants may help.
- All legislation regarding medication use and disposal must be followed.

Prevention

- Prevention should be focused on high-risk species and high-risk procedures.
- Catch and transport plans must be designed to limit the risk of exertional myopathy in susceptible species (see Chapter A14).
- Manual and chemical restraint should be planned carefully; monitoring of blood gases may be indicated in susceptible species (see Chapter A10).
- Ample recovery time should be provided to fish after an exertional stressor; this may take days or weeks.

Bibliography

Cooper, A.R. and Morris, S. (1998). The blood respiratory, haematological, acid-base and ionic status of Port Jackson shark, *Heterodontus portus jacksoni*, during recovery from anaesthesia and surgery: a comparison with sampling by direct caudal puncture. *Comparative Biochemistry and Physiology A* 119: 895–903.

Currey, L.M., Heupel, M.R., Simpfendorfer, C.A., and Clark, T.D. (2013). Blood lactate loads of redthroat emperor *Lethrinus miniatus* associated with angling stress and exhausting exercise. *Journal of Fish Biology* 83: 1401–1406.

Frick, L.H., Reina, R.D., and Walker, T.I. (2010). Stress related physiological changes and post-release survival of Port Jackson sharks (*Heterodontus portusjackson*) and gummy sharks (*Mustelus antarcticus*) following gill-net and longline capture in captivity. *Journal of Experimental Biology and Ecology* 385: 29–37.

Gallagher, A.J., Frick, L.H., Bushnell, P.G. et al. (2010). Blood gas, oxygen saturation, pH, and lactate values in elasmobranch blood measured with a commercially available portable clinical analyser and standard laboratory instruments. *Journal of Aquatic Animal Health* 22: 229–234.

Hanley, C.S., Clyde, V.L., Wallace, R.S. et al. (2010). Effects of anesthesia and surgery on serial blood gas values and lactate concentrations in yellow perch (*Perca flavescens*), walleye pike (*Sander vitreus*), and koi (*Cyprinus carpio*). *Journal of the American Veterinary Medical Association* 236: 1104–1108.

Hyatt, M.W., Anderson, P.A., O'Donnell, P.M., and Berzins, I.K. (2011). Assessment of acid-base derangements among bonnethead (*Sphyrna tiburo*), bull (*Carcharhinus leucas*), and lemon (*Negaprion brevirostris*) sharks from gill net and longline capture and handling methods. *Comparative Biochemistry and Physiology A* 162: 113–120.

Mandelman, J.W. and Skomal, G.B. (2009). Differential sensitivity to capture stress assessed by blood acid-base status in five carcharhinid sharks. *Journal of Comparative Physiology B* 3: 267–277.

Mylniczenko, N.D., Kinsel, M., Young, F. et al. (2003). Lessons from a case of capture myopathy in a pelagic silky shark (*Carcharhinus falciformis*). *Proceedings of the American Association of Zoo Veterinarians Conference*, Minneapolis, MN.

Naples, L.M., Mylniczenko, N.D., Zachariah, T.T. et al. (2012). Evaluation of critical care blood analytes assessed with a point-of-care portable blood analyser in wild and aquarium-housed elasmobranchs and the influence of phlebotomy site on results. *Journal of the American Veterinary Medical Association* 241: 117–125.

Abbreviations/Acronyms

- ICe: Intracoelomic
- IV: Intravenous
- PRN: As needed

Lateral Line Depigmentation

Overview

- Lateral line depigmentation (LLD) is a chronic ulcerative dermatopathy of bony fish. Lesions start on the head and lateral line and do not progress deeper than the dermis.
- It is known under several names, including head and lateral line erosion (HLLE), chronic erosive dermatopathy, and hole-in-the-head, although the last term is also used for other syndromes.
- Some species are particularly susceptible, such as surgeonfish and tangs (*Acanthuridae*).
- LLD can be associated with low levels of micronutrients in the water or diet.
- Prognosis is good if underlying stressors can be resolved.

Etiology

- LLD appears to be associated with damage to sensory canals in the skin. A variety of etiologies are suspected and the syndrome is likely multifactorial.
- Nutritional
  - Vitamin C, carotenoids, or other micronutrient deficiencies.
  - Calcium, phosphorus, or other macronutrient deficiencies.
  - Lack of green algae in the diet.
  - Prolonged fasting.
  - Inappropriate or prolonged storage of food items.
  - Soaking of food items.
- Infectious
  - Reovirus-like agent.
  - *Hexamita* and *Spironucleus* spp. in freshwater bony fish.
- Toxic
  - Heavy metals (e.g. copper).
  - Nitrates.
- Life support system/environmental
  - Granular activated carbon, likely through loss of micronutrients in the water.
  - Excessive UV or ozone disinfection.
  - Lack of full spectrum artificial light or sunlight.
  - Stray voltage.
  - Ground water (e.g. wells).

Signalment

- LLD is most likely in teleosts within established aquariums (>3 mo).
- Among saltwater fish, surgeonfish and tangs, tropical angelfish (*Pomacanthidae*), and butterflyfish (*Chaetodontidae*) are particularly susceptible.
- Among freshwater fish, discus (*Symphysodon* spp.), freshwater angelfish (*Pterophyllum scalare*), oscars (*Astronotus ocellatus*), and gouramis (*Anabantidae* and *Osphronemidae*) are particularly susceptible.
- Grossly similar lesions have been reported in some food fish, including Atlantic cod (*Gadus morhua*) and Murray cod (*Maccullochella peelii*).
- There have been no reports in elasmobranchs.

Signs/Clinical Findings

- Several conspecifics are usually affected.
- Symmetric depigmentation and pitting around the sensory canals of the head and/or lateral line are seen. There is little to no hemorrhage. Lesions can coalesce and progress until most of the epithelium is affected (Figure C2.3). Permanent scarring is possible, but the lesions do not deepen.
- Appetite and behavior are normal.
- Mortalities are not typically associated with LLD.

Differential Diagnoses

- Superficial skin ulcers in teleosts with no associated inflammation or erythema are most commonly due to LLD, but trauma, infection, and neoplasia should be considered.

Diagnosis

- This syndrome is usually diagnosed on visual examination in susceptible species, but additional diagnostics are helpful to rule out differentials and look for possible etiologies.
- Skin scrapes of the ulcerated area should be examined using direct microscopy and stained impression smears to rule out some infectious diseases.

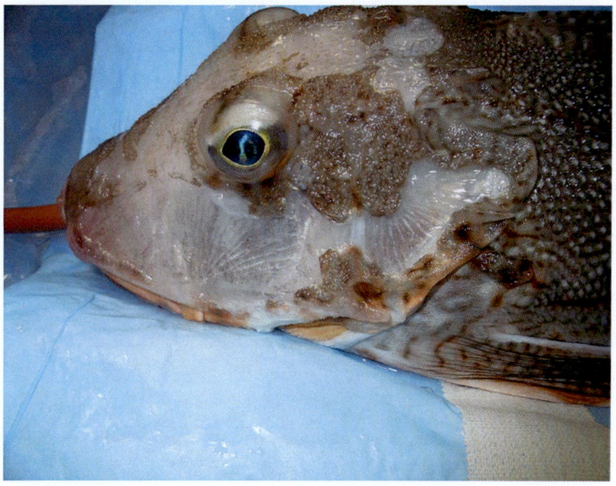

Figure C2.3 Lateral line depigmentation in a northern sea robin (*Prionotus carolinus*).

- Fecal samples may be examined under direct microscopy to look for flagellates, although these can be normal intestinal flora.
- Histology may show thinning, ulceration, or hyperplasia of the epithelium of the skin and lateral line canals. Evidence of re-epithelialization may be seen. The inflammatory response is typically limited. Internal lesions have not been associated with LLD.

Husbandry Management

- If lesions are identified early and stressors can be resolved, the prognosis for full healing is good. Lesions typically resolve over weeks to months depending on the severity and treatments.
- Resolve any environmental stressors.
- Remove any activated carbon filtration.
- Review and improve the diet and feeding if needed.
- Consider grounding the system to reduce the risk of stray voltage.

Medical Management

- Common treatments (see Chapters A12 and A13 for more details):
  - Becaplermin 0.01% gel (Regranex) is effective if underlying stressors are resolved. It is applied topically after gentle debridement of the edges and surfaces, followed by drying with a contact time of one to five minutes. Dilutions in 0.9% sodium chloride to 50 or 25% of the original concentration appear to produce similar healing rates. Repeated treatments are common (e.g. once weekly). However, single applications have been as effective as repeated treatments in ocean surgeonfish (*Acanthurus bahianus*). Suitable PPE should be used to prevent human exposure.
  - Vitamin C oral supplementation at 500–1000 mg/kg of body weight may be beneficial.
  - Metronidazole may be used to treat flagellates. Doses include 6 mg/L immersion every 48 hours or 50 mg/kg body weight orally every 24 hours for 3 treatments.
- Other reported treatments (see Chapters A12 and A13 for more details):
  - Naltrexone 0.03% cream topically has shown similar wound closure rates to becaplermin in mammalian models and may be effective in fish.
  - Collagen products topically (e.g. Collasate) may be effective.
  - Misoprostol 0.0024% and phenytoin 2% powder compounded with a gelling agent and applied topically may be effective. Suitable PPE should be used to prevent human exposure.
- All legislation regarding medication use and disposal must be followed.

Prevention

- Activated carbon filtration should only be used on closed systems for short periods of time.
- Closed systems should receive regular water changes using suitable water.
- Diets should be varied and provide appropriate sources of micronutrients. Food and supplements should be stored correctly (typically in airtight containers at the appropriate temperature and humidity and for a maximum of 6–12 mo). Frozen foods should be thawed in covered containers in a refrigerator and used in <24 hours. Foods should be eaten soon after feeding.
- Susceptible species should not be added to systems with a history of LLD.

Bibliography

Baily, J.E., Bretherton, M.J., Gavine, F.M. et al. (2005). The pathology of chronic erosive dermatopathy in Murray cod, *Maccullochella peelii peelii* (Mitchell). *Journal of Fish Diseases* 28: 3–12.

Boerner, L., Dube, K., Peterson, K. et al. (2003). Angiogenic growth factor therapy using recombinant platelet-derived growth factor (Regranex) for lateral line disease in marine fish. *Proceedings of the International Association for Aquatic Animal Medicine conference*, Kohala, HI.

Clarke, E.O., Hulse, C., Ripley, L. et al. (2014). My collasate is better than your honor roll Regranex: the use of collasate for gross resolution of head lateral line erosion syndrome in an orange shouldered tang (*Acanthurus olivaceus*). *Proceedings of the Eastern Fish Health Workshop*, Shepherdstown, WV.

Corrales, J., Ullal, A., and Noga, E.J. (2009). Lateral line depigmentation (LLD) in channel catfish, *Ictalurus punctatus* (Rafinesque). *Journal of Fish Diseases* 32: 705–712.

Fleming, G.J., Corwin, A., McCoy, A.J., and Stamper, M.A. (2008). Treatment factors influencing the use of recombinant platelet-derived growth factor (Regranex) for head and lateral line erosion syndrome in ocean surgeonfish (*Acanthurus bahianus*). *Journal of Zoo and Wildlife Medicine* 39: 155–160.

McLaughlin, P.J., Cain, J.D., Titunick, M.B. et al. (2017). Topical naltrexone is a safe and effective alternative to standard treatment of diabetic wounds. *Advanced Wound Care* 6: 279–288.

Morrison, C.M., O'Neil, D., and Wright, J.R. (2007). Histolopathology of "hole-in-the-head" disease in the Nile tilapia, *Oreochromis niloticus*. *Aquaculture* 273: 427–433.

Paull, G.C. and Matthews, R.A. (2001). *Spironucleus vortens*, a possible cause of hole-in-the-head disease in cichlids. *Diseases of Aquatic Organisms* 45: 197–202.

Stamper, M.A., Kittell, M.M., Patel, E.E., and Corwin, A.L. (2011). Effects of full-stream carbon filtration on the development of head and lateral line erosion syndrome (HLLES) in ocean surgeon. *Journal of Aquatic Animal Health* 23: 111–116.

Abbreviations/Acronyms

- LLD: Lateral line depigmentation
- HLLE: Head and lateral line erosion
- PPE: Personal protective equipment

Thyroid Hyperplasia (Goiters)

Overview

- Thyroid hyperplasia or hypertrophy, also known as goiters, are common in fish.
- The typical presentation is a mass effect in the opercular cavity in bony fish or a ventral gular mass in elasmobranchs.
- The cause is often low iodide or dissolved organic iodine in the water or diet. These nutrients are readily oxidized to iodate which is not available to fish.
- Ozone disinfection increases the rate of conversion to iodate and the risk of goiters.
- Goiters can usually be resolved by correcting the deficiency.

Etiology

- In bony fish, the thyroid is diffuse and located primarily along the gill arches and within the submucosal tissue of the oropharynx.
- In elasmobranchs, the thyroid is a distinct, encapsulated organ in the gular area, ventral to the coracohyal muscles and medial to the coracomandibular muscles.
- Iodide is required by fish for the synthesis of triiodothyronine (T3) and thyroxine (T4) in response to thyroid-stimulating hormone. T3 is the active form but T4 can be used to assess the activity of the thyroid.
- Iodine exists in three principle forms in water: iodide (I^-), dissolved organic iodine (DOI), and iodate (IO_3^-). Iodide and DOI are absorbed through the gills and gastrointestinal tract. Iodate is not available to fish.
- Known or suspected etiologies are environmental or nutritional:
  - Low iodide or DOI in the water or diet.
  - Ozone disinfection.
  - Nitrates, which inhibit uptake of iodide by the thyroid.
  - Organophosphates, organochlorines, sodium perchlorate, thiocyanates, thiourea, polychlorinated biphenyls (PCBs).
  - High manganese.
  - Poor water quality.
  - Raw brassicas in the diet (e.g. kale, cabbage, broccoli).

Signalment

- Goiters are typically seen in elasmobranchs and tropical marine teleosts that are under long-term human care.
- Within elasmobranchs, bamboo sharks (*Chiloscyllium* spp.), swell sharks (*Cephaloscyllium ventriosum*), and demersal rays (*Myliobatiformes*) may be over-represented.
- Within tropical marine teleosts, grunts (*Haemulidae*) may be over-represented.

Signs/Clinical Findings

- Several conspecifics are usually affected.
- Bony fish:
  - Slowly progressive opercular flaring is common, and often unilateral.
  - Dyspnea or tachypnea may be seen.
  - Reduced appetite may be seen.
  - A pink, yellow, or tan soft tissue mass is usually visible at the base of the gill arches (Figure C2.4a).
- Elasmobranchs:
  - A slowly progressive soft swelling in the ventral midline just caudal to the mouth is common (Figure C2.4b).
  - Abnormal prehension and swallowing of food may be seen.
- Mortality is usually low but may be seen secondary to mass effects on food intake or respiration.

Differential Diagnoses

- Differentials for an opercular or gular mass include neoplasia (e.g. carcinoma, adenoma, papilloma), infectious or inflammatory lesions (e.g. thyroiditis), hematoma, parasitic cysts (e.g. myxozoan pseudocysts, microsporidian xenomas, larval nematodes), and focal trauma or foreign body penetration.

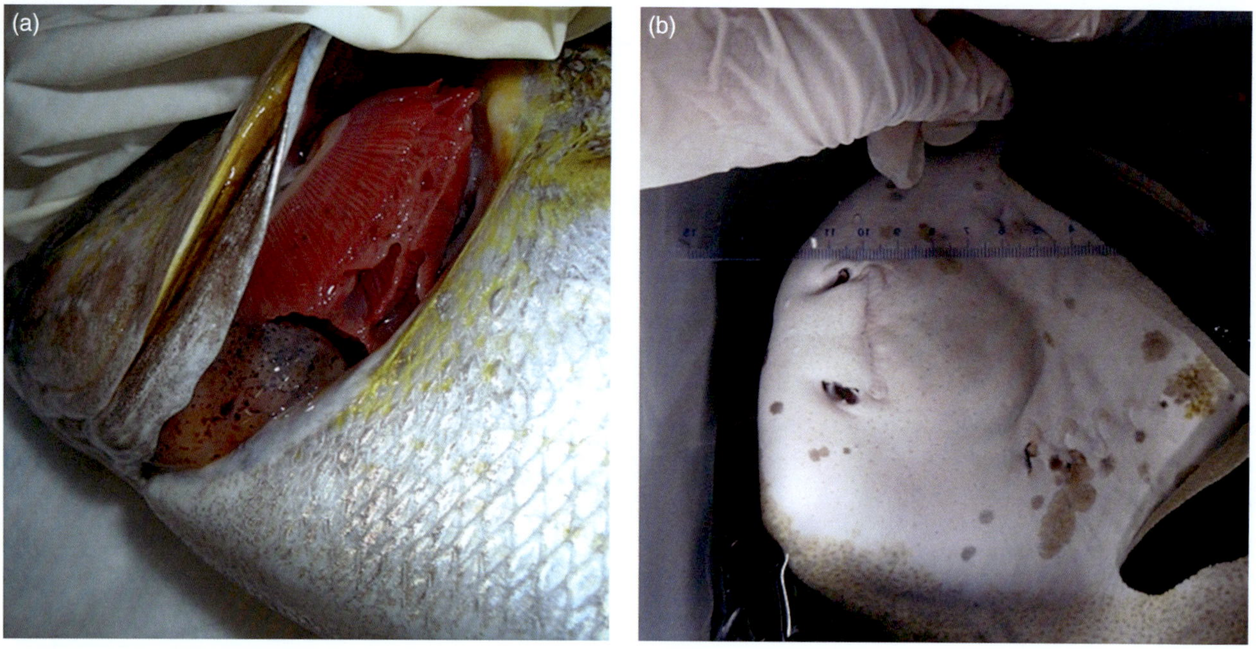

Figure C2.4 Goiters presenting as a ventral opercular mass in a grunt (*Haemulon* sp.) (a) and a ventral gular swelling in a yellow stingray (*Urobatis jamaicensis*) (b).

Diagnosis

- Goiters are typically diagnosed based on clinical signs in susceptible species and response to treatment, but additional diagnostics can help understand the etiology.
- Iodide and nitrate should be measured in the water.
  - Iodide should be 0.03–0.06 mg/L in seawater. Clinical signs have been reported at <0.006 mg/L.
  - Nitrate should be <70 mg/L NO_3–N. Values >100 mg/L should be a concern.
  - This is a chronic disease; comparisons with previous values are helpful.
- Ultrasound imaging of the thyroid is helpful in elasmobranchs to measure the size and assess the type of goiter (e.g. hyperplastic or colloidal).
- Plasma T4 may be low. Assays should be validated for the taxonomic group. Reported values of T4 measured by radioimmunoassay in unaffected animals include:
  - Whitetip reef sharks (*Triaenodon obesus*) in natural seawater: mean 4.9 ± 0.2 ng/mL (range 1.3–9.2 ng/mL).
  - White-spotted bamboo sharks (*Chiloscyllium plagiosum*) in natural seawater: mean 14.8 ng/mL (range 9.6–30.5 ng/mL).
  - Atlantic stingrays (*Hypanus sabinus*) from the wild: mean 17 ± 3 ng/mL (range 13–26 ng/mL).

  Reported values in clinically affected sharks include 0.93–0.99 ng/mL in whitetip reef sharks and 4.6 ng/mL in a white-spotted bamboo shark.
- T3 and TSH levels are typically low in fish and assays may be unreliable.
- Fine-needle aspirates and biopsy may be used to confirm a diagnosis but are not usually needed and morbidity from surgery has been reported anecdotally.
- On histology, goiters are categorized as diffuse hyperplastic (thyroid epithelial cell proliferation with small amounts of colloid), diffuse colloid (most follicles are distended by colloid), or multinodular colloid (follicles of different sizes, usually more chronic). Colloid stains positively with periodic acid–Schiff. Histologic diagnostic criteria in teleosts are described in Fournie et al. (2005).

Husbandry Management

- With husbandry management changes, improvement is usually seen in weeks to months.
- If iodide is low, add potassium iodide to the water using Reef Iodide (Seachem, Madison, GA) or Lugol's solution. Target iodide concentration in salt water should be 0.03–0.06 mg/L. Values above 0.1 mg/L should be avoided because of a potential for toxicity.
- Reduce nitrate levels through water changes or denitrification if >70 mg/L.
- Review ozone disinfection to assess if the dose can be reduced or if ozone disinfection can be taken off-line for one to two months to assess the response.

Medical Management

- Common treatments (see Chapters A12 and A13 for more details):
  - Iodide supplementation is the most common treatment in elasmobranchs, usually with potassium iodide (KI). Reported doses are 1–30 mg/kg of body weight PO once weekly.
- Other reported treatments (see Chapters A12 and A13 for more details):
  - Levothyroxine orally.
  - Methimazole orally.
- Thyroidectomy is not a reported treatment in fish.
- All legislation regarding medication use and disposal must be followed.

Prevention

- All elasmobranchs should receive dietary supplementation with KI at 1–30 mg/kg body weight once weekly (e.g. Mazuri Vita-Zu Shark/Ray tablets, Purina, Richmond, IN), ideally with monitoring of serum iodide.
- Bony fish may also benefit from some oral iodide supplementation.
- Closed systems should receive regular water changes to replenish nutrients and remove nitrates.
- Nitrate should be measured routinely (e.g. every two to four weeks) and maintained at <70 mg/L.
- In systems with ozone disinfection and/or artificial saltwater, iodide levels in the water should be measured routinely and supplemented if needed.

Bibliography

Borucinska, J.D. and Tafur, M. (2009). Comparison of histological features, and description of histopathological lesions in thyroid glands from three species of free-ranging sharks from the northwestern Atlantic, the blue shark, *Prionace glauca* (L.), the shortfin mako, *Isurus oxyrhinchus* Rafinesque, and the thresher, *Alopias vulpinus* (Bonnaterre). *Journal of Fish Diseases* 32: 785–793.

Crow, G.L., Atkinson, M.J., Ron, B. et al. (1998). Relationship of water chemistry to serum thyroid hormones in captive sharks with goiters. *Aquatic Geochemistry* 4: 469–480.

Crow, G.L., Ron, B., Atkinson, S., and Rasmussen, L.E.L. (1999). Serum T_4 and serum T_3 concentrations in immature captive whitetip reef sharks, *Triaenodon obesus*. *Journal of Experimental Zoology* 284: 500–504.

Fournie, J.W., Wolfe, M.J., Wolf, J.C. et al. (2005). Diagnostic criteria for proliferative thyroid lesions in bony fishes. *Toxicologic Pathology* 53: 540–551.

Morris, A., Hamlin, H.J., Francis Floyd, R. et al. (2011). Nitrate-induced goiter in captive whitespotted bamboo sharks *Chiloscyllium plagiosum*. *Journal of Aquatic Animal Health* 23: 92–99.

Morris, A.L., Stremme, D.W., Sheppard, B.J. et al. (2012). The onset of goiter in several species of sharks following the addition of ozone to a touch pool. *Journal of Zoo and Wildlife Medicine* 43: 621–624.

Parkinson, L., Noblitt, S.D., Campbell, T. et al. (2018). Comparison of two iodine quantification methods in an artificial system housing white-spotted bamboo sharks (*Chiloscyllium plagiosum*). *Journal of Zoo and Wildlife Medicine* 49: 952–958.

Sherrill, J., Whitaker, B.R., and Wong, G.T.F. (2004). Effects of ozonation on the speciation of dissolved iodine in artificial seawater. *Journal of Zoo and Wildlife Medicine* 35: 347–355.

Vokoff, H., Wourms, J.P., Amesbury, E., and Snelson, F.F. (1999). Structure of the thyroid gland, serum thyroid hormones, and the reproductive cycle of the Atlantic stingray *Dasyatis sabina*. *Journal of Experimental Zoology* 284: 505–516.

Abbreviations/Acronyms

- PO: Orally

Mucometra and Ovarian Cysts

Overview

- Uterine and ovarian pathology, particularly mucometra and cystic ovaries, are common in female rays (*Myliobatiformes*).
- Affected animals usually present with coelomic distension.
- Ultrasonography is required for diagnosis.
- Treatment may require surgery, hormone therapy, or breeding.

Etiology

- Rays show ovoviviparity (also known as aplacental viviparity) and appear to be induced ovulators. Without males present or without copulation, the females' ovaries

constantly produce follicles and become large and cystic. Ovarian cysts may rupture leading to hemorrhage or coelomitis. The uterus never involutes and continues to produce histotroph. Over time, the uterus becomes filled with dense histotroph (mucometra) and the uterine trophonemata become large and irregular.
- Housing females without access to mature male conspecifics for prolonged periods is a common risk factor.
- Infectious agents may be found such as visceral larval migrans, mycobacteriosis, or fungi (e.g. *Paecilomyces* spp.).

Signalment
- This is a disease of female elasmobranchs, particularly rays.
- Southern stingrays (*Hypanus americanus*) and other dasyatid rays, cownose rays (*Rhinoptera bonasus*), and white-spotted eagle rays (*Aetobatus narinari*) appear over-represented.
- Female skates seem less susceptible.
- Older animals are likely more susceptible.

Signs/Clinical Findings
- One or a few female conspecifics may be affected.
- Generalized coelomic distension is common. This is initially visible from the ventral aspect but it becomes visible dorsally when severe. Skin ulcers and petechiae may develop on the ventrum.
- Lethargy may be seen.
- Inappetence or reduced feeding may be seen.
- Rays can often live for several years with significant pathology, but the disease usually progresses and sporadic, chronic mortalities may be seen.

Differential Diagnoses
- Differentials for coelomic distension in female elasmobranchs include pregnancy, mucometra, pyometra, uterine neoplasia, hepatomegaly, obesity, and coelomic effusion.

Diagnosis
- This is usually diagnosed based on single or serial ultrasound examinations.
- Typical ultrasound findings include a significant increase in hypoechoic uterine fluid and an abnormally thick and irregular uterine wall (Figure C2.5). Sloughing of the trophonemata may be seen. The more active ovary (the left one in many rays) is often large and cystic (Figure C2.5); normal ovaries have an echogenicity similar to soft tissue. There may be obvious coelomic effusion.
- Transcutaneous or per cervical aspiration of abnormal uterine fluid can help determine the cause. However, there is some risk of iatrogenic infection. Histotroph is normally thick and yellow. In cases of mucometra, the histotroph may be thick and yellow, clear, or bloody. Leukocytes, bacteria, parasites, or fungi are abnormal findings.
- Hormone levels can be assessed, but there is limited information available on normal ranges and inaccurate results may result from protein binding in the blood. In general, estradiol concentrations have been higher in affected females.

Husbandry Management
- Consider allowing breeding to resolve signs if the pathology is mild.

Medical Management
- Common treatments (see Chapters A12 and A13 for more details):
  - Catheterization or cannulation of the oviduct through the cloaca and cervix allows removal of the uterine fluid for diagnostic and treatment purposes, but the

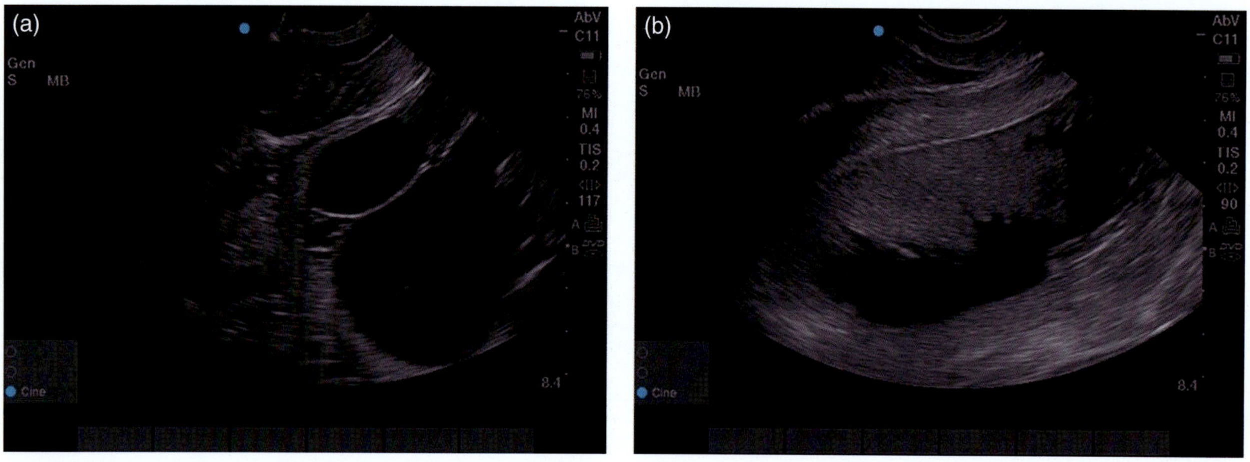

Figure C2.5 Ultrasound images of cystic ovaries (a) and mucometra (b) in a southern stingray (*Hypanus americanus*). *Source*: Images courtesy of Robert George, Ripley's Aquariums.

fluid usually recurs over weeks to months and there is a risk of iatrogenic infection.
  - Medroxyprogesterone acetate at 20 mg/kg IM every 30 days for 2–3 treatments has improved ovarian and uterine pathology; no effect was seen at 5 mg/kg.
- Other reported treatments (see Chapters A12 and A13 for more details):
  - Leuprolide acetate IM may be useful.
  - GnRH vaccines may be useful.
  - Ovariectomy has been reported in many southern stingrays and cownose rays. A dorsal paralumbar approach to each ovary is recommended (see Chapter A11).
  - Ovariohysterectomy has been extremely challenging because of the close association of the uterus to the body wall and kidney.
  - Bilateral vasectomy of male rays has been discussed to allow copulation while also controlling population numbers. However, an effective surgical technique has not been described and it is not clear if copulation without pregnancy would reduce disease incidence.
- All legislation regarding medication use and disposal must be followed.

Prevention

- Allowing female rays to breed periodically may reduce overall incidence, but the reproductive management plan must consider the care and welfare of the pups.
- Prophylactic ovariectomy may be considered in female rays in single-sex groups, although regrowth of ovarian tissue is possible.

Bibliography

Borucinska, J.D. and Adams, D.H. (2014). Parasitic metritis and oophoritis associated with nematode larvae in an Atlantic sharpnose shark, *Phizoprionodon terraenovae* (Richardson), collected in the western Atlantic off Florida. *Journal of Fish Diseases* 36: 811–817.

George, R.H., Gangler, R., Steeil, J., and Baine, K. (2014). Ovariectomy of sub-adult southern stingrays (*Dasyatis americana*) as a tool for managing an exhibit population. *Drum and Croaker* 45: 19–23.

George, R.H., Steeil, J., and Baine, K. (2017). Diagnosis and treatment of common reproductive problems in elasmobranchs. In: The Elasmobranch Husbandry Manual II: Recent Advances in the Care of Sharks, Rays and their Relatives (eds. M. Smith, D. Warmolts, D. Thoney, et al.), 357–362. Columbus: Ohio Biological Survey.

Gore, S.R., Hadfield, C.A., and Clayton, L.A. (2007). Fungal endometritis in a pelagic stingray (*Dasyatis violacea*). *Proceedings of the International Association of Aquatic Animal Medicine Conference*, Orlando, FL.

Mylniczenko, N. and Penfold. L.M. (2012a). Ultrasound findings in southern stingray (*Dasyatis americana*) with and without reproductive disease. *Proceedings of the International Association of Aquatic Animal Medicine Conference*, Atlanta, GA.

Mylniczenko, N. and Penfold. L.M. (2012b). Uterine and ovarian disease in single gender housed southern stingrays (*Dasyatis americana*). *Proceedings of the American Association of Zoo Veterinarians Conference*, Oakland, CA.

Mylniczenko, N.D., Sumigama, S., Wyffels, J.T. et al. (2019). Ultrasonographic and hormonal characterization of reproductive health and disease in wild, semiwild, and aquarium-housed southern stingrays (*Hypanus americanus*). *American Journal of Veterinary Research* 80: 931–942.

Sumigama, S., Penfold, L.M., and Mylniczenko, N.D. (2014). Development of criteria for categorizing ultrasonographic images of uterine health assessments in the southern stingray (*Dasyatis americana*). *Proceedings of the American Association of Zoo Veterinarians Conference*, Orland, FL.

Abbreviations/Acronyms

- IM: Intramuscular

Egg Retention (Egg Binding)

Overview

- Egg retention or egg binding refers to an inability to release eggs from the ovaries, oviducts, or uteri. It is a common problem in fish under human care.
- It is often due to insufficient environmental or social cues for spawning. It may be associated with primary or secondary oophoritis.
- Oviposition can sometimes be triggered by providing suitable environmental cues or hormones, but surgical ovariectomy is often required to resolve the signs.

Etiology

- Life support system/environmental

  - Inappropriate water temperature or flow, or lack of seasonal variation.
  - Inappropriate hardness, pH, or salinity, or lack of seasonal variation.
  - Inappropriate photoperiod or lack of seasonal variation.
  - Inappropriate substrate or décor.
  - Inclement weather if outdoors.
  - Inappropriate social groups.
  - High activity around the system.
  - Noise or vibration.
- Nutritional
  - Low essential fatty acids in the diet.
  - Inadequate food intake.
  - Obesity.
- Neoplasia, particularly of the ovaries, oviducts, uteri, intestines, or cloaca
- Inflammation/infection
  - Oophoritis, salpingitis or adhesions of the oviduct, metritis.
  - Cloacitis.
- Toxic
  - Heavy metals.
  - Endocrine disruptors such as estrogens (theoretically).

Signalment

- This affects oviparous and ovoviviparous female fish.
- Some teleosts are particularly susceptible.
  - Groupers (*Epinephelinae*).
  - Irish lords (*Hemilepidotus* spp.).
  - Flatfish (*Pleuronectiformes*).
  - Tetras (particularly *Paracheirodon* spp.).
- This is less common in elasmobranchs, but specific examples exist.
  - Sand tigers (*Carcharias taurus*) where ova are not released from the uteri.
  - Some skate species (*Rajidae*) where eggs can become entangled in the uteri.

Signs/Clinical Findings

- One or a few female conspecifics may be affected.
- Lethargy may be seen.
- Inappetence or reduced feeding is common.
- Generalized coelomic distension is common (Figure C2.6). Affected fish may be thin or obese.
- Cloacal/anal distension or prolapse is common and a discharge may be seen.
- Cutaneous ulcers or draining fistulas may be seen, particularly in elasmobranchs.
- Sporadic, chronic mortalities may be seen.
- If signs resolve, recurrence is common.

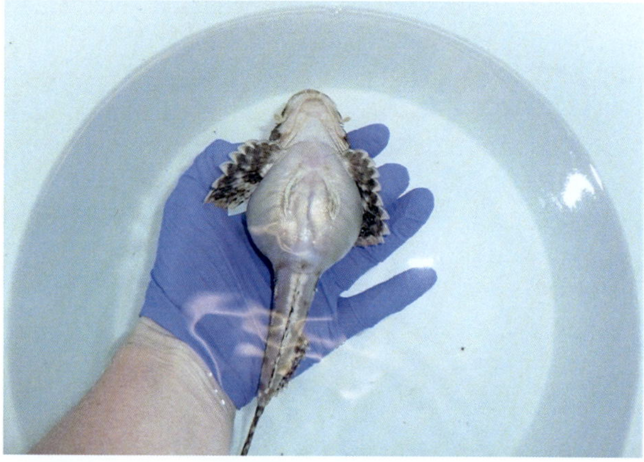

Figure C2.6 Severe coelomic distension due to egg retention in an oyster toadfish (*Opsanus tau*).

Differential Diagnoses

- Coelomic distension and cloacal/anal prolapses in fish have a long list of differentials (see Chapter B4). Where soft tissue is identified as the cause, the most likely differentials include egg retention, obesity, hepatomegaly, neoplasia, and pregnancy.

Diagnosis

- Egg retention is usually suspected from the history, but diagnosis is typically based on aspirates or surgery in bony fish and ultrasound in elasmobranchs.
- Ultrasonography can be used to identify and determine the size of the ovaries, oviducts, or uteri and to look for signs of further pathology (e.g. changes in echogenicity, debris in the oviducts, coelomic effusion).
- In bony fish, a fine-needle aspirate or tru-cut biopsy through the body wall can be used to identify and assess follicles on cytology, culture, or histology. Normal follicles are spherical and relatively uniform. Old follicles show increased translucency, denser cortical cytoplasm, and increased variability in size and content. Degenerative follicles show disintegration and fragmentation within the follicle, lipofuscin deposits, and leukocytes. Bacteria or other pathogens (particularly myxozoans and microsporidians) may be seen. In some bony fish, the ovary can be biopsied using a thin red-rubber tube or IV catheter inserted into the genital pore and rotated gently through the oviduct to collect some follicles.
- Radiology and computed tomography can be helpful to assess coelomic pathology but the ovaries are not usually visible without contrast.

- Coelomic endoscopy or coeliotomy with biopsies provides a definitive diagnosis.
- Hematology may show an inflammatory leukogram due to local or systemic inflammation.

Husbandry Management
- If the tissues look normal, try to stimulate natural spawning.
- Review any known spawning parameters and what has been used to trigger spawning of that species under human care (e.g. in koi, water temperature is increased to 22–25°C (72–77°F) and daylight hours are increased to 16L:8D).
- Provide potential areas for egg-laying based on the natural history (e.g. grasses, brushes, logs, mats, rocks, shells).
- Provide appropriate social groups for egg-laying based on the natural history.
- Consider moving fish to an alternative, suitable system; in some cases, the move can trigger spawning.

Medical Management
- In bony fish, if the ovaries are mature and normal, spawning can be induced and/or eggs can be manually stripped.
- Common treatments to induce spawning in bony fish (see Chapters A12 and A13 for more details):
  - Gonadotropin releasing hormone agonists (e.g. salmonid GnRH and domperidone; Ovaprim, Syndel Laboratories Ltd., Nanaimo, BC, Canada) at 0.5–1.0 mL/kg IM or ICe once may induce spawning. Lower doses are sometimes effective.
  - Chorulon (human chorionic gonadotropin) at variable doses (e.g. 20–2300 IU/kg) IM or by inoculation through the genital pore may induce spawning. It is approved by the FDA for use in finfish in the United States, as of 2020.
- Other reported treatments to induce spawning in bony fish (see Chapters A12 and A13 for more details):
  - Carp pituitary extract.
  - Channel catfish pituitary extract.
  - Prostaglandin PGF-2α (e.g. dinoprost).
- In bony fish, stripping can be tried under anesthesia by applying cranial to caudal pressure along the flanks to milk the roe.
- If induction or stripping is ineffective in bony fish, or if the ovaries are known to be abnormal, surgical or endoscopic ovariectomy is usually required. It is important to try to remove all the ovarian membranes and any loose follicles by curettage or flushing. Recurrence may be seen, even with apparently complete ovariectomy.
- In elasmobranchs, treatment typically requires removal of ova from the uteri by per-cervical aspiration and lavage with saline. If the cervix or cervices are closed, gentle digital pressure will often allow passage of a lubricated tube. Gentle external compression in a cranial to caudal direction can accelerate removal of uterine contents. Systemic antibiotics are often indicated to cover for opportunistic bacterial infections. Surgical removal of uterine contents and ovariectomy may be considered.
- All legislation regarding medication use and disposal must be followed.

Prevention
- Surgical or endoscopic ovariectomy may be considered for prophylaxis. Ovarian regeneration may still be seen after apparent ablation.

Bibliography

George, R.H., Steeil, J., and Baine, K. (2017). Diagnosis and treatment of common reproductive problems in elasmobranchs. In: The Elasmobranch Husbandry Manual II: Recent Advances in the Care of Sharks, Rays and their Relatives (eds. M. Smith, D. Warmolts, D. Thoney, et al.), 357–362. Columbus: Ohio Biological Survey.

Watson, C.A., Hill, J.E., Graves, J.S. et al. (2009). Use of a novel induced spawning technique for the first reported captive spawning of *Tetraodon nigroviridis*. *Marine Genomics* 2: 143–146.

Abbreviations/Acronyms
- FDA: Food and Drug Administration
- GnRH: Gonadotropin release hormone
- ICe: Intracoelomic
- IM: Intramuscular

Dystocia

Overview

- Dystocia means an abnormal or difficult birth. It includes slow passage of a fetus or inability to pass a fetus in a viviparous or ovoviviparous species. It is sometimes used to refer to slow passage of eggs, but in this text, that will be referred to as egg retention.
- In fish, dystocia is most commonly reported in rays (*Myliobatiformes*).
- It is a medical emergency that can lead to death if untreated.

Etiology

- Nutritional
  - Inappropriate diet.
  - Inadequate food intake.
  - Obesity.
- Inflammation/infection, particularly metritis or systemic disease
- Idiopathic
  - Idiopathic uterine inertia.
  - Maternal-fetal disproportion (e.g. large fetus, abnormal fetus).
  - Malpresentation.
- Life support system/environmental
  - Inappropriate water temperature or lack of seasonal variation.
  - Inappropriate salinity or lack of seasonal variation.
  - Inappropriate substrate or décor.
  - Inappropriate photoperiod or lack of seasonal variation.
  - Inappropriate social groups.
  - Other environmental stressors.

Signalment

- Dystocias are most commonly reported in rays, particularly cownose rays (*Rhinoptera bonasus*) and yellow stingrays (*Urobatis jamaicensis*).

Signs/Clinical Findings

- Signs of parturition may not be appreciable in fish.
- Lethargy or other behavioral changes may be seen.
- Acute collapse may be seen.
- Coelomic distension is common if late in gestation.
- Cloacal edema, hyperemia, or discharge may be seen. Fetal parts may be visible at the cloaca.
- Untreated, a true dystocia will often lead to mortality.

Differential Diagnoses

- It may be difficult to distinguish dystocia from other causes of morbidity in late gestation. However, dystocia should be the primary differential if there are no signs of fetal viability.

Diagnosis

- Dystocia may be suspected if the anticipated gestation length has been exceeded.
- Palpation of the cloaca in elasmobranchs may reveal a fetus and allows assessment of the relaxation of the cervix.
- Ultrasound and radiology are essential to assess the number of fetuses and their viability. Viability is typically based on heart rate, movement, and obvious signs of degeneration (e.g. gas, fragmentation).
- Endoscopic evaluation of the cloaca or coelom may be required for diagnosis.

Husbandry Management

- If the animal is otherwise healthy and the fetuses appear to be viable, management changes may help induce parturition.
- Minimize any environmental stressors.
- Review the natural history to check environmental conditions at parturition and make changes if needed.
- Seek advice from other institutions that have bred the species.

Medical Management

- If there are other signs of pathology or management changes have had no effect, intervention is often indicated.
- Common treatments (see Chapters A12 and A13 for more details):
  - Handling and anesthesia may be enough to stimulate parturition in some cases.
  - If a fetus is visible in the cervix or cloaca, it can often be pulled manually. Stingray pups do have a venomous spine and caution is indicated to avoid envenomation.
  - If a fetus is more cranial, the cervix can be dilated with gentle digital pressure or cannulated (e.g. with a sterile syringe case) to allow insertion of padded forceps or hemostats.
  - Cesarean sections have been reported using ventral or paralumbar approaches.
  - Induction of labor has been attempted with various combinations of oxytocin, relaxin, PGE-1/misoprostol, estradiol, or PGF-2α/dinoprost. Doses are anecdotal and overall success has been poor.
- All legislation regarding medication use and disposal must be followed.

Prevention

- Suitable environmental conditions and diets for breeding should be provided.
- Gravid rays should receive regular ultrasound monitoring to assess pup viability, number, and gestation length. Positive reinforcement training can allow these ultrasounds to be done without restraint.

Bibliography

Gearhart, S.A., Croft, L.A., and Swider, D.A. (2014). Cesarian section in the whitetip reef shark (*Triaenodon obesus*). *Proceedings of the International Association of Aquatic Animal Medicine Conference*, Gold Coast, Australia.

Stamper, M.A., Lewbart, G.A., and Wrangell, B.S. (1998). Manually induced parturition of two yellow spotted stingrays (*Urolophus jamaicensis*) with dystocias. *Proceedings of the the American Association of Zoo Veterinarians Conference*, Omaha, NE.

Abbreviations/Acronyms

- PG: Prostaglandin

Cataracts

Overview

- A cataract is an opacity of any part of the ocular lens or its capsule.
- Cataracts are common in fish.
- They may cause reduced feeding, increased predation, and loss of marketability.
- Lens removal or phacoemulsification is usually effective where treatment of individual fish is possible.

Etiology

- Developmental
  - Genetic factors.
  - Age.
- Nutritional
  - Deficiency of vitamin A, C, riboflavin (B2).
  - Deficiency of tryptophan, methionine, histidine.
  - Deficiency of manganese or zinc.
  - Replacement of dietary fish oils with vegetable oils.
  - Phytate-phosphorous in diets.
- Inflammatory, particularly uveitis
- Infectious; any local or systemic infection
  - Bacterial, including vibriosis, *Yersinia*, *Edwardsiella*, *Streptococcus* spp.
  - Fungal.
  - Parasitic, particularly encysted digenes (e.g. *Diplostomum* spp.).
- Toxic
  - Polycyclic aromatic hydrocarbons.
- Trauma
  - Inappropriate enclosure or décor.
  - Recent transport.
- Life support system/environmental
  - Excessive or sudden increase in UV or light exposure.
  - Rapid change in salinity.
  - Excessive ozone disinfection.
  - High, low, or fluctuating water temperature.
  - Gas supersaturation.
  - High carbon dioxide in the water.

Signalment

- All fish are susceptible.

Signs/Clinical Findings

- One or several fish may be affected.
- Lens opacities are usually readily visible on observation; these may remain stable or worsen over time. In rare cases, they can improve over time; this is most likely with cataracts caused by osmotic imbalances or extreme cold.
- There may be no other clinical signs.
- Reduced feeding response, weight loss, or poor growth rates may be seen.
- Skin darkening may be seen.
- Other ocular pathology may be visible (e.g. gas bubbles, inflammation).
- Traumatic wounds may be more common.
- Visual impairment may be appreciable on observation, particularly during feeding or catching.
- Mortality is typically low.

Differential Diagnoses

- It is important to distinguish lens opacities from corneal opacities, anterior uveitis, or an intraocular mass.

Diagnosis

- Cataracts can be diagnosed on slit lamp examination and direct or indirect ophthalmoscopy.
- Fluorescein stain can be used to identify ulcerative keratitis.
- Intraocular pressure (IOP) may be useful to identify increased IOP (possible glaucoma) or decreased IOP (possible uveitis); results are best compared to normal conspecifics. Reported values for teleosts have typically been 10–20 mmHg.

Husbandry Management

- Provide appropriate feeding opportunities and protect from predators.
- Reduce or resolve any water quality or life support system concerns.

Medical Management

- Surgical treatment may be considered, particularly if welfare is affected.

- Treatment typically consists of lens removal (phakectomy) or emulsification (phacoemulsification) under suitable anesthesia and analgesia. An electroretinogram may be considered prior to surgery to ensure that the retina does respond to light (described in Bakal et al. 2005).
- If ocular pathology is severe, enucleation may be considered.
- All legislation regarding medication use and disposal must be followed.
- Prognosis following surgical phakectomy, phacoemulsification, or enucleation is typically good if there is no other pathology.

Prevention

- Suitable environmental conditions and diets should be provided.
- Exposure to any underlying causes should be minimized (e.g. controlling snails to prevent digenes, suitable lighting for the species).

Bibliography

Bakal, R.S., Hickson, B.H., Gilger, B.C. et al. (2005). Surgical removal of cataracts due to *Diplostomum* species in Gulf sturgeon (*Acipenser oxyrinchus desotoi*). *Journal of Zoo and Wildlife Medicine* 36: 504–508.

Link, B.A., Gray, M.P., Smith, R.S., and John, S.W. (2004). Intraocular pressure in zebrafish: comparison of inbred stains and identification of a reduced melanin mutant with raised IOP. *Investigative Ophthalmology & Visual Science* 45: 4415–4422.

Neves, K.J. and Brown, N.P. (2015). Effects of dissolved carbon dioxide on cataract formation and progression in juvenile Atlantic cod, *Gadus morhua* L. *Journal of the World Aquaculture Society* 46: 33–44.

Remø, S.C., Hevrøy, E.M., Olsvik, P.A. et al. (2014). Dietary histidine requirement to reduce the risk and severity of cataracts is higher than the requirement for growth in Atlantic salmon smolts, independently of the dietary lipid source. *British Journal of Nutrition* 111: 1759–1772.

Welk, T., Barrows, F., Overturf, K. et al. (2016). Optimizing zinc supplementation levels of rainbow trout (*Oncorhynchus mykiss*) fed practical type fishmeal- and plant-based diets. *Aquaculture Nutrition* 22: 91–108.

Abbreviations/Acronyms

- UV: Ultraviolet

Lipid Keratopathy (Corneal Lipidosis)

Overview

- Lipid deposition in the cornea or overlying dermal layer is seen in fish under human care, particularly moray eels (*Muraenidae*).
- It is typically associated with systemic lipid abnormalities.
- Dietary management or surgical resection of lesions can improve signs.

Etiology

- Lipid keratopathy is classically associated with a diet high in fat (including cholesterols) and high in total calories. Common seafood items that are particularly high in fat usually include Atlantic mackerel (*Scomber scombrus*), Spanish mackerel (*Scomberomorus* spp.), northern anchovy (*Engraulis mordax*), and herring (*Clupea* spp.).
- Other risk factors may play a role:
  - A lack of normal fasting periods.
  - Low dietary vitamin C.
  - Lack of activity/exercise.
  - Genetics.

Signalment

- The most susceptible groups are carnivorous teleosts under human care, particularly moray eels.
- In other vertebrate classes, females are more prone to lipid keratopathy because of higher plasma triglycerides and cholesterols associated with vitellogenesis, but this has not yet been demonstrated in fish.

Signs/Clinical Findings

- Several conspecifics may be affected.
- Irregular, gray to white plaque-like opacities within the cornea or dermal layer (spectacle) are seen and may be unilateral or bilateral (Figure C2.7). Silver, sparkling or shiny crystalline structures may be visible under magnification. Lesions often worsen over time without intervention and vascularization of the cornea develops. When severe, visualization of the anterior chamber becomes impossible. Other ocular abnormalities (inflammation, ulceration) are usually absent.
- Visual impairment may be appreciable on observation, particularly during feeding or catching.

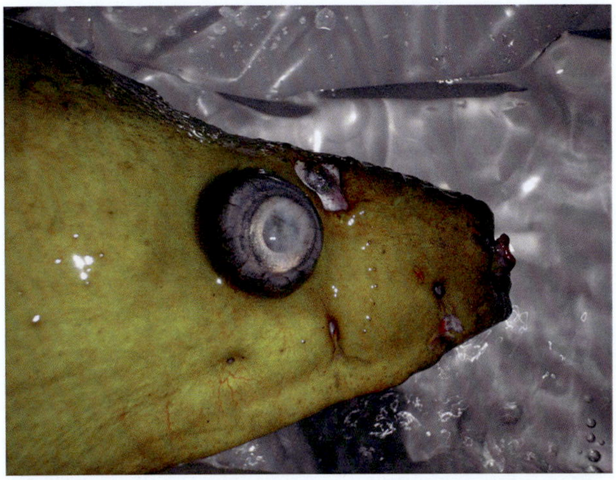

Figure C2.7 Corneal lipidosis in a green moray (*Gymnothorax funebris*). *Source*: Image courtesy of Craig Harms, North Carolina State University.

- Affected fish may be obese.
- Mortality is typically low.

Differential Diagnoses

- It is important to distinguish corneal opacities from lens opacities, anterior uveitis, or an intraocular mass.
- Differentials for corneal opacities include mineral deposition (crystalline opacities), edema (blue, more diffuse opacities, sometimes with a cobblestone appearance), fibrosis (gray or white feathery opacities), and keratitis (yellow, green, or tan stromal opacities). Some drugs can also cause corneal opacities.

Diagnosis

- A tentative diagnosis is usually made following ophthalmic examination.
- On biochemistry, total protein, triglycerides, cholesterol, and aspartate aminotransferase (AST) may be increased.
- Definitive diagnosis is based on histology. Typical lesions include extracellular intrastromal cholesterol clefts, lipid vacuoles, and abundant foamy macrophages. Special stains such as oil red O and Sudan IV can be used to confirm the presence of red-staining lipids.

Husbandry Management

- Reduce fat and cholesterol in the diet. Fat composition of prey items varies significantly based on catch season and location, so a diet analysis with full lipid profiles is recommended to help with decisions.
- Gradually introduce fasting periods, if appropriate for the species.
- Review the natural history and gradually transition to a more wild-type diet.
- Minimize scavenging opportunities, particularly on high-fat foods.
- Provide increased foraging opportunities and other species-appropriate enrichment.

Medical Management

- Possible treatments (see Chapters A12 and A13 for more details):
  - Surgical resection of lesions can improve ocular clarity and feeding behavior. Resected spectacle can be left to heal by second intention, while primary closure is more common following full thickness resection of spectacle and cornea. Suitable analgesia should be provided.
  - Photodynamic therapy may be used.
- All legislation regarding medication use and disposal must be followed.

Prevention

- Diet and feeding intervals should be based on the natural history of the species and life stage, and fish should be maintained at an appropriate body condition.
- Teleost diets that rely heavily on fatty fish should be reviewed.

Bibliography

Clode, A.B., Harms, C., Fatzinger, M.H. et al. (2012). Identification and management of ocular lipid deposition in association with hyperlipidaemia in captive moray eels, *Gymnothorax funebris* Ranzani, *Gymnothorax moringa* (Cuvier) and *Muraena retifera* Goode and Bean. *Journal of Fish Diseases* 35: 683–693.

Ehrlacher-Reid, C., Hoffman, W.E., Priede, M. et al. (2011). Plasma biochemistry values of recently wild-caught purple mouth moray eels (*Gymnothorax vicinus*). *Journal of Zoo and Wildlife Medicine* 42: 671–679.

Raizman, M.B., Hamrah, P., Holland, E.J. et al. (2017). Drug-induced corneal epithelial changes. *Survey of Ophthalmology* 62: 286–301.

Obesity

Overview

- Obesity is common in fish under human care.
- Bony fish deposit fat in their coelomic cavity, viscera, and muscle. Elasmobranchs deposit fat primarily in their liver.
- Obese fish typically have distended coeloms and heavy muscling.
- It is important to rule out other causes of coelomic distension (e.g. egg retention).
- Husbandry management can be effective at reducing body condition and improving overall health.

Etiology

- Obesity typically occurs when food intake chronically exceeds energy expenditure.
- Environmental factors
  - Lack of activity.
  - Lack of enrichment.
- Nutritional factors
  - Excess food intake (e.g. heavy feeding of large groups to support fish that are slow to eat).
  - Lack of appropriate fasting periods.
  - Inappropriate diets (e.g. diets high in pelagic fish to species that normally feed on benthic crustaceans).
  - High-fat diets or inappropriate fatty acid profiles, particularly high levels of long-chain polyunsaturated fatty acids (PUFAs).
  - High-carbohydrate diets or inappropriate carbohydrate profiles.
  - Scavenging or predation opportunities.
- Other factors
  - Hormonal effects.
  - Lipomas.
  - Steatitis.
- Hepatic lipidosis (or hepatosteatosis) refers to abnormal fatty infiltration of the liver and is a common histologic diagnosis of fish, although differentiating normal from abnormal fat levels in the liver can be difficult. Hepatic lipidosis may be associated with high fat levels, mobilization of fat stores during a period of inappetence or stress, micronutrient deficiency, or other liver disease.

Signalment

- All fish are susceptible.
- Older fish may be more susceptible.

Signs/Clinical Findings

- Multiple fish from one or more species are usually affected.
- Obese fish typically show coelomic distension and increased muscling along the epaxial muscles. Skates and rays also show increased muscling in the pelvic fins and over the pelvis.
- Bilateral exophthalmos may be seen in bony fish due to fat deposition in the orbit.
- Feeding response varies.
- Poor reproductive success may be seen.
- Sporadic, chronic mortalities may be seen due to liver failure, pressure effects, trauma to the liver, or secondary disease.

Differential Diagnoses

- There are many differentials for coelomic distension in fish. Where soft tissue is identified as the cause, the most likely differentials include egg retention, obesity, hepatomegaly, neoplasia, and pregnancy.
- Differentials for hepatomegaly include infectious hepatitis (e.g. mycobacteriosis, digenes, myxozoans), hepatic lipidosis, hepatic neoplasia, hepatotoxins, polycystic liver disease, cardiac disease, and drug-induced hepatomegaly.

Diagnosis

- Obesity is typically diagnosed on visual examination, but additional diagnostics (e.g. coelomic aspirate and ultrasound) may be indicated to rule out other differentials.
- A comprehensive diet history is essential. This should include what food is offered and what other food is available, what is eaten, supplements, food sources, storage time and temperatures, method and timing of preparation, method and timing of feeding, length of time this diet has been fed, and other historical trends.
- Obese fish may not be able to navigate well or handle chasing; this should be considered if manual or chemical restraint is needed.
- Ultrasonography will show hepatomegaly and changes in liver echogenicity. In normal bony fish, the liver should have sharp edges and usually fills <1/3 of the coelom, and there should be little fat in the coelom. In normal elasmobranchs, the liver should not extend beyond the pelvic girdle or wrap dorsally around the viscera.
- Liver biopsies are useful to distinguish between obesity and the presence of additional pathology (e.g. hepatitis, hepatic lipidosis).
- Hypertriglyceridemia may be seen.
- At necropsy, abundant coelomic fat is seen in bony fish (Figure C2.8). Enlarged, pale, and friable livers with rounded edges are seen in all fish, with a high hepatosomatic index. Wet mounts and impression smears of the liver show abundant fat droplets, although this can be hard to distinguish from normal fat storage, particularly in elasmobranchs.

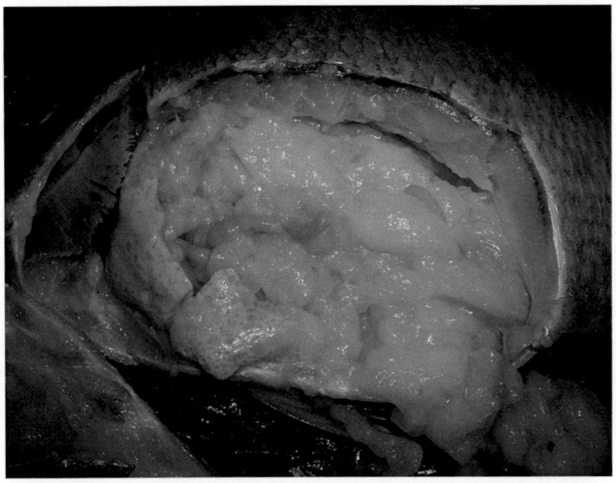

Figure C2.8 Obese grunt (*Haemulon* sp.) on necropsy showing excess fat throughout the coelom and liver.

- Histology of the liver typically shows hepatocyte swelling with vacuoles of varying sizes. Special stains such as oil red O and Sudan IV can be used to confirm the presence of red-staining lipids. Steatitis or hepatitis may be seen. A diagnosis of hepatic lipidosis should be based on normal cohorts at the same life stage and the presence of cellular deterioration (e.g. coalescing vacuoles, necrosis, calcification). To try to increase objectivity, a fractal dimension approach has been suggested by Bianco et al. (2013).

Husbandry Management

- Husbandry changes are often effective, but recovery usually takes several months. Routine weights or body condition scoring can be used to assess improvements.
- Slowly restrict the total diet (e.g. 20% decrease repeated in two weeks). Sudden fasting should be avoided, as this may potentially increase the risk of hepatic lipidosis.
- Split feeds to allow more frequent feeding.
- Gradually introduce a variety of more appropriate food items, if needed, ideally based on the wild-type diet (e.g. crustaceans, bivalves, annelids, vascular plants, algae). Switch to food items from the same environment if not already the case, i.e. marine prey for marine predators. Transitioning fish to new food items can take months, and initial lack of success should not stop attempts to convert animals onto more appropriate food items. Techniques include hiding novel food items within the fish's preferred foods and feeding novel food items at the start of a feed.
- Increase enrichment, particularly foraging opportunities to encourage activity (e.g. prey items frozen in ice or other blocks, food items hidden inside of enrichment). Target training can provide enrichment and help control food intake.
- If on commercial feeds, evaluate the composition and quality. Consider slowly converting fish over to feeds with lower simple carbohydrates and fat, and based on appropriate fish, aquatic invertebrates, and/or algae.
- Reduce opportunities for predation and scavenging.
- Consider increasing enclosure size, if a suitable enclosure exists.
- It is important to return a restricted diet to a maintenance level once the target weight or condition is achieved.

Medical Management

- Medical management is rarely indicated. However, if obese fish become inappetent, nutritional support (e.g. force feeding or tube feeding) may be needed.
- If hepatic lipidosis is a concern, hepatoprotectants such as silymarin, *S*-adenosyl-methionine (SAMe), or milk thistle may help. Ursodeoxycholic acid may help but is less commonly used due to possible side effects. Doses are usually based on conservative mammalian doses. Additional vitamin supplementation may be indicated, including vitamin B complex, E, and K1. Glucocorticoids are likely contraindicated.
- All legislation regarding medication use and disposal must be followed.

Prevention

- Suitable, targeted feeding should be provided based on the natural history, life stage, and activity level of the fish.
- Suitable space, social situations, and enrichment should be provided in order to encourage movement.

Bibliography

Bianco, C., Sirri, R., Sarli, G. et al. (2013). How severe is the lipid accumulation in fish liver? A fractal answer. *The Fractal Laboratory Journal* 2: 3. ISSN2280-3769.

Forn-Cuni, G., Varela, M., Fernández-Rodríguez, C.M. et al. (2015). Liver immune responses to inflammatory stimuli in diet-induced obesity model of zebrafish. *Journal of Endocrinology* 224: 159–170.

Oka, T., Nishmiura, Y., Zang, L. et al. (2010). Diet-induced obesity in zebrafish shares common pathophysiological pathways with mammalian obesity. *BMC Physiology* 10: 21–33.

Twibell, R.G., Gannam, A.L., Barron, J.M. et al. (2017). Effects of dietary lipid and light source on steatitis in steelhead, *Oncorhynchus mykiss*. *Journal of Aquacultures* 479: 370–377.

Micronutrient Deficiency

Overview

- Macronutrients consist of protein, lipid, carbohydrate (including fiber), and the macrominerals calcium, phosphorous, sodium, potassium, and magnesium. Macrominerals are typically available from the water.
- Micronutrients include vitamins, trace, and ultra-trace minerals and are the focus of this section.
- Signs of micronutrient deficiencies are often nonspecific and can be hard to attribute to nutritional imbalances. Response to diet changes (e.g. improved coloration or reduced morbidity) is often how a deficiency is appreciated.
- Nutritional needs are affected by species, environmental parameters, physiologic state, and activity level. For most fish species, nutritional requirements are not known, and diets should try to match the wild-type diet for that species and life stage.
- Diversity and choice are important considerations to help provide a range of micronutrients.
- Storage and preparation of food items should always be considered.

Etiology

- Details on vitamins and minerals in fish are provided in Chapter A4.
- Dietary deficiencies may be due to inappropriate diet, food storage, or preparation.
- Risk factors for nutritional deficiencies include:
  - Inappropriate food items (e.g. fish fillets rather than whole fish, fish high in thiaminase such as alewives (*Alosa pseudoharengus*) and capelin (*Mallotus villosus*), whole fish to demersal skates and rays).
  - Inappropriate food amounts.
  - Inappropriate fatty acid profiles.
  - Lack of variety (e.g. a diet based on capelin and shrimp only).
  - Feeding of freshwater items to saltwater fish and vice versa.
  - Inadequate feeding of live food items (e.g. brine shrimp, rotifers) prior to use.
  - Prolonged storage of food items (e.g. >6 mo for fatty foods, past use-by date for commercial foods).
  - Thawing or holding seafood in water.
  - Food not eaten within a few minutes.
  - Prolonged exposure of supplements to air or water.
  - Competition for food.
  - Adsorption of micronutrients by activated carbon filters.

Signalment

- Any species may be affected, particularly in systems with low organic loads where alternative food sources (e.g. algae, invertebrates) are limited.
- Species with diets that are difficult to provide under human care are most likely to be affected, for example some angelfish (*Pomacanthidae*) feed on sponges, corals, tunicates, and algae in the wild and meeting nutritional needs when using other food sources is difficult.
- Animals under physiologic stress are more susceptible (e.g. breeding females).

Signs/Clinical Findings

- Multiple fish from one or more species may be affected.
- Lethargy may be seen.
- Inappetence, reduced feeding, weight loss, or poor growth rates may be seen.
- Pallor or darkening of the skin, poor coloration, skin ulcers, fin erosions, lateral line depigmentation, or poor wound healing may be seen.
- Petechiae or ocular hemorrhages may be due to deficiency of vitamin A, thiamine (B1), riboflavin (B2), C, or K.
- Exophthalmos may be due to deficiency of vitamin A, pyridoxine (B6), folate (B9), C, or E.
- Cataracts may be due to deficiency of vitamin A, C, riboflavin (B2), tryptophan, methionine, histidine, manganese, or zinc.
- Retinal blindness may be due to deficiency of vitamin A or E.
- Coelomic distension due to ascites and edema may be seen with deficiency of vitamin A, C, or E.
- Gill hyperplasia and clubbing may be due to deficiency of pantothenate (B5).
- Opercular deformity may be due to deficiency of vitamin C or pantothenate (B5) and excess vitamin A.
- Gill pallor may be seen due to anemia from deficiency of vitamin A, C, E, K, and several vitamin Bs (e.g. folate, niacin, pantothenate, pyridoxine).
- Poor reproductive success is common.
- Spinal or other skeletal deformities may be seen with deficiency of vitamin A, C, E, thiamine (B1), riboflavin (B2), tryptophan, phosphorus, potassium, selenium, or zinc and with excess vitamin A or selenium.
- Neurologic signs including ataxia may be seen with deficiency of vitamin E and several vitamin Bs (e.g. thiamine, riboflavin, niacin, folate, pyridoxine, cyanocobalamin).
- Secondary infectious disease may be seen with vitamin C deficiency.
- The squamous metaplasia commonly reported in other vertebrates secondary to hypovitaminosis A has not been reported in fish.

- Mortalities are possible, including epizootics (e.g. salmonid early mortality syndrome from thiamine deficiency).

Differential Diagnoses

- Signs of micronutrient deficiencies are nonspecific. Differentials based on presenting signs are provided in Section B.

Diagnosis

- A comprehensive diet history is essential. This should include what food is offered, what other food is available, what is eaten, supplements used, food sources, storage time and temperatures, method and timing of preparation, method and timing of feeding, length of time this diet has been fed, and other historical trends.
- Good observation during feeding can help to confirm what foods animals are eating and to look for any social factors affecting food intake.
- Radiography or computed tomography may show skeletal abnormalities.
- Hepatic lipidosis, hepatocyte swelling, and necrosis may be identified on histology of liver biopsies or postmortem sampling, particularly with deficiency of vitamin D, E, biotin (B7), or selenium.
- Skeletal muscle histology may show atrophy, necrosis, and ceroidosis, particularly with deficiency of vitamin E or selenium.
- Micronutrient levels in whole blood, serum, or plasma may be useful. Assays are routinely available for vitamin A, β-carotene, vitamin D3, and α-tocopherol. Some reference levels exist (e.g. smooth dogfish (*Mustelus canis*) under human care). Some levels are hard to assess (e.g. thiamine and vitamin C due to poor stability). Some units are unusual (e.g. retinal equivalence, ascorbate equivalence).
- Micronutrient levels in tissues may be assayed by some nutritional laboratories.
- Dietary analyses are helpful in assessing problems and in monitoring management changes.
- Where analyses are not possible, published information on the composition of many common food items is available in the literature and Chapter A4.

Husbandry Management

- Long-term diet improvements are required to resolve the issue.
- Gradually introduce a variety of more appropriate food items, if needed, ideally using whole foods that match the wild-type diet (e.g. change 20–25% of the diet every two weeks). Switch to food items from the same environment if not already the case, i.e. marine prey for marine predators.
- If on commercial feeds, evaluate the composition and quality.
- Improve food storage, preparation, and presentation, if needed.
- Consider supplementation with individual micronutrients but improving the overall diet is preferred.
- If hepatic lipidosis is identified, slowly reduce the total caloric content and fat and carbohydrate in the diet.

Medical Management

- Common treatments (see Chapters A12 and A13 for more details):
  - Nutritional support may be indicated.
  - A wide variety of oral supplements are available. Injectable supplements include vitamin A, thiamine, vitamin B complex, vitamin C, vitamin D3, vitamin E, and selenium. Local injection site reactions have been reported.
- All legislation regarding medication use and disposal must be followed.

Prevention

- Most fish benefit from a diet that closely matches the wild-type, either based on whole foods or compounded.
- Good quality commercial diets designed for the species have several benefits. They should use water-stabilized forms of vitamins such as L-ascorbate polyphosphate (LAPP).
- Diets must be labeled and stored appropriately. Storage usually includes airtight containers at the appropriate temperature and humidity. Labels should include date of production (if known), date received, date opened, and date to discard.
- Fatty foods should have a maximum frozen storage time of 6 mo. Other foods should have a maximum frozen storage time of 6–12 mo.
- Thawing should always be done in air under refrigeration at 4°C (39°F), with foods used within 24 h.
- Supplements should be added immediately before feeding.
- Diet analyses on a regular or risk-assessment basis are helpful in assessing content.

Bibliography

Bowater, R.O. and Burren, B. (2007). Lateral muscular myopathy associated with vitamin E deficiency in farmed barramundi, *Lates calcarifer* (Bloch). *Journal of Fish Diseases* 30: 117–121.

Kupsco, A. and Schlenk, D. (2016). Molecular mechanisms of selenium-induced spinal deformities in fish. *Aquatic Toxicology* 179: 143–150.

Moreau, R. and Dabrowski, K. (2001). Gulonolactone oxidase presence in fishes: activity and significance. In: Ascorbic Acid in Aquatic Organisms (ed. K. Dabrowski), 13–32. Boca Raton, FL: CRC Press LLC.

Persky, M.E., Williams, J.J., Burks, R.E. et al. (2012). Hematologic, plasma biochemistry, and select nutrient values in captive smooth dogfish (*Mustelus canis*). *Journal of Zoo and Wildlife Medicine* 43: 842–851.

Wang, K.Y., Peng, C.Z., Huang, J.L. et al. (2013). The pathology of selenium deficiency in *Cyprinus carpio* L. *Journal of Fish Diseases* 36: 609–615.

Gastrointestinal Foreign Bodies

Overview

- Gastrointestinal (GI) foreign bodies are reported sporadically from fish.
- They are usually an individual fish problem.
- It can be hard to assess if GI foreign bodies need to be removed, as fish may be able to regurgitate or pass them.
- If indicated, removal follows similar protocols to other vertebrate classes.

Etiology

- Foreign bodies may consist of sand, stones, coral, cable ties, pieces of screens, fish hooks, bolts, pieces of décor, fish spines, undigestible food items (e.g. crab exoskeletons), or objects dropped into systems (e.g. sunglasses).
- Lack of enrichment and macro- or micronutrient deficiencies may be risk factors.
- Some foreign bodies can lead to partial or complete GI obstruction, ulceration, or perforation.
- Some can also result in systemic toxicity (e.g. pennies minted since 1983 contain more zinc).

Signalment

- Fish with larger mouths and active predators are more likely to be affected.
- Some species are particularly susceptible (e.g. large pufferfish (*Tetraodontidae*) tend to eat décor).

Signs/Clinical Findings

- Lethargy may be seen.
- Inappetence or reduced feeding response may be seen.
- Regurgitation of food may be seen.
- Oropharyngeal distension may be seen.
- Coelomic distension may develop and is often localized to the cranioventral coelom.
- Abnormal fecal output may be appreciated.
- Gill pallor due to anemia is possible secondary to lead or zinc exposure.
- Neurologic signs may be seen secondary to toxin exposure.
- Mortalities may be seen.

Differential Diagnoses

- Differentials for apparent GI pathology include gastroenteritis (parasitic, other), foreign body ingestion, and neoplasia.

Diagnosis

- In some cases, ingestion of foreign bodies may have been seen.
- Observation of the enclosure may show potential contenders for foreign bodies.
- Physical examination may allow palpation of foreign bodies in some species.
- Radiography or computed tomography may show radiopaque foreign bodies (e.g. gravel, metal). Positive contrast may be needed to show other materials.
- Ultrasonography may show the foreign body, GI fluid, or coelomic effusion.
- Endoscopy of the GI tract may be needed to identify foreign material and can be used to remove the material.
- Measuring lead (in whole blood) or zinc (in plasma) may be indicated. Check with the diagnostic laboratory about sampling requirements prior to collection.

Husbandry Management

- Many esophageal and gastric foreign bodies can be regurgitated by fish unless they are adhered to or penetrate the wall. Many foreign bodies also pass through the intestines normally. If fish are asymptomatic and the objects might be regurgitated or passed, it is often appropriate to monitor.
- Prevent ongoing exposure to foreign bodies through management changes.

Medical Management

- Common treatments (see Chapters A12 and A13 for more details):
  - Foreign bodies can be retrieved from the gastric chamber using forceps, endoscopy, or by hand if the fish is large enough.
  - Foreign bodies that are within the intestines often require surgical retrieval, with appropriate anesthesia and analgesia.

- Supportive care, including fluid and nutritional support, may be indicated.
- Gastroprotectants may be indicated (e.g. sucralfate, ranitidine, famotidine, omeprazole).
- Other reported treatments (see Chapters A12 and A13 for more details):
  - Fluids orally or parenterally.
  - Psyllium (Metamucil) orally.
  - Mineral oil orally or per rectum.
- NSAIDs and corticosteroids are likely contraindicated.
- All legislation regarding medication use and disposal must be followed.

Prevention
- An appropriate diet fed in a manner to promote normal feeding patterns and appropriate enrichment can reduce the incidence of foreign body ingestion.
- Foreign material in systems (e.g. objects dropped into aquariums by visitors) should be removed as soon as possible.

Bibliography

Lloyd, R. and Lloyd, C. (2011). Surgical removal of a gastric foreign body in a sand tiger shark, *Carcharias taurus* Rafinesque. *Journal of Fish Diseases* 34: 951–953.

McDermott, A.J., Field, C.L., Hoopes, L.A., and Clauss, T.M. (2016). Medical management of coelomic distention, abnormal swimming, substrate retention, and hematologic changes in a reef manta ray (*Manta alfredi*). *Journal of Zoo and Wildlife Medicine* 47: 927–930.

Abbreviations/Acronyms
- GI: Gastrointestinal

Neoplasia

Overview
- A wide variety of neoplasms have been reported from fish.
- Common presenting signs are cutaneous masses, ocular masses, or coelomic distension.
- Cutaneous (especially papillomas), ocular, peripheral nerve, gonadal, and renal tumors (especially nephroblastomas) are common in fish.
- Neoplasms of the gills, skeletal system, and gastrointestinal tract tend to be rare in fish.
- Benign neoplasms are more common than malignant. Where malignant neoplasms are seen in fish, they often show malignant morphology and local invasion, but metastases are rare.
- Prognosis is largely unknown.

Etiology
- A variety of etiologies have been identified for fish neoplasms.
  - Viruses, particularly *Retroviridae* (e.g. walleye dermal sarcomas, salmon swim bladder leiomyosarcomas, damselfish neurofibromas); also *Herpesviridae* (e.g. *Oncorhynchus masou* virus) and *Adenoviridae* (e.g. red seabream leukemia).
  - Parasites, e.g. pseudobranch tumors/X cell disease in Atlantic cod (*Gadus morhua*), plasmacytoid leukemia in salmonids (*Salmonidae*) associated with the microsporidian *Nucleospora salmonis*, intestinal carcinomas in zebrafish (*Danio rerio*) associated with the nematode *Pseudocapillaria tomentosa*.
  - Water or feed contaminants, e.g. hepatic neoplasia due to mycotoxins from *Aspergillus flavus* in food, or hepatic and cutaneous tumors due to polycyclic aromatic hydrocarbons (PAHs).
  - Excessive light, UV, or gamma exposure, e.g. retinal neoplasia due to blue light from metal halides in nocturnal pajama cardinal fish (*Sphaeramia nematoptera*).
  - Trauma, particularly papillomas.
  - Immersion medications, including formalin and malachite green.
- Some proposed risk factors include:
  - Water temperature and season.
  - Chronic inflammation.
  - Age.
  - Genetics.

Signalment
- All species are susceptible to neoplasia, although there are more reports in bony fish than elasmobranchs.
- They are reported from wild fish and fish under human care.
- Some species seem to be prone to particular neoplasms, e.g.:
  - Fibromas, also called odontogenic hamartomas, in freshwater angelfish (*Pterophyllum scalare*).

- Aggressive melanomas in platies and swordtails (*Xiphophorus* spp.).
- Ovarian neoplasms in sexually mature female koi (*Cyprinus carpio*).
- Papillomas in sand tigers (*Carcharias taurus*), guitarfish (*Rhinobatidae*), and bamboo sharks (*Hemiscylliidae*).

Signs/Clinical Findings

- Neoplasms typically affect individual animals, although epizootics have been reported, e.g. ameloblastomas in wild and cultured Chinook salmon (*Oncorhynchus tshawytscha*) and renal papillary cystic adenomas and adenocarcinomas in oscars (*Astronotus ocellatus*).
- Any clinical signs are possible.
- Lethargy may be seen.
- Inappetence, reduced feeding, or weight loss may be seen.
- Single or multiple dermal or oral nodules or plaques are common and often ulcerate over time. Masses may be yellow, pink, red, tan, black, or multicolored. Dermal neoplasms in fish are most commonly papillomas. Other dermal or oral neoplasms include fibromas, neurofibromas, schwannomas, ameloblastomas, pigment-cell tumors, lipomas, squamous cell carcinomas, and odontomas, and their associated sarcomas. The color or appearance does not tend to help with diagnosis, but black masses are often melanomas, neurofibromas, or fibromas.
- Exophthalmos or buphthalmos may be seen with ocular neoplasms (intraocular or retrobulbar). Lesions are usually unilateral. Reported ocular neoplasms include fibrosarcomas, adenocarcinomas, retinoblastomas, and melanosarcomas.
- Dyspnea or tachypnea may be seen with oral, gular, or branchial neoplasms.
- Focal or diffuse coelomic distension may be due to internal masses or coelomic effusion. These may also change behavior, buoyancy, or swimming. Coelomic masses have been reported due to adenomas, carcinomas, fibromas, sarcomas, hemangiomas, mesotheliomas, and dysgerminomas.
- Hemorrhage from the cloaca may be seen with gastrointestinal, genital, urinary, or coelomic neoplasms.

Differential Diagnoses

- Differentials for distinct masses include acute or granulomatous inflammation, hyperplasia (e.g. goiter, carp pox, lymphocystis), cysts (e.g. digenes, myxozoan pseudocysts, microsporidian xenomas, mesomycetozoeans), hematomas, xanthomas, and organomegaly (e.g. hepatomegaly, egg retention). Some structures reported as masses are normal, e.g. nuptial tubercles on goldfish (*Carassius auratus*).
- These differentials are more common than neoplasms in fish.

Diagnosis

- Diagnosis is often made at necropsy, but premortem testing can often provide a definitive diagnosis.
  - For discrete masses, aspiration cytology may give an indication of the cause (wet mounts and stained impression smears). Dif-Quik remains a good general-purpose stain, although Wright–Giemsa gives better cellular detail.
  - Incisional or excisional biopsies are often required for diagnosis. For internal masses, exploratory or endoscopic surgery may be used to obtain suitable samples. Tissues should be fixed as needed and submitted for histology, IHC, and potentially ultrastructure studies.
  - For hematopoietic neoplasms, diagnosis is typically based on blood smears.
  - Ultrasound, radiology, CT, and MRI are useful to identify masses and to look for infiltration or dissemination.
- Typical neoplastic indicators include cellular and nuclear pleomorphism, multiple nuclei with irregular margins, increased nuclear to cytoplasm ratios, and mitotic figures. Cells that are foreign to the tissue sampled may be neoplastic. There may be no inflammatory response, although some fish can have a prominent inflammatory response secondary to neoplasia. Other diseases should be ruled out (e.g. granulomas, parasites).
- Cell categories are the same in fish as in other vertebrates.
  - Individual round cells (e.g. lymphomas, lymphosarcomas, melanomas).
  - Scattered individual spindle cells with indistinct cell margins (e.g. fibromas, osteomas, hemangiomas, leiomyomas, myxomas, seminomas, teratomas, odontomas, pigment-cell tumors such as chromatophoromas, peripheral nerve sheath tumors, as well as their associated sarcomas).
  - Clusters of cuboidal epithelial cells (e.g. carcinomas, adenomas, papillomas).
- Differentiation between benign and malignant neoplasia is usually based on cellular differentiation/anaplasia, rate of growth, local invasion, and metastases.
  - Benign neoplasms are usually well-differentiated with a slow rate of growth.
  - Malignant neoplasms usually show variable cellular differentiation, greater mitotic activity, local invasion, and more rapid growth. Metastases are rare, but if seen, are generally in the kidney and spleen.
- A tentative diagnosis can often be made based on cytology and histology by a pathologist with fish experience. For more definitive classification, IHC for specific piscine cell markers or TEM for ultrastructure studies is

often needed. Antibodies validated as cell markers in mammals should be used with caution as they have not been validated in fish.
- If histology or TEM is suggestive of a viral cause, proving a viral etiology requires viral isolation, sequencing, and transmission trials.
- Results can be reported to Stanford University's Exotic Species Cancer Research Alliance to help advance our understanding of fish neoplasia.

Husbandry Management

- If a viral etiology is possible, consider isolation of affected animal(s) or temperature modification if the viruses tend to be temperature-sensitive (e.g. *Herpesviridae*).

Medical Management

- Treatment may be indicated to improve prognosis, reduce mass effects, or for cosmetic reasons.
- Common treatments (see Chapters A12 and A13 for more details):
  - Surgical debulking or surgical removal is common. They often provide at least temporary remission, even with neoplasms where surgical treatment would not be indicated in mammals. Excision can be curative, but suitable surgical margins can be impractical and recurrence is common.
  - Analgesia and supportive care should be provided.
  - Euthanasia may be indicated if quality of life is poor and cannot be improved.
- Other reported treatments (see Chapters A12 and A13 for more details):
  - Cryosurgery or cryotherapy may be used. Cryosurgery for cutaneous neoplasms in goldfish produced more scarring but less hemorrhage and a lower recurrence rate compared to surgical excision. For cryotherapy, liquid nitrogen shows more reliable results than over-the-counter products that rely on dimethyl ether.
  - Chemotherapy has been described in a few case reports (e.g. local infiltration of carboplatin, cisplatin, 5-flurouracil, cyclophosphamide, mitomycin C, bleomycin). Suitable PPE is required. Treatment plans must include how to dispose of water that may be contaminated with the chemotherapeutic drugs. Electrochemotherapy has not been reported in fish.
  - Radiation therapy may be used but reports are rare. In mammals, this is most effective against hematopoietic and epithelial neoplasms.
- All legislation regarding medication use and disposal must be followed.
- There is little information available on prognosis for most fish neoplasms, and prognosis should not be extrapolated from similar neoplasms in other vertebrates.
  - Some are more typically locally invasive (e.g. some squamous cell carcinomas, walleye dermal sarcomas, melanomas in platies and swordtails, and gonadal neoplasms in goldfish and koi).
  - A few are more typically metastatic (e.g. melanomas in butterflyfish (*Chaetodon* spp.) and nurse sharks (*Ginglymostoma cirratum*), hemangiomas and hemangiosarcomas, some carcinomas, some nephroblastomas, and some lymphosarcomas).

Prevention

- Stressors should be minimized, particularly exposure to toxins and inappropriate lighting.

Bibliography

Coffee, L.L., Casey, J.W., and Bower, P.R. (2013). Pathology of tumors in fish associated with retroviruses: a review. *Veterinary Pathology Online* 50: 390–403.

Grim, K.C., Wolfe, M.J., Edwards, M. et al. (2009). Epizootic ameloblastomas in chinook salmon (*Oncorhynchus tshawytscha*) of the Northwestern United States. *Veterinary Pathology* 46: 622–635.

Hochwartner, O., Loupal, G., Wildgoose, W.H., and Schmidt-Posthaus, H. (2010). Occurrence of spontaneous tumours of the renal proximal tubules in oscars *Astronotus ocellatus*. *Diseases of Aquatic Organisms* 89: 185–189.

Johnson, D.H. and Lane, S.L. (2007). Cryosurgery versus excision for removal of peripheral nerve sheath tumors in goldfish. *Exotic DVM* 9: 14–16.

Knüsel, F.O., Doherr, M.G., Knüsel, R. et al. (2015). Risk factors for development of internal neoplasms in koi carp *Cyprinus carpio koi*. *Diseases of Aquatic Organisms* 114: 199–207.

Knüsel, F.O., Knüsel, R., Doherr, M.G., and Schmidt-Posthaus, H. (2016). Frequency and histologic characterization of coelomatic neoplasms in koi *Cyprinus caprio koi*. *Diseases of Aquatic Organisms* 119: 219–229.

Pinkney, A.E., Harshbarger, J.C., and Rutter, M.A. (2009). Tumors in brown bullheads in the Chesapeake Bay watershed: analysis of survey data from 1992 through 2006. *Journal of Aquatic Animal Health* 21: 71–81.

Scala, C., Lair, S., and Marvin, J. (2016). Clusters of retinal neoplasms in aquarium-housed Atlantic striped bass (*Morone saxatilis*) and pajama cardinalfish (*Sphaeramia nematoptera*). Presented at the

International Aquatic Animal Medicine Conference, Virginia Beach, VA.

Sokkar, S.M., Mahmoud, A.M., and Mahrous, K.F. (2001). Histopathological and ultrastructural studies on melanomas in xiphophorus fish. *Bulletin of the European Association of Fish Pathologists* 21: 56–62.

Vergneau-Grosset, C., Summa, N., Rodriguez, C.O. et al. (2016). Excision and subsequent treatment of a leiomyoma from the periventiduct of a koi (*Cyprinus carpio koi*). *Journal of Exotic Pet Medicine* 25: 194–202.

Vergneau-Grosset, C., Nadeau, M.-E., and Groff, J.M. (2017). Fish oncology: diseases, diagnostics, and therapeutics. *Veterinary Clinics of North America: Exotic Animals* 20: 21–56.

Abbreviations/Acronyms

- CT: Computed tomography
- IHC: Immunohistochemistry
- MRI: Magnetic resonance imaging
- PPE: Personal protective equipment
- TEM: Transmission electron microscopy
- UV: Ultraviolet

C3

Viral Diseases

Catherine A. Hadfield

Seattle Aquarium, Seattle, WA, USA

Introduction

Most of the common known viral pathogens of fish are from three families (*Herpesviridae*, *Rhabdoviridae*, and *Iridoviridae*). Novel viral diseases are being identified frequently due to improved diagnostic techniques. This chapter starts with a general overview of viral diseases of fish. Subsequent sections cover herpesviruses, rhabdoviruses, birnaviruses, pox viruses, lymphocystiviruses, ranaviruses, megalocytiviruses, orthomyxoviruses, and betanodaviruses. Where available, information is provided on etiologic agent, life cycle and transmission, signalment, risk factors, clinical signs, diagnosis, husbandry and medical management, and prevention.

Viral Diseases (General)

Overview

- Reports of viral diseases in fish are increasingly common as diagnostic techniques improve.
- Most research has focused on viruses that have economic impacts on important food fish.
- Most viruses reported as fish pathogens are from three families: *Herpesviridae*, *Rhabdoviridae*, and *Iridoviridae*.
- Some viral diseases are reportable to regional and national groups. As of 2020, the following fish viral diseases are reportable to the OIE: koi herpes virus, viral hemorrhagic septicemia, infectious hematopoietic necrosis, spring viremia of carp, epizootic hematopoietic necrosis, red seabream iridovirus, infectious salmon anemia, and salmonid alphavirus. In the United States, this reporting is done through the USDA.
- It can be challenging to definitively diagnose a novel viral disease. A combination of clinical signs with consistent lesions and associated viral agents needs to be shown to identify a possible pathogen. Merely identifying a virus in tissue is insufficient to diagnose a pathogen; similarly, lack of identification does not rule out a viral etiology.
- The risk of introducing novel viruses into a collection can be reduced using appropriate isolation and quarantine.

Etiology

- The following viruses are well-described in fish and detailed information is provided in this section:
  - Cyprinid and ictalurid herpesviruses.
  - Rhabdoviruses.
  - Birnaviruses.
  - Pox viruses.
  - Lymphocystiviruses.
  - Ranaviruses.
  - Iridoviruses.
  - Megalocytivirus.
  - Orthomyxoviruses.
  - Betanodaviruses.
- It is not possible to cover all the viruses reported as pathogenic in fish. Examples of viruses that are less frequently reported include:
  - Adenoviruses (e.g. smooth-hound dogfish dermatitis).
  - Nidoviruses (e.g. fathead minnow nidovirus).
  - Picornaviruses or picorna-like viruses (e.g. bluegill picornavirus).
  - Reoviruses (e.g. grass carp hemorrhage virus, piscine orthoreovirus).
  - Togaviruses (e.g. salmonid alphavirus causing sleeping disease and pancreas disease).
  - Totiviruses (e.g. piscine myocarditis virus).

Clinical Guide to Fish Medicine, First Edition. Edited by Catherine A. Hadfield and Leigh Ann Clayton.

Transmission

- Horizontal transmission is seen with all fish viral diseases.
- Vertical transmission is an important route in some (e.g. IPNV).
- Viruses can be carried by fomites such as containers and nets, particularly non-enveloped viruses.
- Mechanical and biological vectors, particularly aquatic invertebrates and piscivorous birds, can transmit viruses. Mechanical vectors physically transfer pathogens unchanged, while biological vectors can support viral replication or development. Vectors are not susceptible to disease.
- Carriers are an important consideration for many viruses. These are susceptible but asymptomatic animals that shed the virus continuously or intermittently. Survivors of clinical disease may become lifelong carriers (e.g. IPNV and CCV).
- Latency is an important feature of some viruses (e.g. herpesviruses). These are susceptible but asymptomatic animals where the virus is "dormant" within cells and there is no shedding. However, viral replication may restart, often in response to stressors, causing shedding and clinical disease.
- Transmission to and from wild and cultured fish is likely with all viruses; this is often known as spill-over and spill-back.
- Increased global movement of humans and other animals has been important in the spread of several viral diseases (e.g. viral hemorrhagic septicemia through ship ballast water).

Signalment

- All fish species should be considered susceptible to viral diseases.
- Host ranges tend to be narrow, but are wider with experimental infections.
- Younger fish are often more likely to show clinical signs.

Risk Factors

- Exposure and stressors are the most important risk factors.
- General risk factors are described here; specific examples are provided for each viral group.
- Exposure:
  - Poor biosecurity (e.g. lack of suitable quarantine, use of surface water, exposure to wild fish).
  - Permissive water temperature.
  - Permissive salinity.
  - High organic loads.
  - Low water flow-rate or turnover.
  - Exposure of naïve fish.
  - Trauma to the mucus, skin, or gills.
- Stressors:
  - High stocking density.
  - Inappropriate social structure.
  - Inappropriate environment.
  - Aggression or displacement.
  - Poor water quality, particularly low dissolved oxygen and high ammonia.
  - Contaminants.
  - Inappropriate water temperature or changes in water temperature.
  - Poor nutrition.
  - Recent handling.
  - Recent transport.
  - Recent spawning.
  - Other diseases.
  - Immune-suppressive therapy (e.g. copper sulfate immersion).

Signs/Clinical Findings

- Clinical signs are nonspecific in most cases.
- Systemic infections may present with reduced appetite, lethargy, erratic swimming, erythema, ulcers, congestion, dyspnea, tachypnea, or coelomic distension.
- Prognosis depends on the virus, fish species, and underlying stressors.
- Secondary infections are common (e.g. bacterial or parasitic).

Differential Diagnoses

- The clinical signs associated with a systemic viral infection are hard to distinguish from other causes of systemic inflammation (e.g. bacterial, fungal, toxic, parasitic).
- Full differentials are described in Section B; common differentials are highlighted for each viral group.

Diagnosis

- Viral testing is similar to other vertebrate classes (see Chapter A7).
- Necropsy, coeliotomy, and histology lesions are often nonspecific. Systemic infections often present with organomegaly and necrosis. Inclusion bodies may be seen.
- Virus isolation on cell lines is often the gold standard, but is challenging for some viruses (e.g. carp edema virus).
- Molecular tests such as PCR, qPCR, and sequencing are becoming more available for common viral pathogens in fish (Box A6.9).
- IHC or ISH and antibody tests such as FA or ELISA may be available.
- EM can be used to identify viral particles.

- The OIE provides diagnostic recommendations for all reportable diseases. In the United States, the USDA can be contacted to determine sampling recommendations based on the OIE, usually through the state veterinary authority.

Husbandry Management
- Husbandry management typically relies on reducing or resolving stressors and reducing exposure. In a few rare cases, such as some notifiable diseases, management relies on depopulation and disinfection, as directed by the regulatory agency.
- Increase aeration; target dissolved oxygen may be 95–100%.
- Consider isolating affected fish in some cases (e.g. koi herpes virus).
- Consider changing the water temperature to within the preferred range for fish and outside of the preferred range for the virus.
- Increase water flow-rate or turnover.
- Increase cleaning and disinfection of water. Most viruses are sensitive to UV disinfection at ~10–30 mJ/cm^2 or mWs/cm^2. A few viruses are more resistant and require doses of ~100–250 mJ/cm^2, particularly viruses with large double-stranded genomes (e.g. IPNV and adenoviruses). Most viruses are sensitive to ozone disinfection, although results vary across studies. Dose depends on the pathogen and organic load, but common doses for fish are often TRO 0.1–0.2 mg/L for several minutes contact time with a system ORP of 300–350 mV. Higher doses have greater disinfection power but increase risk of damage to fish, particularly with continuous use. UV and ozone disinfection are synergistic and lower applied doses can be used when combined. UV and ozone are most effective after mechanical and biological filtration.
- Increase cleaning and disinfection of fomites. Viruses vary in their sensitivity to disinfectants such as sodium hypochlorite and other chlorine-based disinfectants, alcohols, iodophors, peroxygen compounds (e.g. Virkon® Aquatic), chlorhexidine gluconate, phenols (e.g. Lysol®), and quaternary ammonium compounds (e.g. benzalkonium chloride) (see Appendix 2). Viruses with envelopes are usually susceptible to disinfectants at routine doses; non-enveloped viruses are more resistant (e.g. adenoviruses, betanodaviruses, birnaviruses, picornaviruses, reoviruses). Fomite disinfection is most effective after mechanical cleaning and when followed by drying, particularly in sunlight. High pH may be used for disinfection between groups of fish in commercial pond systems (e.g. draining, cleaning, then liming with calcium oxide to a pH of >12). Heating to >60°C (140°F) for >15 minutes may also be effective.

Medical Management
- For reportable diseases, management recommendations provided by the regulatory agency (e.g. USDA) must be followed.
- Common treatments (see Chapters A12 and A13 for more details):
  - Supportive care may be indicated (e.g. fluid therapy, nutritional support).
  - Management of other infectious diseases is often important.
- Other reported treatments (see Chapters A12 and A13 for more details):
  - Antiviral use is rarely reported in fish.
  - Vaccines are sometimes administered during an outbreak, but are most effective when given prior to exposure or morbidity.
- All legislation regarding medication use and disposal must be followed.

Prevention
- Good biosecurity can reduce the risk of exposure to novel viruses; unlike bacteria, viral pathogens of fish are less likely to be ubiquitous.
- The general preventative measures below relate to all viruses. Specific examples are provided for each viral group.
- Reduce or resolve stressors, particularly when disease is likely (e.g. after transport or at permissive water temperatures).
  - Low stocking density.
  - Suitable social groups and habitats.
  - Excellent water quality and preferred temperature.
  - Good nutrition.
  - Suitable handling and transport protocols, including avoiding routine handling and transport during permissive temperatures.
  - No other disease issues.
- Reduce exposure and transmission through good biosecurity.
  - Isolation with no contact with free-ranging animals, particularly fish and aquatic invertebrates.
  - Pathogen-free water source (e.g. municipal water or ground water that has gone through fine filtration then UV and/or ozone disinfection). Avoid using untreated surface water.
  - Disinfection of recirculating water with fine filtration then UV and/or ozone.
  - High water flow rate or turnover.
  - Removal of dead or moribund fish as soon as possible with appropriate disposition.

- Good cleaning and disinfection protocols.
- Limits on visitors and potential fomites.
- All-in-all-out management of cultured populations, with separation of age classes.
- Specific pathogen-free (SPF) fish, where available.
- Suitable quarantine with isolation, monitoring, and diagnostic testing. This should apply to new animals as well as animals returning from shows or loans.
- Disinfection of fish eggs.
- Avoid using disease survivors as broodstock.
- Frozen-thawed or commercial feeds, with no live feeds.
- Routine monitoring of diseases of concern.
- Disinfection of discharge water to reduce the risk of spill-back to wild populations.

- Reduce severity of disease.
  - Vaccination for some viruses (e.g. infectious salmon anemia).
  - Selective breeding of more resistant fish strains.
  - A healthy and diverse microbiome should reduce the probability of colonization by virulent strains; this might be most easily achieved with native species, local water, natural substrates, and suitable and stable environmental conditions.
- Regularly review morbidity and mortality trends.

Zoonotic Reports
- Fish viruses have no known zoonotic potential.

Bibliography

Crane, M. and Hyatt, A. (2011). Viruses of fish: an overview of significant pathogens. *Viruses* 3: 2025–2046.

Kibenge, F.S.B. and Godoy, M.G. (2016). Aquaculture Virology, 568. Academic Press.

OIE (2017). *Manual of Diagnostic Tests for Aquatic Animals* [online]. http://www.oie.int/international-standard-setting/aquatic-manual/access-online/ (accessed 29 July 2017).

Woo, P.T.K. and Cipriano, R.C. (2017). Fish Viruses and Bacteria: Pathobiology and Protection, 370. CABI.

Abbreviations/Acronyms
- CCV: Channel catfish virus
- ELISA: Enzyme linked immunosorbent assay
- EM: Electron microscopy
- FA: Fluorescent antibody
- IHC: Immunohistochemistry
- IPNV: Infectious pancreatic necrosis virus
- ISH: In situ hybridization
- OIE: World Organisation for Animal Health
- ORP: Oxidation–reduction potential
- PCR: Polymerase chain reaction
- qPCR: Quantitative polymerase chain reaction
- USDA: United States Department of Agriculture
- UV: Ultraviolet

Cyprinid Herpesviruses

Overview
- There are three herpesviruses reported from cyprinids.
- Cyprinid herpesvirus-1 (CyHV-1) causes skin plaques known as carp pox in common carp (*Cyprinus carpio*), subspecies such as koi, and goldfish (*Carassius auratus*); these are primarily a cosmetic concern but can cause mortalities in young fish and affect the value of koi.
- Cyprinid herpesvirus-2 (CyHV-2) causes necrosis of hematopoietic tissues with high mortalities in goldfish and other *Carassius* spp.
- Cyprinid herpesvirus-3 (CyHV-3), also known as koi herpes virus (KHV), causes necrosis of gills and hematopoietic tissues with high mortalities in common carp and koi. Goldfish and grass carp (*Ctenopharyngodon idella*) can be asymptomatic carriers.
- As with other herpesviruses, latency is seen.

Etiology
- Family *Alloherpesviridae*.
- All fish herpesviruses are within *Alloherpesviridae*. This group differs taxonomically from herpesviruses of mammals, birds, and reptiles (*Herpesviridae*), and mollusks (*Metacoherpesviridae*).
- Cyprinid herpesviruses are in a taxonomic clade with anguillid herpesviruses.
- CyHV-1 causes carp pox (although this is not a poxvirus).
- CyHV-2 is also known as herpesviral hematopoietic necrosis virus (HVHNV), as well as goldfish hematopoietic necrosis virus.
- CyHV-3 or KHV was previously known as carp interstitial nephritis and gill necrosis virus. Several genotypes exist.

- These are enveloped, double-stranded DNA viruses with icosahedral capsids.

Transmission
- Horizontal transmission is seen and vertical transmission seems likely.
- All three cyprinid herpesviruses are highly contagious through direct contact or water, particularly if the skin or mucus is damaged.
- Survival of the viruses in water varies from hours to weeks.
- Mechanical vectors may include benthic invertebrates and piscivorous birds.
- Carriers for KHV include goldfish and grass carp. Mixing these species with koi can lead to disease in the koi.
- Latency is common with herpesviruses. Stressors can cause latently infected animals to show overt disease and shed the virus, putting naïve animals in the same systems at risk.
- The international trade of pet fish has contributed to the spread of KHV.

Geographic Distribution
- Carp pox is found worldwide.
- HVHNV was first found in Japan in the 1990s and is now probably worldwide.
- KHV was first found in Israel and the United Kingdom in the 1990s and is now probably worldwide.

Signalment
- Host ranges are narrow.
- Carp pox: Common carp and subspecies including koi, and goldfish, often >1 year old.
- HVHNV: Goldfish, Crucian carp (*Carassius carassius*), and Prussian carp (*Carassius gibelio*), usually <1 year old.
- KHV: Common carp and subspecies including koi and ghost carp (*C. carpio goi*). All ages are susceptible, but particularly young fish <1 year old.

Risk Factors
- General risk factors are described under C3: *Viral Diseases (General)*.
- Permissive water temperatures are often high for HVHNV and KHV (e.g. 15–28°C or 59–82°F).
- Recent introduction of new carp, koi, or goldfish is a common risk factor.

Signs/Clinical Findings
- Carp pox:
  - Usually a few carp, koi, or goldfish in the group are affected.
  - Translucent, tan or white plaques on the head, body, and fins are typical (Figure C3.1). Lesions look like melted candle wax.
  - Lesions regress over time, particularly during the summer in outdoor ponds. There is usually little to no scarring. If the lesions take longer to heal, scarring may occur.
  - It is rare but possible to see systemic signs in young fish including inappetence, erratic swimming, erythema, or mortalities.
- HVHNV:
  - Several goldfish are affected, particularly younger fish.
  - Lethargy is common.
  - Inappetence or reduced appetite is common.
  - Tachypnea and dyspnea are common.
  - Gill pallor is common. Gill necrosis may be seen in some cases.
  - Erythema or ulcerative dermatitis may be seen.
  - Exophthalmos or enophthalmos may be seen.
  - Coelomic distension due to effusion may be seen.
  - Secondary diseases may be seen (e.g. *Flavobacterium columnare*).
  - Peracute, acute, or chronic mortalities may be seen. Mortality can reach 100%.
- KHV
  - Several carp or koi are affected.
  - Tachypnea and dyspnea are common.
  - Gill necrosis is a consistent sign, with multifocal white to brown discoloration (Figure C3.2).
  - Lethargy, erratic swimming, head-down swimming, or other neurologic signs may be seen.
  - Inappetence or reduced appetite may be seen.
  - Enophthalmos may be seen.
  - Profound erythema, congestion, or ulceration on the skin and fins and increased mucus may be seen.

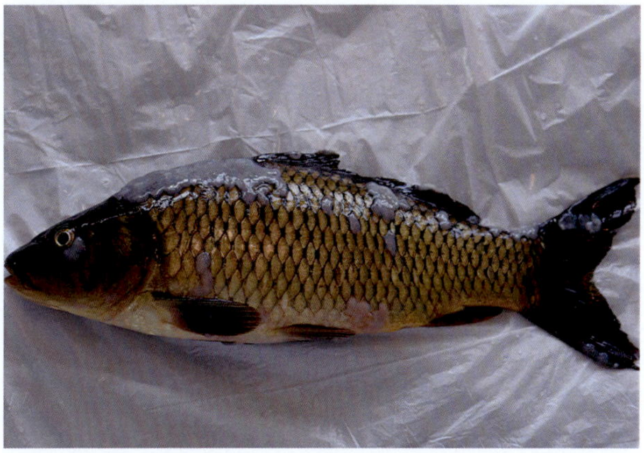

Figure C3.1 Carp pox (Cyprinid herpesvirus-1) lesions on the skin and fins of a koi (*Cyprinus carpio koi*). *Source*: Image courtesy of Eva Lewisch, University of Veterinary Medicine, Vienna.

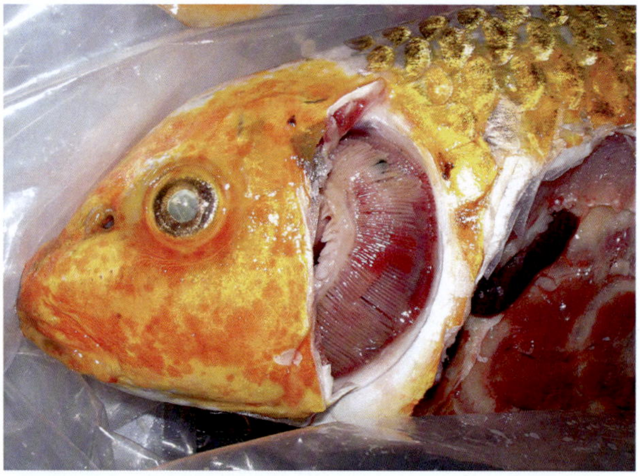

Figure C3.2 Koi herpes virus (cyprinid herpesvirus-3) gill lesions in koi (*Cyprinus carpio koi*). *Source*: Image courtesy of Lance Adams, Aquarium of the Pacific.

  - Secondary diseases may be seen.
  - Acute mortalities are seen one to three weeks post-infection. Mortality is often 70–100%.

Differential Diagnoses
- Full differentials are described in Section B.
- Common differentials for white to tan plaques on the skin of koi or carp include carp pox, lymphocystivirus, epitheliocystis, and neoplasia.
- Common differentials for erythema, skin ulcers, and gill changes in koi or carp include KHV, spring viremia of carp, carp edema virus, viral hemorrhagic septicemia, motile aeromonad septicemia, and *Flavobacterium columnare*.

Diagnosis
- Signalment, necropsy, and histology are suggestive, but PCR is the gold standard for identification.
- Commercial PCR tests are available for carp pox (skin swabs) and KHV (gill swabs, spleen, or kidney). Experimental PCR tests are available for HVHNV on spleen and caudal kidney. Sensitivity is high in clinically affected fish. For carriers, qPCR or nested PCR is usually needed to increase sensitivity.
- For KHV, ELISA and SN tests on blood samples may be available commercially to look for evidence of prior exposure. The ELISA test can detect antibodies for months to a year but may not reliably detect asymptomatic carriers.
- Rapid tests that can detect asymptomatic carriers are being assessed (e.g. recombinase polymerase amplification and loop mediated isothermal amplification).
- Necropsy, coeliotomy, and histology can support the diagnosis.
  - Carp pox: Epithelial hyperplasia.
  - HVHNV: Visceral pallor, renomegaly, splenomegaly, with white nodules, necrosis, or congestion in the cranial kidney and spleen, with or without skin and gill necrosis and hyperplasia.
  - KHV: Gill necrosis and hyperplasia with visceral pallor, edema, and widespread petechiae, ecchymoses, and congestion, with or without skin necrosis. Renomegaly and splenomegaly may be seen in young fish.
  - Intranuclear inclusion bodies may be seen in affected tissues with all three viruses.
- Virus isolation is challenging but some success has been reported using tissue samples (e.g. caudal kidney or spleen) on cell lines such as Koi Fin.
- The OIE Manual of Diagnostic Tests for Aquatic Animals provides specific guidance on the diagnosis of KHV.
- KHV is reportable to some state and national groups and the OIE.

Husbandry Management
- General husbandry management is described under C3: *Viral Diseases (General)*.
- For carp pox, consider slowly increasing water temperature by 5°C (10°F) or to >25°C (77°F).
- For HVHNV and KHV, isolate affected fish, increase dissolved oxygen, and slowly decrease water temperature by ~5°C (10°F) or to <15°C (59°F), if possible. Depopulation and disinfection may be considered but is not typically implemented as the diseases are widespread and carriers make it extremely challenging to ensure new animals are negative.

Medical Management
- Possible treatments (see Chapters A12 and A13 for more details):
  - Low-dose hypersalinity may be used for HVHNV and KHV to reduce osmotic stress (e.g. 1–3 g/L).
  - Other supportive care may be helpful.
  - Treatment of secondary infections may be needed.
  - Antivirals may provide benefits.
- All legislation regarding medication use and disposal must be followed.

Prevention
- General preventative measures are described under C3: *Viral Diseases (General)*.
- Specific examples for KHV include:
  - Avoid keeping goldfish, koi, or other carp in the same system.
  - Consider purchasing carp or koi that are seronegative for KHV with no history of clinical signs when housed at permissive water temperatures.

- ○ Suitable isolated quarantine at a permissive water temperature (e.g. 22°C (72°F); a prolonged quarantine duration may help (e.g. 60–90 days).
- ○ Avoid handling or transport of carp or koi when water temperature is 15–28°C (59–82°F).
- ○ Test for KHV by PCR in carp or koi showing morbidity or mortality.
- ○ Do not mix survivors with susceptible fish or use as broodstock.
- ○ At shows, house fish from different sources in independent water systems and quarantine fish on return.
- ○ A modified-live vaccine (Cavoy, Novartis Animal Health) was approved for KHV in the United States but it has since been removed from the market.
- ○ Exposing koi to KHV outside of the permissive temperature to help with immunity is often described, but can produce latent infections and should be avoided.

Zoonotic Reports

- These viruses have no known zoonotic potential.

Bibliography

Baumer, A., Fabian, M., Wilkens, M.R. et al. (2013). Epidemiology of cyprinid herpesvirus-3 infection in latently infected carp from aquaculture. *Diseases of Aquatic Organisms* 105: 101–108.

Coulthier, S.C., McClure, C., Schroeder, T. et al. (2017). Diagnostic validation of three test methods for detection of cyprinid herpesvirus 3 (CyHV-3). *Diseases of Aquatic Organisms* 123: 101–122.

El-Matbouli, M. and Soliman, H. (2011). Transmission of *Cyprinid herpesvirus*-3 (CyHV-3) from goldfish to naïve common carp by cohabitation. *Research in Veterinary Science* 90: 536–539.

Fichi, G., Susini, F., Cocumelli, C. et al. (2016). New detection of Cyprinid herpesvirus 2 in mass mortality event of *Carassius carassius* (L.) in Italy. *Journal of Fish Diseases* 39: 1523–1527.

Flamm, A., Fabian, M., Runge, M. et al. (2016). Draining and liming of ponds as an effective measure for containment of CyHV-3 in carp farms. *Diseases of Aquatic Organisms* 120: 255–260.

Giovannini, S., Bergmann, S.M., Keeling, C. et al. (2016). Herpesviral hematopoietic necrosis in goldfish in Switzerland: early lesions in clinically normal goldfish (*Carassius auratus*). *Veterinary Pathology* 53: 847–852.

Goodwin, A.E., Merry, G.E., and Sadler, J. (2006). Detection of the herpesviral hematopoietic necrosis disease agent (cyprinid herpesvirus 2) in moribund and healthy goldfish: validation of a quantitative PCR. *Diseases of Aquatic Organisms* 69: 137–143.

Ito, T., Kurita, J., and Haenen, O.L.M. (2017). Importation of CyHV-2 infected goldfish into the Netherlands. *Diseases of Aquatic Organisms* 126: 51–62.

Lu, J., Lu, H., and Cao, G. (2016). Hematological and histological changes in Prussian carp *Carassius gibelio* infected with cyprinid herpesvirus 2. *Journal of Aquatic Animal Health* 28: 150–160.

OIE (2017). *Manual of Diagnostic Tests for Aquatic Animals* [online]. http://www.oie.int/international-standard-setting/aquatic-manual/access-online/ (accessed 29 July 2017).

Prescott, M.A., Reed, A.N., Jin, L., and Pastey, M.K. (2016). Rapid detection of cyprinid herpesvirus 3 in latently infected koi by recombinase polymerase amplification. *Journal of Aquatic Animal Health* 28: 173–180.

Shimizu, T., Yoshida, N., Kasai, H., and Yoshimizu, M. (2006). Survival of koi herpes virus (KHV) in environmental water. *Fish Pathology* 41: 153–157.

Waltzek, T.B., Kelley, G.O., Alfaro, M.E. et al. (2009). Phylogenetic relationships in the family *Alloherpesviridae*. *Disease of Aquatic Organisms* 84: 179–194.

Weber, E.P.S., Malm, K.V., Yun, S.C. et al. (2014). Efficacy and safety of a modified-live cyprinid herpesvirus 3 vaccine in koi (*Cyprinus carpio koi*) for prevention of koi herpes virus disease. *American Journal of Veterinary Research* 75: 899–904.

Abbreviations/Acronyms

- ELISA: Enzyme linked immunosorbent assay
- HVHNV: Herpesviral hematopoietic necrosis virus
- KHV: Koi herpes virus
- OIE: World Organisation for Animal Health
- PCR: Polymerase chain reaction
- qPCR: Quantitative polymerase chain reaction
- SN: Serum neutralization

Ictalurid Herpesviruses

Overview

- There are two commonly reported ictalurid herpesviruses (IcHV-1 and 2).
- IcHV-1 is also known as channel catfish virus (CCV) and causes hemorrhagic septicemia in fry or fingerling channel catfish (*Ictalurus punctatus*) in aquaculture during warm weather.
- IcHV-2 causes similar disease in black bullhead catfish (*Ameiurus melas*) in aquaculture. It is not found in North America and its introduction is considered a high risk to catfish aquaculture.

Etiology

- Family *Alloherpesviridae*.
- Ictalurid herpesviruses are in a different clade from the cyprinid and anguillid herpesviruses. The ictalurid clade is grouped with acipenserid herpesviruses.
- These are enveloped, double-stranded DNA viruses.

Transmission

- Horizontal and vertical transmission are reported.
- The viruses do not survive long in the environment (e.g. two days at 25°C (77°F) and 28 days at 4°C (39°F) in pond water). They survive for longer in dechlorinated tap water.
- Fish that resolve clinical signs probably become lifelong carriers.
- Latency is common with herpesviruses. Stressors can cause latently infected animals to show overt disease and shed the virus, putting naïve animals in the same systems at risk.

Geographic Distribution

- IcHV-1 is found where channel catfish aquaculture is common, including Alabama, Arkansas, Mississippi, Louisiana, and California. It is also reported from Central America and Russia.
- IcHV-2 was first found in Italy in the 1990s. As of 2019, it has not been reported in North America.

Signalment

- IcHV-1 natural infection is only found in channel catfish, blue catfish (*Ictalurus furcatus*), and their hybrids; disease is most severe in channel catfish. Fry and fingerlings are susceptible; disease is rare if >6 mo old or >10 g in weight.
- IcHV-2 natural infection is only found in black bullhead catfish.
- Experimental infection with high mortalities is possible in other catfish species.

Risk Factors

- General risk factors are described under C3: *Viral Diseases (General).*
- Permissive water temperature is often high for IcHV-1 (e.g. with highest losses at 25–28°C or 77–82°F); IcHV-2 shows wider temperature tolerances.
- Recent introduction of new catfish is a common risk factor.

Signs/Clinical Findings

- Both ictalurid herpesviruses cause similar signs.
- Multiple conspecifics are usually affected.
- Inappetence or reduced feeding is typically the first sign.
- Fish may swim near the surface or show abnormal swimming with a head-up position or erratic spirals. There may be periods of excitability followed by lethargy.
- Coelomic distension due to effusion or organomegaly is common.
- Gill petechiae or pallor may be seen.
- Exophthalmos may be seen.
- Erythema or petechial hemorrhages may be seen, particularly at the base of the fins and along the ventrum.
- Morbidity and mortality are typically low but can reach 100% in populations under other stressors.
- Recurrence is common.

Differential Diagnoses

- Full differentials are described in Section B.
- Common differentials for systemic inflammation in channel catfish include CCV, *Edwardsiella ictaluri*, motile aeromonad septicemia, and *Yersinia ruckeri*.

Diagnosis

- A tentative diagnosis is typically based on signalment, time of year, and clinical signs. Confirmation is by virus isolation and identification of characteristic cytopathic effect. The best samples are kidney tissue from freshly dead fish with clinical signs.
- Necropsy or coeliotomy usually show visceral pallor, serosanguinous coelomic effusion, organomegaly, and petechial hemorrhages, particularly in the kidneys.
- Histology typically shows multifocal necrosis and may show intranuclear inclusions.
- SN, FA, ELISA, and PCR tests may be available.

Husbandry Management

- General husbandry management is described under C3: *Viral Diseases (General).*
- Consider isolating affected fish to reduce transmission.
- Slowly reduce water temperature by ~5°C (10°F) or to below 19°C (66°F) to reduce mortality, if possible.

- Depopulation may be considered but these viruses are widespread.

Medical Management

- No antiviral treatments are reported, but supportive care may be helpful.
- Control of concurrent infections is important (e.g. antibiotics for *E. ictaluri* or *Flavobacterium columnare*)
- All legislation regarding medication use and disposal must be followed.

Prevention

- General preventative measures are described under C3: *Viral Diseases (General)*.
- Specific examples include:
  - Avoid handling or transport of channel catfish when water temperature is >20°C (68°F).
  - Bullhead catfish (*Ameiurus* spp.), European catfish (*Silurus glanis*), and African and Asian catfish (*Clarius* spp.) may be considered for culture in IcHV-1-endemic areas.
  - Vaccine experiments have been largely ineffective.

Zoonotic Reports

- These viruses have no known zoonotic potential.

Bibliography

Boon, J.H., McDowell, T., and Hedrick, R.P. (1988). Resistance of the African (*Clarias gariepinus*) and the Asian catfish (*Clarias batrachus*) to channel catfish virus. *Aquaculture* 74: 191–194.

Borzák, R., Haluk, T., Bartha, D., and Doszpoli, A. (2018). Compete genome sequence and analysis of ictalurid herpesvirus 2. *Archives of Virology* 163: 1083–1085.

Silverstein, P.S., Bosworth, B.G., and Gaunt, P.S. (2007). Differential susceptibility of blue catfish, *Ictalurus furcatus* (Valenciennes), channel catfish, *I. punctatus* (Rafinesque), and blue x channel catfish hybrids to channel catfish virus. *Journal of Fish Diseases* 31: 77–79.

Waltzek, T.B., Kelley, G.O., Alfaro, M.E. et al. (2009). Phylogenetic relationships in the family *Alloherpesviridae*. *Disease of Aquatic Organisms* 84: 179–194.

Abbreviations/Acronyms

- CCV: Channel catfish virus
- ELISA: Enzyme linked immunosorbent assay
- FA: Fluorescent antibody
- PCR: Polymerase chain reaction
- SN: Serum neutralization
- UV: Ultraviolet

Rhabdoviruses

Overview

- Several rhabdoviruses are important pathogens of fish, particularly in commercial aquaculture.
- Viral hemorrhagic septicemia viruses (VHSV) and infectious hematopoietic necrosis viruses (IHNV) cause hemorrhagic septicemia in salmonids and other teleosts. They have been responsible for epizootics in wild and cultured fish.
- Spring viremia of carp virus (SVCV) causes hemorrhagic septicemia in cyprinids and is a serious disease of cultured cyprinids including koi.

Etiology

- Family *Rhabdoviridae*.
- Genus *Novirhabdovirus* and *Sprivivirus*.
- There are three important fish rhabdoviruses:
  - VHSV, also known as egtved disease viruses, with four genotypes based on N and G genes (I to IV), subdivided by geography.
  - IHNV, with various genotypes and serotypes. IHNV should not be confused with the similarly named epizootic hematopoietic necrosis virus (EHNV), which is a ranavirus.
  - SVCV, also known as rubella, infectious dropsy, swim bladder inflammation, or *Rhabdovirus carpio* virus.
- These are enveloped RNA viruses with the classic bullet shape.

Transmission

- These viruses are highly contagious.
- Horizontal transmission is common.
- Vertical transmission is possible but appears to be rare.

- The viruses typically persist for days to weeks in water or sediment but can persist for months, particularly in freshwater habitats. They survive freezing.
- Fomites have been implicated in disease spread, including fishing gear and boats.
- Mechanical and biological vectors are probably common, including invertebrates, turtles, and birds.
- Fish that resolve clinical signs are often resistant to the disease, but some do become carriers.
- Other carriers are common (e.g. invasive round gobies (*Neogobius melanostomus*) in the Great Lakes region).

Geographic Distribution

- VHSV genotypes are found across the northern hemisphere, subdivided by geography:
  - VHSV-I predominantly includes the European freshwater isolates, particularly of cultured rainbow trout (*Oncorhynchus mykiss*).
  - VHSV-II consists of marine isolates from the Baltic Sea.
  - VHSV-III consists of marine isolates from the North Atlantic Ocean.
  - VHSV-IVa consists of North Pacific, Japanese, and Korean marine isolates.
  - VHSV-IVb consists of North American freshwater isolates endemic to the Great Lakes region and Saint Lawrence River and shows a particularly wide host range.
- IHNV is endemic in salmonids off the west coast of North America. Other reports include mainland Europe and Asia.
- SVCV is endemic to parts of Europe and Asia. The Americas were considered SVCV-free until 1998; it has since been reported in Brazil, United States, and Canada. It is likely found worldwide, particularly in temperate regions.

Signalment

- Host ranges are wide.
- VHSV can infect freshwater, brackish, and saltwater teleosts.
  - Rainbow trout are particularly susceptible, but all salmonids can show clinical signs.
  - Epizootics have been reported in round gobies, freshwater drum (*Aplodinotus grunniens*), muskellunge (*Esox masquinongy*), gizzard shad (*Dorosoma cepedianum*), yellow perch (*Perca flavescens*), haddock (*Melanogrammus aeglefinus*), turbot (*Scophthalmus maximus*), olive flounder (*Paralichthys olivaceus*), Pacific cod (*Gadus macrocephalus*), and wrasse commonly used as biological controls in salmon aquaculture (*Labrus* spp., *Centrolabrus exoletus*, *Symphodus melops*).
- IHNV typically infects cold freshwater and saltwater salmonids.
  - *Oncorhynchus* and *Salmo* spp. are particularly susceptible, especially rainbow trout.
  - Lake trout (*Salvelinus namaycush*), brook trout (*Salvelinus fontinalis*), arctic char (*Salvelinus alpinus*), and coho salmon (*Oncorhynchus kisutch*) are considered more resistant, although infections are possible.
  - Infection has occasionally been reported in non-salmonids.
- SVCV typically infects cyprinids.
  - Koi and common carp (*Cyprinus carpio*), goldfish (*Carassius auratus*), crucian carp (*Carassius carassius*), minnows (*Leuciscinae*), tench (*Tinca tinca*), and zebrafish (*Danio rerio*) are particularly susceptible.
  - The virus has been isolated from non-cyprinid species including sheatfish (*Silurus glanis*) and northern pike (*Esox lucius*).

Risk Factors

- General risk factors are described under C3: *Viral Diseases (General).*
- Permissive water temperature varies. VHSV shows highest mortalities at 3–12°C (37–54°F), with no clinical signs at >22°C (>72°F); IHNV typically causes disease at 8–15°C (46–59°F); SVCV typically causes disease at 11–18°C (52–65°F), with no clinical signs at >21°C (>70°F).
- Recent introduction of new salmonids or cyprinids is a common risk factor.

Signs/Clinical Findings

- VHSV, IHNV, and SVCV show similar, nonspecific clinical signs of systemic inflammation.
- Multiple conspecifics are usually affected
- Lethargy, loss of equilibrium, sporadic hyperexcitability, spiral swimming, or circling may be seen.
- Reduced food intake or inappetence is common.
- Petechiae, hyphema, and diffuse congestion are common. Skin darkening may be seen.
- Coelomic distension due to coelomic effusion or organomegaly is common.
- Cloacal or anal prolapse may be seen.
- Exophthalmos may be seen.
- Gill pallor and edema may be seen.
- Pale or mucoid fecal casts may be present.
- Secondary bacterial infections are common, particularly with SVCV.
- Mortality varies but can reach 100% in young fish, naïve populations, or under other stressors.

Differential Diagnoses

- Full differentials are provided in Section B.
- Common differentials for systemic inflammation in teleosts are broad and include a variety of viral, bacterial, fungal, parasitic, and toxic etiologies.

Diagnosis

- The signalment, necropsy, and histology can be suggestive but viral isolation and molecular tests are required for definitive identification.
- Necropsy, coeliotomy, and histology show hemorrhagic septicemia with hematopoietic necrosis.
  - Necropsy or coeliotomy usually show widespread hemorrhage and serosanguinous ascites, visceral pallor, renomegaly, splenomegaly, and enteritis (Figure C3.3). Petechiae and hemorrhages in the swim bladder in cyprinids are almost pathognomonic for SVCV.
  - Histology often shows multifocal necrosis, degeneration, and vasculitis. Intranuclear or intracytoplasmic inclusions may be seen. IHNV is commonly associated with pancreatic necrosis and inclusions.
- ELISA or PNT can be used to identify seropositive fish that have been exposed to the virus.
- TEM can show the classic bullet shape of the virus.
- The OIE Manual of Diagnostic Tests for Aquatic Animals provides specific guidance on the diagnosis of VHSV, IHNV, and SVCV. It recommends sampling fresh spleen, cranial kidney, heart, and brain for virus isolation and FA, ELISA, or RT-PCR. Rhabdoviruses are usually easy to isolate and culture. In the United States, the USDA can be contacted to determine sampling recommendations based on the OIE.
- VHSV, IHNV, and SVCV are reportable to the OIE.

Husbandry Management

- General husbandry management is described under C3: *Viral Diseases (General)*.
- Depopulation and disinfection programs exist for these viruses in many countries.
- In the United States, management recommendations provided by the USDA must be followed for VHSV, IHNV, and SVCV.

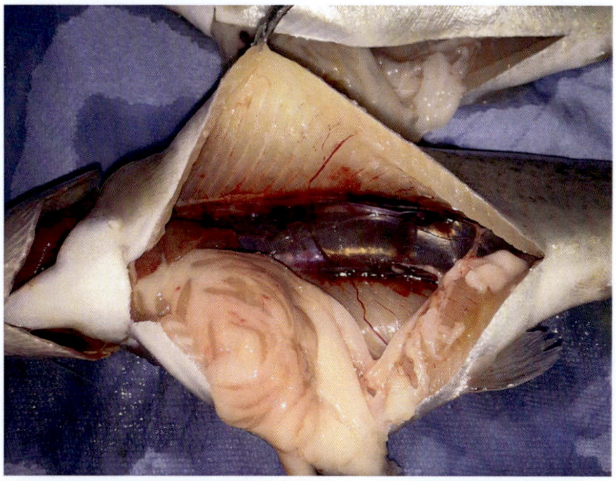

Figure C3.3 Typical necropsy findings of viral hemorrhagic septicemia in rainbow trout (*Oncorhynchus mykiss*). *Source*: Image courtesy of Pierre-Marie Boitard, Fili@vet.

Medical Management

- No antiviral treatments are reported.
- All legislation regarding medication use and disposal must be followed.

Prevention

- General preventative measures are described under C3: *Viral Diseases (General)*.
- Specific examples include:
  - Consider surveying female broodstock through ELISAs or VI on ovaries and disinfection of eggs using iodophors.
  - There are no commercial vaccines for fish rhabdoviruses in the United States. There are licensed vaccines in other countries.

Zoonotic Reports

- These viruses have no known zoonotic potential.

Bibliography

Emmenegger, E.J. and Kurath, G. (2008). DNA vaccine protects ornamental koi (*Cyprinus carpio*) against North American spring viremia of carp virus. *Vaccine* 26: 6415–6421.

Goodwin, A.E. and Merry, G.E. (2011). Replication and persistence of VHSV IVb in freshwater turtles. *Diseases of Aquatic Organisms* 94: 173–177.

Groocock, G.H., Getchell, R.G., Wooster, G.A. et al. (2007). Detection of viral hemorrhagic septicemia in round gobies in New York State (USA) waters of Lake Ontario and the St. Lawrence River. *Diseases of Aquatic Organisms* 76: 187–192.

OIE (2017). *Manual of Diagnostic Tests for Aquatic Animals* [online]. http://www.oie.int/international-standard-setting/aquatic-manual/access-online/ (accessed 29 July 2017).

Munro, E.S., McIntosh, R.E., Weir, S.J. et al. (2015). A mortality event in wrasse species (Labridae) associated with the presence of viral hemorrhagic septicaemia virus. *Journal of Fish Diseases* 38: 335–341.

Phelps, N.B.D., Goodwin, A.E., Marecaux, E., and Goyal, S.M. (2013). Comparison of treatments to inactivate viral hemorrhagic septicemia virus (VHSV-IVb) in frozen baitfish. *Diseases of Aquatic Organisms* 102: 211–216.

Abbreviations/Acronyms

- ELISA: Enzyme linked immunosorbent assay
- FA: Fluorescent antibody
- IHNV: Infectious hematopoietic necrosis virus
- OIE: World Organisation for Animal Health
- PNT: Plaque neutralization tests
- RT-PCR: Reverse transcriptase polymerase chain reaction
- SVCV: Spring viremia of carp virus
- TEM: Transmission electron microscopy
- USDA: United States Department of Agriculture
- VHSV: Viral hemorrhagic septicemia virus
- VI: Virus isolation

Birnaviruses

Overview

- The most commonly reported birnavirus in fish is infectious pancreatic necrosis virus (IPNV).
- It is an important pathogen of young salmonids in aquaculture, particularly rainbow trout (*Oncorhynchus mykiss*).
- It causes acute septicemic disease.
- Birnaviruses are particularly hardy and can be challenging to eliminate.

Etiology

- Family *Birnaviridae.*
- Genus *Aquabirnavirus.*
- IPNV has several serogroups and serotypes.
- Other examples of birnaviruses in fish include yellowtail ascites virus and many IPN-like viruses.
- These are non-enveloped RNA viruses.

Transmission

- These viruses are highly contagious.
- Horizontal and vertical transmissions are reported. Unlike most other viruses that may be carried on the egg surface, IPNV can be carried inside the egg.
- Birnaviruses are hardy and can survive days to weeks in surface water and months in frozen tissues.
- Mechanical and biological vectors may include mollusks, crustaceans, leeches, and piscivorous birds.
- Fish that resolve clinical signs probably become lifelong carriers.
- Other carriers include brook trout (*Salvelinus fontinalis*), striped bass (*Morone saxatilis*), and their hybrids.

Geographic Distribution

- Freshwater and saltwater habitats, probably worldwide.

Signalment

- IPNV is only pathogenic in salmonids, particularly young rainbow trout and brook trout. Fry and fingerlings in freshwater are typically affected, although fish can be affected within three months of transfer to salt water.
- IPNV has been found in wild fish such as brown trout (*Salmo trutta*).
- IPN-like viruses have been reported in a variety of teleosts.

Risk Factors

- General risk factors are described under C3: *Viral Diseases (General).*
- Permissive water temperature is often 10–14°C (50–57°F).
- High number of salmonid farms within a 10 km radius is a known risk factor.
- Identification of IPNV in the previous production cycle makes disease more likely.

Signs/Clinical Findings

- Multiple conspecifics are usually affected.
- Clinical course is typically acute.
- Erratic swimming is common (e.g. spiraling).
- Skin darkening or hemorrhages are common.
- Coelomic distension due to organomegaly or effusion is common.
- White fecal casts may be seen.
- Exophthalmos may be seen.
- Gill pallor due to anemia may be seen.
- Appetite is usually normal.
- Mortality varies depending on the presence of stressors but can reach 100%.

Differential Diagnoses

- Full differentials are provided in Section B.
- Common differentials for septicemic disease in salmonids include IPN, infectious hematopoietic necrosis virus, viral hemorrhagic septicemia, salmonid alphavirus, infectious salmon anemia, *Aeromonas salmonicida*, and *Yersinia ruckeri.*

Diagnosis

- Diagnosis is typically confirmed by virus isolation from the posterior kidney or pyloric ceca, characteristic cytopathic changes, and consistent clinical signs.
- Necropsy or coeliotomy may show tissue pallor and white or clear mucus in the stomach and intestines.
- Histology usually shows pancreatic necrosis and basophilic intracytoplasmic inclusions. McKnight cells (karyolitic and necrotic epithelial cells) may be present

in the pyloric ceca. Other findings may include necrosis of the anterior intestines and renal tubules.
- FA, CF, ELISA may be available.

Husbandry Management
- General husbandry management is described under C3: *Viral Diseases (General).*
- In the United States, some state regulations exist for IPNV and must be followed. Management typically includes depopulation and disinfection.
- Birnaviruses are hardy and disinfection can be challenging, e.g. IPNV is resistant to air drying and requires UV doses of 100–330 mJ/cm^2.

Medical Management
- No antiviral treatments are reported.
- All legislation regarding medication use and disposal must be followed.

Prevention
- General preventative measures are described under C3: *Viral Diseases (General).*
- Specific examples include:
  - Test for IPNV prior to acquisition of young salmonids.
  - Acquire salmonids at >6 mo of age.
  - Consider disinfection of eggs with iodophors to reduce transmission; this does not eliminate it, as IPNV can be carried inside eggs.

Zoonotic Reports
- These viruses have no known zoonotic potential.

Bibliography

Escobar-Dodero, J., Kinsley, A., Perez, A.M. et al. (2018). Risk factors for infectious pancreatic necrosis in farmed Chilean Atlantic salmon (*Salmo salar*) from 2010 to 2013. *Preventative Veterinary Medicine* 167: 182–189.

Liltved, H., Vogelsang, C., Modahl, I., and Dannevig, B.H. (2006). High resistance of fish pathogenic viruses to UV irradiation and ozonated seawater. *Aquacultural Engineering* 34: 72–82.

Roberts, R.J. and Pearson, M.D. (2005). Infectious pancreatic necrosis in Atlantic salmon, *Salmo salar*. *Journal of Fish Diseases* 28: 383–390.

Salimi, B. and Abdi, K. (2016). Detection of infectious pancreatic necrosis virus from the leeches *Hemiclepsis marginata* and *Hirudo medicinalis*. *Journal of Aquatic Animal Health* 28: 209–213.

Abbreviations/Acronyms
- CF: Complement fixation
- ELISA: Enzyme linked immunosorbent assay
- FA: Fluorescent antibody
- IPNV: Infectious pancreatic necrosis virus
- UV: Ultraviolet

Pox Viruses

Overview
- Pox viruses are rarely reported in fish.
- Carp edema virus (CEV) is an emerging pox virus that affects common carp (*Cyprinus carpio*) and subspecies such as koi (*C. carpio koi*).
- The disease has also been called koi sleepy disease due to the profound lethargy.

Etiology
- Family *Poxviridae.*
- CEV is an emerging pox virus in fish.
- Several genogroups exist.
- These are enveloped, double-stranded DNA viruses.

Transmission
- Horizontal transmission is reported.
- Fish that resolve clinical signs may become carriers; fish typically remain PCR-positive for up to five to six months.
- The international trade in koi likely contributed to spread of the disease.

Geographic Distribution
- CEV was first found in Japanese koi breeding facilities in the 1970s, with reports from Europe and United States starting in the late 1990s. It was identified in Brazil in 2015.
- The virus appears to be spreading worldwide.

Signalment
- CEV only infects common carp and subspecies such as koi.
- Epizootics have been seen in wild and cultured common carp.

Risk Factors

- General risk factors are described under C3: *Viral Diseases (General).*
- Outbreaks are more common at 15–25°C (59–77°F), but some strains in Europe show disease at lower water temperatures, e.g. 6–15°C (43–59°F).

Signs/Clinical Findings

- Multiple conspecifics are usually affected.
- Adult fish show severe lethargy, often laterally recumbent on the substrate with minimal response to stimulation (Figure C3.4a). Younger fish may congregate at the surface or sides of a pond.
- Inappetence or reduced feeding is common.
- Skin edema and generalized edema are common in young fish and may be seen in adults.
- Pale, edematous gills with white or gray areas of necrosis are common, similar to koi herpes virus (Figure C3.4b).
- Dyspnea and tachypnea are common.
- Ulcerative or hemorrhagic skin lesions, particularly around the mouth and the base of the fins, and increased mucus may be seen.
- Enophthalmos may be seen in adult fish, similar to koi herpes virus.
- Mortality varies but may reach 70–100%.
- Secondary infections are common.

Differential Diagnoses

- Full differentials are provided in Section B.
- Common differentials for systemic inflammation in carp include CEV, spring viremia of carp, koi herpes virus, viral hemorrhagic septicemia, motile aeromonad septicemia, and vibriosis.

Diagnosis

- Diagnosis is typically based on clinical signs, histology, and PCR.
- Gill wet mounts examined under direct microscopy will often show severe hyperplasia, edema, and increased mucus. There are no gross internal lesions.
- Histology usually shows branchitis with severe epithelial hyperplasia, necrosis, lamellar fusion, interstitial edema, and increased mucus. Large intracytoplasmic inclusions are common.
- PCR assays are best on gill tissue from animals early in the disease process. Nested PCR and qPCR tests are available experimentally and show higher sensitivity and specificity.
- TEM may show viral particles or mature virions.
- Virus isolation is not available as CEV has not yet been cultured.

Husbandry Management

- General husbandry management is described under C3: *Viral Diseases (General).*

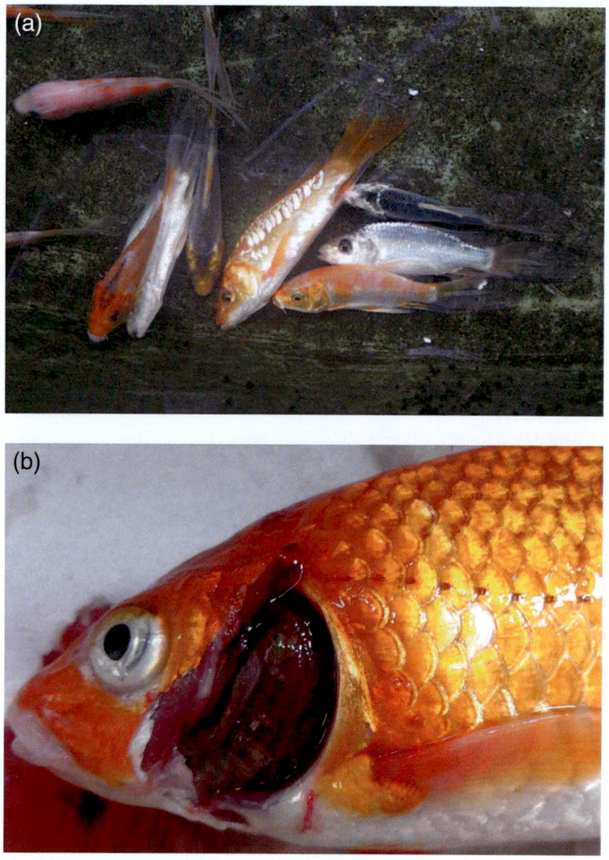

Figure C3.4 Koi (*Cyprinus carpio koi*) recumbent on the substrate due to carp edema virus infection (a) and image of focal necrosis on the gills of a koi with CEV (b). *Source*: Image (a) courtesy of Johnny Shelley, USDA-ARS Aquatic Animal Health Research Unit. Image (b) courtesy of Pierre-Marie Boitard, Fili@vet.

- Isolate affected animals to reduce transmission.
- Reduce or resolve stressors, in particular, maintain adequate dissolved oxygen.

Medical Management

- Common treatments (see Chapters A12 and A13 for more details):
  - Increasing salinity to 5 g/L can significantly reduce morbidity and mortality. A saltwater mix is best. Treatment should continue for at least four weeks.
  - Other supportive care may be helpful.
- All legislation regarding medication use and disposal must be followed.

Prevention

- General preventative measures are described under C3: *Viral Diseases (General).*
- Specific examples include:
  - Evaluate the history of CEV disease or testing in suppliers of carp and koi.

- Increase salinity to 5 g/L during quarantine of carp or koi.
- Consider PCR testing for CEV prior to carp or koi clearing quarantine.
- At shows, house fish from different sources in independent water systems and quarantine fish on return.

Zoonotic Reports
- These viruses have no known zoonotic potential.

Bibliography

Adamek, M., Jung-Schroers, V., Hellmann, J. et al. (2016). Concentration of carp edema virus (CEV) DNA in koi tissues affected by koi sleepy disease (KSD). *Diseases of Aquatic Organisms* 119: 245–251.

Adamek, M., Matras, M., Jung-Schroers, V. et al. (2017). Comparison of PCR methods for the detection of genetic variants of carp edema virus. *Diseases of Aquatic Organisms* 126: 75–81.

Lovy, J., Friend, S.E., Al-Hussinee, L., and Waltzek, T.B. (2018). First report of carp edema virus in the mortality of wild common carp *Cyprinus carpio* in North America. *Diseases of Aquatic Organisms* 131: 177–186.

Miyazaki, T., Isshiki, T., and Katsuyuki, H. (2005). Histopathological and electron microscopy studies on sleepy disease of koi *Cyprinus carpio koi* in Japan. *Diseases of Aquatic Organisms* 65: 197–207.

Seno, R., Hata, N., Oyamatzu, T., and Fukuda, H. (2003). Curative effect of 0.5% salt water treatment on carp, *Cyprinus carpio*, infected with carp edema virus (CEV) results mainly from reviving the physiological condition of the host. *Suisanzoshoku* 51: 123–124.

Way, K., Haenen, O., Stone, D. et al. (2017). Emergency of carp edema virus (CEV) and its significance to European common carp and koi *Cyprinus carpio*. *Diseases of Aquatic Organisms* 126: 155–166.

Abbreviations/Acronyms
- CEV: Carp edema virus
- PCR: Polymerase chain reaction
- qPCR: Quantitative polymerase chain reaction
- TEM: Transmission electron microscopy

Lymphocystiviruses

Overview
- Lymphocystis disease viruses (LCDVs) cause hypertrophy of fibroblastic cells leading to plaques or nodules on the skin and sometimes the viscera.
- Tropical teleosts are particularly susceptible.
- The disease is a cosmetic concern and an indicator of stressors. The visible lesions can cause economic losses in aquaculture.
- Unlike the other genera of *Iridoviridae* in fish, lymphocystiviruses rarely cause systemic disease.

Etiology
- Family *Iridoviridae*.
- Genus *Lymphocystivirus*.
- Several types exist (e.g. LCDV-1, LCDV-2, LCDV-3).
- These are large, enveloped or non-enveloped DNA viruses.

Transmission
- Horizontal transmission is common, primarily by direct contact.
- Vertical transmission (on egg surfaces) is reported.

Geographic Distribution
- Freshwater and saltwater habitats, particularly tropical and subtropical.

Signalment
- Lymphocystis is common in tropical and subtropical marine and freshwater teleosts (>125 species and >42 families). It is less common but also reported in temperate teleosts.
- Susceptible marine species include spotted scats (*Scatophagus* spp.), silver moonies (*Monodactylus* spp.), hamlets (*Hypoplectrus* spp.), Banggai cardinalfish (*Pterapogon kauderni*), groupers (*Epinephelus* spp.), gilthead seabream (*Sparus aurata*), amberjacks (*Seriola* spp.), red drum (*Sciaenops ocellatus*), and olive flounder (*Paralichthys olivaceus*).
- Susceptible freshwater species include many gouramis (*Anabantoidei*), cichlids (*Cichlidae*), and guppies, swordtails, mollies, and platies (*Poeciliidae*).
- While the host range seems wide, many strains seem relatively host-specific.

Risk Factors
- General risk factors are described under C3: *Viral Diseases (General)*.

Signs/Clinical Findings
- These viruses can be carried asymptomatically.
- One or several conspecifics are usually affected.

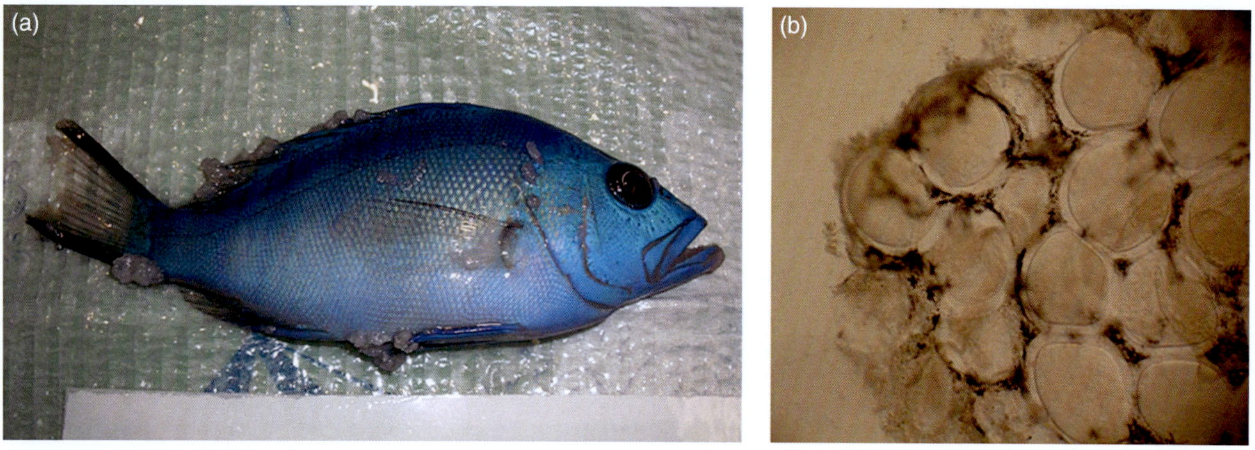

Figure C3.5 Plaques due to lymphocystivirus in a blue hamlet (*Hypoplectrus gemma*) (a) and hypertrophied cells on a skin scrape under direct microscopy (b).

- White or tan plaques or nodules on the skin and fins are typical, particularly on the rostrum, over the operculum, and near the lateral line (Figure C3.5a).
- Systemic signs are rare, but poor growth rates and increased susceptibility to secondary infections have been reported.
- Morbidity and mortality are low.
- Where lesions occur during breeding, they usually resolve then recur the following cycle.

Differential Diagnoses

- Full differentials are provided in Section B.
- Common differentials for plaques or nodules on the skin include lymphocystivirus, carp pox, papillomas, granulomatous inflammation, chlamydia-like organisms, microsporidial xenomas, and calcinosis cutis.

Diagnosis

- Diagnosis is usually based on examination of skin scrapes under direct microscopy.
- The wet mounts show extremely large, round cells with thickened outer membranes (Figure C3.5b). Skin biopsies can be used for confirmation but are rarely necessary.
- Necropsy or coeliotomy findings may include plaques or nodules on viscera such as kidney and spleen.
- Histology shows encapsulated hypertrophied cells on routine hematoxylin and eosin staining. There is no inflammatory response. Feulgen-positive intracytoplasmic inclusion bodies are common.
- Virus isolation in fish cell lines has been challenging.
- PCR tests may be available experimentally.
- EM can demonstrate the characteristic icosahedral virions.

Husbandry Management

- General husbandry management is described under C3: *Viral Diseases (General)*.
- Reduction or resolution of stressors is the most effective management. Lesions regress over days to months if stressors are removed.

Medical Management

- Surgical debridement under anesthesia and analgesia followed by second intention healing can speed resolution in the author's experience.
- All legislation regarding medication use and disposal must be followed.

Prevention

- General preventative measures are described under C3: *Viral Diseases (General)*.

Zoonotic Reports

- These viruses have no known zoonotic potential.

Bibliography

Cano, I., Valverde, E.J., Garcia-Rosado, E. et al. (2013). Transmission of lymphocystis disease virus to cultured gilthead seabream, *Sparus aurata* L., larvae. *Journal of Fish Diseases* 36: 569–576.

Xu, L., Feng, J., and Huang, Y. (2014). Identification of lymphocystis disease virus from paradise fish *Macropodus opercularis* (LDVD-PF). *Archives of Virology* 159: 2445–2449.

Abbreviations/Acronyms
- EM: Electron microscopy
- LCDV: Lymphocystis disease virus
- PCR: Polymerase chain reaction

Ranaviruses

Overview
- A wide variety of ranaviruses have been identified in fish. Most have relatively wide host ranges.
- They can cause severe inflammatory disease and epizootics have been reported in wild and cultured fish.
- They are considered important emerging pathogens of fish, amphibians, and reptiles.
- Epizootic hematopoietic necrosis virus (EHNV) is endemic to Australia and can cause epizootic disease in redfin perch (*Perca fluviatilis*). It should not be confused with similarly-named infectious hematopoietic necrosis virus (IHNV), which is a rhabdovirus.

Etiology
- Family *Iridoviridae*.
- Genus *Ranavirus*.
- The taxonomy is complicated due to classification changes and because fish viruses with "iridovirus" in the name are from the family *Iridoviridae*, but may be from the genus *Ranavirus* or *Megalocytivirus*. The genus *Iridovirus* consists of invertebrate viruses.
- Three fish ranaviruses are considered as exemplar viruses by the International Committee on Taxonomy of Viruses:
  - Epizootic hematopoietic necrosis virus (EHNV), also known as perch ranavirus.
  - Santee-Cooper ranavirus/largemouth bass virus (LMBV), which may be synonymous with doctor fish virus and guppy virus 6.
  - Singapore grouper iridovirus (SGIV).
- Two amphibian ranaviruses can cause disease in fish:
  - Frog virus 3 (FV3).
  - Bohle iridovirus (BIV).
- Multiple other fish ranaviruses are reported in the literature, but many are not yet classified or have been reclassified within *Megalocytivirus*.
- These are large, enveloped or non-enveloped DNA viruses with icosahedral capsids.

Transmission
- Horizontal transmission is common, via water or ingestion.
- Vertical transmission is suspected.
- Carriers may include fish or amphibians.
- The viruses are resistant to drying and can survive for months in water and sediment and >two years in frozen fish tissues.

Geographic Distribution
- Distribution of each virus depends on the range or culture location of the host species.
- EHNV: Australia.
- LMBV: Southeast and eastern United Sates; a similar virus has been reported in China.

Signalment
- Host ranges are often wide, almost always in freshwater.
- EHNV: Natural infection in redfin perch. Cultured rainbow trout (*Oncorhynchus mykiss*) also show infection but disease is mild. Experimental infection has been possible in a wider variety of freshwater fish. Goldfish (*Carassius auratus*) and common carp (*Cyprinus carpio*) appear to be resistant.
- LMBV: Largemouth bass (*Micropterus salmoides*), smallmouth bass (*Micropterus dolomieu*), and other centrarchids, predominantly in the wild.
- FV3: Predominantly in amphibians and reptiles, but mortalities have been reported in pallid sturgeon (*Scaphirhynchus albus*), Russian sturgeon (*Acipenser gueldenstaedtii*), and white sturgeon (*Acipenser transmontanus*).
- BIV: Predominantly in amphibians, but mortalities have been reported in tilapia (*Oreochromis mossambicus*).

Risk Factors
- General risk factors are described under C3: *Viral Diseases (General)*.
- Permissive water temperatures are often high (e.g. 11–20°C (52–68°F) for EHNV or >30°C (86°F) for LMBV).
- Trauma to the mucus or skin is a common risk factor.

Signs/Clinical Findings
- Many of these viruses can be carried asymptomatically or with mild nonspecific signs (e.g. EHNV in rainbow trout).
- If signs are seen, they are typically acute and systemic.
- Multiple conspecifics are usually affected.
- Lethargy is common.

- Skin darkening, petechiae, erythema, skin ulcers, or fin erosions are common.
- Erratic swimming, spiraling, loss of equilibrium, or floating near the surface may be seen.
- Fish may be found dead without other clinical signs.
- LMBV is unusual in that signs are often mild and limited to positive buoyancy. It has a low mortality rate and fish can recover over days or weeks.
- EHNV has a high mortality rate in redfin perch but a low mortality rate (e.g. <4%) in rainbow trout.

Differential Diagnoses

- Full differentials are provided in Section B.
- Common differentials for systemic inflammation in teleosts are broad and include a variety of viral, bacterial, fungal, parasitic, and toxic etiologies.

Diagnosis

- Diagnosis is typically based on histology and virus isolation.
- Necropsy or coeliotomy findings usually include petechial hemorrhages, splenomegaly, and renomegaly.
- Histology findings consist of systemic, necrotizing inflammation with occasional basophilic, intranuclear inclusion bodies. Hematopoietic tissue in the liver, spleen, and cranial kidney are often the worst affected.
- Virus isolation is straightforward; the viruses grow readily in various cell lines and have characteristic cytopathic effects.
- LMBV is unusual in that lesions are limited to swim bladder hyperinflation with few histologic changes. PCR is available commercially for LMBV from the gills, muscle, or swim bladder.
- Antigen-capture ELISA tests are available but cross-react with other ranaviruses.
- TEM can show the large, icosahedral virions.
- The OIE Manual of Diagnostic Tests for Aquatic Animals provides guidance on the diagnosis of EHNV. It recommends frozen liver, kidney, and spleen for virus isolation followed by molecular tests or sequencing.
- EHNV is reportable to the OIE.

Husbandry Management

- General husbandry management is described under C3: *Viral Diseases (General)*.
- Depopulation and disinfection may be considered if there is significant morbidity and mortality.
- Routine disinfectants at standard doses should be effective, including 0.75% chlorhexidine, 70% isopropyl alcohol, or 0.5–1.0% Virkon-Aquatic for one minute.
- Ineffective options have included potassium permanganate (3–5% for five minutes), drying, and freezing.

Medical Management

- No antiviral treatments are reported, but supportive care may be helpful.
- All legislation regarding medication use and disposal must be followed.

Prevention

- General preventative measures are described under C3: *Viral Diseases (General)*.
- Risk assessments are important when sourcing fish from endemic areas (e.g. freshwater fish from Australia).

Zoonotic Reports

- These viruses have no known zoonotic potential.

Bibliography

Bryan, L.K., Baldwin, C.A., Gray, M.J., and Miller, D.L. (2009). Efficacy of select disinfectants at inactivating *Ranavirus*. *Diseases of Aquatic Organisms* 84: 89–94.

Chinchar, V.G. and Waltzek, T.B. (2014). Ranaviruses: not just for frogs. *PLoS Pathogy* 10: e1003850.

OIE (2017). *Manual of Diagnostic Tests for Aquatic Animals* [online]. http://www.oie.int/international-standard-setting/aquatic-manual/access-online/ (accessed 29 July 2017).

Langdon, J.S. (1989). Experimental transmission and pathogenicity of epizootic haematopoietic necrosis virus (EHNV) in redfin perch, *Perca fluviatilis* L., and 11 other teleosts. *Journal of Fish Diseases* 12: 295–310.

Price, S.J., Ariel, E., Maclaine, A. et al. (2017). From fish to frogs and beyond: impact and host range of emergency ranaviruses. *Virology* 511: 272–279.

Waltzek, T.B., Miller, D.L., Gray, M.J. et al. (2014). Expansion of the host range of Frog Virus 3 into hatchery-reared pallid sturgeon (*Scaphirhynchus albus*). *Diseases of Aquatic Organisms* 111: 219–227.

Whittington, R.J., Becker, J.A., and Dennis, M.M. (2010). Iridovirus infections in finfish – critical review with emphasis on ranaviruses. *Journal of Fish Diseases* 33: 95–122.

Abbreviations/Acronyms

- BIV: Bohle iridovirus
- EHNV: Epizootic hematopoietic necrosis virus
- ELISA: Enzyme linked immunosorbent assay
- FV3: Frog virus 3
- LMBV: Largemouth bass virus
- OIE: World Organisation for Animal Health
- PCR: Polymerase chain reaction
- TEM: Transmission electron microscopy

Megalocytiviruses

Overview

- Megalocytiviruses include infectious spleen and kidney necrosis virus (ISKNV) and scale drop disease virus (SDDV).
- They are important pathogens of freshwater and marine teleosts.
- They typically cause systemic inflammatory disease.
- Epizootics have been reported.

Etiology

- Family *Iridoviridae*.
- Genus *Megalocytivirus*.
- The taxonomy is complicated due to classification changes and because fish viruses with "iridovirus" in the name are from the family *Iridoviridae*, but may be from the genus *Ranavirus* or *Megalocytivirus*. The genus *Iridovirus* consists of invertebrate viruses.
- Two species are recognized by the International Committee on Taxonomy of Viruses:
  - ISKNV which is phylogenetically similar to a number of other viruses.
  - SDDV.
- Many closely related viruses are reported in the literature, including red seabream iridovirus (RSIV).
- These are large, enveloped or non-enveloped DNA viruses.

Transmission

- Horizontal transmission is reported.
- Vertical transmission is suspected.

Geographic Distribution

- ISKNV and RSIV were first found in Southeast Asia and Japan and are now probably worldwide.
- SDDV is reported from Singapore, Malaysia, and Indonesia.

Signalment

- ISKNV epizootics have been reported in:
  - Freshwater aquarium teleosts e.g. gouramis (*Trichogaster* spp.); tetras (*Characidae*); guppies, swordtails, mollies, platies (*Poeciliidae*); freshwater angelfish (*Pterophyllum scalare*); oscars (*Astronotus ocellatus*).
  - Freshwater cultured food fish, e.g. Nile tilapia (*Oreochromis niloticus*), Murray cod (*Maccullochella peelii*), marble goby (*Oxyeleotris marmorata*).
  - Marine aquarium teleosts, e.g. mandarin fish (*Siniperca chuatsi*), bangaii cardinalfish (*Pterapogon kaudernii*), orbicular batfish (*Platax orbicularis*).
- SDDV epizootics have only been reported in cultured barramundi (*Lates calcarifer*).
- RSIV tends to infect marine and estuarine teleosts such as red seabream (*Pagrus major*), amberjacks (*Seriola* spp.), grouper (*Epinephelus* spp.), and other *Perciformes* and *Pleuronectiformes*.

Risk Factors

- General risk factors are described under C3: *Viral Diseases (General)*.
- Permissive water temperature varies, e.g. RSIV causes morbidity in rock bream (*Oplegnathus fasciatus*) at 18–30°C (64–86°F) but not at <13°C (55°F).

Signs/Clinical Findings

- The viruses may be carried asymptomatically.
- Multiple conspecifics may be affected.
- Lethargy, abnormal swimming, or abnormal position in the water column may be seen.
- Inappetence or reduced appetite may be seen.
- Skin darkening or pallor, petechiae, erythema, ulcers, or other skin lesions may be seen. Scale loss is common with SDDV.
- Exophthalmos may be seen.
- Dyspnea or tachypnea may be seen.
- Gill pallor due to anemia is common with RSIV. Gill petechiae may also be seen.
- White feces may be seen.
- Coelomic distension due to effusion may be seen.
- Mortality can vary from 0 to 100%. Mortalities may be seen over days to weeks.

Differential Diagnoses

- Full differentials are provided in Section B.
- Common differentials for systemic inflammation in teleosts are broad and include a variety of viral, bacterial, fungal, parasitic, and toxic etiologies.

Diagnosis

- Diagnosis is typically based on characteristic inclusions on histology and virus isolation or PCR.
- Clinical pathology may show hemolytic anemia; erythrocytes may show large eosinophilic intracytoplasmic inclusion bodies.
- Necropsy or coeliotomy may show pallor, petechiae, splenomegaly, renomegaly, hepatomegaly, and serosanguinous coelomic effusion.
- Histology often shows necrosis and inflammation with large, disseminated mesenchymal cells with high cytoplasm to nuclear ratios and large, basophilic or amphophilic intracytoplasmic inclusions. The spleen and kidney are most commonly affected, although any viscera may be affected. Inclusions are less common with SDDV.

- Virus isolation can be useful, usually from spleen and cranial kidney samples. Sequencing of the major capsid protein is required for identification.
- FA, PCR, and qPCR may be available.
- TEM can demonstrate characteristic icosahedral virions.
- The OIE Manual of Diagnostic Tests for Aquatic Animals provides guidance on the diagnosis of RSIV. It recommends kidney and spleen for histology and FA, virus isolation, or PCR. In the United States, the USDA can be contacted to determine sampling recommendations based on the OIE.
- RSIV is reportable to the OIE.

Husbandry Management

- General husbandry management is described under C3: *Viral Diseases (General)*.
- Consider isolating affected groups.
- Consider slowly decreasing the water temperature to slow disease progression, although this may not reduce the mortality rate.
- In the United States, management recommendations for RSIV are provided by the USDA.

Medical Management

- No antiviral treatments are reported, but supportive care may be helpful.
- All legislation regarding medication use and disposal must be followed.

Prevention

- General preventative measures are described under C3: *Viral Diseases (General)*.
- A commercial vaccine for RSIV is available in parts of Asia.

Zoonotic Reports

- These viruses have no known zoonotic potential.

Bibliography

De Groof, A., Guelen, L., Deijs, M. et al. (2015). A novel virus causes scale drop disease in *Lates calcarifer*. *Plos Pathogens* 11(8): e1005074.

Jun, L.J., Jeong, J.B., Kim, J.H. et al. (2009). Influence of temperature shifts on the onset and development of red sea bream iridoviral disease in rock bream *Oplegnathus fasciatus*. *Diseases of Aquatic Organisms* 84: 201–208.

Jung-Schroers, V., Adamek, M., Wohlsein, P. et al. (2016). First outbreak of an infection with infectious spleen and kidney necrosis virus in ornamental fish in Germany. *Diseases of Aquatic Organisms* 119: 239–244.

OIE (2017). *Manual of Diagnostic Tests for Aquatic Animals* [online]. http://www.oie.int/international-standard-setting/aquatic-manual/access-online/ (accessed 29 July 2017).

Sriwanayos, P., Francis-Floyd, R., Stidworthy, M.F. et al. (2013). Megalocytivirus infection in orbiculate batfish *Platax orbicularis*. *Diseases of Aquatic Organisms* 105: 1–8.

Subramaniam, K., Gotesman, M., Smith, C.E. et al. (2016). Megalocytivirus in cultured Nile tilapia *Oreochromis niloticus*. *Disease of Aquatic Organisms* 119: 253–358.

Abbreviations/Acronyms

- FA: Fluorescent antibody
- ISKNV: Infectious spleen and kidney necrosis virus
- OIE: World Organisation for Animal Health
- PCR: Polymerase chain reaction
- qPCR: Quantitative polymerase chain reaction
- RSIV: Red seabream iridovirus
- SDDV: Scale drop disease virus
- TEM: Transmission electron microscopy
- USDA: United States Department of Agriculture

Orthomyxoviruses

Overview

- The most commonly reported orthomyxovirus in fish is infectious salmon anemia virus (ISAV).
- It causes severe hemolytic anemia in Atlantic salmon (*Salmo salar*).
- Infectious salmon anemia virus is the only member of the genus *Isavirus*.
- There are other putative orthomyxoviruses in fish (e.g. tilapia lake virus) but this section will refer to ISAV.
- These are enveloped RNA viruses.

Etiology

- Family *Orthomyxoviridae*.
- Genus *Isavirus*.

Transmission

- Horizontal transmission is reported.
- Vertical transmission is suspected.

- The viruses only survive for hours to days in seawater.
- Vectors probably include sea lice (*Lepeophtheirus salmonis*).
- Carriers include brown trout (*Salmo trutta*), pollock (*Pollachius virens*), and Atlantic cod (*Gadus morhua*).
- Fish that resolve clinical signs usually have lifelong immunity and are resistant to reinfection.

Geographic Distribution

- ISAV is found across North America, South America, and Europe. The European and North American viruses are divided into separate groups.

Signalment

- Natural infection seems limited to Atlantic salmon, mostly in salt water.
- All life stages are susceptible.
- Experimental infection is possible in other salmonids.

Risk Factors

- General risk factors are described under C3: *Viral Diseases (General)*.
- Permissive water temperature is often ~15°C (59°F) with no viral replication at 25°C (77°F).

Signs/Clinical Findings

- Clinical course is typically chronic.
- Multiple Atlantic salmon are usually affected.
- Lethargy is common.
- Affected fish are usually in good condition.
- Tachypnea, dyspnea, and gill pallor are common due to severe anemia.
- Exophthalmos, hyphema, or coelomic distension may be seen due to hemorrhage.
- The daily mortality rate is usually low (<1%) with a cumulative mortality that is typically <50% but may reach 100%.

Differential Diagnoses

- Full differentials are provided in Section B.
- Common differentials for anemia and hemorrhages in Atlantic salmon include ISAV, erythrocytic inclusion body syndrome, infectious hematopoietic necrosis virus, infectious pancreatic necrosis virus, *Moritella viscosa*, *Yersinia ruckeri*, and cardiomyopathy syndrome.

Diagnosis

- Diagnosis is typically based on virus isolation and PCR from Atlantic salmon with severe anemia and hemorrhages.
- Clinical pathology shows severe anemia, with a packed cell volume of <10% in late stages.
- Necropsy or coeliotomy may show visceral pallor, coelomic effusion, renomegaly, splenomegaly, or hepatomegaly with necrosis, petechiae, and hemorrhages.
- The OIE Manual of Diagnostic Tests for Aquatic Animals provides guidance on the diagnosis of ISAV. It recommends virus isolation and RT-PCR on blood or heart. The virus should be differentiated from a nonpathogenic form of ISAV (HPR0). In the United States, the USDA can be contacted to determine sampling recommendations based on the OIE.
- ISAV is reportable to the OIE.

Husbandry Management

- In the United States, management recommendations provided by the USDA must be followed. Depopulation and disinfection, along with movement restrictions, are often implemented.

Medical Management

- Common treatments (see Chapters A12 and A13 for more details):
  - Nucleotide analog ribavirin orally at 6.5 μmol/kg body weight SID for 10 days reduced mortality of experimentally infected salmon.
- All legislation regarding medication use and disposal must be followed.

Prevention

- General preventative measures are described under C3: *Viral Diseases (General)*.
- Atlantic salmon sea pens should be far from wild stocks, other farmed Atlantic salmon (>5 km), and salmon processing plants.
- A USDA-approved vaccine is available, although the protection is variable.

Zoonotic Reports

- These viruses have no known zoonotic potential.

Bibliography

Liltved, H., Vogelsang, C., Modahl, I., and Dannevig, B.H. (2006). High resistance of fish pathogenic viruses to UV irradiation and ozonated seawater. *Aquacultural Engineering* 34: 72–82.

OIE (2017). *Manual of Diagnostic Tests for Aquatic Animals* [online]. http://www.oie.int/international-standard-setting/aquatic-manual/access-online/ (accessed 29 July 2017).

Rivas-Aravena, A., Vallegjos-Vidal, E., Cortez-San Martin, M. et al. (2011). Inhibitory effect of a nucleotide analog on infectious salmon anemia virus infection. *Journal of Virology* 85: 8037–8045.

Abbreviations/Acronyms

- ISAV: Infectious salmon anemia virus
- OIE: World Organisation for Animal Health
- PCR: Polymerase chain reaction
- RT-PCR: Reverse transcriptase polymerase chain reaction
- USDA: United States Department of Agriculture

Betanodaviruses

Overview

- Several betanodaviruses have been identified in fish, particularly marine teleosts.
- The diseases are typically known as vacuolating encephalopathy and retinopathy (VER) or viral nervous necrosis (VNN) because of the vacuolar lesions in the brain and retina.
- The viruses represent a risk to global aquaculture, particularly Mediterranean mariculture.

Etiology

- Family *Nodaviridae*.
- Genus *Betanodavirus*.
- Viruses are typically identified based on common name followed by nervous necrosis virus (NNV). Four species are recognized by the International Committee on Taxonomy of Viruses; each now includes viruses originally named for other species:
  - Striped jack NNV.
  - Tiger puffer NNV.
  - Red-spotted grouper NNV.
  - Barfin flounder NNV.
- These are small, non-enveloped RNA viruses with icosahedral capsids.

Transmission

- Horizontal transmission is reported.
- Vertical transmission seems likely in some species.
- Nodaviruses can survive freezing and extended periods in saltwater, particularly at low temperatures.
- Invertebrate vectors have been reported (e.g. Manila clams (*Ruditapes philippinarum*) for red-spotted grouper NNV). The viruses have been found in common live feeds such as brine shrimp (*Artemia*) and copepods.
- Carriers include gilthead sea bream (*Sparus aurata*) and other species.

Geographic Distribution

- Betanodaviruses in fish were first reported from Australia and the Caribbean in the 1990s and are now probably worldwide.

Signalment

- Each virus is named after a species, but host ranges are wide.
- Infection is typically in marine teleosts, e.g. striped trumpeter (*Latris lineata*), white trevally (*Pseudocaranx dentex*), halibut (*Hippoglossus* spp.), turbot (*Scophthalmus maximus*), red-spotted grouper (*Epinephelus akaara*), seven-band grouper (*Epinephelus septemfasciatus*), barred knifefish (*Oplegnathus fasciatus*), wrasses (*Labridae*), and European bass (*Dicentrarchus labrax*).
- Some predominantly euryhaline fish are susceptible, e.g. barramundi (*Lates calcarifer*), orange-spotted grouper (*Epinephelus coioides*), and Australian bass (*Macquaria novemaculeata*).
- Some freshwater fish are susceptible, e.g. sleepy cod (*Oxyeleotris lineolata*) and Nile tilapia (*Oreochromis niloticus*).

Risk Factors

- General risk factors are described under C3: *Viral Diseases (General)*.

Signs/Clinical Findings

- Multiple conspecifics are usually affected.
- Clinical course is typically acute.
- Abnormal swimming is often the predominant sign (e.g. spiraling, darting, or inverted swimming). Flatfish may be recumbent on the wrong side.
- Inappetence or reduced feeding is common.
- Apparent blindness may be seen.
- Progressive changes in coloration may be seen, including pallor or darkening.
- Mortality may reach 100%.

Differential Diagnoses

- Full differentials are provided in Section B.
- Common differentials for neurologic signs in multiple bony fish include a variety of bacterial, viral, and toxic etiologies.

Diagnosis

- The disease is tentatively diagnosed based on histology of the central nervous system.

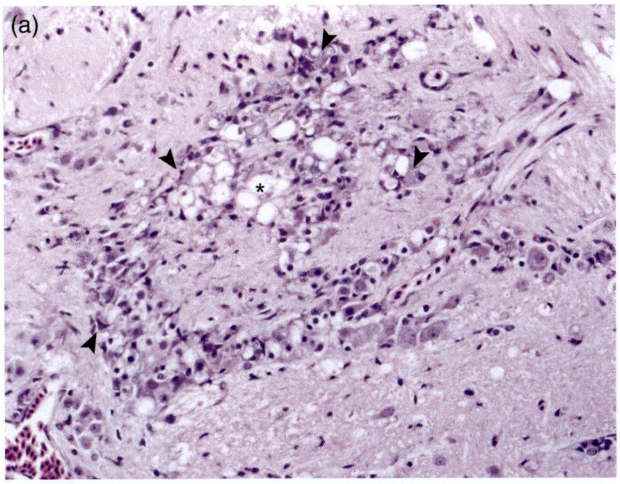

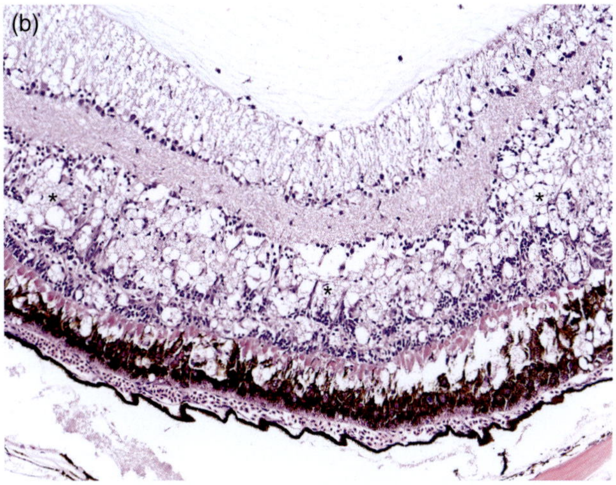

Figure C3.6 Signs of vacuolation (*) and necrosis (arrowheads) on histology of the brain (a) and retina (b) from a Bartletts' anthias (*Pseudanthias bartlettorum*), consistent with viral nervous necrosis. H&E x400 and x200. *Source*: Images courtesy of Justin Stilwell, University of Georgia.

- Histology shows vacuolating necrosis of neural cells of the spinal cord, brain, and retina (Figure C3.6). Intracytoplasmic inclusion bodies may be seen.
- TEM can show the shape of the virions.
- The OIE Manual of Diagnostic Tests for Aquatic Animals provides guidance on the diagnosis of nervous necrosis viruses. It recommends sampling brain and eyes for a combination of histology, RT-PCR, virus isolation, and sequencing.

Husbandry Management

- General husbandry management is described under C3: *Viral Diseases (General).*
- Nodaviruses are relatively resistant to UV. Barfin flounder NNV and red-spotted grouper NNV required 105 and 211 mJ/cm^2, respectively. Nodaviruses have shown a variable response to ozone disinfection, often needing high doses.
- Routine chemical disinfectants may need higher doses or longer contact times. Prolonged drying is helpful (>7 days).

Medical Management

- No antiviral treatments are reported, but supportive care may be helpful.
- All legislation regarding medication use and disposal must be followed.

Prevention

- General preventative measures are described under C3: *Viral Diseases (General).*

Zoonotic Reports

- These viruses have no known zoonotic potential.

Bibliography

Bigarré, L., Cabon, J., Baud, M., and Heimann, M. (2009). Outbreak of betanodavirus infection in tilapia, *Oreochromis niloticus* (L.) in fresh water. *Journal of Fish Diseases* 32: 667–673.

Costa, J.Z. and Thompson, K.D. (2016). Understanding the interaction between Betanodavirus and its host for the development of prophylactic measures for viral encephalopathy and retinopathy. *Fish and Shellfish Immunology* 53: 35–49.

Korsnes, K., Karlsbakk, E., Skår, C.K. et al. (2017). High nervous necrosis virus (NNV) diversity in wild wrasse (Labridae) in Norway and Sweden. *Diseases of Aquatic Organisms* 126: 43–50.

Liltved, H., Vogelsang, C., Modahl, I., and Dannevig, B.H. (2006). High resistance of fish pathogenic viruses to UV irradiation and ozonated seawater. *Aquacultural Engineering* 34: 72–82.

OIE (2017). *Manual of Diagnostic Tests for Aquatic Animals* [online]. http://www.oie.int/international-standard-setting/aquatic-manual/access-online/ (accessed 29 July 2017).

Toffan, A., Pascoli, F., Pretto, T. et al. (2017). Viral nervous necrosis in gilthead sea bream (*Sparus aurata*) caused by reassortant betanodavirus RGNNV/SJNNV: an emerging threat for Mediterranean aquaculture. *Scientific Reports* 7: 1–12.

Volpe, E., Pagnini, N., Serratore, P., and Ciulli, S. (2017). Fate of redspotted grouper nervous necrosis virus (RGNNV) in experimentally challenged Manila clam *Rudipates philippinarum*. *Diseases of Aquatic Organisms* 125: 53–61.

Abbreviations/Acronyms

- NNV: Nervous necrosis virus
- OIE: World Organisation for Animal Health
- RT-PCR: Reverse transcriptase polymerase chain reaction
- TEM: Transmission electron microscopy
- UV: Ultraviolet
- VER: Vacuolating encephalopathy and retinopathy

C4

Bacterial Diseases

Catherine A. Hadfield

Seattle Aquarium, Seattle, WA, USA

Introduction

Most bacterial diseases of fish are due to opportunistic infections by ubiquitous bacteria. Most are Gram-negative bacilli. The chapter starts with a general overview. Subsequent sections include *Aeromonas*, *Vibrio*, *Edwardsiella*, *Flavobacterium*, *Yersinia*, *Streptococcus*, *Renibacterium*, *Mycobacterium*, *Nocardia*, *Francisella* spp., epitheliocystis, and piscirickettsial-like organisms. Where available, information is provided on etiologic agent, life cycle and transmission, signalment, risk factors, clinical signs, diagnosis, husbandry and medical management, and prevention.

Bacterial Diseases (General)

Overview

- Most bacterial diseases of fish are caused by opportunistic Gram-negative bacilli (rods).
- Some significant Gram-positive bacterial infections are reported (e.g. *Streptococcus* and *Renibacterium* spp.; *Mycobacterium* spp. may also take up Gram stain).
- Morbidity and mortality are often secondary to stressors.
- Systemic infections are most common, although local infections may be seen.
- Clinical signs are often nonspecific and definitive diagnosis requires ancillary testing.
- Antibiotic treatment should be based on culture and sensitivity results.

Etiology

- The bacteria that cause disease in fish can usually be grouped based on Gram stain and morphology, although some staining variability exists.
- Gram-negative bacilli are commonly reported to cause disease in fish.
  - *Acinetobacter* spp.
  - *Aeromonas* spp.
  - Chlamydia-like organisms.
  - *Chryseobacterium* spp.
  - *Citrobacter* spp.
  - *Edwardsiella* spp.
  - *Flavobacterium* spp.
  - *Francisella* spp.
  - *Moritella* spp.
  - *Pasteurella* spp.
  - *Photobacterium* spp.
  - *Piscirickettsia* spp. and piscirickettsial-like organisms.
  - *Pseudomonas* spp.
  - *Shewanella* spp.
  - *Tenacibaculum* spp.
  - *Vibrio* spp.
  - *Yersinia* spp.
- Gram-positive bacilli are less commonly reported.
  - *Erysipelothrix piscisicarius* sp. nov. (although Gram stain uptake is variable).
  - *Mycobacterium* spp. (although Gram stain uptake is variable).
  - *Nocardia* spp. (although Gram stain uptake is variable)
  - *Renibacterium* spp.
- Gram-positive cocci are emerging fish pathogens.
  - *Enterococcus* spp.
  - *Lactococcus* spp.
  - *Streptococcus* spp.
  - *Vagococcus* spp.

Clinical Guide to Fish Medicine, First Edition. Edited by Catherine A. Hadfield and Leigh Ann Clayton.

- Obligate anaerobic bacteria are rarely reported, although this may be because fewer anaerobic diagnostic procedures are used in fish.

Transmission

- Horizontal transmission is seen with all bacteria, typically through ingestion and contact.
- Vertical transmission is an important route in a few (e.g. *Renibacterium salmoninarum*, *Flavobacterium psychrophilum*).
- Many are ubiquitous in the environment and are normal components of the biofilm, which can provide protection from immersion treatments and disinfectants.
- Pathogenic bacteria can be carried by fomites such as containers and nets.
- Bacteria can also be transmitted by mechanical and biological vectors and asymptomatic carriers, including aquatic invertebrates, fish, amphibians, and piscivorous birds.

Geographic Distribution

- Most bacterial pathogens of fish are ubiquitous and probably found worldwide.

Signalment

- All individuals are susceptible.
- Juvenile and geriatric fish are often more likely to show clinical signs.
- Species that are common in aquaculture dominate the literature, but bacterial diseases are common in all fish.
- Disease and epizootics are reported in both wild and managed fish populations.

Risk Factors

- Most bacterial pathogens are opportunistic and morbidity and mortality are primarily seen in fish under additional stressors. Increased exposure, such as from poor biosecurity, increases the probability of transmission.
- General risk factors are described here; specific examples are provided for each bacterial group.
- Stressors:
  - High stocking density.
  - Inappropriate social structure.
  - Inappropriate environment.
  - Aggression or displacement.
  - Poor water quality, particularly low dissolved oxygen and high ammonia.
  - Contaminants.
  - Inappropriate water temperature or changes in water temperature.
  - Poor nutrition.
  - Recent handling.
  - Recent transport.
  - Recent spawning.
  - Other diseases, particularly where they damage physical or physiological defenses (e.g. *Ichthyophthirius multifiliis*).
  - Immune-suppressive therapy (e.g. copper sulfate immersion).
- Exposure factors:
  - Poor biosecurity (e.g. use of surface water, exposure to wild fish).
  - Permissive water temperature.
  - Permissive salinity.
  - High organic loads.
  - Low water flow rate or turnover.
  - Trauma to the mucus, skin, or gills.

Signs/Clinical Findings

- Clinical course may be peracute, acute, or chronic.
- Clinical signs are typically nonspecific but can help differentiate between acute and chronic presentations. This delineation affects differentials and prognosis.
- Lethargy, increased hiding, or abnormal behavior is common.
- Inappetence or reduced appetite is common.
- Acute infections often present with erythema, petechiae, skin ulcers, and fin erosions. Ulcerative keratitis or uveitis may be seen.
- Chronic infections may present with poor body condition and change in coloration.
- Coinfections (e.g. viral, fungal, parasitic) are common.
- Some bacterial diseases of fish are cyclical.

Differential Diagnoses

- The clinical signs associated with a systemic bacterial infection are hard to distinguish from other causes of systemic inflammation (e.g. viral, fungal, toxic, parasitic).
- Full differentials are described in Section B; common differentials are highlighted for each bacterial group.

Diagnosis

- Diagnosis must be based on multiple consistent results, including history, clinical signs, cytology, necropsy, histology, culture, and molecular diagnostics. Mixed infections, autolysis, and contaminants are common and can create false impressions of a bacterial infection.
- Cytology (e.g. effusions, blood smears, tissue aspirates, tissue impressions) may show bacteria. Motility, morphology, and staining characteristics can help narrow down the differentials.
- Necropsy or coeliotomy and histology may show organomegaly, congestion, or necrosis. Chronic inflammation may cause granulomas. Intralesional bacteria may be

seen. Morphology and staining characteristics can help narrow down the differentials.

- Culture has been the mainstay of diagnosis but is limited to bacteria that grow in culture. Routine media such as trypticase soy agar with blood, brain–heart infusion agar, or MacConkey agar are particularly useful for *Aeromonas*, *Pseudomonas*, *Vibrio*, *Edwardsiella*, *Streptococcus*, and *Yersinia* spp. Selective media are needed for a number of fish pathogens (e.g. *Flavobacterium*, *Renibacterium*, *Francisella* spp.). False positives are possible from postmortem overgrowth and contaminants. False negatives are common, due to insufficient sample size, inappropriate temperature or media, and antibiotic treatment. It is best to use laboratories that are familiar with fish pathogens and to discuss possible differentials prior to sample collection and submission. Laboratories in the United States with expertise in fish pathogens are listed in Appendix 3.
- Molecular testing and sequencing allow definitive species identification. Identification based on phenotype alone (appearance and biochemical tests) may not be reliable for bacteria in fish.

Husbandry Management

- General management is described here; specific examples are provided for each bacterial group.
- Husbandry management typically relies on reducing or resolving stressors.
  - Increase aeration; target dissolved oxygen may be 95–100%.
  - Resolve any water quality issues.
  - Resolve any temperature stressors.
  - Increase water flow rate or turnover.
  - Reduce social stressors (e.g. add visual barriers).
  - Review the diet and consider additional vitamin C supplementation.
  - Minimize any additional stressors (e.g. transport).
- Husbandry changes can also reduce exposure and transmission rates.
  - Remove dead or moribund fish as soon as possible with appropriate disposition.
  - For virulent infections, isolate affected systems (e.g. limit access, use dedicated equipment).
  - Increase cleaning and disinfection of water. Many bacteria are sensitive to UV disinfection. Recommended doses are typically ~3–10 mJ/cm^2 or mWs/cm^2, but higher doses are reported for some, such as *Flavobacterium* and *Renibacterium* spp. Many bacteria are sensitive to ozone disinfection, although results vary across the studies. Dose depends on the pathogen and organic load, but common doses for fish are often TRO 0.1–0.2 mg/L for several minutes contact time with a system ORP of 300–350 mV. Higher doses have greater disinfection power but increase the risk of damage to fish. UV and ozone disinfection are synergistic and lower applied doses can be used when combined. UV and ozone are most effective after mechanical and biological filtration.
  - Increase cleaning and disinfection of fomites. Most bacteria are susceptible to routine disinfectants such as sodium hypochlorite and other chlorine-based disinfectants, alcohols, iodophors, peroxygen compounds (e.g. Virkon® Aquatic), chlorhexidine gluconate, phenols (e.g. Lysol®), and quaternary ammonium compounds (e.g. benzalkonium chloride) (see Appendix 2). All disinfectants are concentration-, time-, and temperature-dependent. Fomite disinfection is most effective after mechanical cleaning and when followed by drying, particularly in sunlight. Some bacteria are particularly resistant (e.g. *Mycobacterium* spp. and spore-forming bacteria).

Medical Management

- Treatment of an individual may differ from treatment or management of a group.
- Common treatments (see Chapters A12 and A13 for more details):
  - Antibiotic therapy is usually indicated and should be based on culture and sensitivity results.
  - For an individual, injectable or targeted oral medications may be considered along with supportive care such as fluid and nutritional support.
  - For a group of fish, medicated feed or immersion treatments are often required.
  - The effectiveness of oral treatments can be limited by reduced appetites.
  - Some formulations of the antibiotics florfenicol, oxytetracycline, and sulfadimethoxine/ormetoprim are FDA-approved in the United States for specific conditions in some fish species. Dose instructions and withdrawal periods must be followed.
  - Enrofloxacin, ceftazidime, amikacin, and sulfamethoxazole/trimethoprim are commonly used in aquarium fish but are not FDA-approved for use in food fish.
  - Low dose hypersalinity can be used to reduce the osmotic stress in freshwater fish (e.g. 1–3 g/L).
- Other reported treatments (see Chapters A12 and A13 for more details):
  - Anti-inflammatory doses of steroids may limit overstimulation of the immune system and improve prognosis.
- All legislation regarding medication use and disposal must be followed.

Prevention

- Morbidity and mortality can be prevented by reducing stressors, exposure, and severity of disease. While many bacterial pathogens are ubiquitous opportunists, good biosecurity can reduce the risk of introducing virulent strains.
- The general preventative measures below relate to all bacteria. Specific examples are provided for each bacterial group.
- Reduce or resolve stressors, particularly when disease is likely (e.g. after transport or at permissive water temperatures).
  - Low stocking density.
  - Suitable social groups and habitats.
  - Excellent water quality and preferred water temperature.
  - Good nutrition.
  - Suitable handling and transport protocols.
  - No other disease issues.
- Reduce exposure and transmission.
  - Isolation with no contact with free-ranging animals, particularly fish and aquatic invertebrates.
  - Pathogen-free water source (e.g. municipal water or ground water that has gone through fine filtration then UV and/or ozone disinfection). Avoid using untreated surface water.
  - Disinfection of recirculating water with fine filtration then UV and/or ozone.
  - High water flow rate or turnover.
  - Removal of dead or moribund fish as soon as possible with appropriate disposition.
  - Good cleaning and disinfection protocols.
  - Limits on visitors and potential fomites.
  - All-in-all-out management.
  - Suitable quarantine with isolation, monitoring, and diagnostic testing. This should apply to new animals as well as animals returning from shows or loans.
  - Frozen-thawed or commercial feeds, with no live feeds.
  - Routine monitoring of diseases of concern.
  - Disinfection of discharge water to reduce the risk of spill-back to wild populations.
- Reduce severity of disease.
  - Vaccination, where available.
  - High vitamin C in the diet; 500–1000 mg/kg of ascorbic acid equivalent in the diet consistently improves response to disease. Vitamin C is easily degraded by food processing, storage, light, oxygen, and high temperatures.
  - Immune-stimulants can be used prior to a known stressor (e.g. transport) or following an acute stressor (e.g. temperature change) to provide additional protection against extracellular bacteria such as *Aeromonas*, *Vibrio*, *Yersinia*, *Edwardsiella*, and *Streptococcus* spp. The range of products and doses is wide; examples of doses that are commonly effective in teleosts include: beta glucans at 1 g/kg of diet (0.1%) PO for one to two weeks; allicin or crushed garlic at 5–10 g/kg of diet (0.5–1%) PO for four weeks; or propolis ethanol extract at 5–10 g/kg of diet (0.5–1%) PO for four weeks.
  - Selective breeding of more resistant fish strains.
  - A healthy and diverse microbiome should reduce the probability of colonization by virulent strains; this might be most easily achieved with native species, local water, natural substrates, and suitable and stable environmental conditions.
- Regularly review morbidity and mortality trends and response to treatments.

Zoonotic Reports

- Several fish bacterial pathogens have zoonotic potential, but transmission is much more common from ingestion of raw or inadequately cooked or processed fish than from contact with fish.
- The highest risk from contact with fish is direct wound inoculation (e.g. fish spine injury or bite wound).
- Most fish bacterial pathogens are also common in the environment and transmission is possible through water contact with mucosal surfaces, open wounds, or food, although this appears to be rare.
- Disease is more likely with immune suppression.

Bibliography

Austin, B. and Austin, D.A. (2012). Bacterial Fish Pathogens: Diseases of Farmed and Wild Fish, 652. Springer Science.

Barros, M.M., Falcon, D.R., Orsi, R.O. et al. (2015). Immunomodulatory effects of dietary β-glucan and vitamin C in Nile tilapia, *Oreochromis niloticus* L., subjected to cold-induced stress or bacterial challenge. *Journal of the World Aquaculture Society* 46: 363–380.

Lee, J.Y. and Gao, Y. (2012). Review of the application of garlic, *Allium sativum*, in aquaculture. *Journal of the World Aquaculture Society* 43: 447–458.

Meena, D.K., Das, P., Kumar, S. et al. (2013). Beta-glucan: an ideal immunostimulant in aquaculture (a review). *Fish Physiology and Biochemistry* 39: 431–457.

Pomaranski, E.K., Reichley, S.R., Yanong, R. et al. (2018). Characterization of *spaC*-type *Erysipelothrix* sp. isolates causing systemic disease in ornamental fish. *Journal of Fish Diseases* 41: 49–60.

Sakai, M. (1999). Current research status of fish immunostimulants. *Aquaculture* 172: 63–92.

Sharrer, M.J., Summerfelt, T., Bullock, G.L. et al. (2005). Inactivation of bacteria using ultraviolet irradiation in a recirculating salmonid culture system. *Aquacultural Engineering* 33: 135–149.

Woo, P.T.K. and Cipriano, R.C. (2017). Fish Viruses and Bacteria: Pathobiology and Protection, 370. CABI.

Abbreviations/Acronyms

- FDA: Food and Drug Administration
- ORP: Oxidation–reduction potential
- PO: Orally
- TRO: Total residual oxidant
- UV: Ultraviolet

Aeromonas salmonicida

Overview

- *Aeromonas salmonicida* subsp. *salmonicida* causes furunculosis, a serious disease of salmonids in aquaculture.
- Other *Aeromonas salmonicida* subspecies can cause atypical furunculosis in a variety of fish species.
- Both cause septicemia; skin ulcers and hemorrhages are common clinical signs.

Etiology

- Family *Aeromonadaceae.*
- *Aeromonas salmonicida* has several subspecies:
  - Typical furunculosis: *A. salmonicida* subsp. *salmonicida.*
  - Atypical furunculosis: *A. salmonicida* subsp. *achromogenes* (previously *Haemophilus piscium*), *A. salmonicida* subsp. *masoucida*, *A. salmonicida* subsp. *smithia*.
- This division of typical and atypical furunculosis is likely oversimplified, but remains a common categorization.
- *A. salmonicida* can be associated with other diseases, e.g. in carp (*Cyprinus* spp.), *A. salmonicida* is commonly associated with rhabdovirus carpio as part of infectious dropsy of carp (known as carp erythrodermatitis in Europe).
- These are nonmotile, Gram-negative bacilli and facultative anaerobes.

Transmission

- Transmission is typically horizontal, through ingestion and contact.
- The bacteria can survive for months in freshwater and sediment and for days in salt water.

Geographic Distribution

- Freshwater and saltwater habitats.

Signalment

- Typical furunculosis infects wild and cultured freshwater salmonids such as brown trout (*Salmo trutta*), Atlantic salmon (*Salmo salar*), and Pacific salmon (*Oncorhynchus* spp.), although rainbow trout (*Oncorhynchus mykiss*) seem less susceptible.
- Atypical furunculosis can infect a variety of freshwater and saltwater teleosts including salmonids (*Salmonidae*), sand eels (*Ammodytes lancea*), flatfish such as turbot (*Scophthalmus maximus*), plaice (*Pleuronectes platessa*), and halibut (*Hippoglossus* spp.), cyprinids such as goldfish (*Carassius auratus*) and koi (*Cyprinus carpio koi*), and Atlantic cod (*Gadus morhua*, causing ulcer disease of cod).

Risk Factors

- General risk factors are described under C4: *Bacterial Diseases (General).*
- Permissive water temperature is often >22°C (>72°F).

Signs/Clinical Findings

- Multiple fish from one or more species are usually affected.
- Clinical course may be peracute, acute, or chronic.
- Peracute death is common in juvenile fish.
- Lethargy may be seen.
- Inappetence or reduced appetite may be seen.
- Erythema, ecchymoses (particularly at the base of fins), hemorrhages, skin ulcers, or fin erosions are common.
- Boils (furuncles) or nodules may be seen prior to skin ulcers, although furuncles are not common, despite the name of the disease.
- Skin darkening may be seen.
- Exophthalmos may be seen.
- Coelomic distension and cloacal/anal distension may be seen.

- Gill pallor or gill edema may be seen.
- Generalized edema may be seen.
- Mortality is often high, up to 90%.

Differential Diagnoses

- Full differentials are described in Section B.
- Common differentials for bacterial septicemia include vibriosis, *Aeromonas*, *Citrobacter*, *Pseudomonas*, *Edwardsiella*, *Flavobacterium*, *Yersinia*, *Streptococcus*, and *Francisella* spp.

Diagnosis

- Diagnosis is typically based on a combination of cytology, histology, and culture.
- Short Gram-negative bacilli may be seen on blood smears, effusions, tissue cytology, or histology. They are nonmotile on wet mounts.
- Necropsy or coeliotomy and histology typically show petechiae, congestion, serosanguinous coelomic effusion, tissue pallor, organomegaly, or focal necrosis of any tissues with intralesional Gram-negative bacilli.
- Culture of affected tissues or blood is often successful. Routine or selective media (e.g. TSA with Coomassie brilliant blue) can be used aerobically at ~18–25°C (64–77°F). However, bacteria are easily killed by high temperatures, antibiotic treatment, and faster growing aeromonads.
- Biochemical identification schemes are often used, but species identification is rarely definitive. Even molecular techniques have limited ability to differentiate between species and subspecies.
- PCR tests are available commercially.
- ELISAs can be used to assess antibody response.

Husbandry Management

- General husbandry management is described under C4: *Bacterial Diseases (General).*

Medical Management

- Common treatments (see Chapters A12 and A13 for more details):
  - Antibiotic therapy is indicated. Treatment should be based on culture and sensitivity as antibiotic resistance is common and published reports show different antibiotic susceptibilities.
  - Oxytetracycline dihydrate (Terramycin® 200) orally is approved in the United States for salmonids with furunculosis at 55–83 mg/kg every 24 hours for 10 days, with a 21-day withdrawal, as of 2020.
  - Sulfadimethoxine and ormetoprim (Romet® 30) orally is approved in the United States for salmonids with furunculosis at 50 mg/kg every 24 hours for five days, with a 42-day withdrawal, as of 2020.
  - Florfenicol (Aquaflor®) orally is approved in the United States for freshwater-reared salmonids with furunculosis at 10–15 mg/kg every 24 hours for 10 days, with a 15-day withdrawal, as of 2020.
- Other reported treatments (see Chapters A12 and A13 for more details):
  - Potassium permanganate immersion if infection is limited to the skin.
- All legislation regarding medication use and disposal must be followed.

Prevention

- General preventative measures are described under C4: *Bacterial Diseases (General).*
- Effective commercial vaccines are available for typical furunculosis in salmonids, usually by intraperitoneal injection. Vaccines with mineral oil adjuvants provide the greatest protection but often cause adverse reactions including coelomic pigmentation, adhesions, and granulomas.
- Autogenous vaccines may be considered for other *A. salmonicida* subspecies; commercial vaccines are unlikely because of antigenic diversity.
- Immune-stimulants such as allicin, glucans, chitosan, and probiotics (e.g. *Lactobacillus*, *Lactococcus*, *Carnobacterium* spp.) can increase resistance to *A. salmonicida*. They are most effective at specific doses, short courses, and when given prior to infection.

Zoonotic Reports

- This disease has no known zoonotic potential.

Bibliography

Beaz-Hidalgo, R., Alperi, A., Bujan, N. et al. (2010). Comparison of phenotypic and genetic identification of *Aeromonas* strains isolated from diseased fish. *Systematic Applied Microbiology* 33: 149–153.

Breyer, K.E., Getchell, R.G., Cornwell, R.E. et al. (2015). Efficacy of an extract from garlic, *Allium sativum*, against infection with the furunculosis bacterium, *Aeromonas salmonicida*, in rainbow trout, *Oncorhynchus mykiss*. *Journal of the World Aquaculture Society* 46: 273–282.

Meinelt, T., Phan, T.-M., Behrens, S. et al. (2015). Growth inhibition of *Aeromonas salmonicida* and *Yersinia ruckeri* by disinfectants containing peracetic acid. *Diseases of Aquatic Organisms* 113: 207–213.

Menanteau-Ledouble, S., Kumar, G., Saleh, M., and El-Matbouli, M. (2016). *Aeromonas salmonicida*: updates on an old acquaintance. *Diseases of Aquatic Organisms* 120: 49–68.

Ngamkala, S., Futami, K., Endo, M. et al. (2010). Immunological effects of glucan and *Lactobacillus rhamnosus* GG, a probiotic bacterium, on Nile tilapia *Oreochromis niloticus* intestine with oral *Aeromonas* challenges. *Fish Science* 76: 833–840.

Villumsen, K.R., Koppang, E.O., and Raida, M.K. (2015). Adverse and long-term protective effects following oil-adjuvanted vaccination against *Aeromonas salmonicida* in rainbow trout. *Fish and Shellfish Immunology* 42: 193–203.

Abbreviations/Acronyms

- ELISA: Enzyme linked immunosorbent assay
- PCR: Polymerase chain reaction
- TSA: Trypticase soy agar

Motile Aeromonad Septicemia

Overview

- Several *Aeromonas* species are opportunists that can cause motile aeromonad septicemia (MAS).
- MAS is the most commonly reported bacterial infection of fish.
- The bacteria grow readily in culture and may be secondary infections or contaminants. This can result in a misdiagnosis or masking of the primary disease.

Etiology

- Family *Aeromonadaceae.*
- *Aeromonas hydrophila (liquefaciens), Aeromonas sobria*, *Aeromonas caviae*, *Aeromonas veronii*, and *Aeromonas dhakensis* are all reported in fish, although a variety of strains exist and the taxonomy changes frequently.
- The bacteria are common in the environment and many aeromonad species are nonpathogenic.
- Some *Aeromonas* species are normal commensals on fish skin.
- These are motile, short, straight, Gram-negative bacilli and facultative anaerobes.

Transmission

- Transmission is typically horizontal, through ingestion and contact.
- Amphibians and reptiles may act as carriers or vectors.

Geographic Distribution

- Predominantly in freshwater and brackish water habitats, probably worldwide.

Signalment

- Predominantly found in cultured and wild freshwater fish, including carp (*Cyprinus carpio*), goldfish (*Carassius auratus*), channel catfish (*Ictalurus punctatus*), tilapia (*Oreochromis* spp.), striped bass (*Morone saxatilis*), largemouth bass (*Micropterus salmoides*), and European eel (*Anguilla anguilla*).
- Infections are less common in marine teleosts. Examples include cod (*Gadus morhua*) and marine elasmobranchs.

Risk Factors

- General risk factors are described under C4: *Bacterial Diseases (General).*
- Permissive water temperature is often ~10–22°C (50–72°F) or higher.

Signs/Clinical Findings

- Individual or multiple fish from one or more species may be affected.
- Inappetence or reduced appetite may be seen.
- Lethargy may be seen.
- Erythema, petechiae, skin ulcers and fin erosions, scale loss, cutaneous edema, or boils (furuncles) are common.
- Exophthalmos may be seen.
- Coelomic distension may be seen.
- Gill pallor or edema may be seen.
- Neurologic signs may be seen.
- Mortality is typically low but can reach 100% in fry or fingerlings.

Differential Diagnoses

- Full differentials are described in Section B.
- Common differentials for bacterial septicemia include vibriosis, *Aeromonas*, *Citrobacter*, *Pseudomonas*, *Edwardsiella*, *Flavobacterium*, *Yersinia*, *Streptococcus*, and *Francisella* spp.

Diagnosis

- Diagnosis should be based on multiple consistent findings (e.g. clinical signs, cytology, necropsy, histology, and culture) and not culture alone.
- Short (1–3 μm), straight, Gram-negative bacilli may be seen on blood smears, effusions, tissue cytology, or histology. They are motile on wet mounts.

- Necropsy or coeliotomy and histology typically show petechiae, congestion, serosanguinous coelomic effusion, tissue pallor, organomegaly, or focal necrosis of any tissues with intralesional Gram-negative bacilli.
- Culture of affected tissues or blood is often successful. Routine or selective media (e.g. Coomassie brilliant blue) can be used aerobically at ~18–25°C (64–77°F). Bacteria are easily killed by high temperatures and concurrent antibiotic treatments.
- Traditional biochemical identification tests are often used, but species identification is frequently debated; definitive identification requires sequencing.
- PCR and ELISA tests may be available.

Husbandry Management

- General husbandry management is described under C4: *Bacterial Diseases (General)*.
- Reduction of stressors can be sufficient to control signs.

Medical Management

- Common treatments (see Chapters A12 and A13 for more details):
  - Antibiotic therapy may be indicated. Treatment should be based on culture and sensitivity as antibiotic resistance is common and published reports show different antibiotic susceptibilities.
  - Oxytetracycline dihydrate (Terramycin® 200) orally is approved in the United States for catfish and salmonids with *A. hydrophila* at 55–83 mg/kg every 24 hours for 10 days, with a 21-day withdrawal, as of 2020.
  - Enrofloxacin, ceftazidime, amikacin, florfenicol, and trimethoprim-sulfamethoxazole are commonly used in aquarium fish.
  - Low-dose hypersalinity can be used to reduce the osmotic stress in freshwater fish (e.g. 1–3 g/L).
- Other reported treatments (see Chapters A12 and A13 for more details):
  - Surgical debridement of lesions.
  - Potassium permanganate immersion if the disease is limited to the skin.
- All legislation regarding medication use and disposal must be followed.

Prevention

- General preventative measures are described under C4: *Bacterial Diseases (General)*.
- Motile aeromonads are ubiquitous and cannot be eliminated. Disease is usually secondary to other issues and prevention should focus on reducing stressors and reducing severity of disease.
- Autogenous vaccines can help with recurrent outbreaks; commercial vaccines are unlikely because of antigenic diversity.
- Immune-stimulants, such as beta glucans, allicin, and propolis, can increase resistance to MAS. They are most effective at specific doses, short courses, and when given prior to infection.

Zoonotic Reports

- Some aeromonad species and strains are zoonotic.
- Transmission may be foodborne, waterborne, or by inoculation.
- *A. hydrophila*, *A. sobria*, and *A. caviae* are implicated in foodborne and waterborne diarrhea from consumption of raw or inadequately cooked or processed fish and shellfish or contaminated food or water.
- Infection by inoculation can lead to local infection or septicemia.
- With a healthy immune system, no damage to the skin barrier, and good food hygiene, risk of transmission to humans from contact with fish or aquarium water appears to be low.

Bibliography

Beaz-Hidalgo, R., Alperi, A., Bujan, N. et al. (2010). Comparison of phenotypic and genetic identification of *Aeromonas* strains isolated from diseased fish. *Systematic and Applied Microbiology* 33: 149–153.

El-Asey, A.M., Abbass, A.A., and Austin, B. (2014). Honey bee pollen improves growth, immunity and protection of Nile tilapia (*Oreochromis niloticus*) against infection with *Aeromonas hydrophila*. *Fish and Shellfish Immunology* 40: 500–506.

Harikrishnan, R., Balasundaram, C., and Heo, M. (2010). Potential use of probiotic- and triherbal extract-enriched diets to control *Aeromonas hydrophila* infection in carp. *Diseases of Aquatic Organisms* 92: 41–49.

Ngamkala, S., Futami, K., Endo, M. et al. (2010). Immunological effects of glucan and *Lactobacillus rhamnosus* GG, a probiotic bacterium, on Nile tilapia *Oreochromis niloticus* intestine with oral *Aeromonas* challenges. *Fish Science* 76: 833–840.

Nya, E.J. and Austin, B. (2011). Development of immunity in rainbow trout (*Oncorhynchus mykiss*, Walbaum) to *Aeromonas hydrophila* after the dietary application of garlic. *Fish and Shellfish Immunology* 30: 845–850.

Abbreviations/Acronyms

- ELISA: Enzyme linked immunosorbent assay
- MAS: Motile aeromonad septicemia
- PCR: Polymerase chain reaction

Vibriosis

Overview

- Vibriosis is caused by a variety of bacteria within the genus *Vibrio* and bacteria that used to be within the genus (e.g. *Aliivibrio*, *Moritella*, and *Photobacterium*).
- Some can be primary pathogens, but most are ubiquitous in the environment and cause disease secondary to other stressors.
- They can cause bacterial septicemia in a wide range of fish species.
- *Aliivibrio salmonicida* is particularly common in salmonid and cod aquaculture in Canada, Norway, and the United Kingdom.
- They are part of normal fish intestinal flora. Intestinal *Vibrio* flora closely resembles the populations in the water.
- These are common commensals (autochthonous bacteria) in elasmobranch tissues and blood, particularly *V. alginolyticus*, *V. harveyi*, and *P. damselae*.
- *Vibrio* spp. are present in light-emitting organs of marine fish and cephalopods.
- These are curved to spiral-shaped, Gram-negative bacilli that are usually motile and are facultative anaerobes.

Etiology

- Family *Vibrionaceae*.
- More than 20 *Vibrio* spp. may cause disease. Two are reported most commonly:
  - *Vibrio* (*Listonella*, *Beneckea*) *anguillarum*, causing saltwater furunculosis.
  - *Vibrio ordalii* (previously atypical strain of *V. anguillarum* biotype 2).
- Other *Vibrio* spp. that can cause disease are listed in alphabetical order below.
  - *V. alginolyticus*.
  - *V. cholera*.
  - *V. fischeri*.
  - *V. harveyi* (including previous *V. carchariae* and *V. trachuri*).
  - *V. ichthyoenteri*.
  - *V. logei*.
  - *V. parahaemolyticus*.
  - *V. pelagius*.
  - *V. splendidus*.
  - *V. tapetis*.
  - *V. vulnificus*.
- Several *Vibrio* spp. have been renamed but are still considered to cause vibriosis.
  - *Aliivibrio salmonicida*, causing hitra or cold-water vibriosis.
  - *Moritella viscosa*.
  - *Moritella marina*.
  - *Photobacterium damselae* subsp. *damselae*.
  - *Photobacterium* (*Pasteurella*) *damselae* subsp. *piscicida* (pseudotuberculosis, pasteurellosis, photobacteriosis).

Transmission

- Horizontal transmission is common; vertical transmission seems possible.
- Aquatic invertebrates (e.g. bivalves, penaeid shrimp) may act as carriers or vectors.

Geographic Distribution

- Predominantly in saltwater and brackish water habitats, probably worldwide.

Signalment

- Disease is likely possible in any marine or brackish fish, including elasmobranchs.
- Vibriosis is commonly reported in some groups:
  - Salmon and trout (*Salmonidae*).
  - Striped bass (*Morone saxatilis*), European bass (*Dicentrarchus labrax*).
  - Cod (*Gadus morhua*).
  - Yellowtail (*Seriola quinqueradiata*).
  - Seahorses (*Syngnathidae*).
  - Requiem sharks (*Carcharhinidae*).
- Disease is occasionally reported in freshwater fish (e.g. guppies, *Poecilia reticulata*).

Risk Factors

- General risk factors are described under C4: *Bacterial Diseases (General)*.
- Permissive water temperature is high for most *Vibrio* spp. and low for *Aliivibrio salmonicida*, e.g. 15°C (59°F).

Signs/Clinical Findings

- Individual or multiple fish from one or more species may be affected.
- Clinical course may be peracute, acute, or chronic.
- Lethargy may be seen.

- Inappetence or reduced appetite may be seen.
- Skin darkening or pallor, erythema, petechiae, ecchymoses, skin ulcers, or fin erosions may be seen.
- Coelomic distension due to ascites or organomegaly or a pinched coelom due to loss of body condition may be seen.
- Corneal edema, keratitis, or exophthalmos may be seen.
- Gill pallor due to anemia may be seen.
- Neurologic or respiratory signs may be seen.
- Mortality can be >50%, up to 90% in rare cases.

Differential Diagnoses

- Full differentials are described in Section B.
- Common differentials for bacterial septicemia include vibriosis, *Aeromonas*, *Citrobacter*, *Pseudomonas*, *Edwardsiella*, *Flavobacterium*, *Yersinia*, *Streptococcus*, and *Francisella* spp.

Diagnosis

- Diagnosis should be based on multiple consistent findings (e.g. clinical signs, cytology, necropsy, histology, and culture) and not culture alone.
- Short (1–3 μm), curved to spiral-shaped, Gram-negative bacilli may be seen on blood smears, effusions, tissue cytology, or histology (Figure C4.1). They may be motile on wet mounts.
- Necropsy or coeliotomy and histology typically show petechiae, congestion, serosanguinous coelomic effusion, tissue pallor, organomegaly, or focal necrosis of any tissues (particularly kidney and spleen) with intralesional Gram-negative bacilli. In more chronic cases, inflammation may be granulomatous, particularly with *P. damselae*.
- Culture of affected tissues (especially the kidney and spleen) or blood is often successful. Routine or selective media (e.g. thiosulfate citrate bile salts) can be used. Culture success may be improved in marine species with 10 g/L sodium chloride. Incubation temperature needs to be low for *Aliivibrio salmonicida*. Autochthonous bacteria are present in elasmobranchs and blood cultures may be positive in healthy animals.
- Species identification using biochemical profiles can be difficult and PCR or sequencing is recommended.
- Serology is not routinely available.

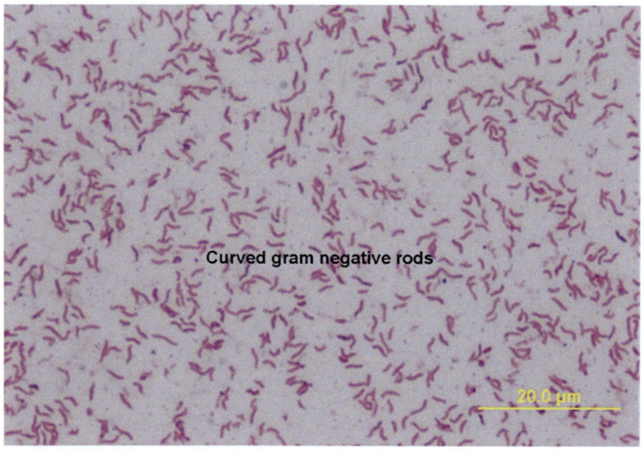

Figure C4.1 Cytologic appearance of curved Gram-negative bacilli, consistent with *Vibrio* spp. *Source*: Image courtesy of Jill Arnold, National Aquarium.

Husbandry Management

- General husbandry management is described under C4: *Bacterial Diseases (General)*.
- Reduction of stressors or other disease issues is sometimes enough to control signs.
- In aquaculture, regulations may require movement restrictions, depopulation, and disinfection.

Medical Management

- Common treatments (see Chapters A12 and A13 for more details):
  - Antibiotic therapy is usually indicated and should be based on culture and sensitivity results.
- All legislation regarding medication use and disposal must be followed.

Prevention

- General preventative measures are described under C4: *Bacterial Diseases (General)*.
- A healthy, diverse microbiome may reduce exposure to more pathogenic *Vibrio* spp. (e.g. survival of *V. ordalii* is reduced by the presence of other microbiota).
- Commercial immersion vaccines are available for some species (e.g. *V. anguillarum* and *V. ordalii* in salmonids).
- Autogenous vaccines may be considered.
- Immune-stimulants, such as beta glucans, can increase resistance to vibriosis. They are most effective at specific doses, short courses, and when given prior to infection.

Zoonotic Reports

- Vibriosis is predominantly a foodborne zoonosis through ingestion of raw or inadequately cooked shellfish (particularly oysters) or contaminated food and water. Species implicated in human disease include *V. parahaemolyticus*, *V. vulnificus*, *V. harveyi*, *V. alginolyticus*, and *P. damselae*. Signs may include nausea, vomiting, abdominal cramps, and pyrexia.
- Transmission is possible though inoculation into wounds, either from water or fish. This can cause local infections or septicemia, particularly if associated with immune suppression.
- The CDC estimates that vibriosis causes 80 000 human illnesses in the United States each year, of which two thirds are due to eating contaminated food.
- The species that causes cholera (*Vibrio cholerae*) is not found in fish.
- With a healthy immune system, no damage to the skin barrier, and good food hygiene, risk of transmission to humans from contact with fish or aquarium water appears to be low.

Bibliography

Blanch, A.R., Hispano, C., Bulto, P. et al. (2009). Comparison of *Vibrio* spp. populations found in seawater, in exhibition aquaria, in fish intestine and in fish feed. *Journal of Applied Microbiology* 106: 57–65.

Mylniczenko, N., Harris, B., Wilborn, R.E., and Young, F.A. (2007). Blood culture results from healthy captive and free-ranging elasmobranchs. *Journal of Aquatic Animal Health* 19: 159–167.

Ruiz, P., Poblete-Morales, M., Irgang, R. et al. (2016). Survival behaviour and virulence of the fish pathogen *Vibrio ordalii* in seawater microcosms. *Diseases of Aquatic Organisms* 120: 27–38.

Tao, Z., Bullard, S.A., and Arias, C.R. (2014). Diversity of bacteria cultured from the blood of lesser electric rays caught in the northern Gulf of Mexico. *Journal of Aquatic Animal Health* 26: 225–232.

Abbreviations/Acronyms

- CDC: Centers for Disease Control and Prevention
- PCR: Polymerase chain reaction

Enteric Septicemia of Catfish

Overview

- *Edwardsiella ictaluri* is the causative agent of enteric septicemia of catfish.
- It is a primary pathogen that causes significant economic losses in aquaculture of channel catfish (*Ictalurus punctatus*).
- It causes enteric, neurologic, and septicemic disease.

Etiology

- Family *Enterobacteriaceae.*
- The causative agent is *Edwardsiella ictaluri.* Several strains exist.
- *E. ictaluri* is a primary, obligate pathogen, unlike *Edwardsiella tarda* and *Edwardsiella piscicida*, which are opportunists.
- These are motile, short, pleomorphic, Gram-negative bacilli and facultative anaerobes.

Transmission

- Transmission is primarily by ingestion, often feco-oral or through scavenging. Transmission can also be waterborne through the gills and nares.
- *E. ictaluri* does not survive long in water but can survive in pond mud for >3 mo at 25°C (77°F).
- Fish that resolve clinical signs can become carriers.
- Piscivorous birds may act as vectors.

Geographic Distribution

- *E. ictaluri* has been reported in all areas of the United States where catfish aquaculture is common, including Alabama, Arkansas, Mississippi, Louisiana, and California.
- Other reports have included Japan, southeast Asia, Australia, and Europe.

Signalment

- Epizootic disease is seen primarily in channel catfish in aquaculture.
- Disease is also seen in blue catfish (*Ictalurus furcatus*), brown bullhead (*Ameiurus nebulosus*), and white catfish (*Ameiurus catus*), but signs are typically less severe.
- Hybrid catfish are typically more resistant, although reports of disease may be increasing.
- More recently, natural infection and clinical signs have been reported in a wider range of species, including wild ayu (*Plecoglossus altivelis*), cultured zebrafish (*Danio rerio*), and cultured Nile tilapia (*Oreochromis niloticus*), although these appear to be different strains.
- *E. ictaluri* has been isolated from a wider variety of freshwater fish without morbidity or mortality.

Risk Factors

- General risk factors are described under C4: *Bacterial Diseases (General).*
- Permissive water temperature is often 22–28°C (72–82°F).

Signs/Clinical Findings

- Multiple conspecifics are usually affected.
- Most presentations are neurologic or enteric/septicemic, although the signs can overlap.
- The neurologic form is typically more chronic.
  - Spiral swimming, circling, and inappetence are common.
  - Lethargy or hanging in the water with a low tail position is also seen.
  - Fingerlings may show skin ulcers on the head (known as hole in the head).
- The enteric/septicemic form is typically more acute.
  - Erythema, petechiae, ecchymoses, hemorrhages, and skin ulcers are common.
  - Exophthalmos may be seen.

  - Coelomic distension may be seen.
  - Gill pallor due to anemia may be seen.
- A biphasic pattern is common with disease typically seen in the spring and fall.
- Mortality varies but can reach >50%, particularly with acute disease. Mortalities can increase rapidly if additional stressors are introduced, such as handling.

Differential Diagnoses
- Full differentials are described in Section B.
- Major differentials for septicemic disease in young channel catfish include *E. ictaluri*, *E. piscicida*, and channel catfish virus.
- Common differentials for bacterial granulomatous lesions in teleosts include *Mycobacterium*, *Nocardia*, *Edwardsiella*, *Francisella*, *Streptococcus*, *Photobacterium* spp., and piscirickettsial-like organisms.

Diagnosis
- Diagnosis should be based on multiple consistent findings (e.g. clinical signs, cytology, necropsy, histology, and culture) and not culture alone.
- Short (~1.25 μm) Gram-negative bacilli may be seen on blood smears, effusions, tissue cytology, or histology. They are motile on wet mounts.
- Necropsy or coeliotomy may show petechiae, congestion, serosanguinous coelomic effusion, tissue pallor, splenomegaly and renomegaly with nodules.
- Histology typically shows hemorrhagic enteritis and granulomatous splenitis, nephritis, and encephalitis with intralesional Gram-negative bacilli.
- Culture of affected tissues (particularly spleen, anterior kidney, liver, and brain) or blood is often successful. Routine media works well, usually at ~25–30°C (77–86°F).
- Biochemical tests (e.g. API 20E) can be used for tentative identification.
- PCR tests are available commercially and offer higher sensitivity; sequencing is required for confirmation.
- FA and ELISA may be available.

Husbandry Management
- General husbandry management is described under C4: *Bacterial Diseases (General).*
- Consider slowly taking the water temperature out of the permissive range of 22–28°C (72–82°F), if possible.
- In catfish aquaculture, food is often reduced or withheld for 3–28 days to reduce fecal shedding of the bacteria. This is typically started immediately after identification of infection or when water temperature reaches >22°C (72°F). Withholding food can reduce mortality and antibiotic use, but does reduce growth rates, increase the risk of columnaris, and has welfare implications.

Medical Management
- Common treatments (see Chapters A12 and A13 for more details):
  - Antibiotic therapy is indicated if water temperature is likely to remain in the permissive range for weeks. Antibiotic resistance is common and choice should be based on culture and sensitivity results.
  - Sulfadimethoxine and ormetoprim (Romet® TC) orally is approved in the United States for catfish with *E. ictaluri* at 50 mg/kg every 24 hours for five days, with a three-day withdrawal, as of 2020.
  - Florfenicol (Aquaflor®) orally is approved in the United States for catfish with *E. ictaluri* at 10–15 mg/kg every 24 hours for 10 days, with a 15-day withdrawal, as of 2020.
- All legislation regarding medication use and disposal must be followed.

Prevention
- General preventative measures are described under C4: *Bacterial Diseases (General).*
- Effective commercial immersion vaccines are available.
- Immune-stimulants, such as beta glucans, can increase resistance to *E. ictaluri*. They are most effective at specific doses, short courses, and when given prior to infection.

Zoonotic Reports
- This disease has no known zoonotic potential.
- A different *Edwardsiella* sp. (*E. hoshinae*) is reported in mammals.

Bibliography

Buján, N., Toranzo, A.E., and Magariños, B. (2018). *Edwardsiella piscicida*: a significant bacterial pathogen of cultured fish. *Diseases of Aquatic Organisms* 131: 59–71.

Gaunt, P.S., Chatakondi, N., Gao, D., and Endris, R. (2015). Efficacy of florfenicol for control of mortality associated with *Edwardsiella ictaluri* in three species of catfish. *Journal of Aquatic Animal Health* 27: 45–49.

Hawke, J.P., Kent, M., Rogge, M. et al. (2013). Edwardsiellosis caused by *Edwardsiella ictaluri* in laboratory populations of zebrafish, *Danio rerio*. *Journal of Aquatic Animal Health* 25: 171–183.

Mainous, M.E., Smith, S.A., and Kuhn, D.D. (2010). Effect of common aquaculture chemicals against *Edwardsiella ictaluri* and *E. tarda*. *Journal of Aquatic Animal Health* 22: 224–228.

Nagai, T., Iwamoto, E., Sakai, T. et al. (2008). Characterization of *Edwardsiella ictaluri* isolated from wild ayu *Plecoglossus altivelus* in Japan. *Fish Pathology* 43: 158–163.

Soto, E., Griffin, M., Arauz, M. et al. (2012). *Edwardsiella ictaluri* as the causative agent of mortality in cultured Nile Tilapia. *Journal of Aquatic Animal Health* 24: 81–90.

Wise, D.J., Greenway, T., Li, M.H. et al. (2008). Effects of variable periods of food deprivation on the development of enteric septicemia in channel catfish. *Journal of Aquatic Animal Health* 20: 39–44.

Abbreviations/Acronyms

- API: Analytical profile index
- ELISA: Enzyme linked immunosorbent assay
- FA: Fluorescent antibody
- PCR: Polymerase chain reaction

Edwardsiellosis

Overview

- *Edwardsiella tarda*, *Edwardsiella piscicida*, and *Edwardsiella anguillarum* are enteric bacteria that can cause bacterial septicemia known as edwardsiellosis.
- All bony fish seem susceptible.
- The response may be suppurative and in catfish, the disease is also known as emphysematous putrefactive disease.
- Clinical management is similar for all three species.

Etiology

- Family *Enterobacteriaceae.*
- *Edwardsiella tarda* was the original causative agent of edwardsiellosis.
- *Edwardsiella piscicida* and *E. piscicida*-like bacteria have been identified since 2013. Molecular diagnostics have shown that some infections previously reported as *E. tarda* were more likely *E. piscicida*.
- *Edwardsiella anguillarum* was first identified in 2015.
- Differentiation between the species requires molecular diagnostics.
- These are small, straight, Gram-negative bacilli that may be motile and are facultative anaerobes.

Transmission

- Transmission is typically oral.
- The bacteria are also found in invertebrates, amphibians, reptiles, and mammals, including humans; their role in transmission is unknown.

Geographic Distribution

- Ubiquitous in freshwater and saltwater habitats, probably worldwide.

Signalment

- Disease is likely possible in many marine and freshwater fish.
- Epizootics have been reported in several species in aquaculture, including eels (*Anguilla* spp.), tilapia (*Oreochromis* spp.), red seabream (*Pagrus major*), striped bass (*Morone saxatilis*), largemouth bass (*Micropterus salmoides*), channel catfish (*Ictalurus punctatus*), Amur catfish (*Silurus asotus*), olive flounder (*Paralichthys olivaceus*), and turbot (*Scophthalmus maximus*).
- Infection is common in marine aquarium teleosts but there are fewer reports in the literature.
- There is one report of disease in an elasmobranch: a round ribbontail ray (*Taeniura meyeni*).

Risk Factors

- General risk factors are described under C4: *Bacterial Diseases (General).*

Signs/Clinical Findings

- Individual or multiple fish from one or more species may be affected.
- Clinical course may be acute or chronic; chronic is more common.
- Lethargy, spiral swimming, or positive buoyancy may be seen.
- Inappetence or reduced feeding may be seen.
- Erythema, petechiae, ecchymoses, skin ulcers, fin erosions, or loss of color are common. Some species, particularly catfish, may show skin abscesses or fistulas.
- Gill pallor due to anemia may be seen.
- Coelomic distension and cloacal/anal distension may be seen.
- Keratitis, uveitis, hypopyon, or exophthalmos may be seen.
- Mortality is usually low and chronic.

Differential Diagnoses

- Full differentials are described in Section B.
- Common differentials for bacterial septicemia include vibriosis, *Aeromonas*, *Citrobacter*, *Pseudomonas*,

Edwardsiella, *Flavobacterium*, *Yersinia*, *Streptococcus*, and *Francisella* spp.

Diagnosis

- Diagnosis to genus is typically based on signs, cytology, histology, and culture.
- Small, straight, Gram-negative bacilli may be seen on blood smears, effusions, tissue cytology, or histology. They may be motile on wet mounts.
- Necropsy or coeliotomy may show petechiae, congestion, serosanguinous coelomic effusion, tissue pallor, organomegaly, or nodules in any tissues. Malodorous abscesses may be found in the viscera or skeletal muscle, particularly in catfish.
- Histology typically shows suppurative inflammation, but it may be granulomatous. Intralesional Gram-negative bacilli are common.
- Culture of affected tissues (particularly kidney and spleen) or blood is often successful. Routine media works well, typically at ~30–35°C (86–95°F).
- FA can be used to highlight *Edwardsiella* sp. on histology or impression smears.
- PCR, qPCR, ELISA, LAMP assays, and sequencing may be available, but should be used in conjunction with other diagnostics.

Husbandry Management

- General husbandry management is described under C4: *Bacterial Diseases (General)*.

Medical Management

- Common treatments (see Chapters A12 and A13 for more details):
  - Antibiotics are usually indicated and should be based on culture and sensitivity.
  - In vitro testing usually shows a wide range of sensitivities, including tetracyclines, aminoglycosides, and fluoroquinolones. Resistance to macrolides and lincosamides is common.
- All legislation regarding medication use and disposal must be followed.

Prevention

- General preventative measures are described under C4: *Bacterial Diseases (General)*.
- Autogenous vaccines can help with recurrent outbreaks; commercial vaccines are unlikely because of antigenic diversity.
- Immune-stimulants, such as beta glucans, allicin, and propolis, can increase resistance to edwardsiellosis. They are most effective at specific doses, short courses, and when given prior to infection.

Zoonotic Reports

- *E. tarda* is zoonotic, although human disease is rare.
- Transmission is typically oral through ingestion of raw or inadequately cooked or processed fish. Gastroenteritis is the most common sequela, with several days of nausea, vomiting, diarrhea, and pyrexia.
- Inoculation into wounds is possible and can result in local wound infection with abscessation and necrosis.
- Septicemia and meningitis are rare sequelae.
- Humans can be asymptomatic carriers.

Bibliography

Abayneh, T., Colquhoun, D.J., and Sorum, H. (2012). *Edwardsiella piscicida* sp. nov., a novel species pathogenic to fish. *Journal of Applied Microbiology* 114: 644–654.

Camus, A., Dill, J., McDermott, A. et al. (2016). *Edwardsiella piscicida*-associated septicaemia in a blotched fantail stingray *Taeniura meyeni* (Müeller and Henle). *Journal of Fish Disease* 39: 1125–1131.

Fogelson, S.B., Petty, B.D., Reichley, S.R. et al. (2016). Histologic and molecular characterization of *Edwardsiella piscicida* infection in largemouth bass (*Micropterus salmoides*). *Journal of Veterinary Diagnostic Investigation* 28: 338–344.

Griffin, M.J., Quiniou, S.M., Cody, T. et al. (2013). Comparative analysis of *Edwardsiella* isolates from fish in the eastern United States identifies two distinct genetic taxa amongst organisms phenotypically classified as *E. tarda*. *Veterinary Microbiology* 165: 358–372.

Mainous, M.E., Smith, S.A., and Kuhn, D.D. (2010). Effect of common aquaculture chemicals against *Edwardsiella ictaluri* and *E. tarda*. *Journal of Aquatic Animal Health* 22: 224–228.

Reichley, S.R., Ware, C., Greenway, T.E. et al. (2015). Real-time polymerase chain reaction assays for the detection and quantification of *Edwardsiella tarda*, *Edwardsiella piscicida*, and *Edwardsiella piscicida*-like species in catfish tissues and pond water. *Journal of Veterinary Diagnostic Investigation* 27: 130–139.

Shao, S., Lai, Q., Wu, H. et al. (2015). Phylogenomics characterization of a highly virulent *Edwardsiella* strain ET080813(T) encoding two distinct T2SS and three T6SS gene clusters: propose a novel species as *Edwardsiella anguillarum* sp. nov. *Systematic and Applied Microbiology* 38: 36–47.

Stock, I. and Widemann, B. (2001). Natural antibiotic susceptibilities of *Edwardsiella tarda*, *E. ictaluri*, and *E. hoshinae*. *Antimicrobial Agents and Chemotherapy* 45: 2245–2255.

Abbreviations/Acronyms

- ELISA: Enzyme linked immunosorbent assay
- FA: Fluorescent antibody
- LAMP: Loop-mediated isothermal amplification
- PCR: Polymerase chain reaction
- qPCR: Quantitative polymerase chain reaction

Columnaris and Flexibacteriosis

Overview

- *Flavobacterium columnare* is the causative agent of columnaris disease, sometimes known as saddle-back or peduncle disease.
- Columnaris is particularly common in freshwater ponds.
- Lesions are typically on the skin, fins, and gills, but the infection can become systemic.
- The marine counterpart is *Tenacibaculum maritimum*. Lesions are similar but systemic spread is less common.

Etiology

- Family *Flavobacteriaceae.*
- *Flavobacterium* (*Flexibacter*, *Bacillus*, *Cytophaga*) *columnare* is the cause of columnaris in freshwater fish.
- *Tenacibaculum* (*Flexibacter*, *Cytophaga*) *maritimum* (*marina*, *marinus*, *marimus*) is the cause of marine flexibacteriosis.
- These are motile, long, thin Gram-negative bacilli.

Transmission

- Horizontal transmission is common, through ingestion, contact, or inoculation.
- The bacteria are highly contagious.
- Data on survival in the environment varies from days to months depending on the conditions.
  - Survival of columnaris is increased in warm, hard, alkaline freshwater, and high organic loads. Water temperature of <5°C (<41°F) reduces survival.
  - Columnaris may be a component of the biofilm, which can provide protection for the bacteria.

Geographic Distribution

- *F. columnare* is ubiquitous in freshwater habitats worldwide.
- *T. maritimum* is ubiquitous in salt water habitats worldwide.

Signalment

- Columnaris is likely possible in all freshwater bony fish.
  - In aquariums and ornamental aquaculture, it is particularly common in goldfish (*Carassius auratus*), common carp and koi (*Cyprinus carpio*), mollies and guppies (*Poecilia* spp.), swordtails and platies (*Xiphophorus* spp.).
  - In food fish aquaculture, it is particularly common in channel catfish (*Ictalurus punctatus*), tilapia (*Oreochromis* spp.), sockeye salmon (*Oncorhynchus nerka*), and rainbow trout (*Oncorhynchus mykiss*).
- Marine flexibacteriosis is likely possible in all marine teleosts.
  - It is particularly common in several cultured food fish, including marine-reared Atlantic salmon (*Salmo salar*), barramundi (*Lates calcifer*), gilthead seabream (*Sparus auratus*), European bass (*Dicentrarchus labrax*), yellowtail amberjack (*Seriola lalandi*), olive flounder (*Paralichthys olivaceus*), and turbot (*Scophthalmus maximus*).
- Marine flexibacteriosis has also been identified in elasmobranchs under human care, including skates (*Rajidae*) and a sand tiger shark (*Carcharias taurus*).

Risk Factors

- General risk factors are described under C4: *Bacterial Diseases (General).*
- Permissive water temperature is usually high (e.g. >15°C or 59°F, with morbidity and mortality highest at 24–32°C or 75–90°F), but is low for salmonid winter ulcer disease (e.g. <8°C or 46°F).
- High nitrite, alkalinity, hardness, and calcium are known risk factors.

Signs/Clinical Findings

- Individual or multiple fish from one or more species may be affected.
- An acute presentation may be seen, particularly in young fish.
  - Mortalities may be seen with no other signs.
  - Yellow-white or dark brown discoloration of the gills, particularly at the distal aspect of the primary lamellae, may be seen.
  - Dyspnea and tachypnea often develop.
  - Pruritus may be seen.

- A chronic presentation is more common.
  - Inappetence or reduced feeding is common.
  - Lesions on the skin, fins, and oral cavity are common. Multifocal skin pallor develops into ulcers covered with white or yellow cotton-like mucus plaques. Lesions often have a hyperemic, yellow, or white rim (Figure C4.2a). Skeletal muscle may be exposed.
  - Fin lesions often start at the base of the fin and progress distally, unlike typical bacterial fin rot.
  - Pruritus may be seen.
  - Edema, diffuse pallor, or darkening of the gills may be seen.
- Mortality is variable, but morbidity can be high.

Differential Diagnoses
- Full differentials are described in Section B.
- Common differentials for ulcers and mucus plaques on the skin of bony fish include oomycetes and scuticociliates, although a variety of skin pathogens and irritants can cause similar lesions.

Diagnosis
- Diagnosis is typically based on direct microscopy of skin scrapes or gill biopsies.
- Long (2–10 μm), thin, Gram-negative bacterial bacilli are seen, often grouped together in "haystacks" (Figure C4.2b and c). These show a slow, gliding and flexing motion on wet mounts.
- Wet mounts also often show increased mucus, opportunist pathogens (e.g. scuticociliates), gill hyperplasia and fusion of secondary filaments.
- Histology typically shows necrotizing, ulcerative dermatitis or branchitis with intralesional long, thin Gram-negative bacilli. Columnaris can become systemic with bacteremia and renomegaly. Marine flexibacteriosis rarely becomes systemic.
- Culture is possible, often collected from the edge of active lesions. However, contaminants are common with external cultures and the organisms are fastidious and inhibited by the high-nutrient content of routine media. Columnaris grows best with low-nutrient media (e.g. Shieh, Cytophaga, Hsu–Shotts), often at 25–30°C (77–86°F). Marine flexibacteriosis benefits from additional sodium chloride. Sensitivities can be problematic as the organisms do not grow well in Mueller–Hinton agar and other methodologies are needed (e.g. Gieseker et al. 2012).
- PCR and qPCR tests on gill, skin, or cranial kidney are available and provide specific, sensitive, and faster results than culture.
- LAMP from gills, skin, or cranial kidneys is used commonly in channel catfish.

Husbandry Management
- General husbandry management is described under C4: *Bacterial Diseases (General)*.
- Resolving environmental stressors can result in significant improvement.
- Slowly reduce the water temperature to <24°C (<75°F) and ideally <15°C (<59°F), if possible.
- In freshwater, consider low-dose hypersalinity treatment to reduce physiologic stress (e.g. 2–3 g/L).

Medical Management
- Common treatments (see Chapters A12 and A13 for more details):
  - Antibiotic therapy can improve morbidity and mortality but elimination is unlikely. Drug choice should be based on culture and sensitivity, but difficulties getting sensitivities mean that empirical therapy is common.
  - Florfenicol (Aquaflor®) orally is approved in the United States for freshwater-reared finfish with columnaris at 10–15 mg/kg every 24 hours for 10 days, with a 15-day withdrawal, as of 2020.
  - Oxytetracycline dihydrate (Terramycin® 200) orally is approved in the United States for freshwater-reared rainbow trout with columnaris at 83 mg/kg every 24 hours for 10 days, with a 21-day withdrawal, as of 2020.
  - Other antibiotics used in aquarium fish include enrofloxacin and trimethoprim sulfamethoxazole immersion.
  - Chloramine-T (HALAMID Aqua®) immersion is approved in the United States for walleye (*Sander vitreus*) and freshwater-reared salmonids and warm-water finfish with external columnaris under various treatment protocols, with a 0-day withdrawal, as of 2020.
  - Hydrogen peroxide (35% Perox-Aid®) immersion is approved in the United States for use in freshwater-reared cool-water and warm-water finfish with external columnaris at 50–75 mg/L for one hour every 48 hours for three treatments, with a 0-day withdrawal, as of 2020.
  - Potassium permanganate ($KMnO_4$) immersion treatment at 2 mg/L above the permanganate demand has been effective.
- Other reported treatments (see Chapters A12 and A13 for more details):
  - Oxolinic acid immersion.
  - Copper sulfate immersion.
- All legislation regarding medication use and disposal must be followed.

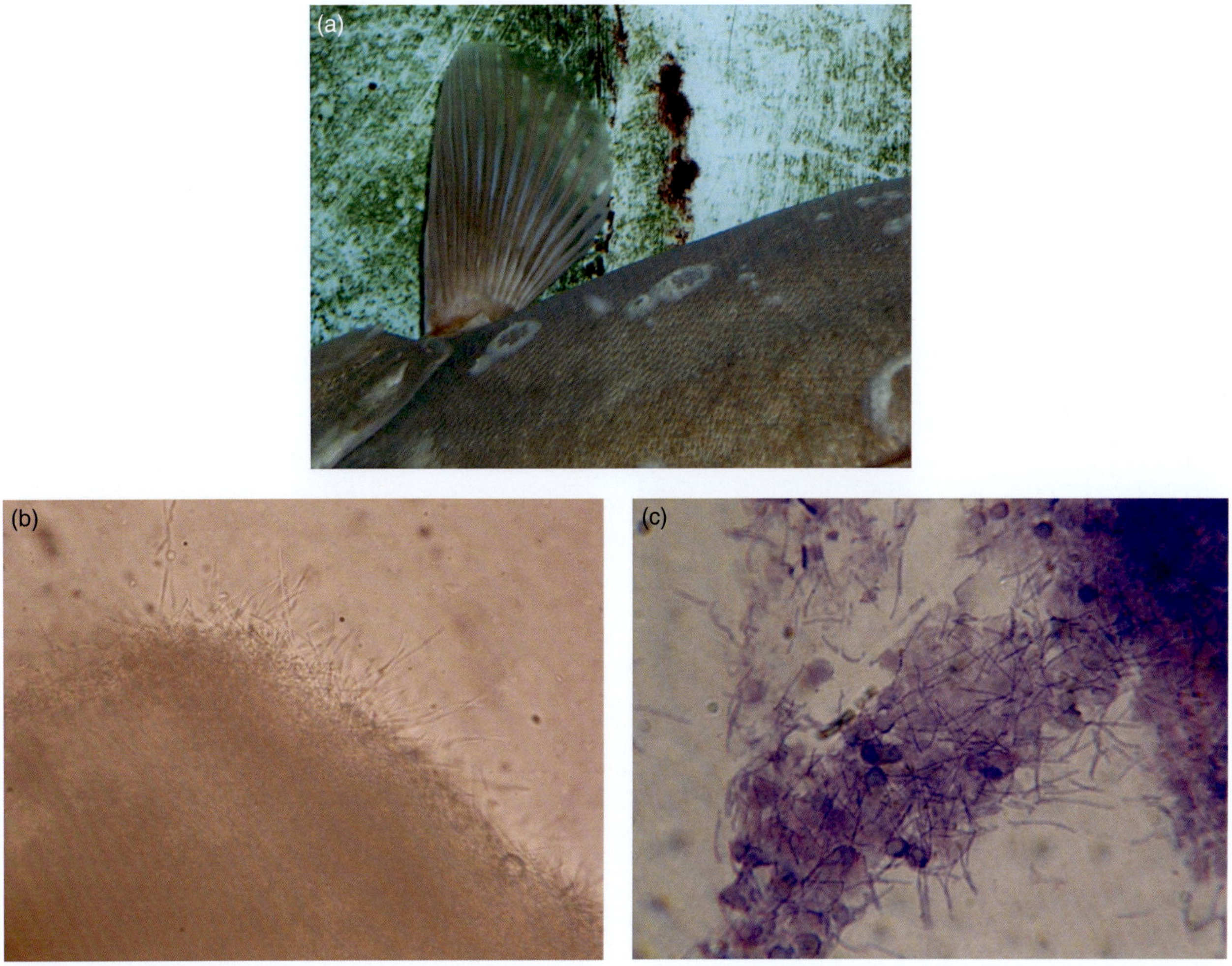

Figure C4.2 Gross appearance of columnaris lesions on a grouper (*Epinephelus* sp.) (a) and typical haystack structures on skin scrapes examined as a wet mount (b) and on Dif-Quik stain (c).

Prevention

- General preventative measures are described under C4: *Bacterial Diseases (General)*.
- High salinity (>5 g/L) and low hardness (<70 mg/L) reduce columnaris survival.
- Vaccination studies have shown variable success. A USDA-approved attenuated immersion vaccine is available for channel catfish.

Zoonotic Reports

- This disease has no known zoonotic potential.

Bibliography

Cai, W., De La Fuente, L., and Arisas, C.R. (2013). Biofilm formation by the fish pathogen *Flavobacterium columnare*: development and parameters affecting surface attachment. *Applied and Environmental Microbiology* 79: 5633–5642.

Declerq, A.M., Haesebrouck, F., den Broech, W.V. et al. (2013). Columnaris disease in fish: a review with emphasis on bacterium-host interactions. *Veterinary Research* 44: 27–44.

Farmer, B.D., Mitchell, A.J., and Straus, D.L. (2011). The effect of high total ammonia concentration on the survival of channel catfish experimentally infected with *Flavobacterium columnare*. *Journal of Aquatic Animal Health* 23: 162–168.

Florio, D., Gridelli, S., Fioravanti, M.L., and Zanoni, R.G. (2016). First isolation of *Tenacibaculum maritimum* in a captive sand tiger shark (*Carcharias taurus*). *Journal of Zoo and Wildlife Medicine* 47: 351–353.

Gaunt, P.S., Gao, D., Sun, F., and Endris, R. (2010). Efficacy of florfenicol for control of mortality caused by

Flavobacterium columnare infection in channel catfish. *Journal of Aquatic Animal Health* 22: 115–122.

Gieseker, C.M., Mayer, T.D., Crosby, T.C. et al. (2012). Quality control ranges for testing broth microdilution susceptibility of *Flavobacterium columnare* and *F. psychrophilum* to nine antimicrobials. *Diseases of Aquatic Organisms* 101: 207–215.

Thomas-Jinu, S. and Goodwin, A.E. (2004). Acute columnaris infection in channel catfish, *Ictalurus punctatus* (Rafinesque): efficacy of practical treatments for warmwater aquaculture ponds. *Journal of Fish Disease* 27: 23–28.

Abbreviations/Acronyms

- IM: Intramuscular
- LAMP: Loop-mediated isothermal amplification
- PCR: Polymerase chain reaction
- qPCR: Quantitative polymerase chain reaction
- PO: Orally
- USDA: United States Department of Agriculture

Flavobacterium psychrophilum

Overview

- *Flavobacterium psychrophilum* causes two serious diseases of salmonids.
- Bacterial cold-water disease (BCWD) is also known as peduncle or saddle-back disease and is typically seen in salmonid adults and fingerlings.
- Rainbow trout fry syndrome (RTFS) is also known as fry anemia syndrome and is typically seen in salmonid fry.
- Disease is seen when water temperature falls below 15°C (59°F).
- The diseases continue to be a significant problem in salmonid aquaculture and restocking programs.

Etiology

- Family *Flavobacteriaceae*.
- The causative agent is *Flavobacterium* (*Cytophaga*, *Flexibacter*) *psychrophilum*.
- These are motile, long, thin Gram-negative bacilli.

Transmission

- Horizontal and vertical transmission are reported.
- The bacteria are found in water and soil, as well as within the biofilm, which can provide protection for the bacteria.

Geographic Distribution

- Cold freshwater habitats.
- BCWD was first reported in the United States and RTFS was first reported in Europe, but they are now widespread.

Signalment

- Freshwater teleosts in cold-water only.
- This is a common problem in freshwater salmonids, particularly rainbow trout (*Oncorhynchus mykiss*) and coho salmon (*Oncorhynchus kisutch*).
  - BCWD is more common in adults and fingerlings.
  - RTFS is more common in fry.
- The disease has also been reported from other teleosts, including European eels (*Anguilla anguilla*), tench (*Tinca tinca*), common carp (*Cyprinus carpio*), Crucian carp (*Carassius carassius*), and ayu (*Plecoglossus altivelis*).

Risk Factors

- General risk factors are described under C4: *Bacterial Diseases (General)*.
- Permissive water temperature is usually low, e.g. 3–15°C (37–59°F).

Signs/Clinical Findings

- Multiple conspecifics are usually affected.
- In both BCWD and RTFS, lethargy, inappetence, reduced feeding, or gradual weight loss may be seen. Coelomic distension and cloacal/anal distension may be seen. Bilateral exophthalmos or gill pallor may be seen.
- BCWD:
  - Skin darkening and large cutaneous ulcers and erosions, particularly around the dorsal fins, are common. Erosions can be deep enough to expose vertebrae.
  - Mortality can reach 70–90%.
- RTFS:
  - Skin darkening or asymmetrical coloration may be seen, with the right and left side varying in color.
  - Neurologic signs are possible, particularly abnormal position in the water and spiral swimming.
  - Mortality is usually low.
- Chronic spinal deformities may be seen in survivors.

Differential Diagnoses

- Full differentials are described in Section B.
- Common differentials for skin ulcers in salmonids with long thin bacterial rods include *Flavobacterium columnare* and *F. psychrophilum*.

Diagnosis

- A tentative diagnosis is often possible from direct microscopy of skin scrapes or gill biopsies.
- Long (~2–6 μm), thin, Gram-negative bacilli may be seen on skin or gill samples; the bacilli are shorter than *F. columnare*. They are motile on wet mounts.
- Necropsy or coeliotomy may show splenomegaly, serosanguinous coelomic effusion, and tissue pallor.
- Histology typically shows pyogranulomatous inflammation and necrosis extending into muscle, bone, and cartilage with intralesional Gram-negative bacilli, particularly in the spleen, heart, gills, muscle, bone, and cartilage.
- Diagnosis is usually confirmed by PCR.
- Culture from blood or tissues (e.g. spleen, kidney) is possible, but the organisms are fastidious and inhibited by the high-nutrient content of routine media. Growth usually requires low-nutrient media (e.g. tryptone yeast extract salts), often at ~15–16°C (59–61°F).
- ELISA and FA tests have been developed for screening salmonid broodstock using kidney and ovarian tissues.

Husbandry Management

- General husbandry management is described under C4: *Bacterial Diseases (General).*
- Environmental management alone can resolve morbidity and mortality.
- Slowly increase the water temperature, if possible. Clinical signs will typically resolve as temperature increases.
- Consider transferring fish to systems that have been cleaned and disinfected with sodium hypochlorite (e.g. 100 mg/L chlorine for one hour followed by sodium thiosulfate).
- Increase cleaning and disinfection; while *F. psychrophilum* is susceptible to most routine disinfectants, it is slightly less sensitive than *F. columnare.*

Medical Management

- Medical management has poor success due to reduced appetites limiting intake of oral medications and immune suppression at lower water temperatures.
- Common treatments (see Chapters A12 and A13 for more details):
  - Antibiotic therapy may be indicated and should be based on culture and sensitivity results.
  - Florfenicol (Aquaflor®) orally is approved in the United States for freshwater-reared salmonids with BCWD at 10–15 mg/kg every 24 hours for 10 days, with a 15-day withdrawal, as of 2020.
  - Oxytetracycline dihydrate (Terramycin® 200) orally is approved in the United States for freshwater-reared salmonids with BCWD at 83 mg/kg every 24 hours for 10 days, with a 21-day withdrawal, as of 2020.
- Other reported treatments (see Chapters A12 and A13 for more details):
  - Oxytetracycline immersion.
  - Potassium permanganate immersion.
  - Copper sulfate immersion.
  - Chloramine-T immersion.
- All legislation regarding medication use and disposal must be followed.

Prevention

- General preventative measures are described under C4: *Bacterial Diseases (General).*
- Broodstock should be screened using diagnostic assays (e.g. ELISA).
- Disinfection of eggs (e.g. with iodophors) can reduce vertical transmission, but high doses may be needed.
- Experimental vaccines are reported but success has been inconsistent.

Zoonotic Reports

- This disease has no known zoonotic potential.

Bibliography

Bebak, J.A., Welch, T.J., Starliper, C.E. et al. (2007). Improved husbandry to control an outbreak of rainbow trout fry syndrome caused by infection with *Flavobacterium psychrophilum*. *Journal of the American Veterinary Medical Association* 231: 114–116.

Lindstrom, N.M., Call, D.R., House, M.L. et al. (2008). A quantitative enzyme-linked immunosorbent assay and filtration-based fluorescent antibiotic test as potential tools to screen broodstock for infection with *Flavobacterium psychrophylum*. *Journal of Aquatic Animal Health* 21: 43–56.

Mainous, M.E., Kuhn, D.D., and Smith, S.A. (2012). Efficacy of common aquaculture compounds for disinfection of *Flavobacterium columnare* and *F. psychrophilum*. *Journal of Applied Aquaculture* 24: 262–270.

Oplinger, R.W. and Wagner, E. (2010). Disinfection of contaminated equipment: evaluation of benzalkonium chloride exposure time and solution age and the ability of air-drying to eliminate *Flavobacterium psychrophilum*. *Journal of Aquatic Animal Health* 22: 248–253.

Oplinger, R.W. and Wagner, E.J. (2012). Effects of media ingredient substitution and comparison of growth of *Flavobacterium psychrophilum* among four media. *Journal of Aquatic Animal Health* 24: 49–57.

Starliper, C.E. (2011). Bacterial coldwater disease of fishes caused by *Flavobacterium psychrophilum*. *Journal of Advanced Research* 2: 97–108.

Abbreviations/Acronyms

- BCWD: Bacterial cold water disease
- ELISA: Enzyme linked immunosorbent assay
- FA: Fluorescent antibody
- PCR: Polymerase chain reaction
- RTFS: Rainbow trout fry syndrome

Yersiniosis

Overview

- *Yersinia ruckeri* can cause hemorrhagic septicemia known as yersiniosis or enteric red mouth.
- It is an obligate pathogen of freshwater salmonids and has caused significant losses in aquaculture.

Etiology

- Family *Enterobacteriaceae*.
- The causative agent is *Yersinia ruckeri*.
- It was originally identified as a *Salmonella* sp.
- It is genetically similar to *Salmonella* spp., *Yersinia enterocolitis*, and *Yersinia pseudotuberculosis*.
- Several serotypes and biotypes exist. Serotypes are more relevant to virulence than biotypes. Serotype O1a is the cause of most epizootics.
- These are short, straight, Gram-negative bacilli that are usually motile.

Transmission

- Horizontal transmission is reported, predominantly feco-oral but waterborne transmission via the gills may also occur.
- There is some evidence of vertical transmission.
- The bacteria can survive for at least 4 mo outside the host, particularly within the biofilm, which can provide protection for the bacteria.
- Carriers include fathead minnows (*Pimephales promelas*). Fish that resolve clinical signs continue to shed the bacteria for up to 2 mo.
- *Y. ruckeri* is also found in aquatic invertebrates, reptiles, birds, and mammals, and these may be vectors.

Geographic Distribution

- Predominantly in freshwater habitats, probably worldwide.

Signalment

- Freshwater teleosts are most susceptible, particularly salmonids in aquaculture such as rainbow trout (*Oncorhynchus mykiss*) and Atlantic salmon (*Salmo salar*).
- *Y. ruckeri* has been isolated from other freshwater fish, including goldfish (*Carassius auratus*), common carp and koi (*Cyprinus carpio*), eels (*Anguilla* spp.), channel catfish (*Ictalurus punctatus*), and turbot (*Scophthalmus maximus*).

Risk Factors

- General risk factors are described under C4: *Bacterial Diseases (General)*.
- Permissive water temperature is often 20–28°C (68–82°F).

Signs/Clinical Findings

- Multiple conspecifics are usually affected.
- Clinical course is usually acute presentation, particularly in juveniles. A more chronic course is seen in adults.
- Lethargy or swimming near the surface may be seen.
- Inappetence or reduced feeding may be seen.
- Petechiae, erythema, or hemorrhages are common, particularly in and around the oral cavity and eyes. This often progresses to severe oral ulceration.
- Skin darkening may be seen.
- Hyphema, keratitis, and exophthalmos (unilateral or bilateral) may be seen; fish may appear to be blind.
- Gill edema or pallor may be seen.
- Coelomic distension and cloacal/anal distension may be seen.
- Mortality rate is usually low, but cumulative losses can be high.

Differential Diagnoses

- Full differentials are described in Section B.
- Common differentials for bacterial septicemia include vibriosis, *Aeromonas*, *Citrobacter*, *Pseudomonas*, *Edwardsiella*, *Flavobacterium*, *Yersinia*, *Streptococcus*, and *Francisella* spp.

Diagnosis

- Diagnosis is typically based on clinical signs in susceptible species and culture results.

- Short (1–3 μm), straight, Gram-negative bacilli may be seen on blood smears, effusions, tissue cytology, or histology. They are typically motile on wet mounts.
- Necropsy or coeliotomy and histology typically show petechiae, congestion, yellow to serosanguinous coelomic effusion, tissue pallor, splenomegaly, with intralesional Gram-negative bacilli. Enteritis with intestines filled with thick, yellow fluid may be seen.
- Culture of affected tissues (particularly kidney in acutely sick fish and intestines in carriers) is often successful. Routine or selective media (e.g. Shotts–Waltman) can be used, often at ~20–28°C (68–82°F).
- PCR, RFLP, ELISA, FA, and LAMP tests may be available on blood, fecal, or tissue samples.

Husbandry Management

- General husbandry management is described under C4: *Bacterial Diseases (General).*

Medical Management

- Common treatments (see Chapters A12 and A13 for more details):
  - Antibiotic therapy is usually indicated and should be based on culture and sensitivity results.
  - Commonly used antibiotics include oxytetracycline, potentiated sulfonamides, and florfenicol.
- All legislation regarding medication use and disposal must be followed.

Prevention

- General preventative measures are described under C4: *Bacterial Diseases (General).*
- Restrict access by birds and mammals as they may act as vectors.
- A USDA-approved, monovalent vaccine is available for biotype 1 in rainbow trout and usually provides good protection, but outbreaks of biotype 2 remain possible. Bivalent vaccines are less commonly available.
- Autogenous vaccines may be considered.

Zoonotic Reports

- This disease has no known zoonotic potential.
- The *Yersinia* sp. that causes plague (*Y. pestis*) has not been identified in fish.
- The *Yersinia* spp. that cause yersiniosis in humans (*Y. enterocolitica* and *Y. pseudotuberculosis*) have not been identified in fish.

Bibliography

Ghosh, B., Nguyen, T.D., Crosbie, P.B.B. et al. (2016). Oral vaccination of first-feeding Atlantic salmon, *Salmo salar* L., confers greater protection against yersiniosis than immersion vaccination. *Vaccine* 34: 599–608.

Kumar, G., Menanteau-Ledouble, S., Saleh, M., and El-Matbouli, M. (2015). *Yersinia ruckeri*, the causative agent of enteric redmouth disease in fish. *Veterinary Research* 46: 103–113.

Meinelt, T., Phan, T.-M., Behrens, S. et al. (2015). Growth inhibition of *Aeromonas salmonicida* and *Yersinia ruckeri* by disinfectants containing peracetic acid. *Diseases of Aquatic Organisms* 113: 207–213.

Abbreviations/Acronyms

- ELISA: Enzyme linked immunosorbent assay
- FA: Fluorescent antibody
- LAMP: Loop-mediated isothermal amplification
- PCR: Polymerase chain reaction
- RFLP: Restriction fragment length polymorphism
- USDA: United States Department of Agriculture

Streptococcosis

Overview

- *Streptococcus* spp. are emerging pathogens of bony fish, often causing meningoencephalitis, panophthalmitis, and septicemia.
- They are one of the few Gram-positive bacterial infections of fish.
- They are a common cause of epizootics in wild and cultured fish.

Etiology

- Family *Streptococcaceae.*
- Two streptococcal species are most commonly reported to cause disease in fish:
  - *S. agalactiae* (also known as group B *Streptococcus*, GBS, and very similar to *Streptococcus difficilis*); there are several serotypes and biotypes.
  - *S. iniae.*
- Several other streptococcal species have been reported to cause disease in fish and may be increasing in importance.
  - *S. dysgalactiae.*

- S. ictaluri.
- S. milleri.
- S. parauberis.

- These are aerobic Gram-positive cocci.

Transmission

- Transmission is typically horizontal through ingestion and contact.
- The bacteria survive well in organics and suspended solids.
- Feed can remain a source of infection after >6 mo of freezing.

Geographic Distribution

- Predominantly in saltwater and brackish water habitats, probably worldwide.

Signalment

- Disease is reported from marine, brackish, and freshwater fish, particularly teleosts.
- The majority of reports are from cultured fish including tilapia (*Oreochromis* spp.), striped bass and hybrids (*Morone saxatilis*), gilthead seabream (*Sparus auratus*), golden shiners (*Notemigonus crysoleucas*), coho salmon (*Oncorhynchus kisutch*), rainbow trout (*Oncorhynchus mykiss*), sea trout (*Cynoscion nebulosus*), mullet (*Mugilidae*), sturgeon (*Acipenseridae*), yellowtail (*Seriola quinqueradiata*), pinfish (*Lagodon rhomboides*), rabbitfish (*Siganidae*), bluefish (*Pomatomus saltatrix*), zebrafish (*Danio rerio*), olive flounder (*Paralichthys olivaceus*), barramundi (*Lates calcarifer*), golden pompano (*Trachinotus ovatus*), and channel catfish (*Ictalurus punctatus*, although some reports suggest this species can be resistant).
- Reports from aquarium fish are less common. They include red-tail black sharks (*Epalzeorhynchos bicolor*), rainbow sharks (*Epalzeorhynchos erythrurus*), rosy barbs (*Pethia conchonius*), tetras (*Characidae*), and cichlids (*Cichlidae*).
- Reports from elasmobranchs are rare. They include stingrays (*Hypanus* spp.), mangrove whiprays (*Himantura granulata*), and shovelnose rays (*Glaucostegus* and *Aptychotrema* spp.).
- Epizootics have been reported in wild teleosts, including Queensland grouper (*Epinephelus lanceolatus*), striped bass (*Morone saxatilis*), and Caribbean reef fish.
- Common carp and koi (*Cyprinus carpio*) and goldfish (*Carassius auratus*) may be resistant.

Risk Factors

- General risk factors are described under C4: *Bacterial Diseases (General)*.

Signs/Clinical Findings

- Individual or multiple fish from one or more species may be affected.
- Clinical course may be acute or chronic.
- Spiraling, circling, or erratic swimming, and loss of buoyancy are common signs as the bacteria tend to localize in the central nervous system. Fish may lose their flight response.
- Reduced appetite or weight loss may be seen.
- Darkening of the skin, petechiae, erythema (particularly on the ventrum and fin bases), skin ulcers, or fin erosions may be seen. There may be abscess-like swellings, particularly along the peduncle.
- Exophthalmos (unilateral or bilateral), periocular and periorbital hemorrhage, corneal hypopyon, or corneal opacity may be seen.
- Coelomic distension due to ascites may be seen.
- Spinal deformities may be seen.
- Poor reproductive success may be seen.
- Acute mortalities are common, usually in a few days. Mortality is usually low (<10%), but may reach 50–70%. Large-scale epizootics have been reported for *S. iniae*.
- Signs can be cyclic.

Differential Diagnoses

- Full differentials are described in Section B.
- Differentials for Gram-positive bacterial cocci in fish include *Streptococcus*, *Vagococcus*, *Enterococcus*, and *Lactococcus* spp.

Diagnosis

- Diagnosis is typically based on a combination of cytology, histology, and culture.
- Gram-positive cocci that form chains may be seen on blood smears, effusions, cerebrospinal fluid, tissue cytology, or histology (Figure C4.3).
- Necropsy or coeliotomy may show petechiae, congestion, serosanguinous coelomic effusion, and organomegaly.
- Histology typically shows granulocytic, pyogranulomatous, or granulomatous inflammation in the central nervous system, vertebrae, and eyes. Meningoencephalitis, panophthalmitis, and septicemia are common. There are usually abundant intralesional Gram-positive cocci that form long chains. *S. ictaluri* in channel catfish is unusual in that it does not show tropism for the central nervous system and causes epidermal necrosis, myositis, and arthritis.
- Culture of affected tissue (particularly brain or kidney) or blood can be done on routine or selective media (e.g. Todd Hewitt or thallium acetate).
- Sequencing is required for definitive identification.

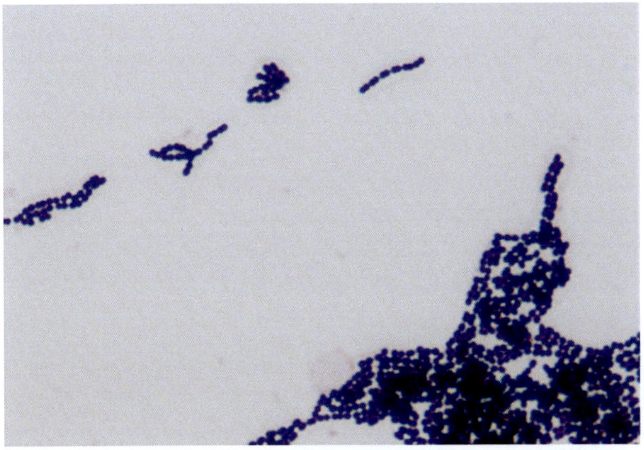

Figure C4.3 Typical appearance of *Streptococcus* spp. on Gram stain showing chains of Gram-positive cocci. *Source*: Image courtesy of Jill Arnold, National Aquarium.

Husbandry Management

- General husbandry management is described under C4: *Bacterial Diseases (General)*.

Medical Management

- Common treatments (see Chapters A12 and A13 for more details):
  - Antibiotic therapy is usually indicated and should be based on culture and sensitivity results.
  - Florfenicol (Aquaflor®) orally is approved in the United States for freshwater-reared warm-water finfish with *S. iniae* at 10–15 mg/kg every 24 hours for 10 days, with a 15-day withdrawal, as of 2020.
  - Other commonly used antibiotics include erythromycin, enrofloxacin, oxytetracycline, ampicillin, and amoxicillin.
- All legislation regarding medication use and disposal must be followed.

Prevention

- General preventative measures are described under C4: *Bacterial Diseases (General)*.
- Experimental vaccines have been challenging because of the rapid emergence of new strains. Autogenous vaccines show the most promise.

Zoonotic Reports

- Many *S. agalactiae* and *S. iniae* strains are zoonotic and can be associated with neonatal septicemia, pneumonia, and meningitis in humans. However, fish strains of these bacteria are different from the typical human isolates.
- Zoonotic transmission from fish has been reported rarely. Cases have been associated with processing infected tilapia, likely via inoculation through a wound. Cellulitis, endocarditis, and arthritis developed. All reported cases resolved.
- The *Streptococcus* spp. that cause strep throat, scarlet fever, impetigo, and pneumococcal disease have not been identified in fish.

Bibliography

Bowater, R.O., Forbes-Faulkner, J., Anderson, I.G. et al. (2012). Natural outbreak of *Streptococcus agalactiae* (GBS) infections in wild giant Queensland grouper, *Epinephelus lanceolatus* (Bloch), and other wild fish in northern Queensland, Australia. *Journal of Fish Diseases* 35: 173–186.

Bowker, J.E., Ostland, V.E., Carty, D., and Bowman, M.P. (2010). Effectiveness of Aquaflor (50% florfenicol) to control mortality associated with *Streptococcus iniae* in freshwater-reared subadult sunshine bass. *Journal of Aquatic Animal Health* 22: 254–265.

Camus, A.C., Shewmaker, P.L., Mauel, M.J., and Wise, D.J. (2008). *Streptococcus ictaluri* arthritis, osteolysis, myositis, and spinal meningitis in channel catfish broodstock. *Journal of Aquatic Animal Health* 20: 54–62.

Darwish, A.M. (2007). Laboratory efficacy of florfenicol against *Streptococcus iniae* infection in sunshine bass. *American Fisheries Society* 19: 1–7.

Gaunt, P.S., Endris, R., McGinnis, A. et al. (2010). Determination of florfenicol dose rate in feed for control of mortality in Nile tilapia infected with *Streptoccus iniae*. *Journal of Aquatic Animal Health* 22: 158–166.

Keirstead, N.D., Brake, J.W., Griffin, M.J. et al. (2014). Fatal septicemia caused by the zoonotic bacterium *Streptococcus iniae* during an outbreak in Caribbean reef fish. *Veterinary Pathology* 51: 1035–1041.

Liu, G., Zhu, J., Chen, K. et al. (2016). Development of *Streptococcus agalactiae* vaccines for tilapia. *Diseases of Aquatic Organisms* 122: 163–170.

Renibacterium salmoninarum

Overview

- *Renibacterium salmoninarum* is the cause of bacterial kidney disease (BKD) in salmonids.
- BKD is a slowly progressive, systemic disease that has been reported from wild and cultured salmonids.

- Typical pathology consists of granulomatous renomegaly with Gram-positive diplobacilli.
- It is a significant concern for salmonid culture and restoration projects.
- Medical treatment is rarely effective.

Etiology

- Family *Micrococcaceae.*
- The causative agent is *Renibacterium salmoninarum*, an obligate pathogen.
- These are nonmotile, small, Gram-positive diplobacilli that are facultatively intracellular.

Transmission

- Horizontal and vertical transmission are reported.
- The bacteria survive for up to a few weeks in the environment.
- Asymptomatic carriers are common.
- Transmission to and from wild and cultured fish is likely.

Geographic Distribution

- Freshwater and saltwater salmonid habitats, probably worldwide.

Signalment

- BKD infects freshwater and marine salmonids.
- Pacific salmonid species are the most susceptible, such as coho salmon (*Oncorhynchus kisutch*), Chinook salmon (*Oncorhynchus tshawytscha*), sockeye salmon (*Oncorhynchus nerka*), brook trout (*Salvelinus fontinalis*), brown trout (*Salmo trutta*), and Arctic char (*Salvelinus alpinus*).
- Disease is most likely in fish <6–12 months of age.

Risk Factors

- General risk factors are described under C4: *Bacterial Diseases (General).*
- Permissive water temperature is usually low, with signs seen in fall and winter.
- Recent transfer to salt water and spawning are known risk factors.

Signs/Clinical Findings

- BKD is usually a chronic disease that is slowly progressive.
- Multiple salmonids are usually affected.
- Lethargy is common.
- Poor growth rates are common.
- Coelomic distension is common.
- Darkening of the skin, petechiae, erythema, ulcers, or pustules along the lateral line, often known as spawning rash, may be seen.
- Exophthalmos may be seen.
- Mortality rate is typically low but chronic, sporadic mortalities tend to continue.

Differential Diagnoses

- Full differentials are described in Section B.
- Common differentials for bacterial granulomatous inflammation in salmonids include *Renibacterium salmoninarum*, *Flavobacterium psychrophilum*, *Mycobacterium*, *Nocardia*, *Streptococcus*, *Francisella*, *Photobacterium* spp., and piscirickettsial-like organisms.
- Differentials for Gram-positive bacterial rods in fish include *Mycobacterium* and *Lactobacillus* spp.

Diagnosis

- Diagnosis is typically based on gross necropsy in susceptible species and molecular diagnostics.
- Small (1–2 μm), Gram-positive diplobacilli may be seen on blood smears, effusions, tissue cytology, or histology (Figure C4.4). They are nonmotile on wet mounts. The bacteria stain positively with periodic acid–Schiff.
- Necropsy findings usually include renomegaly with granulomas (Figure C4.4). Granulomas may also be present in the spleen, liver, and heart. Serosanguinous ascites and pseudodiphtheritic serosal membranes may be present. Cavernous lesions in the skeletal muscle adjacent to the kidney may be seen.
- Culture from tissues (particularly kidney) is possible, but the organisms are fastidious, requiring kidney disease media with cysteine and growth is slow, taking several weeks. Media may need antibiotics and antifungals to prevent overgrowth.
- Nested PCR has a high sensitivity and is a common test outside of hatcheries.
- Standard ELISAs are used commonly to screen broodstock in hatcheries, although quantitative ELISAs have a higher sensitivity and specificity. Samples are usually serum, ovarian fluid, or kidney supernatant.
- FA tests can show organisms on kidney slides.
- LAMP may provide a faster, simpler, cheap test with a similar sensitivity to nested PCR.
- The disease may be reportable to national, regional, or local agencies (as of 2020, it is not notifiable to the OIE).

Husbandry Management

- Control measures may be dictated by national, regional, or local agencies to prevent spread.
- Consider culling of fish with clinical signs to reduce further transmission, as medical management often shows limited success.

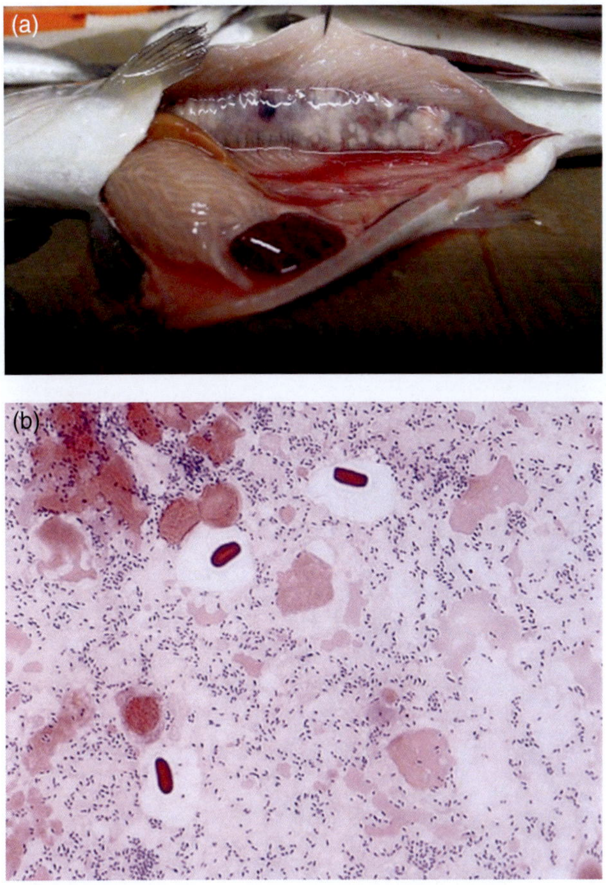

Figure C4.4 Severe granulomatous renomegaly due to bacterial kidney disease (a) and Gram stain of a kidney impression smear showing abundant Gram-positive bacilli at x1000 (b). *Source*: Images courtesy of Aimee Reed, Oregon Department of Fish and Wildlife, Fish Health Services.

Medical Management

- Common treatments (see Chapters A12 and A13 for more details):
  - Antibiotic therapy may reduce morbidity and mortality if early in the disease process, but signs often recur after treatment. Choice should be based on culture and sensitivity results.
  - Macrolide antibiotics are commonly used, particularly erythromycin.
- All legislation regarding medication use and disposal must be followed.

Prevention

- General preventative measures are described under C4: *Bacterial Diseases (General)*.
- Good biosecurity has been shown to reduce prevalence in aquaculture, including isolation from other farms, all-in-all-out management, and separation of generations.
- Regular examination of broodstock is helpful, so that fish with clinical signs can be excluded from breeding.
- ELISAs on ovarian fluid in broodstock prior to breeding allows affected fish to be excluded.
- Erythromycin injection of females pre-spawning can reduce vertical transmission.
- Erythromycin immersion treatment of eggs can reduce transmission.
- Experimental live vaccines have shown some promise.

Zoonotic Reports

- This disease has no known zoonotic potential.

Bibliography

Faisal, M. and Eissa, A.E. (2009). Diagnostic testing patterns of *Renibacterium salmoninarum* in spawning salmonid stock. *Journal of Wildlife Diseases* 45: 447–456.

Faisal, M., Schulz, C., Eissa, A. et al. (2012). Epidemiological investigation of *Renibacterium salmoninarum* in Michigan from 2001 to 2010. *Preventative Veterinary Medicine* 107: 260–274.

Purcell, M.K., McKibben, C.L., Pearman-Gillman, S. et al. (2016). Effects of temperature on *Renibacterium salmoninarum* infection and transmission potential in chinook salmon *Oncorhynchus tshawytscha* (Walbaum). *Journal of Fish Diseases* 39: 787–798.

Saleh, M., Soliman, H., and El-Matbouoli, M. (2008). Loop-mediated isothermal amplification (LAMP) for rapid detection of *Renibacterium salmoninarum*, the causative agent of bacterial kidney disease. *Diseases of Aquatic Organisms* 81: 143–151.

Abbreviations/Acronyms

- BKD: Bacterial kidney disease
- ELISA: Enzyme linked immunosorbent assay
- FA: Fluorescent antibody
- LAMP: Loop-mediated isothermal amplification
- OIE: World Organisation for Animal Health
- PCR: Polymerase chain reaction

Mycobacteriosis

Overview

- Mycobacteriosis is a common chronic disease of teleosts.
- It is caused by non-tuberculous mycobacteria (NTM), particularly *Mycobacterium fortuitum*, *Mycobacterium marinum*, and *Mycobacterium chelonae*. These are ubiquitous bacteria, common in water and biofilms.
- Almost all fish are susceptible, particularly *Cichlidae*, *Syngnathidae*, and *Cyprinidae*.
- Lesions are usually granulomatous. The acid-fast bacteria are readily identified on cytology and histology.
- Identification to species level is not essential, but can be helpful if control options, antigenic variation, or zoonotic potential need to be assessed.
- Medical treatment is rarely effective.

Etiology

- Family *Mycobacteriaceae*.
- These are NTM, also known as atypical mycobacteria. This is an important differentiation from the tuberculous mycobacteria such as *Mycobacterium tuberculosis* and *Mycobacterium bovis*.
- Species classification changes rapidly, and new genera are being proposed. The three predominant *Mycobacterium* spp. remain:
  - *M. fortuitum*, typically in freshwater.
  - *M. marinum*, typically in salt water but also in freshwater; this may include isolates previously reported as *M. piscium*.
  - *M. chelonae*, particularly in zebrafish (*Danio rerio*).
- Less commonly reported mycobacterial species:
  - *M. abscessus* (previously *M. chelonae* subsp. *abscessus*).
  - *M. avium*; identified on rare occasions in fish.
  - *M. gordonae* (previously *M. aquae*).
  - *M. haemophilum*, particularly in zebrafish.
  - *M. hippocampi* novel sp., in seahorses (*Hippocampus* spp.).
  - *M. montefiorense*, particularly in moray eels (*Gymnothorax* spp.) and rockfish (*Sebastes* spp.).
  - *M. neoaurum*.
  - *M. peregrinum*.
  - *M. poriferae*.
  - *M. pseudoshottsii*, particularly in striped bass (*Morone saxatilis*).
  - *M. salmoniphilum*, particularly in marine salmonids (*Salmonidae*).
  - *M. shottsii*, particularly in striped bass.
  - *M. simiae*.
  - *M. triplex*.
- These are nonmotile, acid-fast positive, non-spore forming, pleomorphic and often beaded bacilli. They may take up Gram stain.
- They are aerobic, facultatively intracellular, and slow-growing.

Transmission

- Transmission is typically horizontal, often through ingestion (e.g. from live prey such as rotifers, unpasteurized dead prey, scavenging, picking at the biofilm). Other routes include inoculation and immersion.
- Vertical transmission can occur but does not seem to be common.
- NTM are frequently found in water, sediment, and biofilms.
- NTM are common in amphibians and reptiles and these may act as carriers or vectors.
- NTM are occasionally reported from invertebrates.
- Fomites may carry NTM, including sterilized medical equipment.

Geographic Distribution

- Ubiquitous in freshwater and saltwater habitats, probably worldwide.

Signalment

- Mycobacteriosis is reported from a wide range of fish (>180 spp.).
- It is common in teleosts, with some species and groups appearing to be particularly susceptible.
  - Bettas and gouramis (*Anabantidae*).
  - Sunfish (*Centrarchidae*).
  - Tetras (*Characidae*).
  - Cichlids (*Cichlidae*).
  - Zebrafish (*Danio rerio*), goldfish (*Carassius auratus*), and other cyprinids (*Cyprinidae*).
  - Cod (*Gadus morhua*).
  - Striped bass (*Morone saxatilis*).
  - Flatfish (*Pleuronectiformes*).
  - Yellowtail (*Seriola quinqueradiata*).
  - Rabbitfish (*Siganus rivulatus*).
  - Seahorses, pipefish, and seadragons (*Syngnathidae*).
- Some teleosts seem relatively resistant to clinical disease, such as catfish (*Siluriformes*).
- Mycobacteriosis is rare in elasmobranchs. It has been limited to individual animals under long-term human care, including an Atlantic guitarfish (*Rhinobatos lentiginosus*), an epaulette shark (*Hemiscyllium ocellatum*), and a yellow stingray (*Urobatis jamaicensis*).
- Disease is more common in adult and geriatric fish.

Risk Factors

- General risk factors are described under C4: *Bacterial Diseases (General)*.
- Permissive water temperature is often high (e.g. 28–30°C (82–86°F) for *M. marinum*).
- Low pH, high humic and fulvic acids, and contaminants (e.g. zinc, iron) are known risk factors.

Signs/Clinical Findings

- Fish are often asymptomatic.
- Where disease is seen, it is usually chronic (weeks, months, or years following infection) and progressive, although an acute presentation is possible.
- Inappetence, reduced appetite, weight loss, or poor growth rates are common.
- Lethargy, abnormal swimming, or abnormal buoyancy may be seen.
- Pigment changes (hyper- and hypopigmentation), petechiae, skin ulcers, scale loss, cutaneous nodules, or firm or soft cutaneous masses with possible exudate may be seen (Figure C4.5a).
- Coelomic distension may be seen.
- Exophthalmos, or less commonly enophthalmos, may be seen.
- Spinal deformities may be seen.
- Chronically low fecundity or poor breeding success may be seen.
- Mortalities are typically sporadic, but epizootics are possible.

Differential Diagnoses

- Full differentials are described in Section B.
- Common differentials from granulomatous dermatitis include *Mycobacterium* spp., *Nocardia* spp., *Renibacterium salmoninarum*, *Exophiala* spp., and *Mesomycetozoea*.
- Common differentials for granulomatous inflammation associated with acid-fast positive structures include *Mycobacterium* spp., *Nocardia* spp., myxozoans, and *Cryptosporidium* spp., although stain artifacts should also be considered.

Diagnosis

- Presumptive diagnosis is usually based on granulomas with acid-fast beaded bacilli on cytology or histology. Definitive diagnosis requires culture and PCR.
- Variable length (1–10 μm), beaded bacilli may be seen on blood smears, effusions, scrapes from lesions, tissue cytology, or histology, but staining depends on species and growth phase. They are Gram-positive but do not stain reliably. On Romanowsky (e.g. Diff-Quik) and Gram stains, they often take up no stain ("ghosting"). Acid-fast stains (e.g. Ziehl–Neelsen, Kinyoun, Fite) show pink to red beaded rods. Sensitivity of cytology is often higher than culture.
- Necropsy or coeliotomy and histology typically show organomegaly, granulomas, congestion, and necrosis (particularly the liver, spleen, kidney, and gonads) with intralesional acid-fast bacilli (Figure C4.5b–d). If bacilli are only found within the gastrointestinal tract, they may be transient. In rare cases, granulomas are not seen and a more acute inflammatory response is noted. 10% formalin, Bouin's, and Dietrich's fixatives do not affect cytology outcome, but Cal-Ex decalcifier may cause false negatives.
- Diagnostic imaging may show organomegaly particularly splenomegaly, hepatomegaly, renomegaly, or large gonads. Mineralization is rare.
- Culture is possible using some routine media, but selective media is often preferred (e.g. Lowenstein–Jensen, Middlebrook 7H10, Mitchison 7H11). Homogenization of tissues facilitates recovery. The growth rate and ease of culture vary significantly by species. Some (e.g. *M. chelonae*, *M. fortuitum*, *M. abscessus*) have a short generation time, while others require months to grow in culture (e.g. *M. marinum*, *M. haemophilum*, *M. pseudoshottsii*).
- PCR or nested PCR is recommended for slow-growing species and should be followed by sequencing for species identification.
- Mycolic acid or fatty acid profiles can be used for species identification.
- RFLP shows inconsistent results. PCR-RFLP (also known as terminal-RFLP) can provide more reliable identification.

Husbandry Management

- The best way to reduce morbidity and mortality is to minimize exposure and stressors.
- Minimize environmental stressors.
- Consider reducing the water temperature to reduce morbidity and mortality from *M. marinum*.
- Consider culling of fish with clinical signs to reduce further transmission.
- With virulent strains or to protect valuable collections, isolate affected systems. Consider depopulation and disinfection. If done, all substrate and filter media must be disposed of and the biofilm must be removed. Biosecurity must be strict to prevent reintroduction of virulent strains. Reintroduction of some strains via fish or water will happen.
- Increase cleaning and disinfection, with thorough mechanical cleaning to remove any organic material. In vitro testing has shown some effect from:
  - Heat (e.g. reports of >60–121°C or 140–250°F).
  - Sunlight.
  - Chlorine at >500 mg/L for 30 minutes.

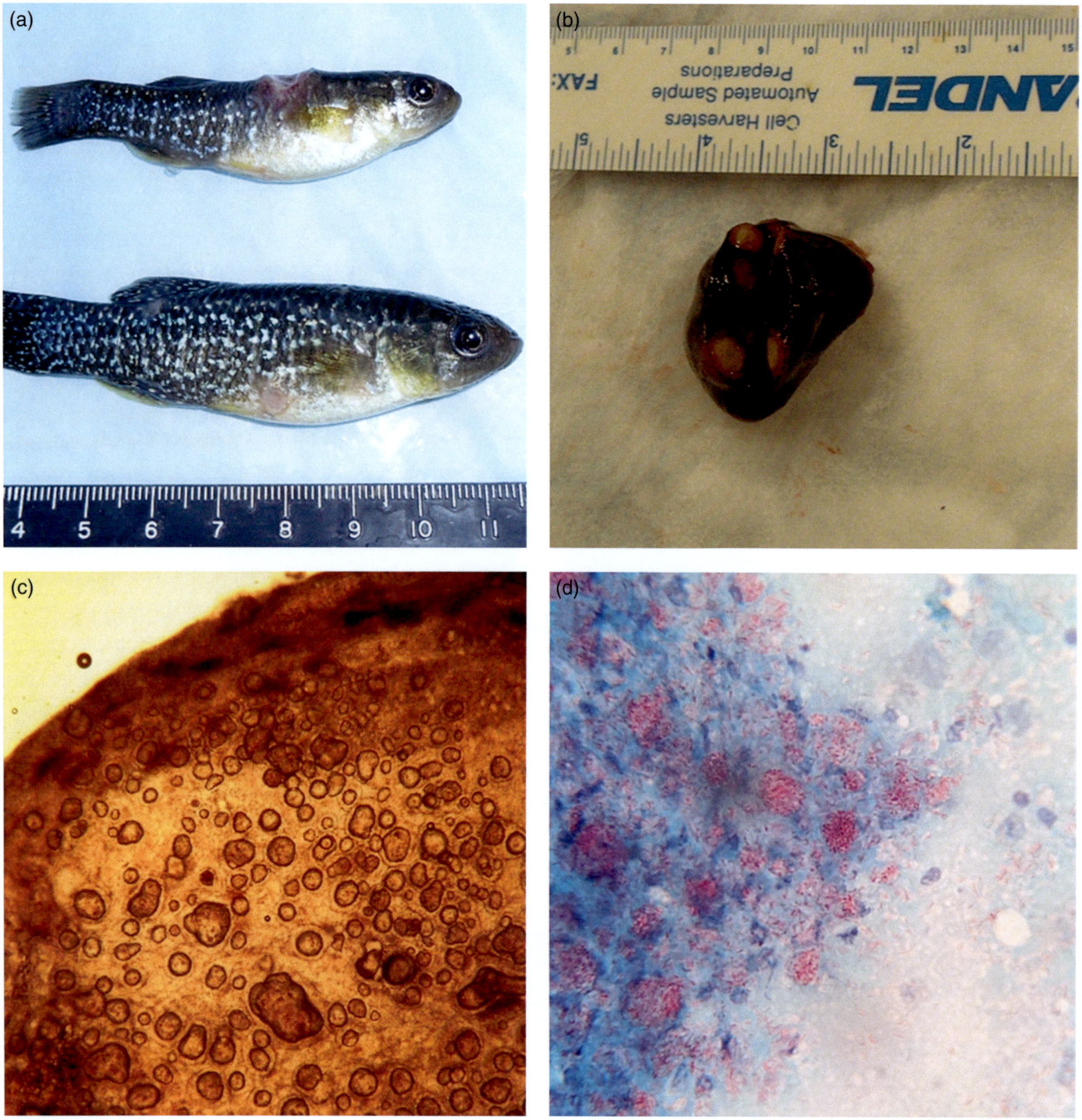

Figure C4.5 Mycobacterial lesions: cutaneous ulceration in mummichogs (*Fundulus* sp.) (a), granulomas visible grossly on a spleen (b), granulomas on a liver wet mount (c), and acid-fast positive beaded bacilli on a tissue impression smear at x400 (d).

 - Phenols (e.g. benzyl-4-chlorophenol/phenylphenol (Lysol) 1% for one minute).
 - Ethyl alcohol 70% for one minute.
 - UV disinfection with high applied doses (e.g. >90 mJ/cm^2).
- No effective disinfection has been seen from ammonium chloride, peroxymonosulfate, or freezing.

Medical Management

- Reported treatments (see Chapters A12 and A13 for more details):
 - Medical treatment is rarely recommended due to the poor response and risk of resistance.
 - If antibiotic therapy is pursued (e.g. for valuable genetic stock), it should be based on culture and sensitivity results.

  - Reported antibiotics include azithromycin, kanamycin, tobramycin, and amikacin.
  - Medications routinely used for human treatment of mycobacterial diseases should be avoided, including isoniazid, rifampin, and clarithromycin.
  - Multidrug therapy is more likely to be helpful than single-drug therapy.
- All legislation regarding medication use and disposal must be followed.

Prevention

- General preventative measures are described under C4: *Bacterial Diseases (General).*
- Routine monitoring should include acid-fast staining at necropsy and histology.
- Pasteurization of fish feeds can reduce transmission.
- Elderly fish should not be used as broodstock.
- Sentinel programs are used in zebrafish colonies to monitor for virulent strains.
- Routine disinfection of eggs and larvae is used in zebrafish colonies.
- No commercial vaccines are available. Experimental live attenuated vaccines (including BCG) and DNA vaccines given by ICe or IM injection can provide some protection. Killed vaccines have shown no effect.

Zoonotic Reports

- About one-third of NTM are zoonotic.
- The fish NTM that is most commonly zoonotic is probably *M. marinum*. It is usually transmitted by inoculation into wounds. The typical presentation is a nonhealing skin lesion on an extremity. The lesion may include papules, nodules, plaques, or exudate. Lesions may progress slowly over months.
- Systemic infections are possible with NTM species that can tolerate higher temperatures (e.g. *M. fortuitum*, *M. gordonae*), usually in immune-suppressed individuals. These cases may be fatal.
- Gloves should be worn when working with high-risk fish or systems. It is essential to avoid contamination of wounds.
- Immune-suppressed individuals should not work with high-risk fish or systems.
- There are extremely rare reports of fish infection with *M. avium* complex and *M. ulcerans*. Human infections with these bacteria are possible, but are much more likely from other sources.
- *Mycobacterium* spp. within the tuberculous complex (e.g. *M. tuberculosis* and *M. leprae*) have not been identified in fish.

Bibliography

Babb, J., Bradley, C., and Friase, A. (1997). Glutaraldehyde-resistant *Mycobacterium chelonae* from endoscope washer disinfectors. *Journal of Applied Microbiology* 82: 519–526.

Balcázar, J.L., Planas, M., and Pintado, J. (2011). Novel *Mycobacterium* species in seahorses with tail rot. *Emerging Infectious Diseases* 17: 1770–1772.

Chang, C.T. and Whipps, C.M. (2015). Activity of antibiotics against *Mycobacterium* species commonly found in laboratory zebrafish. *Journal of Aquatic Animal Health* 27: 88–95.

Chang, C.T., Lewis, J., and Whipps, C.M. (2018). Source or sink: examining the role of biofilms in transmission of *Mycobacterium* spp. in laboratory zebrafish. *Zebrafish* 16: 197–206.

Clarke, E.O., Dorn, B., Boone, A. et al. (2013). Mycobacteriosis, *Mycobacterium chelonae*, in a captive yellow stingray (*Urobatis jamaicensis*). *Journal of Zoo and Wildlife Medicine* 44: 470–474.

Cui, Z., Samuel-Shaker, D., Watral, V., and Kent, M.L. (2010). Attenuated *Mycobacterium marinum* protects zebrafish against mycobacteriosis. *Journal of Fish Diseases* 33: 371–375.

Grimm, C., Huntsberger, C., Markey, K. et al. (2016). Identification of a *Mycobacterium* sp. as the causative agent of orange nodular lesions in the Atlantic sea scallop *Placopecten magellanicus*. *Diseases of Aquatic Organisms* 118: 247–258.

Janse, M. and Kik, M.J.L. (2012). *Mycobacterium avium* granulomas in a captive epaulette shark, *Hemiscyllium ocellatus* (Bonnaterre). *Journal of Fish Diseases* 35: 935–940.

Jeon, S.J., Gonsalves, L.C., Jacobs, J.M. et al. (2011). Short-term infection of striped bass *Morone saxatilis* with *Mycobacterium marinum*. *Diseases of Aquatic Organisms* 94: 117–124.

Kato, G., Kato, K., Saito, K. et al. (2011). Vaccine efficacy of *Mycobacterium bovis* BCG against *Mycobacterium* sp. infection in amberjack *Seriola dumerili*. *Fish and Shellfish Immunology* 30: 467–472.

Mainous, M.E. and Smith, S.A. (2005). Efficacy of common disinfectants against *Mycobacterium marinum*. *Journal of Aquatic Animal Health* 17: 284–288.

Miyamoto, M., Yamaguchi, Y., and Sasatsu, M. (2000). Disinfectant effects of hot water, ultraviolet light, silver ions and chlorine on strains of *Legionella* and nontuberculous *Mycobacteria*. *Microbios* 101: 7–13.

Yanong, R.P.E., Curtis, E.W., Terrell, S.P., and Case, G. (2003). Atypical presentation of mycobacteriosis in a collection of frogfish. *Journal of Zoo and Wildlife Medicine* 34: 400–407.

Abbreviations/Acronyms

- BCG: Bacillus Calmette and Guérin
- ICe: Intracoelomic
- IM: Intramuscular
- NTM: Non-tuberculous mycobacteria
- PCR: Polymerase chain reaction
- RFLP: Restriction fragment length polymorphism
- UV: Ultraviolet

Nocardiosis

Overview

- Nocardiosis is a poorly understood disease in fish.
- It is similar to mycobacteriosis, with a chronic presentation, systemic granulomatous inflammation, and acid-fast positive rods. However, *Nocardia* spp. are long, branching rods that look like fungal hyphae.
- Medical treatment is rarely effective.

Etiology

- Order *Actinomycetales*.
- Family *Nocardiaceace*.
- Several *Nocardia* species cause disease in fish:
  - *N. seriolae* (previously *N. kampachi*) in marine fish.
  - *N. asteroides* in freshwater fish.
  - *N. salmonicida* (previously *Streptomyces salmonicida*).
  - *N. crassostreae* in fish and oysters.
- These are nonmotile, Gram-positive and acid-fast positive, slender, filamentous, branching bacterial rods that are facultatively intracellular.

Transmission

- Transmission is typically horizontal through contact, although ingestion has been reported.
- These are often found in invertebrates, which may act as carriers or vectors. Fish pathogens can cause severe disease in some species such as oysters.

Geographic Distribution

- Ubiquitous in freshwater and saltwater habitats, probably worldwide.

Signalment

- Disease is likely possible in many freshwater and saltwater fish.
- Susceptible aquarium fish include neon tetras (*Paracheirodon innesi*) and seahorses (*Hippocampus* spp.).
- Susceptible cultured fish include salmonids (*Oncorhynchus*, *Salmo*, *Salvelinus* spp.), largemouth bass (*Micropterus salmoides*), Japanese seabass (*Lateolabrax japonicus*), three-striped tiger fish (*Terapon jarbua*), yellow croaker (*Larimichthys crocea*), yellowtail (*Seriola quinqueradiata*), and greater amberjacks (*Seriola dumerili*).

Risk Factors

- General risk factors are described under C4: *Bacterial Diseases (General)*.

Signs/Clinical Findings

- Individual fish are usually affected at one time.
- Lethargy may be seen.
- Inappetence, reduced feeding, or weight loss may be seen.
- Later signs include skin ulcers, nodules, or boils (furuncles).
- Coelomic distension may be seen.
- Mortalities are seen intermittently, but because of the chronic nature, cumulative mortality may reach 30%.

Differential Diagnoses

- Full differentials are described in Section B.
- Common differentials for granulomatous inflammation with hyphae or rod-like structures include mycobacteriosis and systemic fungal disease, although stain artifacts should be considered.

Diagnosis

- Presumptive diagnosis is typically based on cytology and histology, although additional testing is required for species identification.
- Long, thin branching rods that resemble fungal hyphae may be seen on blood smears, scrapes from lesions, or tissue cytology or histology (Figure C4.6). The rods are Gram-positive, but do not take up stain well. The rods are acid-fast positive, with better stain uptake using Fite's stains than Ziehl–Neelsen stains.
- Necropsy or coeliotomy and histology typically show multiple white to yellow nodules due to granulomatous inflammation within the viscera, especially the gills, heart, spleen, liver, kidney, and swim bladder.
- Culture from affected tissues can be successful. *Nocardia* spp. will grow on blood agar, as well as mycobacterial and fungal media (e.g. Sabouraud's).

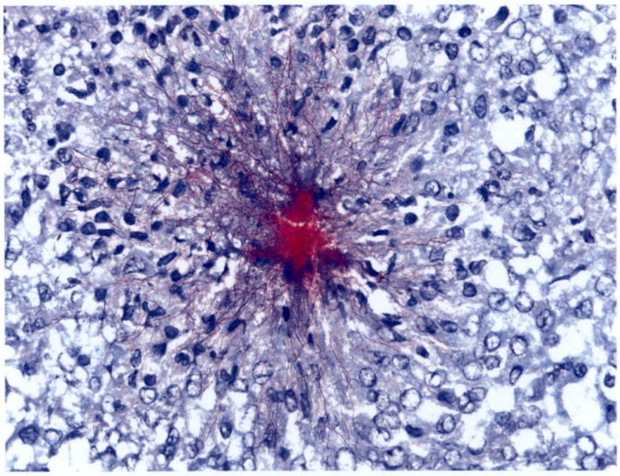

Figure C4.6 Long, branching, acid-fast rods consistent with *Nocardia* sp. on histology of the skeletal muscle of an Atlantic salmon (*Salmo salar*); acid-fast x1000. *Source*: Image courtesy of David Groman, University of Prince Edward Island.

- PCR testing may be available.
- Serological tests are not routinely available.

Husbandry Management

- General husbandry management is described under C4: *Bacterial Diseases (General)*.
- *Nocardia* spp. are relatively resistant to disinfection; benzalkonium chloride is considered most effective.

Medical Management

- Common treatments (see Chapters A12 and A13 for more details):
  - Medical treatment is rarely recommended due to the poor response and risk of resistance.
  - If antibiotic therapy is pursued (e.g. for valuable genetic stock), it should be based on culture and sensitivity results.
  - In vitro, trimethoprim sulfamethoxazole is often effective.
  - Long-term therapy is recommended, ideally for several months.
- All legislation regarding medication use and disposal must be followed.

Prevention

- General preventative measures are described under C4: *Bacterial Diseases (General)*.

Zoonotic Reports

- *N. asteroides* is zoonotic and systemic disease has been reported in humans with immune suppression.
- In humans, nocardiosis is typically transmitted by aerosolization of bacteria in soil, standing water, or decaying plants. It usually presents as a slowly progressive pneumonia with chronic cough. In some cases, endocarditis or encephalitis can develop.
- Inoculation into a wound or surgical site can result in cellulitis or abscessation.
- The CDC estimates that there are 500–1000 new cases in the United States each year.
- The author can find no reports of disease transmission from fish.

Bibliography

Brosnahan, C.L., Humphrey, S., Knowles, G. et al. (2017). Nocardiosis in freshwater reared chinook salmon (*Oncorhynchus tshawytscha*). *New Zealand Veterinary Journal* 65: 214–218.

Dill, J., Sanchez, S., McDermott, A., and Camus, A. (2017). Disseminated nocardiosis associated with the isolation of *Nocardia nova* in a longsnout seahorse *Hippocampus reidi* (Ginsburg). *Journal of Fish Diseases* 40: 1235–1239.

Wang, G.L., Yuan, S.P., and Jin, S. (2009). Nocardiosis in large yellow croaker, *Larimichthys crocea* (Richardson). *Journal of Fish Diseases* 28: 339–345.

Abbreviations/Acronyms

- CDC: Centers for Disease Control and Prevention
- PCR: Polymerase chain reaction

Epitheliocystis

Overview

- Epitheliocystis is an emerging bacterial disease that often infects fish gills.
- The Gram-negative bacilli have been hard to classify. They are considered chlamydia-like, but they may be *Proteobacteria*.
- Pathology is usually identified on histology; lesions are characterized by large hypertrophied cells that look like spherical cysts.
- Morbidity and mortality are rare but have been reported in cultured freshwater and marine fish.

Etiology

- The taxonomy is complicated.
- They were historically grouped within the phylum *Chlamydiae* and reported as chlamydia-like organisms (CLOs).
- Most of the species found in fish are described under the term *Candidatus*, e.g. *Candidatus* Piscichlamydia salmonis, *Candidatus* Clavichlamydia salmonicola, *Candidatus* Renichlamydia lutjani.
- More recent analyses suggest these may instead belong within the phylum *Proteobacteria*. Isolates from elasmobranchs appear to cluster within *Gammaproteobacteria*.
- These are obligate intracellular, Gram-negative bacteria.

Transmission

- Fish CLOs appear to show the typical developmental cycle of *Chlamydiales* with three forms: elemental, reticular, and intermediate bodies.
- Horizontal transmission following rupture of the infected cells seems likely.
- Amoeba and other protists can harbor environmental chlamydiae and it is suspected that fish CLOs may use amoeba as intermediate hosts.

Geographic Distribution

- Their distribution has not been determined.

Signalment

- CLOs have been reported from >90 species of freshwater and marine teleosts, including several cultured species such as Atlantic salmon (*Salmo salar*), brown trout (*Salmo trutta*), Arctic charr (*Salvelinus alpinus*), lake trout (*Salvelinus namaycush*), white sturgeon (*Acipenser transmontanus*), barramundi (*Lates calcarifer*), European bass (*Dicentrarchus labrax*), largemouth bass (*Micropterus salmoides*), yellowtail (*Seriola quinqueradiata*), greater amberjack (*Seriola dumerili*), gilthead seabream (*Sparus aurata*), carp (*Cyprinus carpio*), and pacu (*Piaractus mesopotamicus*).
- CLOs have been reported from aquarium species including leafy sea dragons (*Phycodurus eques*).
- In Atlantic salmon, a CLO is considered a possible etiological agent of proliferative gill inflammation, seen around 3–5 mo after transfer to salt water.
- There have been increasing reports in elasmobranchs including spiny dogfish (*Squalus acanthias*), smooth dogfish (*Mustelus canis*), leopard sharks (*Triakis semifasciata*), spotted eagle rays (*Aetobatus narinari*), and bonnethead sharks (*Sphyrna tiburo*).

Risk Factors

- General risk factors are described under C4: *Bacterial Diseases (General)*.

Signs/Clinical Findings

- Fish are often asymptomatic.
- Individual fish are usually affected.
- Small, white, spherical nodules up to 0.5 mm diameter may be seen on the gills, oral cavity, and skin, often with no other signs.
- Lethargy may be seen.
- Reduced appetite or poor growth rates may be seen.
- Exophthalmos may be seen.
- Abnormal swimming may be seen.
- Skin ulcers may be seen.
- Dyspnea, tachypnea, or bradypnea may be seen.
- Morbidity and mortality are highest in young fish in culture.
- Disease may be cyclic.

Differential Diagnoses

- Full differentials are described in Section B.
- Common differentials for nodules on the gills include herpesviruses, papillomas, granulomatous inflammation, epitheliocystis or other CLOs, *Mesomycetozoea*, microsporidial xenomas (e.g. *Loma* spp.), *Ichthyophthirius multifiliis*, and *Cryptocaryon irritans*.

Diagnosis

- Tentative diagnosis may be based on cytology and histology of the gills or skin (Figure C4.7). Definitive diagnosis requires PCR and sequencing.
- Small bacteria may be seen within cells on cytology or histology; they may be bacilli or cocci and typically stain Gram-negative and Giemsa-positive.
- Histology of epithelial tissue shows large hypertrophied cells that resemble spherical cysts with a single intracytoplasmic, basophilic inclusion or vacuole (10–30 μm) that contains the bacteria. There is usually minimal inflammatory response, but there may be a mild granulocytic or lymphocytic response and local tissue necrosis.
- Culture has been unsuccessful to date. This means that Koch's postulates have not been met and little is known about pathogenesis.
- TEM shows homogeneous bacteria and typical elementary, reticular, and intermediate bodies.
- PCR and sequencing are commonly used.
- ISH and IHC may be available.

Husbandry Management

- General husbandry management is described under C4: *Bacterial Diseases (General)*.

Medical Management

- This may be an incidental finding with no treatment needed.
- Reported treatments (see Chapters A12 and A13 for more details):

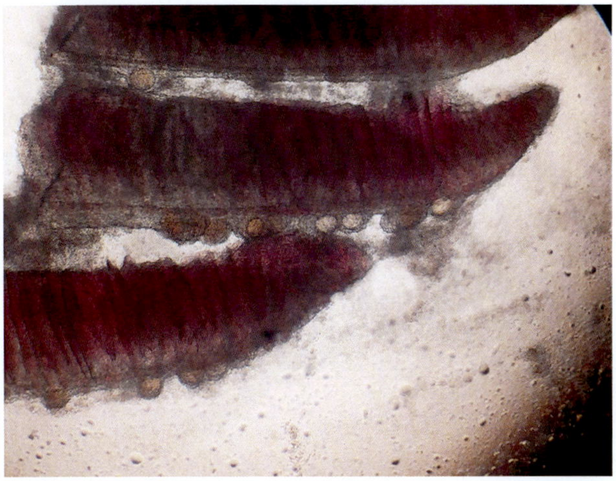

Figure C4.7 Nodules due to epitheliocystis on direct microscopy of a gill biopsy in a yelloweye rockfish (*Sebastes ruberrimus*).

- CLOs are often susceptible to macrolides (e.g. azithromycin) and tetracyclines (e.g. doxycycline, oxytetracycline).
- Oxytetracycline immersion at 25 mg/L every 12 hours for three days in largemouth bass in freshwater raceways resolved clinical signs. This is likely to be less effective in salt water.

- Enrofloxacin has been largely ineffective.
- All legislation regarding medication use and disposal must be followed.

Prevention

- General preventative measures are described under C4: *Bacterial Diseases (General).*

Zoonotic Reports

- There are no reports of zoonotic transmission from fish, but this is an emerging disease and its true status is not known.
- The *Chlamydiales* that commonly infect humans (*Chlamydia trachomatis*, *Chlamydophila pneumoniae*, and *Chlamydia psittaci*) are phylogenetically distinct from the species in fish.

Bibliography

Blandford, M.I., Taylor-Brown, A., Schlacher, T.A. et al. (2018). Epitheliocystis in fish: an emerging aquaculture disease with a global impact. *Transboundary and Emerging Diseases* 65:1436–1446.

Camus, A., Soto, E., Berliner, A. et al. (2013). Epitheliocystis hyperinfection in captive spotted eagle rays *Aetobatus narinari* associated with a novel *Chlamydiales* 16S rDNA signature sequence. *Diseases of Aquatic Organisms* 104: 13–21.

Goodwin, A.E., Park, E., and Nowak, B.F. (2005). Successful treatment of largemouth bass, *Micropterus salmoides* (L.), with epitheliocystis hyperinfection. *Journal Fish Diseases* 28: 623–625.

Goy, G. and Greub, G. (2009). Antibiotic susceptibility of *Waddlia chondrophila* in *Acanthamoeba castellanii* amoebae. *Antimicrobial Agents and Chemotherapy* 53: 2663–2666.

Pawlikowska-Warych, M. and Deptula, W. (2016). Characteristics of chlamydia-like organisms pathogenic to fish. *Journal of Applied Genetics* 57: 135–141.

Polkinghorne, A., Schmidt-Posthaus, H., Meijer, A. et al. (2010). Novel *Chlamydiales* associated with epitheliocystis in a leopard shark *Triakis semifasciata*. *Diseases of Aquatic Organisms* 91: 75–81.

Abbreviations/Acronyms

- CLO: Chlamydia-like organism
- IHC: Immunohistochemistry
- ISH: In situ hybridization
- PCR: Polymerase chain reaction
- TEM: Transmission electron microscopy

Francisellosis

Overview

- *Francisella* species are emerging, global pathogens that can cause septicemia and granulomatous inflammation in multiple fish species.
- *Francisella noatunensis* subsp. *noatunensis* and *Francisella noatunensis* subsp. *chilensis* are reported from cold-water marine teleosts and are serious pathogens of cultured Atlantic cod (*Gadus morhua*).
- *Francisella orientalis* is reported from warm-water teleosts and is a serious pathogen of cultured tilapia (*Oreochromis* spp.).

Etiology

- Family *Francisellaceae.*
- These are piscirickettsial-like organisms (PLOs).
- Taxonomy is debated, but the proposed taxonomy is:

- *Francisella noatunensis* subsp. *noatunensis* (previously *F. philomiragia* subsp. *noatunensis* and *F. piscicida*).
- *Francisella noatunensis* subsp. *chilensis* (previously within *F. noatunensis* subsp. *noatunensis*).
- *Francisella orientalis* (previously *F. noatunensis* subsp. *orientalis*, *F. asiatica*, and *F. victoria*).

- These are nonmotile, small, pleomorphic, Gram-negative and acid-fast negative coccobacilli that are facultatively intracellular and strictly aerobic.

Transmission

- Transmission is typically horizontal, predominantly feco-oral; vertical transmission has not been reported.
- Survival in the environment is reported as days to months. Survival rates seem highest in mud and brackish water.
- Invertebrates such as mussels and crabs may act as vectors.

Geographic Distribution

- *F. noatunensis* in saltwater habitats in Europe and Chile.
- *F. orientalis* in freshwater and saltwater habitats including South, Central, and North America, Southeast Asia, and the United Kingdom.

Signalment

- *F. noatunensis*: Marine teleosts in cold water, particularly Atlantic cod and Atlantic salmon (*Salmo salar*).
- *F. orientalis*: Freshwater, brackish, and marine teleosts in warm water. This is a particular problem for tilapia in aquaculture. It is also reported from ornamental cichlids (*Cichlidae*), striped bass and hybrids (*Morone* spp.), chicken grunts (*Parapristipoma trilineatum*), French and Caesar grunts (*Haemulon* spp.), fairy wrasses (*Cirrhilabrus* spp.), and green chromis (*Chromis viridis*).

Risk Factors

- General risk factors are described under C4: *Bacterial Diseases (General)*.
- Mortalities from *F. orientalis* are higher at 20–28°C (68–82°F).

Signs/Clinical Findings

- Individual or multiple fish from one or more species may be affected.
- Clinical course may be acute or chronic.
- Lethargy may be seen.
- Inappetence, reduced feeding, or poor growth rates may be seen.
- Abnormal swimming (e.g. spiraling or circling) may be seen.
- Erythema, petechiae, or raised hemorrhagic nodules are common. Skin ulcers are less common but may be seen. Dark coloration may be seen.
- Exophthalmos may be seen.
- White gill nodules, hyperplasia, or pallor may be seen.
- The acute form may have a mortality of up to 90% with few clinical signs.
- The chronic form may have a mortality of up to 20%.

Differential Diagnoses

- Full differentials are described in Section B.
- Common differentials for bacterial granulomatous lesions in teleosts include *Mycobacterium*, *Nocardia*, *Edwardsiella*, *Francisella*, *Streptococcus*, *Photobacterium* spp., and other piscirickettsial-like organisms.

Diagnosis

- Diagnosis is difficult and usually relies on consistent signs and molecular testing.
- Small (1.5 μm), Gram-negative coccobacilli may be seen. The bacteria are acid-fast negative and Giemsa-positive. They are nonmotile on wet mounts.
- Necropsy and histology usually show severe splenomegaly and renomegaly with white-tan nodules that consist of granulomas and intracellular bacteria. Adjacent muscle and skin are often affected. Granulomas are rare in the brain. Generalized pallor may be seen. More acute systemic signs may be seen.
- Culture is limited as the organisms are fastidious and need additional cysteine and iron to grow. Specialized media include cysteine heart or Thayer–Martin agar. They can also be grown in cell lines. False negatives are still common due to antibiotic therapy and low bacterial loads. Homogenization of tissues in saline or phosphate buffered saline can improve recovery. A recommended protocol for sensitivity testing is provided by Soto et al. (2016).
- PCR, qPCR, IHC, and ISH tests on fresh spleen or kidney are available experimentally. Sequencing is required to confirm identification.

Husbandry Management

- General husbandry management is described under C4: *Bacterial Diseases (General)*.
- For *F. orientalis*: Slowly increase water temperature if possible; mortalities stop rapidly at >28°C (>82°F).

Medical Management

- Common treatments (see Chapters A12 and A13 for more details):
  - Antibiotic therapy is usually indicated and should be based on culture and sensitivity results, but results are variable.
  - In vitro antibiotic sensitivity has been high for florfenicol and oxolinic acid, variable for oxytetracycline and enrofloxacin, and low for potentiated sulfonamides and erythromycin.
  - Florfenicol orally at 15–20 mg/kg every 24 hours for 10 days reduced mortalities from *F. orientalis* in Nile

tilapia at 25°C (77°F); 10 mg/kg every 24 hours was less effective.

- All legislation regarding medication use and disposal must be followed.

Prevention

- General preventative measures are described under C4: *Bacterial Diseases (General).*

Zoonotic Reports

- These bacteria have no known zoonotic potential, but other *Francisella* spp. do.
- The *Francisella* sp. that causes tularemia (*F. tularensis*) is genetically similar, but has never been identified in fish.

Bibliography

Camus, A.C., Dill, J.A., McDermott, A.J. et al. (2013). *Francisella noatunensis* subsp. *orientalis* infection in Indo-Pacific reef fish entering the United States through the ornamental fish trade. *Journal of Fish Diseases* 36: 681–684.

Dong, H.T., Gangnonngiq, W., Phiwsaiya, K. et al. (2016). Duplex PCR assay and in situ hybridization for detection of *Francisella* spp. and *Francisella noatunensis* subsp. *orientalis* in red tilapia. *Diseases of Aquatic Organisms* 120: 39–47.

Isachsen, C.H., Vagnes, O., Jakobsen, R.A., and Samuelsen, O.B. (2012). Antimicrobial susceptibility of *Francisella noatunensis* subsp. *noatunensis* strains isolated from Atlantic cod *Gadus morhua* in Norway. *Diseases of Aquatic Organisms* 98: 57–62.

Ramirez-Paredes, J.G., Larsson, P., Thompson, K.D. et al. (2020). Reclassification of *Francisella noatunensis* subsp. *orientalis* Ottem et al. 2009 as *Francisella orientalis* sp. nov., *Francisella noatunensis* subsp. *chilensis* subsp. nov. and emended description of *Francisella noatunensis*. *International Journal of Systematic and Evolutionary Microbiology* 73: 2034–2048.

Soto, E., Kidd, S., Gaunt, P.S., and Endris, R. (2013). Efficacy of florfenicol for control of mortality associated with *Franciscella noatunensis* subsp. *orientalis* in Nile tilapia, *Oreochromis niloticus* (L.). *Journal of Fish Diseases* 36: 411–418.

Soto, E., Primus, A.E., Pouder, D.B. et al. (2014). Identification of *Francisella noatunensis* in novel host species French grunt (*Haemulon flavolineatum*) and Caeser grunt (*Haemulon carbonarium*). *Journal of Zoo and Wildlife Medicine* 45: 727–731.

Soto, E., Halliday-Simmonds, I., Francis, S. et al. (2016). Improved broth microdilution method for antimicrobial susceptibility testing of *Francisella noatunensis orientalis*. *Journal of Aquatic Animal Health* 28: 199–207.

Abbreviations/Acronyms

- IHC: Immunohistochemistry
- ISH: In situ hybridization
- PCR: Polymerase chain reaction
- qPCR: Quantitative polymerase chain reaction

Piscirickettsiosis

Overview

- *Piscirickettsia salmonis* causes rickettsial septicemia, also known as piscirickettsiosis and salmon rickettsia syndrome.
- Pacific salmonids in seawater are the most susceptible.
- It is a major concern for salmonid culture and restoration projects in some areas.

Etiology

- Family *Piscirickettsiaceae.*
- These are piscirickettsial-like organisms (PLOs).
- The first species identified in fish was *Piscirickettsia salmonis*. The taxonomy for other species is unclear and this section will focus on *P. salmonis*.
- These are nonmotile, Gram-negative and acid-fast negative pleomorphic coccobacilli that are facultatively intracellular.

Transmission

- Transmission is typically horizontal, through contact with fish or water. Vertical transmission seems uncommon.
- Crustaceans may act as vectors, as with other rickettsials.

Geographic Distribution

- Freshwater and saltwater habitats along the west coast of North America, South America, and Europe. Epidemics have been common in Chile.

Signalment

- *P. salmonis* is reported from coho salmon (*Oncorhynchus kisutch*), pink salmon (*Oncorhynchus gorbuscha*), Chinook salmon (*Oncorhynchus tshawytscha*), rainbow

trout (*Oncorhynchus mykiss*), and Atlantic salmon (*Salmo salar*).
- Other PLOs are reported from a variety of freshwater and marine bony fish.

Risk Factors
- General risk factors are described under C4: *Bacterial Diseases (General).*
- Specific examples for *P. salmonis* include:
  - Transfer to salt water within the previous 6 mo.
  - Season: fall or spring.
  - High prevalence of infected stock within a 7–10 km radius.

Signs/Clinical Findings
- The incubation period is thought to be weeks to months following natural infection.
- Several conspecifics are usually affected.
- Lethargy is common, with fish often seen swimming at the surface or edges of enclosures.
- Inappetence or reduced feeding is common.
- Dark coloration is common.
- Gill pallor due to anemia is common.
- Erythema, petechiae, skin ulcers, and fin erosions are common. Nodules may be seen.
- Coelomic distension may be seen.
- Mortality rate can reach 90% but is typically lower.

Differential Diagnoses
- Full differentials are described in Section B.
- Common differentials for bacterial septicemia include vibriosis, *Aeromonas*, *Citrobacter*, *Pseudomonas*, *Edwardsiella*, *Flavobacterium*, *Yersinia*, *Streptococcus*, and *Francisella* spp.

Diagnosis
- Diagnosis is typically made based on a combination of clinical signs, cytology, necropsy, histology, and serologic or molecular testing.
- Gram-negative and acid-fast negative pleomorphic coccobacilli that are often found in pairs or ring-shaped structures up to 1.5 μm in diameter may be seen in cells on blood smears, effusions, tissue cytology, or histology. The bacteria stain positively on Giemsa, methylene blue, and acridine orange staining. They are nonmotile on wet mounts.
- Necropsy or coeliotomy may show serosanguinous coelomic effusion, tissue pallor, hepatomegaly, splenomegaly, renomegaly, along with pathognomonic gray to yellow ring-shaped foci on the liver. There may be nodules in the viscera.
- Histology of the liver, spleen, kidney, and intestines often show the intracellular bacteria within macrophages. The bacteria may be associated with necrosis and granulomatous inflammation.
- Culture is limited as the organisms are fastidious and need additional cysteine or specific eukaryotic cell lines at low temperatures, typically ~15–18°C (59–64°F). Highest culture rates are from liver, spleen, or kidney tissue during acute infection. The growth rate is slow.
- FA, ELISA, IHC, or PCR tests may be available.

Husbandry Management
- General husbandry management is described under C4: *Bacterial Diseases (General).*

Medical Management
- Common treatments (see Chapters A12 and A13 for more details):
  - Clinical response to medical treatment is often limited, likely due to the intracellular nature of the bacteria, antibiotic resistance, and reduced feeding responses. Treatment success is highest if started early in the disease process.
  - In vitro sensitivity is typically highest for aminoglycosides, tetracyclines, macrolides, and quinolones.
- All legislation regarding medication use and disposal must be followed.

Prevention
- General preventative measures are described under C4: *Bacterial Diseases (General).*
- A variety of commercial vaccines are in use, but efficacy is debated.
- Early harvesting of cultured salmonids, less than 6 mo after transfer to salt water or prior to high water temperatures in summer, may reduce the risk.

Zoonotic Reports
- These bacteria have no known zoonotic potential.

Bibliography

Henríquez, P., Kasier, M., Bohle, H. et al. (2016). Comprehensive antibiotic susceptibility profiling of Chilean *Piscirickettsia salmonis* field isolates. *Journal of Fish Diseases* 39: 441–448.

Jakob, E., Stryhn, H., Yu, J. et al. (2014). Epidemiology of Piscirickettsiosis on selected Atlantic salmon (*Salmo salar*) and rainbow trout (*Oncorhynchus mykiss*) saltwater aquaculture farms in Chile. *Aquaculture* 433: 288–294.

Price, D., Stryhn, H., Sánchez, J. et al. (2016). Retrospective analysis of antibiotic treatments against piscirickettsiosis in farmed Atlantic salmon *Salmo salar* in Chile. *Diseases of Aquatic Organisms* 118: 227–235.

Rees, E.E., Ibarra, R., Medina, M. et al. (2014). Transmission of *Piscirickettsia salmonis* among saltwater salmonid farms in Chile. *Aquaculture* 428–429: 189–194.

Rozas, M. and Enríquez, R. (2014). Piscirickettsiosis and *Piscirickettsia salmonis* in fish: a review. *Journal of Fish Diseases* 37: 163–188.

Abbreviations/Acronyms

- ELISA: Enzyme linked immunosorbent assay
- FA: Fluorescent antibody
- IHC: Immunohistochemistry
- PCR: Polymerase chain reaction
- PLO: Piscirickettsial-like organism

C5

Fungal and Fungal-Like Diseases

Catherine A. Hadfield

Seattle Aquarium, Seattle, WA, USA

Introduction

Fish are susceptible to a variety of fungal and fungal-like diseases. Oomycetes, *Exophiala* spp., *Fusarium* spp., microsporidians, and mesomycetozoeans are reviewed in this chapter. Where available, information is provided on etiologic agent, life cycle and transmission, signalment, risk factors, clinical signs, diagnosis, husbandry and medical management, and prevention.

Oomycota (Saprolegniasis)

Overview

- *Oomycota*, commonly known as oomycetes or water molds, are fungal-like organisms that can infect the skin or gills of fish, fish eggs, and any decaying matter.
- They are common opportunistic pathogens of freshwater and brackish fish and are a particular issue for catfish in aquaculture.
- Infection is often secondary to trauma or temperature stressors.
- Typical oomycetes can be treated using medical and husbandry management, although recurrence is common.
- Atypical oomycetes are more invasive and result in severe chronic inflammation.
- *Aphanomyces invadans* is an atypical oomycete that can cause seasonal epizootics in wild and cultured freshwater and brackish fish.

Etiology

- Phylum *Oomycota*.
- Families *Saprolegniaceae* and *Leptolegniellaceae*.
- Oomycetes were originally classified within the kingdom *Fungi*, because their appearance, feeding, filamentous growth, and reproduction are similar to fungi. However, they are more closely related to diatoms, brown algae, and golden-brown algae.
- Taxonomy of the group remains complicated and is likely to change as more molecular data are published.
- Typical oomycetes primarily infect the skin, fins, or gills:
  - *Achlya* spp.
  - *Branchiomyces sanguinis* and *Branchiomyces demigrans* (gills only).
  - *Dictyuchus* spp.
  - *Leptolegnia* spp.
  - *Saprolegnia ferax*, *Saprolegnia diclina*, *Saprolegnia parasitica*.
- One species that shows deeper tissue invasion and is often known as an atypical oomycete is *Aphanomyces invadans* (syn. *piscicida*). The disease is also known as ulcerative mycosis, epizootic ulcerative syndrome, mycotic granulomatosis, epizootic granulomatous aphanomycosis, and red spot disease.

Life Cycle and Transmission

- Horizontal transmission through direct and indirect contact is seen.
- Oomycetes show sexual and asexual reproduction.
  - Sexual reproduction is by fusion of two gametes to produce a thick-walled oospore. This stage is important for morphological identification.
  - Asexual reproduction is via biflagellated zoospores released from the tip of the sporangium. The zoospores can encyst in the environment if there is no suitable host.

Clinical Guide to Fish Medicine, First Edition. Edited by Catherine A. Hadfield and Leigh Ann Clayton.

- Unlike true fungi, oomycetes require water for growth and sporulation.
- Oomycetes can survive within the biofilm, which can provide protection from immersion treatments and disinfectants.

Geographic Distribution

- Typical oomycetes are ubiquitous in freshwater and can be found in brackish water habitats, probably worldwide.
- *A. invadans* has been implicated in epizootics in the Atlantic and Gulf coasts of the United States, southern Africa, south and southeast Asia, Japan, and Australia. It has not been reported in Europe, as of 2019.

Signalment

- Typical oomycetes are common in all freshwater bony fish and are reported in brackish water bony fish.
  - Commonly affected aquarium fish include goldfish (*Carassius auratus*), guppies (*Poecilia reticulata*), and swordtails (*Xiphophorus* spp.). *Branchiomyces* spp. are particularly common in cyprinids (*Cyprinidae*).
  - Commonly affected species in food fish aquaculture include channel catfish (*Ictalurus punctatus*, where the disease may be known as winter kill), brook trout (*Oncorhynchus mykiss*), and brown trout (*Salmo trutta*).
  - Freshwater fish eggs are susceptible, particularly clumped, unfertilized eggs.
- *A. invadans* is less common but has been reported in a variety of freshwater and brackish fish.
  - Natural infections in wild fish include Atlantic menhaden (*Brevoortia tyrannus*), sheepshead (*Archosargus probatocephalus*), striped mullet (*Mugil cephalus*), white mullet (*Mugil curema*), silver perch (*Bairdiella chrysoura*), black drum (*Pogonias cromis*), largemouth bass (*Micropterus salmoides*), American shad (*Alosa sapidissima*), great snakehead (*Channa marulius*), and bluegill (*Lepomis macrochirus*).
  - Natural infections in aquarium species include the three-spot gourami (*Trichogaster trichopterus*).
  - Juveniles may be more susceptible than adults.
  - Some fish are considered resistant to natural infection, including common carp (*Cyprinus carpio*), milk fish (*Chanos chanos*), European eel (*Anguilla anguilla*), and Nile tilapia (*Oreochromis niloticus*).

Risk Factors

- Exposure:
  - Trauma to the mucus, skin, fins, or gills (e.g. recent handling, transport, or surgery).
  - Permissive water temperature (e.g. 18–25 °C or 64–77 °F for *A. invadans*).
  - Permissive salinity.
  - Poor storage or quality of food items.
  - Excess food not removed.
  - High organic loads, particularly decaying matter.
  - Low water flow rate or turnover.
- Stressors:
  - High stocking density.
  - Inappropriate social groups or habitats.
  - Poor water quality, particularly high ammonia.
  - Changes in water temperature, particularly a sudden decrease.
  - Other diseases, particularly ectoparasites, viruses, or bacteria that damage the skin (e.g. *Flavobacterium* spp.).

Signs/Clinical Findings

- Typical oomycetes:
  - Individual or multiple fish from one or more species may be affected.
  - Skin lesions typically start on wounds or on the peduncle or head.
  - Early lesions are gray-white, circular, and raised, with a cotton wool appearance (Figure C5.1a). Lesions become brown or green as debris and algae accumulate.
  - Lesions can be focal or multifocal and coalescing. Lesions rarely extend below superficial muscle.
  - Dyspnea or tachypnea may be seen if gill lesions are severe.
  - Systemic signs (e.g. inappetence) are rare.
  - Morbidity and mortality are typically low but may occur. Mortality may be higher with *Branchiomyces* spp. due to gill damage.
- *A. invadans:*
  - Multiple fish from one or more species are usually affected.
  - Deep, irregular, multifocal skin ulcers develop rapidly, often behind the head and in the perianal region. Fin erosions, petechiae, or depigmentation of the skin are often seen.
  - Inappetence, reduced feeding, or weight loss is common.
  - Erratic swimming or loss of equilibrium may be seen.
  - Corneal opacity due to edema or keratitis may be seen.
  - Dyspnea or tachypnea may be seen in late stages.
  - Morbidity and mortality are high (>50%) and start within 10–30 days post-infection.

Differential Diagnoses

- Full differentials are described in Section B.
- Common differentials for white "cotton wool" lesions on the skin, fins, or gills of freshwater or brackish fish include oomycetes, *Flavobacterium* spp., and sessile ciliates.

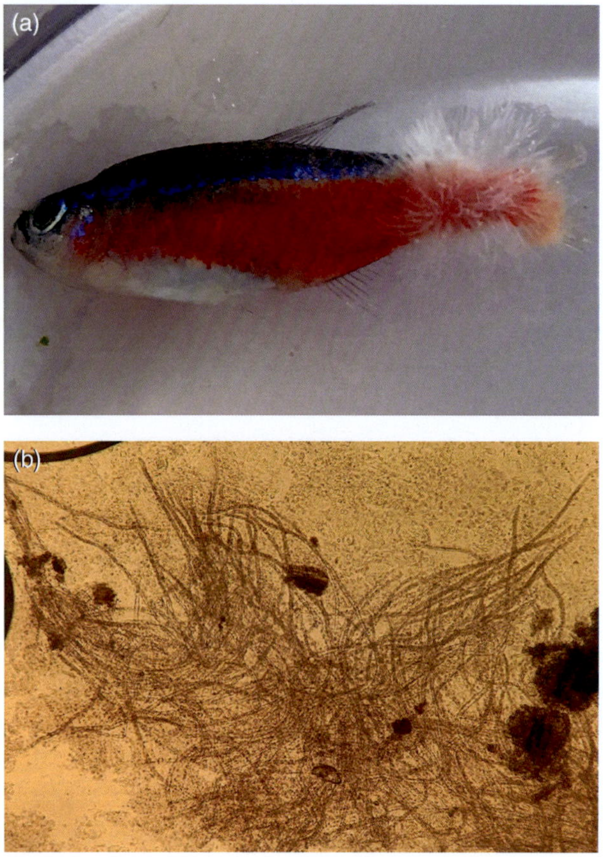

Figure C5.1 Oomycete infection on a cardinal tetra (*Paracheirodon axelrodi*); gross appearance (a) and cytologic appearance on direct microscopy of a skin scrape (b).

Diagnosis

- Oomycetes are usually diagnosed based on fungal hyphae seen on skin scrape or gill biopsy under direct microscopy. Atypical oomycetes require histology, culture, or PCR for identification.
- Hyphae vary but are generally broad (7–25 μm), transparent, with thick, irregular walls, occasional branching, and asexual zoosporangia (Figure C5.1b). The hyphae are aseptate, unlike true fungi. On rare occasions, the oogonia are visible and these are helpful if further identification is required. In cyprinids, if infection is limited to the gills, *Branchiomyces* spp. are most likely.
- Histology of the affected tissues may show hyphae as described above. Hyphae stain positively with periodic acid–Schiff and silver stains.
  - For typical oomycetes infections, superficial hyphae may be lost in processing, but some hyphae, along with necrosis and edema of the tissues, are usually seen. There may be little to no inflammatory response.
  - Atypical oomycetes are readily visible on histology with hyphae invading into muscle and viscera with associated granulomatous inflammation and necrosis.
- Fungal cultures from lesions may be used to grow oogonia for further identification. Sabouraud, potato dextrose, or glucose-peptone media can be used. Antibacterials may be added to the media to reduce bacterial growth.
- PCR and ISH assays are available for *A. invadans*.
- The OIE Manual of Diagnostic Tests for Aquatic Animals provides specific guidance on the diagnosis of *A. invadans*. It recommends histology, culture, and PCR.
- *A. invadans* is reportable in some states within the United States and to the OIE.

Husbandry Management

- Where clinical signs are seen, husbandry and medical management are indicated; fish will not usually recover without them.
- Typical oomycetes can be managed in a variety of ways.
  - Reduce or avoid sources of trauma (e.g. by modifying the habitat or social group).
  - Remove any excess organic material as soon as possible, particularly dead or moribund fish, uneaten food, and unfertilized eggs.
  - Increase mechanical cleaning and disinfection.
  - Increase water flow rate and turnover.
  - Improve water quality, if needed.
  - Resolve any temperature stressors.
  - Fish moves are not typically indicated unless the source of trauma cannot be removed or treatment is not possible in the current system.
- For *A. invadans*, there is no effective treatment.
  - Euthanasia followed by cleaning and disinfection should be considered to prevent further spread.
  - Drying in sunlight after cleaning and disinfection is helpful.

Medical Management

- Common treatments for typical oomycetes (see Chapters A12 and A13 for more details):
  - Where individual fish are affected, sedation and debridement of the fungal material are recommended. Bleeding is rarely seen and lesions typically heal well if risk factors have been eliminated.
  - Where groups of fish are affected, husbandry management and immersion treatments are recommended.
  - Formalin (Formalin-FTM, Formacide-B, Parasite-S®) immersion is approved in the United States for treatment of finfish and their eggs with *Saprolegniaceae* under various immersion treatment protocols with 0-day withdrawal, as of 2020.
  - Increased salinity is common used. Salinity of 3–4 g/L may decrease loads and reduce osmotic stress on the fish. However, higher levels such as 10–20 g/L are usually

needed to clear oomycetes and may not be tolerated by freshwater fish.
  - Hydrogen peroxide immersion (Perox-aid®) is approved in the United States for treatment of freshwater finfish and their eggs with *Saprolegniaceae*; the dose for fish is 75 mg/L for 1 hour every 48 hours for three treatments with 0-day withdrawal, as of 2020.
  - If lesions are severe, systemic antibiotics should be considered to limit secondary bacterial infections.
  - If lesions are treated and risk factors are resolved, prognosis is good and lesions should heal over several days.
  - However, lack of response to immersion treatment and recurrence are common if risk factors are still present or if the oomycetes are able to survive in protected sites (e.g. deep within the gill lamellae or the biofilm).
- Other reported treatments for typical oomycetes (see Chapters A12 and A13 for more details):
  - Copper sulfate immersion.
  - Sodium percarbonate immersion, which slowly releases hydrogen peroxide.
  - Photodynamic surgery; this cleared superficial infections with a different *Oomycota* in rabbits (*Oryctolagus cuniculus*).
- Azole antifungal agents have limited effect because oomycetes do not synthesize ergosterol (the target for azole drugs) and have cellulose in their cell walls, limiting drug penetration. However, combined azole treatments have still shown some effect.
- All legislation regarding medication use and disposal must be followed.

Prevention

- Reduce or resolve stressors.
  - Low stocking density.
  - Suitable social groups and habitats.
  - Excellent water quality and preferred water temperature.
  - Good nutrition.
  - Suitable handling and transport protocols.
- Reduce exposure and transmission.
  - Pathogen-free water source (e.g. municipal water or ground water that has gone through fine filtration then UV and/or ozone disinfection). Avoid using untreated surface water.
  - Disinfection of recirculating water with fine filtration then UV and/or ozone. UV doses reported to inactivate *Saprolegnia* spp. hyphae and zoospores are 10–40 mJ/cm^2 or mWs/cm^2.
  - High water flow rate or turnover.
  - Removal of dead fish or eggs, uneaten food, and decaying plants as soon as possible with appropriate disposition.
  - Good cleaning and disinfection protocols, including disinfection of eggs (e.g. with formalin or hydrogen peroxide).
  - Good food storage and inspection protocols.
- Reduce severity of disease.
  - Where *A. invadans* is endemic, culture of more resistant fish species such as common carp could be considered.

Zoonotic Reports

- Oomycetes from fish have no known zoonotic potential.
- One species of *Oomycota* (*Pythium insidiosum*) can infect humans. It has never been reported from fish, but infection is usually associated with exposure to infected freshwater or soil in endemic areas, including tropical and subtropical areas within the southern United States.

Bibliography

Giseker, C.M., Serfling, S.G., and Reimschuessel, R. (2006). Formalin treatment to reduce mortality associated with *Saprolegnia parasitica* in rainbow trout, *Oncorhynchus mykiss*. *Aquaculture* 253: 120–129.

Latijnhouwers, M., de Wit, P.J.G.M., and Govers, F. (2003). Oomycetes and fungi: similar weaponry to attack plants. *Trends in Microbiology* 11: 462–469.

OIE (2017). *Manual of Diagnostic Tests for Aquatic Animals*. http://www.oie.int/international-standard-setting/aquatic-manual/access-online/ (accessed 29 July 2017).

Pires, L., Bosco, S.M.G., da Silva, N.F., and Kurachi, C. (2013). Photodynamic therapy for pythiosis. *Veterinary Dermatology* 24: 130–136.

Saylor, R.K., Miller, D.L., Vandersea, M.W. et al. (2010). Epizootic ulcerative syndrome caused by *Aphanomyces invadans* in captive bullseye snakehead *Channa marulius* collected from south Florida, USA. *Diseases of Aquatic Organisms* 88: 169–175.

Small, B.C. (2009). Evaluation of sodium carbonate peroxyhydrate as a potential catfish egg disinfectant. *Journal of Aquatic Animal Health* 21: 117–123.

Sosa, E.R., Landsberg, J.H., Stephenson, C.M. et al. (2007). *Aphanomyces invadans* and ulcerative mycosis in estuarine and freshwater fish in Florida. *Journal of Aquatic Animal Health* 19: 14–26.

Sun, Q., Hu, K., and Yang, X. (2014). Efficacy of copper sulfate in controlling infection of *Saprolegnia parasitica*. *Journal of the World Aquaculture Society* 45: 220–225.

Sutela, T., Pasanen, P., Louhi, P., and Mäki-Petäys, A. (2007). Impacts of water quality and hand-picking of dead eggs on the survival of brown trout and Atlantic salmon eggs. *North America Journal of Aquaculture* 69: 235–238.

Warrilow, A.G.S., Hull, C.M., Rolley, N.J. et al. (2014). Clotrimazole as a potent agent for treatment the oomycete fish pathogen *Saprolegnia parasitica* through inhibition of sterol 14a-demethylase (CYP51). *Applied and Environmental Microbiology* 80: 6154–6166.

Abbreviations/Acronyms

- ISH: In situ hybridization
- OIE: World Organisation for Animal Health
- PCR: Polymerase chain reaction
- UV: Ultraviolet

Exophiala spp.

Overview

- *Exophiala* spp. are opportunistic fungal pathogens.
- They typically cause chronic necrotizing granulomatous disease.
- In aquariums, *Exophiala* is usually a sporadic problem for individual fish or small groups of the same species.
- In aquaculture, epizootics have been reported.
- Successful treatment has not been reported.

Etiology

- Phylum or division *Ascomycota*.
- Order *Chaetothyriales*.
- Family *Herpotrichiellaceae*.
- These are true fungal organisms.
- They are referred to as dematiaceous, phaeoid, or melanized fungi, or black yeast.
- Species are grouped within clades.
- Most waterborne species are found within the *salmonis*-clade. Species that most commonly infect fish include *Exophiala salmonis*, *Exophiala pisciphila*, and *Exophiala psychrophila*.
- Other waterborne species that can infect fish include *Exophiala angulospora* in the *dermatitidis*-clade, *Exophiala lacus* in the *bantiana*-clade, and *Exophiala xenobiotica* in the *jeanselmei*-clade.
- *Exophiala* spp. are one of the many causes of phaeohyphomycosis; this term refers to a local or systemic infection by several genera of melanized fungi. Other fungi that can cause phaeohyphomycosis include *Phoma*, *Wangiella*, and *Veronaea* spp.

Life Cycle and Transmission

- The primary route of transmission is probably inoculation. Ingestion of contaminated food is another route.
- They are not highly contagious.
- The species that infect fish have also been reported in amphibians and aquatic invertebrates; these may play a role in transmission.

Geographic Distribution

- Ubiquitous in all aquatic habitats and soil, probably worldwide.

Signalment

- Reports are primarily from farmed salmonids, demersal teleosts, and syngnathids.
  - Susceptible salmonids include cutthroat trout (*Oncorhynchus clarkii*) and Atlantic salmon (*Salmo salar*).
  - Susceptible demersal or demersopelagic teleosts include olive flounder (*Paralichthys olivaceus*), American plaice (*Hippoglossoides platessoides*), Atlantic halibut (*Hippoglossus hippoglossus*), Atlantic cod (*Gadus morhua*), King George whiting (*Sillaginodes punctatus*), and lumpfish (*Cyclopterus lumpus*).
  - Susceptible syngnathids include weedy sea dragons (*Phyllopteryx taeniolatus*) and leafy sea dragons (*Phycodurus eques*).
  - Other reports in bony fish include channel catfish (*Ictalurus punctatus*) and striped jacks (*Caranx vinctus*).
  - Reports in elasmobranchs are less common but include smooth dogfish (*Mustelus canis*), a zebra shark (*Stegostoma tigrinum*), a swell shark (*Cephaloscyllium ventriosum*), and a thornback guitarfish (*Platyrhinoidis triseriata*).
- Each report has been limited to a single fish species, suggesting that *Exophiala* spp. or strains may be species-specific.

Risk Factors

- Exposure:
  - Trauma to the mucus, skin, or gills.
  - Permissive water temperature; most *Exophiala* spp. have narrow temperature ranges.
  - Poor storage or quality of food items.
  - High organic loads.

- Stressors:
  - High stocking density.
  - Inappropriate environment.
  - Poor water quality.
  - Inappropriate water temperature or changes in water temperature.
  - Recent transport.
  - Salmonids following transfer to seawater.

Signs/Clinical Findings

- An individual or several conspecifics may be affected.
- This is typically a chronic disease lasting weeks to months.
- Lethargy may be seen.
- Inappetence, reduced feeding, or weight loss may be seen.
- Dyspnea or tachypnea may be seen.
- Abnormal buoyancy or swimming (e.g. spiraling or circling) may be seen due to neurologic or swim bladder involvement.
- Coelomic distension may be seen.
- Skin lesions may include changes in pigmentation, dermal masses, or chronic skin ulcers, sometimes crateriform in shape. Lesions may have black margins. In some cases, skin lesions are the only clinical signs with no systemic changes.
- Lesions typically progress slowly but may remain static.
- Overall morbidity and mortality are usually low. In olive flounder, infection is limited to the skin and mortalities are rare. Salmonids may show epizootics with up to 50% mortality. In aquarium fish, sporadic mortalities may continue to occur.

Differential Diagnoses

- Full differentials are described in Section B.
- Common differentials for granulomatous inflammation with hyphae in fish include atypical oomycetes, *Exophiala*, *Fusarium*, and *Paecilomyces* spp.

Diagnosis

- Diagnosis is typically based on cytology, histology, culture, and sequencing.
- Useful samples include skin (if lesions are present), gill, brain, and kidney.
- Cytology shows thin fungal hyphae that are dark yellow to brown, 2–3 μm in diameter, thin-walled, irregularly septate or aseptate, with acute or right-angled branching (Figure C5.2).
- Necropsy or coeliotomy may show organomegaly or multifocal coalescing foci throughout the viscera; these foci are often black, but may be tan or white. They can develop into large multinodular masses. Coelomic effusion may be present.
- Histology shows necrotizing, granulomatous inflammation with intralesional fungal hyphae as described above. Hyphae stain positively with periodic acid–Schiff and silver stains, and the melanin stains positively on Fontana–Masson stain. Numerous giant cells and mineralization may be seen within the granulomas. The inflammatory response varies: in sea dragons, there is often little inflammatory response and the predominant histologic change is necrosis, while in Atlantic salmon, a granulocytic response with microabscesses has been reported.
- Fungal culture is slow but *Exophiala* spp. grow readily on fungal media (e.g. Sabouraud or potato dextrose agar). Warm temperatures may be needed. Antimicrobial agents may be added to the media.
- PCR and sequencing are required for species identification. Identification should be carried out by a laboratory that specializes in fungal organisms of fish.

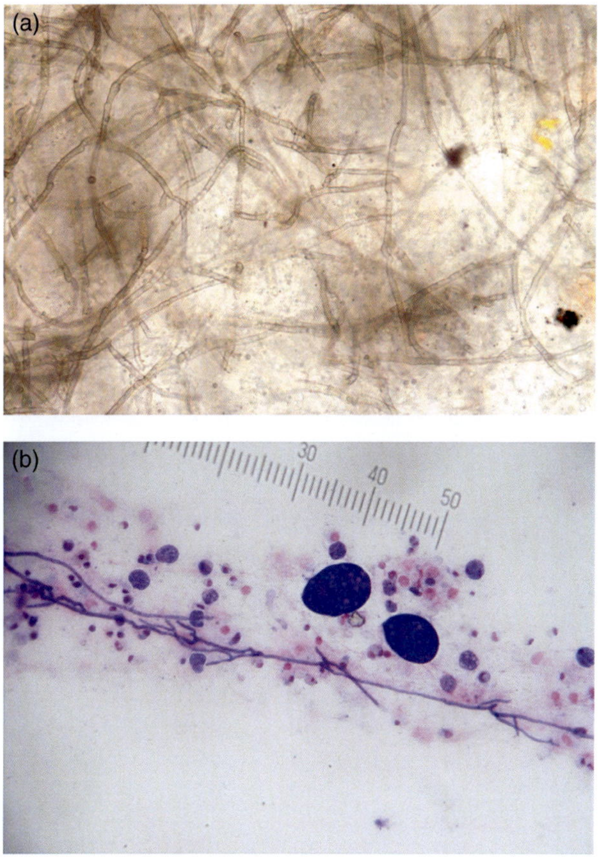

Figure C5.2 Cytologic appearance of *Exophiala* sp. under wet mount (a) and on Dif-Quik stain (b); ciliates are also visible on (b). *Source:* Images courtesy of New England Aquarium.

Husbandry Management
- Husbandry management options are limited.
- Reduce or resolve stressors, particularly water quality and temperature issues.

Medical Management
- No effective treatments have been reported.
- If antifungal therapy is used, it should be based on culture and sensitivity and continue for several months.
- Itraconazole and posaconazole showed greater in vitro activity against *Exophiala* spp. than voriconazole, fluconazole, caspofungin, or amphotericin B. Griseofulvin showed no effect.
- Supportive care and surgical debridement of lesions may help.
- All legislation regarding medication use and disposal must be followed.

Prevention
- Reduce or resolve stressors.
  - Low stocking density.
  - Suitable social groups and habitats.
  - Excellent water quality and preferred water temperature.
  - Good nutrition.
  - Suitable handling and transport protocols.
- Reduce exposure and transmission.
  - Suitable quarantine with isolation, monitoring, and diagnostic testing, particularly necropsy, cytology, and histology.
  - Disinfection of recirculating water with fine filtration then UV and/or ozone.
  - High water flow rate or turnover.
  - Removal of dead or moribund fish as soon as possible with appropriate disposition.
  - Good food storage and inspection protocols.

Zoonotic Reports
- Some *Exophiala* spp. have significant zoonotic potential, but these are generally species that are not found in fish and prefer or tolerate higher temperatures (e.g. *E. dermatitidis*, *E. spinifera*, *E. asiatica*, *E. oligosperma*).
- The zoonotic potential of the species identified in fish is lower, although rare cases of cutaneous lesions in immune-suppressed humans have been reported (e.g. *E. salmonis*, *E. xenobiotica*). Exposure was thought to be through contaminated water.

Bibliography

Gjessing, M.C., Davey, M., Kvellestad, A., and Vralstad, T. (2011). *Exophiala angulospora* causes systemic inflammation in Atlantic cod *Gadus morhua*. *Diseases of Aquatic Organisms* 96: 209–219.

DeHoog, G.S., Vicente, V.A., Najafzadeh, M.J. et al. (2011). Waterborne *Exophiala* species causing disease in cold-blooded animals. *Persoonia* 27: 46–72.

Erlacher-Reid, C.D., Hendrick, H.N., Schmitt, T.L. et al. (2016). Phaeohyphomycosis associated with ossification of the skull and cervical vertebrae in a swell shark (*Cephaloscyllium ventriosum*). *Journal of Zoo and Wildlife Medicine* 47: 1081–1085.

Fothergill, A.W., Rinaldi, M.G., and Sutton, D.A. (2009). Antifungal susceptibility testing of *Exophiala* spp.: a head-to-head comparison of amphotericin B, itraconazole, posaconazole and voriconazole. *Medical Mycology* 47: 41–43.

Madan, V., Bisset, D., and Harris, P. (2006). Phaeohypomycosis caused by *Exophiala salmonis*. *British Journal of Dermatology* 32: 329–349.

Marancik, D.P., Berliner, A.L., Cavin, J.M. et al. (2011). Disseminated fungal infection in two species of captive sharks. *Journal of Zoo and Wildlife Medicine* 42: 686–693.

Nyaoke, A., Weber, E.S., Innis, C. et al. (2009). Disseminated phaeohyphomycosis in weedy sea dragons (*Phyllopteryx taeniolatus*) and leafy seadragons (*Phycodurus eques*) caused by species of *Exophiala*, including a novel species. *Journal of Veterinary Diagnostic Investigation* 21: 69–79.

Steckler, N.K., Yanong, R.P.E., Pouder, D.B., and Nyaoke, A. (2014). New disease records for hatchery-reared sturgeon. II. Phaeohyphomycosis due to *Veronaea botryosa*. *Diseases of Aquatic Organisms* 111: 229–238.

Abbreviations/Acronyms
- PCR: Polymerase chain reaction
- UV: Ultraviolet

Fusarium spp.

Overview
- *Fusarium* spp. are environmental saprophytes commonly isolated from soil and plants.
- Opportunistic infections are seen sporadically in fish, particularly marine fish.
- They are usually an individual animal problem.

- Lesions start as necrotizing, granulomatous dermatitis.
- Treatment is rarely successful once the fungi have invaded deeper tissues.

Etiology

- Phylum or division *Ascomycota.*
- Order *Hypocreales.*
- Family *Nectriaceae.*
- These are true fungal organisms.
- They are often referred to as non-dematiaceous fungi or hyphomycetes.
- *Fusarium solani* species complex (FSSC) is the most common *Fusarium* infection in fish. It includes >60 members that can only be identified by sequence data. It has recently been divided into three clades. Most of the species of veterinary importance are in clade 3.
- *Fusarium oxysporum* is also reported.
- *Fusarium* spp. produce mycotoxins such as trichothecenes, zearalenone, fumonisins, enniatins, deoxynivalenol, and beauvericin. Fish can be exposed to the mycotoxins through contaminated feeds, particularly grain- and legume-based feeds. Some effects on fish have been shown experimentally (e.g. developmental abnormalities and reduced growth rates), but they will not be covered in this infectious disease section.

Life Cycle and Transmission

- Horizontal transmission is seen, primarily through inoculation.
- FSSC and other *Fusarium* spp. have been identified in plants, invertebrates, amphibians, aquatic reptiles, and mammals; these may play a role in transmission.

Geographic Distribution

- FSSC and other *Fusarium* spp. are considered ubiquitous in all aquatic habitats, probably worldwide.
- Reports of disease in fish are mostly from marine habitats, with rare reports from freshwater aquaculture.

Signalment

- Marine elasmobranchs are susceptible, particularly bonnethead sharks (*Sphyrna tiburo*), scalloped hammerheads (*Sphyrna lewini*), and Port Jackson sharks (*Heterodontus portusjacksoni*). There is a report in a round ribbontail ray (*Taeniura meyeni*).
- Marine teleosts are susceptible, particularly parrotfish (*Scaridae*), pufferfish (*Tetraodontidae*), and lined seahorses (*Hippocampus erectus*).
- This is one report in freshwater fish, in farmed tilapia fry (*Oreochromis niloticus*).
- This is a problem of managed fish; it has not been reported from wild fish.

Risk Factors

- Exposure:
  - Trauma to the mucus, skin, fins, or eyes.
- Stressors:
  - High stocking density.
  - Inappropriate enclosure design.
  - Poor water quality.
  - Inappropriate water temperature, particularly low temperature for tropical sharks.
  - Recent transport.

Signs/Clinical Findings

- An individual fish is usually affected, although several conspecifics may be affected.
- Lethargy and abnormal swimming (e.g. slow swimming interspersed with burst swimming and spiral swimming) are common.
- Inappetence, reduced appetite, or weight loss may be seen.
- Skin lesions are common, particularly along the head, lateral line, fin edges, and tail. Reports include white, pink, or red pustules, swollen lateral line pores, erythema, or depigmentation. A white viscous fluid or blood may be seen from within the lesions. The lesions ulcerate and may expose muscle, cartilage, or bone.
- Exophthalmos may be seen.
- Mortalities have been reported days to months after the appearance of external lesions.

Differential Diagnoses

- Full differentials are described in Section B.
- Common differentials for fungal hyphae associated with skin ulcers include *Fusarium* spp. and other causes of hyphalomycosis (e.g. *Aspergillus*, *Paecilomycosis*, *Penicillium* spp.) and phaeohyphomycosis (e.g. *Exophiala* spp.).

Diagnosis

- Diagnosis is typically made on cytology or histology of gill, skin, or tissue and culture followed by molecular testing.
- Cytology shows thin-walled fungal hyphae, 1–7 μm diameter, variably septate, with acute and right-angled branching, and characteristic large, sickle-shaped macroconidia with numerous septa (Figure C5.3).
- Necropsy and histology usually show necrotizing, hemorrhagic dermatitis. Intralesional fungi often invade into the underlying skeletal muscle, nerves, and blood vessels and can invade cartilage and bone. Hyphae stain positively with periodic acid–Schiff and silver stains. Lesions may be granulomatous or there may be no inflammatory response. Lesions in the coelomic viscera are uncommon.
- *Fusarium* spp. grow slowly but readily on fungal media (e.g. Sabouraud or potato dextrose agar). Sodium chloride and antimicrobials may be added to the media.

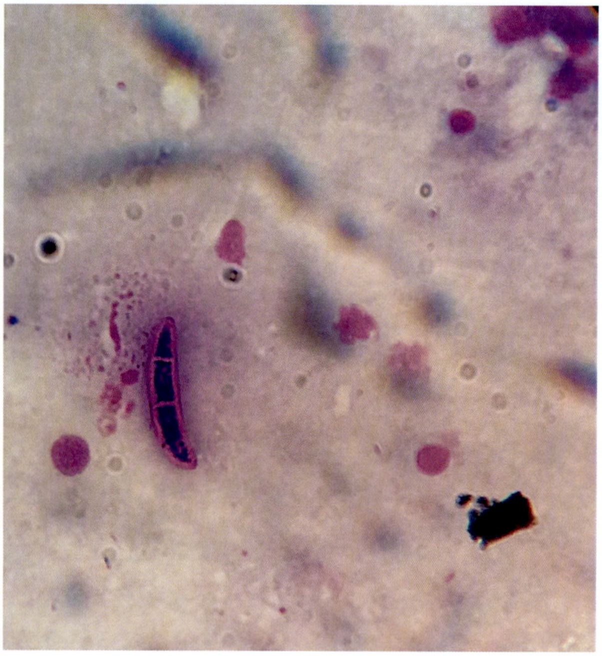

Figure C5.3 Cytologic appearance of characteristic sickle-shaped macroconidia of *Fusarium* spp.

- PCR followed by sequencing is needed for definitive identification.
- Diagnostic imaging, particularly MRI, may help to determine the extent of the infection.

Husbandry Management

- Remove sources of skin trauma.
- Reduce or resolve other stressors.
- Consider slowly increasing the water temperature (e.g. >28 °C or 82 °F for bonnethead sharks).

Medical Management

- Treatment is rarely successful due to limited penetration and high minimum inhibitory concentrations of antifungals.
- Common treatments (see Chapters A12 and A13 for more details):
  - Supportive care with fluid and nutritional therapy is usually indicated.
  - Voriconazole is the most commonly recommended treatment (e.g. 10–50 mg/kg PO every 24 hours or 6 mg/kg slow IV). Monitoring of serum levels is the best way to ensure therapeutic levels in fish; therapeutic plasma levels in humans are 2–6 μg/mL. Treatment should likely continue for months.
- Other reported treatments (see Chapters A12 and A13 for more details):
  - In vitro testing tends to show highest sensitivity to voriconazole, posaconazole, and amphotericin B. Low sensitivity is seen to fluconazole, itraconazole, flucytosine, and echinocandins.
  - Itraconazole also showed poor in vivo sensitivity in lined seahorses.
  - Amphotericin B and clotrimazole are reported treatments in humans.
- All legislation regarding medication use and disposal must be followed.

Prevention

- Reduce or resolve stressors.
  - Low stocking density.
  - Suitable social groups and habitats; in particular, pelagic sharks should be housed in large, oval systems, with smooth, clearly marked walls.
  - Excellent water quality and preferred water temperature.
  - Good nutrition.
  - Suitable handling and transport protocols.
- Reduce exposure and transmission.
  - Pathogen-free water source (e.g. municipal water or ground water that has gone through fine filtration then UV and/or ozone disinfection). Avoid using untreated surface water.
  - Disinfection of recirculating water with fine filtration then UV and/or ozone.
  - High water flow rate or turnover.

Zoonotic Reports

- FSSC and *F. oxysporum* are zoonotic, but have not historically been reported from fish exposure. Keratitis is seen from contaminated contact lenses or contact lens solution, or ocular trauma in immune-competent humans. Nail infections may be seen following trauma. Systemic spread has been reported rarely in immune-suppressed humans. The disease is known as fusariosis.

Bibliography

Cutuli, M.T., Gibello, A., Rodriguez-Bertos, A. et al. (2015). Skin and subcutaneous mycoses in tilapia (*Oreochromis niloticus*) caused by *Fusarium oxysporum* in coinfection with *Aeromonas hydrophila*. *Medical Mycology Case Reports* 9: 7–11.

Fernando, N., Hui, S.-W., Tsang, C.-C. et al. (2015). Fatal *Fusarium solani* species complex infections in elasmobranchs: the first case report for black spotted stingray (*Taeniura melanopsila*) and a literature review. *Mycoses* 58: 422–431.

Pirarat, N., Sahatrakul, K., Lacharoje, S. et al. (2016). Molecular and pathological characterization of *Fusarium solani* species complex infection in the head and lateral line system of *Sphyrna lewini*. *Diseases of Aquatic Organisms* 120: 195–204.

Salah, H., Al-Hatmi, A.M.S., Theelen, B. et al. (2015). Phylogenetic diversity of human pathogenic *Fusarium* and emergency of uncommon virulent species. *Journal of Infection* 71: 658–666.

Salter, C.E., O'Donnell, K., Sutton, D.A. et al. (2012). Dermatitis and systemic mycosis in lined seahorses *Hippocampus erectus* associated with a marine-adapted *Fusarium solani* species complex pathogen. *Diseases of Aquatic Organisms* 101: 23–31.

Tolosa, J., Font, G., Manes, J., and Ferrer, E. (2014). Natural occurrence of emerging *Fusarium* mycotoxins in feed and fish from aquaculture. *Journal of Agricultural and Food Chemistry* 62: 12462–12470.

Abbreviations/Acronyms

- FSSC: *Fusarium solani* species complex
- IV: Intravenous
- MRI: Magnetic resonance imaging
- PO: Orally
- PCR: Polymerase chain reaction
- UV: Ultraviolet

Microsporidia

Overview

- Microsporidians are a large group of obligate, intracellular parasites that typically infect invertebrates and fish.
- They are grouped taxonomically with fungi.
- Most microsporidians are species-, tissue-, and/or cell-specific.
- Microsporidians often form spore-filled cysts (xenomas), but some can cause diffuse infections.
- They are often carried asymptomatically but may cause morbidity and mortality.

Etiology

- Kingdom *Fungi*.
- Division *Microsporidia*.
- These are considered to be highly specialized fungi, but they were historically grouped with protozoa.
- More than 160 species infect fish. Some commonly reported genera of microsporidia are:
  - *Glugea*
  - *Heterosporis*
  - *Loma*
  - *Nucleospora*
  - *Ovipleistophora*
  - *Pleistophora*
  - *Pseudoloma*
  - *Spraguea*
  - *Tetramicra*

Life Cycle and Transmission

- Microsporidians have a direct life cycle in fish.
- Horizontal transmission is common. Vertical transmission is important for some (e.g. *Loma*, *Ovipleistophora*, *Pleistophora* spp.).
- Spores are released when the fish dies or lesions rupture, typically weeks to months post-infection.
- Spores are hardy and can survive in the environment for months, particularly at low temperatures.
- When spores identify a suitable host cell, the polar tubule is extruded and the sporoplasm is injected into the host cell. In the host cell, multiplication occurs by merogony (binary fission) or schizogony (multiple fission), then sporogony to produce mature spores with a thick wall. Xenomas may form; these are giant cells each with one nucleus, filled with spores.

Geographic Distribution

- Microsporidians are found in freshwater and saltwater habitats, probably worldwide.
- Species often have narrower ranges, e.g. *Heterosporis sutherlandae* n. sp. in the Great Lakes region of North America.

Signalment

- Microsporidians are particularly common in temperate, freshwater teleosts.
- Most infect only one species or a closely related group, e.g.:
  - *Glugea heraldi* in seahorses (*Syngnathidae*).
  - *Loma salmonae* and *Nucleospora salmonis* in salmonids, particularly Chinook (*Oncorhynchus tshawytscha*) and coho (*Oncorhynchus kisutch*).
- A few have wider host ranges, e.g. *Pleistophora hyphessobryconis* in tetras (*Characidae*), cyprinids (*Cyprinidae*), guppies, mollies, and swordtails (*Poeciliidae*), and cichlids (*Cichlidae*).
- *Dasyatipora levantinae* is the first microsporidian reported in elasmobranchs, identified in common stingrays (*Dasyatis pastinaca*).

Risk Factors

- Exposure:

  - Poor biosecurity (e.g. lack of suitable quarantine, use of surface water, exposure to wild fish).
  - Permissive water temperature (e.g. *L. salmonae* prefers 13–17 °C or 55–63 °F).
  - Low water flow rate or turnover.
  - Exposure of naïve fish.
- Stressors:
  - High stocking density.
  - Poor water quality.
  - Recent handling.
  - Recent transport.

Signs/Clinical Findings

- Microsporidians are usually carried asymptomatically.
- If signs are seen, lesions develop weeks to months after infection.
- Multiple conspecifics may be affected.
- Lethargy may be seen.
- Inappetence, reduced feeding, weight loss, or poor growth may be seen.
- Dark coloration may be seen, which may be focal.
- Dyspnea or tachypnea may be seen.
- Coelomic distension may be seen.
- Some microsporidians can cause white, yellow, brown, or black cysts known as xenomas (e.g. *Ichthyosporidium*, *Loma*, *Microgemma*, *Pseudoloma*, *Spraguea*, *Tetramicra*, and most *Glugea* spp.). These vary from microscopic to several millimeters in diameter.
  - *L. salmonae* affects the gills causing visible nodules and congestion.
  - *Pseudoloma* spp. primarily affect the brain and spinal cord causing scoliosis, weight loss, or decreased fecundity.
  - *D. levantinae* affects skeletal muscle producing long thin swellings filled with caseous material.
- Other microsporidians cause a local, diffuse infection (e.g. *Heterosporis*, *Nucleospora*, *Ovipleistophora*, and *Pleistophora* spp.).
  - *Ovipleistophora ovariae* affects the ovaries, causing reduced fecundity.
  - *P. hyphessobryconis* affects skeletal muscle, causing muscle wasting and abnormal swimming.
- Morbidity and mortality rates vary.
- Resolution of signs over time is seen in some cases.
- Protective immunity following exposure is seen in some cases.

Differential Diagnoses

- Full differentials are described in Section B.
- Common differentials for nodules include granulomatous inflammation, abscesses, cysts, hyperplasia, and neoplasia.

Diagnosis

- Xenomas are usually grossly visible (Figure C5.4a). Wet mounts or impression smears of ruptured xenomas or histology of lesions is typically sufficient to confirm the presence of microsporidian spores. Microsporidians that cause diffuse disease can be identified on impression smears or histology of affected tissues.
- Microsporidian parasites look similar on cytology and histology. Spores are small, often 1–6 μm in length and ~2 μm in width, egg-shaped, each with a prominent, clear posterior vacuole creating a clog-like appearance (Figure C5.4b and c). Spores are visible on hematoxylin and eosin, Romanowsky, Giemsa, and Luna stains. Depending on the stage of development, spores can be Gram-positive, PAS-positive, and acid-fast positive. The walls of most spores are birefringent.
- The type and degree of inflammation vary.
- Tentative species identification is often based on host species and tissue location, but definitive identification requires molecular testing or EM.
- Some PCR and ISH tests are available commercially and show the highest sensitivity after tissue sonification to break up spores.

Husbandry Management

- Husbandry management can help reduce clinical signs, if present.
- Consider isolating affected fish to reduce transmission rates, if a suitable environment is available.
- Increase aeration; target dissolved oxygen may be 95–100%.
- Consider slowly taking the temperature outside of the preferred range of the parasites but within the preferred range of the fish.
- Increase water flow rate and turnover.
- Increase cleaning and disinfection of water; some species are sensitive to UV and ozone disinfection at common doses.
- Increase cleaning and disinfection of fomites, but sensitivity varies. Some reports show inactivation of spores using 70% isopropyl alcohol or 2–100 mg/L chlorine for 15 minutes.
- With a virulent infection and valuable colonies, consider depopulation of affected groups and disinfection.

Medical Management

- Treatment can reduce the production of new xenomas and improve clinical signs but has limited effect on existing xenomas. Recurrence after treatment ends is common.

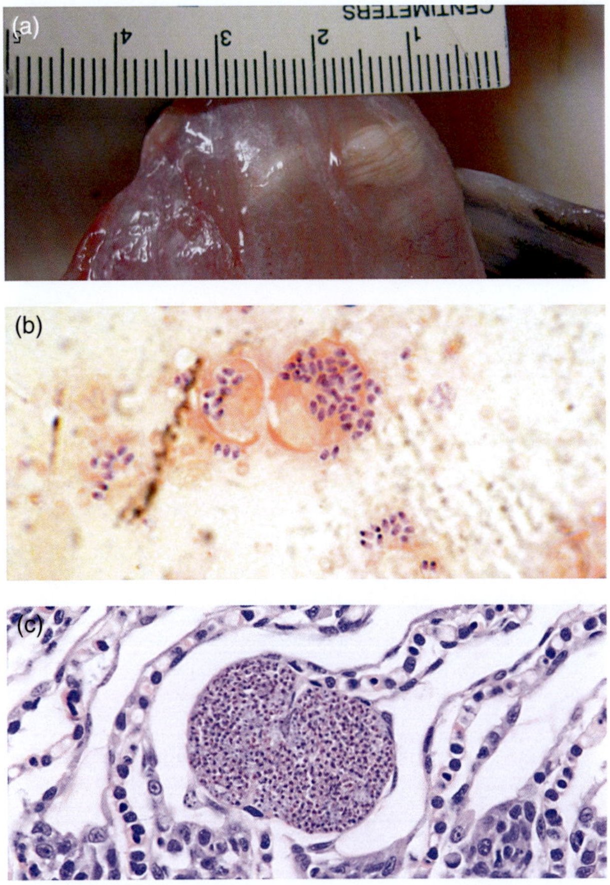

Figure C5.4 Microsporidial xenoma in the muscle of a shorthorn sculpin (*Myoxocephalus scorpius*) (a) and cytologic appearance of microsporidia on Dif-Quik stain of an impression smear (b) and on H&E stain of gill histology (c); ×1000. *Source:* Image (a) courtesy of New England Aquarium and image (c) courtesy of David Groman, University of Prince Edward Island.

- Common treatments (see Chapters A12 and A13 for more details):
  - Fumagillin orally is the most effective treatment in comparative studies. Toxicity to fumagillin is also reported. Doses are often 3–15 mg/kg body weight every 24 hours for 3–4 weeks.
  - Supportive care with fluid and nutritional therapy may help.
- Other reported treatments (see Chapters A12 and A13 for more details):
  - Albendazole orally.
  - Toltrazuril orally.
  - Monensin orally.
  - Pyrimethamine and sulfaquinoxaline orally.
  - Nitazoxanide orally.
  - Salinomycin and amprolium orally.
  - Quinine hydrochloride orally.
  - Since inflammation is highest after rupture of xenomas, anti-inflammatory therapy may reduce morbidity and mortality. The nonsteroidal anti-inflammatory agent indomethacin showed potential in rainbow trout (*Oncorhynchus mykiss*), but was associated with gastric ulceration and granulomatous peritonitis.
- Metronidazole has generally been ineffective.
- All legislation regarding medication use and disposal must be followed.

Prevention

- Reduce or resolve stressors.
  - Low stocking density.
  - Suitable social groups and habitats.
  - Excellent water quality and preferred water temperature.
  - Good nutrition.
- Reduce exposure and transmission.
  - Isolation with no contact with free-ranging animals.
  - Pathogen-free water source (e.g. municipal water or ground water that has gone through fine filtration then UV and/or ozone disinfection). Avoid using untreated surface water or choose a specific pathogen-free source (e.g. *L. salmonae*-free water may be pulled from a lake with no salmonids).
  - Disinfection of recirculating water with fine filtration then UV and/or ozone.
  - High water flow rate or turnover.
  - Acquire specific pathogen-free (SPF) fish, where available (e.g. zebrafish).
  - Suitable quarantine with isolation, necropsy, PCR, and histology.
  - Fallowing between batches may be helpful, although spore viability is often unknown.
  - Frozen-thawed or commercial feeds, with no live feeds, although some spores survive freezing.
  - Avoid using infected fish as broodstock.
  - Disinfection of eggs is typically ineffective at stopping transmission. Safe doses of iodine or chlorine for disinfection of salmonid and zebrafish eggs rarely affect these parasites.
- Reduce severity of disease.
  - Experimental vaccines to *L. salmonae* in salmonids show promise.
  - Immune stimulants such as beta glucans can decrease severity of signs from *L. salmonae*. They are most effective at specific doses, short courses, and when given prior to exposure or prior to onset of clinical signs.

Zoonotic Reports

- Fish are not a common source of microsporidiosis in humans.
- Some microsporidians have been found in humans, usually associated with severe immune suppression. Some have been found in immune-competent humans.
  - Most of the genera reported in humans are not found in fish (e.g. *Encephalitozoon* and *Anncaliia*).
  - There have been a few reports of *Pleistophora ronneafiei* myositis in humans. While the genus is reported in fish, the source and route of transmission in humans are unknown.

Bibliography

Becker, J.A., Speare, D.J., Daley, J., and Dick, P. (2002). Effects of monensin dose and treatment time on xenoma reduction in microsporidial gill disease in rainbow trout, *Oncorhynchus mykiss* (Walbaum). *Journal of Fish Diseases* 25: 673–680.

Diamant, A., Goren, M., Yokes, M.B. et al. (2010). *Dasyatipora levaninae* gen. et sp. nov., a new microsporidian parasite from the common stingray *Dasyatis pastinaca* in the eastern Mediterranean. *Diseases of Aquatic Organisms* 91: 137–150.

Ferguson, J.A., Watral, V., Schwindt, A.R., and Kent, M.L. (2007). Spores of two fish microsporidia (*Pseudoloma neurophilia* and *Glugea anomala*) are highly resistant to chlorine. *Disease of Aquatic Organisms* 76: 205–214.

Kent, M.L., Buchner, C., Watral, V.G. et al. (2011). Development and maintenance of a specific pathogen-free (SPF) zebrafish research facility for *Pseudoloma neurophilia*. *Diseases of Aquatic Organisms* 95: 73–79.

Leiro, J.M., Piazzon, C., Domínguez, B. et al. (2012). Evaluation of some physical and chemical treatments for inactivating microsporidian spores isolated from fish. *International Journal of Food Microbiology* 156: 152–160.

Lovy, J., Wright, G.M., and Speare, D.J. (2007). Pathological effects caused by chronic treatment of rainbow trout with indomethacin. *Journal of Aquatic Animal Health* 19: 94–98.

Mathis, A., Weber, R., and Deplazes, P. (2005). Zoonotic potential of the Microsporidia. *Clinical Microbiology Reviews* 18: 423–445.

Speare, D.J., Athanassopoulou, F., Daley, J., and Sanchez, J.G. (1999). A preliminary investigation of alternatives to fumagillin for the treatment of *Loma salmonae* infection in rainbow trout. *Journal of Comparative Pathology* 121: 241–248.

Abbreviations/Acronyms

- EM: Electron microscopy
- ISH: In situ hybridization
- PAS: Periodic acid–Schiff
- PCR: Polymerase chain reaction
- UV: Ultraviolet

Mesomycetozoea (DRIPs)

Overview

- *Mesomycetozoea* are an unusual group of fungal-like organisms with a complicated taxonomy.
- The disease is usually chronic.
- They may be associated with white nodules that consist of thin-walled cysts containing characteristic spores.
- There is no specific treatment, but lesions may resolve over time.

Etiology

- Class *Mesomycetozoea.*
- DRIP clade.
- These are fungal-like organisms that are clustered together taxonomically.
- The literature is complicated, but they are currently placed in the class *Mesomycetozoea* (previously *Ichthyosporea*). This was previously referred to as the DRIP clade (*Dermocystidium*, rosette agent, *Ichthyophonus*, *Psorospermium*).
- *Sphaerothecum destruens* was previously known as the rosette agent.
- Other parasitic genera include *Rhinosporidium.*
- Many are identified based on gross appearance and host species rather than genetic data. The taxonomy is likely to change as more molecular studies are reported.

Life Cycle and Transmission

- Horizontal transmission is seen. There is no evidence of vertical transmission.
- Infection may be from ingestion of viable spores in prey, particularly scavenging on dead fish. Waterborne transmission has also been reported.

- The life cycle, where identified, usually includes intracellular spores and free-living, flagellated zoospores that are likely to be the infectious stage.
- They can survive in salt water for up to two years.
- *S. destruens* is known to have asymptomatic carriers including the topmouth gudgeon (*Pseudorasbora parva*), an invasive species in Europe.

Geographic Distribution

- Freshwater and saltwater habitats, probably worldwide.

Signalment

- *Mesomycetozoea* are reported in a wide range of marine and freshwater teleosts, such as:
  - Koi (*Cyprinus carpio koi*), e.g. *Dermocystidium koi*.
  - Chinook salmon (*Oncorhynchus tshawytscha*), e.g. *Dermocystidium salmonis*.
  - European eels (*Anguilla anguilla*), e.g. *Dermocystidium anguillae*.
  - Marine and anadromous teleosts such as Atlantic herring (*Clupea harengus*), Pacific herring (*Clupea pallasii*), and rainbow trout (*Oncorhynchus mykiss*), e.g. *Ichthyophonus hoferi*.

Risk Factors

- Risk factors are largely unknown but stressors and exposure likely play a role.

Signs/Clinical Findings

- Several conspecifics are likely to be affected.
- The presentation is usually chronic, but may be acute.
- Skin and fin lesions are common, typically white nodules, plaques, papules, or linear tracts (Figure C5.5a). Lesions may be red and ulcerative and tend to progress. Similar gill lesions may be seen.
- Weight loss may be seen.
- Exophthalmos may be seen and white nodules or linear tracts may be noted within the conjunctiva.
- Neurologic signs may be seen.
- Spinal curvature may be seen.
- Morbidity and mortality are usually low but may reach 50–80%.
- Signs may resolve over several months in some cases.

Differential Diagnoses

- Full differentials are described in Section B.
- Common differentials for nodules include granulomatous inflammation, abscesses, cysts, hyperplasia, and neoplasia.

Diagnosis

- *Mesomycetozoea* are usually initially identified on direct microscopy of the lesions, after rupturing the thin cyst wall. This releases abundant spores.
- Spores are uniform, round to elliptical, 2–15 μm in diameter, thick or double-walled, and signet-ring shaped with a prominent central refractile body (Figure C5.5b). The central body is negative on acid-fast stain and positive on periodic acid–Schiff and silver stains. Spores may germinate after host death producing hyphae.
- Histology shows thin-walled cysts within the hypodermal tissue contain spores as described above. Granulomatous inflammation and necrosis are possible, particularly associated with ruptured cysts. Systemic spread is less common but is seen with some species and strains (e.g. *D. salmonis* and *S. destruens* in salmonids).
- Culture is possible using fungal media (e.g. Sabouraud or potato dextrose agar) or cell lines, but sensitivity is low.
- Identification to genus or species requires molecular diagnostics.

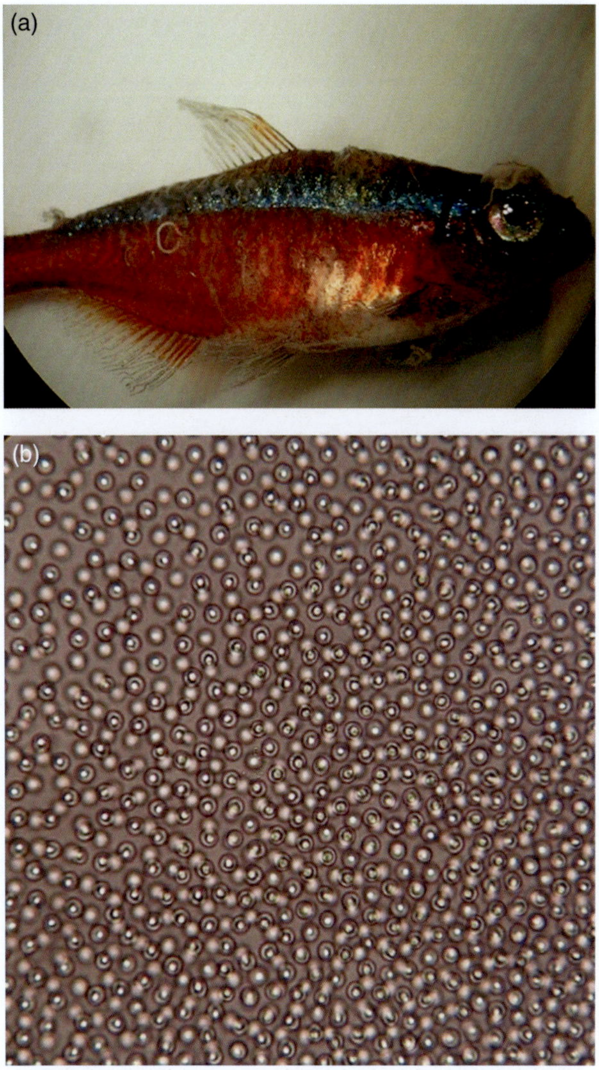

Figure C5.5 *Mesomycetozoea* infection in a cardinal tetra (*Paracheirodon axelrodi*): gross lesions (a) and cytologic appearance of the uniform spores under direct microscopy (b).

Husbandry Management

- Reduce or resolve stressors.

Medical Management

- Treatment is not indicated in incidental infections.
- Surgical removal may be helpful for individual fish if the mass is causing secondary issues or if there are cosmetic concerns.
- Antifungals may be considered; ketoconazole has shown some potential against *Ichthyophonus* sp. but toxicity was seen.
- All legislation regarding medication use and disposal must be followed.

Prevention

- Reduce or resolve stressors.
  - Low stocking density.
  - Suitable social groups and habitats.
  - Excellent water quality and preferred water temperature.
  - Good nutrition.
- Reduce exposure and transmission.
  - Isolation with no contact with free-ranging animals.
  - Pathogen-free water source (e.g. municipal water or ground water that has gone through fine filtration then UV and/or ozone disinfection). Avoid using untreated surface water.
  - Disinfection of recirculating water with fine filtration then UV and/or ozone.
  - High water flow rate or turnover.
  - Removal of dead or moribund fish as soon as possible with appropriate disposition.
  - Suitable quarantine with isolation, monitoring, and diagnostic testing, particularly cytology and histology.
  - Frozen-thawed or commercial feeds, with no live feeds.
  - Good food inspection protocols.

Zoonotic Reports

- Most of these organisms have no known zoonotic potential.
- *Rhinosporidium seeberi* can cause slow-growing nasal or conjunctival polyps in humans, but disease transmission from fish has not been reported. Disease is most commonly identified in India and Sri Lanka.

Bibliography

Andreous, D., Gozlan, R.E., Stone, D. et al. (2011). *Sphaerothecum destruens* pathology in cyprinids. *Diseases of Aquatic Organisms* 95: 145–151.

Arkush, K.D., Mendoza, L., Adkison, M.A., and Hedrick, R. (2003). Observations on the life stages of *Sphaerothecum destruens* n. g., n. sp., a mesomycetozoan fish pathogen formally referred to as the rosette agent. *Journal of Eukaryotic Microbiology* 50: 430–438.

Fredricks, D.N., Jolley, J.A., Lepp, P.W. et al. (2000). *Rhinosporidium seeberi*: a human pathogen from a novel group of aquatic protistan parasites. *Emerging Infectious Diseases* 6: 273–282.

Hershberger, P.K., Hart, L.M., MacKenzie, A.H. et al. (2015). Infecting Pacific herring with *Ichthyophonus* sp. in the laboratory. *Journal of Aquatic Animal Health* 27: 217–221.

Hontoria, F., González, M.A., Sitjà-Bobadilla, A. et al. (2013). Ketoconazole modulates the infectivity of *Ichthyophonus* sp. (Mesomycetozoa) in vivo in experimentally injected European seabass. *Diseases of Aquatic Organisms* 105: 225–235.

C6

Protozoal Diseases

Catherine A. Hadfield

Seattle Aquarium, Seattle, WA, USA

Introduction

Protozoa is an informal term for single-celled eukaryotes. Common ciliate, flagellate, dinoflagellate, and amoebic diseases of fish are reviewed in this chapter. Where available, information is provided on the etiologic agent, life cycle and transmission, signalment, risk factors, clinical signs, diagnosis, husbandry and medical management, and prevention.

Ichthyophthirius multifiliis

Overview

- *Ichthyophthirius multifiliis* is a ciliated protozoan ectoparasite that infects the skin and gills of freshwater bony fish.
- The disease is often called freshwater ich or white spot.
- It is a common cause of morbidity and mortality in freshwater aquarium fish and food fish aquaculture.
- It is typically treated with long-term immersion medications.
- It is often considered the freshwater equivalent of *Cryptocaryon irritans*, because the life cycle and clinical signs are similar, but the organisms are not closely related.

Etiology

- Phylum *Ciliophora.*
- Family *Icthyophthiriidae.*
- *Ichthyophthirius multifiliis* is the only reported species, although characteristics of different isolates vary.

Life Cycle and Transmission

- The life cycle is direct.
  - The trophont is the feeding stage that burrows under the epithelium, triggering an inflammatory response in the host. This stage is resistant to treatment.
  - Trophonts mature and grow, leave the host, attach to a solid surface (e.g. gravel, plants, nets) and encyst, becoming reproductive tomonts within which tomites develop.
  - The tomonts rupture asynchronously and each release 100–2000 tomites that differentiate into free-swimming theronts. This stage is most sensitive to immersion treatments.
  - Theronts are immediately infectious and must find a host within 48 hours at ~25 °C (77 °F). They burrow into fish skin or gills.
- The life cycle is faster than *Cryptocaryon.* Times vary across different studies and isolates, but general ranges are:
  - 1.5–7 days at 20–25 °C (68–77 °F).
  - 10–14 days at 15 °C (59 °F).
  - 20–90 days at 5–10 °C (41–50 °F).
- The optimum temperature range for theront production has been reported as 12–25 °C (54–77 °F).
- There is little to no development at <3 °C (37 °F) and >30–32 °C (86–90 °F).
- Horizontal transmission through water, fomites (e.g. nets), and aerosolization (as far as 90 cm with static airflow) have all been seen.

Geographic Distribution

- Freshwater habitats, probably worldwide.

Signalment

- All freshwater bony fish may be susceptible.

Clinical Guide to Fish Medicine, First Edition. Edited by Catherine A. Hadfield and Leigh Ann Clayton.

- In aquaculture, rainbow trout (*Oncorhynchus mykiss*), grass carp (*Ctenopharyngodon idella*), common carp (*Cyprinus carpio*), and channel catfish (*Ictalurus punctatus*) are commonly reported hosts.
- In aquariums, infection is common in most freshwater species.
- Most strains have wide host ranges, affecting multiple species in the same system, although some strains are species-specific.
- These do not infect elasmobranchs or invertebrates, although they can likely act as mechanical vectors.

Risk Factors

- Exposure and stressors are the most important risk factors.
- Exposure:
  - Poor biosecurity (e.g. lack of suitable quarantine, untreated surface water).
  - Permissive water temperature, typically 12–25 °C (54–77 °F).
  - Permissive salinity, typically <5 g/L.
  - High organic loads.
  - Low water flow rate or turnover.
  - Exposure of naïve fish (e.g. following introduction of new fish).
  - Established infection; once established in a large habitat, this becomes a recurrent issue.
- Stressors:
  - High stocking density.
  - Inappropriate social structure.
  - Inappropriate environment.
  - Aggression or displacement.
  - Poor water quality, particularly low dissolved oxygen and high ammonia.
  - Contaminants.
  - Inappropriate water temperature or changes in water temperature.
  - Poor nutrition.
  - Recent handling.
  - Recent transport.
  - Recent spawning.
  - Other diseases.

Signs/Clinica l Findings

- Signs are often seen 5–10 days after new fish are added to a system.
- Multiple fish from one or more species are usually affected.
- Initial signs are subtle and may include reduced feeding, increased hiding, and skin darkening.
- White spots up to 1 mm diameter develop on the skin, fins, and gills (Figure C6.1a). Good lighting (e.g. a flashlight with a focal beam) helps to show early changes. The spots are slightly larger than with *Cryptocaryon*.
- Late signs include lethargy or pruritus (e.g. flashing, hyperactivity), dyspnea, tachypnea, keratitis, opaque fins, inappetence, and mortalities.
- Gill pallor due to anemia may be seen.
- Secondary infections may be seen.
- Mortalities typically start within days. Mortality varies but is often high and can reach 100%.

Differential Diagnoses

- Full differentials are described in Section B.
- The most common differential for white spots on the skin or gills of freshwater fish is *Ichthyophthirius*. Other differentials include monogeneans, sessile ciliates, *Flavobacterium* spp., lymphocystis, and herpesviruses (e.g. carp pox). Granulomatous lesions and gas bubble disease can resemble white spots.

Diagnosis

- A tentative diagnosis can often be made based on clinical signs in susceptible species with a history of recent fish additions or acute stressors.
- Diagnosis is usually confirmed by identification of trophonts on direct microscopy of skin scrapes or gill or fin biopsies (Figure C6.1b and c).
- Trophonts often vary in size but some are large (up to 500–1000 μm). They are round, clear to tan, slowly rolling ciliates. The cilia are short and evenly distributed across the whole cell. A C-shaped macronucleus is readily visible in most trophonts. Some parasites may be within the gill epithelium. Even one trophont should be considered significant.
- Theronts are rarely seen, but are 20–45 μm motile ciliates.
- Cytology may also show increased mucus and gill hyperplasia, clubbing, and telangiectasia.
- Histology of skin, gill, or fin shows ciliates. It can be hard to distinguish ciliate morphology on histology, but the large size of some of the trophonts in a freshwater bony fish is usually an indicator of *Ichthyophthirius*.
- Experimental PCR assays are reported and may be helpful in learning more about the different strains.

Husbandry Management

- This parasite has a fast life cycle; start treatment as soon as possible to minimize morbidity and mortality.
- Use an integrated management approach, incorporating husbandry and medical management.
- Isolate affected system(s). This parasite is easily transmitted by fish, fomites, and aerosolization.
- Increase aeration; target dissolved oxygen may be 95–100%.
- Reduce or resolve any environmental stressors.

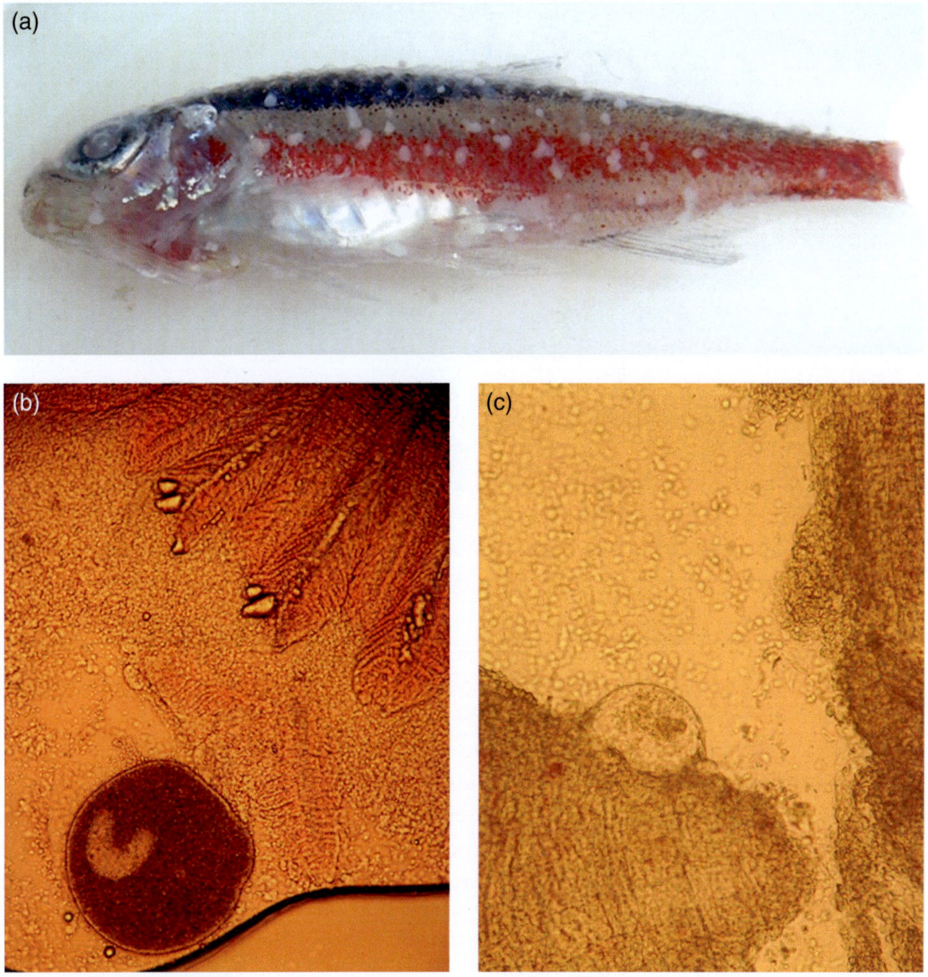

Figure C6.1 *Ichthyophthirius multifiliis* infection producing white spots in a cardinal tetra (*Paracheirodon axelrodi*) (a), and trophonts on direct microscopy of gill wet mounts at ×40 that are live (b) and dead (c).

- Remove dead or moribund fish as soon as possible with appropriate disposition.
- Increase mechanical cleaning; where possible, the substrate should be frequently siphoned to remove parasites.
- Remove unnecessary substrate or reduce the depth.
- Increase cleaning and disinfection of water and fomites, although high doses may be needed. The UV doses required to inactivate *Ichthyophthirius* tomites have been reported as >100 mJ/cm^2 or mWs/cm^2. Drying is likely to be effective.
- Regularly back-wash filters, such as sand filters.
- Increase the flow rate of flow-through systems.
- Increase the turnover of recirculating systems (e.g. > one exchange per hour) to try to reduce reinfection rates, although results have been inconsistent.
- If the fish species can tolerate the upper temperature limit for the parasite, slowly increase the water temperature, e.g. by ~5 °C (10 °F) per day to 30–32 °C (86–90 °F) for 5–14 days. This can eliminate the parasite, but it may be necessary to use immersion treatments to reduce clinical signs as the water temperature is brought up.
- Consider reducing the stocking density.
- For chronic or recurrent infections, consider biological control, e.g. leopard pleco (*Pterygoplichthys gibbiceps*) reduced parasite loads on blue tilapia (*Oreochromis aureus*), potentially by grazing on the biofilm.

Medical Management

- Therapy must be maintained or repeated for several weeks as treatment primarily targets theronts.
- Treatment success depends on the species, parasite strain, and abiotic factors; what has worked in one situation may not be effective in another.
- Common treatments (see Chapters A12 and A13 for more details):
  - Formalin immersion (37%) is the most commonly reported treatment. Most studies recommend 40–100 mg/L for 1–2 hours (0.16–0.4 mL/gallon). The doses must be repeated, and effective courses have included five to seven treatments every 48 hours at 9–11 °C (48–52 °F) and every 24 hours at 17–20 °C (63–68 °F). At higher temperatures, the dosing frequency

may need to be at least twice daily. Higher doses (up to 200 mg/L for one hour) have been reported where they can be tolerated by the fish. Lower doses (e.g. 10–30 mg/L) are almost always ineffective. Formalin levels should be assayed to assess actual drug concentration. Supplemental aeration should be provided and DO and biological filtration should be monitored closely. Some fish and invertebrate species or life stages may be sensitive to formalin. Suitable PPE should be used. Formalin (Formalin-FTM, Formacide-B, Parasite-S®) is approved in the United States for use in finfish with *Ichthyophthirius* under various immersion treatment protocols with a 0-day withdrawal, as of 2020.
  - Copper sulfate immersion is common in pond systems. Alkalinity and system volume must be known for accurate dosing. Alkalinity should be >50 mg/L of $CaCO_3$ as copper is more toxic at low alkalinity. The applied dose in mg/L is 1% of alkalinity, to a maximum of 2.5 mg/L, although this calculation may be an overestimate and some studies have shown effects at 0.5% of alkalinity. It is often redosed every 48 hours for four doses. Copper levels should be monitored daily. Supplemental aeration should be provided and DO should be monitored. Where DO is low or turbidity or plant load are high, there is a greater risk of adverse effects. Some species and life stages are sensitive to copper, including most elasmobranchs, invertebrates, and plants.
- Other reported treatments (see Chapters A12 and A13 for more details):
  - Salinity may be increased to reduce osmotic stress (e.g. 2–3 g/L). Higher levels may reduce parasite loads, but some strains can survive and breed at 7.5–10 g/L, which is above the level tolerated by most stenohaline freshwater teleosts.
  - Potassium permanganate ($KMnO_4$) immersion.
  - Potassium ferrate (VI) immersion, an oxidizing agent similar to $KMnO_4$.
  - Hydrogen peroxide immersion.
  - Sodium percarbonate or peracetic acid immersion, which slowly releases hydrogen peroxide.
  - Chlorophyllin immersion, which releases reactive oxygen species, has shown effects in vitro.
  - Potentiated sulfonamides orally.
  - Malachite green immersion, particularly in combination with formalin, is effective, but malachite green is banned in many countries and should be avoided for safety and regulatory reasons.
- Chloroquine diphosphate has not been effective in in vitro trials.
- If the parasite loads are heavy, consider antibiotics to help protect against secondary bacterial infections.
- Recurrence is common; keep fish isolated and monitor for at least three weeks after treatment has ended.
- If treatment is unsuccessful, keep the system empty of fish for at least six to nine weeks to allow time for tomonts encysted in the environment to release theronts.
- All legislation regarding medication use and disposal must be followed.

Prevention

- Reduce or resolve stressors.
  - Low stocking density.
  - Suitable social groups and habitats.
  - Excellent water quality and preferred water temperature.
  - Good nutrition.
  - Suitable handling and transport protocols.
- Reduce exposure and transmission.
  - Isolation with no contact with free-ranging freshwater fish.
  - Pathogen-free water source (e.g. municipal water or ground water that has gone through fine filtration then UV and/or ozone disinfection). Avoid using untreated surface water.
  - Disinfection of recirculating water with fine filtration then UV and/or ozone.
  - High water flow rate or turnover.
  - Removal of dead or moribund fish as soon as possible with appropriate disposition.
  - Good cleaning and disinfection protocols.
  - Suitable quarantine of fish for at least 30 days with isolation, monitoring, and diagnostic testing, particularly skin scrapes and gill biopsies. Prophylactic treatment for *Ichthyophthirius* may be indicated for freshwater bony fish.
  - Quarantine of freshwater plants prior to addition to fish systems (e.g. thorough rinsing then holding them without fish for a week or longer). Aquarium plants are often grown in ponds with fish and the plants may be mechanical carriers of pathogens.
  - Frozen-thawed or commercial feeds, with no live feeds.
- Reduce severity of disease.
  - Experimental vaccines using intracoelomic injection of live theronts show promise, but protection will likely be strain-specific. Vaccination using killed theronts, trophonts, cilia, or recombinant vaccines has had limited success.

- Immune stimulants such as beta glucans can decrease severity of clinical signs. They are most effective at specific doses, short courses, and when given prior to clinical signs.
- Selective breeding of more resistant fish strains may reduce susceptibility.

Zoonotic Reports

- These parasites have no known zoonotic potential.

Bibliography

Abdel-Hafez, G., Lahnsteiner, F., Mansour, N., and Licek, E. (2014). Pathophysiology of *Ichthyophthirius multifiliis* infection in rainbow trout (*Oncorhynchus mykiss*) and chub (*Leuciscus cephalus*). *Journal of Comparative Pathology* 151: 394–399.

Forwood, J.M., Harris, J.O., Landos, M., and Deveney, R. (2015). Life cycle and settlement of an Australian isolate of *Ichthyophthirius multifiliis* Fouquet, 1876 from rainbow trout. *Folia Parasitologica* 62: 13.

Kawano, F. and Hirazawa, N. (2012). Antiparasitic effect of in-feed inhibitors of folic acid synthesis and dihydrofolate reductase against ciliate *Cryptocaryon irritans* infection in the red sea bream *Pagrus major* and against ciliate *Ichthyophthirius multifiliis* infection in black pop-eye goldfish *Carassius auratus*. *Aquaculture* 330-333: 1–7.

Lahnsteiner, F. and Weismann, T. (2007). Treatment of ichthyophthiriasis in rainbow trout and common carp with common and alternative therapeutics. *Journal of Aquatic Animal Health* 19: 186–194.

Lauridsen, J.H. and Buchmann, K. (2010). Effects of short- and long-term glucan feeding of rainbow trout (Salmonidae) on the susceptibility to *Ichthyophthirius multifiliis* infections. *Acta Ichthyologica et Piscatoria* 40: 61–66.

Ling, F., Wang, J.-G., Lui, Q.-F. et al. (2010). Prevention of *Ichthyophthirius multifiliis* infestation in goldfish (*Carassius auratus*) by potassium ferrate (VI) treatment. *Veterinary Parasitology* 168: 212–216.

Picón-Camacho, S.M., Leclercq, E., Bron, J.E., and Shinn, A.P. (2012). The potential utility of the leopard pleco (*Glyptoperichthys gibbiceps*) as a biological control of the ciliate protozoan *Ichthyophthirius multifiliis*. *Pest Management Science* 68: 557–563.

Picón-Camacho, S.M., Marcos-Lopez, M., Bron, J.E., and Shinn, A.P. (2012). An assessment of the use of drug and non-drug interventions in the treatment of *Ichthyophthirius multifiliis* Fouquet, 1876, a protozoan parasite of freshwater fish. *Parasitology* 139: 149–190.

Rowland, S.J., Mifsud, C., Nixon, M. et al. (2009). Use of formalin and copper to control ichthyophthiriosis in the Australian freshwater silver perch (*Bidyanus bidyanus* Mitchell). *Aquaculture Research* 40: 44–54.

Straus, D.L., Hossain, M.M., and Clark, T.G. (2009). Copper sulfate toxicity to two isolates of *Ichthyophthirius multifiliis* relative to alkalinity. *Diseases of Aquatic Organisms* 83: 31–36.

Sudová, E., Straus, D.L., Wienke, A., and Meinelt, T. (2010). Evaluation of continuous 4-day exposure to peracetic acid as a treatment for *Ichthyophthirius multifiliis*. *ParasitologyResearch* 106: 539–542.

Wohllebe, S., Richter, P., and Häder, D.-P. (2012). Chlorophyllin for the control of *Ichthyophthirius multifiliis* (Fouquet). *Parasitology Research* 111: 729–733.

Xu, D.-H., Zhang, Q.-Z., Shoemaker, C.A. et al. (2016). Molecular immune response of channel catfish immunized with live theronts of *Ichthyophthirius multifiliis*. *Fish and Shellfish Immunology* 54: 86–92.

Abbreviations/Acronyms

- DO: Dissolved oxygen
- PCR: Polymerase chain reaction
- PPE: Personal protective equipment
- UV: Ultraviolet

Cryptocaryon irritans

Overview

- *Cryptocaryon irritans* is a ciliated protozoan ectoparasite that infects the skin and gills of marine bony fish.
- The disease is often called marine ich or marine white spot.
- It is a common cause of morbidity and mortality in aquarium fish and mariculture.
- It is typically treated with long-term immersion medications.
- It is often considered the saltwater equivalent of *Ichthyophthirius multifiliis*, because the life cycle and clinical signs are similar, but the organisms are not closely related.

Etiology
- Phylum *Ciliophora.*
- Family *Holophryidae.*
- *Cryptocaryon irritans* is the only reported species, although characteristics of different isolates vary.

Life Cycle and Transmission
- The life cycle is direct.
  - The trophont is the feeding stage that burrows under the epithelium, triggering an inflammatory response in the host. This stage is resistant to treatment.
  - Trophonts mature and grow, leave the host, attach to a solid surface and encyst, becoming reproductive tomonts within which tomites develop.
  - The tomonts rupture asynchronously, typically after dark, and each release 100–1000 tomites that differentiate into free-swimming theronts. This stage is most sensitive to immersion treatments.
  - Theronts are the infective stage but do not swim well – it is likely that most infections are acquired close to the substrate. Theronts must find a host within 6–48 hours. Theronts burrow into fish skin or gills.
- The life cycle is slower than *Ichthyophthirius.*
  - 7 days at 27 °C (81 °F).
  - 11–15 days at 24 °C (75 °F).
- There is little development at <12 °C (54 °F) and >30 °C (86 °F).

Geographic Distribution
- Saltwater habitats, particularly tropical and subtropical.

Signalment
- All marine bony fish may be susceptible, particularly tropical species.
- In aquaculture, olive flounder (*Paralichthys olivaceus*), red seabream (*Pagrus major*), and obscure pufferfish (*Takifugu obscurus*) are commonly reported hosts.
- There are no reports in brackish water fish.
- These do not infect elasmobranchs or invertebrates, although they can likely act as mechanical vectors.

Risk Factors
- Exposure and stressors are the most important risk factors.
- Exposure:
  - Poor biosecurity (e.g. lack of suitable quarantine, untreated surface water).
  - Preferred water temperature, typically 19–26 °C (66–79 °F).
  - Permissive salinity, typically 25–50 g/L.
  - High organic loads.
  - Low water flow rate or turnover.
  - Exposure of naïve fish.
  - Established infection; once established in a large habitat, this becomes a recurrent issue.
- Common stressors are described under C6: *Ichthyophthirius multifiliis.*

Signs/Clinical Findings
- Signs are often seen one to three weeks after new fish are added to a system.
- Multiple fish from one or more species are usually affected.
- Initial signs are subtle and may include reduced feeding, increased hiding, skin darkening, and subtle tachypnea.
- Fine white spots up to 0.5 mm in diameter develop on the skin, fins, and gills. Good lighting (e.g. a flashlight with a focal beam) helps to show early changes.
- Later signs include lethargy or pruritus (e.g. flashing, hyperactivity), dyspnea, tachypnea, keratitis, opaque and twitchy fins, inappetence, and mortalities.
- Secondary infections may be seen.
- Mortalities may start within days. The rate varies widely: this can be a chronic condition in established systems with a low mortality rate, but it can also cause acute disease with mortality of up to 100%.

Differential Diagnoses
- Full differentials are described in Section B.
- The most common differential for white spots on the skin or gills of tropical marine fish is *Cryptocaryon.* Other differentials include monogeneans, *Tenacibaculum* spp., and lymphocystis. Granulomatous lesions and gas bubble disease can resemble white spots.

Diagnosis
- A tentative diagnosis can often be made based on clinical signs in susceptible species with a history of recent fish additions or acute stressors.
- Diagnosis is usually confirmed by identification of trophonts on direct microscopy of skin scrapes or gill or fin biopsies (Figure C6.2).
- Trophonts often vary in size but some are large (up to 500–700 μm). They are round, clear to tan, slowly rolling ciliates. The cilia are short and cover the whole cell. A macronucleus may be visible and looks slightly lobulated. Some parasites may be within the gill epithelium. Even one trophont should be considered significant.
- Cytology may also show increased mucus and gill hyperplasia, clubbing, and telangiectasia.
- Histology of skin, gill, or fin shows ciliates. It can be hard to distinguish ciliate morphology on histology, but the large size of some of the trophonts in a marine bony fish is usually an indicator of *Cryptocaryon.*

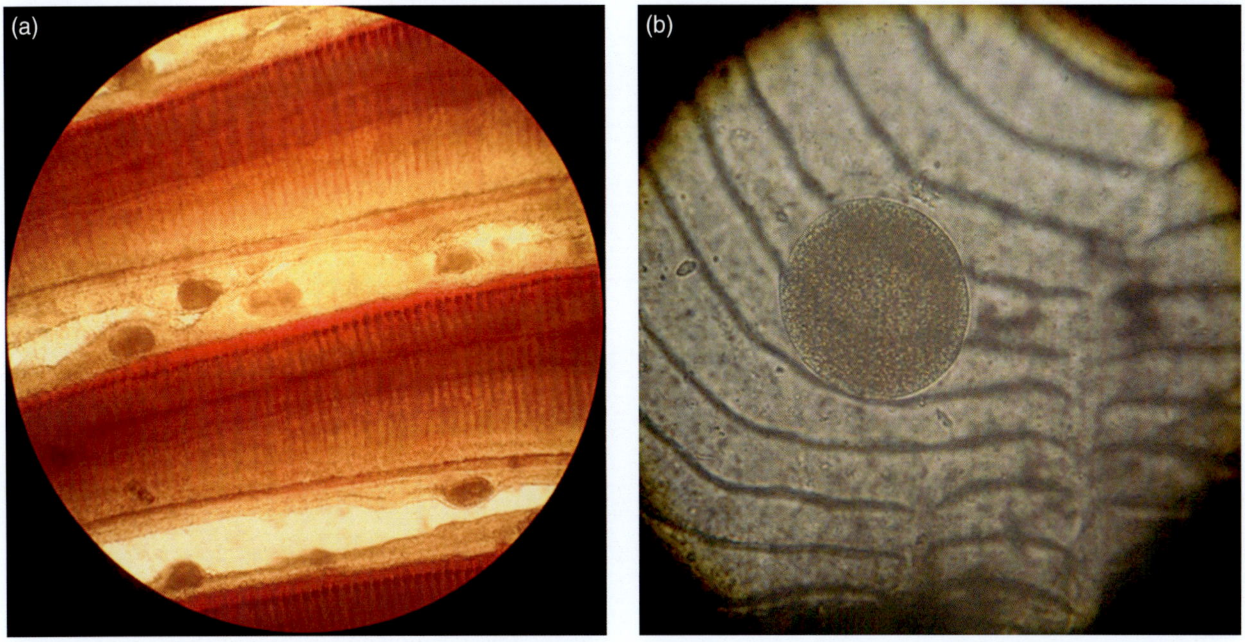

Figure C6.2 *Cryptocaryon irritans* trophont on a gill biopsy under direct microscopy at ×40 (a) and on a skin scrape at ×100 (b).

- Experimental PCR assays are reported and may be helpful in learning more about the different strains.

Husbandry Management

- Use an integrated management approach, incorporating husbandry and medical management.
- Isolate affected system(s).
- Increase aeration; target dissolved oxygen may be 95–100%.
- Reduce or resolve any environmental stressors.
- Remove dead or moribund fish as soon as possible with appropriate disposition.
- Increase mechanical cleaning; where possible, the substrate should be frequently siphoned to remove parasites.
- Remove unnecessary substrate or reduce the depth.
- Increase cleaning and disinfection of water and fomites, although high doses may be needed. For fomites, the following have been shown to reduce cyst hatching:
  - Sodium hypochlorite at 60 mg/L chlorine for 24 hours.
  - Benzalkonium chloride at 100 mg/L for 1 hour.
  - Hot water (e.g. 40 °C, 104 °F) for 1 hour.
  - Drying for >24 hours.
- Freshwater has shown no effect on cyst hatching after 24 hours.
- Regularly back-wash filters, such as sand filters.
- Increase the flow rate of flow-through systems.
- Increase the turnover of recirculating systems (e.g. >one exchange per hour) to try to reduce reinfection rates, although results have been inconsistent.
- Consider rotation of tank mats; in aquaculture, replacement of tarpaulin mats to remove parasites every three days for four rotations improves survival rates.
- Consider reducing the stocking density.
- Consider rotation of fish. Typical recommendations are to move the fish every three days at least four times, ideally into clean systems but transferring from one system then back again three days later can help.
- For chronic or recurrent infections, consider biological control, e.g. cleaner wrasse (*Labridae*) and cleaner shrimp.

Medical Management

- Therapy must be maintained or repeated for several weeks as treatment primarily targets theronts.
- Treatment success depends on the species, parasite strain, and abiotic factors; what has worked in one situation may not be effective in another.
- Immersion treatments may be most effective when applied late in the day to target the theront release at night.
- Common treatments (see Chapters A12 and A13 for more details):
  - Copper sulfate immersion is the most common treatment. Using ionized copper sulfate, the typical course is a slow increase over 5–7 days to 0.16–0.21 mg/L of ionized copper (Cu^{2+}), maintained for 21 days at 22–26 °C (72–79 °F). Ionized copper has a narrow safety margin. Alkalinity should be >50 mg/L of

$CaCO_3$ (alkalinity in marine systems is usually much higher). System volume must be known for accurate dosing. Ionized copper forms complexes readily, so $[Cu^{2+}]$ should be assayed every 12–24 hours to determine redosing needs. Some species and life stages are sensitive to copper, including most elasmobranchs, invertebrates, and plants. Biological filtration should be monitored.

  - Chelated copper products (e.g. Coppersafe™) may have a wider safety margin but drug levels can be less predictable. Label instructions should be followed. Alkalinity should be >50 mg/L of $CaCO_3$. System volume must be known for accurate dosing. Total copper should be assayed every 12–24 hours to determine redosing needs.
  - Formalin immersion (37%) is a common treatment. Many studies suggest a minimum of 50 mg/L (0.2 mL/gallon) every 24 hours until no clinical signs are seen then every 48 hours for >21 days. Doses <50 mg/L are typically ineffective. Supplemental aeration should be provided and DO and biological filtration should be monitored closely. Some fish and invertebrate species or life stages may be sensitive to formalin. Suitable PPE should be used.
  - Chloroquine diphosphate immersion is a common treatment, often at 10–15 mg/L maintained for three to four weeks, but recurrence may be more common than with copper treatment. A UV spectrophotometric assay can be used to assess drug concentration in the water. Some fish and invertebrate species or life stages may be sensitive to chloroquine; it cannot be used in reef aquariums.
  - Hyposalinity can be effective where tolerated. This may be a long-term treatment (e.g. maintaining at 18–20 g/L salinity) or pulse-treatments, e.g. gilthead seabream (*Sparus aurata*) with three-hour baths at 10 g/L salinity (by gradual acclimation at a rate of 5 g/L/hr in both directions) repeated four times, three days apart. This treatment may not be tolerated by some stenohaline species, including many elasmobranchs and corals.
- Other reported treatments (see Chapters A12 and A13 for more details):
  - Hydrogen peroxide immersion.
  - Salinomycin orally.
  - Potentiated sulfonamides orally.
- If the parasite loads are heavy, consider antibiotics to help protect against secondary bacterial infections.
- Elasmobranchs and invertebrates are sensitive to many of the treatments and are not susceptible to the disease.
  - For *Cryptocaryon* in coral systems, the best option is often to remove the susceptible teleosts and treat them in an isolated system.
  - For *Cryptocaryon* in systems with teleosts and elasmobranchs, the best option is often to remove the elasmobranchs while the system is treated.
- Recurrence is common; keep fish isolated and monitor for at least three weeks after treatment has ended.
- Some fish develop protective immunity to the parasite following sublethal exposure.
- If treatment is unsuccessful, keep the system empty of fish for at least six to nine weeks to allow time for tomonts encysted in the environment to release theronts.
- All legislation regarding medication use and disposal must be followed.

Prevention

- Reduce or resolve stressors.
  - Common stressors are described under C6: *Ichthyophthirius multifiliis.*
- Reduce exposure and transmission.
  - Isolation with no contact with free-ranging marine fish.
  - Pathogen-free water source (e.g. municipal water or ground water that has gone through fine filtration, then UV and/or ozone disinfection). Avoid using untreated surface water. If using natural seawater, store the water for at least 48 hours prior to use to allow any theronts to die.
  - Disinfection of recirculating water with fine filtration, then UV and/or ozone.
  - High water flow rate or turnover.
  - Removal of dead or moribund fish as soon as possible with appropriate disposition.
  - Good cleaning and disinfection protocols.
  - Suitable quarantine for at least 30 days with isolation, monitoring, and diagnostic testing, particularly skin scrapes and gill biopsies. Prophylactic treatment of *Cryptocaryon* is often recommended for tropical marine teleosts.
  - Frozen-thawed or commercial feeds, with no live feeds.
- Reduce severity of disease.
  - Experimental vaccines show promise but are hard to develop and protection will likely be strain-specific.
  - Immune stimulants such as allicin can decrease severity of clinical signs. They are most effective at specific doses, short courses, and when given prior to clinical signs.

Zoonotic Reports

- These parasites have no known zoonotic potential.

Bibliography

Hirazawa, N., Goto, T., and Shirasu, K. (2003). Killing effects of various treatments on the monogenean *Heterobothrium okamotoi* eggs and oncomiracidia and the ciliate *Cryptocaryon irritans* cysts and theronts. *Aquaculture* 223: 1–13.

How, K.H., Zenke, K., and Yoshinaga, T. (2015). Dynamics and distribution properties of theronts of the parasitic ciliate *Cryptocaryon irritans*. *Aquaculture* 438: 170–175.

Jang, B., Li, Y.W., Abdullahi, A.Y. et al. (2016). Placemat and rotational culturing: a novel method to control *Cryptocaryon irritans* infection by removing tomonts. *Aquaculture* 456: 84–88.

Kawano, F. and Hirazawa, N. (2012). Antiparasitic effect of in-feed inhibitors of folic acid synthesis and dihydrofolate reductase against ciliate *Cryptocaryon irritans* infection in the red sea bream *Pagrus major* and against ciliate *Ichthyophthirius multifiliis* infection in black pop-eye goldfish *Carassius auratus*. *Aquaculture* 330–333: 1–7.

Kawano, F., Hirazawa, N., Gravningen, K., and Brentsen, J.O. (2012). Antiparasitic effect of Romet30 against ciliate *Cryptocaryon irritans* infection in red sea bream *Pagrus major* and tiger puffier *Takifugu rubripe*. *Aquaculture* 344–349: 35–39.

Luo, X., Xie, M., Zhu, X., and Li, A. (2007). Protective immunity in grouper (*Epinephelus coioides*) following exposure to or injection with *Cryptocaryon irritans*. *Fish and Shellfish Immunology* 22: 427–432.

Picon-Camacho, S.M., de Ybáñez, R., Holzer, A.S. et al. (2011). In vitro treatments for the theront stage of the ciliate protozoan *Cryptocaryon irritans*. *Diseases of Aquatic Organisms* 94: 167–172.

Priya, T.A.J., Lin, Y.H., Wang, Y.C. et al. (2012). Codon changed immobilization antigen (iAg), a potent DNA vaccine in fish against *Cryptocaryon irritans* infection. *Vaccine* 30: 893–903.

Yoshinaga, T., Im, H.J., Nishida, S., and Ogawa, K. (2011). In vitro and in vivo efficacies of ionophores against *Cryptocaryon irritans*. *Aquaculture* 321: 167–172.

Abbreviations/Acronyms

- DO: Dissolved oxygen
- PCR: Polymerase chain reaction
- PPE: Personal protective equipment
- UV: Ultraviolet

Chilodonella spp.

Overview

- *Chilodonella* spp. are ciliated protozoan ectoparasites that infect the skin and gills of freshwater and brackish bony fish.
- The parasites are relatively common. Severe disease is rare, but epizootics have been reported in freshwater fish in aquaculture, aquariums, and in the wild.
- The infection can usually be cleared with a single immersion treatment.
- *Chilodonella* spp. are considered the freshwater equivalent to *Brooklynella* spp., due to a similar appearance and life cycle.

Etiology

- Phylum *Ciliophora.*
- Family *Chilodonellidae.*
- There are many species within the genus and most are free-living.
- *Chilodonella piscicola* and *Chilodonella hexasticha* are the most common species identified in epizootics.

Life Cycle and Transmission

- The life cycle is direct with no encysted stages.
- Transmission is horizontal, through direct or indirect contact.

Geographic Distribution

- Freshwater and brackish water habitats, probably worldwide.

Signalment

- Freshwater and brackish water bony fish are susceptible.
- Severe disease has been reported in a wide range of cultured and wild fish, including channel catfish (*Ictalurus punctatus*), Australian cod (*Maccullochella* spp.), carp (*Carassius* spp.), silver perch (*Bidyanus bidyanus*), freshwater salmonids (*Oncorhynchus* and *Salmo* spp.), and barramundi (*Lates calcarifer*).
- Examples from aquarium fish include freshwater angelfish (*Pterophyllum* spp.), discus (*Symphysodon* spp.), platies (*Xiphophorus maculatus*), and guppies (*Poecilia reticulata*).
- They may be found on invertebrates.
- There are no reports from elasmobranchs.

Risk Factors

- Exposure and stressors are the most important risk factors.

- Exposure includes:
  - Poor biosecurity (e.g. lack of suitable quarantine, untreated surface water).
  - Permissive water temperature, although values vary by species and strain; *C. piscicola* can tolerate 4–20 °C (39–68 °F).
  - Permissive salinity.
  - Low water flow rate or turnover.
  - Exposure of naïve fish.
- Common stressors are described under C6: *Ichthyophthirius multifiliis*.

Signs/Clinical Findings

- Multiple fish from one or more species are usually affected.
- Signs are often subtle and may include lethargy, increased hiding, reduced feeding, skin darkening or pallor, gray skin coloration, skin ulcers, dyspnea, or tachypnea.
- The disease may present peracutely, with sudden death as the first clinical sign.
- Mortality is usually low but can be high in fish under other stressors.

Differential Diagnoses

- Full differentials are described in Section B.
- Common differentials for skin and gill ciliates in freshwater bony fish include *Ichthyophthirius multifiliis*, *Chilodonella* spp., scuticociliates, trichodinids, and sessile ciliates.

Diagnosis

- Diagnosis is typically by direct microscopy of skin scrapes or gill biopsies.
- The ciliates are oval or heart-shaped (30–70 × 20–50 μm), dorsoventrally flattened, translucent, and some show a notched anterior end (Figure C6.3). Parallel rows of cilia are sometimes visible, but are not as obvious as with *Brooklynella* spp. The parasites show slow, mostly straight, gliding movements.

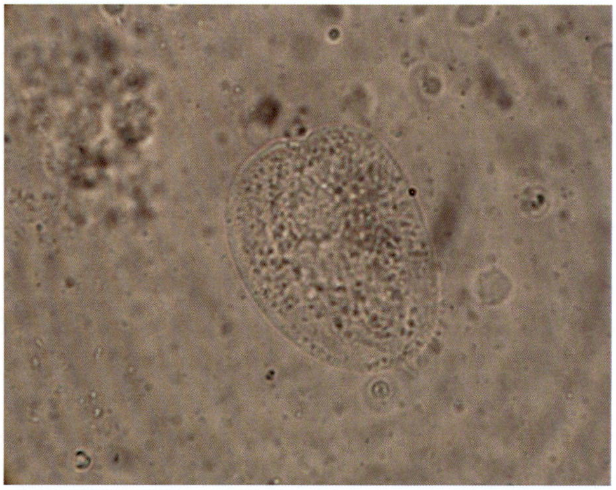

Figure C6.3 *Chilodonella* sp. ciliate on skin scrape under direct microscopy at ×400.

- Increased mucus and gill hyperplasia, necrosis, and edema may also be seen.
- A high load is indicative of a problem. A single organism may not be significant.
- For definitive identification, morphologic data following silver staining and molecular diagnostics are recommended.

Husbandry Management

- Consider isolating affected system(s).
- Reduce or resolve any environmental stressors.
- Remove any unnecessary organic material.
- Increase cleaning and disinfection.

Medical Management

- Common treatments (see Chapters A12 and A13 for more details):
  - Formalin immersion (37%) at 25–50 mg/L once is often effective. Supplemental aeration should be provided. The biological filtration should be monitored closely. Some fish and invertebrate species or life stages may be sensitive to formalin. Suitable PPE should be used. Formalin (Formalin-FTM, Formacide-B, Parasite-S®) is approved in the United States for use in finfish with *Chilodonella* under various immersion treatment protocols with a 0-day withdrawal, as of 2020.
  - Saltwater dips, matched to pH and temperature, followed by a move to an uninfected system can be effective.
- Other reported treatments (see Chapters A12 and A13 for more details):
  - Long-term hypersalinity.
  - Potassium permanganate immersion.
  - Hydrogen peroxide immersion.
- All legislation regarding medication use and disposal must be followed.

Prevention

- Reduce or resolve stressors.
  - Common stressors are described under C6: *Ichthyophthirius multifiliis*.
- Reduce exposure and transmission.
  - Isolation with no contact with free-ranging fish.
  - Pathogen-free water source (e.g. municipal water or ground water that has gone through fine filtration, then UV and/or ozone disinfection). Avoid using untreated surface water.

- ○ Disinfection of recirculating water with fine filtration, then UV and/or ozone.
- ○ High water flow rate or turnover.
- ○ Removal of dead or moribund fish as soon as possible with appropriate disposition.
- ○ Good cleaning and disinfection protocols.
- ○ Suitable quarantine for at least 30 days with isolation, monitoring, and diagnostic testing, particularly skin scrapes and gill biopsies if morbidity is seen.
- ○ Frozen-thawed or commercial feeds, with no live feeds.

Zoonotic Reports
- These parasites have no known zoonotic potential.

Bibliography

Bowater, R.O. and O'Donoghue, P.J. (2015). An epizootic of chilodonelliasis in farmed barramundi *Lates calcarifer* (Bloch), a case report. *Journal of Fish Diseases* 38: 931–936.

Gomes, G.B., Jerry, D.R., Miller, T.L., and Kutson, K.S. (2017). Current status of parasitic ciliates *Chilodonella* spp. (Phyllopharyngea: Chilodonellidae) in freshwater fish aquaculture. *Journal of Fish Diseases* 40: 703–715.

Pádua, S.B., Martins, M.L., Carrijo-Mauad, J.R. et al. (2013). First record of *Chilodonella hexasticha* (Ciliophora: Chilodonellidae) in Brazilian cultured fish: a morphological and pathological assessment. *Veterinary Parasitology* 191: 154–160.

Abbreviations/Acronyms
- PPE: Personal protective equipment
- UV: Ultraviolet

Brooklynella spp.

Overview
- *Brooklynella* spp. are ciliated protozoan ectoparasites that typically infect the gills of marine bony fish, although they can infect the skin.
- They are common pathogens that can occasionally cause high morbidity and mortality in aquarium fish and aquaculture.
- *Brooklynella* spp. are considered the saltwater equivalent of *Chilodonella* spp., due to similar appearance and life cycle.

Etiology
- Phylum *Ciliophora.*
- Family *Hartmannulidae.*
- *Brooklynella hostilis* is the type species; there are likely many others.

Life Cycle and Transmission
- The life cycle is direct with no encysted stages.
- Transmission is horizontal, through direct or indirect contact.

Geographic Distribution
- Saltwater habitats, probably worldwide.

Signalment
- Tropical and temperate marine bony fish are susceptible.
- Seahorses and pipefish (*Syngnathidae*), marine angelfish (*Pomacanthidae*), and clownfish (*Amphiprioninae*) may be particularly susceptible.
- These do not infect elasmobranchs or invertebrates.

Risk Factors
- Exposure and stressors are the most important risk factors.
- Exposure includes:
  - ○ Poor biosecurity (e.g. lack of suitable quarantine, untreated surface water).
  - ○ Permissive salinity.
  - ○ Low water flow rate or turnover.
  - ○ Exposure of naïve fish.
- Common stressors are described under C6: *Ichthyophthirius multifiliis.*

Signs/Clinical Findings
- Multiple fish from one or more species are usually affected.
- Initial signs are subtle and may include lethargy, increased hiding, reduced feeding, skin darkening, or pallor.
- Later signs include dyspnea, tachypnea, gray skin coloration, opaque fins, and mortalities.
- The disease may present peracutely, with sudden death as the first clinical sign.
- Mortality can be high.

Differential Diagnoses
- Full differentials are described in Section B.
- Common differentials for skin and gill ciliates in marine bony fish include *Cryptocaryon irritans*, *Brooklynella hostilis*, and scuticociliates.

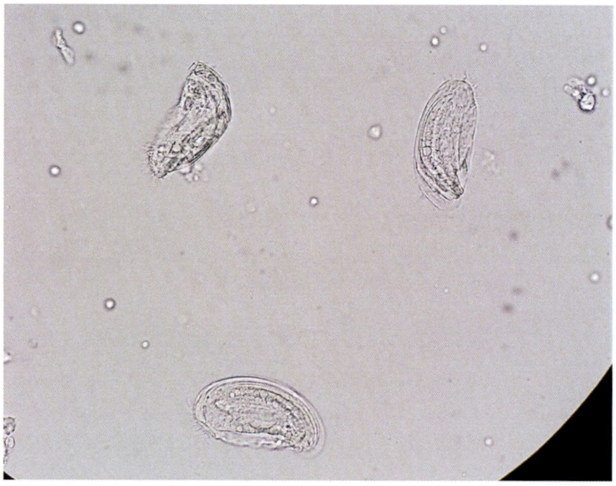

Figure C6.4 *Brooklynella* sp. ciliates under direct microscopy of a skin scrape at ×100. Source: Image courtesy of Johnny Shelley, USDA-ARS Aquatic Animal Health Research Unit.

Diagnosis

- Diagnosis is typically by direct microscopy of gill biopsies or skin scrapes.
- The ciliates are oval or heart-shaped (55–80 × 25–50 μm), dorsoventrally flattened, translucent, and some show a notched anterior end (Figure C6.4). Rows of cilia are typically visible across the organism. The parasites show fast, gliding movements.
- Increased mucus and gill hyperplasia, necrosis, and edema may also be seen.
- A high or moderate load is indicative of a problem. A single organism may not be significant.
- For definitive identification, molecular diagnostics are recommended.

Husbandry Management

- Isolate affected system(s).
- Reduce or resolve any environmental stressors.
- Remove any unnecessary organic material.
- Increase cleaning and disinfection.
- Increase water flow-rate and turnover.

Medical Management

- Common treatments (see Chapters A12 and A13 for more details):
  - Formalin immersion (37%) at 25–100 mg/L once or repeated in two to three days is usually effective, although recurrence is seen. Supplemental aeration should be provided and DO and biological filtration should be monitored closely. Some fish and invertebrate species or life stages may be sensitive to formalin. Suitable PPE should be used.
- Other reported treatments (see Chapters A12 and A13 for more details):
  - Long-term hyposalinity.
  - Freshwater dips, matched to pH and temperature.
- This ciliate is not susceptible to copper sulfate immersion at routine doses.
- All legislation regarding medication use and disposal must be followed.

Prevention

- Reduce or resolve stressors.
  - Common stressors are described under C6: *Ichthyophthirius multifiliis*.
- Reduce exposure and transmission.
  - Isolation with no contact with free-ranging fish.
  - Pathogen-free water source (e.g. municipal water or ground water that has gone through fine filtration, then UV and/or ozone disinfection). Avoid using untreated surface water.
  - Disinfection of recirculating water with fine filtration, then UV and/or ozone.
  - High water flow rate or turnover.
  - Removal of dead or moribund fish as soon as possible with appropriate disposition.
  - Good cleaning and disinfection protocols.
  - Suitable quarantine for at least 30 days with isolation, monitoring, and diagnostic testing, particularly gill biopsies and skin scrapes if morbidity is seen.
  - Formalin dips (e.g. 50 mg/L for 2 hours) after acclimation and prior to introduction to a quarantine system can prevent the introduction of this parasite, in the author's experience.
  - Frozen-thawed or commercial feeds, with no live feeds.

Zoonotic Reports

- These parasites have no known zoonotic potential.

Bibliography

Diamant, A. (1998). *Brooklynella hostilis* (Hartmannulidae), a pathogenic ciliate from the gills of maricultured seabream. *Bulletin of the European Association of Fish Pathologists* 18: 33–36.

Abbreviations/Acronyms

- PPE: Personal protective equipment
- UV: Ultraviolet

Scuticociliates

Overview

- Scuticociliates are ciliated, histophagous protozoa that are typically free-living but can be pathogenic.
- If present in heavy loads on live fish, they are likely to be pathogenic.
- If found in necrotic tissue or on dead fish, interpretation can be difficult as these rapidly colonize damaged tissues.
- Differentiation of genera and species requires molecular techniques.
- *Uronema*, *Miamiensis*, and *Philasterides* spp. are common pathogens in marine aquariums and flatfish aquaculture.
- *Tetrahymena corlissi* is a common pathogen of guppies (*Poecilia reticulata*).
- Scuticociliates are emerging pathogens of elasmobranchs.

Etiology

- Phylum *Ciliophora.*
- Subclass *Scuticociliata.*
- There are a variety of species and the taxonomy is complicated.
- The most commonly reported scuticociliates in salt water are *Uronema marinum*, *Uronema nigricans*, *Miamiensis avidus*, and *Philasterides dicentrarchi*, although the last two may be synonymous.
- The most commonly reported scuticociliates in freshwater are *Tetrahymena corlissi*, also known as tet disease or guppy killer, and *Tetrahymena pyriformis.*
- Other species that have been reported include *Mesanophrys* and *Pseudocohnilembus* spp.

Life Cycle and Transmission

- The life cycle is direct with no encysted stages.
- These are predominantly facultative parasites that can be free-living in the environment.
- Transmission is horizontal, through direct or indirect contact.
- The parasites can spread hematogenously (e.g. through the nasal cavity or ampullary system to the brain).
- Several species that affect fish have been identified in crustaceans and mollusks; these may play a role in transmission.

Geographic Distribution

- Freshwater and saltwater habitats, probably worldwide.

Signalment

- Marine scuticociliates (*Uronema*, *Miamiensis*, *Philasterides* spp.) affect a wide variety of fish. Particularly susceptible species and groups include:
  - Seahorses, pipefish, and sea dragons (*Syngnathidae*).
  - Flatfish such as turbot (*Scophthalmus maximus*) and olive flounder (*Paralichthys olivaceus*).
  - European bass (*Dicentrarchus labrax*).
  - Southern bluefin tuna (*Thunnus maccoyii*).
  - Zebra and horn sharks (*Stegostoma* and *Heterodontus* spp.).
- Freshwater scuticociliates (*Tetrahymena* spp.) have been reported most commonly from:
  - Guppies, swordtails, mollies, and platies (*Poeciliidae*).
  - Tetras (*Characidae*).
  - Cichlids (*Cichlidae*).
  - Carp, goldfish, and zebrafish (*Cyprinidae*).
- Juveniles are more susceptible.

Risk Factors

- Exposure and stressors are the most important risk factors.
- Exposure includes:
  - Permissive water temperature; epizootics have been reported at a wide range of temperatures (8–28 °C or 46–82 °F) but in aquaculture, disease is more common at higher summer temperatures.
  - Permissive salinity, although epizootics of marine scuticociliates have been reported at a wide range of salinities; 15–35 g/L.
  - High organic loads.
  - Low water flow rate or turnover.
  - Trauma to the mucus, skin, or gills.
- Common stressors are described under C6: *Ichthyophthirius multifiliis.*

Signs/Clinical Findings

- One or more fish may be affected.
- Typical clinical signs include increased mucus, skin darkening, rough gray, white, or brown skin lesions, petechiae and erythema particularly around the base of the fins and the mouth, muscle swelling, or skin ulcers. However, some infections are not associated with skin lesions (e.g. *P. dicentrarchi* in European bass and *U. nigricans* in bluefin tuna).
- Inappetence or reduced feeding may be seen.
- Lethargy may be seen.
- Abnormal swimming (e.g. spiraling) is common if the infection becomes systemic.
- Exophthalmos or keratitis may be seen.
- Gill pallor, dyspnea, or tachypnea may be seen with heavy infections, particularly in flatfish.
- Enteritis with yellow, mucoid fecal material may be seen.
- Coelomic distension from serosanguinous coelomic effusion may be seen.
- Mortality may reach 100%.

Differential Diagnoses

- Full differentials are described in Section B.
- Common differentials for skin and gill ciliates in freshwater bony fish include *Ichthyophthirius multifiliis*, *Chilodonella* spp., scuticociliates, trichodinids, and sessile ciliates.
- Common differentials for skin and gill ciliates in marine bony fish include *Cryptocaryon irritans*, *Brooklynella hostilis*, and scuticociliates.

Diagnosis

- Diagnosis is typically by direct microscopy of gill biopsies or scrapes of skin lesions. If invasive, ciliates may be identified on wet mounts of the brain and viscera, particularly the gonads, kidney, liver, or intestines. They may be found in the cerebrospinal fluid or coelomic effusion.

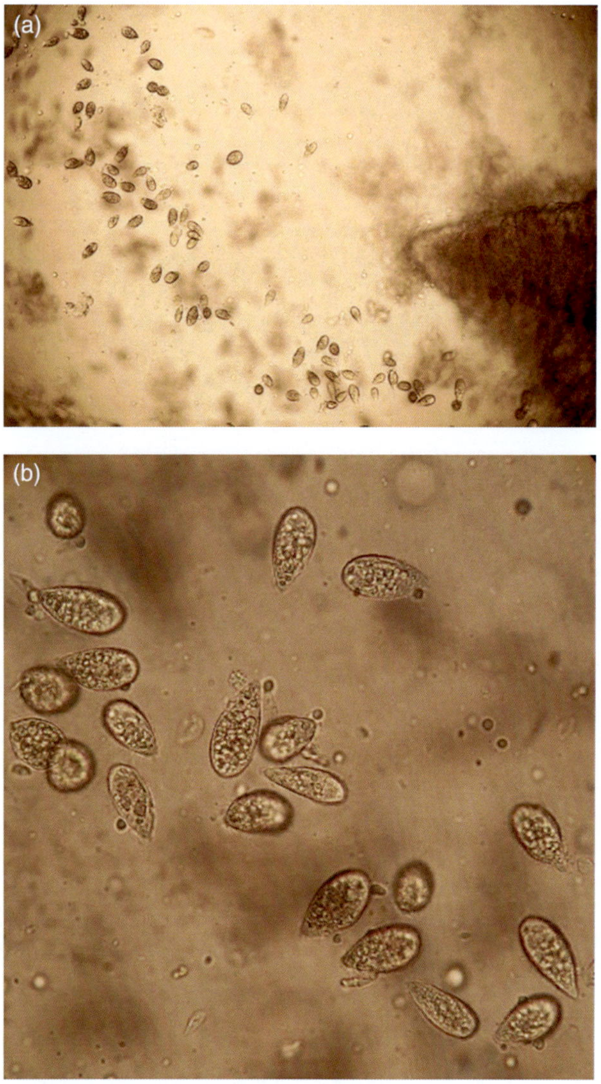

Figure C6.5 Scuticociliates under direct microscopy of skin scrapes at ×40 (a) and ×100 (b).

- The ciliates are small (*Uronema*, *Miamensis*, and *Philasterides* spp. ~20×40 µm, *Tetrahymena* ~30–40×55–80 µm), and teardrop (pyriform) to oval in shape (Figure C6.5). Cilia are just visible and evenly spaced. The parasites show fast, forward, spinning movements. They can be present in very high numbers.
- On necropsy, coeliotomy, or histology, affected tissues such as the skin, brain, or viscera may be edematous, hemorrhagic, or necrotic. Intralesional ciliates are often vascular or perivascular. Meningoencephalitis is common in bluefin tuna and elasmobranchs, while systemic infections seem common in syngnathids.
- Molecular testing is required to distinguish the genera, although this is rarely necessary for clinical management. PCR and IHC may be available experimentally.

Husbandry Management

- It can be hard to judge if scuticociliates are clinically significant, as free-living forms often colonize necrotic tissue (e.g. skin ulcers) and can rapidly colonize tissues postmortem. Indications for management changes may include identification on several live or recently euthanized fish or signs of invasive infection.
- Reduce or resolve any environmental stressors.
- Remove any unnecessary organic material.
- Remove dead or moribund fish as soon as possible with appropriate disposition.
- Avoid overfeeding.
- Increase cleaning and disinfection. The UV doses required to inactivate scuticociliates have been reported as $>30\,mJ/cm^2$.
- Increase water flow rate and turnover.
- Consider depopulation and disinfection for virulent strains.

Medical Management

- Treatment of external scuticociliates is usually straightforward. Invasive scuticociliates carry a poor prognosis and treatment is rarely successful.
- Common treatments (see Chapters A12 and A13 for more details):
  - Formalin immersion (37%) is commonly reported, with doses ranging from 25 mg/L for six hours to 250 mg/L for one hour. Supplemental aeration should be provided and DO and biological filtration should be monitored closely. Some fish and invertebrate species or life stages may be sensitive to formalin. Increased toxicity may be seen in fish with skin ulcers and respiratory signs. Suitable PPE should be used.
  - Metronidazole immersion may be used, e.g. at 50 mg/L every 24 hours for 10 days. A spectrophotometric assay can be used to assess drug level in water.

- Surgical debridement of necrotic tissue can improve healing.
- Antibiotics may be used with antiparasitics to prevent secondary bacterial infections. They should be based on culture and sensitivity.
- Other reported treatments (see Chapters A12 and A13 for more details):
  - Potassium permanganate immersion.
  - Saltwater dips for freshwater fish, matched to pH and temperature.
  - Freshwater dips for saltwater fish, matched to pH and temperature.
  - Chloroquine diphosphate immersion or orally.
  - Hydrogen peroxide immersion.
  - Niclosamide orally.
  - Nitroimidazole or dimetridazole orally.
- All legislation regarding medication use and disposal must be followed.

Prevention

- Reduce or resolve stressors.
  - Common stressors are described under C6: *Ichthyophthirius multifiliis*.
- Reduce exposure and transmission.
  - Good mechanical filtration and disinfection of water with UV and/or ozone.
  - High water flow rate or turnover.
  - Removal of dead or moribund fish as soon as possible with appropriate disposition.
  - Good cleaning and disinfection protocols.
  - With seasonal epizootics in aquaculture, fish can be harvested at a smaller size prior to onset of disease or not stocked until after the summer water temperatures have resolved.

Zoonotic Reports

- These parasites have no known zoonotic potential.

Bibliography

DiCicco, E., Paradis, E., Stephen, C. et al. (2013). Scuticociliatid ciliate outbreak in Australian pot-bellied seahorse, *Hippocampus abdominalis* (Lesson, 1827): clinical signs, histopathologic findings, and treatment with metronidazole. *Journal of Zoo and Wildlife Medicine* 44: 435–440.

Leibowitz, M.P., Chettri, J.K., Ofir, R., and Zilberg, D. (2010). Treatment development for systemic *Tetrahymena* sp. infection in guppies, *Poecilia reticulata* Peters. *Journal of Fish Diseases* 33: 473–480.

Li, W.-T., Lo, C., Su, C.-Y. et al. (2017). Locally extensive meningoencephalitis caused by *Miamensis avidus* (syn. *Philasterides dicentrarchi*) in a zebra shark. *Diseases of Aquatic Organisms* 126: 167–172.

Stidworthy, M.F., Garner, M.M., Bradway, D.S. et al. (2014). Systemic scuticociliatosis (*Philasterides dicentrarchi*) in sharks. *Veterinary Pathology* 51: 628–632.

Webb, D.H., Marrero, C., Ellis, H. et al. (2013). A simple reagent-free spectrophotometric assay for monitoring metronidazole therapy in aquarium water. *Journal of Aquatic Animal Health* 25: 165–170.

Abbreviations/Acronyms

- IHC: Immunohistochemistry
- PCR: Polymerase chain reaction
- PPE: Personal protective equipment
- UV: Ultraviolet

Trichodinids

Overview

- Trichodinids are ectoparasitic ciliates commonly found on the skin, fins, gills, and eyes of bony fish.
- Low loads are usually incidental.
- Heavy loads are usually indicative of poor environmental quality; improving the environment will usually resolve the problem.

Etiology

- Phylum *Ciliophora*.
- Family *Trichodinidae*.
- Several genera have been identified in fish (e.g. *Trichodina*, *Trichodinella*, *Dipartiella*, *Paratrichodina*, *Tripartiella*).

Life Cycle and Transmission

- The life cycle is direct with no encysted stages.
- Transmission is horizontal.

Geographic Distribution

- Freshwater and saltwater habitats, probably worldwide.

Signalment

- Freshwater, brackish, and marine bony fish are susceptible, although the parasites are more common in freshwater fish, particularly carp (*Cyprinus carpio*), goldfish (*Carassius auratus*), Nile tilapia (*Oreochromis niloticus*), and other cichlids.
- There are rare, older reports of *Trichodina* spp. in skates (*Raja* spp.).

Risk Factors

- Stressors are the most important risk factors, particularly high nitrogenous wastes and high organic loads.

Signs/Clinical Findings

- These are usually carried asymptomatically.
- Dyspnea or tachypnea may be seen.
- Pruritus (e.g. flashing) or increased mucus may be seen.
- Gills may look edematous.
- Lethargy may be seen.
- Reduced appetite or growth rates may be seen.
- Secondary infections may be seen.
- Mortality is usually low.

Differential Diagnoses

- Full differentials are described in Section B.
- Common differentials for skin and gill ciliates in freshwater bony fish include *Ichthyophthirius multifiliis*, *Chilodonella* spp., scuticociliates, trichodinids, and sessile ciliates.
- Common differentials for skin and gill ciliates in marine bony fish include *Cryptocaryon irritans*, *Brooklynella hostilis*, and scuticociliates.

Diagnosis

- Diagnosis is typically by direct microscopy of skin scrapes or gill biopsies. Some species are more likely on skin (e.g. *Trichodina* spp.), while others are more likely on the gills (e.g. *Trichodinella*, *Tripartiella* spp.).
- The ciliates are round, radially symmetric, flat or dome shaped, 30–130 μm in diameter, with rings of cilia and denticles (Figure C6.6). The ciliates show steady gliding or erratic rotating movements.
- On cytology and histology, gills may show hyperplasia, edema, inflammatory infiltrate, and necrosis, as well as intralesional ciliates.
- Trichodinids may be found on direct microscopy or histology of the urogenital system (e.g. kidney, urinary bladder, oviduct, copulatory sac).
- Speciation is not common as it does not affect management, but is typically based on denticle morphology. Silver staining of fixed samples helps with further identification.

Husbandry Management

- Improving the environment is often enough to resolve signs.
- Reduce or resolve any environmental stressors, particularly poor water quality.
- Remove any unnecessary organic material.
- Increase cleaning and disinfection. The UV doses required to inactivate *Trichodina* spp. have been reported as 35–159 mJ/cm^2.
- Increase water flow rate and turnover.

Medical Management

- Medication may be warranted if signs are severe or environmental problems cannot be resolved. A single treatment is often enough unless organic load remains high.
- Common treatments (see Chapters A12 and A13 for more details):
  - Formalin immersion (37%) using a single treatment at a low dose (e.g. 25–50 mg/L for 1–2 hours). Supplemental aeration should be provided. Suitable PPE should be used. Formalin (Formalin-FTM, Formacide-B, Parasite-S®) is approved in the United States for use in finfish with *Trichodina* under various immersion treatment protocols with a 0-day withdrawal, as of 2020.
  - Long-term hypersalinity, but susceptibility varies and salinity of 3 to >10 g/L may be needed.
  - Copper sulfate immersion is common in pond systems. Alkalinity and system volume must be known for accurate dosing. Alkalinity should be >50 mg/L of $CaCO_3$ as copper is more toxic at low alkalinity. The dose in mg/L may be 0.5% of alkalinity, to a maximum of 2.0 mg/L. Copper levels should be monitored. Supplemental aeration should be provided and DO should be monitored. Where DO is low or turbidity or plant load are high, there is a greater risk of adverse effects. Some species and life stages are sensitive to copper, including most elasmobranchs, invertebrates, and plants.
- Other reported treatments (see Chapters A12 and A13 for more details):
  - Chelated copper immersion.
  - Saltwater dips for freshwater fish, matched to pH and temperature.
  - Freshwater dips for saltwater fish, matched to pH and temperature.
  - Potassium permanganate immersion.
  - Teflubenzuron immersion.
- All legislation regarding medication use and disposal must be followed.

Prevention

- Reduce or resolve stressors.
  - Common stressors are described under C6: *Ichthyophthirius multifiliis*.
- Reduce exposure and transmission.
  - Good mechanical filtration and disinfection of water with UV and/or ozone.
  - High water flow rate or turnover.

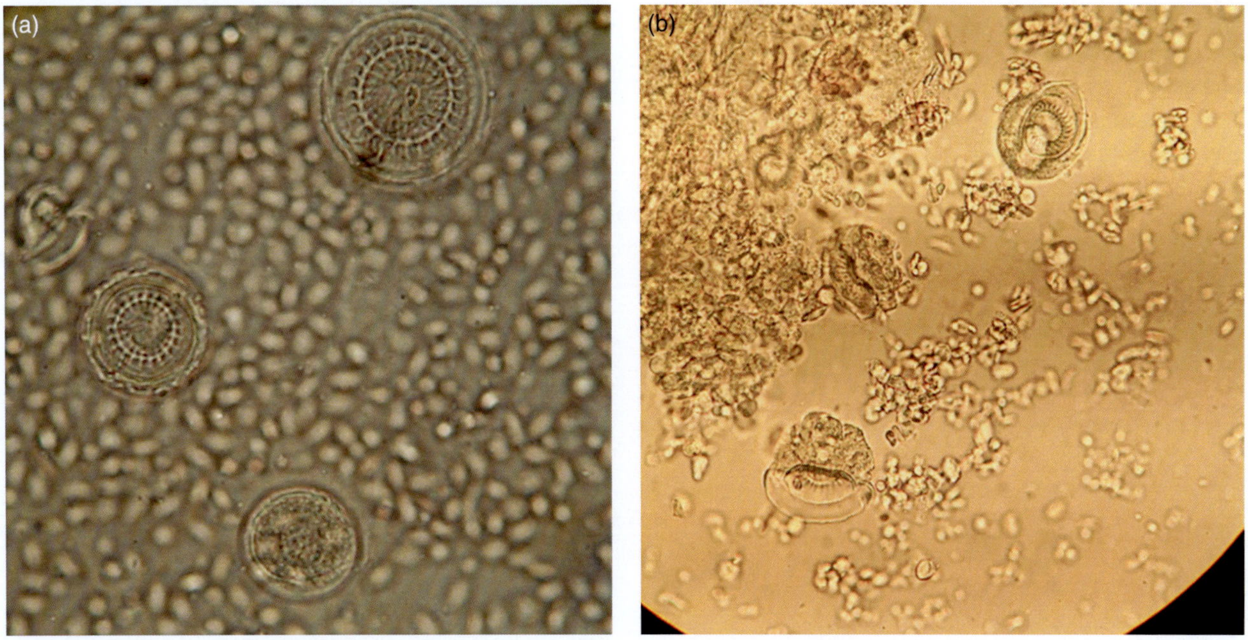

Figure C6.6 Trichodinid ciliates under direct microscopy of skin scrapes (a and b); ×100.

- Removal of dead or moribund fish as soon as possible with appropriate disposition.
- Good cleaning and disinfection protocols.

Zoonotic Reports

- These parasites have no known zoonotic potential.

Bibliography

Bruno, D.W., Nowak, B., and Elliott, D.G. (2006). Guide to the identification of fish protozoan and metazoan parasites in stained tissue sections. *Diseases of Aquatic Organisms* 70: 1–36.

Gong, Y., Yu, Y., Feng, W., and Shen, Y. (2005). Phylogenetic relationships among *Trichodinidae* (Ciliophora: Peritricha) derived from the characteristic values of denticles. *Acta Protozoology* 44: 237–243.

Ikefuti, C.V., Carraschi, S.P., Barbuio, R. et al. (2015). Teflubenzuron as a tool for control of trichodinids in freshwater fish: acute toxicity and in vivoefficacy. *Experimental Parasitology* 154: 108–112.

Khan, R.A. (1972). Taxonomy, prevalence, and experimental transmission of a protozoan parasite, *Trichodina oviducti* Poylanskii (Ciliata: Peritrichida) of the thorny skate, *Raja radiata* Donovan. *Journal of Parasitology* 58: 680–685.

Abbreviations/Acronyms

- DO: Dissolved oxygen
- PPE: Personal protective equipment

Sessile Ciliates

Overview

- A variety of sessile ciliates can be found on fish, particularly freshwater fish.
- They typically attach to the skin and gills.
- They are often found where organic load is high.
- They are rarely pathogenic, unless fish are under significant stressors. An exception to this is *Heteropolaria* spp. (red sore disease), which tend to be more pathogenic.

Etiology

- Phylum *Ciliophora*.
- Subclasses *Peritrichia* and *Suctoria.*
- A variety of ciliates with a sessile adult stage are reported in fish:
  - *Ambiphrya* (previously *Scyphidia*) spp.
  - *Apiosoma* (previously *Glossatella*) spp.
  - *Capriniana* (synonymous with *Trichophrya*) spp.
  - *Heteropolaria* (synonymous with *Epistylis*) spp.
  - *Vorticella* spp.

Life Cycle and Transmission

- The life cycle is direct with no encysted stages.

- Transmission is horizontal, through direct or indirect contact.
- These typically reproduce by binary fission, producing free-swimming juveniles. They attach and become sessile when a suitable host is found.

Geographic Distribution

- Freshwater and saltwater habitats, probably worldwide.

Signalment

- Freshwater fish are commonly reported hosts, particularly in ponds, e.g. carp and koi (*Cyprinus carpio*), goldfish (*Carassius auratus*), and catfish (*Siluriformes*).
- They may be found on saltwater fish.

Risk Factors

- Stressors are the most important risk factors, particularly high nitrogenous wastes and high organic loads.

Signs/Clinical Findings

- These are usually carried asymptomatically.
- Signs may include reduced appetite, pruritus (e.g. flashing), dyspnea, or tachypnea.
- Skin lesions may include ulcers, white spots, or white, gray, or brown fluffy lesions, particularly on the fin margins and around the mouth.
- *Capriniana* spp. are more likely to cause respiratory signs than skin changes.
- Secondary infections may be seen, particularly with *Aeromonas hydrophila*.
- Mortality is usually low.

Differential Diagnoses

- Full differentials are described in Section B.
- The most common differentials for small structures attached to the skin or gills by a stalk are sessile ciliates and flagellates (e.g. *Ichthyobodo* spp.).

Diagnosis

- Diagnosis is typically by direct microscopy of skin scrapes or fin or gill biopsies.
- The parasites are all small (<100 μm), with an attachment stalk that may contract and oral rings of cilia.
- *Ambiphrya* spp. are ~50–100 × ~50 μm, solitary, barrel-shaped with two rows of cilia (oral and mid-body) and no stalk (Figure C6.7a). Only the cilia move.
- *Apiosoma* spp. are ~70–100× ~50 μm, solitary or colonial, shaped like a long vase or cup with a wide, noncontractile stalk and oral cilia at the distal end (Figure C6.7b). Only the cilia and oral disc move.
- *Capriniana* spp. are ~40–110 ×~30–50 μm, solitary, with an amorphous-shaped body and long, straight feeding tentacles that look like pins (Figure C6.7c). They attach to gills via a sucker. They are not typically found on the skin.
- *Heteropolaria* spp. are ~40–80 × ~20 μm, solitary or colonial, shaped like a long vase with a wide, noncontractile stalk and oral cilia at the distal end (Figure C6.7d). Only the cilia move.
- *Vorticella* spp. are ~50–100 × ~30–50 μm, solitary, and spherical, conical, or bell-shaped, with a long, thin contractile stalk (Figure C6.7e).
- Parasites on smears can be air-dried, fixed in methanol, then stained with Giemsa for morphologic identification.

Husbandry Management

- Management changes are only indicated if the parasite load is high or morbidity is seen.
- Improving the environment is often enough to resolve signs.
- Reduce or resolve any environmental stressors, particularly poor water quality.
- Remove any unnecessary organic material.
- Increase mechanical cleaning.
- Increase water flow rate and turnover.

Medical Management

- Where needed, a single immersion treatment is often enough to reduce parasite loads if organic load is low.
- Common treatments (see Chapters A12 and A13 for more details):
  - Formalin immersion (37%) using a single treatment at a low dose (e.g. 25–50 mg/L for 2 hours). Supplemental aeration should be provided. Suitable PPE should be used. Formalin (Formalin-FTM, Formacide-B, Parasite-S®) is approved in the United States for use in finfish with *Heteropolaria* spp. under various immersion treatment protocols with a 0-day withdrawal, as of 2020.
  - Long-term hypersalinity in freshwater fish, where the fish can tolerate the treatment.
  - Saltwater dips in freshwater fish, matched to pH and temperature.
- Other treatments (see Chapters A12 and A13 for more details):
  - Hydrogen peroxide immersion.
  - Copper sulfate immersion.
  - Potassium permanganate immersion.
- All legislation regarding medication use and disposal must be followed.

Prevention

- Reduce or resolve stressors.
  - Common stressors are described under C6: *Ichthyophthirius multifiliis*.
- Reduce exposure and transmission.

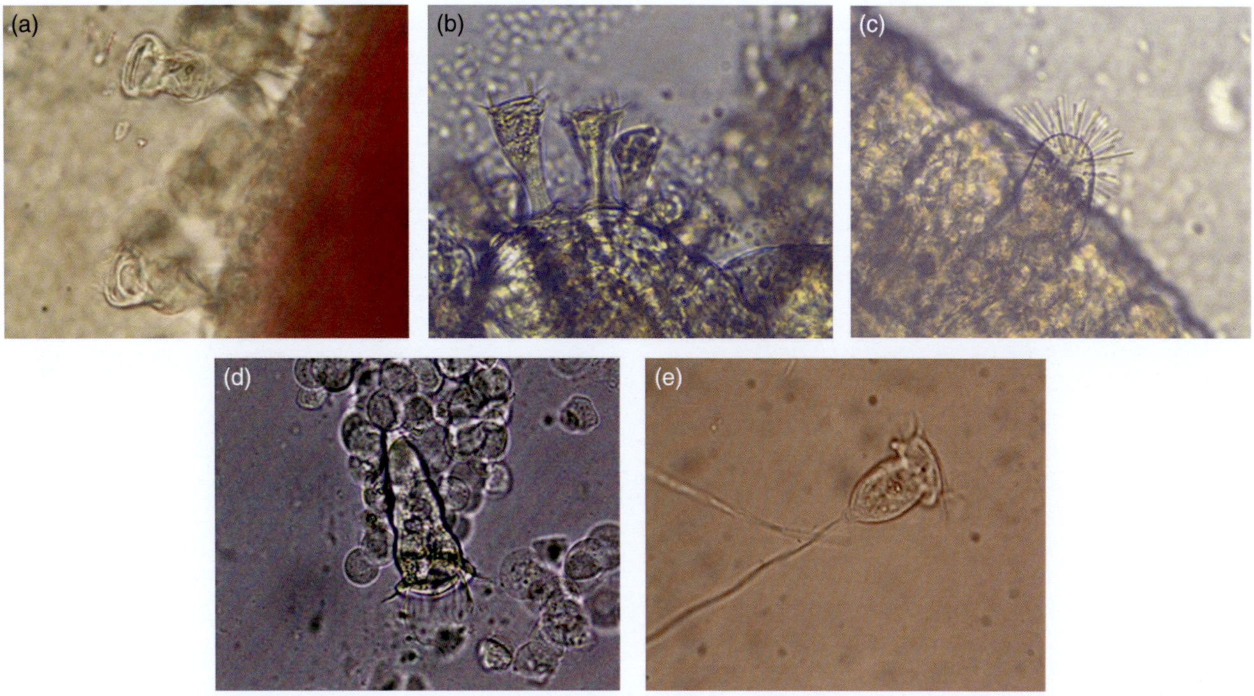

Figure C6.7 Direct, bright-field microscopy of sessile ciliates: *Ambiphrya* sp. (a), *Apiosoma* sp. (b), *Capriniana* sp. (c), *Heteropolaria* sp. (d), and *Vorticella* sp. (e). *Source*: Images (b and c) courtesy of John Drennan, Aquatic Animal Health Laboratory, Colorado Parks and Wildlife. Image (d) courtesy of Bartolomeo Gorgoglione, University of Veterinary Medicine, Vienna.

  - Good mechanical filtration and disinfection of recirculating water with UV and/or ozone.
  - High water flow rate or turnover.
  - Removal of dead or moribund fish as soon as possible with appropriate disposition.
  - Good cleaning and disinfection protocols.

Zoonotic Reports

- These parasites have no known zoonotic potential.

Bibliography

Abdel-Baki, A.S., Gewik, M.M., and Al-Quraishy, S. (2014). First records of *Ambiphrya* and *Vorticella* spp. (Protozoa, Ciliophora) in cultured Nile tilapia (*Oreochromis niloticus*) in the central region of Saudi Arabia. *Saudi Journal of Biological Sciences* 21: 520–523.

Li, M., Wang, J., Zhu, D. et al. (2008). Study of *Apiosoma piscicola* (Blanchard 1885) occurring on fry of freshwater fishes in Hongze, China with consideration of the genus *Apiosoma*. *Parasitology Research* 102: 931–937.

Rach, J.J., Gaikowski, M.P., and Ramsay, R.T. (2000). Efficacy of hydrogen peroxide to control parasitic infestations on hatchery-reared fish. *Journal of Aquatic Animal Health* 12: 267–273.

Abbreviations/Acronyms

- PPE: Personal protective equipment

Cryptobia spp.

Overview

- *Cryptobia* spp. are flagellates. Some can be pathogenic in fish.
- *Cryptobia iubilans* is commonly found in the gastrointestinal tract of discus (*Symphysodon* spp.) and other cichlids and can cause granulomatous gastritis.
- *Cryptobia branchialis* predominantly infects the gills of freshwater fish.
- Some *Cryptobia* (often classified as *Trypanoplasma*) spp. are hemoparasites that can cause high mortality. They have been a particular problem for Pacific salmonid broodstock (*Oncorhynchus* spp.).

- Gastrointestinal cryptobiosis may not result in morbidity or mortality; branchial, systemic, and hematozoic cryptobiosis are more likely to be pathogenic.

Etiology
- Phylum *Euglenozoa.*
- Class *Kinetoplastea.*
- Typical species are non-hematozoic, e.g. *Cryptobia iubilans*, *Cryptobia branchialis.*
- Hematozoic *Cryptobia* include *Cryptobia* (*Trypanoplasma*) *salmositica*, *Cryptobia* (*Trypanoplasma*) *bullocki*, and *Cryptobia* (*Trypanoplasma*) *borreli.*

Life Cycle and Transmission
- Non-hematozoic species show direct life cycles.
- Hematozoic species usually show indirect life cycles involving leeches but can show direct transmission.
- For *C. salmositica*, brook trout (*Salvelinus fontinalis*) and sculpin (*Cottus* spp.) can act as carriers.

Geographic Distribution
- Predominantly in freshwater habitats, probably worldwide, with some in saltwater habitats.
- Each species has a narrower range (e.g. *C. salmositica* off the Pacific coast of North America).

Signalment
- Non-hematozoic species are often reported from African and Central American cichlids, particularly discus, oscars (*Astronotus ocellatus*), and tilapia (*Oreochromis* spp.).
- Hematozoic species have been reported from:
  - Wild and cultured Pacific salmonids and sculpin – *C. salmositica*.
  - Flatfish (*Paralichthys* and *Pleuronectes* spp.), hogchokers (*Trinectes maculatus*), and croaker (*Micropogonias undulatus*) – *C. bullocki*.
  - Cyprinids (*Cyprinidae*) – *C. borreli*.
- Younger fish may be more susceptible.

Risk Factors
- Stressors are the most important risk factors.
  - Common stressors are described under C6: *Ichthyophthirius multifiliis*.
- Exposure to leeches and other hematophagous parasites is important for hematozoic species, so wild-caught and pond-reared fish are at higher risk.

Signs/Clinical Findings
- Multiple conspecifics may be affected.
- Inappetence, reduced feeding, or weight loss is common.
- Lethargy, increased hiding, or lateral or ventral recumbency may be seen.
- Skin darkening or increased mucus production may be seen.
- Dyspnea or tachypnea may be seen.
- Abnormal fecals may be seen.
- *Cryptobia* (*Trypanoplasma*) spp. can also cause gill pallor, generalized edema, exophthalmos, or coelomic distension. Disease progress is slower with hematozoic forms.
- Mortality rate is usually low but may reach 100%.

Differential Diagnoses
- Full differentials are described in Section B.
- Common differentials for gastrointestinal flagellates include *Cryptobia* and *Spironucleus*/*Hexamita* spp.
- Common differentials for small gill flagellates include *Cryptobia* and *Ichthyobodo* spp.
- Common differentials for hemoparasites in fish include *Cryptobia* spp. (trypanoplasms), trypanosomes, hemogregarines, and piroplasms.

Diagnosis
- *C. iubilans* is usually identified on direct microscopy or histology of gastric samples and *C. branchialis* on direct microscopy or histology of gill samples.
  - The flagellates are small ($10–20 \times 2–4\,\mu m$), teardrop to oval in shape, with an anterior and posterior flagellum. The flagellates show slow, undulating movements, different from the flickering motion of *Ichthyobodo* spp.
  - Cytology and histology will often show granulomas with intralesional flagellates. The infection can become systemic, affecting any viscera.
  - Acid-fast staining, culture, and PCR are useful to rule out mycobacteriosis, another common cause of granulomas.
- *C. salmositica* is usually identified on blood samples or at necropsy.
  - During acute disease, the flagellates are typically found on direct microscopy or Giemsa-stained blood smears or coelomic effusion (Figure C6.8).
  - The flagellates are $6–25\,\mu m$ in length and have two anterior flagella (only one of which may be visible) and a posterior flagellum.
  - On exam, coeliotomy, and necropsy, microcytic and hypochromic anemia and splenomegaly are common findings.
  - Histology may show generalized hemorrhage, congestion, and necrosis, with flagellates within the capillaries.
  - During chronic disease, examination of the buffy coat from chilled hematocrit tubes increases sensitivity.

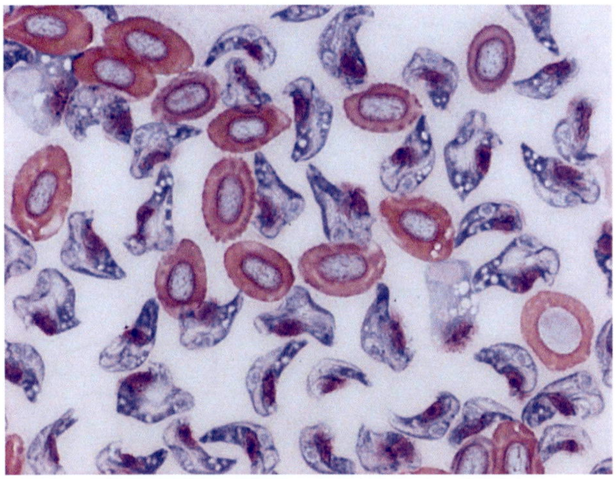

Figure C6.8 *Cryptobia* (*Trypanoplasma*) sp. on a blood smear; Leishman and Giemsa ×600. *Source*: Image courtesy of Craig Olson, Northwest Indian Fisheries Commission.

  - Cell-mediated and serological assays may be available.
- EM is needed for definitive identification.

Husbandry Management

- Treatment is rarely effective but improving environmental conditions can reduce morbidity and mortality.
- Increase aeration; target dissolved oxygen may be 95–100%.
- Reduce or resolve any environmental stressors.
- Consider adjusting the water temperature; slowly increasing temperature from 10 °C (50 °F) to 20 °C (68 °F) reduced mortality in rainbow trout (*Oncorhynchus mykiss*) and sockeye salmon (*Oncorhynchus nerka*) with *C. salmositica*.

Medical Management

- Common treatments (see Chapters A12 and A13 for more details):
  - Isometamidium chloride at 1 mg/kg IM as a single dose may reduce parasitemia in salmonids; toxicity has been seen at higher doses.
  - Dimetridazole immersion at 80 mg/L 24 hours immersion every 24 hours for three days may reduce clinical signs. This is more soluble than metronidazole but is typically under greater regulatory control.
- Other reported treatments (see Chapters A12 and A13 for more details):
  - 2-amino-5-nitrothiazole orally or by immersion.
- Many treatments have proven ineffective, including metronidazole, albendazole, fenbendazole, chloroquine, primaquine, and sulfonamides.
- All legislation regarding medication use and disposal must be followed.

Prevention

- Reduce or resolve stressors.
  - Common stressors are described under C6: *Ichthyophthirius multifiliis*.
- Reduce exposure and transmission.
  - Isolation with no contact with free-ranging fish.
  - Reduce or eliminate leeches in the habitat.
  - Pathogen-free water source (e.g. municipal water or ground water that has gone through fine filtration, then UV and/or ozone disinfection). Avoid using untreated surface water.
  - Disinfection of recirculating water with fine filtration then UV and/or ozone.
  - High water flow rate or turnover.
  - Removal of dead or moribund fish as soon as possible with appropriate disposition.
  - Good cleaning and disinfection protocols.
  - Suitable quarantine for at least 30 days with isolation, monitoring, and diagnostic testing, particularly necropsy, cytology, and histology.
  - Frozen-thawed or commercial feeds, with no live feeds.
- Reduce severity of disease.
  - *C. salmositica* vaccines for salmonid broodstock.
  - Selective breeding of more resistant fish strains.

Zoonotic Reports

- These parasites have no known zoonotic potential.

Bibliography

Ardelli, B.F. (2001). Therapeutic and prophylactic effects of isometamidium chloride (Samorin) against the haemoflagellate *Cryptobia salmositica* in chinook salmon (*Oncorhynchus tshawytscha*). *Parasitology Research* 87: 18–26.

Bower, S.M. and Margolis, L. (1983). Direct transmission of the hemoflagellate *Cryptobiasalmositica* among Pacific salmon (*Oncorhynchus* spp.). *Canadian Journal of Zoology* 61: 1242–1250.

Burreson, E.M. (2007). Hemoflagellates of Oregon marine fishes with the description of new species of *Trypanosoma* and *Trypanoplasma*. *Journal of Parasitology* 93: 1442–1451.

Woo, P.T.K. (2001). *Cryptobia (Trypanoplasma) salmositica* and salmonid cryptobiosis. *Journal of Fish Diseases* 26: 627–646.

Yanong, R.P.E., Curtis, E., Russo, R. et al. (2004). *Cryptobia iubilans* infection in juvenile discus. *Journal of the American Veterinary Medical Association* 224: 1644–1650.

Abbreviations/Acronyms
- EM: Electron microscopy
- IM: Intramuscular
- PCR: Polymerase chain reaction

Ichthyobodo spp.

Overview
- *Ichthyobodo necator* is a small ectoparasitic flagellate.
- The parasites can be found on the skin, fins, or gills of bony fish.
- They can cause epizootic disease in cultured fish.

Etiology
- Phylum *Euglenozoa*.
- Class *Kinetoplastea*.
- *Ichthyobodo necator* (*Costia necatrix*) is the type species, but others are reported (e.g. *Ichthyobodo salmonis*).
- The disease is sometimes referred to as costiosis.

Life Cycle and Transmission
- *I. necator* has a direct life cycle with a motile and sessile stage; there is no encysted stage. Both the motile and sessile stages are susceptible to immersion medications.

Geographic Distribution
- Freshwater and saltwater habitats, probably worldwide.

Signalment
- All bony fish may be susceptible.
- They are commonly reported from rainbow trout (*Oncorhynchus mykiss*).
- Juvenile fish may be more susceptible.

Risk Factors
- Exposure and stressors are the most important risk factors.
- Exposure includes:
  - Poor biosecurity (e.g. lack of suitable quarantine, untreated surface water).
  - Permissive water temperature, typically low, although some can tolerate a wide range (8–30 °C or 46–86 °F).
  - Low water flow rate or turnover.
  - Exposure of naïve fish.
- Common stressors are described under C6: *Ichthyophthirius multifiliis*.

Signs/Clinical Findings
- Multiple fish from one or more species are usually affected.
- Inappetence, reduced feeding, or poor body condition may be seen.
- Lethargy, increased hiding, or swimming at the surface may be seen.
- Pruritus (e.g. flashing) may be seen.
- Skin ulcers or dull gray-blue coloration may be seen.
- Dyspnea, tachypnea, or gill pallor due to anemia may be seen.
- Mortality is typically low but may be high with other stressors.

Differential Diagnoses
- Full differentials are described in Section B.
- Common differentials for small gill flagellates include *Cryptobia* and *Ichthyobodo* spp.

Diagnosis
- Diagnosis is typically by direct microscopy or histology of skin or gill samples. High magnification with immersion oil is usually needed.
- They are small flagellates, 10–20 × 5 μm, similar in size to a red blood cell, and often shaped like a comma or teardrop (Figure C6.9). The parasites have two pairs of flagella that are rarely visible on direct microscopy, although the characteristic flicking, tumbling motion is usually obvious. When attached to the epithelium, the cilia flick erratically, similar to a candle flame.
- Cytology and histology may show increased mucus, gill hyperplasia or edema, and flagellates.
- Poorly buffered tricaine methanesulfonate (MS222) anesthesia can cause the parasites to detach and reduces the sensitivity of direct microscopy and histology.
- PCR and qPCR tests may be available commercially.

Husbandry Management
- Management changes are indicated if the parasite load is high or morbidity is seen.
- Increase aeration; target dissolved oxygen may be 95–100%.
- Reduce or resolve any environmental stressors, particularly poor water quality.
- Increase cleaning and disinfection. The UV doses required to inactivate *I. necatrix* have been reported as >318 mJ/cm^2.

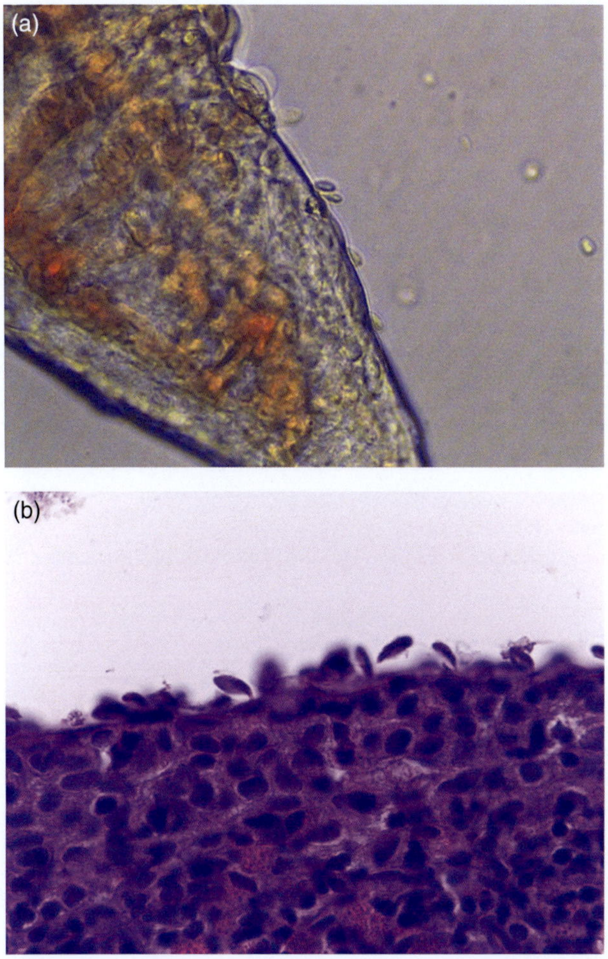

Figure C6.9 *Ichthyobodo* sp. from a gill biopsy under direct microscopy (a) and on histology (H&E) (b). *Source*: Image (a) courtesy of John Drennan, Aquatic Animal Health Laboratory, Colorado Parks and Wildlife; image (b) courtesy of Rubén López, National Autonomous University of Mexico.

Medical Management

- Common treatments (see Chapters A12 and A13 for more details):
  - Formalin immersion (37%) at low doses (e.g. 25–80 mg/L for 2 hours) is usually effective. Supplemental aeration should be provided. Suitable PPE should be used. Formalin (Formalin-FTM, Formacide-B, Parasite-S®) is approved in the United States for use in finfish with costiosis under various immersion treatment protocols with a 0-day withdrawal, as of 2020.
  - Copper sulfate immersion can reduce parasite load and improve survival. This may be effective at lower doses and shorter courses than needed for *Cryptocaryon* and *Ichthyophthirius*. Alkalinity and system volume must be known for accurate dosing. Alkalinity should be >50 mg/L of $CaCO_3$. Copper levels should be monitored daily. Supplemental aeration should be provided and DO should be monitored. Some species and life stages are sensitive to copper, including most elasmobranchs, invertebrates, and plants.
- Other reported treatments (see Chapters A12 and A13 for more details):
  - Metronidazole orally or by immersion.
  - Triclabendazole orally.
  - Hydrogen peroxide immersion.
  - Sodium percarbonate or peracetic acid immersion.
  - Potassium permanganate immersion.
- All legislation regarding medication use and disposal must be followed.

Prevention

- Reduce or resolve stressors.
  - Common stressors are described under C6: *Ichthyophthirius multifiliis*.
- Reduce exposure and transmission.
  - Isolation with no contact with free-ranging fish.
  - Pathogen-free water source (e.g. municipal water or ground water that has gone through fine filtration, then UV and/or ozone disinfection). Avoid using untreated surface water.
  - Disinfection of recirculating water with fine filtration then UV and/or ozone.
  - High water flow rate or turnover.
  - Removal of dead or moribund fish as soon as possible with appropriate disposition.
  - Good cleaning and disinfection protocols.
  - Suitable quarantine for at least 30 days with isolation, monitoring, and diagnostic testing, particularly gill biopsies and histology.
  - Frozen-thawed or commercial feeds, with no live feeds.

Zoonotic Reports

- These parasites have no known zoonotic potential.

Bibliography

Callahan, H.A. and Noga, E.J. (2002). Tricaine dramatically reduces the ability to diagnose the protozoan ectoparasite (*Ichthyobodo necator*) infections. *Journal of Fish Diseases* 25: 433–437.

Farmer, B.D., Straus, D.L., Beck, B.H. et al. (2013). Effectiveness of copper sulfate, potassium permanganate and peracetic acid to reduce mortality and infestation of *Ichthyobodo necator* in channel catfish *Ictalurus punctatus* (Rafinesque 1818). *Aquaculture Research* 44: 1103–1109.

Jaafar, R.M., Kuhn, J.A., Chettri, J.K., and Buchmann, K. (2013). Comparative efficacies of sodium percarbonate, peracetic acid, and formaldehyde for control of *Ichthyobodo necator*-an ectoparasitic flagellate from rainbow trout. *Ichthyologica et Piscatoria* 43: 139–143.

Mitchell, A.J., Darwish, A., and Fuller, A. (2008). Comparison of tank treatments with copper sulfate and potassium permanganate for sunshine bass with ichthyobodosis. *Journal of Aquatic Animal Health* 20: 202–206.

Mizuno, S., Urawa, S., Miyamoto, M. et al. (2017). Epizootiology of the ectoparasitic protozoans *Ichthyobodo salmonis* and *Trichodina truttae* on wild chum salmon *Oncorhynchus keta*. *Diseases of Aquatic Organisms* 126: 99–109.

Abbreviations/Acronyms

- PCR: Polymerase chain reaction
- PPE: Personal protective equipment
- qPCR: Quantitative polymerase chain reaction
- UV: Ultraviolet

Spironucleus and *Hexamita* spp.

Overview

- *Spironucleus* and *Hexamita* spp. are diplomonad flagellates that are often found in the intestinal tract of cichlids, cyprinids, and salmonids.
- They are typically commensal, but they can cause enterocolitis and weight loss, particularly in angelfish (*Pterophyllum* spp.) and discus (*Symphysodon* spp.). Affected fish are usually chronic poor-doers.
- Treatment with metronidazole can often improve signs.

Etiology

- Phylum *Metamonada.*
- Family *Hexamitidae.*
- Common parasitic species include:
  - *Spironucleus (Hexamita) salmonis, Spironucleus salmonicida, Spironucleus vortens, Spironucleus elegans.*
  - *Hexamita truttae, Hexamita intestinalis.*

Life Cycle and Transmission

- The life cycle is direct with no encysted stages.
- Transmission is horizontal, through direct and indirect contact.

Geographic Distribution

- Predominantly in freshwater habitats. Also found in cold-water marine habitats.

Signalment

- Freshwater teleosts are commonly reported hosts, but cold-water marine teleosts can be affected.
- They are particularly common in cichlids such as angelfish and discus, as well as cyprinids (*Cyprinidae*), salmon and trout (*Salmonidae*), and bettas and gouramis (*Anabantoidei*).

Risk Factors

- Stressors are the most important risk factors.
  - Common stressors are described under C6: *Ichthyophthirius multifiliis.*

Signs/Clinical Findings

- These are often carried asymptomatically.
- Where clinical signs are seen, inappetence, reduced feeding, and weight loss are the most common.
- Lethargy or agitated swimming may be seen.
- Coelomic distension due to coelomic effusion and enteritis may be seen.
- Exophthalmos may be seen.
- Skin ulcers or skin darkening may be seen.
- Stringy, mucoid, or pale fecal material or erythema at the vent may be seen.
- Poor reproductive success may be seen.
- *Spironucleus* spp. have been associated with lateral line depigmentation (also known as head and lateral line erosion) in discus and angelfish, but their role is unclear.
- Mortality is usually low.

Differential Diagnoses

- Full differentials are described in Section B.
- Common differentials for gastrointestinal flagellates include *Cryptobia* and *Spironucleus/Hexamita* spp.

Diagnosis

- Diagnosis is typically by direct microscopy of intestinal contents or scrapes at necropsy, although the parasites may be seen on fecal samples or cloacal washes. The parasites are usually more caudal in the GI tract than *Cryptobia* spp.
- These are small (~10×4 μm), elongated, pear-shaped flagellates with paired nuclei and six anterior and two posterior flagella, although the flagella are rarely visible on light microscopy (Figure C6.10). The parasites show fast, jerky movements.
- Necropsy may also show fluid-filled intestines and coelomic effusion.

- Histology may show flagellates and enteritis, which can be severe.
- The parasites may spread systemically with associated hemorrhage and edema. Lesions may be granulomatous or suppurative, although granulomatous lesions are less common than with *Cryptobia* spp. In rare cases, parasites may be visible on blood smears or buffy coat smears.
- EM is needed to differentiate between *Hexamita* and *Spironucleus* spp.

Husbandry Management

- Reduce or resolve any environmental stressors, particularly poor water quality.
- Remove any unnecessary organic material.
- Increase mechanical cleaning.

Medical Management

- Medical treatment is indicated where clinical signs are seen.
- Unlike *Cryptobia* spp., these are easily controlled.
- Common treatments (see Chapters A12 and A13 for more details):
  - Metronidazole orally is considered more effective than by immersion. High doses are often needed, e.g. 50–100 mg/kg body weight every 24 hours for three to five days.
  - Metronidazole immersion is used routinely. Common dose regimens are 5–7 mg/L every 24 hours for five days or 25 mg/L for 6 hours every 48 hours for three treatments. A spectrophotometric assay can be used to measure drug concentration in the water.
- Other reported treatments (see Chapters A12 and A13 for more details):
  - Other nitroimidazoles may be considered (e.g. benznidazole, ronidazole, triclabendazole, albendazole, mebendazole).
  - Magnesium sulfate orally.

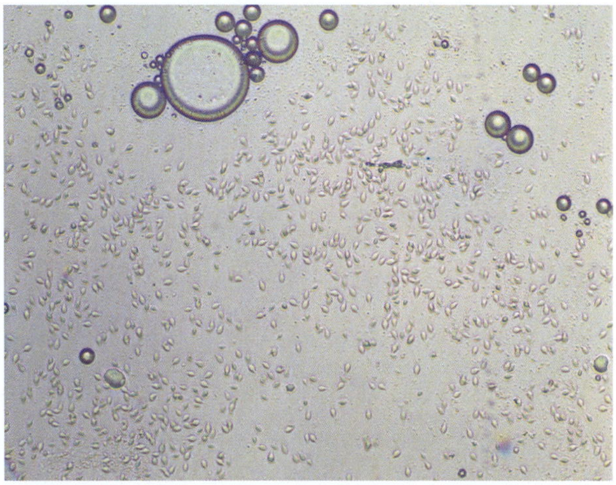

Figure C6.10 Abundant *Hexamita* sp. under direct microscopy of an intestinal wet mount. *Source*: Image courtesy of John Drennan, Aquatic Animal Health Laboratory, Colorado Parks and Wildlife.

- All legislation regarding medication use and disposal must be followed.

Prevention

- Reduce or resolve stressors.
  - Common stressors are described under C6: *Ichthyophthirius multifiliis*.
- Reduce exposure and transmission.
  - Good mechanical filtration and disinfection of recirculating water with UV and/or ozone.
  - High water flow rate or turnover.
  - Good cleaning and disinfection protocols.
  - Prophylactic metronidazole may be given to cichlid broodstock.

Zoonotic Reports

- These parasites have no known zoonotic potential.

Bibliography

O'Brien, G.M., Ostland, V.E., and Ferguson, H.W. (1993). *Spironucleus*-associated necrotic enteritis in angelfish (*Pterophyllum scalare*). *Canadian Veterinary Journal* 34: 301–303.

Paull, G.C. and Matthews, R.A. (2001). *Spironucleus vortens*, a possible cause of hole-in-the-head disease in cichlids. *Diseases of Aquatic Organisms* 45: 197–202.

Webb, D.H., Marrero, C., Ellis, H., and Merriweather, L. (2013). A simple reagent-free spectrophotometric assay for monitoring metronidazole therapy in aquarium water. *Journal of Aquatic Animal Health* 25: 165–170.

Whaley, J., and Francis-Floyd, R. (1991) A comparison of metronidazole treatments for hexamitiasis in angelfish. *Proceedings of the International Association for Aquatic Animal Medicine*, Augustine, FL.

Abbreviations/Acronyms

- EM: Electron microscopy
- GI: Gastrointestinal

Amyloodinium and *Piscinoodinium* spp.

Overview

- *Amyloodinium ocellatum* and *Piscinoodinium* spp. are ectoparasitic dinoflagellates found on the skin and gills of various fish species.
- *A. ocellatum* is found on marine and brackish fish and has caused high morbidity and mortality in aquaculture and display aquariums. It is sometimes known as marine velvet or gold dust disease.
- *Piscinoodinium* spp. are found on freshwater fish and are typically less pathogenic than *A. ocellatum*.

Etiology

- Phylum *Myzozoa (Miozoa)*.
- Infraphylum *Dinoflagellata*.
- Family *Oodiniaceae*.
- These are dinoflagellates that photosynthesize using zooxanthellae.
- Three genera appear to be parasitic in fish:
  - *Amyloodinium ocellatum* is the only reported member of the genus.
  - *Piscinoodinium* (*Oodinium*) spp.
  - *Crepidoodinium* spp.

Life Cycle and Transmission

- The life cycle is direct with three stages.
  - Nonmotile, parasitic trophonts attach and feed on the gills and skin of fish.
  - Trophonts detach and encyst in the environment to become nonmotile reproductive tomonts.
  - Tomonts produce free-swimming, infective dinospores. These are most infective for the first 24 hours, but can be infective for 6–15 days.
- Dinospores are susceptible to immersion treatment.
- Dinospores can be transmitted through water, fomites, and aerosolization (up to 44 cm in static air and 3 m with fans).
- The life cycle is often reported as three to six days at 20 °C (68 °F).

Geographic Distribution

- Freshwater and saltwater habitats, probably worldwide.

Signalment

- *A. ocellatum* is found in tropical and temperate fish in marine and brackish environments. It has been particularly problematic for red drum (*Sciaenops ocellatus*), gilthead seabream (*Sparus aurata*), striped bass (*Morone saxatilis*), European bass (*Dicentrarchus labrax*), and clownfish (*Amphiprion* spp.). It has also been reported in elasmobranchs (e.g. bonnethead sharks, *Sphyrna tiburo*).
- *Piscinoodinium* spp. are found in tropical freshwater bony fish.
- *Crepidoodinium* spp. are found in marine and brackish bony fish.

Risk Factors

- Exposure and stressors are the most important risk factors.
- Exposure includes:
  - Poor biosecurity (e.g. lack of suitable quarantine, untreated surface water).
  - Permissive water temperature, often >15 °C (>59 °F).
  - Permissive or preferred salinity, e.g. 15–32 g/L for *A. ocellatum*, although individual strains have narrower ranges.
  - High organic loads.
  - Low water flow rate or turnover.
  - Exposure of naïve fish.
  - Established infection; once established in a large habitat, this becomes a recurrent issue.
- Common stressors are described under C6: *Ichthyophthirius multifiliis*.

Signs/Clinical Findings

- Multiple fish from one or more species are usually affected.
- Inappetence or reduced feeding may be seen.
- Lethargy or increased hiding may be seen.
- Gray, golden, or dark coloration may be seen. Skin lesions can become almost granular in appearance. Skin ulcers are rare.
- Pruritus (e.g. flashing) may be seen.
- Dyspnea, tachypnea, or gill edema may be seen.
- The disease may present peracutely, with sudden death as the first clinical sign.
- Without treatment, mortality from *A. ocellatum* can reach 100% in days. Mortality from *Piscinoodinium* spp. is typically lower.

Differential Diagnoses

- Full differentials are described in Section B.
- More common differentials for protozoa on the skin or gills are *Cryptocaryon irritans* (saltwater) and *Ichthyophthirius multifiliis* (freshwater), but these are motile when alive and lighter in color.

Diagnosis

- Diagnosis is typically by direct microscopy of skin scrapes or fin or gill biopsies. The parasites may not be seen on autolyzed specimens.
- Trophonts are nonmotile, golden-brown, and round, oval, or hexagonal in shape (Figure C6.11). They look

more dense than other common ectoparasites. Different size trophonts are usually present on a single sample (50–300 μm).

- Cytology and histology can also show increased mucus, branchitis, or dermatitis with focal hyperplasia, hemorrhage, inflammation, or necrosis with intralesional trophonts, although sensitivity is highest with direct microscopy. Lugol's iodine stains can help visualize the parasites.
- Freshwater dips, matched to pH and temperature, can be used for diagnosis of *A. ocellatum*. The sediment from the dips can be spun down and examined under direct microscopy.
- Species identification depends on the structure of the attachment organelle and molecular diagnostics such as PCR.

Husbandry Management

- Isolate affected system(s).
- Increase aeration; target dissolved oxygen may be 95–100%.
- Reduce or resolve any environmental stressors.
- Remove dead or moribund fish as soon as possible with appropriate disposition.
- Increase mechanical cleaning.
- Remove any unnecessary organic material.
- Increase cleaning and disinfection of water and fomites. Quaternary ammonium compounds may be most effective for inanimate fomites.
- Increase water flow rate and turnover.
- Consider adjusting the water temperature; clinical signs may resolve if <15 °C (<59 °F), although disease often recurs when water temperature increases.
- For chronic or recurrent infections, consider biological control (e.g. shrimp, wrasse, or gobies).

Medical Management

- Treatment is recommended, particularly for *Amyloodinium* spp., and usually resolves signs readily.
- Treatment only affects the free-swimming dinospore stage, so needs to be long-term (i.e. continuous or pulse therapy for >10 days) or followed by a move to an uninfected system. Recurrence may still be seen.
- Common treatments (see Chapters A12 and A13 for more details):
  - Copper sulfate immersion for saltwater fish, usually at lower doses than needed for *Cryptocaryon* (e.g. 0.10–0.15 mg/L ionic copper in salt water for 10–21 days). Ionic copper should be assayed every 12–24 hours. Some species and life stages are sensitive to copper, including most elasmobranchs, invertebrates, and plants.
  - Chloroquine diphosphate immersion (e.g. 5–10 mg/L for 10 days). A UV spectrophotometric assay can be used to assess drug level in water. Some fish and invertebrate species or life stages may be sensitive to chloroquine; it cannot be used in reef aquariums.
  - Freshwater dips for saltwater fish, matched to pH and temperature. A possible schedule is to repeat every three days for three treatments, moving fish to an uninfected system after each dip.
  - Long-term hypersalinity for freshwater fish (e.g. 3–5 g/L).
- Other reported treatments (see Chapters A12 and A13 for more details):
  - Hydrogen peroxide immersion.
  - Long-term hyposalinity for saltwater fish.
  - Acriflavine immersion.
  - Formalin immersion.
  - Magnesium restriction in seawater may prevent completion of the life cycle of *A. ocellatum*.
- If treatment is unsuccessful, the system should be kept empty of fish for at least two weeks, although longer may be needed.
- Survivors may become subclinical carriers that can infect other fish.
- Some fish develop protective immunity to the parasite following sublethal exposure; protective antibodies have been found for up to 6 months in clownfish.
- All legislation regarding medication use and disposal must be followed.

Prevention

- Reduce or resolve stressors.
  - Common stressors are described under C6: *Ichthyophthirius multifiliis*.

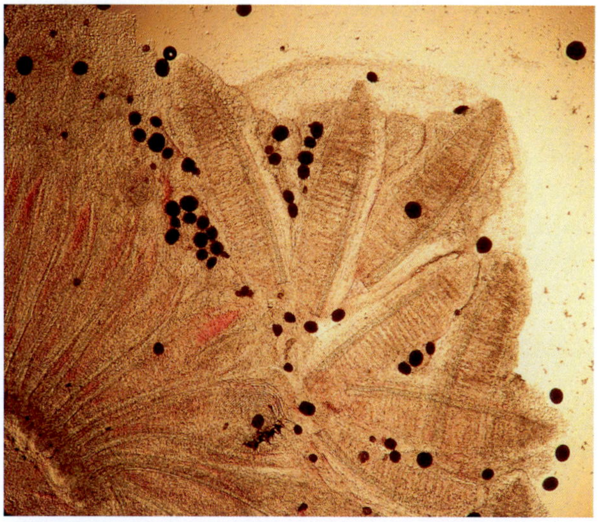

Figure C6.11 *Amyloodinium* sp. and increased mucus on a gill biopsy under direct microscopy.

- Reduce exposure and transmission; good biosecurity can prevent this parasite.
  - Isolation with no contact with free-ranging fish.
  - Pathogen-free water source (e.g. municipal water or ground water that has gone through fine filtration, then UV and/or ozone disinfection). Avoid using untreated surface water. If using surface water, consider storing the water prior to use.
  - Disinfection of recirculating water with fine filtration then UV and/or ozone.
  - High water flowrate or turnover.
  - Removal of dead or moribund fish as soon as possible with appropriate disposition.
  - Good cleaning and disinfection protocols.
  - Suitable quarantine for at least 30–60 days with isolation, monitoring, and diagnostic testing, particularly skin scrapes and gill biopsies.
  - Frozen-thawed or commercial feeds, with no live feeds.

Zoonotic Reports

- These parasites have no known zoonotic potential.

Bibliography

Bessat, M. and Fadel, A. (2018). Amyloodiniosis in cultured *Dicentrarchus labrax*: parasitological and molecular diagnosis, and an improved treatment protocol. *Diseases of Aquatic Organisms* 129: 41–51.

Boylan, S.M., Skoy, J., and Ellis, H. (2014) Who needs the foul-line when you have the 'trifecta' of bonnethead (*Sphyrna tiburo*) infectious diseases in captivity: *Erpocotyle* monogeneans, *Fusarium solani*, and *Amyloodinium*. *Proceedings of the Eastern Fish Health Workshop*, Shepherdstown, WV.

Levy, M.G., Litaker, R.W., Goldstein, R.J. et al. (2007). *Piscinoodinium*, a fish-ectoparasitic dinoflagellate, is a member of the class Dinophyceae, subclass Gymndiniphycidae: convergent evolution with *Amyloodinium*. *Journal of Parasitology* 93: 1006–1015.

Levy, M.G., Poore, M.F., Colorni, A. et al. (2007). A highly specific PCR assay for detecting the fish ectoparasite *Amyloodinium ocellatum*. *Diseases of Aquatic Organisms* 73: 219–226.

Montgomery-Brock, D., Sato, V.T., Brock, J.A., and Tamaru, C.S. (2001). The application of hydrogen peroxide as a treatment for the ectoparasite *Amyloodinium ocellatum* (Brown 1931) on the Pacific threadfin *Polydactylus sexfilis*. *Journal of the World Aquaculture Society* 32: 250–254.

Roberts-Thomson, A., Barnes, A., Fielder, D.S. et al. (2006). Aerosol dispersal of the fish pathogen, *Amyloodinium ocellatum*. *Aquaculture* 257: 118–123.

Abbreviations/Acronyms

- PCR: Polymerase chain reaction
- UV: Ultraviolet

Amoebic Gill Disease

Overview

- *Neoparamoeba* and *Paramoeba* spp. are marine amoebae with that are typically commensal and free-living but can be pathogenic.
- They can invade the gills and cause amoebic gill disease (AGD) in marine teleosts.
- *Neoparamoeba perurans* is the only organism for which Koch's postulates have been fulfilled. *N. perurans* is responsible for significant losses in Atlantic salmon (*Salmo salar*) and turbot (*Scophthalmus maximus*) in aquaculture.

Etiology

- Phylum *Amoebozoa*.
- Three species are typically reported from marine fish, although the taxonomy is complicated and *Neoparamoeba* and *Paramoeba* are sometimes considered synonymous.
  - *Neoparamoeba (Paramoeba) perurans.*
  - *Neoparamoeba (Paramoeba) pemaquidensis.*
  - *Neoparamoeba branchiphila.*
- There are freshwater amoeba species that may cause disease in fish (e.g. *Acanthamoeba, Thecamoeba* spp.).

Life Cycle and Transmission

- Transmission is horizontal through direct or indirect contact with infected fish and potentially invertebrates.
- The life cycle is unknown, but the trophozoite is believed to be the only stage.
- Amoebae survive on the gills of dead fish for at least 30 hours.

Geographic Distribution

- Predominantly saltwater habitats.

- AGD was first identified off Tasmania in the 1980s. It is now common in areas where Atlantic salmon are cultured (e.g. United States, Chile, Japan).

Signalment

- *N. perurans* primarily affects Atlantic salmon but has caused disease in other salmonids (particularly rainbow trout, *Oncorhynchus mykiss*), turbot, European bass (*Dicentrarchus labrax*), and ayu (*Plecoglossus altivelis*).
- *Neoparamoeba* and other spp. have been identified from other marine, estuarine, and freshwater teleosts.
- They are usually isolated from fish in culture; they are rarely found in wild fish.

Risk Factors

- Exposure and stressors are the most important risk factors.
- Exposure includes:
  - Poor biosecurity (e.g. lack of suitable quarantine, untreated surface water).
  - Permissive water temperature, typically 12–20 °C (54–68 °F).
  - Permissive salinity, often >32 g/L in salmonids and >22 g/L in turbot.
  - Exposure of naïve fish.
  - High calcium and magnesium ions in the water.
- Common stressors are described under C6: *Ichthyophthirius multifiliis*.

Signs/Clinical Findings

- Multiple conspecifics may be affected.
- Lethargy is common.
- Dyspnea or tachypnea is common.
- Gills may show white or gray spots, focal pallor, edema, or increased mucus. Lesions often start at the base of the gills.
- Morbidity is high. Mortality is usually low but can reach 50–70%.

Differential Diagnoses

- Full differentials are described in Section B.
- Common differentials for gill lesions in marine salmonids include piscirickettsial-like organisms, *Tenacibaculum*, *Ichthyobodo*, and *Gyrodactylus* spp., Atlantic salmon paramyxovirus, environmental toxins, and harmful algal blooms.

Diagnosis

- A tentative diagnosis can often be made based on typical gill lesions in susceptible species, along with cytology and histology.
- Amoebae are often abundant, 10–50 µm in size, and almost spherical. Some show pseudopodia, but with no obvious motility on direct microscopy. They contain endosymbiotic organisms that are often visible on microscopy.
- Cytology and histology may also show gill epithelial hyperplasia, fusion of lamellae, and prominent vesicles containing trophozoites.
- In rare cases, some amoeba infections can become systemic and granulomatous.
- There are few morphological differences between the species.
- The parasites have proven difficult to culture; only *N. perurans* has been cultured.
- PCR, ISH, or FA tests on gill tissue, gill swabs, or water samples are needed for confirmation and species identification.

Husbandry Management

- Isolate affected system(s).
- Increase aeration; target dissolved oxygen may be 95–100%.
- Reduce or resolve any environmental stressors.
- Remove dead or moribund fish as soon as possible with appropriate disposition.
- Increase mechanical cleaning.
- Reduce the stocking density, if possible.

Medical Management

- Common treatments (see Chapters A12 and A13 for more details):
  - Freshwater immersion (bath) is the most common treatment for Atlantic salmon and turbot (e.g. two to three hours oxygenated, soft freshwater in a liner-filled production enclosure).
- Other reported treatments (see Chapters A12 and A13 for more details):
  - Long-term hyposalinity.
  - Levamisole immersion.
  - Hydrogen peroxide immersion.
- All legislation regarding medication use and disposal must be followed.

Prevention

- Reduce or resolve stressors.
  - Common stressors are described under C6: *Ichthyophthirius multifiliis*.
- Reduce exposure and transmission, although this is challenging for Atlantic salmon in sea pens.
  - Routine gill examinations by experienced personnel.
  - Routine freshwater baths during the marine stage of salmon production, either every few weeks or based on gill examination scores.
  - Removal of dead or moribund fish as soon as possible with appropriate disposition.

- Good cleaning and disinfection protocols.
- All-in-all-out management with fallowing between groups.
- Consider keeping salmon sea pens below the surface.

Zoonotic Reports

- These parasites have no known zoonotic potential.

Bibliography

Douglas-Helders, M., Nowak, B., Zilberg, D., and Carson, J. (2000). Survival of *Paramoeba pemaquidensis* on dead salmon: implications for management of cage hygiene. *Bulletin of European Association of FishPathologists* 20: 167–169.

Douglas-Helders, G.M., Weird, I.J., O'Brien, D.P. et al. (2004). Effects of husbandry on prevalence of amoebic gill disease and performance of reared Atlantic salmon (*Salmo salar* L.). *Aquaculture* 241: 21–30.

Douglas-Helders, M., Nowak, B., and Butler, R. (2005). The effect of environmental factors on the distribution of *Neoparamoeba pemaquidensis* in Tasmania. *Journal of Fish Diseases* 38: 583–592.

Florent, R.L., Becker, J.A., and Powell, M.D. (2010). *In vitro* toxicity of bithionol and bithionol sulphoxide to *Neoparamoeba* spp., the causative agent of amoebic gill disease (AGD). *Diseases of Aquatic Organisms* 91: 257–262.

Kim, W., Kong, K., Kim, J., and Oh, M. (2016). Amoebic gill infection in coho salmon *Oncorhynchus kisutch* farmed in Korea. *Diseases of Aquatic Organisms* 121: 75–78.

Munday, B.L., Zilberg, D., and Findlay, V. (2001). Gill disease of marine fish caused by infection with *Neoparamoeba pemaquidensis*. *Journal of Fish Diseases* 24: 497–507.

Nash, G., Nash, M., and Schlotfeldt, H.-J. (1988). Systemic amoebiasis in cultured European catfish *Silurus glanis* L. *Journal of Fish Diseases* 11: 57–71.

Young, N.D., Dyková, I., Snekvik, K. et al. (2008). *Neoparamoeba perurans* is a cosmopolitan aetiological agent of amoebic gill disease. *Diseases of Aquatic Organisms* 78: 217–223.

Abbreviations/Acronyms

- AGD: Amoebic gill disease
- FA: Fluorescent antibody
- ISH: In situ hybridization
- PCR: Polymerase chain reaction

C7

Metazoan Diseases

Catherine A. Hadfield

Seattle Aquarium, Seattle, WA, USA

Introduction

Metazoa are multicellular eukaryotic organisms. Common metazoan diseases of fish are reviewed in this chapter, including monogeneans, digenes, turbellaria, cestodes, leeches, nematodes, pentastomids, acanthocephalans, copepods, isopods, and branchiurans. Where available, information is provided on etiologic agent, life cycle and transmission, signalment, risk factors, clinical signs, diagnosis, husbandry and medical management, and prevention.

Monogeneans (General)

Overview

- Monogeneans are flatworms (flukes) that are common ectoparasites of fish.
- They can cause significant morbidity and mortality in aquariums and aquaculture.
- They have direct life cycles.
- Most fish monogeneans (other than gyrodactylids) are oviparous. Eggs are relatively resistant to treatment and oviparous species are harder to eradicate than viviparous species.
- Prevention is more effective than treatment.
- One species, *Gyrodactylus salaris*, is currently reportable to the OIE.

Etiology

- Phylum *Platyhelminthes*.
- Class *Monogenoidea*.
- Subclasses *Monopisthocotylea* and *Polyopisthocotylea*.
- These are metazoan flatworms that typically have prominent hooks (*Monopisthocotylea*) or multiple suckers with small hooks (*Polyopisthocotylea*) to attach to the host.
- Most monogeneans are monopisthocotyles. Families include *Capsalidae, Gyrodactylidae, Dactylogyridae*, and *Microbothriidae*.
- Polyopisthocotyle monogeneans are less commonly reported.

Life Cycle and Transmission

- All monogeneans have direct life cycles.
- All monogeneans are hermaphroditic and are probably capable of self-fertilization.
- Most are oviparous. Gyrodactylids are an exception and are viviparous.
- Within oviparous species, eggs are produced singly but continuously, so total egg production is high.
- Transmission is horizontal, through direct or indirect contact. Vectors may be seen.
- The infective stage is the oncomiracidium (larva) that moves using cilia or by crawling.
- Once the oncomiracidium finds a host, it migrates to the preferred tissue site, then matures.
- Maturation usually takes weeks to months; it is longer in polyopisthocotyles than monopisthocotyles.

Geographic Distribution

- Monogeneans are found in freshwater and saltwater habitats, probably worldwide.
- Distribution of each parasite species depends on the range or culture location of the host species.

Signalment

- Host ranges tend to be narrow (e.g. *Dermophthirius*, *Neodermophthirius* spp.).

Clinical Guide to Fish Medicine, First Edition. Edited by Catherine A. Hadfield and Leigh Ann Clayton.

- Host ranges may be narrow in the wild but wider in fish under human care.
- A few have unusually wide host ranges (e.g. *Neobenedenia* spp.).
- Juvenile fish may be more susceptible than adults.

Risk Factors

- Stressors and exposure are the main risk factors for morbidity and mortality.
- Stressors include:
  - High stocking density.
  - Inappropriate social structure.
  - Inappropriate environment.
  - Aggression or displacement.
  - Poor water quality, particularly low dissolved oxygen and high ammonia.
  - Contaminants (e.g. PCBs, hydrocarbons, sewage exposure).
  - Inappropriate water temperature or changes in water temperature.
  - Poor nutrition.
  - Recent handling.
  - Recent transport.
  - Recent spawning.
- Exposure to other hosts or environmental stages can be due to:
  - Poor biosecurity (e.g. lack of suitable quarantine, use of surface water, exposure to wild fish or live feeder fish).
  - Permissive water temperature.
  - Permissive salinity.
  - High organic loads.
  - Low water flow rate or turnover.
  - Limited mechanical cleaning of the habitat.
  - Exposure of naïve fish.
  - Established infection; once established in a large habitat, this becomes a recurrent issue.

Signs/Clinical Findings

- Infected fish may be asymptomatic.
- Clinical signs may initially be seen in one or two individuals, but the entire system should be considered infected.
- Lethargy or increased hiding may be seen.
- Inappetence or reduced feeding may be seen.
- Pruritus (e.g. flashing, erratic swimming) or clamped fins may be seen.
- Dyspnea or tachypnea is common, including signs such as yawning and piping at the surface.
- Erythema, skin ulcers, fin erosions, small plaques, or trailing lines on the skin may be seen.
- Corneal opacity due to ulcerative keratitis is particularly common with *Neobenedenia* spp.
- Secondary bacterial, fungal, or viral infections may be seen.
- Morbidity is often high; mortality can be high.

Differential Diagnoses

- Full differentials are provided in Section B.
- Common differentials are provided for each monogenean group.

Diagnosis

- Monogeneans are usually identified on direct microscopy of skin scrapes or gill biopsies.
- Some are identified on corneal scrapes (*Neobenedenia* spp.) or from other epithelial surfaces such as the oral cavity, nares (olfactory sacs), urinary bladder, anus, or cloaca.
- These are metazoan flatworms with distinct anterior and posterior ends. The anterior end is involved in feeding. The posterior end (haptor) typically has prominent hooks to attach to the host (*Monopisthocotylea*) (Figure C7.1a) or multiple suckers with small hooks (*Polyopisthocotylea*).
- The hooks are still visible after the parasites have died, although they may be in pieces (Figure C7.1b).
- Adults are usually tissue-specific, while larvae and juveniles may have wider tissue distributions.
- If further morphological or molecular identification is required, adults or larvae can be relaxed in near-boiling water or saline followed by fixation in 95% ethanol, or fixed in hot 70% ethanol or hot AFA (ethanol, formalin, acetic acid). Since they are soft-bodied, it is often best to fix them in situ with a small piece of the tissue they were attached to. Freezing is an additional method that works well for monogeneans.
- Quantitative assessments of eggs can be helpful for monitoring oviparous parasites in systems over time and following treatment.
  - Following dips (e.g. freshwater, praziquantel) in a known volume of water, the sediment can be collected and the eggs counted on a McMasters slide.
  - A fine-mesh filter (e.g. 50 μm mesh filter sock) on the skimmer or on a siphon can be examined routinely to count trapped eggs.

Husbandry Management

- Husbandry management typically relies on reducing or resolving stressors and reducing exposure.
- Increase aeration; target dissolved oxygen may be 95–100%.
- Consider isolating affected systems if this is a new or virulent pathogen.
- Reduce or resolve any environmental stressors.

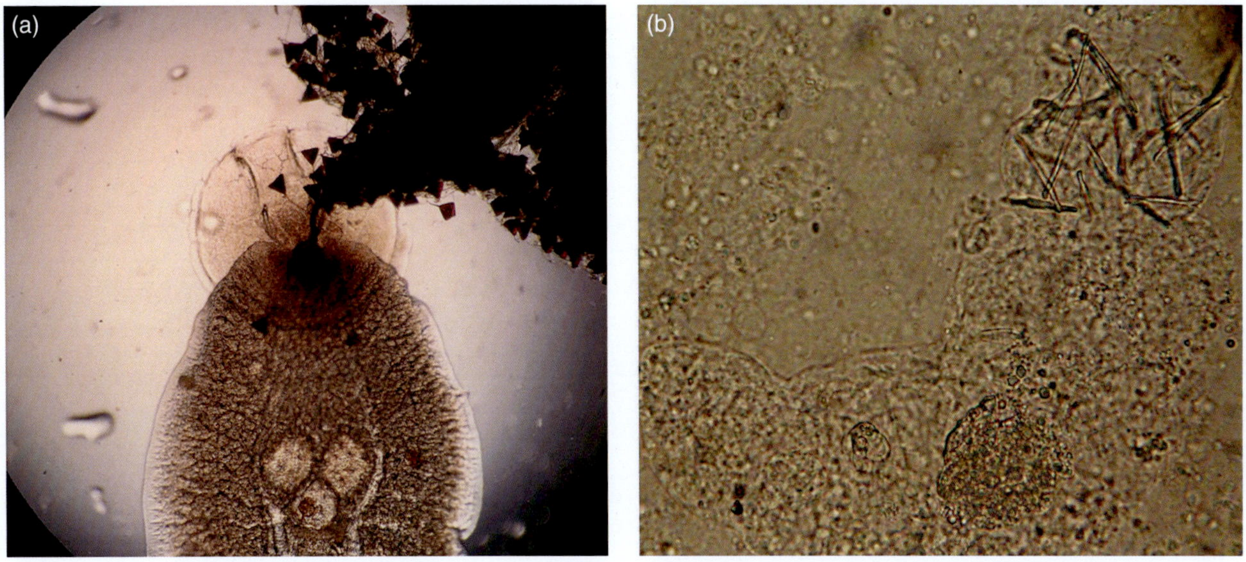

Figure C7.1 Prolific egg production by a capsalid monogenean (a) and skin scrape showing the hooks from a monogenean that has died (b).

- Remove dead or moribund fish as soon as possible with appropriate disposition.
- Increase mechanical cleaning; where possible, the substrate should be regularly siphoned to remove parasites.
- Remove unnecessary substrate or reduce the depth.
- Increase cleaning and disinfection of fomites. Regularly remove and either replace or clean décor and nets that can entangle eggs. This can be targeted strategically to areas of highest egg accumulation.
- Regularly back-wash filters, such as sand filters.
- Increase the flow rate of flow-through systems.
- Increase the turnover of recirculating systems (e.g. >1 exchange/h) to try to reduce reinfection rates.
- Consider slowly taking the water temperature outside of the preferred range of the parasites but within the preferred range of the fish.
- Consider removing susceptible species for treatment and leaving the system without suitable hosts. This is a form of fallowing that may allow the parasites in the original habitat to die off.
- Consider cleaner fish and invertebrates to try to reduce parasite burdens.

Medical Management

- Once introduced into a system with suitable hosts, particularly with heavy organic loads and substrate, eradication of oviparous species is unlikely. If fish are removed for dip treatments, parasites in the environment lead to reinfection. If the system is treated with immersion treatments, eggs that did not hatch while at therapy and adults that were not killed by the treatment can reinfect fish. When deciding on management plans, it is important to discuss if the goal is to reduce the parasite load and clinical signs or to try to eliminate the parasite.
- Treatment should always be combined with husbandry changes as part of an integrated management strategy.
- A particularly effective strategy is to dose-and-move: providing an immersion treatment during the move to a suitable, uninfected system. This reduces the risk of reinfection following treatment.
- Similar drugs are used for all monogeneans, but treatment regimens and prognosis differ between viviparous and oviparous species.
  - Viviparous gyrodactylids are usually easy to eradicate in closed systems.
  - Oviparous species are problematic because treatments have little to no effect on the eggs and egg viability, hatching cues, and maximum time to hatching are largely unknown. Therefore, long-term treatment to kill emerging larvae, either as a pulse therapy or maintained at therapy, is required to try to resolve the infection.
- Common treatments (see Chapters A12 and A13 and each monogenean group for more details):
  - Praziquantel immersion.
  - Praziquantel orally.
  - Trichlorfon immersion.
  - Salinity changes.
  - Supportive care.
  - Treatment of secondary infections.
- Other reported treatments (see Chapters A12 and A13 and each monogenean group for more details):

  - Hydrogen peroxide immersion.
  - Peracetic acid immersion.
  - Formalin dips.
  - Quinacrine orally.
- All legislation regarding medication use and disposal must be followed.

Prevention
- Morbidity and mortality can be prevented by reducing stressors, exposure, and severity of disease.
- The general preventative measures below relate to all monogeneans. Specific examples are provided for each monogenean group.
- Reduce or resolve stressors, particularly when disease is likely (e.g. after transport, at permissive water temperatures).
  - Low stocking density.
  - Suitable social groups and habitats.
  - Excellent water quality and preferred water temperature.
  - Good nutrition.
  - Suitable handling and transport protocols.
- Reduce exposure and transmission through good biosecurity.
  - Isolation with no contact with free-ranging animals, particularly fish. In open systems, physical distance from other susceptible species is important (e.g. distance between sea pens with salmonids).
  - Pathogen-free water source (e.g. municipal water or ground water that has gone through fine filtration (<40 μm) then UV and/or ozone disinfection). Avoid using untreated surface water.
  - Disinfection of recirculating water with fine filtration (<40 μm) then UV and/or ozone.
  - High water flow rate or turnover.
  - Removal of dead or moribund fish as soon as possible with appropriate disposition.
  - Good cleaning and disinfection protocols.
  - Limits on visitors and potential fomites.
  - Specific pathogen-free sources of fish (e.g. *G. salaris*).
  - All-in-all-out management with strict separation of generations and fallowing between groups. This typically means keeping only one generation in one location and leaving it fallow for four to six weeks before the next group is brought in.
  - Suitable quarantine with isolation, monitoring, and diagnostic testing, particularly gill biopsies and skin scrapes. Quarantine may include prophylactic treatment of high-risk pathogens or dose-and-move treatment of susceptible groups. Quarantine should apply to new animals as well as animals returning from shows or loans.
  - Disinfection of eggs.
  - Frozen-thawed or commercial feeds, with no live feeds.
- Reduce severity of disease.
  - Routine monitoring of high-risk species using skin scrapes, gill biopsies, or egg traps to identify changes that might require treatment.
  - Selective breeding of more resistant fish strains (e.g. Baltic Neva strains of Atlantic salmon show greater resistance to *G. salaris*).
  - Vaccine trials have shown no protection.
  - Immune stimulants such as beta glucans and allicin can decrease severity of clinical signs from monogeneans. The effect in vivo is always less than in vitro. They are most effective at specific doses, short courses, and when given prior to infection.
- Regularly review morbidity and mortality trends and response to treatments.

Zoonotic Reports
- These parasites have no known zoonotic potential.

Bibliography

Justine, J., Briand, M.J., and Bray, R.A. (2012). A quick and simple method, usable in the field, for collecting parasites in suitable condition for both morphological and molecular studies. *Parasitology Research* 111: 341–351.

Abbreviations/Acronyms
- OIE: World Organisation for Animal Health
- UV: Ultraviolet

Capsalid Monogeneans

Overview

- Capsalids are large, oval, oviparous monogeneans.
- They infect the skin, eyes, and gills of marine fish.
- These can result in significant morbidity and mortality in aquariums and aquaculture, particularly *Neobenedenia* spp.
- Identification to genus is important because host range and control strategies vary.
- Management is difficult because the egg stage is resistant to treatment. Recurrence is common.

Etiology

- Phylum *Platyhelminthes*.
- Class *Monogenoidea*.
- Subclass *Monopisthocotylea*.
- Family *Capsalidae*.
- Many genera are reported commonly from fish:
  - *Benedenia*.
  - *Benedeniella*.
  - *Capsala*.
  - *Encotyllabe*.
  - *Entobdella*.
  - *Neobenedenia melleni* and *Neobenedenia girellae*, although these may represent larger species complexes or clades, and the term *Neobenedenia* spp. may be more appropriate.
  - *Neoentobdella*.
  - *Nitzschia* [NB there is also a diatom with the genus name *Nitzschia*].
  - *Trilobiodiscus*.
  - *Pseudonitzschia*.

Life Cycle and Transmission

- All monogeneans have a direct life cycle.
- Capsalids are oviparous and produce large numbers of eggs (Figure C7.2); a single *Neobenedenia* can produce 3300 eggs over 17 days.
- Eggs are laid continuously and released into the water where they become tangled in décor or fall to the substrate.
- Eggs hatch into ciliated larvae (oncomiracidia) which infect new hosts close to the site of hatching.
- Larvae attach, lose their cilia, then migrate to their preferred tissue site.
- Hatching typically occurs days after egg-laying and maturation takes a few weeks, depending on species, temperature, and salinity. The life cycle is faster in warm water and high salinities.
- While the larvae cannot survive more than a few days in the environment, it is unclear how long the eggs can survive in the environment. This makes it difficult to coordinate medical treatment with egg hatching.

Geographic Distribution

- Saltwater habitats, probably worldwide.
- Distribution of each parasite species depends on the range or culture location of the host species, e.g.:
  - *Benedenia seriolae* in amberjacks (*Seriola* spp.) in sea pens in Japan, Australia, and New Zealand.
  - *Entobdella soleae* in common sole (*Solae solae*) in Europe.

Signalment

- Marine or brackish fish are susceptible.
- Most reports of morbidity and mortality involve marine teleosts and rays in aquariums and their culture and

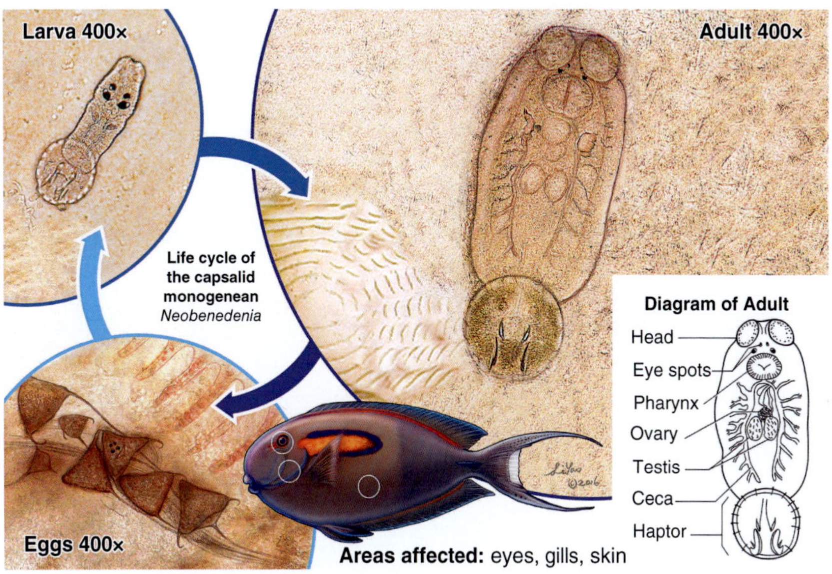

Figure C7.2 Life cycle of *Neobenedenia* spp. *Source*: Image courtesy of Li Yao, copyright reserved.

supply chains. There are reports of epizootics in food fish aquaculture, particularly in sea pens.

- Most have a single host species and strict tissue specificity, e.g.:
  - *Benedeniella posterocolpa* on the skin (particularly the ventrum) of cownose rays (*Rhinoptera bonasus*).
  - *Entobdella bumpusii* on the gills of southern stingrays (*Hypanus americanus*).
- Some have wide host ranges, e.g.:
  - *B. seriolae* on the skin of a variety of amberjacks in aquaculture.
  - *Nitzschia sturionis*, *Nitzschia superba*, and *Nitzschia quadritestes* on the skin of sturgeon (*Acipenseridae*).
  - *Neobenedenia* spp. on the skin, eyes, and gills of >100 species, including surgeonfish (*Acanthuridae*), spadefish (*Ephippidae*), puffers and filefish (*Tetraodontiformes*), butterflyfish (*Chaetodontidae*), marine angelfish (*Pomacanthidae*), grouper (*Epinephalus* spp.), barramundi (*Lates calcarifer*), seabream (*Pagrus* spp.), olive flounder (*Paralichthys olivaceus*), cobia (*Rachycentron canadum*), amberjacks, and marine-cultured tilapia (*Oreochromis* spp.).

Risk Factors

- General risk factors are described under C7: *Monogeneans (General)*.
- Permissive salinity is typically 25–45 g/L.
- Permissive water temperature is usually high, e.g. 21–28°C (70–82°F) for *B. seriolae* and 24–32°C (75–90°F) for *Neobenedenia* spp.

Signs/Clinical Findings

- Infected fish may be asymptomatic.
- Multiple fish from one or more species are usually affected.
- Lethargy and increased hiding are common.
- Inappetence, reduced appetite, or poor growth rates are common.
- Pruritus (e.g. flashing, erratic swimming) is common.
- Skin darkening, poorly demarcated white foci on the skin, grossly visible white to brown plaques or strands on the skin, gills, or around the teeth may be seen (Figure C7.3). Petechiae and skin ulcers are possible. In rare cases, pink nodules may be seen on the gills.
- Ocular opacities from keratitis are common, particularly with *Neobenedenia* spp.
- Dyspnea or tachypnea may be seen.
- Mortality can be high, often due to disruption of osmoregulation or secondary infections.
- Once established in a system, recurrence following stressors is common, although some fish have shown immunity following infection (e.g. olive flounder).

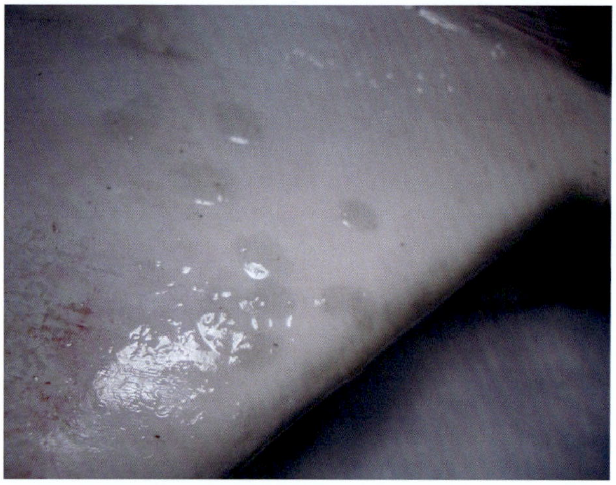

Figure C7.3 *Benedeniella posterocolpa* on the ventrum of a cownose ray (*Rhinoptera bonasus*).

Differential Diagnoses

- Full differentials are provided in Section B.
- Common differentials for external flatworms on marine teleosts include capsalid monogeneans, particularly *Neobenedenia* spp., gyrodactylid monogeneans, and polyopisthocotyles. Leeches can resemble flatworms.
- Common differentials for external flatworms on marine rays include capsalid and monocotylid monogeneans, particularly *Dendromonocotyle* spp. Leeches can resemble flatworms.
- Common differentials for tetrahedral eggs on direct microscopy include all capsalid, and some monocotylid, dactylogyrid, and diplectanid monogeneans.

Diagnosis

- Many capsalids are large enough to be grossly visible. Diagnosis is typically by direct microscopy of parasites pulled from the skin, gills, nares, eyes, anus, or cloaca, or microscopy of skin scrapes, gill biopsies, or eye impression smears.
- Adults are large, oval, unsegmented flatworms that move by stretching and jerking.
  - They are mostly 2–12 mm in length, although some are larger. Capsalids are larger than dactylogyrids and gyrodactylids and usually rounder, although *Entobdella* spp. are slender.
  - They are white, gray, or translucent, which often makes them hard to see. In a freshwater or praziquantel dip, the parasites become more opaque.
  - Four large black eye spots are present at the anterior end, along with two anterior attachment lappets.
  - The attachment organ (opisthaptor) is small relative to body size, round to oval, and aseptate. It has large central hooks (hamuli and accessory sclerites), small

marginal hooklets, and a conspicuous marginal valve around the edge.
  - Exceptions to this description are the less common *Encotyllabe* and *Alloencotyllabe* spp. which are tube-like with a long peduncle.
  - The genera can be distinguished based on host species and morphology of the hamuli and lappets.
- Larvae are smaller, thinner, with large paired eye spots each associated with a large crystalline lens.
- Eggs tend to be identified on gill biopsies and are brown, tetrahedral (although these often look triangular), up to 150 µm in size, each with a trailing filament. Some eggs may have visible eye spots if the larvae within are well-developed.
- If further morphological or molecular identification is required, see C7: *Monogeneans (General).*
- Egg traps are useful for routine monitoring; see C7: *Monogeneans (General).*

Husbandry Management

- General husbandry measures are described under C7: *Monogeneans (General).*
- Many studies have evaluated cleaner fish and invertebrates for capsalid management. Reduced pathogen load has been seen using cleaner fish bred under human care, suggesting this may be an innate behavior. The following have been shown to reduce load:
  - Neon gobies (*Elacatinus oceanops*).
  - Barber gobies (*Elacatinus figaro*).
  - Cleaner gobies (*Elacatinus genie*).
  - Bluestreak cleaner wrasse (*Labroides dimidiatus*).
  - Pacific cleaner shrimp (*Lysmata amboinensis*).
  - Pederson shrimp (*Ancylomenes pedersoni*).
  - Cleaner fish and invertebrates often do best in complex, naturalistic systems with abundant small hides and alternative food sources.
- Consider reducing overall brightness and black-and-white contrast. This can reduce hatching of *Neobenedenia* spp.
- Increase cleaning and disinfection of fomites.
  - Most effective may be mechanical cleaning in hot freshwater, followed by full drying. Water at 50°C (122°F) for 30 seconds or 30°C (86°F) for 48 hours prevented *B. seriolae* egg hatching. However, *Entobdella hippoglossi* eggs survived 50°C for five minutes.
  - Ethanol 25% for three minutes prevented *B. seriolae* egg hatching.
  - Sodium hypochlorite is typically ineffective, even at high doses.

Medical Management

- General information is provided under C7: *Monogeneans (General).*
- In several studies comparing treatments, *Neobenedenia* spp. built up more rapidly and were less sensitive to treatments than *Benedenia* spp. and other capsalids.
- Frequency of medical treatment depends on the species, goals, and practical limitations. A common treatment interval is less than two to three weeks apart at ~18–21°C (64–70°F).
- It may be helpful to apply treatments in the early morning as most oncomiracidia emerge in the first three hours of light.
- Common treatments (see Chapters A12 and A13 for more details):
  - Praziquantel immersion is the most commonly reported treatment. Typical doses are 2–10 mg/L. Drug level may be maintained in the water, but praziquantel can degrade rapidly in the environment and the drug level should be monitored. Alternatively, a pulse therapy can be used, such as 5 mg/L immersion as pulse treatments, dosed every four days for eight treatments without water changes for *Neobenedenia* spp. at ~24°C (75°F). To reduce loads, or when moving animals, higher dose dips can be used (e.g. 20 mg/L).
  - Praziquantel orally is also used. Most reports suggest high doses are needed, e.g. 120–150 mg/kg body weight PO every 24 hours for three days reduced the load of *B. seriolae* in amberjacks and *N. girellae* in chub mackerel (*Scomber japonicus*), although there was little effect on *N. girellae* in jacks; 50–75 mg/kg PO every 24 hours for three to six days reduced the load of *B. seriolae* in yellowtail amberjack (*Seriola lalandi*); and 40 mg/kg PO every 24 hours for 11 days reduced loads of *Neobenedenia* spp. in spotted halibut (*Verasper variegatus*). Poor palatability, leading to reduced intake and vomiting, are common with oral praziquantel at higher doses, which can reduce effectiveness. Microencapsulation, binding to frozen krill, and gavaging medication can help.
  - Freshwater dips for three to five minutes (matched to pH and temperature) can remove many capsalids from affected animals. Reinfection, sometimes with increased parasite loads, may be seen after treatment; so treatment is either repeated regularly (e.g. every 7–28 days) to keep loads down, or used as a dose-and-move strategy to try to prevent reinfection. Freshwater dips are rarely effective alone; *Neobenedenia* spp. required 20 minutes exposure to reduce adult and larval populations by 95% and eggs survived 72–96 hours exposure.
  - Long-term hyposalinity can reduce parasite loads and clinical signs as egg hatching in most reports is reduced by exposure to <18 g/L for more than four to

seven days. However, these salinity levels are not tolerated by many stenohaline fish.
  - Trichlorfon immersion at 0.25–0.70 mg/L active drug level is used, often repeated in 3–14 days. Adverse reactions to trichlorfon are common. Bioassays, close monitoring, and pretreatment with atropine should be considered. Suitable PPE must be used. Drug disposal must be considered.
  - Supportive care, such as fluids, nutritional support, and treatment of secondary infections may be indicated.
- Other reported treatments (see Chapters A12 and A13 for more details):
  - Hydrogen peroxide immersion.
  - Copper sulfate immersion for marine teleosts.
  - Calcium- and magnesium-free saltwater immersion.
- Formalin is rarely effective.
- All legislation regarding medication use and disposal must be followed.

Prevention

- General preventative measures are described under C7: *Monogeneans (General).*
- Good biosecurity is essential to prevent introduction of these parasites.

Zoonotic Reports

- These parasites have no known zoonotic potential.

Bibliography

Brazenor, A.K. and Hutson, K.S. (2015). Effects of temperature and salinity on the life cycle of *Neobenedenia* sp. (Monogenea: Capsalidae) infecting farmed barramundi (*Lates calcarifer*). *Parasitology Research* 114: 1875–1886.

De Souza, R.A.R., Da Annunciação, W.F., Lins, S.M. et al. (2014). Can barber goby *Elacatinus figaro* control *Neobenedenia melleni* infections on dusky grouper *Epinephelus marinatus*? *Aquaculture* 45: 619–628.

Ernst, I., Whittington, I.D., Cornillie, S., and Talbot, C. (2005). Effects of temperature, salinity, desiccation and chemical treatments on egg embryonation and hatching success of *Benedenia seriolae* (Monogenea: Capsalidae), a parasite of farmed *Seriola* spp. *Journal of Fish Diseases* 28: 157–164.

Fajer-Ávila, E.J., Martínez-Rodríguez, I., de la Parra, M.I.A. et al. (2008). Effectiveness of freshwater treatment against *Lepeophtheirus simplex* (Copepoda: Caligidae) and *Neobenedenia* sp. (Monogenea: Capsalidae), skin parasites of bullseye pufferfish, *Sphoeroides annulatus* reared in tanks. *Aquaculture* 284: 277–280.

Forwood, J.M., Bubner, E.J., Landos, M. et al. (2016). Praziquantel delivery via most pellets to treat monogenean parasites of yellowtail kingfish *Seriola lalandi*: efficacy and feed acceptance. *Diseases of Aquatic Organisms* 121: 201–209.

Hirazawa, N., Takano, R., Hagiwara, H. et al. (2010). The influence of different water temperatures on *Neobenedenia girellae* (Monogenea) infection, parasite growth, egg production and emerging second generation on amberjack *Seriola dumerili* (Carangidae) and the histopathological effect of this parasite on fish skin. *Aquaculture* 299: 2–7.

Hirazawa, N., Akiyama, K., and Umeda, N. (2013). Differences in sensitivity to the anthelmintic praziquantel by the skin-parasitic monogeneans *Benedenia seriolae* and *Neobenedenia girellae*. *Aquaculture* 404–405: 59–64.

Hurley-Saunders, J., Harms, C., Christiansen, E. et al. (2016). Exuberant granulation tissue response associated with *Neobenedenia* sp. (Monogenea: Capsalidae) infestation in two cobia, *Rachycentron canadum* (Linnaeus). *Journal of Fish Diseases* 39: 277–283.

Ishida, M., Kawano, F., Umeda, N., and Hirazawa, N. (2007). Response of *Neobenedenia girellae* (Monogenea) oncomiracidia to brightness and black-and-white contrast. *Parasitology* 134: 1823–1830.

McCammon, A., Sikkel, P.C., and Nemeth, D. (2010). Effects of three Caribbean cleaner shrimps on ectoparasitic monogeneans in a semi-natural environment. *Coral Reefs* 29: 419–426.

Militz, T.A. and Hutson, S. (2015). Beyond symbiosis: cleaner shrimp clean up in culture. *PLoSOne* 10: e0117723.

Ohashi, H., Umeda, N., Hirazawa, N. et al. (2007). Antiparasitic effects of calcium and magnesium ion-free buffer treatments against a common monogenean *Neobenedenia girellae*. *Parasitology* 134: 229–236.

Shirakashi, S. and Hirano, C. (2015). Accumulation and distribution of skin fluke *Neobenedenia girellae* eggs on a culture cage. *Aquaculture* 443: 1–4.

Tubbs, L.A., Poortenaar, C.W., Sewell, M.A., and Diggles, B.K. (2005). Effects of temperature on fecundity in vitro, egg hatching and reproductive development of *Benedenia seriolae* and *Zeuxapta seriolae* (Monogenea) parasitic on yellowtail kingfish *Seriola lalandi*. *International Journal of Parasitology* 35: 315–327.

Whittington, I.D. (2004). The Capsalidae (Monogenea: Monoopisthocotylea): a review of diversity, classification and phylogeny with a note about species complexes. *Folia Parasitologica* 51: 109–122.

Williams, R.E., Ernst, I., Chambers, C.B., and Whittington, I.D. (2007). Efficacy of orally administered praziquantel against *Zeuxapta seriolae* and *Benedenia seriolae* (Monogenea) in yellowtail kingfish *Seriola lalandi*. *Diseases of Aquatic Organisms* 77: 199–205.

Yamamoto, S., Shirakashi, S., Morimoto, S. et al. (2011). Efficacy of oral praziquantel treatment against the skin fluke infection of cultured chub mackerel, *Scomber japonicas*. *Aquaculture* 319: 53–57.

Abbrev iations/Acronyms

- PO: Orally
- PPE: Personal protective equipment

Dactylogyrid Monogeneans

Overview

- Dactylogyrids are oviparous monogeneans that typically infect the gills and skin of a variety of bony fish.
- There are also a few unusual examples of endoparasitic dactylogyrids (e.g. *Acolpenteron* spp.).
- Infections are usually asymptomatic, but morbidity and mortality are possible.
- Management is difficult because the egg stage is resistant to treatment. Recurrence is common.

Etiology

- Phylum *Platyhelminthes.*
- Class *Monogenoidea.*
- Subclass *Monopisthocotylea.*
- Order *Dactylogyridea.*
- Multiple genera from several families have been reported in fish:
  - *Dactylogyrus* is the most common, particularly *D. vastator*, *D. extensus*, and *D. intermedius*.
  - *Ancylodiscoides.*
  - *Euryhaliotrema.*
  - *Euryhaliotrematoides.*
  - *Haliotrema.*
  - *Haliotrematoides.*
  - *Pseudodactylogyrus.*
  - *Acolpenteron* and *Kritskyia* are unusual as they are endoparasitic.

Life Cycle and Transmission

- All monogeneans have direct life cycles.
- Dactylogyrids are oviparous (Figure C7.4).
- Ectoparasitic species shed eggs directly into the water. Endoparasitic species are found within the kidneys and ureters of fish and shed eggs in the urine.
- The life cycle is temperature-dependent. Generation times for *D. vastator* and *D. extensus* are reported as:
  - 6–13 days at 24–28°C (75–82°F).
  - 5–6 months at 1–2°C (34–36°F).

Geographic Distribution

- Predominantly in freshwater habitats, probably worldwide; can be found in saltwater habitats.

Signalment

- *Dactylogyrus* spp. are common in freshwater bony fish. Some fish species seem over-represented:
  - Cyprinids, particularly goldfish (*Carassius auratus*), common carp and koi (*Cyprinus carpio*), and grass carp (*Ctenopharyngodon idella*).
  - Cichlids, particularly discus (*Symphysodon* spp.) and freshwater angelfish (*Pterophyllum* spp.).
- Some common examples from other parasite genera include:
  - Eels (*Anguilla* spp.) with *Pseudodactylogyrus bini* and *Pseudodactylogyrus anguillae.*
  - Various tropical marine teleosts, particularly butterflyfish (*Chaetodontidae*), surgeonfish (*Acanthuridae*), and grouper (*Serranidae*) with *Haliotrema* spp.
  - Bass (*Micropterus* spp.) with *Acolpenteron ureteroecetes.*

Risk Factors

- General risk factors are described under C7: *Monogeneans (General).*

Signs/Clinical Findings

- Infected fish are often asymptomatic.
- Multiple fish from one or more species may be affected.
- Lethargy may be seen.
- Reduced appetite, weight loss, or poor growth rates may be seen.
- Dark coloration, gray sheen, poorly demarcated gray or white foci, edema, or hyperemia may be seen on the skin.
- Dyspnea or tachypnea may be seen.
- Gill pallor or edema may be seen.
- Compared to other monogeneans, this tends to have a slow course over months.
- Mortality is typically low but can reach 50%.

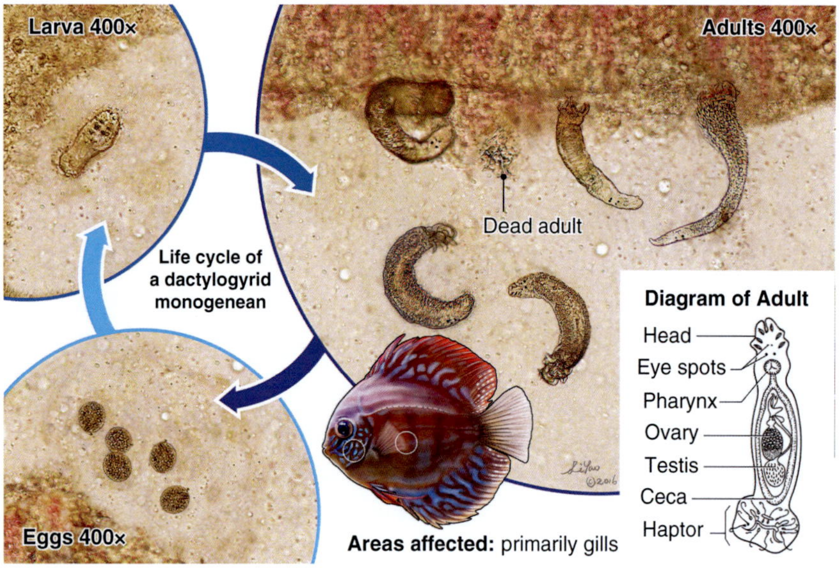

Figure C7.4 Life cycle of *Dactylogyrus* spp. *Source*: Image courtesy of Li Yao, copyright reserved.

Differential Diagnoses

- Full differentials are provided in Section B.
- Common differentials for external flatworms on freshwater bony fish include dactylogyrid and gyrodactylid monogeneans. Leeches can resemble flatworms.
- Common differentials for tetrahedral eggs on direct microscopy include all capsalid, and some monocotylid, dactylogyrid, and diplectanid monogeneans.

Diagnosis

- Dactylogyrids are typically identified on direct microscopy of gill biopsies or skin scrapes. Loads are typically higher on the gills than the skin, although sensitivity is low in asymptomatic animals.
- Adults are usually 0.2–2.0 mm in length with four small eye spots, one pair of large anchor hooks (hamuli), one smaller pair of anchor hooks, marginal hooklets, and a scallop-shaped head. *Haliotrema* spp. have transverse bars between the anchor hooks and some species do not have eye spots.
- Eggs are ~50 μm in size, oval or tetrahedral, with thin walls and a small anopercular process. Some eggs may have visible eye spots and hamuli if the larvae within are well-developed.
- Cytology and histology often also show increased mucus and gill hyperplasia.
- Dactylogyrid adults and eggs are occasionally found on direct microscopy, stained cytology, or histology of the kidneys or ureters. Lesions may include collecting duct hyperplasia and granulomatous inflammation.
- Identification to family is often enough for management. Further identification is usually based on haptor and reproductive morphology, although DNA sequencing is becoming more common. If further morphological or molecular identification is required, see C7: *Monogeneans (General).*

Husbandry Management

- Management changes may not be indicated if parasite load is low and there is no morbidity or mortality, but the parasites should be monitored.
- General husbandry measures are described under C7: *Monogeneans (General).*
- Reducing or resolving stressors can significantly reduce morbidity and mortality.
- Increase cleaning and disinfection of fomites.
  - Sodium hypochlorite at 120 mg/L available chlorine for three hours prevented hatching of *Haliotrema* sp. and *Euryhaliotrema* sp., and 12–36 mg/L chlorine for 24 hours reduced hatching of *P. anguillae*.
  - Desiccation may not be as effective as in other monogeneans (e.g. some *P. anguillae* eggs survived 24 hr drying).

Medical Management

- General information is provided under C7: *Monogeneans (General).*
- Common treatments (see Chapters A12 and A13 for more details):
  - Praziquantel immersion is the most common treatment. Doses and courses vary, but 10 mg/L every two to seven days is often reported. Praziquantel can degrade rapidly in the environment and the drug level should be monitored.
- Other reported treatments (see Chapters A12 and A13 for more details):
  - Praziquantel orally.
  - Levamisole immersion.

- Trichlorfon immersion.
- Emamectin orally.
- Long-term hypersalinity.
- Formalin immersion, but high doses are needed.
- All legislation regarding medication use and disposal must be followed.

Prevention
- General preventative measures are described under C7: *Monogeneans (General)*.

Zoonotic Reports
- These parasites have no known zoonotic potential.

Bibliography

Fajer-Ávila, E.J., Velásquez-Medina, S.P., and Betancourt-Lozano, M. (2007). Effectiveness of treatments against eggs and adults of *Haliotrema* sp. and *Euryhaliotrema* sp. (Monogenea: Ancryocephalinae) infecting red snapper, *Lutjanus gutattus*. *Aquaculture* 264: 66–72.

Forwood, J.M., Harris, J.O., and Deveney, M.R. (2013). Efficacy of bath and orally administered praziquantel and fenbendazole against *Lepidotrema bidyana* Murray, a monogenean parasite of silver perch, *Bidyanus bidyanus* (Mitchell). *Journal of Fish Diseases* 36: 939–947.

Larrat, S., Marvin, J., and Lair, S. (2012). Low sensitivity of antemortem gill biopsies for the detection of subclinical *Pseudodactylogyrus bini* infestations in American eels (*Anguilla rostrata*). *Journal of Zoo and Wildlife Medicine* 43: 190–192.

Reimschuessel, R., Gieseker, C., and Poynton, S. (2011). In vitroeffect of seven antiparasitics on *Acolpenteron ureteroecetes* (Dactylogyridae) from largemouth bass *Micropterus salmoides* (Centrarchidae). *Diseases of Aquatic Organisms* 94: 59–72.

Umeda, N., Nibe, H., Hara, T., and Hirazawa, N. (2006). Effects of various treatments on hatching of eggs and viability of oncomiracidia of the monogenean *Pseudodactylogyrus anguillae* and *Pseudodactylogyrus bini*. *Aquaculture* 253: 148–153.

Gyrodactylid Monogeneans

Overview
- Gyrodactylids are monogeneans that commonly infect the skin and gills of a wide variety of bony fish.
- Unusually for monogeneans, they are viviparous and numbers can escalate rapidly, particularly in closed systems.
- Treatment is usually easier than for oviparous monogeneans.
- *Gyrodactylus salaris* is an important parasite of salmonids in Europe.

Etiology
- Phylum *Platyhelminthes*.
- Class *Monogenoidea*.
- Subclass *Monopisthocotylea*.
- Order *Gyrodactylidea*.
- Family *Gyrodactylidae*.
- Many species have been identified.
- Examples of species where some strains show high pathogenicity include *Gyrodactylus anguillae*, *Gyrodactylus derjavinoides* (*derjavini*), and *G. salaris*.
- Some species exhibit much lower pathogenicity (e.g. *Gyrodactylus thymalli* is nonpathogenic to salmon but its morphology and DNA sequence are similar to *G. salaris*).

Life Cycle and Transmission
- All monogeneans have direct life cycles.
- Gyrodactylids are viviparous, with up to three generations developing inside a single parasite, which makes them prolific breeders (Figure C7.5). There are no eggs or cysts.
- Transmission is more effective from parasites that are attached to live or dead fish than from free-living parasites. The spread of *G. salaris* has been mostly due to transport and restocking of infected fish, rather than contaminated water. Risk of dispersal between surface water systems due to common human activities (e.g. boating, swimming) appears to be low.
- The life cycle is usually fast (e.g. 24–60 hours at 25°C or 77°F).
- Survival time off the host is typically a few days (e.g. usually one to four days in *G. salaris*).

Geographic Distribution
- Freshwater and saltwater habitats, probably worldwide.
- Distribution of each species varies:
  - *G. salaris* is currently limited to northern Europe and has been particularly problematic in Norway. It has the potential to spread to other salmonid areas.

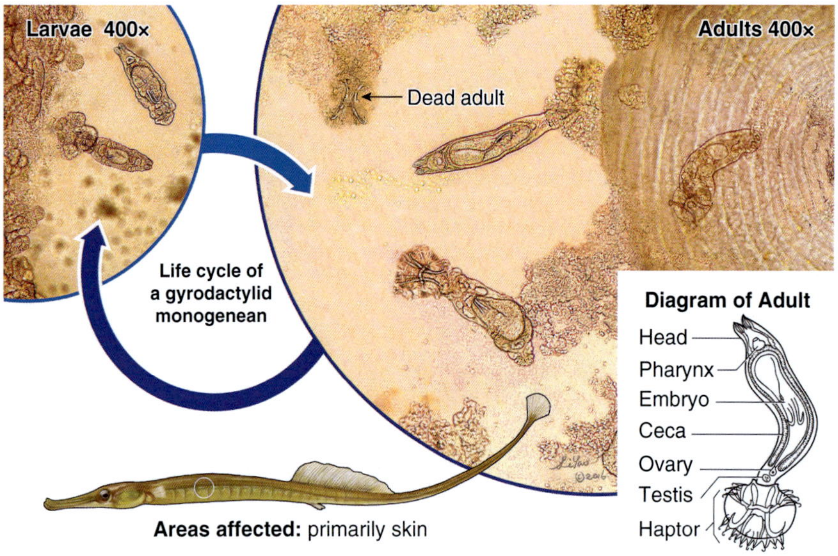

Figure C7.5 Life cycle of *Gyrodactylus* spp. *Source*: Image courtesy of Li Yao, copyright reserved.

- *G. anguillae* is predominantly found in Europe with some reports from Japan.

Signalment

- Freshwater and saltwater bony fish are susceptible.
- The host range of each parasite species is often narrow, e.g.:
  - Wild and cultured Atlantic salmon (*Salmo salar*) in freshwater are particularly susceptible to *G. salaris*. Other hosts include rainbow trout (*Oncorhynchus mykiss*) and Arctic charr (*Salvelinus alpinus*). This parasite is generally nonpathogenic in populations of the original fish host, Baltic Atlantic salmon. Other gyrodactylids also infect salmonids (e.g. *G. derjavinoides*).
  - Pipefish (*Syngnathus* spp.) – *Gyrodactylus shorti*, *Gyrodactylus syngnathi*, and *Gyrodactylus pisculentus*.
  - European eels (*Anguilla anguilla*) – *G. anguillae*.
  - Guppies (*Poecilia reticulata*) – *Gyrodactylus turnbulli* and *Gyrodactylus bullatarudis*.

Risk Factors

- General risk factors are described under C7: *Monogeneans (General)*.

Signs/Clinical Findings

- Infected fish are often asymptomatic.
- Multiple fish from one species or several closely related species may be affected.
- Lethargy and increased hiding may be seen.
- Reduced appetite, weight loss, or poor growth rates may be seen.
- Dark coloration or pallor, gray sheen, or poorly demarcated gray or white foci may be seen on the skin.
- Pruritus (e.g. flashing) may be seen.
- Dyspnea or tachypnea may be seen.
- Mortality is typically low, but can reach 30–45% in recirculating systems and close to 100% in susceptible salmonids with *G. salaris*.

Differential Diagnoses

- Full differentials are provided in Section B.
- Common differentials for external flatworms on freshwater bony fish include dactylogyrid and gyrodactylid monogeneans. Leeches can resemble flatworms.
- Common differentials for external flatworms on marine teleosts include capsalid monogeneans, particularly *Neobenedenia* spp., gyrodactylid monogeneans, and polyopisthocotyles. Leeches can resemble flatworms.

Diagnosis

- Gyrodactylids are typically identified on direct microscopy of skin scrapes. They are less common but can be found on gill biopsy or on scrapes of the eye or oral cavity. Sensitivity is much lower if tissues have dried.
- Adults are 0.3–1 mm in length with no eye spots, two pairs of large central hooks (hamuli) at the opisthaptor, 16 marginal hooklets, and a V-shaped head.
- Larvae look similar to adults. They may be free-living or readily visible within adult parasites, seen as an additional set of smaller hooks in the middle of the adult parasite.
- Identification to species has historically been based on morphology of the opisthaptor and protonephridia. If further morphological or molecular identification is required, see C7: *Monogeneans (General)*.
- *G. salaris* confirmation is by PCR, particularly TaqMan PCR, but ISH and RFLP tests may also be available. It is important for tests to differentiate *G. salaris* from similar gyrodactylids.

- The OIE Manual of Diagnostic Tests for Aquatic Animals provides specific guidance on the diagnosis of *G. salaris*. It recommends fixing of whole fish or freshly cut fin specimens in >95% ethyl alcohol for morphologic examination of the opisthaptor with confirmation by PCR and sequencing.
- *G. salaris* is reportable to many national, regional, or local groups and the OIE. It is not listed under EC directive 2006/88/EC but is covered under "additional guarantees" in some countries.

Husbandry Management

- Management changes may not be indicated if parasite load is low and there is no morbidity or mortality, but the parasites should be monitored as they can build up rapidly.
- General husbandry measures are described under C7: *Monogeneans (General)*.
- *G. salaris* should be susceptible to most common disinfectants at routine doses (e.g. Virkon-S 1% for 15 minutes) and freezing or heating (e.g. >40°C (104°F) for >5 minutes).

Medical Management

- Treatment of gyrodactylids is easier than other monogeneans since they do not produce eggs.
- Common treatments (see Chapters A12 and A13 for more details):
  - Praziquantel immersion is common. Doses range from 2 to 10 mg/L. Single doses may be sufficient, although treatment is often repeated in 7–14 days. The author recommends starting at the low end of the range with heavy infections, as increased morbidity may be seen after treatment if parasite loads are high. Praziquantel can degrade rapidly in the environment and the drug level should be monitored.
  - Formalin immersion can be effective at high doses, such as 250 mg/L for one hour every seven days for three treatments. However, these doses may result in morbidity and mortality. Formalin (Formalin-FTM, Formacide-B, Parasite-S®) is approved in the United States for use in finfish with *Gyrodactylus* spp. under various immersion treatment protocols with a 0-d withdrawal, as of 2020.
  - Hydrogen peroxide immersion (35% Perox-aid®) is approved in the United States for use in freshwater-reared salmonids with *Gyrodactylus* spp. at 50–100 mg/L for 60–30 minutes every 48 hours for three doses with a 0-d withdrawal, as of 2020.
  - Hypersalinity immersion can reduce parasite loads in freshwater fish that can tolerate the treatment. *G. salaris* treatment required 7.5 g/L for ~5–9 weeks, 15 g/L for 24 hours, and 33 g/L for ~10–20 minutes, while 5 g/L had little effect.
- Other reported treatments (see Chapters A12 and A13 for more details):
  - Freshwater dips in marine fish.
  - Levamisole immersion.
  - Sodium percarbonate immersion.
  - Trichlorfon immersion.
  - Triclabendazole orally.
  - Rotenone immersion has been used in rivers, but carries human health and environmental concerns.
  - Aqueous aluminum sulfate immersion has been used in rivers, but carries human health and environmental concerns.
- Chloroquine and metronidazole appear to be ineffective.
- All legislation regarding medication use and disposal must be followed.

Prevention

- General preventative measures are described under C7: *Monogeneans (General)*.

Zoonotic Reports

- These parasites have no known zoonotic potential.

Bibliography

Bakke, T.A., Cable, J., and Harris, P.D. (2007). The biology of gyrodactylid monogeneans: the 'Russian-doll killers'. *Advances in Parasitology* 64: 161–176.

Høgåsen, H.R., Brun, E., and Jansen, P.A. (2009). Quantification of free-living *Gyrodactylus salaris* in an infested river and consequences for inter-river dispersal. *Diseases of Aquatic Organisms* 87: 217–223.

OIE (2017). *Manual of Diagnostic Tests for Aquatic Animals* [online].http://www.oie.int/international-standard-setting/aquatic-manual/access-online/ (accessed 29July2017).

Olstad, K., Cable, J., Robertsen, G., and Bakke, T.A. (2006). Unpredicted transmission strategy of *Gyrodactylus salaris* (Monogenea: Gyrodactylidae): survival and infectivity of parasites on dead hosts. *Parasitology* 133: 33–41.

Rowland, S.J., Nixon, M., Landos, M. et al. (2006). Effects of formalin on water quality and parasitic monogeneans on silver perch (*Bidyanus bidyanus* Mitchell) in earthen ponds. *Aquaculture Research* 37: 869–876.

Schelkle, B., Doetjes, R., and Cable, J. (2011). The salt myth revealed: treatment of gyrodactylid infections on ornamental guppies, *Poecilia reticulata*. *Aquaculture* 311: 74–79.

Soleng, A. and Bakke, T.A. (1997). Salinity tolerance of *Gyrodactylus salaris* (Platyhelminthes, Monogenea): laboratory studies. *Canadian Journal of Fisheries and Aquatic Sciences* 54: 1837–1864.

Williams, S.R., Kritsky, D.C., Dunnigan, B. et al. (2008). *Gyrodactylus pisculentus* sp. n. (Monogenoidea: Gyrodactylidae) associated with mortality of the northern pipefish, *Syngnathus fuscus* (Syngnathiformes: Syngnathidae) at the Woods Hole Science Aquarium. *Folia Parasitologica* 55: 265–269.

Abbreviations/Acronyms

- EC: European Community
- ISH: In situ hybridization
- OIE: World Organisation for Animal Health
- PCR: Polymerase chain reaction
- RFLP: Restriction fragment length polymorphism

Monocotylid Monogeneans

Overview

- Monocotylids are large monogeneans that parasitize the skin or gills of elasmobranchs, particularly rays and skates.
- They are common in public aquariums and can cause recurrent morbidity and mortality.

Etiology

- Phylum *Platyhelminthes*.
- Class *Monogenoidea*.
- Subclass *Monopisthocotylea*.
- Order *Monocotylidea*.
- Family *Monocotylidae*.
- Several genera are reported as fish parasites:
  - *Clemacotyle*.
  - *Decacotyle*.
  - *Dendromonocotyle*.
  - *Dictyocotyle*.
  - *Empruthotrema*.
  - *Heterocotyle*.
  - *Merizocotyle*.
  - *Monocotyle*.
  - *Neoheterocotyle*.

Life Cycle and Transmission

- All monogeneans have direct life cycles.
- Monocotylids are oviparous.
- Eggs usually drop to the substrate and hatch over days to weeks producing ciliated oncomiracidia (larvae) that are the infective stage.
- Hatching may be stimulated by mechanical disturbance, shadows, or host secretions.
- Many monocotylids have an unusually wide temperature tolerance, e.g. *Dendromonocotyle pipinna* eggs start hatching four days post-laying at 30°C (86°F) and 16 days post-laying at 16°C (61°F).

Geographic Distribution

- Saltwater habitats with susceptible elasmobranchs.
- Distribution of each parasite species depends on the range of the host species.

Signalment

- Monocotylids seem largely restricted to marine rays (*Myliobatiformes*), skates (*Rajiformes*), and guitarfish and sawfish (*Rhinopristiformes*).
- Most are host-specific, although host range may be wider under human care.
- *Dendromonocotyle* spp. are reported on the skin of rays, e.g.:
  - *D. californica* in bat rays (*Myliobatis californica*).
  - *D. colorni* in several whipray species (*Himantura* spp.).
  - *D. kuhlii* in bluespotted stingrays (*Neotrygon kuhlii*).
  - *D. octodiscus* in yellow stingrays (*Urobatis jamaicensis*) and several dasyatid stingrays (*Hypanus* spp.).
  - *D. pipinna* in blackblotch stingrays (*Taeniurops meyeni*).
  - *D. torosa* in whitespotted eagle rays (*Aetobatus narinari*).
- Other genera are reported, e.g.:
  - *Clemacotyle australis* in whitespotted eagle rays.
  - *Decacotyle octona*, *Decacotyle floridana*, and *Decacotyle elpora* in whitespotted eagle rays.
  - *Dictyocotyle coeliaca* in skates (*Raja* spp.).
  - *Heterocotyle taeniuropi* in blackblotch stingrays.

Risk Factors

- General risk factors are described under C7: *Monogeneans (General)*.
- Permissive salinity is typically 30–40 g/L.
- Permissive water temperatures are usually high (e.g. >25°C (77°F) for *D. pipinna*).

Signs/Clinical Findings

- Multiple conspecifics are usually affected.
- White, translucent, or dark flatworms may be grossly visible on the skin, particularly the dorsal skin for *Dendromonocotyle* spp. Other genera are more cryptic and may be found deep within the gills (*Clemacotyle*, *Decacotyle*, *Heterocotyle*, *Monocotyle*, and *Neoheterocotyle*

spp.) or within the nasal tissue (*Empruthotrema* and *Merizocotyle* spp.), and some unusual ones are endoparasitic (*Dictyocotyle* spp.).

- In several reports, parasites were not readily visible until three to six months post-infection.
- There may be no other clinical signs.
- If loads are high, the skin may look slightly dull or gray due to increased mucus, particularly around the eyes and spiracles.
- Lethargy may be seen.
- Pruritus may be seen (e.g. flashing, erratic swimming, increased jumping, lifting of the pectoral fin tips and tail).
- Reduced appetite may be seen.
- Mortality rate is usually low.

Differential Diagnoses

- Full differentials are provided in Section B.
- Common differentials for external flatworms on marine rays include capsalid and monocotylid monogeneans. Leeches can resemble flatworms.
- Tetrahedral eggs in elasmobranchs are most likely due to capsalid, microbothriid, or monocotylid monogeneans.

Diagnosis

- Many monocotylids are large enough to be grossly visible. Diagnosis is typically by direct microscopy of parasites pulled from the skin, gills, or nares, or microscopy of a skin scrape or gill biopsy. Endoscopic examination may be helpful in species where the gills and nasal tissue are not visible grossly. *Dictyocotyle* spp. are unusual since they are endoparasitic, e.g. *D. coeliaca* is typically found in the coelom or liver.

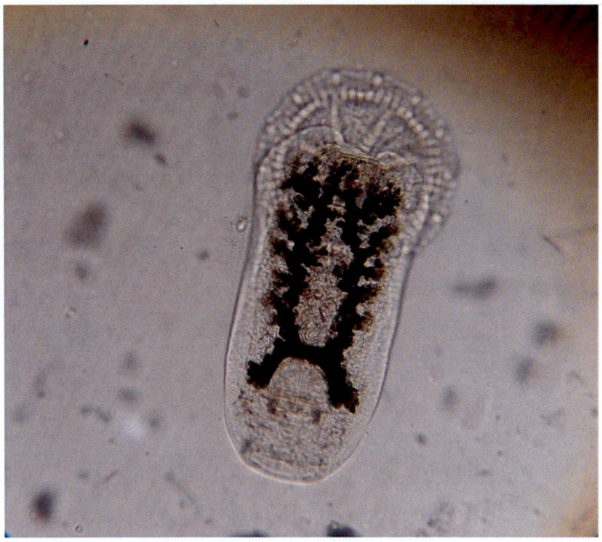

Figure C7.6 *Dendromonocotyle* sp. on direct microscopy of a skin scrape at x100.

- Adults are large, unsegmented flatworms, 1–6 mm in length. The attachment organ (opisthaptor) is large relative to body size and divided into one central and eight peripheral sections by septa with small sclerites (resembling a wagon-wheel). Small hooks (hamuli) may be present and are used for species identification. Most have highly dendritic intestinal ceca that often look dark and obscure some of the anatomy (Figure C7.6).
- Larvae are smaller, with a small haptor and two pairs of large eye spots each associated with a large crystalline lens. There are visible bands of cilia that allow steady movement.
- Eggs are brown, tetrahedral (although these often look triangular), 70–100 μm in size, each with a trailing filament. Some eggs may have visible eye spots if the larvae within are well-developed.
- Identification to species level is usually based on morphology of the male copulatory organ, hamuli, and terminal sclerites on the marginal papillae. If further morphological or molecular identification is required, see C7: *Monogeneans (General).*
- Egg traps are useful for routine monitoring; see C7: *Monogeneans (General).*

Husbandry Management

- General husbandry measures are described under C7: *Monogeneans (General).*
- Morbidity and mortality resolved in blackblotch stingrays without medical treatment by resolving environmental stressors.
- Increase cleaning and disinfection of fomites.
  - Full drying for >10 minutes prevented egg hatching of *D. pipinna*.
  - Sodium hypochlorite at >10 mg/L available chlorine for 18 hours prevented egg hatching of *D. pipinna;* 5 mg/L was ineffective even after 24 hours.
  - Freshwater is likely to have an effect, but the required duration is unknown.
- Cleaner fish have been shown to reduce load in some cases, e.g. bluehead wrasse (*Thalassoma bifasciatum*) and bluestreak cleaner wrasse (*Labroides dimidiatus*), although they have less impact on the more cryptic monocotylids.

Medical Management

- General information is provided under C7: *Monogeneans (General).*
- Because of the narrow host range, the most effective management may be to remove susceptible species for treatment. Treatment should be targeted during the move, then for a prolonged time in a suitable alternative habitat, effectively fallowing the original system.

However, since duration of egg viability is unknown, reinfection risk is also unknown.

- Common treatments (see Chapters A12 and A13 for more details):
  - Praziquantel immersion at 10 mg/L for two hours is often effective for skin monocotylids. Longer duration and/or higher doses may be required for monocotylids in the gills or nasal tissue. Intervals vary from every two days to two weeks. For routine maintenance to reduce parasite load, the interval may be extended to every two to six months. Praziquantel can degrade rapidly in the environment and the drug level should be monitored.
  - Praziquantel orally at 100–150 mg/kg body weight reduced parasite load in lesser guitarfish (*Acroteriobatus annulatus*) and whitespotted eagle rays. When gavaging meds, endoscopic guidance under sedation has been recommended to ensure the drug is delivered into the stomach.
  - Freshwater dips (matched to pH and temperature) can reduce the parasite load. They are a common form of long-term management and may be used weekly to monthly as needed. They are not tolerated by all marine elasmobranchs.
  - Long-term hyposalinity treatment can be effective where tolerated by the fish. Salinity of <15 g/L prevented egg hatching of *D. pipinna*.
- Other reported treatments (see Chapters A12 and A13 for more details):
  - Trichlorfon immersion, but safety index is low with many elasmobranch species.
  - Praziquantel by intramuscular injection.
- All legislation regarding medication use and disposal must be followed.

Prevention

- General preventative measures are described under C7: *Monogeneans (General)*.
- Good biosecurity can prevent the introduction of these parasites. This includes suitable quarantine of elasmobranchs with examination of the skin and gills (often endoscopic) and prophylactic treatment with praziquantel.
- In blackblotch stingrays infected with *D. pipinna*, prohibiting staff members from going into a shallow pool for visitor-interactive feedings when the water temperature was >25°C (77°F) resolved the clinical signs.

Zoonotic Reports

- These parasites have no known zoonotic potential.

Bibliography

Chen, H.-G., Chen, H.-Y., Wang, C.-S. et al. (2010). Effects of various treatments on egg hatching of *Dendromonocotyle pipinna* (Monogenea: Monocotylidae) infecting the blotched fantail ray, *Taeniurops meyeni*, in Taiwan. *Veterinary Parasitology* 171: 228–237.

Chisholm, L.A. and Whittington, I.D. (2002). Efficacy of praziquantel bath treatments for monogenean infections of the *Rhinobatos typus*. *Journal of Aquatic Animal Health* 14: 230–234.

Chisholm, L.A., Whittington, I.D., and Fischer, A.B.P. (2004). A review of *Dendromonocotyle* (Monogenea: Monocotylidae) from the skin of stingrays and their control in public aquaria. *Folia Parasitologica* 51: 123–130.

Janse, M. and Borgsteede, F.H.M. (2003). Praziquantel treatment of captive white-spotted eagle rays (*Aetobatus narinari*) infested with monogenean trematodes. *Bulletin of the European Association of Fish Pathologists* 23: 152–156.

Mylniczenko, N., Nolan, E.C., Thomas, A. et al. (2015). Management of monogenes in eagle rays (*Aetobatus narinari*) with high oral praziquantel. Presented at the *International Aquatic Animal Medicine Conference*, Chicago, IL.

Vaughan, D.B. and Chisholm, L.A. (2009). Three *Dendromonocotyle* species (Monogenea: Monocotylidae) reported from captive rays, including *D. lotteri* sp. n. from *Himantura gerrardi* (Elasmobranchii: Dasyatidae) in the public aquarium at the Atlantis resort, Dubai. *Folia Parasitological* 56: 99–106.

Microbothriid Monogeneans

Overview

- Microbothriids are large monogeneans that usually parasitize the skin of elasmobranchs, particularly sharks.
- They are typically host-specific. Management is difficult because the egg stage is resistant to treatment. Recurrence is common.

Etiology

- Phylum *Platyhelminthes*.
- Class *Monogenoidea*.
- Subclass *Monopisthocotylea*.
- Order *Monocotylidea*.
- Family *Microbothriidae*.
- Several genera are reported as fish parasites, including:
  - *Dermophthirioides*.
  - *Dermophthirius*.
  - *Dermopristis*.
  - *Leptocotyle*.
  - *Microbothrium*.
  - *Neodermophthirius*.

Life Cycle and Transmission

- All monogeneans have direct life cycles.
- Microbothriids are oviparous.
- Life cycle details are largely unknown but are probably similar to *Monocotylidae*.

Geographic Distribution

- Saltwater habitats with susceptible elasmobranchs.
- Distribution of each parasite species depends on the range of the host species.

Signalment

- Microbothriids are only found in elasmobranchs, particularly requiem sharks (*Carcharhinidae*).
- Most are highly host-specific. Unlike other monogeneans, their host ranges do not appear to widen under human care.
  - *Dermophthirioides pristidis* in smalltooth sawfish (*Pristis pectinata*).
  - *Dermophthirius carcharhini* in Galapagos sharks (*Carcharhinus galapagensis*), bignose sharks (*Carcharhinus altimus*), and dusky sharks (*Carcharhinus obscurus*).
  - *Dermophthirius melanopteri* in blacktip reef sharks (*Carcharhinus melanopterus*).
  - *Dermophthirius penneri* in blacktip sharks (*Carcharhinus limbatus*).
  - *Leptocotyle minor* in smallspotted catsharks (*Scyliorhinus canicula*).
  - *Neodermophthirius harkemai* in lemon sharks (*Negaprion brevirostris*).

Risk Factors

- General risk factors are described under C7: *Monogeneans (General)*.

Signs/Clinical Findings

- Multiple conspecifics are usually affected.
- Pruritus (e.g. flashing, erratic swimming) is common.
- Multifocal, irregular, white or gray skin plaques or ulcers may be seen and may coalesce. These lesions are particularly common on the head and the trailing edges of the dorsal and caudal fins.
- Dark bands of hemorrhage and mucus may be seen, particularly around the mouth.
- Dyspnea or tachypnea may be seen.
- Mortality rate is usually low.

Differential Diagnoses

- Full differentials are provided in Section B.
- Common differentials for external flatworms on marine sharks include microbothriids, udonellids, and polyopisthocotyles. Leeches can resemble flatworms.

Diagnosis

- Many microbothriids are large enough to be just grossly visible. Diagnosis is typically by direct microscopy of parasites pulled from the skin or skin scrapes.
- They are less common on gills.
- Adults are large, unsegmented flatworms, 2–5 mm in length (Figure C7.7a). Body shapes may be lanceolate (e.g. *Neodermophthirius* spp.) or ovoid to round (e.g. *Dermophthirius* spp.). They are often transparent or opaque and look like wet plaques when the skin is out of the water. They have a small haptor without hooks or suckers, which is unusual for monogeneans; they attach using a cement-like substance. The ovaries are rectangular and anterior to testes. The number of testes can be used to differentiate genera.
  - Single testis in *Microbothrium* spp.
  - Paired testes in *Dermophthirius* spp. and *Dermophthirioides* spp. that are readily visible on routine microscopy.
  - Numerous testes (10–11) in *Neodermophthirius* spp. although these may not be readily visible on routine microscopy.
- Eggs are brown and triangular with short filaments at each pole, ~200 μm in size (Figure C7.7b).
- Identification to species requires detailed light or electron microscopy. If further morphological or molecular identification is required, see C7: *Monogeneans (General)*.
- Egg traps are useful for routine monitoring; see C7: *Monogeneans (General)*.

Husbandry Management

- General husbandry measures are described under C7: *Monogeneans (General)*.
- Consider slowly adjusting the water temperature (e.g. reducing temperature to 19°C (66°F) reduced clinical signs in lemon sharks with *Dermophthirius* spp.).
- Consider manual removal due to resistance to medical treatments.

Medical Management

- General information is provided under C7: *Monogeneans (General)*.

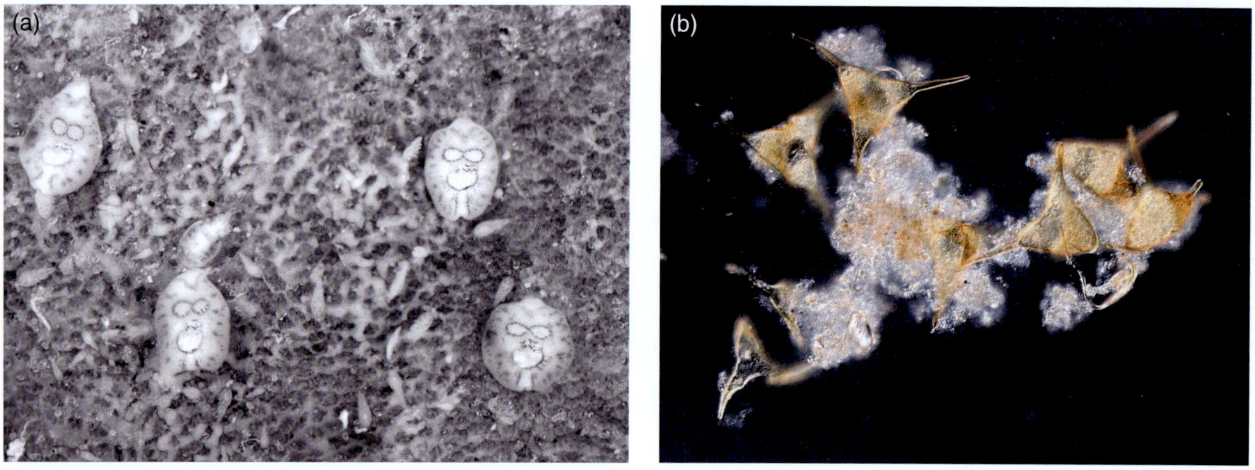

Figure C7.7 *Dermophthirius penneri* from a blacktip shark (*Carcharhinus limbatus*) showing adults (a) and triangular eggs (b). *Source*: Images courtesy of Stephen Bullard, Auburn University.

- Because of the narrow host range, the most effective management may be to remove susceptible species for treatment. Treatment should be targeted during the move, then for a prolonged time in a suitable alternative habitat, effectively fallowing the original system. However, since duration of egg viability is unknown, reinfection risk is also unknown.
- Common treatments (see Chapters A12 and A13 for more details):
  - Praziquantel immersion is reported at ~10 mg/L. Intervals vary from every two weeks to months. However, resistance to drug treatment is commonly reported for this group.
  - Trichlorfon immersion at 0.5 mg/L repeated every three to seven days for three treatments can reduce or resolve clinical signs. Adverse reactions to trichlorfon are common. Bioassays, close monitoring, and pre-treatment with atropine should be considered. Suitable PPE must be used. Drug disposal must be considered.
- Other reported treatments (see Chapters A12 and A13 for more details):
  - Praziquantel orally and via intramuscular injection have been reported as ineffective, but the doses were low.
  - Copper sulfate immersion resolved signs in lemon sharks. Most elasmobranchs cannot tolerate copper treatment.
  - Freshwater dips (matched to pH and temperature) have shown variable success.
- All legislation regarding medication use and disposal must be followed.

Prevention

- General preventative measures are described under C7: *Monogeneans (General)*.

Zoonotic Reports

- These parasites have no known zoonotic potential.

Bibliography

Bullard, S.A., Frasca, S., and Benz, G.W. (2000). Skin lesions caused by *Dermophthirius penneri* (Monogenea: Microbothriidae) on wild-caught blacktip sharks (*Carcharhinus limbatus*). *Journal of Parasitology* 86: 618–622.

Bullard, S.A., Dippenaar, S.M., Hoffmayer, E.R., and Benz, G.W. (2004). New locality records for *Dermophthirius carcharhini* (Monogenea: Microbothriidae) and *Dermophthirius maccalumi* and a list of hosts and localities for species of *Dermophthirius*. *Comparative Parasitology* 71: 78–80.

Poynton, S.L., Campbell, T.W., and Palm, H.W. (1997). Skin lesions in captive lemon sharks *Negaprion brevirostris* (Carcharhinidae) associated with the monogenean *Neodermophthirius harkemai* Price, 1963 (Microbothriidae). *Diseases of Aquatic Organisms* 31: 29–33.

Young, J.M., Frasca, S., Gruber, S.H., and Benz, G.W. (2013). Monogenoid infection of neonatal and older juvenile lemon sharks, *Negaprion brevirostris* (Carcharhinidae), in a shark nursery. *Journal of Parasitology* 99: 1151–1154.

Abbreviations/Acronyms

- PPE: Personal protective equipment

Polyopisthocotyle Monogeneans

Overview

- *Polyopisthocotylea* monogeneans are closely related to the *Monopisthocotylea* monogeneans, but can be hematophagous (blood feeders) and have multiple attachment clamps/suckers.
- They are less commonly reported than *Monopisthocotylea* monogeneans.
- They may be incidental findings but can become problematic when parasite loads are high or under other stressors.
- Typical signs include anemia and dyspnea.
- Treatment is similar to that of *Monopisthocotylea* monogeneans.

Etiology

- Phylum *Platyhelminthes*.
- Class *Monogenoidea*.
- Subclass *Polyopisthocotylea*.
- Many genera are known to infect fish:
  - *Diclidophora*.
  - *Diplozoon*.
  - *Erpocotyle*.
  - *Heterobothrium*.
  - *Microcotyle*.
  - *Neoheterobothrium*.
  - *Sparicotyle*.
  - *Zeuxapta*.

Life Cycle and Transmission

- All monogeneans have direct life cycles.
- Polyopisthocotyles are oviparous.
- Eggs typically drop off the host. Eggs hatch to release ciliated oncomiracidia (larvae) that swim or creep until they find a host. They mature into adult stages on the host.
- Hatching typically takes a few days and the oncomiracidia can survive a few days without a host. Maturation takes weeks to months, depending on the species and temperature. This is longer than for other monogeneans.

Geographic Distribution

- Predominantly in saltwater habitats, probably worldwide, but can be found in freshwater habitats.
- Distribution of each parasite species depends on the range or culture location of the host species.

Signalment

- All fish may be susceptible, particularly marine teleosts.
- The host range of each parasite species is often narrow, e.g.:
  - *Erpocotyle tiburonis* in bonnethead sharks (*Sphyrna tiburo*).
  - *Heterobothrium okamotoi* in tiger puffers (*Takifugu rubripes*).
  - *Microcotyle sebastis* in black and Korean rockfish (*Sebastes melanops* and *schlegelii*).
  - *Neoheterobothrium hirame* in olive flounder (*Paralichthys olivaceus*).
  - *Zeuxapta seriolae* in amberjacks (*Seriola* spp.).

Risk Factors

- General risk factors are described under C7: *Monogeneans (General)*.

Signs/Clinical Findings

- Infected fish may be asymptomatic.
- Multiple fish from one or more closely related species may be affected.
- Lethargy may be seen.
- Inappetence, reduced appetite, or weight loss may be seen.
- Pruritus (e.g. flashing, erratic swimming) may be seen.
- Flounder may show reduced burrowing activity.
- Gill pallor may be seen. In heavy infections, the gills can be white (Figure B2.3c).
- Dyspnea or tachypnea may be seen.
- Mortality rate is usually low but may increase in response to additional stressors (e.g. low dissolved oxygen, handling).

Differential Diagnoses

- Full differentials are provided in Section B.
- Common differentials for external flatworms on marine fish include capsalid, gyrodactylid, monocotylid, and microbothriid monogeneans and polyopisthocotyles. Leeches can resemble flatworms.

Diagnosis

- Diagnosis is typically based on direct microscopy of skin scrapes or gill biopsies. The parasites may also be found on scrapes of the oral or branchial cavities.
- Adults are unsegmented flatworms up to 0.5 mm in length, although some species are larger (e.g. *N. hirame*). Caudally, there are several pairs (often three to four pairs) of small clamps or suckers, each with small hooks for attachment; the hooks are barely visible on direct microscopy (Figure C7.8a–c). These clamps may be symmetric or asymmetric. They may be embedded in host tissues. Adults are less motile than monopisthocotyles.
- Eggs may be visible inside the parasites or free (Figure C7.8d). They may be oval or spindle-shaped and form long strings or tangled bunches.
- Necropsy or coeliotomy may show severe anemia. Histology may show the parasites and hyperplasia, inflammation, or necrosis at the insertion points.

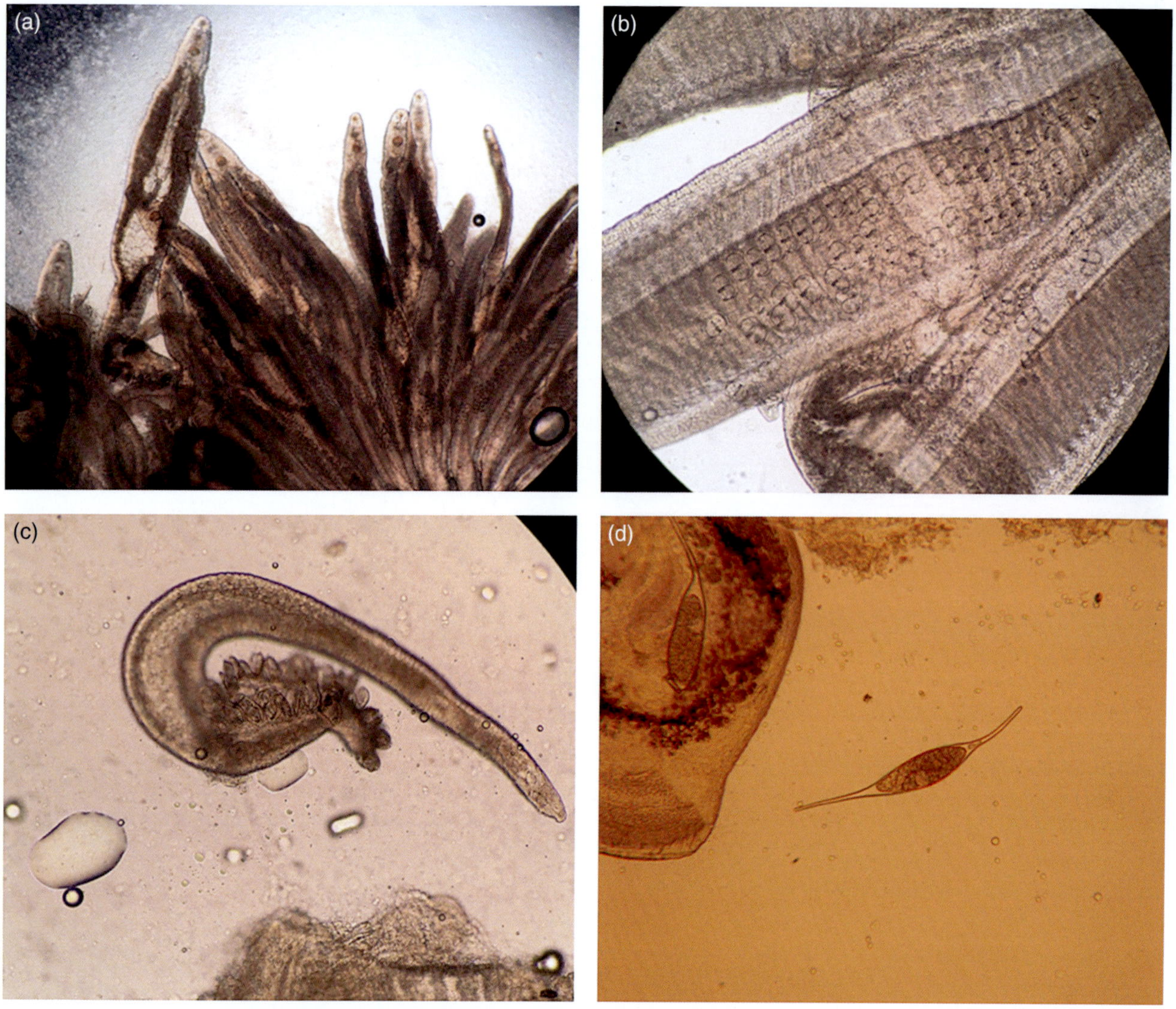

Figure C7.8 Polyopisthocotyles tightly embedded in gill tissue (a); examination of the attachment points shows the multiple clamps (b). Free-swimming adults are easier to identify (c). Some eggs are spindle-shaped, as seen here with *Erpocotyle tiburonis* (d). *Source*: Image (d) courtesy of Shane Boylan, South Carolina Aquarium.

- If further morphological or molecular identification is required, see C7: *Monogeneans (General)*.
- Egg traps are useful for routine monitoring; see C7: *Monogeneans (General)*.

Husbandry Management

- Management changes may not be indicated if parasite load is low and there is no morbidity or mortality, but the parasites should be monitored.
- General husbandry measures are described under C7: *Monogeneans (General)*.
- Control strategies can be tailored to the species, e.g.:
  - *Heterobothrium* spp. eggs tangle in décor, and mechanical removal of egg stages should accompany medical management (e.g. scrubbing or changing nets or décor).
  - *Neoheterobothrium* spp. eggs are loose in the water column and increased water turnover may reduce loads.
- Consider slowly adjusting the water temperature, e.g. *Z. seriolae* showed reduced egg production and prolonged embryonation times at 13°C (55°F) compared to 18–21°C (64–70°F).
- Increase cleaning and disinfection of fomites.
  - Hot water may be effective, e.g. 40°C (104°F) for one hour suppressed hatching of *H. okamotoi* eggs.
  - Drying for one to five hours prevented hatching of *H. okamotoi* and *Z. seriolae* eggs.
  - Sodium hypochlorite at 60 mg/L available chlorine for 24 hours prevented hatching of *H. okamotoi* eggs.
- Freshwater had no effect on *H. okamotoi* eggs, even after 24 hours.

Medical Management

- General information is provided under C7: *Monogeneans (General)*.
- Common treatments (see Chapters A12 and A13 for more details):
  - Praziquantel immersion is used, but the few reported doses are high (e.g. 100 mg/L for four minutes reduced the load of *M. sebastis*).
  - Praziquantel orally at high doses such as 50–400 mg/kg body weight every 24 hours can reduce or resolve infection in individual animals, but reinfection is common so long courses are recommended (e.g. every 24–48 hours for 30 days). The addition of cimetidine at 200 mg/kg PO increased the effectiveness of oral praziquantel in Korean rockfish, allowing lower applied doses (likely through inhibiting the rapid metabolism of praziquantel by cytochrome P_{450} isoenzymes).
  - Trichlorfon immersion at doses of 0.25–0.50 mg/L can be used, but adverse reactions to trichlorfon are common. Bioassays, close monitoring, and pretreatment with atropine should be considered. Suitable PPE must be used. Drug disposal must be considered.
  - Long-term hyposalinity immersion (e.g. 18–20 g/L) may reduce parasite loads but some polyopisthocotyle adults and eggs can tolerate low salinity.
  - Febantel orally at 25–50 mg/kg every 24 hours for three to five days is often used to reduce *Heterobothrium* spp. load in tiger puffers.
- Other reported treatments (see Chapters A12 and A13 for more details):
  - Formalin immersion.
  - Hydrogen peroxide immersion.
  - Quinacrine orally.
- All legislation regarding medication use and disposal must be followed.

Prevention

- General preventative measures are described under C7: *Monogeneans (General)*.

Zoonotic Reports

- These parasites have no known zoonotic potential.

Bibliography

Bullard, S.A., Frasca, S., and Benz, G.W. (2001). Gill lesions associated with *Erpocotyle tiburonis* (Monogenea: Hexabothriidae) on wild and aquarium-held bonnethead sharks (*Sphyrna tiburo*). *Journal of Parasitology* 87: 972–977.

Forwood, J.M., Bubner, E.J., Landos, M. et al. (2016). Praziquantel delivery via most pellets to treat monogenean parasites of yellowtail kingfish *Seriola lalandi*: efficacy and feed acceptance. *Diseases of Aquatic Organisms* 121: 201–209.

Hirazawa, N., Goto, T., and Shirasu, K. (2003). Killing effects of various treatments on the monogenean *Heterobothrium okamotoi* eggs and oncomiracidia and the ciliate *Cryptocaryon irritans* cysts and theronts. *Aquaculture* 223: 1–13.

Kang, Y.J., Wakabayashi, C., and Kim, K.H. (2016). Anthelmintic potential of quinacrine and oxyclozanide against gill parasite *Microcotyle sebastis* in black rockfish *Sebastes schlegeli*. *Diseases of Aquatic Organisms* 119: 259–263.

Kim, K.H. and Cho, J.B. (2000). Treatment of *Microcotyle sebastis* (Monogenea: Polyopisthocotylea) infestation with praziquantel in an experimental cage simulating commercial rockfish *Sebastes schlegeli* culture conditions. *Diseases of Aquatic Organisms* 40: 229–231.

Kim, K.H., Lee, E.H., Kwon, S.R., and Cho, J.B. (2001). Treatment of *Microcotyle sebastis* infestation in cultured rockfish *Sebastes schlegeli* by oral administration of praziquantel in combination with cimetidine. *Diseases of Aquatic Organisms* 44: 133–136.

Kimura, T., Nomura, Y., Kawakami, H. et al. (2009). Field trials of febantel against gill fluke disease caused by the monogenean *Heterobothrium okamotoi* in cultured tiger puffer *Takifugu rubripes*. *Fish Pathology* 44: 67–71.

Shirakashi, S., Teruya, K., and Ogawa, K. (2008). Altered behavior and reduced survival of juvenile olive flounder, *Paralichthys olivaceus*, infected by an invasive monogenean, *Neoheterobothrium hirame*. *InternationalJournal for Parasitology* 38: 513–1522.

Tubbs, L.A., Poortenaar, C.W., Sewell, M.A., and Diggles, B.K. (2005). Effects of temperature on fecundity in vitro, egg hatching and reproductive development of *Benedenia seriolae* and *Zeuxapta seriolae* (Monogenea) parasitic on yellowtail kingfish *Seriola lalandi*. *International Journal of Parasitology* 35: 315–327.

Williams, R.E., Ernst, I., Chambers, C.B., and Whittington, I.D. (2007). Efficacy of orally administered praziquantel against *Zeuxapta seriolae* and *Benedenia seriolae* (Monogenea) in yellowtail kingfish *Seriola lalandi*. *Diseases of Aquatic Organisms* 77: 199–205.

Abbreviations/Acronyms

- PO: Orally
- PPE: Personal protective equipment

Digenes (Excluding Blood Flukes)

Overview

- Digenes other than blood flukes are unsegmented endoparasitic flatworms. Adults have one or two obvious suckers and no hooks.
- Fish can be the intermediate or definitive host (IH or DH).
- When fish are the IH, encysted stages can be found in any tissues. These are usually clinically insignificant, but they can cause morbidity and mortality if critical tissues have been damaged.
- When fish are the DH, adult parasites can be found in the gastrointestinal tract, coelom, or viscera. Morbidity is more common when fish are the definitive host.
- Digenes have been particularly problematic in pond culture of catfish (*Siluriformes*).

Etiology

- Phylum *Platyhelminthes*.
- Class *Trematoda*.
- Subclass *Digenea*.
- A wide range of families, genera, and species can parasitize fish.
- Fish are typically reported as the IH with encysted metacercariae in the tissues:
  - *Bolbophorus* spp. in muscle and viscera.
  - *Clinostomum* spp. in muscle and viscera.
  - *Cryptocotyle* spp. in skin and gills.
  - *Diplostomum* spp. in the eyes, typically the lenses.
  - *Nanophyetus* spp. in muscle; *N. salmonicola* is the vector for a rickettsial disease of dogs.
  - *Neascus* spp. in skin and muscle.
  - *Posthodiplostomum* spp. in skin, muscle, and corneas.
- Fish can also be the DH with adult digenes in the gastrointestinal tract and viscera. This is under-reported in the literature.
  - *Crepidostomum* spp. in the gastrointestinal tract.
  - *Hemiurus* spp. in the stomach.

Life Cycle and Transmission

- All digenes have an indirect life cycle.
- Digenes, except for blood flukes, have two intermediate hosts (Figure C7.9).
  - The first IHs are typically mollusks (often lymnaeid or planorbid snails).
  - The second IHs are typically fish or amphibians.
  - The DH can be fish or piscivorous birds (e.g. gulls, pelicans, herons, egrets, bitterns).
- Some life cycles have been elucidated. For example, for *Bolbophorus damnificus*, the first IH is the rams-horn snail (*Planorbella trivolvis*), the second IH is the channel catfish (*Ictalurus punctatus*), and the DH is the American white pelican (*Pelecanus erythrorhynchos*).
- Sexual reproduction takes place in the DH. Large opercular eggs are produced within a few days and are passed in feces. The eggs hatch to form ciliated miracidia (larvae) that swim to and penetrate the first IH. Where known, this can take one to two weeks during summer temperatures. In the IH, the miracidia settle to become sporocysts, which asexually produce rediae or more sporocysts. Some rediae develop into cercariae. These crawl out of the IH into the water. Cercariae burrow into the second IH where they migrate rapidly to their preferred tissue site and encyst as metacercariae. Metacercarial maturation takes several weeks. Metacercariae remain viable in fish for several years. The life cycle is completed when the second IH is eaten by the DH and the metacercariae invade the gastrointestinal tract of the DH.
- The parasites cannot be transmitted directly between fish.

Geographic Distribution

- Freshwater and saltwater habitats, probably worldwide.
- Distribution of each parasite species depends on the range or culture location of the host species (e.g. *Clinostomum* and *Bolbophorus* spp. are common in southern United States and California where channel catfish are farmed).

Signalment

- All bony fish are likely susceptible. There are rare reports from elasmobranchs.
- Some digenes have narrow host ranges, e.g.:
  - *B. damnificus* in channel catfish and their hybrids.
  - *N. salmonicola* in Pacific salmonids, particularly Chinook (*Oncorhynchus tshawytscha*).
- Other digenes have wider host ranges, e.g.:
  - *Crassiphiala bulboglossa* and *Clinostomum marginatum* in North American freshwater fish such as sunfish (*Lepomis* spp.) and killifish (*Fundulus* spp.).
  - *Diplostomum spathaceum* in a variety of brackish and freshwater fish such as channel catfish, salmonids, and Atlantic sturgeon (*Acipenser oxyrinchus*).

Risk Factors

- Exposure and stressors are the most important risk factors.
- Exposure includes:
  - Poor biosecurity (e.g. lack of suitable quarantine, exposure to birds, particularly wading birds).

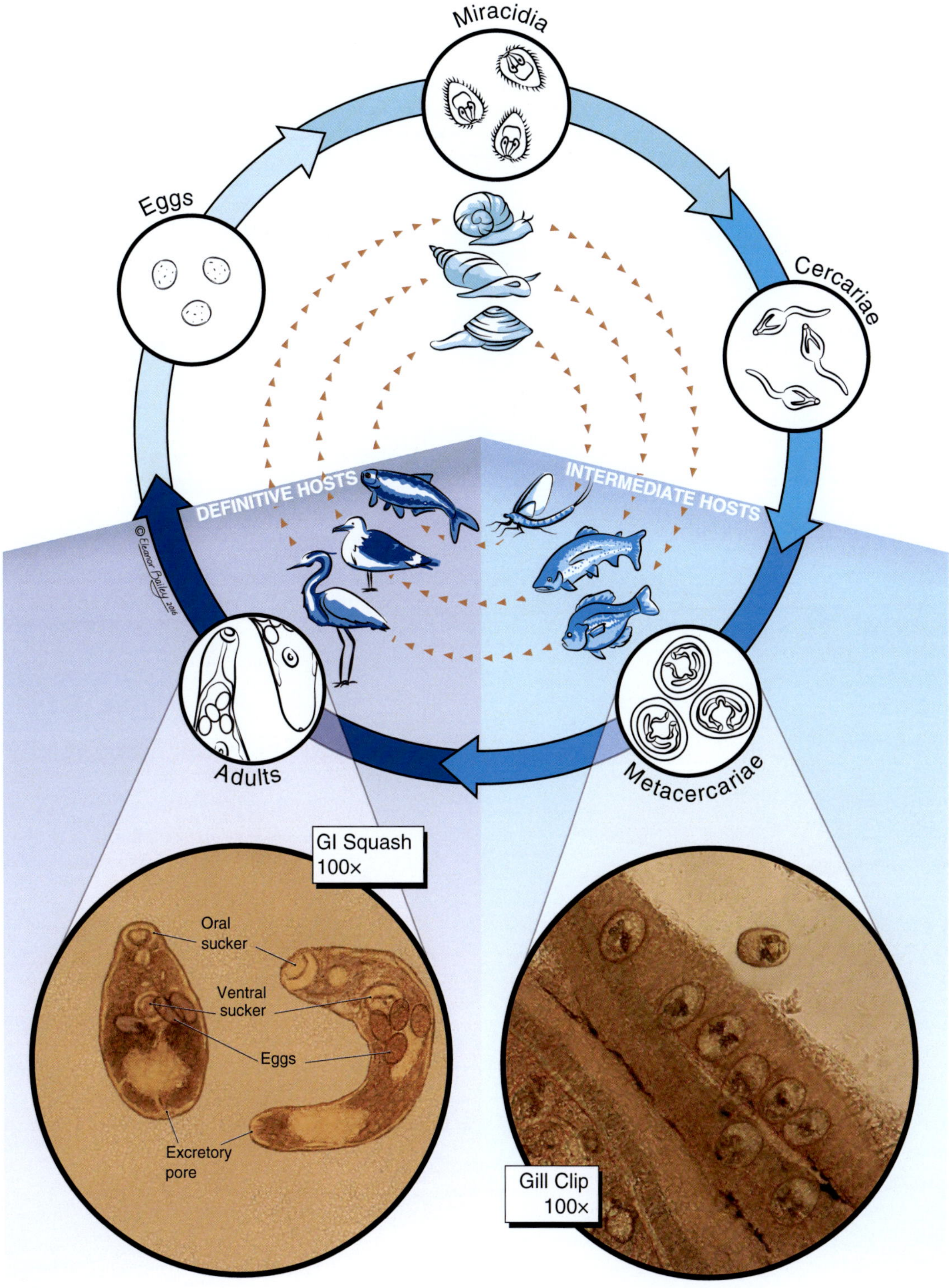

Figure C7.9 Diagram of the life cycle of digenes with fish as the definitive or second intermediate hosts. *Source*: Image courtesy of Eleanor Bailey, copyright reserved.

  - Permissive temperature; infection rates are highest in the summer.
  - Outdoor or wild-caught fish.
  - High organic loads.
  - Abundant habitat for snails (e.g. mud substrate, shallow systems with macrophytes, shallow banks).
- Common stressors are described under C7: *Monogeneans (General)*.

Signs/Clinical Findings

- Where fish are the IH:
  - Infected fish are usually asymptomatic.
  - If seen, signs depend on the location and burden of the metacercariae.
  - Inappetence, reduced feeding, poor growth, or weight loss may be seen.
  - Black, white, or yellow foci on the skin or gills are often seen, providing the common names of black spot disease, white grubs, or yellow grubs.
  - Corneal opacities or cataracts may be seen (e.g. *Diplostomum* spp.).
  - Abnormal behavior or swimming may be seen.
  - Increased predation may be seen.
  - Mortalities are rare but possible.
- Where fish are the DH:
  - Signs are more common.
  - Multiple conspecifics are usually affected.
  - Inappetence, reduced feeding, poor growth, or weight loss may be seen.
  - Abnormal buoyancy may be seen.
  - Dark coloration may be seen.
  - Mortalities are more likely.

Differential Diagnoses

- Full differentials are provided in Section B.
- Common differentials for thin-walled cysts in the tissues of bony fish include digenes, cestodes, nematodes, leeches, pentastomids, acanthocephalans, and mussel glochidia.

Diagnosis

- Adults may be found on gross exam, direct microscopy, or histology of the gastrointestinal tract, fecal material, coelom, swim bladder, liver, or bile ducts. Adults are multicellular, flat, and 0.2–5.0 mm in length. They have a distinct anterior and posterior pole, no segmentation, one to two obvious suckers (anterior/oral and ventral), and no hooks. They move with a jerking motion.
- Encysted metacercariae may be found in any tissues. They may produce grossly visible white, yellow, or black nodules or cysts. On direct microscopy or histology, they are oval, thin-walled, and often bilaterally symmetric. Further identification is difficult from encysted metacercaria, but host species and tissue location can provide a tentative genus or species.
- Eggs are typically 15–20 μm in length, opercular, and thin-walled. They may have bipolar filaments.
- Several digene species may be present concomitantly.
- Inflammation may be present on cytology or histology and may be granulomatous.
- If further morphological or molecular identification is required, adults (or gastrointestinal contents) can be relaxed in near-boiling water or saline followed by fixation in 95% ethanol, or rinsed in water or saline followed by fixation in hot 70% ethanol or hot AFA (ethanol–formalin–acetic acid).

Husbandry Management

- Husbandry management relies on disrupting the life cycle and reducing or resolving stressors.
- Reduce contact with snails and birds. This is particularly important where affected fish are the IH, e.g.:
  - Cover outdoor systems with nets.
  - Reduce vegetation at the edges of outdoor systems.
  - Reduce the depth or extent of mud substrate.
  - Use dogs to deter birds. Note that some bird species are protected by national, state, or local agencies.
  - Consider molluscicide treatment (e.g. niclosamide, hydrated lime, copper sulfate). These are usually applied to pond edges at night, when there is no wind or rainfall. They typically need to be repeated several times through the growing season.
  - Consider biological control of snails (e.g. with black carp (*Mylopharyngodon piceus*) or redear sunfish (*Lepomis microlophus*) in freshwater, or gilthead seabream (*Sparus aurata*) in salt water). Regulations may apply to the use of these species.

Medical Management

- Treatments work best on adult parasites in the DH. They may reduce metacercarial load in the IH, but they do not resolve signs such as cataracts.
- Common treatments (see Chapters A12 and A13 for more details):
  - Praziquantel immersion, typically reported at 1–10 mg/L for one to nine hours, repeated several times.
  - Praziquantel orally at 35–330 mg/kg. The higher doses are likely more effective but are less palatable.
  - Praziquantel by intramuscular injection (e.g. at 25 mg/kg IM).
- Trichlorfon immersion has not been effective.

- Cataracts can be managed surgically. If possible, retinal function should be checked prior to surgery using electroretinograms (described in Bakal et al. 2005). Surgical options include phacoemulsification and aspiration or lens removal (phakectomy). Further information is available in Chapter A11.
- All legislation regarding medication use and disposal must be followed.

Prevention

- Reduce or resolve stressors.
  - Common stressors are described under C7: *Monogeneans (General)*.
- Reduce exposure and transmission.
  - Limit access to snails. This is the most effective control measure.
  - Monitor snail loads.
  - Eliminate or limit access by birds.
  - Removal of dead or moribund fish as soon as possible with appropriate disposition.
  - High water flow rate or turnover and turbulence.
  - Frozen-thawed or commercial feeds, with no live feeds.

Zoonotic Reports

- There are no reports of zoonotic transmission from fish by contact or inhalation.
- There are reports of infection in humans following ingestion of raw or inadequately cooked or processed fish. They can lead to gastroenteritis (e.g. *Echinostoma*, *Nanophyetus* spp.) or hepatitis (e.g. *Clonorchis*, *Metorchis*, *Opisthorchis* spp.).

Bibliography

Bakal, R.S., Hickson, B.H., Gilger, B.C. et al. (2005). Surgical removal of cataracts due to *Diplostomum* species in Gulf sturgeon (*Acipenser oxyrinchus desotoi*). *Journal of Zoo and Wildlife Medicine* 36: 504–508.

Chai, J.-Y., Murrell, K.D., and Lymbery, A.J. (2005). Fish-borne parasitic zoonoses: Status and issues. *International Journal of Parasitology* 35: 1233–1254.

Justine, J., Briand, M.J., and Bray, R.A. (2012). A quick and simple method, usable in the field, for collecting parasites in suitable condition for both morphological and molecular studies. *Parasitology Research* 111: 341–351.

Køie, M. (1995). The life-cycle and biology of *Hemiurus communis* Odhner, 1905 (Digenea, Hemiuridae). *Parasite* 2: 195–202.

McKeown, C.A. and Irwin, S.W.B. (1995). The life cycle stages of three *Diplostomum* species maintained in the laboratory. *International journal for Parasitology* 25: 897–906.

Ondračková, M., Šimková, A., Gelnar, M., and Jurajda, P. (2004). *Posthodiplostomum cuticola* (Digenea: Diplostomatidae) in intermediate fish hosts: factors contributing to the parasite infection and prey selection by the definitive bird host. *Parasitology* 129: 761–770.

Tkach, V.V., Curran, S.S., Bell, J.A., and Overstreet, R.M. (2013). A new species of *Crepidostomum* (Digenea: Allocreadiidae) from *Hiodon tergisus* in Mississippi and molecular comparison with three congeners. *Journal of Parasitology* 99: 1114–1121.

Abbreviations/Acronyms

- DH: Definitive host
- IH: Intermediate host
- SEM: Scanning electron microscopy

Digenes (Blood Flukes)

Overview

- Blood flukes are unsegmented flatworms within the *Digenea* that lack suckers and are found within the vasculature.
- Unlike typical digenes, there is only one intermediate host (IH) and no encysted metacercarial stage. Fish are the definitive host (DH).
- Some are serious pathogens in aquaculture, particularly in sea pens, e.g. *Cardicola* spp. in bluefin tuna (*Thunnus maccoyii* and *Thunnus orientalis*).
- They are currently classified as aporocotylids but are sometimes referred to as sanguinicolids based on a previous family name.

Etiology

- Phylum *Platyhelminthes*.
- Class *Trematoda*.
- Subclass *Digenea*.
- Superfamily *Schistosomatoidea*.
- Family *Aporocotylidae*.

- Many genera and species are known to infect fish. *Cardicola forsteri* and *Sanguinicola inermis* are two of the more commonly reported species.

Life Cycle and Transmission

- The life cycle is indirect, similar to other digenes.
- Blood flukes only have one IH, usually a mollusk or polychaete.
- Adults are dioecious (with separate sexes), unlike other digenes and unlike mammalian blood flukes.
- Adults are found within the major blood vessels or heart. Mature adults copulate and eggs are released into the vascular system. Most eggs reach the gill capillaries, where the accumulation causes the blood vessels to rupture, releasing the eggs. Miracidia hatch from the eggs then swim to and penetrate the IH. In the IH, some of the miracidia develop asexually into sporocysts with cercariae that become free-swimming. These leave the IH in the evening and burrow into the fish DH, where they migrate to the vascular system.
- The prepatent period is usually one to three months.

Geographic Distribution

- Freshwater and saltwater habitats, probably worldwide.
- Distribution of each parasite species depends on the range or culture location of the host species.

Signalment

- Freshwater, brackish, and marine fish are susceptible, including elasmobranchs.
- The host range of each parasite species is often narrow, e.g.:
  - *C. forsteri* in southern bluefin tuna.
  - *Cardicola orientalis* and *Cardicola opisthorchis* in Pacific Bluefin tuna.
  - *S. inermis* in freshwater cyprinids, particularly common carp and koi (*Cyprinus carpio*).
- Young fish are more susceptible to disease.

Risk Factors

- Exposure and stressors are the most important risk factors.
- Exposure includes:
  - Poor biosecurity (e.g. lack of suitable quarantine, use of surface water).
  - Outdoor or wild-caught fish.
  - Abundant habitat for other hosts.
- Common stressors are described under C7: *Monogeneans (General).*

Signs/Clinical Findings

- Infected fish may be asymptomatic.
- Multiple conspecifics may be affected.
- Inappetence, reduced feeding, poor growth, or weight loss may be seen.
- Dyspnea or tachypnea is common.
- Gill pallor, edema, or increased mucus is common; gill pallor may be severe.
- Dark skin coloration may be seen.
- Mortalities are possible and may start weeks to months post-infection. Mortalities may occur after increased activity (e.g. feeding or handling).

Differential Diagnoses

- Full differentials are provided in Section B.
- Common differentials for anemia in fish include blood flukes, polyopisthocotyles, leeches, hemorrhagic and hemolytic viruses, trauma, nutritional deficiencies, and toxins.

Diagnosis

- Diagnosis is typically based on finding eggs in the vasculature, particularly on direct microscopy or histology of gill biopsies (Figure C7.10). Eggs may also be found in other viscera, often within granulomas.
- Eggs are thin-walled, oval, triangular, or crescent-shaped, and 25–50 μm in size.
- Histology may also show significant branchitis with necrosis, thrombi, and epithelial hyperplasia. Inflammation may be granulocytic or granulomatous.
- Adults are less commonly identified but are usually in large blood vessels or heart chambers. They can reach 20 cm in length but are often translucent and easy to miss at necropsy. They may be associated with endocardial thickening and thrombi. Unlike other digenes, the adults do not have the typical oral or ventral suckers, although the pre-esophageal muscular organ can look like a sucker.

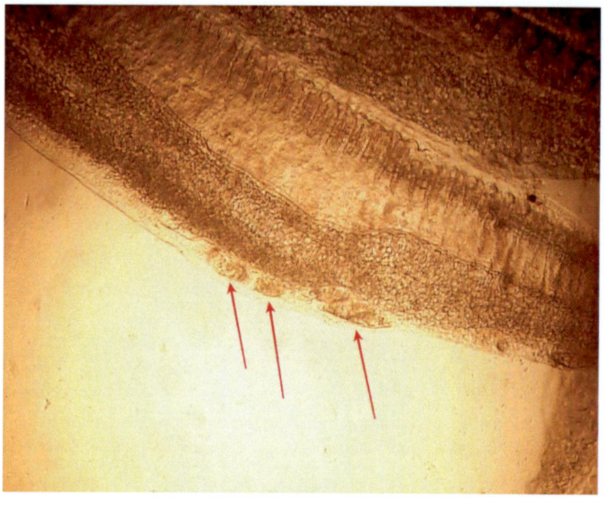

Figure C7.10 Eggs from blood flukes on direct microscopy of a gill biopsy at x100.

- If further morphological or molecular identification is required, adults can be relaxed in near-boiling water or saline followed by fixation in 95% ethanol, or rinsed in water or saline followed by fixation in hot 70% ethanol or hot AFA (ethanol–formalin–acetic acid).

Husbandry Management

- Reduce or resolve stressors.
- Increase aeration; target dissolved oxygen may be 95–100%.
- Reduce exposure to the intermediate hosts (e.g. mollusks, polychaetes).

Medical Management

- Reported treatments (see Chapters A12 and A13 for more details):
  - Praziquantel orally at 7.5–15 mg/kg of body weight every 24 hours for three days eradicated adult worms and reduced mortalities in Pacific bluefin tuna with *Cardicola* spp., although recurrence was reported in one study three to five weeks after treatment.
- All legislation regarding medication use and disposal must be followed.

Prevention

- Reduce or resolve stressors.
  - Common stressors are described under C7: *Monogeneans (General)*.
- Reduce exposure and transmission.
  - Limit access to intermediate hosts.
  - Suitable quarantine with isolation, monitoring, and diagnostic testing, particularly gill biopsies.

Zoonotic Reports

- These parasites have no known zoonotic potential.

Bibliography

Dennis, M.M., Landos, M., and D'Antignana, T. (2011). Case-control study of epidemic mortality and *Cardicola forsteri*-associated disease in farmed southern bluefin tuna (*Thunnus maccoyii*) of South Australia. *Veterinary Pathology* 46: 846–855.

Ishimaru, K., Ryoma, M., Shirakashi, S. et al. (2013). Praziquantel treatment against *Cardicola* blood flukes; determination of the minimal effective dose and pharmacokinetics in juvenile Pacific bluefin tuna. *Aquaculture* 402–403: 24–27.

Justine, J., Briand, M.J., and Bray, R.A. (2012). A quick and simple method, usable in the field, for collecting parasites in suitable condition for both morphological and molecular studies. *Parasitology Research* 111: 341–351.

Shirakashi, S., Andrews, M., Kishimoto, Y. et al. (2012). Oral treatment of praziquantel as an effective control measure against blood fluke infection in Pacific Bluefin tuna (*Thunnus orientalis*). *Aquaculture* 326–329: 15–19.

Warren, M.B., Orélis-Ribeiro, R., Ruiz, C.F. et al. (2017). Endocarditis associated with blood fluke infections (Digenea: Aporocotylidae: *Psettarium* cf. *anthicum*) among aquacultured cobia (*Rachycentron canadum*) from Nha Trang Bay, Vietnam. *Aquaculture* 468: 549–555.

Abbreviations/Acronyms

- DH: Definitive host
- IH: Intermediate host

Turbellaria

Overview

- Turbellaria are metazoan flatworms that are lined with cilia.
- Most turbellaria are free-living, but some can be pathogenic to tropical marine fish.
- The disease is sometimes known as black ich or black spot disease.

Etiology

- Phylum *Platyhelminthes*.
- Subphylum *Rhabditophora*.
- The class *Turbellaria* is now considered obsolete and this paraphyletic group is found within *Rhabditophora*, which includes cestodes, monogenes, and digenes.
- The common name remains turbellaria.
- Several are reported as fish parasites:
  - *Paravortex* spp.
  - *Piscinquilinus* (*Ichthyophaga*) *subcutaneous*.
  - *Micropharynx* spp.

Life Cycle and Transmission

- *Paravortex* spp. are viviparous with a direct life cycle that can be completed in around 10 days.
- The life cycles of the other genera may differ.

Geographic Distribution

- Saltwater habitats, particularly tropical and temperate.

Signalment

- Turbellarians are commonly reported from tropical marine teleosts, although there are reports from elasmobranchs.
  - *Paravortex* spp. on marine teleosts including butterflyfish (*Chaetodontidae*); surgeonfish (*Acanthuridae*), particularly yellow tangs (*Zebrasoma flavescens*); and carangids (*Carangidae*), particularly lookdowns (*Selene vomer*) and Florida pompano (*Trachinotus carolinus*).
  - *P. subcutaneous* on temperate and tropical marine teleosts including surgeonfish, lookdowns, parrotfish (*Scarinae*), and kelp greenlings (*Hexagrammos decagrammus*).
  - *Micropharynx* spp. on skates and rays (*Batoidea*).

Risk Factors

- Exposure and stressors are the most important risk factors.
- Exposure includes:
  - Poor biosecurity (e.g. lack of suitable quarantine, use of surface water).
  - Permissive salinity.
- Common stressors are described under C7: *Monogeneans (General)*.

Signs/Clinical Findings

- Infected fish may be asymptomatic.
- Multiple fish from one or more species may be affected.
- Typical clinical signs are black or white foci or linear masses on the skin.
- Lethargy may be seen.
- Inappetence or reduced feeding may be seen.
- Acute mortalities are possible.

Differential Diagnoses

- Full differentials are provided in Section B.
- Common differentials for black foci on the skin of marine fish include digenes, turbellarians, and *Huffmanela* spp.

Diagnosis

- Turbellaria are typically diagnosed on direct microscopy of skin scrapes or gill biopsies.
- Ciliated flatworms may be free or within a thin-walled cyst; gentle pressure can be used to rupture the cyst and show the flatworms (Figure C7.11). They are typically <0.5 mm in length, but can be up to 3 mm. Cilia are just visible at the margins and there are two obvious anterior eye spots. The pharynx is anterior in *Paravortex* spp. and posterior in *Piscinquilinus* spp. Turbellaria move with a smooth gliding motion, unlike the jerking motion of monogeneans.
- The parasites are often visible on histology usually with little or no associated inflammation.

Husbandry Management

- Reduce or resolve stressors.
- Increase aeration; target dissolved oxygen may be 95–100%.
- Increase water flow rate and turnover.
- Increase mechanical cleaning.

Medical Management

- There are few reports of treatment (see Chapters A12 and A13 for more details):

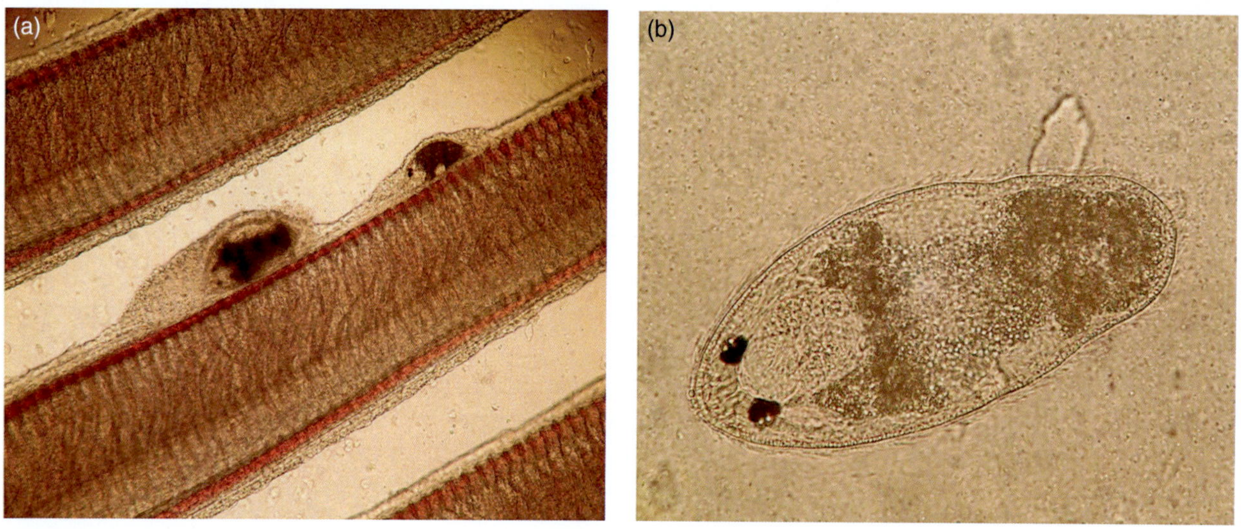

Figure C7.11 Turbellarians on direct microscopy of a gill biopsy (a) and following rupture of a cyst to show the ciliated flatworm at x400 (b).

  - Formalin immersion at >50 mg/L.
  - Praziquantel immersion at 10–20 mg/L.
  - Praziquantel by intramuscular injection at ~20–40 mg/kg repeated in ~30 days.
- Freshwater dips were not effective in bluespine unicornfish (*Naso unicornis*) but there are anecdotal reports of success.
- Copper sulfate immersion has typically not been effective.
- All legislation regarding medication use and disposal must be followed.

Prevention
- Reduce or resolve stressors.
  - Common stressors are described under C7: *Monogeneans (General)*.
- Reduce exposure and transmission.
  - Isolation with no contact with free-ranging animals, particularly fish.
  - Pathogen-free water source (e.g. municipal water or ground water that has gone through fine filtration (<40 μm) then UV and/or ozone disinfection). Avoid using untreated surface water.
  - Disinfection of recirculating water with fine filtration (<40 μm), then UV and/or ozone.
  - High water flow rate or turnover.
  - Removal of dead or moribund fish as soon as possible with appropriate disposition.
  - Suitable quarantine with isolation, monitoring, and diagnostic testing, particularly gill biopsies.
  - Frozen-thawed or commercial feeds, with no live feeds.

Zoonotic Reports
- These parasites have no known zoonotic potential.

Bibliography

Cannon, L.R.G. and Lester, R.J.G. (1988). Two turbellarians parasitic in fish. *Diseases of Aquatic Organisms* 5: 15–22.

Justine, J.-L., Leblanc, P., Keller, F., and Lester, R.J.G. (2009). Turbellarian black spot disease in bluespine unicornfish *Naso unicornis* in New Calendonia, caused by the parasitic turbellarian *Piscinguilinus* sp. *Diseases of Aquatic Organisms* 85: 245–249.

Noga, E.J., Smith, J., and Smith, S.A. (1999). Turbellarian infection of carangids. *Journal of Fish Diseases* 22: 489–491.

Cestodes

Overview
- Cestodes, also known as tapeworms, are segmented endoparasitic flatworms.
- They are obligate parasites but rarely cause significant morbidity and mortality in fish.
- Fish can be the intermediate or definitive host (IH or DH). As IH, fish can have encysted plerocercoids in any tissues. As the DH, fish have adult parasites within the gastrointestinal tract.
- *Schyzocotyle acheilognathi*, also known as the Asian tapeworm, has an unusually wide host range and is a threat to aquaculture and reintroduction programs.

Etiology
- Phylum *Platyhelminthes*.
- Class *Cestoda*.
- Most cestodes that infect fish are within the subclass *Eucestoda*. Commonly reported genera include:
  - *Schyzocotyle (Bothriocephalus)*.
  - *Diphyllobothrium*.
  - *Eubothrium*.
  - *Khawia*.
  - *Proteocephalus*.
  - *Schyzocotyle*.

Life Cycle and Transmission
- The life cycle is indirect with one or two IHs.
- IHs can be invertebrates (e.g. copepods, amphipods, isopods, mollusks) or fish. DHs can be fish or other vertebrates, e.g. *Triaenophorus nodulus* has a copepod as first IH, fish like the redfin perch (*Perca fluviatilis*) as the second IH, and northern pike (*Esox lucius*) as the DH.
- Adults are found within the GI tract of the DH. Gravid proglottids or eggs are passed in feces. Motile coracidiae emerge after embryonation. Eggs or coracidiae are eaten by the IH. Plerocercoids develop and encyst in the tissues of the IH. When the IH is ingested by the DH, the parasites mature into adults.

Geographic Distribution
- Ubiquitous in freshwater and saltwater habitats worldwide.

- There are reports of low pathogenicity in endemic regions with increased pathogenicity following introduction to naïve populations (e.g. *S. acheilognathi* after introduction to Europe, Americas, South Africa, and Australia).

Signalment

- All fish are likely susceptible.
- The host range of each parasite species is often narrow, e.g.:
  - *Khawia sinensis* in common carp (*Cyprinus carpio*).
  - *Prochristianella tenuispine* in nurse sharks (*Ginglymostoma cirratum*).
  - *Proteocephalus ambloplitis* in largemouth bass (*Micropterus salmoides*).
- A few cestodes have wider host ranges, e.g.:
  - *Diphyllobothrium dendriticus* in salmonids (*Salmonidae*).
  - *S. acheilognathi* in cyprinids (*Cyprinidae*) and mosquitofish (*Gambusia affinis*).

Risk Factors

- Exposure and stressors are the most important risk factors.
- Exposure includes:
  - Poor biosecurity (e.g. lack of suitable quarantine, use of surface water, exposure to wild invertebrates).
  - Outdoor or wild-caught fish.
  - Abundant habitat for intermediate hosts.
- Common stressors are described under C7: *Monogeneans (General)*.

Signs/Clinical Findings

- Infected fish are usually asymptomatic.
- Inappetence, reduced feeding, or weight loss may be seen.
- Abnormal fecal output or intestinal obstruction may be seen.
- Gill pallor due to anemia may be seen.
- Coelomic distension may be seen.
- Sporadic, chronic mortalities are possible.

Differential Diagnoses

- Full differentials are provided in Section B.
- Common differentials for flatworms in fish that look segmented include cestodes and leeches.
- Common differentials for thin-walled cysts in the tissues of fish include digenes, cestodes, nematodes, leeches, pentastomids, acanthocephalans, and mussel glochidia.

Diagnosis

- Adult cestodes are usually found in the intestinal tract on gross examination. Adults, segments (proglottids), or eggs may be seen. Encysted larvae can be found in any tissues on direct microscopy or histology.
- Adults are usually several centimeters in length but can be longer. They are multicellular, flat, truly segmented, with no GI tract, and a distinctive head (scolex) with hooks or suckers (Figure C7.12). They may be associated with erythema and erosions. Inflammation may be granulocytic or granulomatous.
- Larvae can be found in the gills, muscle, coelom, or viscera. They are usually encysted and may form small nodules. On direct microscopy, movement within the cyst and the characteristic scolex may be seen.
- Eggs are round to oval, often thick-walled, and hooks may be visible on microscopy.
- If further morphological or molecular identification is required, cestodes can be relaxed in near-boiling water or saline followed by fixation in 95% ethanol, or relaxed with cold water or saline for two to five minutes then fixed in hot 70% ethanol or hot AFA (ethanol, formalin, acetic acid). Agitation of these solutions can break up adult cestodes; larval cestodes hold together better.

Husbandry Management

- Management changes are usually not indicated if parasite load is low, only encysted parasites are seen, and there is no morbidity or mortality.
- Reduce or resolve stressors.
- Try to identify and disrupt the life cycle.

Medical Management

- Medical treatment of fish cestodes is rarely reported. It is likely to be most effective against adult cestodes in the DH.
- Possible treatments (see Chapters A12 and A13 for more details):
  - Praziquantel by intramuscular injection.

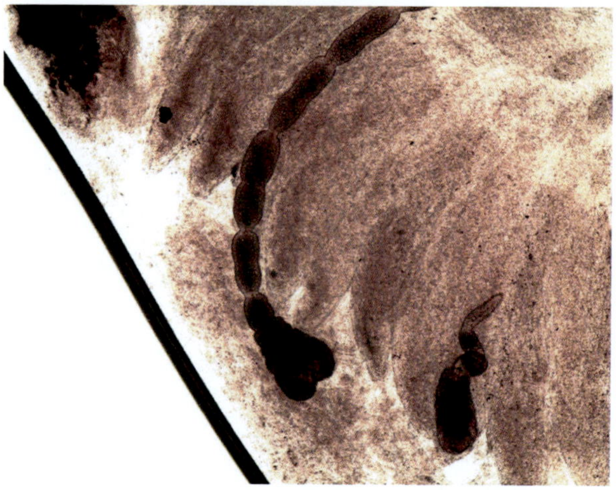

Figure C7.12 Cestodes on direct microscopy of a squash prep of a hake fry (*Merluccius* sp.); x40. *Source*: Image courtesy of New England Aquarium.

- Praziquantel orally.
- Albendazole orally.
- All legislation regarding medication use and disposal must be followed.

Prevention

- Reduce or resolve stressors.
  - Common stressors are described under C7: *Monogeneans (General).*
- Reduce exposure and transmission.
  - Isolation with no contact with free-ranging animals.
  - Limit access to invertebrate IHs.
  - High water flow rate or turnover.
  - Removal of dead or moribund fish as soon as possible with appropriate disposition.
  - Suitable quarantine with isolation, monitoring, and diagnostic testing.
  - Frozen-thawed or commercial feeds, with no live feeds.

Zoonotic Reports

- There are no reports of zoonotic transmission from fish by contact or inhalation.
- There are reports of infection in humans following ingestion of raw or inadequately cooked or processed fish (e.g. *Diphyllobothrium* spp.). Mild gastroenteritis may be seen.

Bibliography

Chai, J.-Y., Murrell, K.D., and Lymbery, A.J. (2005). Fish-borne parasitic zoonoses: status and issues. *International Journal of Parasitology* 35: 1233–1254.

Dexfuli, B.S., Manera, M., and Giari, L. (2015). Ultrastructural assessment of granulomas in the liver of perch (*Perca fluviatilis*) infected by tapeworm. *Journal of Comparative Pathology* 152: 97–102.

Justine, J., Briand, M.J., and Bray, R.A. (2012). A quick and simple method, usable in the field, for collecting parasites in suitable condition for both morphological and molecular studies. *Parasitology Research* 111: 341–351.

Abbreviations/Acronyms

- DH: Definitive host
- IH: Intermediate host
- GI: Gastrointestinal

Leeches

Overview

- Leeches are hematophagous metazoan parasites.
- They are often visible on the skin, fins, and eyes, but some are found in more cryptic sites.
- They typically have wide host ranges.
- High loads can cause severe anemia and secondary infections.
- Leeches are common vectors for a variety of diseases.

Etiology

- Phylum *Annelida*.
- Class *Clitellata*.
- Subclass *Hirudinea*.
- Most leeches that infect fish are within the family *Piscicolidae*, although some are within *Glossiphoniidae*. Commonly reported genera include:
  - *Branchellion.*
  - *Hemibdella.*
  - *Myxobdella.*
  - *Piscicola.*
  - *Pontobdella.*

Life Cycle and Transmission

- The life cycle is direct.
- Some stay on the host for the life of the parasite (e.g. *Branchellion torpedinis*). Eggs within cocoons are shed from the host into the environment and hatch in weeks. They climb up substrate, reach up, and attach to any fish within range. These may be responsible for greater morbidity and mortality than temporary parasites.
- In other species, gravid adults leave the host after a blood meal and deposit eggs within cocoons in the substrate and vegetation (e.g. *Piscicola salmositica*).
- Fecundity is normally low, but some are more prolific breeders (e.g. *B. torpedinis*).

Geographic Distribution

- Freshwater and saltwater habitats, probably worldwide.

Signalment

- Most fish are probably susceptible.
- Examples of leeches in bony fish include:
  - *Myzobdella lugubris* in clupeids (*Clupeidae*), drums (*Sciaenidae*), and catfish (*Ictaluridae*).

- *Piscicola salmositica* in freshwater Pacific salmonids (*Oncorhynchus* spp.).
- Examples of leeches that have been problematic in elasmobranchs include:
  - *B. torpedinis* in the oropharyngeal cavity of demersal elasmobranchs including whitespotted eagle rays (*Aetobatus narinari*), cownose rays (*Rhinoptera bonasus*), yellow stingrays (*Urobatis jamaicensis*), porcupine rays (*Urogymnus asperrimus*), and zebra sharks (*Stegostoma tigrinum*).
  - *Branchellion lobata* in the spiral valve and reproductive tract of Pacific angelsharks (*Squatina californica*).

Risk Factors

- Exposure and stressors are the most important risk factors.
- Exposure includes:
  - Poor biosecurity (e.g. lack of suitable quarantine, use of surface water, exposure to wild fish or live feeder fish).
  - Outdoor or wild-caught fish.
- Common stressors are described under C7: *Monogeneans (General)*.

Signs/Clinical Findings

- Infected fish may be asymptomatic.
- Multiple fish from one or more species may be affected.
- Leeches may be visible externally on the skin, fins, mouth, and eyes.
- Lethargy may be seen and can be severe.
- Inappetence, reduced appetite, or poor growth may be seen.
- Gill pallor due to anemia may be seen and can be severe.
- Pruritus (e.g. flashing, erratic swimming) may be seen.
- Skin ulcers can be seen; these may not be associated with leeches as the parasites may have moved.
- Secondary disease may be seen due to tissue damage or disease transmission.
  - Leeches are known vectors of infectious hematopoietic necrosis virus, viral hemorrhagic septicemia, infectious pancreatic necrosis virus, *Cryptobia* (*Trypanoplasma*) spp., *Trypanosoma* spp., hemogregarines, and piroplasmas.
  - Leeches are probably mechanical vectors of a wide variety of viruses, bacteria, and fungi.
- Mortalities may be seen.
- Survivors can show some immunity against reinfection.

Differential Diagnoses

- Full differentials are provided in Section B.
- Common differentials for linear tags on fish include copepods, leeches, monogeneans, egg strands, and mucus strands.
- Common differentials for flatworms in fish that look segmented include cestodes and leeches.

Diagnosis

- Leeches can be grossly visible on external surfaces, but they can also be found in the gills, oropharynx, nares, anus, or cloaca (Figure C7.13a). Some of the more cryptic sites may require endoscopy. Leeches can be removed with forceps and examined under direct microscopy.
- Adults are multicellular, long and thin, flat or round, typically up to 5 cm in length. They look segmented with setae present on the cephalic segments (Figure C7.13b). They have anterior and posterior suckers and move with a looping or wave-like motion. Eye spots may be present. Red may be readily visible within the ceca due to a recent blood meal (Figure C7.13c). The narrow proboscis may be visible at the oral sucker.
- Encysted stages are thin-walled, oval, and large. They are hard to differentiate from other encysted parasites.
- Cocoons may be grossly visible and are often round to oval, dark, and may look gelatinous or foamy.
- Hematology may show anemia and hypoproteinemia.
- Fixing leeches for further identification is an involved process. They can be fixed in 95% ethanol, but it may be easier to transport them live to a taxonomist for proper handling.

Husbandry Management

- Reduce or resolve stressors.
- Increase aeration; target dissolved oxygen may be 95–100%.
- Increase mechanical cleaning.
- Increase water flow rate and turnover.
- Consider mechanical removal from affected fish, but this is labor-intensive.
- Consider salinity or temperature trials to identify conditions that may affect the life cycle or survival of the parasites.

Medical Management

- Treatment should always be combined with husbandry changes as part of an integrated management strategy.
- Cocoons are resistant to treatment and egg viability and hatching cues are largely unknown. Therefore, long-term treatment to kill emerging larvae, either as a pulse therapy or maintained at therapy, is required to try to resolve the infection. A more effective treatment plan might be to dose and move to a clean system, but recurrence remains common.
- Common treatments (see Chapters A12 and A13 for more details):
  - Trichlorfon immersion at 0.25–0.50 mg/L (active ingredient) for 1–24 hours repeated in 10–14 days can be effective. Adverse reactions to trichlorfon are common. Bioassays, close monitoring, and pretreatment

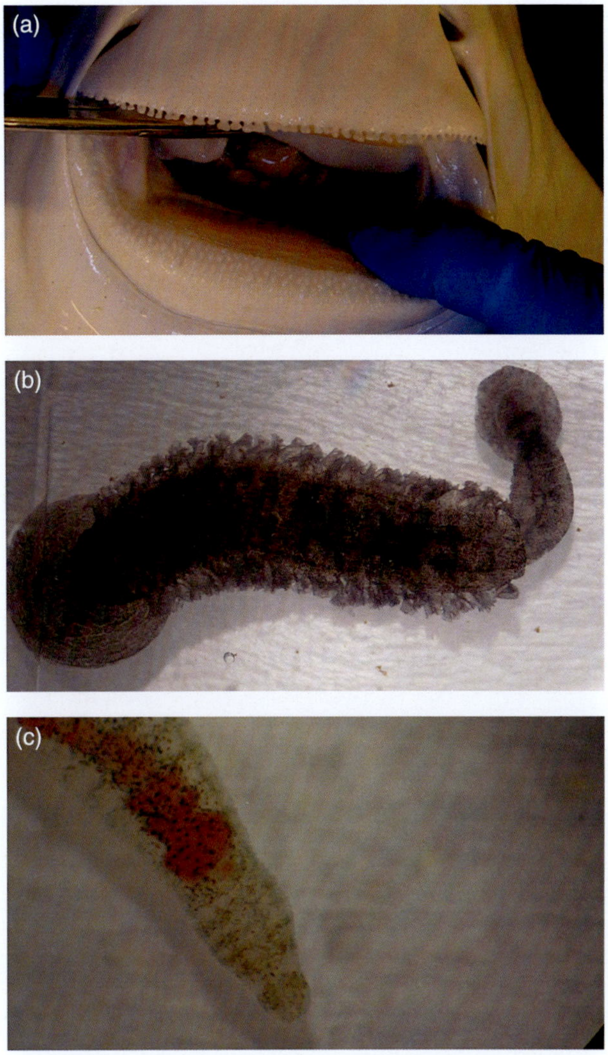

Figure C7.13 Leeches visible in the oral cavity of a cownose ray (*Rhinoptera bonasus*) (a). Leeches on direct microscopy showing the apparent segmentation (b) and blood ingestion (c). *Source:* Image (a) courtesy of Tonya Clauss, Georgia Aquarium.

with atropine should be considered. Suitable PPE must be used. Drug disposal must be considered.

  - Individual animals may need intravenous fluids, whole blood transfusion from a healthy conspecific (ideally after cross-matching), erythropoietin therapy, iron dextran supplementation, and other supportive care.
  - Treatment of secondary infections may be indicated.
- Other reported treatments (see Chapters A12 and A13 for more details):
  - Copper sulfate immersion at high doses.
  - Formalin immersion at high doses.
  - Diflubenzuron immersion may be effective against leeches with chitinous jaws, but marine leeches tend to lack jaws and rely on a muscular proboscis.
- All legislation regarding medication use and disposal must be followed.

Prevention

- Reduce or resolve stressors.
  - Common stressors are described under C7: *Monogeneans (General).*
- Reduce exposure and transmission.
  - Isolation with no contact with free-ranging animals, particularly fish.
  - Good mechanical cleaning.
  - High water flow rate or turnover.
  - Suitable quarantine with isolation, monitoring, and diagnostic testing. Good visual examinations can reduce the risk of introducing leeches that are visible externally. For species that commonly harbor leeches in cryptic locations (e.g. *Myliobatiformes*), endoscopic examination of the oral and branchial cavity of each individual may be indicated.
  - Frozen-thawed or commercial feeds, with no live feeds.

Zoonotic Reports

- These parasites have no known zoonotic potential.

Bibliography

Dove, A.D.M., Clauss, T.M., Marancik, D.P., and Camus, A.C. (2017). Emerging diseases of elasmobranchs in aquaria. In: The Elasmobranch Husbandry Manual II: Recent Advances in the Care of Sharks, Rays, and their Relatives (eds. M. Smith, D. Warmolts, D. Thoney, et al.), 263–275. Ohio Biological Survey.

Kua, B.C., Choong, F.C., and Leaw, Y.Y. (2014). Effect of salinity and temperature on marine leech. *Zeylanicobdella arugamensis* (De Silva) under laboratory conditions. *Journal of Fish Diseases* 37: 201–207.

Marancik, D.P., Dove, A.D., and Camus, A.C. (2012). Experimental infection of yellow stingrays *Urobatis jamaicensis* with the marine leech *Branchellion torpedinis*. *Diseases of Aquatic Organisms* 101: 51–60.

Salimi, B. and Abdi, K. (2016). Detection of infectious pancreatic necrosis virus from the leeches *Hemiclepsis marginata* and *Hirudo medicinalis*. *Journal of Aquatic Animal Health* 28: 209–213.

Abbreviations/Acronyms

- PPE: Personal protective equipment

Ascarid Nematodes

Overview

- Ascarid nematodes have indirect life cycles. Fish are usually the intermediate hosts (IH) or paratenic hosts, showing encysted larvae in the coelom, muscle, or viscera. Marine mammals and piscivorous birds are typically the definitive hosts (DH).
- The most commonly reported ascarid nematode in fish is *Anisakis simplex*.
- In aquariums, ascarid nematodes are usually incidental findings.
- In food fish aquaculture and fisheries, these present cosmetic, zoonotic, and hypersensitivity concerns to humans.

Etiology

- Phylum *Nematoda*.
- Order *Rhabditida*.
- Superfamily *Ascaridoidea*.
- Family *Anisakidae* and *Raphidascarididae*.
- Several genera are reported commonly from fish:
  - *Anisakis*.
  - *Contracaecum*.
  - *Hysterothylacium*.
  - *Pseudoterranova*.
  - *Terranova*.

Life Cycle and Transmission

- The life cycle is indirect.
- Fish are usually the IH (where larvae can continue to develop) or paratenic host (where no development occurs), but may be the DH.
- The life cycle typically involves four larval stages (L1 to L4) and one adult stage. Gravid females in the DH lay eggs that are passed in feces. Eggs hatch and larvae start to develop. IHs or paratenic hosts may ingest eggs, L1, L2, or L3 stages; the parasites migrate into various tissues and become encapsulated. Several IHs may be involved. The life cycle can be completed when IHs or paratenic hosts with L3 larvae are ingested by the DH.
- *A. simplex*
  - DHs are typically cetaceans or pinnipeds with parasites in the stomach.
  - First IHs are planktonic or pelagic crustaceans (e.g. copepods, krill).
  - Second IHs and paratenic hosts are marine teleosts or squid (*Decapodiformes*).
- *Contracaecum* spp.
  - DHs are typically piscivorous birds or pinnipeds.
  - IHs are typically fish or planktonic crustaceans.
- *Terranova* spp.
  - DHs include elasmobranchs.
  - IHs include bony fish.

Geographic Distribution

- *A. simplex* sensu stricto is found in saltwater habitats, mainly in the northern Atlantic and Pacific Oceans.
- Other ascarids are found in various saltwater habitats and, less commonly, freshwater habitats.

Signalment

- Most fish can likely be IHs or paratenic hosts for ascarids, particularly marine fish.
- *A. simplex* can infect a variety of marine teleosts, including Atlantic cod (*Gadus morhua*), hake (*Merluccius* spp.), Atlantic mackerel (*Scomber scombrus*), herring (*Clupea* spp.), capelin (*Mallotus villosus*), monkfish (*Lophius* spp.), European sardine (*Sardina pilchardus*), Atlantic salmon (*Salmo salar*), and Pacific salmon (*Oncorhynchus* spp.).
- Some species can be DHs for ascarids, e.g. sharks and rays with *Terranova* spp.

Risk Factors

- Exposure and stressors are the most important risk factors.
- Exposure includes:
  - Poor biosecurity (e.g. access to wild fish and invertebrates, use of surface water).
  - Outdoor or wild-caught fish.
  - Abundant habitat for intermediate or paratenic hosts.
- Common stressors are described under C7: *Monogeneans (General)*.

Signs/Clinical Findings

- Infected fish are usually asymptomatic.
- Reduced appetite or growth rates may be seen, although even high loads had no adverse effects on body condition in herring.
- Reduced fecundity may be seen.
- Coelomic distension may be seen with large ascarids (e.g. *Contracaecum* spp.).
- Hemorrhage and swelling at the vent have been associated with some *A. simplex* infections in wild Atlantic salmon (red vent syndrome).
- Mortalities are rare.

Differential Diagnoses

- Full differentials are provided in Section B.
- Common differentials for roundworms in fish include ascarids, camallanids, capillarids, eustrongylids, and

philometrids. Leeches, pentastomids, and acanthocephalans can resemble roundworms.

Diagnosis

- Ascarids are typically diagnosed at necropsy or during processing of fillets from food fish by finding encysted larvae in the tissues.
- Larvae are often on serosal surfaces within the coelom or in striated muscle, particularly the ventral body wall. Encysted larvae may also be found in the liver or swim bladder. Encysted larvae are coiled in a flat spiral within thin-walled cysts up to 5 mm in size. The larvae are usually translucent or white. When the cyst is ruptured, the larvae are up to 3 cm long and may be motile.
- Adults are less common but may be identified in the stomach or intestines. They are multicellular, long and thin, round in cross-section, unsegmented, with a full gastrointestinal tract and no setae, suckers, or hooks.
- On histology, the parasites may be associated with increased pigmented macrophage aggregates but little other inflammatory response unless they are actively migrating.
- If further morphological or molecular identification is required, nematodes can be relaxed in near-boiling water or saline followed by fixation in 95% ethanol (particularly for molecular studies), or washed in water or saline followed by fixation in hot 70% ethanol or hot AFA (ethanol, formalin, acetic acid). Definitive identification is difficult if adult stages are not available.

Husbandry Management

- Management changes are not usually indicated if parasite load is low, only encysted parasites are seen, and there is no morbidity or mortality.
- Reduce or resolve stressors.
- Disrupt the life cycle by reducing access to other hosts.

Medical Management

- Medical treatments can affect adults and migrating larvae but have little to no effect on encysted larvae or eggs.
- Morbidity and mortality have been reported secondary to deworming. This may be from direct toxicity of the medication or due to an inflammatory response to dead or dying parasites.
- Reported treatments (see Chapters A12 and A13 for more details):
  - Albendazole orally.
  - Emamectin orally.
  - Fenbendazole orally.
  - Ivermectin orally.
  - Mebendazole orally.
- All legislation regarding medication use and disposal must be followed.

Prevention

- Reduce or resolve stressors.
  - Common stressors are described under C7: *Monogeneans (General).*
- Reduce exposure and transmission.
  - Eliminate or limit access to other hosts.
  - High water flow rate or turnover.
  - Removal of dead or moribund fish as soon as possible with appropriate disposition.
  - Suitable quarantine with isolation, monitoring, and diagnostic testing.
  - Frozen-thawed or commercial feeds, with no live feeds.
- Since these can be a zoonotic concern following ingestion, monitoring of food fish during processing and cooking is an essential part of prevention.

Zoonotic Reports

- There are no reports of zoonotic transmission from fish by contact or inhalation.
- There are reports of infection in humans following ingestion of L3 larvae in raw or inadequately cooked or processed fish.
  - The most common foodborne pathogens in this group are *A. simplex* and *Pseudoterranova* (*Phocanema*) *decipiens.* Less common pathogens include *Contracaecum osculatum.*
  - Gastroenteritis may be seen and the parasites can invade the intestinal wall causing nodules.
  - Allergic reactions have also been reported.
  - Prevention of zoonotic spread is by adequate freezing (>seven days) and cooking of fish. Gutting of fish does not prevent transmission since the L3 larvae can be within the musculature (Figure C7.14). Larval loads may be higher on the ventrum and those tissues may be trimmed to reduce the risk.

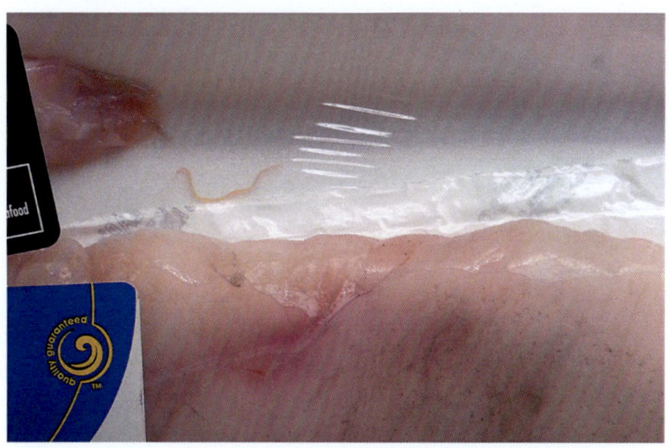

Figure C7.14 Live anisakid larva seen in a monkfish (*Lophius americanus*) fillet for sale in a supermarket. *Source*: Image courtesy of Bartolomeo Gorgoglione, Michigan State University.

Bibliography

Arias-Diaz, J., Zuloaga, J., Vara, E. et al. (2006). Efficacy of albendazole against *Anisakis simplex* larvae in vitro. *Digestive and Liver Disease* 38: 24–26.

Audicana, M.T. and Kennedy, M.W. (2008). *Anisakis simplex* from obscure infectious worms to inducer of immune hypersensitivity. *Clinical Microbiological Reviews* 21: 360–379.

Chai, J.-Y., Murrell, K.D., and Lymbery, A.J. (2005). Fish-borne parasitic zoonoses: status and issues. *International Journal of Parasitology* 35: 1233–1254.

Justine, J., Briand, M.J., and Bray, R.A. (2012). A quick and simple method, usable in the field, for collecting parasites in suitable condition for both morphological and molecular studies. *Parasitology Research* 111: 341–351.

Karl, H., Baumann, F., Ostermeyer, U. et al. (2011). *Anisakis simplex* (s.s.) larvae in wild Alaska salmon: no indication of post-mortem migration from viscera into flesh. *Diseases of Aquatic Organisms* 94: 201–209.

Larrat, S., Bouchard, F., Séguin, G., and Lair, S. (2013). Relationship between red vent syndrome and anisakid larvae burden in wild Atlantic salmon (*Salmo salar*). *Journal of Wildlife Diseases* 49: 229–234.

Levsen, A. and Lunestad, B.T. (2010). *Anisakis simplex* third stage larvae in Norwegian spring spawning herring (*Clupea harengus* L.), with emphasis on larval distribution in the flesh. *Veterinary Parasitology* 171: 247–253.

Tanzola, R.D. and Sardella, N.H. (2006). *Terranova galeocerdonis* (Thwaite, 1927) (Nematoda: Anisakidae) from *Carcharias taurus* (*Chondrichthyes*: *Odontaspididae*) off Argentina, with comments on some related species. *Systematic Parasitology* 64: 27–36.

Abbreviations/Acronyms

- DH: definitive host
- IH: intermediate host

Camallanid Nematodes

Overview

- Camallanid nematodes have indirect life cycles with fish as the definitive hosts.
- Camallanids are one of several groups of "red worms" in fish, with the distinction that they are considered ovoviviparous.
- They are typically found in the gastrointestinal tract of fish.
- They are usually incidental findings.

Etiology

- Phylum *Nematoda*.
- Superfamily *Camallanoidea*.
- Family *Camallanidae*.
- The most commonly reported species in fish is *Camallanus cotti*.

Life Cycle and Transmission

- The life cycle is indirect.
- Fish are the definitive hosts.
- Invertebrates such as copepods are the intermediate hosts.
- *C. cotti* is ovoviviparous and other camallanid nematodes are considered the same. Eggs may be seen in the uteri, but the females produce live young.

Geographic Distribution

- Freshwater habitats, probably worldwide.

Signalment

- Most freshwater teleosts are likely susceptible, particularly:
  - Cichlids (*Cichlidae*).
  - Guppies, swordtails, mollies, platies (*Poeciliidae*).
  - Gouramis, bettas (*Anabantiformes*).
  - Redfin perch (*Perca fluviatilis*).

Risk Factors

- Exposure and stressors are the most important risk factors.
- Exposure includes:
  - Poor biosecurity (e.g. lack of suitable quarantine, use of surface water).
  - Outdoor or wild-caught fish.
  - Abundant habitat for intermediate hosts.
- Common stressors are described under C7: *Monogeneans (General)*.

Signs/Clinical Findings

- Infected fish are often asymptomatic.
- One or more fish may be affected.
- Inappetence, reduced appetite, or weight loss may be seen.
- Coelomic distension may be seen.
- Red worms may be seen passing through the anus, cloaca, or body wall.
- Mortalities are rare.

Differential Diagnoses

- Full differentials are provided in Section B.
- Common differentials for gastrointestinal roundworms in fish include ascarids, camallanids, capillarids, and philometrids. Acanthocephalans can resemble roundworms

Diagnosis

- Camallanids are typically diagnosed when adults are found within the gastrointestinal tract at necropsy.
- Adults are multicellular, up to 1 cm long, thin, round in cross-section, usually red, unsegmented, with a full gastrointestinal tract and no setae, suckers, or hooks (Figure C7.15). The head looks split due to lateral valves.
- Eggs and larvae may be seen within the adults (free eggs may be seen if parasites ruptured during sample preparation). The eggs have bipolar plugs.
- Necropsy may also show gastrointestinal ulceration or erythema and coelomic effusion.
- If further morphological or molecular identification is required, nematodes can be relaxed in near-boiling water or saline followed by fixation in 95% ethanol, or fixed in hot 70% ethanol or hot AFA (ethanol, formalin, acetic acid).

Husbandry Management

- Management changes are not indicated if parasite load is low and there is no morbidity or mortality.
- Reduce or resolve stressors.
- Disrupt the life cycle by reducing access to other hosts.

Medical Management

- Morbidity and mortality have been reported secondary to deworming. This may be from direct toxicity of the medication or due to an inflammatory response to dead or dying parasites.
- Common treatments (see Chapters A12 and A13 for more details):
  - Fenbendazole orally is the most commonly reported treatment in fish at 25–50 mg/kg or bioencapsulated in live brine shrimp (*Artemia*) (60 minutes at 2 g/L in freshwater, resulting in a fenbendazole concentration of ~4.5 mg/g of shrimp), repeated at variable intervals.

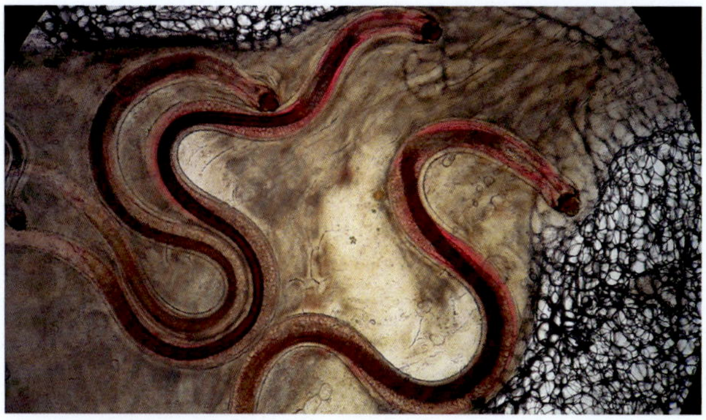

Figure C7.15 Camallanid nematodes on direct microscopy of a coelomic sample. Adipocytes are also visible. *Source*: Image courtesy of Rubén López, National Autonomous University of Mexico.

- Other reported treatments (see Chapters A12 and A13 for more details):
  - Emamectin orally.
  - Fenbendazole immersion.
  - Levamisole immersion.
  - Pyrantel orally.
- All legislation regarding medication use and disposal must be followed.

Prevention

- Reduce or resolve stressors.
  - Common stressors are described under C7: *Monogeneans (General)*.
- Reduce exposure and transmission.
  - Eliminate or limit access to other hosts.
  - High water flow rate or turnover.
  - Removal of dead or moribund fish as soon as possible with appropriate disposition.
  - Suitable quarantine with isolation, monitoring, and diagnostic testing.
  - Frozen-thawed or commercial feeds, with no live feeds.

Zoonotic Reports

- These parasites have no known zoonotic potential.

Bibliography

Allender, M.C., Kastura, M., George, R. et al. (2012). Bioencapsulation of fenbendazole in adult *Artemia*. *Journal of Exotic Pet Medicine* 21: 207–212.

Justine, J., Briand, M.J., and Bray, R.A. (2012). A quick and simple method, usable in the field, for collecting parasites in suitable condition for both morphological and molecular studies. *Parasitology Research* 111: 341–351.

Myers, G.E., Garner, M.M., Barrie, M.T. et al. (2007). Fenbendazole toxicity in sharks. *Proceedings of the American Association of Zoo Veterinarians Conference*, Knoxville, TN.

Reed, A.N., Clayton, L.A., and Hadfield, C.A. (2012). Morbidity and mortality associated with fenbendazole use in teleost fish at the National Aquarium, Baltimore.

Proceedings of the International Association of Aquatic Animal Medicine Conference, Atlanta, GA.

Tavakiol, S., Halajian, A., Smit, W.J. et al. (2017). Guppies (*Poecilia reticulata*) introducing an alient parasite, *Camallanus cotti* (Nematoda: Cammallanidae) to African, the first report. *Parasitology Research* 116: 3441–3445.

Wu, S.G., Wang, G.T., Xi, B.W. et al. (2007). Population dynamics and maturation cycle of *Camallanus cotti* (Nematoda: Camallanidae) in the Chinese hooksnout carp (Osteichthyes: Cyprinidae) from a reservoir in China. *Veterinary Parasitology* 147: 124–131.

Philometrid Nematodes

Overview

- Philometrid nematodes have indirect life cycles with fish as definitive or paratenic hosts.
- They tend to be host- and tissue-specific.
- Often only the larvae are found, making further identification impossible.
- Where adults are found, it is typically only the large, red, hematophagous females.

Etiology

- Phylum *Nematoda*.
- Order *Rhabditida*.
- Superfamily *Dracunculoidea*.
- Family *Philometridae*.
- A variety of species have been reported, all showing high host and tissue specificity, e.g.:
  - *Philometra orbitalensis* in the retrobulbar space and *Philometroides aphanonaris* in the subcutaneous tissues of the head of largemouth bass (*Micropterus salmoides*).
  - *Philometra overstreeti* and *Philometroides paralichthydis* in the teeth, tongue, jaw bones, gills, or muscles of southern flounder (*Paralichthys lethostigma*).
- Presumptive dracunculoid or philometrid nematode larvae have been reported in a variety of sharks. Few are identified to species, but examples include *Phylctainophora* spp.

Life Cycle and Transmission

- The life cycle is likely indirect, although few have been elucidated in detail.
- Intermediate hosts are invertebrates such as copepods, in which larvae molt to the infective L3 stage.
- Definitive and paratenic hosts are usually fish that ingest intermediate hosts.
- Males are rarely found. Males die after mating and females migrate to the definitive tissue site.
- Most are viviparous, which is unusual for nematodes.

Geographic Distribution

- Freshwater and saltwater habitats, probably worldwide.

Signalment

- Many freshwater, brackish, and marine fish are susceptible.
- *Philometra* spp. have been identified in a variety of freshwater and marine teleosts, particularly centrarchid fish in the northeastern US.
- Dracunculoid or philometrid nematode larvae have been reported in Atlantic sharpnose sharks (*Rhizoprionodon terraenovae*), shortfin mako sharks (*Isurus oxyrinchus*), whitetip reef sharks (*Triaenodon obesus*), blacktip sharks (*Carcharhinus limbatus*), nurse sharks (*Ginglymostoma cirratum*), spiny dogfish (*Squalus acanthias*), and blue sharks (*Prionace glauca*).

Risk Factors

- Exposure and stressors are the most important risk factors.
- Exposure includes:
  - Poor biosecurity (e.g. lack of suitable quarantine, use of surface water).
  - Outdoor or wild-caught fish.
  - Abundant habitat for intermediate hosts.
- Common stressors are described under C7: *Monogeneans (General)*.

Signs/Clinical Findings

- Infected fish are usually asymptomatic.
- Multiple conspecifics may be affected.
- Clinical signs depend on the site of infection.
- Lethargy may be seen.
- Inappetence, reduced appetite, or weight loss may be seen.
- Abnormal swimming may be seen.
- Exophthalmos with a red appearance to the conjunctiva is common if the nematodes are retrobulbar.
- Dyspnea or tachypnea may be seen.
- Fecundity may be reduced if the parasites are within the gonads.

Differential Diagnoses

- Full differentials are provided in Section B.
- Common differentials for roundworms in fish include ascarids, camallanids, capillarids, eustrongylids, and philometrids. Leeches, pentastomids, and acanthocephalans can resemble roundworms.

Diagnosis

- Philometrids are usually found on necropsy, cytology, or histology, particularly the larvae. They may be found in the retrobulbar space, subcutaneous tissues, gills, teeth, oral cavity, jaw bones, gastrointestinal tract, gonads, or coelom.
- Larvae are multicellular, round in cross-section, and may be coiled and encapsulated or free. They may be associated with cysts, plaques, nodules, or ulcers.
- Adult females are multicellular, often 10–35 mm long, round in cross-section, usually red, unsegmented, with a full gastrointestinal tract and no setae, suckers, or hooks. The head is rounded and caudal alae are reduced. They are often gravid, with larvae in their uteri. Males are smaller and are rarely found. The inflammatory response varies.
- If further morphological or molecular identification is required, nematodes can be relaxed in near-boiling water or saline followed by fixation in 95% ethanol, or rinsed in water or saline followed by fixation in hot 70% ethanol or hot AFA (ethanol, formalin, acetic acid). Definitive identification is difficult if adult stages are not available.
- SEM and molecular studies may provide more taxonomic information.

Husbandry Management

- Management changes are not indicated if parasite load is low and there is no morbidity or mortality.
- Reduce or resolve stressors.
- Disrupt the life cycle by reducing access to other hosts.

Medical Management

- The effectiveness of treatment will depend on tissue distribution. Parasites in the retrobulbar space or jaw bones are likely to be resistant to drug treatment.
- Morbidity and mortality have been reported secondary to deworming. This may be from direct toxicity of the medication or due to an inflammatory response to dead or dying parasites.
- Common treatments (see Chapters A12 and A13 for more details):
  - Surgical removal has been effective at clearing the infection (Figure C7.16).

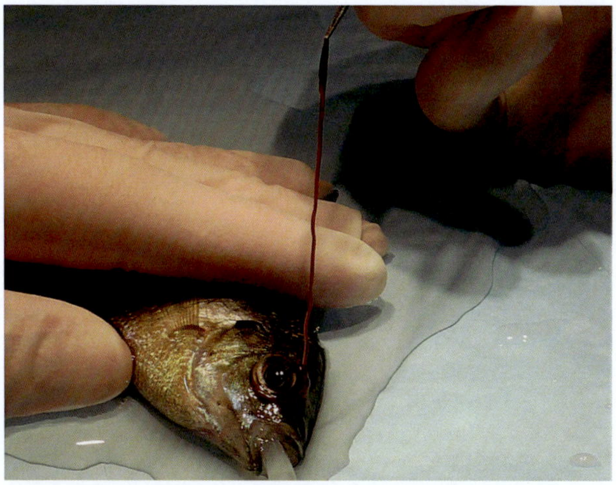

Figure C7.16 An adult female philometrid nematode being removed from the retrobulbar space of a bluegill (*Lepomis macrochirus*).

  - Emamectin benzoate orally at 0.05 mg/kg every 24 hours for seven days killed *Philometra* sp. in a majority of striped bass (*Morone saxatilis*).
- Fenbendazole and levamisole have typically been ineffective.
- All legislation regarding medication use and disposal must be followed.

Prevention

- Reduce or resolve stressors.
  - Common stressors are described under C7: *Monogeneans (General)*.
- Reduce exposure and transmission.
  - Eliminate or limit access to other hosts.
  - High water flow rate or turnover.
  - Removal of dead or moribund fish as soon as possible with appropriate disposition.
  - Suitable quarantine with isolation, monitoring, and diagnostic testing.
  - Frozen-thawed or commercial feeds, with no live feeds.

Zoonotic Reports

- These parasites have no known zoonotic potential.

Bibliography

Borucinska, J.D. and Adams, D.H. (2013). Parasitic metritis and oophoritis associated with nematode larvae in an Atlantic sharpnose shark, *Rixoprionodon terraenovae* (Richardson), collected in the western Atlantic off Florida. *Journal of Fish Diseases* 36: 811–817.

de Buron, I. and Roumillat, W.A. (2010). Histopathology of two philometric parasites of the southern flounder, *Paralichthys lethostigma*. *Journal of Wildlife Diseases* 46: 277–282.

Hadfield, C.A., Clayton, L.A., Brignell, J. et al. (2013). Branchitis and gill nematodiasis in whitetip reef sharks

(*Triaenodon obesus*). *Proceedings of the International Association of Aquatic Animal Medicine*,Sausalito, CA.

Justine, J., Briand, M.J., and Bray, R.A. (2012). A quick and simple method, usable in the field, for collecting parasites in suitable condition for both morphological and molecular studies. *Parasitology Research* 111: 341–351.

Lampen, F., Pearton, D., Christison, K. et al. (2016). Fatal branchitis and acute systemic inflammatory response associated with gill nematodiasis in bowmouth sharks (*Rhina ancylostoma*). *Proceedings of the International Association of Aquatic Animal Medicine Conference*, Virginia Beach, VA.

Moravec, F. (2004). Some aspects of the taxonomy and biology of dracunculoid nematodes parasitic in fishes: a review. *Folia Parasitologica* 51: 1–13.

Moravec, F., Crosby, M.D., de Buron, I. et al. (2008). Three new species of philometrids (Nematoda: Philometridae) from centrarchid fishes in the USA. *Journal of Parasitology* 94: 1103–1113.

Myers, G.E., Garner, M.M., Barrie, M.T. et al. (2007). Fenbendazole toxicity in sharks. *Proceedings of the International Association of Aquatic Animal Medicine*, Orlando, FL.

Séguin, G., Lair, S., Uhland, F.C. et al. (2008). Effectiveness and safety of different anthelmintics for the treatment of the nematode *Philometra* sp. in striped bass (*Morone saxatilis*). *Proceedings of the International Association of Aquatic Animal Medicine*, Rome, Italy.

Abbreviations/Acronyms

- SEM: Scanning electron microscopy

Anguillicolid Nematodes

Overview

- *Anguillicoloides* spp. are nematodes that reproduce in the swim bladder of anguillid eels.
- *Anguillicoloides crassus* can infect several anguillid species and has been introduced into native populations from eel aquaculture. It represents a significant threat to both cultured and wild eel populations.
- Other *Anguillicoloides* spp. are limited to a single anguillid species or geographic area.

Etiology

- Phylum *Nematoda*.
- Order *Rhabditida*.
- Superfamily *Dracunculoidea*.
- Family *Anguillicolidae*.
- *A. crassus* is the most important member of this group, as it has a wide geographic and host range.
- Other *Anguillicoloides* spp. include *A. australiensis*, *A. novaezelandiae*, and *A. papernai*.

Life Cycle and Transmission

- The life cycle is indirect.
- Anguillid eels are the definitive hosts.
- Intermediate hosts include copepods and ostracods.
- Paratenic hosts include mollusks, insects, fish, and tadpoles.
- Adult nematodes live and breed in the swim bladder lumen or wall, feeding on blood. Thin-walled eggs with L2 larvae are passed through the pneumatic duct and gastrointestinal tract and are eaten by intermediate hosts. Eels ingest the intermediate hosts at the advanced elver (glass eel) stage just after moving from the ocean into estuaries. L3 and L4 larvae then migrate to the swim bladder wall or lumen.

Geographic Distribution

- The natural range of *A. crassus* is likely to have been in East Asia. The species has been translocated to freshwater and saltwater habitats around Europe, Africa, and North America, particularly along the east coast.

Signalment

- All anguillid eels are susceptible, e.g. Japanese eels (*Anguilla japonica*), American eels (*Anguilla rostrata*), and European eels (*Anguilla anguilla*). Pathogenicity is higher in American and European eels.

Risk Factors

- Exposure and stressors are the most important risk factors.
- Exposure includes:
  - Poor biosecurity (e.g. lack of suitable quarantine, use of surface water, exposure to wild eels).
  - Geographic location.
  - Recent introduction of eels into a new area.
  - Abundant habitat for intermediate or paratenic hosts.
- Common stressors are described under C7: *Monogeneans (General)*.

Signs/Clinical Findings

- Infected fish may be asymptomatic.
- Several conspecifics may be affected.
- Reduced appetite, weight loss, or poor growth may be seen.

- Negative buoyancy or coelomic distension may be seen.
- Gill pallor may be seen.
- Decreased swimming speed may be seen.
- Migration and breeding may be affected.
- Mortality rate may correlate with tissue damage and dissolved oxygen more than parasite load.
- Mortality may reach 10–20%.

Differential Diagnoses

- Clinical signs are nonspecific, but other diseases of anguillid eels include an aquabirnavirus *eel virus European*, a rhabdovirus *eel virus European X*, anguillid herpesvirus, viral erythrocytic necrosis, *Aeromonas*, *Pseudomonas*, *Vibrio*, *Edwardsiella*, *Trichodina* spp., *Ichthyophthirius multifiliis*, dactylogyrids, gyrodactylids, and *Myxidium* spp. and other myxozoans.
- Nematodes in the swim bladder of anguillid eels are pathognomonic for *Anguillicoloides* spp.

Diagnosis

- Anguillicolids are large and are typically found in the swim bladder at necropsy (Figure C7.17a). They may also be seen on radiography, coeliotomy, or endoscopy (Figure C7.17b). A scoring system based on radiographic changes to the swim bladder is available (Berengi et al. 1998).
- Adults are round, multicellular, unsegmented, long and thin, with a full GI tract and no setae, suckers, or hooks.
- Encysted larvae may be seen in the swim bladder lumen or wall.
- Degenerate eggs and fluid may also be seen within the swim bladder.
- If further morphological or molecular identification is required, nematodes can be relaxed in near-boiling water or saline followed by fixation in 95% ethanol, or fixed in hot 70% ethanol or hot AFA (ethanol, formalin, acetic acid).

Husbandry Management

- Reduce or resolve stressors.
- Increase aeration; target dissolved oxygen may be 95–100%.
- Disrupt the life cycle by reducing access to other hosts, particularly copepods.

Medical Management

- Common treatments (see Chapters A12 and A13 for more details):
  - Levamisole immersion 20 mg/L for six days can reduce parasite loads in salt water. Treatment may need to be

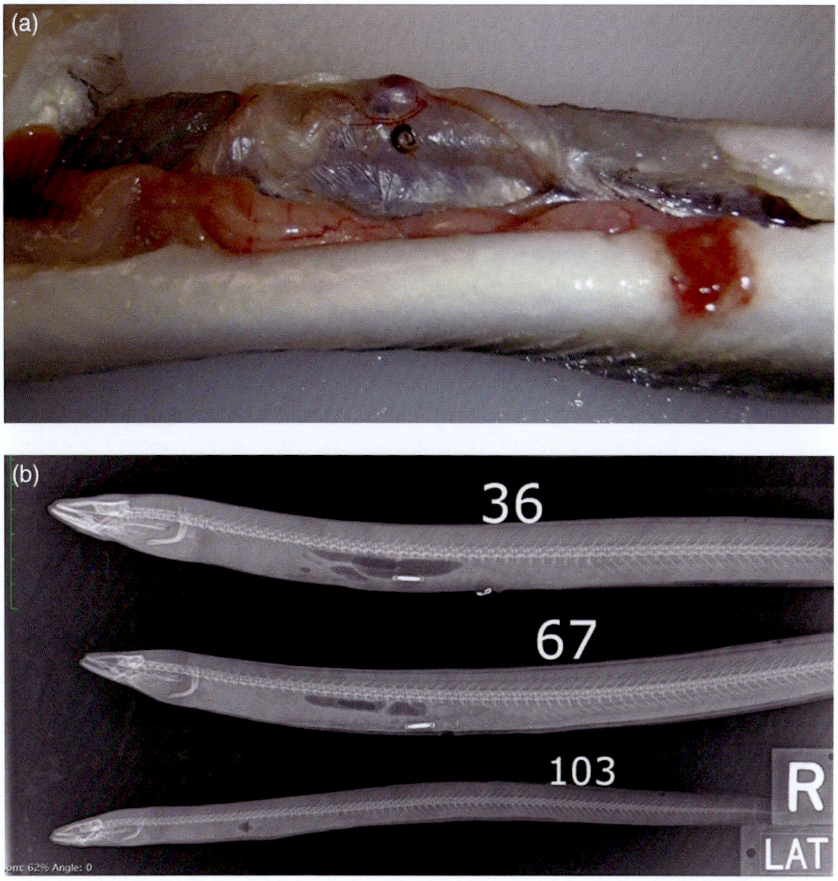

Figure C7.17 Anguillicolid nematodes on necropsy (a) and radiography (b) of American eels (*Anguilla rostrata*). *Source*: Images courtesy of Craig Harms, North Carolina State University.

repeated every three weeks. The effective dose in freshwater may be lower, e.g. 1 mg/L for 24 hours.
- Other reported treatments (see Chapters A12 and A13 for more details):
  - Emamectin orally.
- All legislation regarding medication use and disposal must be followed.

Prevention
- Reduce or resolve stressors.
  - Common stressors are described under C7: *Monogeneans (General)*.
- Reduce exposure and transmission
  - Assess the risks in a pond or lagoon prior to animal acquisition.
  - Acquire eels at the glass eel stage before they start feeding.
  - Suitable quarantine with isolation, monitoring, and diagnostic testing, such as necropsies or radiography.
  - Prevent or limit indirect contact with free-ranging eels.
  - Limit access to other hosts such as copepods.

Zoonotic Reports
- These parasites have no known zoonotic potential.

Bibliography

Berengi, A., Molnar, K., Bekesi, L., and Szekely, C.S. (1998). Radiodiagnostic method for studying swim bladder inflammation caused by *Anguillicola crassus* (Nematoda:Draculuncoidea). *Disease of Aquatic Organisms* 34: 155–160.

Hein, J.L., Arnott, S.A., Roumillat, W.A. et al. (2014). Invasive swimbladder parasite *Anguillicoloides crassus*: infection status 15 years after discovery in wild populations of American eel *Anguilla rostrata*. *Diseases of Aquatic Organisms* 107: 199–209.

Justine, J., Briand, M.J., and Bray, R.A. (2012). A quick and simple method, usable in the field, for collecting parasites in suitable condition for both morphological and molecular studies. *Parasitology Research* 111: 341–351.

Lefebvre, F., Contournet, P., and Crivelli, A.J. (2007). Interaction between severity of the infection by the nematode *Anguillicola crassus* and the tolerance to hypoxia in the European eel, *Anguilla anguilla*. *Acta Parasitologica* 52: 171–175.

Moravec, F. (2004). Some aspects of the taxonomy and biology of dracunculoid nematodes parasitic in fishes: a review. *Folia Parasitologica* 51: 1–13.

Trichosomoidid Nematodes

Overview
- Of the trichosomoidid nematodes, only *Huffmanela* spp. have been reported in fish
- In carcharhinid sharks, *Huffmanela* spp. are typically identified from sinuous, black tracks in the skin formed by the eggs.
- In teleosts, *Huffmanela* spp. are more likely to cause black foci in the muscle or swim bladder wall.
- Adults are rarely found and have never been identified from infections in sharks.
- Treatment with injectable levamisole has resolved signs in sharks.

Etiology
- Phylum *Nematoda*.
- Order *Trichinellida*.
- Family *Trichosomoididae*.
- Species identification is often uncertain, but is based on egg and larval morphology, host species, and tissue site.
- *Huffmanela carcharhini*, *Huffmanela lata*, and *Huffmanela markgracei* have been reported from elasmobranchs.
- A variety of *Huffmanela* species have been reported from teleosts, including *H. huffmani*, *H. branchialis*, *H. canadensis*, and *H. shikokuensis*.

Life Cycle and Transmission
- Information is primarily available for the eggs and larvae; adults have only been found for a few of the teleost parasites (e.g. *H. canadensis*, *H. huffmani*).
- The life cycle is largely thought to be indirect, potentially through a crustacean intermediate host. The life cycle has been completed experimentally for *H. huffmani* using amphipod intermediate hosts (*Hyalella* spp.). The pre-patent period was 7.5 months and the eggs were not infective until several months after shedding, suggesting a prolonged life cycle.
- In some reports, larvae are occasionally seen emerging from eggs, but in other reports, only early larval development stages are seen, suggesting hatching may take place elsewhere.
- With skin infections, it is postulated that epidermal sloughing may release eggs for infection of the subsequent host.
- Eggs are typically negatively buoyant.

Geographic Distribution

- In elasmobranchs, these were initially reported from Atlantic Ocean and Gulf of Mexico sharks. There are now sporadic reports from the Pacific Ocean.
- Reports in marine teleosts have come from the Atlantic and Pacific Oceans.
- Reports in freshwater teleosts have been limited to the San Marcos River in Texas, United States.

Signalment

- Many freshwater and marine fish may be susceptible.
- The host range of each parasite species is often narrow.
- Carcharhinid sharks are the most commonly reported hosts.
  - Sandbar sharks (*Carcharhinus plumbeus*).
  - Gray reef sharks (*Carcharhinus amblyrhynchos*).
  - Atlantic sharpnose sharks (*Rhizoprionodon terraenovae*).
- Marine teleost hosts include pouting (*Trisopterus luscus*), rockfish (*Sebastes* spp.), and swordfish (*Xiphias gladius*).
- Freshwater teleost hosts are centrarchid fish (*Micropterus* and *Lepomis* spp.).

Risk Factors

- Exposure and stressors are the most important risk factors.
- Exposure includes:
  - Permissive salinity; almost all are marine (*H. huffmani* is found in freshwater).
  - Abundant habitat for potential intermediate hosts.
- Common stressors are described under C7: *Monogeneans (General)*.

Signs/Clinical Findings

- Infected fish may be asymptomatic.
- Individuals or multiple conspecifics may be affected.
- In sharks, characteristic gray or black, sinuous, linear tracts or spots on the skin are seen, particularly around the head (Figure C7.18a). They can also be found in the oral and branchial cavities. The band of tracks is often 4–6 cm wide. There is no pruritus.
- In teleosts, some *Huffmanela* spp. cause similar dark, linear tracks or spots on the skin (e.g. *H. canadensis* in rockfish). Others cause no external signs, with eggs found within the muscle or swim bladder wall.

Differential Diagnoses

- Full differentials are provided in Section B.
- Common differentials for black foci on the skin include digenes, turbellarians, and *Huffmanela* spp.

Diagnosis

- Diagnosis is typically based on eggs found on direct microscopy or histology of lesions.
- Eggs are darkly pigmented (golden, brown, or black), ellipsoid, usually 70–90 × 40–50 μm in size but up to 110 × 80 μm in some species (Figure C7.18b). They have large bipolar plugs and coiled larvae within.
- There is often little or no associated inflammatory response. Hyperplasia may be present.
- Adults are rarely seen. They are filariform nematodes that are small and readily missed. They have been found in the swim bladder and skin of teleosts.
- If further morphological or molecular identification is required, eggs are often examined under histology and SEM. Species keys are provided by Moravec and Fajer-Avila (2000).

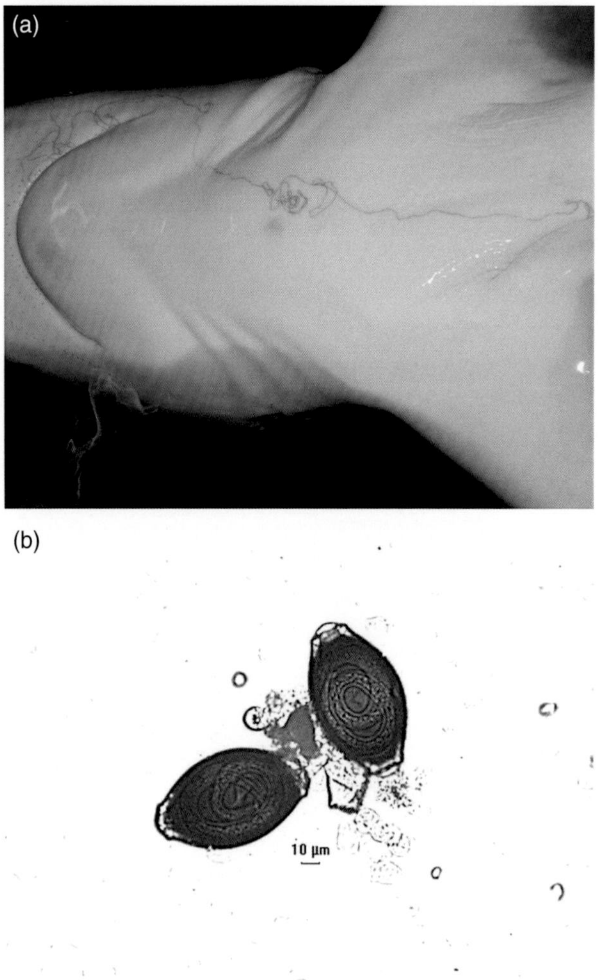

Figure C7.18 Black linear tracts on the skin of a sandbar shark (*Carcharhinus plumbeus*) due to *Huffmanela* sp. (a) and typical appearance of eggs on direct microscopy of a skin scrape (b). *Source*: Image (a) courtesy of Craig Harms, North Carolina State University, and (b) courtesy of Robert MacLean, Audubon Nature Institute.

Husbandry Management

- Reduce or resolve stressors.

Medical Management

- Common treatments (see Chapters A12 and A13 for more details):
  - Levamisole by intramuscular injection at 10 mg/kg repeated at two and four weeks has led to slow resolution of clinical signs in sharks.
  - The lesions may be self-limiting and may resolve without treatment.
- Other reported treatments (see Chapters A12 and A13 for more details):
  - Levamisole orally.
- All legislation regarding medication use and disposal must be followed.

Prevention

- This is largely unknown.

Zoonotic Reports

- These parasites have no known zoonotic potential but *Huffmanela* sp. eggs have been identified in human fecals due to consumption of infected fish.

Bibliography

Bullard, S.A., Ruiz, C.F., McElwain, A. et al. (2012). *Huffmanela* cf. *carcharhini* (Nematoda: Trichosomoididae: Huffmanelinae) from skin of a sandbar shark, *Carcharhinus plumbeus*, in the Pacific Ocean. *Journal of Parasitology* 98: 333–340.

Esteves, A., Seixas, F., Carvalho, S. et al. (2009). *Huffmanela* sp. (Nematoda: Trichosomoididae) muscular parasite from *Trisopterus luscus* captured off the Portuguese coast. *Diseases of Aquatic Organisms* 84: 251–255.

Justine, J., Briand, M.J., and Bray, R.A. (2012). A quick and simple method, usable in the field, for collecting parasites in suitable condition for both morphological and molecular studies. *Parasitology Research* 111: 341–351.

MacLean, R.A., Fatzinger, M.H., Woolard, K.D., and Harms, C.A. (2006). Clearance of a dermal *Huffmanela* sp. in a sandbar shark (*Carcharhinus plumbeus*) using levamisole. *Diseases of Aquatic Organisms* 73: 83–88.

Moravec, F. and Fajer-Avila, E. (2000). *Huffmanela mexicana* n. sp. (Nematoda: Trichosomoididae) from the marine fish *Sphoeroides annulatus* in Mexico. *Journal of Parasitology* 86: 1229–1231.

Ruiz, C.F. and Bullard, S.A. (2013). *Huffmanela markgracei* sp.n. (Nematoda: Trichosomoididae) from buccal cavity of Atlantic sharpnose shark, *Rhisoprionodon terraenovae* (Carcharhiniformes: Carcharhinidae), in the northwestern Gulf of Mexico off Texas. *Folia Parasitologica* 60: 353–358.

Worsham, M.L.D., Huffman, D.G., Moravec, F., and Gibson, J.R. (2016). The life cycle of *Huffmanela huffmani* Moravec, 1987 (Nematode: Trichosomoididae), and endemic marine-relict parasite of Centrarchidae from a Central Texas spring. *Folia Parasitologica* 63: 020.

Abbreviations/Acronyms

- SEM: Scanning electron microscopy

Pentastomids

Overview

- Pentastomids are unusual parasites that are closely related to crustaceans.
- They are obligate endoparasites with an indirect life cycle.
- Fish can be intermediate hosts (IH). The larvae (nymphs) look like coiled worms. They rarely cause morbidity or mortality in fish.
- The definitive hosts (DH) are piscivorous aquatic reptiles, where respiratory signs may be seen.

Etiology

- Phylum *Arthropoda*.
- Subphylum *Crustacea*.
- Subclass *Pentastomida*.
- Pentastomids are closely related to branchiurans.
- A variety of genera have been identified in fish, including:
  - *Agema*.
  - *Alofia*.
  - *Diesingia*.
  - *Leiperia*.
  - *Sebekia*.
  - *Subtriquetra*.
- Pentastomids may be called tongue worms.

Life Cycle and Transmission

- The life cycle is indirect.
- For pentastomids that infect fish, fish are the IH and aquatic reptiles are the DH, particularly crocodilians (*Crocodilia*) and piscivorous turtles such as soft-shell turtles (*Trionychidae*), snapping turtles (*Macrochelys* and *Chelydra* spp.), and mud turtles (*Kinosternon* spp.). Aquatic snakes are less common DHs.
- In the DH, adults are found within the trachea or lungs. Eggs with mite-like, four-legged larvae are coughed up by the DH and passed in the feces. These eggs are typically ingested by the IH but some (*Subtriquetra* spp.) can hatch into free-swimming larvae and attach to the skin of the IH then invade. In the IH, they migrate to various tissues and go through several molts to develop into encysted nymphs. This unusual name is because the nymphs are worm-like. The IH is ingested by the DH, where the parasites migrate to the trachea or lungs.
- The parasites cannot be transmitted directly between fish.

Geographic Distribution

- Predominantly in freshwater habitats.

Signalment

- A variety of teleosts are susceptible, particularly pond and aquarium fish, e.g.:
  - Tilapia (*Oreochromis* and *Tilapia* spp.).
  - Flagfish (*Jordanella floridae*).
  - Danios (*Danio* spp.).
  - Mosquitofish, swordtails, mollies, guppies, and platies (*Poeciliidae*).

Risk Factors

- Exposure and stressors are the most important risk factors.
- Exposure includes:
  - Outdoor or wild-caught fish.
  - Presence of aquatic reptiles.
- Common stressors are described under C7: *Monogeneans (General)*.

Signs/Clinical Findings

- Infected fish are usually asymptomatic.
- One or more fish may be affected.
- Skin nodules, coelomic distension, or abnormal buoyancy may be seen.
- Signs may wax and wane depending on parasite migration.

Differential Diagnoses

- Full differentials are provided in Section B.
- Common differentials for coiled worm-like structures seen in bony fish include cestodes, nematodes, leeches, and pentastomids.

Diagnosis

- Pentastomid larvae are usually found at necropsy or on direct microscopy of the skin, muscle, swim bladder, serosal surfaces, or viscera.
- Larvae are multicellular, round-bodied, short (<1 cm), stout, and coiled (Figure C7.19). Small hooks are present at the anterior end (unlike the oral and ventral suckers of digenes). The larvae look segmented, known as pseudosegmentation or annulation. The larvae do not move but may be seen pulsing because the cuticle is soft. The inflammatory response varies.
- Parasites are typically incidental and further identification is rarely needed or possible from the larvae. Definitive identification is usually based on the morphology of the copulatory spicule in males in the definitive host.

Husbandry Management

- In fish, this is often more of a cosmetic concern than a health concern, but management should be considered if the fish are housed with reptiles.
- Reduce or resolve stressors.
- Disrupt the life cycle by reducing or eliminating access to other hosts.

Medical Management

- No effective treatment has been reported in fish.

Prevention

- Reduce or resolve stressors.
  - Common stressors are described under C7: *Monogeneans (General)*.
- Reduce exposure and transmission.

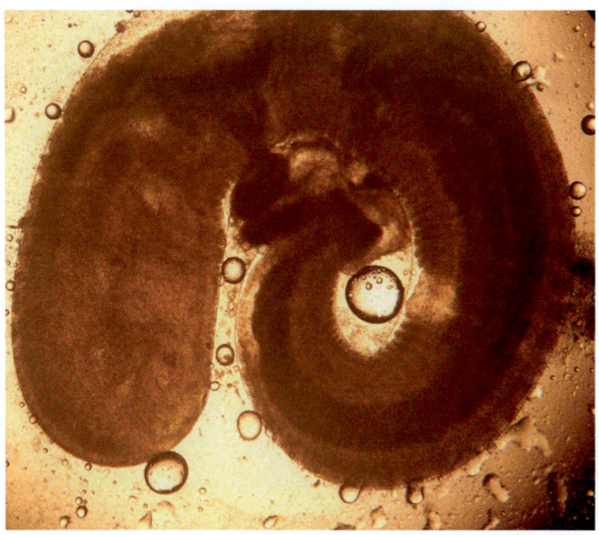

Figure C7.19 Pentastomid larvae on direct examination of a serosal scrape from an Australian rainbowfish (*Melanotaenia* sp.).

- Avoid housing crocodilians and piscivorous turtles in systems with fish.
- Outdoor ponds may benefit from being kept fallow periodically.

Zoonotic Reports

- Zoonotic transmission from fish has not been reported.
- Pentastomids are reported in humans but these have a different life cycle, with mammals as the IH and reptiles as the DH (e.g. *Armillifer*, *Porocephalus* spp.), or with herbivorous mammals as the IH and carnivorous mammals as the DH (e.g. *Linguatula* spp.). Humans can be an aberrant host due to ingestion of eggs from the DH or ingestion of raw or inadequately cooked meat from the IH.

Bibliography

Boyce, W.M., Kazacos, E.A., Kazacos, K.R., and Engelhardt, J.A. (1987). Pathology of pentastomid infections. *Journal of Wildlife Diseases* 23: 689–692.

Paré, J. (2008). An overview of pentastomiasis in reptiles and other vertebrates. *Journal of Exotic Pet Medicine* 17: 285–294.

Abbreviations/Acronyms

- DH: Definitive host
- IH: Intermediate host

Acanthocephalans

Overview

- Acanthocephalans are obligate endoparasites, usually found in the intestines.
- Adults have a distinctive, eversible, spiny proboscis.
- They also known as spiny-headed or thorny-headed worms.
- Fish can be intermediate (IH), definitive (DH), or paratenic hosts.

Etiology

- Phylum *Acanthocephala*.
- A variety of genera have been described in fish, including:
  - *Acanthocephalus*.
  - *Corynosoma*.
  - *Echinorhynchus*.
  - *Pomphorhynchus*.
  - *Sclerocollum*.

Life Cycle and Transmission

- The life cycle is indirect where known, although few have been elucidated in detail.
- There are one or two IHs, typically crustaceans (e.g. amphipods) and fish. Fish can also be the DHs or paratenic hosts.
- In the DH, gravid females lay bipolar eggs that are passed in the feces. The eggs are eaten by the first IH and hatch into acanthellae. These migrate into the body cavity and encyst into the infective cystacanth stage. IHs may then by ingested by a second IH, paratenic host, or DH. In the second IH or paratenic host, the parasite encysts again. In the DH, the parasite excysts, anchors its proboscis in the intestinal wall and matures.

Geographic Distribution

- Freshwater and saltwater habitats, probably worldwide.

Signalment

- Freshwater and marine bony fish are the most commonly reported hosts, e.g. carp, koi, goldfish (*Cyprinidae*), sea breams (*Sparidae*), salmonids (*Salmonidae*), and suckers (*Catostomidae*).
- There have been rare reports from elasmobranchs, e.g. in the spiral valve of spiny dogfish (*Squalus acanthias*).

Risk Factors

- Exposure and stressors are the most important risk factors.
- Exposure includes:
  - Poor biosecurity (e.g. lack of suitable quarantine, use of surface water).
  - Outdoor or wild-caught fish.
  - Abundant crustacean hosts.
- Common stressors are described under C7: *Monogeneans (General)*.

Signs/Clinical Findings

- Infected fish are usually asymptomatic.
- Parasites may be seen dangling from the anus or cloaca.
- Coelomic distension may be seen.
- Mortalities may be seen.

Differential Diagnoses

- Full differentials are provided in Section B.
- Common differentials for round worm-like parasites in fish include nematodes, leeches, acanthocephalans, and pentastomids.

Diagnosis

- Acanthocephalans are typically identified on necropsy or coeliotomy.
- Adults are found within the intestines, particularly the distal intestines (Figure C7.20a). They are multicellular, round to slightly flattened parasites that look segmented (pseudosegmentation). They are typically ~1 cm in length but can be much longer. Each has a large, eversible spiny proboscis that is anchored into the intestinal wall (Figure C7.20b). The other end is tapered. There is no gastrointestinal tract. They are dioecious and females are often larger than males.
- Encysted larvae can be found in any tissues, particularly the mesentery or coelomic wall.
- Eggs may be found in intestinal contents or on fecal sedimentation examination; they are not commonly seen on fecal flotation. Eggs have distinctive poles.
- Histology may show any life stages, but identification is difficult unless the proboscis is identified. There may be ulceration or penetration of the intestinal wall and significant inflammatory response around the proboscis, which may be granulomatous.
- If further morphological or molecular identification is required, adults can be relaxed in near-boiling water or saline followed by fixation in 95% ethanol, or fixed in hot 70% ethanol or hot AFA (ethanol, formalin, acetic acid).

Husbandry Management

- Management changes are not indicated if parasite load is low, only encysted parasites are seen, and there is no morbidity or mortality.
- Reduce or resolve stressors.
- Disrupt the life cycle by reducing access to crustacean intermediate hosts.

Medical Management

- Treatments are not commonly reported. It is likely that benzimidazoles will have some effect on adult worms. However, since adults are typically embedded in the intestinal wall, treatment may be associated with inflammatory sequelae.
- All legislation regarding medication use and disposal must be followed.

Prevention

- Reduce or resolve stressors.
  - Common stressors are described under C7: *Monogeneans (General).*
- Reduce exposure and transmission.
  - Isolation with no contact with free-ranging fish and invertebrates.
  - Pathogen-free water source (e.g. municipal water or ground water that has gone through fine filtration (<40 μm) then UV and/or ozone disinfection). Avoid using untreated surface water.
  - Disinfection of recirculating water with fine filtration (<40 μm) then UV and/or ozone.
  - High water flow rate or turnover.
  - Suitable quarantine with isolation, monitoring, and diagnostic testing.
  - Frozen-thawed or commercial feeds, with no live feeds.

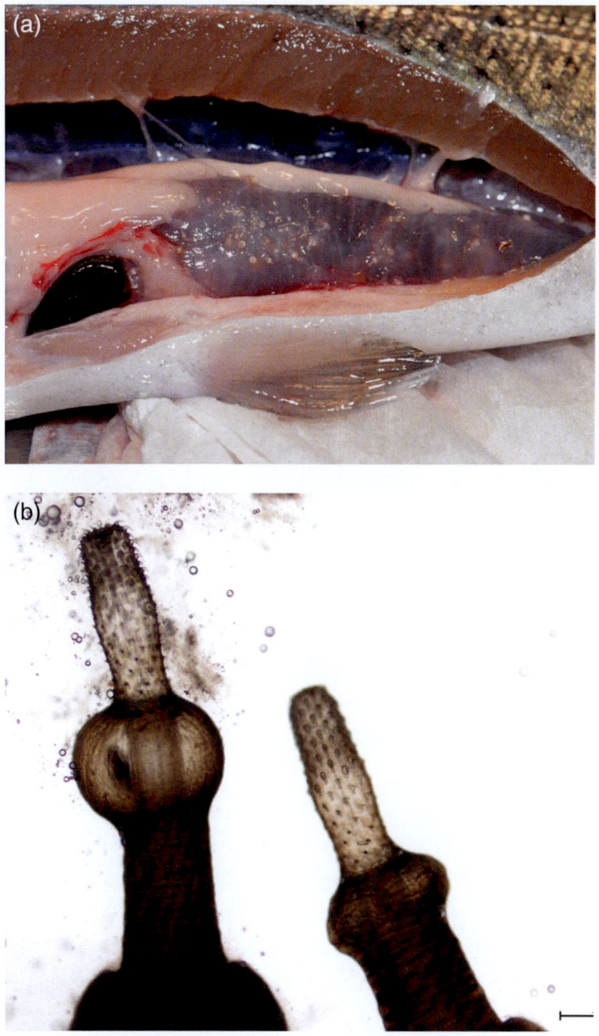

Figure C7.20 The acanthocephalan *Pomphorhynchus laevis* in the gastrointestinal tract of a rainbow trout (*Oncorhynchus mykiss*); encysted parasites seen through the wall of the distal intestines on necropsy (a), and an everted proboscis on brightfield microscopy (b). *Source*: Images courtesy of Bartolomeo Gorgoglione, University of Veterinary Medicine, Vienna.

Zoonotic Reports

- Zoonotic transmission from fish has not been reported.
- Rare cases of acanthocephaliasis are reported in humans but these tend to be terrestrial species (e.g. *Moniliformis* and *Macracanthorhynchus* spp.) with rats, raccoons, and swine as the normal DH, insects as the IH, and humans as an aberrant host.

Bibliography

Heller, N.P., Reyda, F.B., and Heller, A.D. (2016). Histopathology of *Catostomus commersoni* (white sucker) infected with the acanthocephalan *Pomphorhynchus bulbocolli*. *Journal of Parasitology* 102: 533–537.

Justine, J., Briand, M.J., and Bray, R.A. (2012). A quick and simple method, usable in the field, for collecting parasites in suitable condition for both morphological and molecular studies. *Parasitology Research* 111: 341–351.

Yasumoto, S. and Nagasawa, K. (1996). Possible life cycle of *Longicollum pagrasomi*, an acanthocephalan parasite of cultured red sea bream. *Fish Pathology* 31: 235–236.

Copepods

Overview

- Copepods are crustaceans. Most are free-living, but some are parasitic in fish.
- Sea lice (*Lepeophtheirus salmonis*) are significant pathogens of salmonids in aquaculture.
- Other copepods are more commonly incidental findings, but they can cause morbidity and mortality and act as disease vectors.
- Management is difficult because treatment options are limited and the egg stage is relatively resistant to treatment.

Etiology

- Phylum *Arthropoda*.
- Subphylum *Crustacea*.
- Subclass *Copepoda*.
- There are three main orders that parasitize fish.
- Most parasitic copepods are from the order *Siphonostomatoida*.
  - *Caligidae* (e.g. *Alebion*, *Caligus*, and *Lepeophtheirus* spp.).
  - *Dissonidae* (e.g. *Dissonus* spp.).
  - *Eudactylinidae* (e.g. *Eudactylina* spp.).
  - *Kroyeriidae* (e.g. *Kroyeria* spp.).
  - *Lernaeopodidae* (e.g. *Ommatokoita* spp.).
  - *Lernanthropidae* (e.g. *Lernanthropus* spp.).
  - *Pennellidae* (e.g. *Lernaeocera* spp., *Peroderma* spp.).
- Some important species are from the order *Poecilostomatoida*.
  - *Ergasilidae* (e.g. *Ergasilus* spp.).
- Some important species are from the order *Cyclopoida*.
  - *Lernaeidae* (e.g. *Lernaea* spp., also known as anchor worms).

Life Cycle and Transmission

- Life cycles vary depending on the species, but they are usually direct with a single host and multiple life stages. A few species require two hosts.
- Adults are dioecious. Males are temporary parasites and leave the host after sexual reproduction. Mature females stay attached to the host and produce two egg sacs. The eggs hatch into free-living (planktonic) nauplii that develop into infective copepodids that colonize the host and mature into adults.
- Life cycle duration (from egg to adult) varies.
  - *L. salmonis* life cycle varies from 19 days at 17°C (63°F) to 93 days at 5°C (41°F).
  - *Caligus rogercresseyi* life cycle varies from 26 days at 15°C (59°F) to 45 days at 10°C (50°F).
- There are important asymptomatic carriers in some areas (e.g. three-spined sticklebacks, *Gasterosteus aculeatus*, for *L. salmonis*).
- Transmission to and from wild and cultured fish is common.

Geographic Distribution

- Freshwater and saltwater habitats, probably worldwide.
- *L. salmonis* is only found in the northern hemisphere.

Signalment

- All fish are likely susceptible. Some examples of commonly reported fish parasites include:
  - *Alebion* spp. in carcharhinid sharks (*Carcharhinidae*).

- *C. rogercresseyi* in a variety of South American marine fish (e.g. Chilean silverside smelt (*Odontesthes regia*) and introduced salmonids).
- *Lepeophtheirus acutus* in zebra sharks (*Stegostoma tigrinum*), reef sharks (*Carcharhinus* and *Triaenodon* spp.), shovelnose rays (*Rhinobatos typus*), and manta rays (*Manta* spp.).
- *L. salmonis* in salmonids, particularly Atlantic salmon (*Salmo salar*), brown trout (*Salmo trutta*), and some Pacific salmonids such as Chinook salmon (*Oncorhynchus tshawytscha*) and chum salmon (*Oncorhynchus keta*).
- *Lernaea cyprinacea* particularly in cyprinids and freshwater salmonids.

Risk Factors

- Exposure and stressors are the most important risk factors.
- Exposure includes:
  - Poor biosecurity (e.g. lack of suitable quarantine, use of surface water).
  - Permissive water temperature; *Lernaea* spp. prefer 25–30°C (77–86°F).
  - Permissive salinity (e.g. >25 g/L for *L. salmonis*).
  - Low water flow rate or turnover.
  - Low-light conditions.
- Common stressors are described under C7: *Monogeneans (General).*

Signs/Clinical Findings

- Copepods are often grossly visible as small white to gray foci or trailing lines on the skin, fins, gills, eyes, oropharynx, nares, anus, or cloaca.
- Several individuals from one or more closely related species may be affected.
- Lethargy or periods of agitated swimming may be seen.
- Inappetence, reduced appetite, or poor growth rates may be seen.
- Petechiae or skin ulcers may be seen around the sites of attachment. The lesions may coalesce.
- Ulcerative keratitis may be seen.
- Gill pallor due to anemia may be seen.
- Dyspnea or tachypnea are rare but may be seen.
- Mortalities are possible.
- Co-infections are possible (e.g. *Aeromonas*, *Pseudomonas*, *Vibrio*, *Tenacibaculum* spp., infectious salmon anemia virus, infectious hematopoietic necrosis virus, nematodes, cestodes).
- Immunity following infection appears to be limited.

Differential Diagnoses

- Full differentials are provided in Section B.
- Common differentials for linear tags on fish include copepods, leeches, monogeneans, egg strands, and mucus strands.
- Common differentials for crustacean-like ectoparasites on fish include copepods, isopods, branchiurans, amphipods, and mites.

Diagnosis

- Parasite identification is usually confirmed by direct microscopy after gentle removal.
- Adults are usually 1–30 mm in total length. There are several body compartments and usually four pairs of jointed swimming appendages. A single, simple eye is present. Prominent paired eggs sacs are readily visible in mature females (Figure C7.21); males are rarely seen. If ruptured, the released eggs have a uniform appearance. Copepods do not have suckers or compound eyes.
- Some species show other adaptations; e.g. *Lernaea* spp. have a long, thin body and reduced limbs for burrowing (Figure C7.21b).
- Free-living copepods are sometimes seen on skin scrapes and gill biopsies and it is important to differentiate these from parasitic copepods. Free-living copepods do not have large grasping limbs and many males (adult-size copepods without trailing egg sacs) are seen (Figure C7.22).
- Identifying the species can help with management. If further morphological or molecular identification is required, copepods can be fixed in 10% neutral buffered formalin or 70 or 95% ethanol.

Husbandry Management

- Management changes may not be indicated if parasite load is low and there is no morbidity or mortality, but the parasites should be monitored.
- Reduce or resolve stressors.
- Consider isolating affected systems.
- Remove dead or moribund fish as soon as possible with appropriate disposition.
- Increase mechanical cleaning.
- Increase water flow-rate and turnover.
- For chronic or recurrent cases, consider cleaner fish. For *L. salmonis*, these can reduce clinical signs and the need for medical treatments. Cleaner fish should be from the same geographic area as the other fish in the system and provided with good husbandry care. Examples include goldsinny wrasse (*Ctenolabrus rupestris*), rock-cook wrasse (*Centrolabrus exoletus*), corkwing wrasse (*Symphodus melops*), ballan wrasse (*Labrus bergylta*), scale-rayed wrasse (*Acantholabrus palloni*), cunner fish (*Tautogolabrus adspersus*), goldfish (*Carassius auratus*), and lumpfish (*Cyclopterus lumpus*). Hatchery-reared ballan wrasse have been as effective as wild-caught conspecifics.

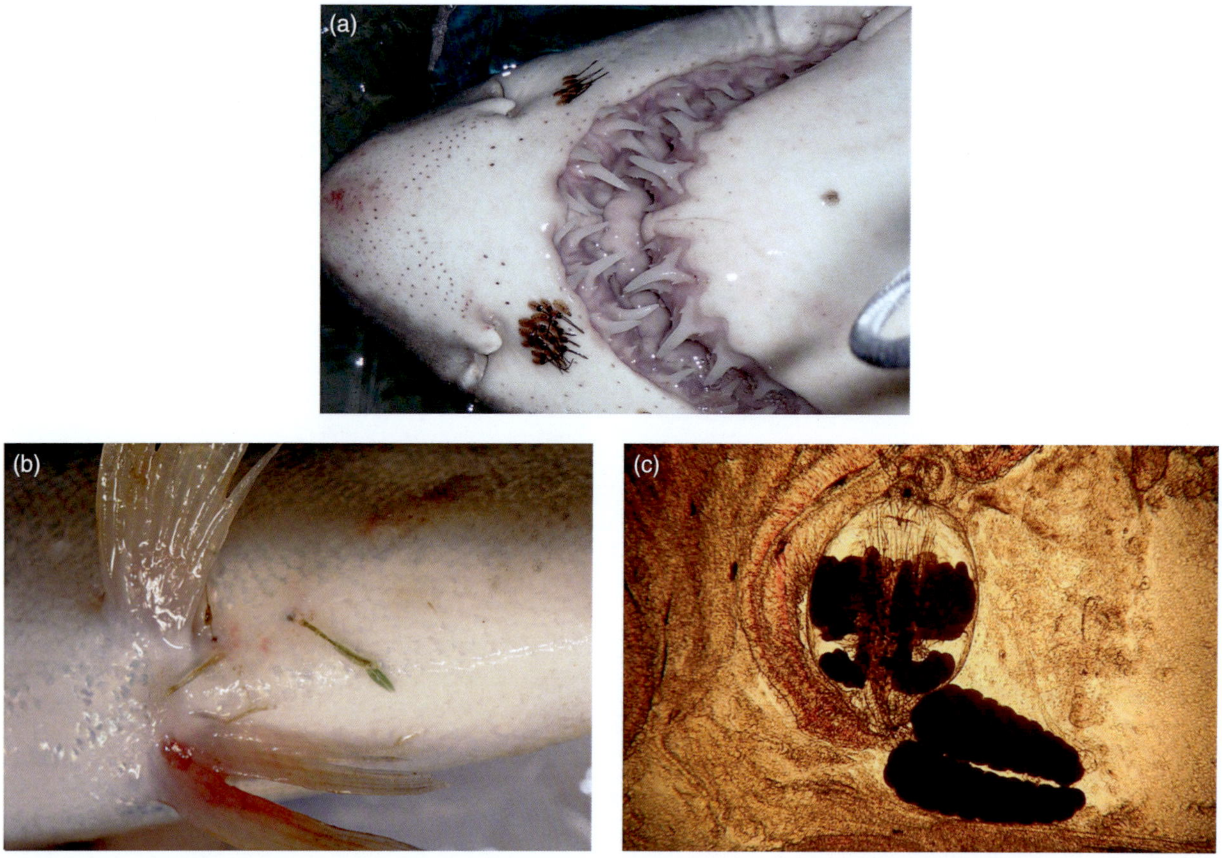

Figure C7.21 Parasitic copepods: unidentified copepods on the skin of a sand tiger (*Carcharias taurus*) (a), *Lernaea* sp. on the skin of a rainbow trout (*Oncorhynchus mykiss*) (b), and a copepod on direct microscopy of a gill biopsy at x40 (c). All show the prominent paired egg sacs. *Source*: Image (b) courtesy of Bartolomeo Gorgoglione, University of Veterinary Medicine, Vienna.

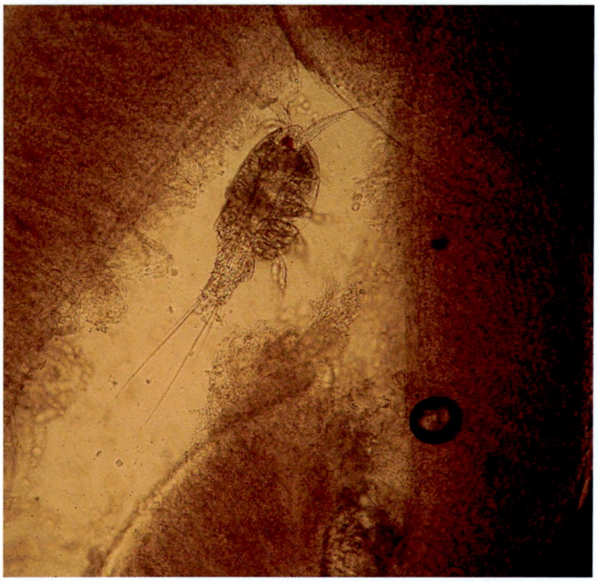

Figure C7.22 Free-living copepod on direct microscopy of a gill biopsy.

Medical Management

- Treatment should always be combined with husbandry changes as part of an integrated management strategy. Specific programs for *L. salmonis* are in place in several countries.
- Permanently attached adults are relatively resistant to treatment, but treatments can be used to kill younger stages, allowing the adults to die over time. Treatment should be continued until no attached females are visible.
- If dips or oral medications are used, the enclosures and décor should be treated within one to two days.
- Common treatments (see Chapters A12 and A13 for more details):
    - Trichlorfon immersion at 0.2–1.0 mg/L 1–24 hours repeated once or twice is commonly reported. Intervals vary from five days at 30°C (86°F) to 12–21 days at ~18°C (64°F). Adverse reactions to trichlorfon are common. Bioassays, close monitoring, and pretreatment with atropine should be considered.

Suitable PPE must be used. Drug disposal must be considered.
  - Diflubenzuron immersion is used, typically at 0.01–0.05 mg/L 8–24 hours, sometimes repeated once or twice within two to three weeks. This drug persists in water and regulatory issues and disposal must be considered prior to use.
  - Lufenuron immersion is used, typically at 0.01 mg/L every seven days. This drug persists in water and regulatory issues and disposal must be considered prior to use.
  - Emamectin benzoate orally has been the primary treatment for *L. salmonis* and other salmonid copepods since 2000. Typical dose is 50 μg/kg body weight every 24 hours for seven days in salmonids and goldfish. Emamectin is approved for use in salmonids with fish lice in Canada, Great Britain, Norway, and Chile; withdrawal periods vary. Resistance is a problem in some areas.
  - Physical removal can be effective, if practical.
- Other reported treatments (see Chapters A12 and A13 for more details):
  - Chitin inhibitors orally (e.g. diflubenzuron, teflubenzuron).
  - Other organophosphate immersion (e.g. dichlorvos, azamethiphos).
  - Pyrethroid immersion (e.g. deltamethrin, cypermethrin).
- Freshwater dips for marine fish are rarely effective. The parasites can tolerate long periods in freshwater.
- All legislation regarding medication use and disposal must be followed.

Prevention

- Reduce or resolve stressors.
  - Common stressors are described under C7: *Monogeneans (General).*
- Reduce exposure and transmission.
  - Isolation with no contact with free-ranging fish or invertebrates.
  - Pathogen-free water source (e.g. municipal water or ground water that has gone through fine filtration (<40 μm) then UV and/or ozone disinfection). Avoid using untreated surface water.
  - Good mechanical cleaning.
  - High water flow rate or turnover.
  - All-in-all-out management with fallowing between groups.
  - Suitable quarantine with isolation, monitoring, and diagnostic testing, particularly physical examinations of the skin, gills, and oropharynx. Prophylactic treatment of copepods in quarantine is rare.
  - Routine monitoring of high-risk groups (e.g. Atlantic salmon in sea pens) with treatment at specified parasite loads.
- Reduce severity of disease.
  - There is work on a vaccine for *L. salmonis.*
  - Selective breeding of more resistant fish strains.

Zoonotic Reports

- These parasites have no known zoonotic potential.

Bibliography

Fajer-Ávila, E.J., Martínez-Rodríguez, I., de la Parra, M.I.A. et al. (2008). Effectiveness of freshwater treatment against *Lepeophtheirus simplex* (Copepoda: Caligidae) and *Neobenedenia* sp. (Monogenea: Capsalidae), skin parasites of bullseye pufferfish, *Sphoeroides annulatus* reared in tanks. *Aquaculture* 284: 277–280.

Groner, M.L., Cox, R., Gettinby, G., and Revie, C.W. (2013). Use of agent-based modelling to predict benefits of cleaner fish in controlling sea lice, *Lepeophtheirus salmonis*, infestations on farmed Atlantic salmon, *Salmo salar* L. *Journal of Fish Diseases* 36: 195–208.

Iqbal, Z., Rani, I., and Pervaiz, K. (2012). Treatment of lernaeasis in carps with Thunder: an organophosphate. *Pakistan Journal of Zoology* 44: 415–420.

Justine, J., Briand, M.J., and Bray, R.A. (2012). A quick and simple method, usable in the field, for collecting parasites in suitable condition for both morphological and molecular studies. *Parasitology Research* 111: 341–351.

Kik, M.J.L., Janse, M., and Benz, G.W. (2011). The sea louse *Lepeophtheirus acutus* (Caligidae, Siphonostomatoida, Copepoda) as a pathogen of aquarium-held elasmobranchs. *Journal of Fish Diseases* 34: 793–799.

Skiftesvik, A.B., Bjelland, R.M., Durif, C.M.F. et al. (2013). Delousing of Atlantic salmon (*Salmo salar*) by cultured vs. wild ballan wrasse (*Labras bergylta*). *Aquaculture* 402-403: 113–118.

Torrissen, O., Jones, S., Asche, F. et al. (2013). Salmon lice – impact on wild salmonids and salmon aquaculture. *Journal of Fish Diseases* 36: 171–194.

Abbreviations/Acronyms

- PPE: Personal protective equipment

Isopods

Overview

- Isopods are crustaceans. Some are ectoparasites of fish, typically found on the skin or in the oral or branchial cavity of marine teleosts.
- Most isopods are incidental findings, with a single isopod found on one or two fish.
- They can cause morbidity in the affected fish, but are rarely a problem for a group.
- Gnathiid isopods are unusual in that the larvae are parasitic; they are more likely to cause morbidity in a group of fish.

Etiology

- Phylum *Arthropoda*.
- Subphylum *Crustacea*.
- Class *Malacostraca*.
- Order *Isopoda*.
- There are two major groups that parasitize fish:
  - Cymothoids (*Cymothoidae*) are typical isopods (e.g. *Ceratothoa*, *Cymothoa* spp.); a previous taxonomic group, *Flabellifera*, has been moved into *Cymothoidae*.
  - Gnathiids (*Gnathidae*), which have a different life cycle from other parasitic isopods (e.g. *Gnathia* spp.).
  - Several other families include fish parasites, but they are less common in the literature (e.g. *Corallanidae*, *Aegidae* spp.).

Life Cycle and Transmission

- The life cycle is direct, usually with only one host.
- Isopods typically have three larval stages (L1, L2, L3); adults do not molt.
- In most cases, the adults are parasitic and reproduce on the definitive host. The larger female is seen most commonly and may have a ventral marsupium filled with larvae.
- In the family *Gnathiidae*, only the larvae are parasitic. The larvae feed on blood and tissue fluids. Larvae alternate between feeding on the skin or gills (praniza phases), and nonfeeding periods off the host to molt (zuphea phases). Adults are non-feeding, free-living, and typically reproduce in the substrate.

Geographic Distribution

- Saltwater habitats, particularly tropical and subtropical.

Signalment

- Tropical and subtropical marine teleosts are the most commonly reported hosts. There are some reports in temperate marine and freshwater bony fish and marine elasmobranchs.
- Host specificity varies, e.g.:
  - *Ceratothoa gaudichaudii* in Atlantic salmon (*Salmo salar*).
  - *Gnathia trimaculata* in teleosts such as triplefins (*Enneapterygius* spp.) (L1 and L2) and a wide range of elasmobranchs, particularly demersal stingrays (L3).
  - *Gnathia maxillaris* in a wide range teleosts, particularly gilthead seabream (*Sparus aurata*) and European bass (*Dicentrarchus labrax*).

Risk Factors

- Exposure and stressors are the most important risk factors.
- Exposure includes:
  - Poor biosecurity (e.g. lack of suitable quarantine, exposure to wild fish).
  - Permissive water temperature (e.g. *G. maxillaris* prevalence is higher at 20°C (68°F) than 18°C (64°F)).
  - Outdoor or wild-caught fish.
- Common stressors are described under C7: *Monogeneans (General)*.

Signs / Clinical Findings

- Individual fish are usually affected by cymothoids.
- The isopods may be grossly visible on the skin or in the oral or branchial cavity (Figure C7.23).
- Dyspnea or tachypnea may be seen. Unilateral distension of a gill operculum is common when an isopod is in the branchial cavity.
- Reduced feeding or weight loss may be seen.
- Gill pallor may be seen due to anemia or from an isopod in the branchial cavity, in which case the pallor is often unilateral.
- Gnathiid isopods are much smaller and may be seen in high numbers on the skin or gills of several conspecifics. They may also be found around the nares, mouth, eyes, anus, or cloaca.
- Secondary infections may be seen. Isopods may be vectors for viruses, bacteria, hemoparasites, nematodes, and cestodes.

Differential Diagnoses

- Full differentials are provided in Section B.
- Common differentials for crustacean-like ectoparasites on fish include copepods, isopods, branchiurans, amphipods, and mites.

Diagnosis

- Parasitic adults are up to 6 cm in length, dorsoventrally compressed or dome-shaped, with obvious segmentation of the body and appendages. They have needle-like mouthparts for feeding.

- Parasitic larvae (*Gnathiidae*) are up to 6 mm in length, thin, slightly dome-shaped, with obvious segmentation of the body and appendages, but the segmentation is lost in the mid-abdominal area.
- Nonparasitic adults (*Gnathiidae*) are unlikely to be seen on animals but may be found if substrate or décor is examined.
- Parasite load of *Gnathiidae* can be monitored using spotlights and 200 μm plankton nets (Hispano et al. 2013). This can be used to evaluate treatments and monitor for recurrence.
- Some isopods are found in unusual sites (e.g. *Natatolana (Cirolana) borealis* migrate into the pericardium of carcharhinid sharks).
- Histology may show erosion at the attachment site. Inflammation is usually limited but some granulomatous inflammation may be present.
- If further morphological or molecular identification is required, isopods can be fixed in 10% neutral buffered formalin, 70 or 95% ethanol, or dehydrated with acetone washes (for SEM).

Husbandry Management

- These are usually an individual animal problem, where physical removal is curative.
- Management changes are only indicated if this becomes a problem for a group (e.g. with gnathiid isopods).
- Increase water flow rate and turnover.
- Increase mechanical cleaning; where possible, the substrate should be regularly siphoned to remove gnathiid isopods.
- Consider biological control; gnathiid isopods are an important food source for several teleost species (e.g. cleaner wrasse, *Labroides dimidiatus*). However, cleaner wrasse have little effect on gill parasites in demersal stingrays.

Medical Management

- Common treatments (see Chapters A12 and A13 for more details):
  - Gentle traction with forceps will usually remove an isopod. Care must be taken to not damage gill arches.

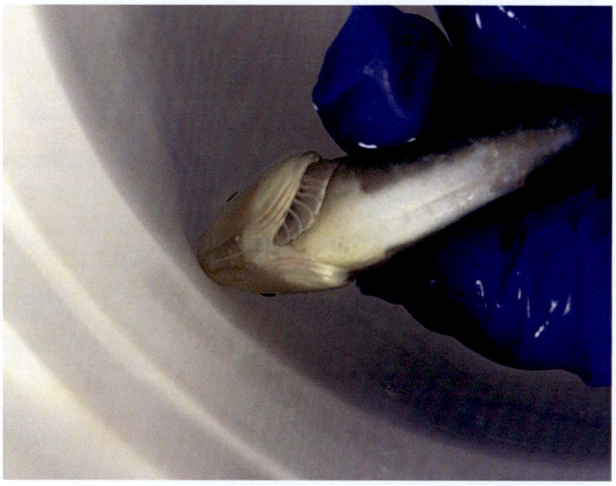

Figure C7.23 Isopod distending the operculum of a killifish (*Fundulus* sp.); ventrodorsal view.

    If the parasite cannot be removed manually, it can be killed by severing or crushing the body; it will subsequently fall off the fish.
  - Trichlorfon immersion has been reported for gnathiids at 0.3–0.5 mg/L for 48 hours every seven days for three treatments, but treatment needed to be repeated every three months. Adverse reactions to trichlorfon are common. Bioassays, close monitoring, and pretreatment with atropine should be considered. Suitable PPE must be used. Drug disposal must be considered.
- Other reported treatments (see Chapters A12 and A13 for more details):
  - Diflubenzuron orally or by immersion.
  - Lufenuron immersion.
  - Deltamethrin immersion.
- All legislation regarding medication use and disposal must be followed.

Prevention

- Isolation with no contact with free-ranging animals and suitable quarantine with close monitoring are usually enough to prevent introducing isopods into a collection.

Zoonotic Reports

- These parasites have no known zoonotic potential.

Bibliography

Bouboulis, D., Athanassopoulou, F., and Tyrpenou, A. (2004). Experimental treatments with diflubenzuron and deltamethrin of sea bass, *Dicentrarchus labrax* L., infected with the isopod, *Ceratothoa oestroides*. *Journal of Applied Ichthyology* 20: 314–317.

Heupel, M.R. and Bennett, M.B. (1999). The occurrence, distribution and pathology associated with gnathiid isopod larvae infection the epaulette shark, *Hemiscyllium ocellatum*. *International Journal for Parasitology* 29: 321–330.

Hispano, C., Bultó, P., and Blanch, A.R. (2013). *Gnathia maxillaris* infestation in exhibit aquaria: control and treatment strategies. *Journal of Applied Ichthyology* 29: 1139–1144.

Justine, J., Briand, M.J., and Bray, R.A. (2012). A quick and simple method, usable in the field, for collecting parasites in suitable condition for both morphological and molecular studies. *Parasitology Research* 111: 341–351.

Ota, Y., Hoshino, O., Hirose, M. et al. (2012). Third-state larva shifts host fish from teleost to elasmobranch in the temporary parasitic isopod, *Gnathia trimaculata* (Crustacea; Gnathiidae). *Marine Biology* 159: 2333–2347.

Rameshkumar, G. and Ravichandran, S. (2014). Problems caused by isopod parasites in commercial fishes. *Journal of Parasitic Disease* 38: 138–141.

Abbreviations/Acronyms

- PPE: Personal protective equipment
- SEM: Scanning electron microscopy

Branchiurans

Overview

- Branchiurans are ectoparasitic crustaceans, often referred to as fish lice.
- *Argulus* is the most commonly reported genus.
- *Argulus* spp. can build-up and become problematic, particularly in cyprinid ponds and salmonid aquaculture.
- Husbandry and medical management often resolve clinical signs, but recurrence is common.

Etiology

- Phylum *Arthropoda*.
- Subphylum *Crustacea*.
- Subclass *Branchiura*.
- Family *Argulidae*.
- The most well-known are *Argulus coregoni*, *Argulus foliaceus*, and *Argulus japonicus*.
- Other branchiurans are reported less commonly in fish (e.g. *Dolops*, *Chonopeltis*, *Dipteropeltis* spp.).

Life Cycle and Transmission

- The life cycle is direct.
- Adults are dioecious. Mating usually occurs on the skin of the host. Females then leave the host and deposit gelatinous strings or clutches of eggs on hard surfaces (e.g. stones) at various depths. A preference for dark substrates and shaded areas has been reported. Eggs may hatch after 10–60 days, depending on water temperature, but can remain dormant for several years. The pelagic larvae are immediately infective and can live up to four days without a host. They attach to the host using claws while adults attach using modified suckers (maxillules). Adults can survive without a host for about two weeks.
- The entire life cycle can take 30–100 days.

Geographic Distribution

- Freshwater and saltwater habitats, probably worldwide.

Signalment

- Host specificity is low.
- *Argulus* spp. are most commonly reported from freshwater bony fish including salmonids, particularly rainbow trout (*Oncorhynchus mykiss*), and cyprinids, particularly goldfish (*Carassius auratus*) and common carp and koi (*Cyprinus carpio*), as well as stingrays (*Potamotrygon* spp.). Many more species may be susceptible.

Risk Factors

- Exposure and stressors are the most important risk factors.
- Exposure includes:
  - Poor biosecurity (e.g. lack of suitable quarantine, use of surface water).
  - Permissive water temperature, often high.
  - High turbidity.
  - Low lighting.
  - Low water flow rate or turnover
  - Limited mechanical cleaning of the habitat.
- Common stressors are described under C7: *Monogeneans (General)*.

Signs/Clinical Findings

- Infected fish may be asymptomatic.
- Multiple fish from one or more species are usually affected.
- Lethargy may be seen.
- Pruritus (e.g. flashing, erratic swimming) may be seen.
- Inappetence, reduced appetite, or poor growth rates may be seen.
- The parasites are usually grossly visible on close examination of the skin, fins, or oropharynx (Figure C7.24a). They are particularly common at the base of the fins and on the head. They resemble white or dark plaques and they move slowly, which can look like shifting fish scales. There may be skin ulcers, petechiae, or increased mucus.
- Gill pallor due to anemia may be seen.

- Secondary infections may be seen.
- Mortalities may be seen.
- *Argulus* spp. may be vectors for bacterial or viral diseases (e.g. spring viremia of carp, carp pox, koi herpes virus).

Differential Diagnoses

- Full differentials are provided in Section B.
- Common differentials for crustacean-like ectoparasites on fish include copepods, isopods, branchiurans, amphipods, and mites.

Diagnosis

- Diagnosis is usually based on gross examination of the skin, fins, or oropharynx and direct microscopy of scrapes. Samples should be collected rapidly, as the parasites may leave the host when disturbed (e.g. when caught in a net).
- Adults are 3–20 mm in length with a dorsoventrally flattened body (Figure C7.24b). The external exoskeleton is obvious, with a large carapace, thorax, and abdomen. There are jointed appendages on the carapace and thorax, although these are largely hidden by the exoskeleton. The abdomen is small and bilobed. There is a pair of small compound eye spots cranially, and a pair of large suckers caudal to the compound eyes which may be mistaken for eyes.
- Eggs are long with thin, gelatinous capsules. They may be free or visible in gravid females.
- Diagnosis to genus is sufficient for management. If speciation is required, it is usually done based on external morphology, particularly the abdominal and cephalothoracic lobes. Branchiurans can be fixed in 10% neutral buffered formalin or 70 or 95% ethanol.

Husbandry Management

- Reduce or resolve stressors.
- Isolate affected systems.
- Remove unnecessary décor with smooth surfaces (e.g. stones) to reduce egg-laying sites.
- Increase water flow rate and turnover.
- Increase mechanical cleaning. Boards can be used as egg traps: they can be regularly placed at various depths then later removed.
- Drying for >24–48 hours can kill eggs; fallowing and drying ponds can be an effective protocol.
- Cleaner fish have been suggested, e.g. mosquitofish (*Gambusia affinis*), white crappies (*Pomoxis annularis*), bluegill (*Lepomis macrochirus*), and longear sunfish (*Lepomis megalotis*).

Medical Management

- Treatment should always be combined with husbandry changes as part of an integrated management strategy.
- Common treatments (see Chapters A12 and A13 for more details):
  - Diflubenzuron immersion is reported, e.g. at 0.01 mg/L every seven days after a partial water change for six weeks. This drug persists in water and regulatory issues and disposal must be considered prior to use.
  - Lufenuron immersion is reported, typically at 0.1–0.3 mg/L every seven days after a partial water change for two to five weeks. This drug persists in water and regulatory issues and disposal must be considered prior to use. Lufenuron may be used in combination with milbemycin oxime at similar doses.
  - Trichlorfon immersion at 0.2–1.0 mg/L may be used, usually repeated at 7–10 days intervals for two to three treatments. Adverse reactions to trichlorfon are common. Bioassays, close monitoring, and pretreatment with atropine should be considered. Suitable PPE must be used. Drug disposal must be considered.

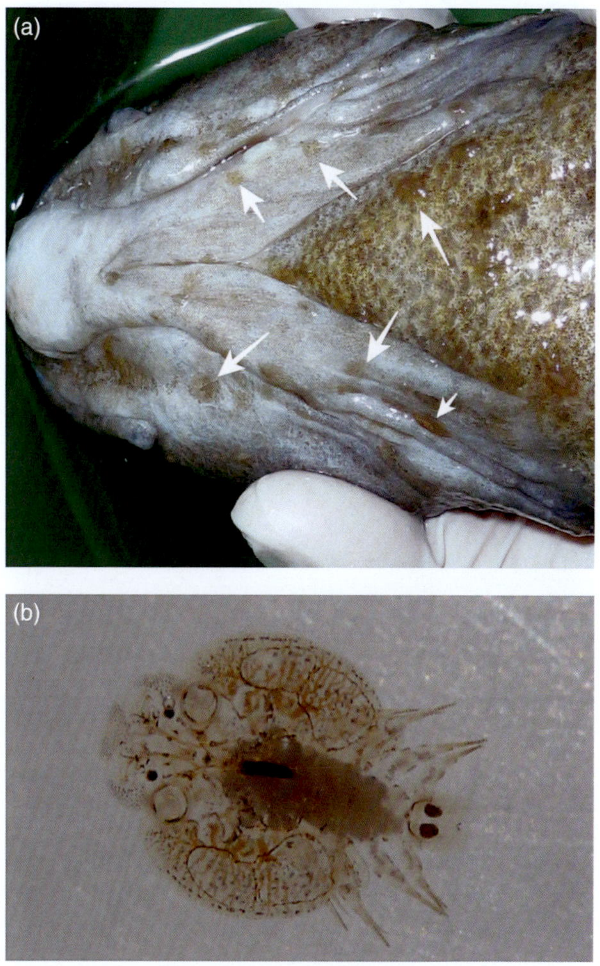

Figure C7.24 *Argulus* sp. on a giant gudgeon (*Oxyeleotris selheimi*) on examination (a; arrows) and direct microscopy at x40 (b).

  - Emamectin benzoate orally is reported, e.g. at 5–50 μg/kg every 24 hours for seven days.
- Other reported treatments (see Chapters A12 and A13 for more details):
  - Teflubenzuron orally.
  - Milbemycin oxime orally.
  - Potassium permanganate immersion.
- Hypersalinity treatment of freshwater hosts (e.g. 20 g/L) is typically not effective.
- Formalin is not effective, even at high doses.
- All legislation regarding medication use and disposal must be followed.

Prevention

- Reduce or resolve stressors.
  - Common stressors are described under C7: *Monogeneans (General)*.
- Reduce exposure and transmission.
  - Isolation with no contact with free-ranging fish.
  - Pathogen-free water source (e.g. municipal water or ground water that has gone through fine filtration (<40 μm) then UV and/or ozone disinfection). Avoid using untreated surface water.
  - Good mechanical cleaning.
  - High water flow rate or turnover.
  - All-in-all-out management with fallowing between groups, including drying.
  - Suitable quarantine with isolation, monitoring, and diagnostic testing. Prophylactic treatment of *Argulus* spp. in quarantine is rare but may be considered for known carriers, as the parasites may not be visible until naïve hosts become available.
  - Once identified, monitor for recurrence for several months following treatment and each spring as water temperatures increase.
- Reduce severity of disease.
  - Vaccination has not been effective.

Zoonotic Reports

- These parasites have no known zoonotic potential.

Bibliography

Hakalahti, T., Pasternak, A.F., and Valtonen, E.T. (2004). Seasonal dynamics of egg laying and egg-laying strategy of the ectoparasite *Argulus coregoni* (Crustacea: Branchiura). *Parasitology* 128: 655–660.

Hakalahti-Sirén, T., Mikheev, V.N., and Valtonen, E.T. (2008). Control of freshwater fish louse *Argulus coregoni*: a step towards an integrated management strategy. *Diseases of Aquatic Organisms* 82: 67–77.

Hanson, S.K., Hill, J.E., Watson, C.A. et al. (2011). Evaluation of emamectin benzoate for the control of experimentally induced infestations of *Argulus* sp. in goldfish and koi carp. *Journal of Aquatic Anial Health* 23: 30–34.

Harrison, A.J., Gault, N.F.S., and Dick, J.T.A. (2006). Seasonal and vertical patterns of egg-laying by the freshwater fish louse *Argulus foliaceus* (Crustacea: Branchiura). *Diseases of Aquatic Organisms* 68: 167–173.

Mayer, J., Hensel, P., Mejia-Fava, J. et al. (2013). The use of lufenuron to treat fish lice (*Argulus* sp) in koi (*Cyprinus carpio*). *Journal of Exotic Pet Medicine* 22: 65–69.

Schram, T.A., Iversen, L., Heuch, P.A., and Sterud, E. (2005). *Argulus* sp (Crustacea: Branchiura) on cod, *Gadus morhua*, from Finnmark, northern Norway. *Journal of the Marine Biological Association of the UK* 85: 81–86.

Tang, K.N., O'Connor, M.R., Landolfi, J., and Van Bonn, W. (2019). Safety and efficacy of milbemycin oxime and lufenuron to treat *Argulus* spp. infestation in smooth back river stingrays (*Potamotrygon orbignyi*) and Magdalena river stingrays (*Potamotrygon magdalenae*). *Journal of Zoo and Wildlife Medicine* 50: 383–388.

Taylor, N.G.H., Wootten, R., and Sommerville, C. (2009). The influence of risk factors on the abundance, egg laying habits and impact of *Argulus foliaceus* in stillwater trout fisheries. *Journal of Fish Diseases* 32: 509–519.

Abbreviations/Acronyms

- PPE: Personal protective equipment

C8

Myxozoan and Coccidial Diseases

Catherine A. Hadfield

Seattle Aquarium, Seattle, WA, USA

Introduction

Microsporidians, myxozoans, and coccidia used to be grouped together under the term sporozoa. Microsporidians are now known to be fungi and are covered in Chapter C5. Myxozoans are now classified under *Cnidaria*. *Apicomplexa* is the current group of unicellular, spore-forming, parasitic alveolates that includes the coccidia, gregarines, piroplasmas, and plasmodia. The chapter starts with a general overview of myxozoans. Several myxozoan genera and two coccidia genera (*Eimeria* and *Cryptosporidium*) are then reviewed. Where available, information is provided on the etiologic agent, life cycle and transmission, signalment, risk factors, clinical signs, diagnosis, husbandry and medical management, and prevention.

Myxozoan (General)

Overview

- Myxozoans are common parasites of wild-caught fish and pond aquaculture.
- Most of these parasites have an indirect life cycle, usually involving an oligochaete, polychaete, or bryozoan.
- Mature spores have characteristic symmetry and prominent polar capsules that are readily visible under microscopy (wet mounts and stained slides).
- In most pet, aquarium, and wild fish, myxozoan spores are usually incidental findings.
- In food fish aquaculture, some myxozoans are common and serious pathogens (e.g. *Myxobolus cerebralis* which causes whirling disease in salmonids), while others are problematic in food fish due to unsightly cysts and post-mortem liquefaction (e.g. *Kudoa thyrsites*).

Etiology

- Phylum *Cnidaria* (previously *Myxozoa*).
- Unranked subphylum *Myxozoa*.
- Class *Myxozoa* and class *Malacosporea*.
- The taxonomy has changed frequently, with "Myxozoa" being used as the phylum, subphylum, and class. The class has also been referred to as "Myxosporean". The terminology used in this publication will be the phylum *Cnidaria*, which also includes anemones and jellyfish, and two classes, *Myxozoa* and *Malacosporea*. The classes *Myxozoa* and *Malacosporea* will be considered together in this general section as the generic term "myxozoan" typically refers to both groups.
- The genera have historically been based on morphology, particularly the number of polar capsules.
- Most genera have two polar capsules. Examples include:
  - *Ceratonova*.
  - *Chloromyxum*.
  - *Enteromyxum*.
  - *Henneguya*.
  - *Hoferellus*.
  - *Myxidium*.
  - *Myxobolus*.
  - *Parvicapsula*.
  - *Sphaerospora*.
- Some genera have other numbers of polar capsules:
  - *Kudoa* – four to seven.
  - *Thelohanellus* – one.
  - *Unicapsula* – one.
- The parasites in the class *Malacosporea* look similar but they have softer spores. This class includes the salmonid parasite *Tetracapsuloides bryosalmonae*.

Clinical Guide to Fish Medicine, First Edition. Edited by Catherine A. Hadfield and Leigh Ann Clayton.

Life Cycle and Transmission

- Most have indirect life cycles.
- The terms definitive host and intermediate host vary across publications; technically the invertebrate is the definitive host and the vertebrate is the intermediate host. For clarity in this publication, the terms vertebrate host and invertebrate host will be used.
- The myxospore stage is found in the vertebrate hosts, typically fish.
- The actinospore stage is found in the invertebrate hosts, typically oligochaetes (e.g. *Tubifex* spp.), polychaetes, and bryozoans.
- Spores are usually transmitted between hosts by ingestion or by release into the water when the host dies or when lesions rupture; some can be released into the water in feces and urine.
- Spores are only infectious for a brief time after release from the invertebrate host, typically <1 day, although up to seven days in some cases.
- When in the vertebrate host, the parasite migrates to a final site of maturation that is either histozoic (intra- or intercellular) or coelozoic (in hollow organs such as the gastrointestinal or urinary tract). At the final site, multinucleate plasmodia (pseudocysts) can develop, and mature spores develop within these.
- Approximately 5% of myxospore stages have been matched with their actinospore stages, e.g.:
  - *Ceratonova shasta* in salmon and *Manayunkia speciosa* in freshwater polychaetes.
  - *Henneguya ictaluri* in channel catfish and *Aurantiactinomyxon ictaluri* in oligochaetes *Dero digitata*.
- Some myzoxoans can show direct life cycles with transmission between fish (e.g. *Enteromyxum*, *Myxobolus* spp.).
- The life cycle varies from days to months.
- Fish that resolve clinical signs probably become carriers.
- Transmission to and from wild and cultured fish is common (also known as spill-forward and spill-back).

Geographic Distribution

- Myxozoans are found in freshwater and saltwater habitats, probably worldwide.
- Distribution of each parasite species depends on the range or culture location of the host species.

Signalment

- Myxozoans typically infect fish that were wild-caught or pond-reared, particularly temperate freshwater teleosts, although all species are likely susceptible.
- Host ranges are usually narrow, e.g. *Sinuolinea phyllopteryxa* in weedy sea dragons (*Phyllopteryx taeniolatus*).
- Myxozoans have been identified sporadically in elasmobranchs (e.g. *Kudoa* and *Chloromyxum* spp.).
- Juvenile fish typically show more severe signs, although some myxozoans initially present in older fish before encompassing all age classes (e.g. enteromyxosis in gilthead seabream, *Sparus aurata*), or present after harvesting (e.g. *K. thyrsites*).

Risk Factors

- Exposure and stressors are the most important risk factors.
- Exposure:
  - Poor biosecurity (e.g. lack of suitable quarantine, use of surface water, exposure to free-ranging fish or invertebrates).
  - Abundant habitat for invertebrate hosts.
  - Permissive water temperature.
  - Permissive salinity.
  - High organic loads.
  - Low water flow rate or turnover.
  - Exposure of naïve fish.
  - Established infection; once established in a large habitat, this becomes a recurrent issue.
- Stressors:
  - High stocking density.
  - Inappropriate social structure.
  - Inappropriate environment.
  - Poor water quality.
  - High water temperature; most myxozoan infections are more likely to be transmitted and progress more rapidly during summer months.
  - Poor nutrition.
  - Recent transport.

Signs/Clinical Findings

- Fish are often asymptomatic.
- If clinical signs are present, they may be seen in individual fish or several conspecifics.
- Clinical signs may develop within weeks of infection (e.g. *Sphaerospora renicola* in common carp) or several months or years later (e.g. *M. cerebralis* in rainbow trout, *K. thyrsites* in Atlantic salmon).
- Inappetence, reduced feeding, weight loss, or poor growth rates are common. The weight loss can be severe.
- Gill pallor due to anemia may be seen.
- Other signs depend on the myxozoan species, its tissue preference, the parasite load, and the host response.
- Most myxozoans are histozoic and can cause white nodules known as pseudocysts or present with a disseminated infection. Most are tissue-specific but some can be distributed more widely. Histozoic myxozoans are usually more pathogenic than coelozoic.

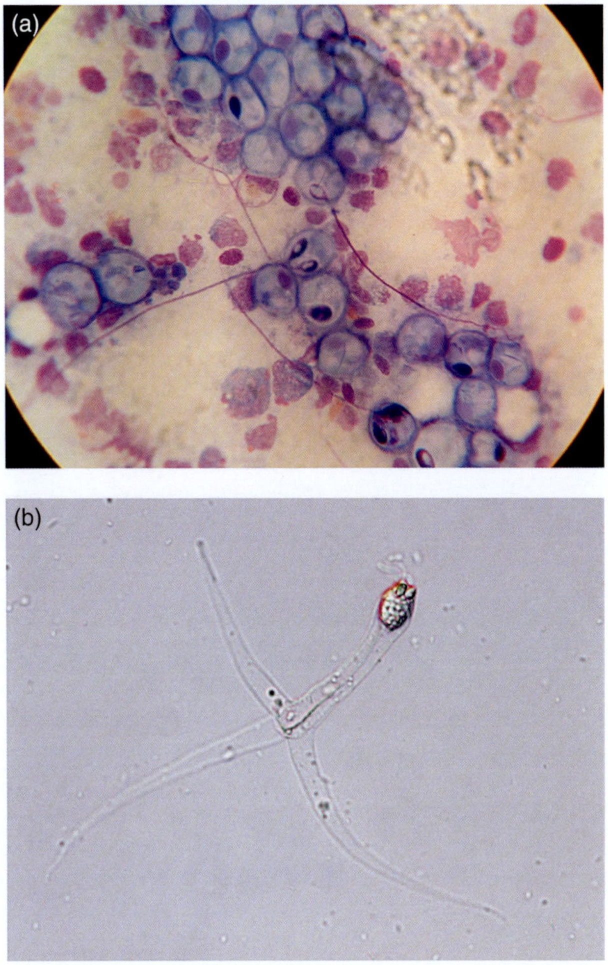

Figure C8.1 "Typical" myxozoan spores with two polar capsules seen on impression smear using Dif-Quik stain (a), and bright-field microscopy of the actinospore stage of a *Myxobolus* sp. (b). *Source*: Image (b) courtesy of Bartolomeo Gorgoglione, University of Veterinary Medicine, Vienna.

  - Gill infections can lead to dyspnea, tachypnea, and nodules or other grossly visible gill abnormalities (e.g. *Henneguya* spp., *Myxobolus koi*).
  - Renal infections may present with coelomic distension or edema (e.g. *Hoferellus carassii*, *T. bryosalmonae*).
  - Neural and cartilaginous infections can cause circling or spiral swimming, skeletal abnormalities, dark tails, or exophthalmos (e.g. *Myxobolus balantiocheili*, *M. cerebralis*).
  - Muscle infections may present with abnormal swimming but may not be noted until nodules or liquefaction is seen at processing, after harvesting the fish.
- Some myxozoans are coelozoic and reside within hollow organs (e.g. intestinal tract, gallbladder, swim bladder, kidney tubules, urinary bladder). Coelozoic myxozoans are usually less pathogenic than histozoic.
  - Intestinal infections can cause lethargy, weight loss, coelomic distension, cloacal, or anal swelling (e.g. *Ceratonova shasta*, *Enteromyxum* spp.).
  - Gallbladder and urinary tract infections are less likely to cause clinical signs (e.g. *Chloromyxum* spp.).
- Mortality is usually low and sporadic but can reach 100% in fish under severe or chronic stressors or under multiple stressors.
- Survivors can show regeneration of damaged tissue, with the rate of improvement dependent on water temperature.
- Survivors are probably carriers that can release viable spores years post-infection, but some survivors show immunity.

Differential Diagnoses

- Differentials are described for each myxozoan group below.

Diagnosis

- Myxozoans are usually identified on direct microscopy, impression smear, or histology of affected tissues. Important features for tentative identification are spore shape, the number of polar capsules, and host and tissue specificity.
- Affected tissues may show visible nodules known as pseudocysts, be diffusely abnormal, or be grossly normal.
- Mature spores are typically 8–24 μm in length and bilaterally or radially symmetric. Most species have two polar capsules (Figure C8.1), although species with one to seven polar capsules are seen. Some spores have one or more caudal processes, also known as a tail (e.g. *Henneguya* spp.).
- Myxozoans are detectable on most routine stains. Mature polar capsules are strongly Gram-positive and Giemsa-positive, and shell valves are acid-fast positive. The spore wall is typically positive on periodic acid-Schiff stain.
- Histologic lesions depend on tissue site, parasite load, and the host response. Inflammation may be present and is typically chronic and granulomatous.
- Culture has not been possible.
- Definitive species identification requires TEM or molecular techniques.
- PCR and ISH tests are available commercially to detect some myxozoans (e.g. *M. cerebralis*, *K. thyrsites*). Tissues are best, but swabs have been effective (e.g. rectal swab for *Enteromyxum leei* PCR). The tests show a higher sensitivity than histology or direct microscopy.
- qPCR tests allow assessment of parasite load and can be done on water samples.

- ELISAs are used experimentally and can detect infection before spores are visible histologically.
- *M. cerebralis* may be reportable to state or national agencies. It is reportable in the United States.

Husbandry Management

- Management changes may not be indicated unless there are clinical signs.
- Increase aeration, particularly if there is gill damage; target dissolved oxygen may be 95–100%.
- Remove dead or moribund fish as soon as possible.
- Remove or reduce mud and increase substrate cleaning to reduce exposure to invertebrate hosts.
- Increase the flow rate of flow-through systems.
- Increase the turnover of recirculating systems (e.g. >1 exchange/h) to try to reduce reinfection rates.
- Regularly back-wash filters, such as sand filters.
- Add a sand filter, fine filtration (<40 µm), ozone (>700 mV for 10 minutes contact time), and/or UV disinfection (>30–40 mWs/cm^2 or mJ/cm^2) to recirculating or incoming water.
- Increase cleaning and disinfection of the habitat and fomites. These target primarily the actinospore stage; the myxospore stage is resistant to most disinfectants, so these practices serve only to reduce parasite load.
  - Small equipment or empty systems can be disinfected with sodium hypochlorite at 130–500 mg/L chlorine for 10–15 minutes, ammonium chloride at 1500 mg/L for 10 minutes, benzalkonium chloride at 1500 mg/L for 10 minutes, hydrogen peroxide (>10%) for 10 minutes, or Virkon-Aquatic 0.5–1.0% for five minutes, followed by full drying.
  - Keeping materials at >20°C (>68°F) for >two months can be effective.
  - Saltwater systems can be cleaned with freshwater, and vice versa, to reduce parasite viability.
- If signs are mild and fish can handle a transport, consider moving them to suitable, uninfected systems.
- If signs are severe, consider depopulation and disinfection.

Medical Management

- Treatment may improve clinical signs but does not resolve the infection and spores are typically carried for the life of the animal.
- In general, combination treatments show more promise than single treatments.
- Many of the reported treatments can cause adverse effects.
- Many of the proposed treatments are under regulatory control.
- Common treatments (see Chapters A12 and A13 for more details):
  - Salinomycin and amprolium orally.
  - Fumagillin orally, where available.
- Other reported treatments (see Chapters A12 and A13 for more details):
  - Toltrazuril orally.
  - Robenidine and sulfonamides orally or by immersion.
  - Furazolidone orally.
  - Acetarsone orally.
  - Narasin and nicarbazine orally.
- Specific treatment protocols are described for each genus.
- Surgical removal has been reported for individual fish.
- All legislation regarding medication use and disposal must be followed.

Prevention

- Reduce or resolve stressors.
  - Low stocking density.
  - Suitable social groups and habitats.
  - Excellent water quality and preferred water temperature.
  - Good nutrition.
  - Suitable handling and transport protocols.
- Reduce exposure through good biosecurity.
  - Isolation with no contact with free-ranging animals, particularly invertebrate hosts (e.g. *Tubifex*, blackworms, red worms).
  - Pathogen-free water source (e.g. municipal water or ground water that has gone through fine filtration then UV and/or ozone disinfection). Avoid using untreated surface water.
  - Disinfection of recirculating water with fine filtration then ozone and/or UV.
  - High water flow rate or turnover.
  - Removal of dead or moribund fish as soon as possible with appropriate disposition.
  - Regular removal of mud and other organic debris. Consider changing to an inorganic substrate if suitable for the species.
  - Good cleaning and disinfection protocols, including frequent changing of nets.
  - All-in-all-out systems, with fallowing and drying of systems between groups.
  - Suitable quarantine with isolation, monitoring, and diagnostic testing, particularly necropsy, cytology, histology, and PCR or qPCR. Quarantine should apply to new animals as well as animals returning from shows or loans. This cannot prevent disease, as infection may not present until months after infection, but it reduces the risk.

  - Freeze seafood to −20°C (−4°F) for more than seven days to reduce parasite load, although some (e.g. *M. cerebralis* spores at high loads) can survive freezing for two to four months. Do not use live feeds.
  - Biological control of invertebrate hosts with juvenile carp (*Cyprinus* spp.), fathead minnows (*Pimephales promelas*), smallmouth buffalofish (*Ictiobus bubalus*), or freshwater shrimp.
- Reduce severity of disease.
  - Sentinel fish or routine PCR or qPCR to catch an outbreak early and prevent introducing naïve fish into a system that is breaking with a myxozoan infection.
  - Careful stock selection (e.g. non-susceptible species or selective breeding for resistance).
  - Only adding susceptible fish after permissive temperatures have passed (e.g. after the summer) or after the fish are more than six months old.
- Immune stimulants have provided no protection from disease following subsequent exposure.

Zoonotic Reports

- There is no known zoonotic potential from inoculation or immersion.
- There are rare reports of myxozoans as potential foodborne pathogens following the consumption of raw or inadequately cooked or processed fish (e.g. *Kudoa septempunctata* causing diarrhea and vomiting). The signs have been self-limiting.

Bibliography

Azevedo, C., Casal, G., Garcia, P. et al. (2009). Ultrastructural and phylogenetic data of the *Chloromyxum riorajum* sp. nov. (Myxozoa), a parasite of the stingray *Rioraja agassizii* in Southern Brazil. *Diseases of Aquatic Organisms* 85: 41–51.

Bobadila, A., Palenzuela, O., Riaza, A. et al. (2006). Risk factors associated with *Enteromyxum scophthalmi* (Myxozoa) infection in cultured turbot (*Scophthalmus maximus* L.). *Parasitology* 13: 433–442.

Cobcroft, J.M. and Battaglene, S.C. (2012). Ultraviolet irradiation is an effective alternative to ozonation as a sea water treatment to prevent *Kudoa neurophila* (Myxozoa: Myxosporea) infection of striped trumpeter, *Latris lineata* (Forster). *Journal of Fish Diseases* 36: 57–65.

Kawai, T., Sekizuka, T., Yahata, Y. et al. (2012). Identification of *Kudoa septempunctata* as the causative agent of novel food poisoning outbreaks in Japan by consumption of *Paralichthys olivaceus* in raw fish. *Clinical Infectious Diseases* 54: 1046–1052.

Kent, M.L., Andree, K.B., Bartholomew, J.L. et al. (2001). Recent advances in our knowledge of the Myxozoa. *Journal of Eukaryotic Microbiology* 48: 395–413.

Shin, S.P., Jee, H., Jan, J.E. et al. (2011). Surgical removal of an anal cyst caused by a protozoan parasite (*Thelohanellus kitauei*) from a koi (*Cyprinus carpio*). *Journal of the American Veterinary Medical Association* 238: 784–786.

Whipps, C.M.K., Murray, K.N., and Kent, M.L. (2015). Occurrence of a myxozoan parasite *Myxidium streisingeri* n. sp. in laboratory zebrafish *Danio rerio*. *Journal of Parasitology* 101: 86–90.

Abbreviations/Acronyms

- ELISA: Enzyme linked immunosorbent assay
- ISH: In situ hybridization
- PCR: Polymerase chain reaction
- qPCR: Quantitative polymerase chain reaction
- TEM: Transmission electron microscopy
- UV: Ultraviolet

Enteromyxum spp.

Overview

- *Enteromyxum* spp. are coelozoic myxozoans that infect the intestines and sometimes the gallbladder of a variety of marine teleosts.
- They typically cause chronic enteritis and severe wasting.
- *Enteromyxum leei* and *Enteromyxum scophthalmi* are serious pathogens in some cultured food fish.

Etiology

- Phylum *Cnidaria.*
- Class *Myxozoa.*
- Family *Myxidiidae.*
- Several species cause disease in fish, including:
  - *Enteromyxum* (*Myxidium*) *leei.*
  - *Enteromyxum scophthalmi.*
  - *Enteromyxum fugu.*
- The disease is known as enteromyxosis.

Life Cycle and Transmission

- General life cycle information is described under C8: *Myxozoa (General).*
- An indirect life cycle with invertebrate and fish hosts seems likely.
- An additional direct life cycle has been shown for *E. leei* and *E. scophthalmi*, with transmission between fish through cohabitation, ingestion, and waterborne exposure. This is unusual for myxozoans.

Geographic Distribution

- *E. leei* has been reported from a variety of saltwater habitats including the Mediterranean, Red Sea, Canary Islands, and Japan. Some Indo-Pacific fish in the aquarium trade have been found to be infected, including in the United States.
- *E. scophthalmi* has been reported from Spain.
- *E. fugu* has been reported from Japan.

Signalment

- *E. leei* has an unusually wide host range affecting >46 species of warm-water marine teleosts.
  - Cultured food fish include gilthead seabream (*Sparus aurata*), sharpsnout seabream (*Diplodus puntazzo*), red seabream (*Pagrus major*), tiger puffer (*Takifugu rubripes*), red drum (*Sciaenops ocellatus*), knifejaw (*Oplegnathus punctatus*), turbot (*Scophthalmus maximus*), European bass (*Dicentrarchus labrax*), and olive flounder (*Paralichthys olivaceus*).
  - Aquarium species include blennies (*Blenniidae*), wrasses (*Labridae*), yellow tangs (*Zebrasoma flavescens*), powder blue tangs (*Acanthurus leucosternon*), and emperor angelfish (*Pomacanthus imperator*).
  - Wild species include mullet (*Liza*, *Mugil*, *Chelon* spp.).
- *E. scophthalmi* is reported from cultured turbot and Senegalese sole (*Solea senegalensis*).
- *E. fugu* is reported from cultured tiger puffers.
- Experimental infection of freshwater teleosts has been possible.
- Disease may show in older fish first, before encompassing all age classes. This is unusual for a myxozoan.

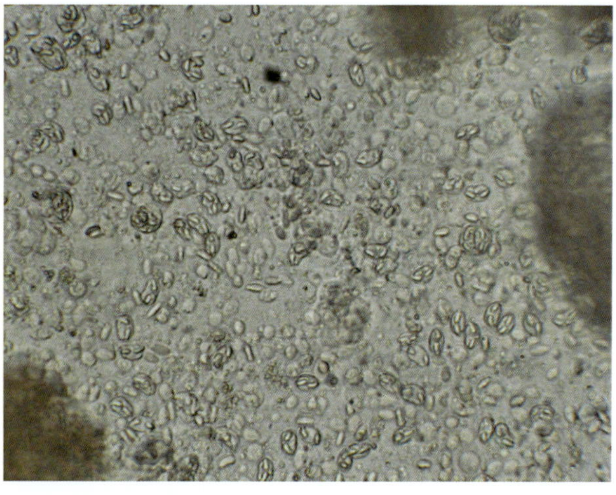

Figure C8.2 *Enteromyxum* sp. spores on direct cytology of the gastrointestinal tract of a yellow tang (*Zebrasoma flavescens*). Fully developed spores with two polar capsules are visible, along with other stages. *Source*: Image courtesy of Michael Hyatt, Wildlife Conservation Society.

Risk Factors

- General risk factors are described under C8: *Myxozoa (General).*
- Permissive water temperature is often 15–22°C (59–72°F).

Signs/Clinical Findings

- Clinical signs may take months to show following infection.
- Inappetence or reduced feeding and severe weight loss are common.
- Coelomic distension is common.
- Cloacal or anal prolapse may be seen.
- Skin discoloration or scale loss may be seen.
- Enophthalmos may be seen.
- Gill pallor due to anemia may be seen.
- Mortalities are usually chronic and intermittent but can reach 100% under other stressors.

Differential Diagnoses

- Full differentials are described in Section B.
- Common differentials for weight loss in a group of teleosts include chronic disease (often viral, bacterial, or parasitic), and nutritional or social factors.

Diagnosis

- Diagnosis is typically from finding characteristic spores in the intestinal tract on cytology or histology or on fecal examination (Figure C8.2). The parasites are occasionally found in the stomach, esophagus, or gallbladder.
- Mature spores are ~15–18 × 6–10 μm and bilaterally symmetrical, with two polar capsules, each ~8 × 3 μm. Sporoblasts are thin-walled and contain a number of spores. The parasites are detectable on most routine stains and the polar capsules stain Gram-positive and shell valves stain acid-fast positive.
- Necropsy usually shows severe emaciation with catarrhal enteritis and an enlarged gallbladder. Viscera may be pale and the liver may be stained green. Edema may be present.
- PCR and ISH tests are available and premortem testing for *E. leei* is possible using rectal swabs.
- False negatives are possible on cytology, histology, and PCR, particularly at <15°C (<59°F).

Husbandry Management

- General husbandry management is described under C8: *Myxozoa (General).*
- Consider slowly increasing water temperature to >25°C (77°F) to reduce clinical signs.

Medical Management

- General medical management is described under C8: *Myxozoa (General).*
- Reported treatments (see Chapters A12 and A13 for more details):
  - Salinomycin and amprolium together orally can reduce clinical signs and mortality. Doses have included salinomycin at 70 mg/kg and amprolium at 100 mg/kg every 24 hours for 56–60 days.
- All legislation regarding medication use and disposal must be followed.

Prevention

- General preventative measures are described under C8: *Myxozoa (General).*

Zoonotic Reports

- These parasites have no known zoonotic potential.

Bibliography

Bobadila, A., Palenzuela, O., Riaza, A. et al. (2006). Risk factors associated with *Enteromyxum scophthalmi* (Myxozoa) infection in cultured turbot (*Scophthalmus maximus* L.). *Parasitology* 13: 43–42.

Golomazou, E., Athanassopoulou, F., Karagouni, E. et al. (2006). Efficacy and toxicity of orally administrated anti-coccidial drug treatment on *Enteromyxum leei* infections in sharpsnout seabream (*Diplodus puntazzo* C.). *Israeli Journal of Aquaculture* 58: 157–169.

Hyatt, M., Waltzek, T.B., Kieran, E.A. et al. (2018). Diagnosis and treatment of multi-species fish mortality attributed to *Enteromyxum leei* while in quarantine at a US aquarium. *Diseases of Aquatic Organisms* 132: 37–48.

Katharios, P., Rigos, G., and Divanach, P. (2011). *Enteromyxum leei* (Myxozoa), a lethal intruder of tropical pet fish: first case in humphead wrasse, *Cheilinus undulatus* (Ruppel, 1835). *Journal of Exotic Pet Medicine* 20: 138–143.

Kent, M.L., Andree, K.B., Bartholomew, J.L. et al. (2001). Recent advances in our knowledge of the Myxozoa. *Journal of Eukaryotic Microbiology* 48: 395–413.

Padrós, F., Palenzuela, O., Hispano, C. et al. (2001). *Myxidium leei* (Myxozoa) infections in aquarium-reared Mediterranean fish species. *Diseases of Aquatic Organisms* 47: 57–62.

Quiroga, M.I., Redondo, M.J., Sitjà-Bobadilla, A. et al. (2006). Risk factors associated with *Enteromyxum scophthalmi* (Myxozoa) infection in cultured turbot, *Scophthalmus maximus* (L.). *Parasitology* 133: 433–442.

Yanagida, T., Yokoyama, H., Palenzuela, O. et al. (2008). Myxosporean emaciation disease of cultured red sea bream *Pagrus major* and spotted knifejaw *Oplegnathus punctatus*. *Fish Pathology* 48: 45–48.

Abbreviations/Acronyms

- ISH: In situ hybridization
- PCR: Polymerase chain reaction

Henneguya spp.

Overview

- *Henneguya* spp. are histozoic myxozoans with a predilection for gill tissue.
- The most commonly reported species is *Henneguya ictaluri.* This is a serious pathogen of channel catfish (*Ictalurus punctatus*) in aquaculture. The disease is called proliferative gill disease or hamburger gill disease.
- Several species cause disease in fish, including:
  - *Henneguya ictaluri.*
  - *Henneguya koi.*
  - *Henneguya salminicola.*
  - *Henneguya zschokkei*, considered synonymous with *H. salminicola* in some texts.
  - *Henneguya exilis.*

Etiology

- Phylum *Cnidaria.*
- Class *Myxozoa.*
- Family *Myxobolidae.*

Life Cycle and Transmission

- General life cycle information is described under C8: *Myxozoa (General).*

- The myxospore and actinospore stages are known for *H. ictaluri*.
  - Channel catfish are the vertebrate host.
  - Benthic oligochaetes (*Dero digitata* and sometimes *Dero furcata*) are the invertebrate host. The actinospore stage is called *Aurantiactinomyxon ictaluri*.

Geographic Distribution

- Freshwater and saltwater habitats, probably worldwide.
- Distribution of each parasite species depends on the range or culture location of the host species (e.g. *H. ictaluri* is found where channel catfish aquaculture is common, including Alabama, Arkansas, Mississippi, Louisiana, and California).

Signalment

- *Henneguya* spp. can affect >30 spp. of warm freshwater and saltwater bony fish, e.g.:
  - *H. ictaluri* in channel catfish and hybrids, although disease may be less severe in hybrids.
  - *H. koi* in carp (*Cyprinus carpio*).
  - *H. salminicola* and *H. zschokkei* in Pacific salmonids, particularly Chinook (*Oncorhynchus tshawytscha*) and coho salmon (*Oncorhynchus kisutch*).

Risk Factors

- General risk factors are described under C8: *Myxozoa (General)*.
- Permissive water temperature is often high (e.g. 16–25°C (61–77°F) for *H. ictaluri*).

Signs/Clinical Findings

- Inappetence, reduced feeding, weight loss, and poor growth rates are common.
- Dyspnea and tachypnea are common, despite adequate dissolved oxygen.
- The gills may look mottled, mashed, edematous, and bleed easily (similar to raw hamburger meat, giving the disease its common name in catfish).
- Mortality can exceed 50% in some outbreaks.
- Following an outbreak in a pond, the disease does not usually recur that season.

Differential Diagnoses

- Full differentials are described in Section B.
- Common differentials for dyspnea and tachypnea in teleosts include hypoxia, ammonia toxicity, and ectoparasites or other gill disease.
- Other common diseases of channel catfish that can present with nonspecific signs are channel catfish virus, *Edwardsiella ictaluri*, *Yersinia ruckeri*, *Flavobacterium columnaris*, *Ichthyophthirius multifiliis*, and monogeneans.
- Differentials for tailed myxozoan spores with two polar capsules include *Henneguya*, *Myxobilatus*, *Hennegoides*, *Thelohanellus*, *Tetrauronema*, *Dicauda*, and *Unicauda*.

Diagnosis

- A tentative diagnosis may be made based on clinical signs in susceptible species. Confirmation is usually by cytology, histology, or molecular testing.
- Mature spores are slender, ~35–50 × 8–11 µm, bilaterally symmetrical, with two polar capsules. Each spore has two caudal processes or tails (Figure C8.3). Spores are seen during the acute phase of the disease but may not be seen with more chronic cases. The parasites are detectable on most routine stains and the polar capsules stain Gram-positive and shell valves stain acid-fast positive.
- Histology is more sensitive than cytology. It can show severe branchitis with epithelial hyperplasia, fusion, and gill cartilage lysis or fractures. These cartilage lesions in pond-reared channel catfish with normal skin are considered pathognomonic for *H. ictaluri*. Multifocal muscle cysts with milky fluid are typical of *H. salminicola* and *H. zschokkei*. Inflammation may be granulomatous.
- PCR and qPCR tests are available and can be run on gill swabs, gill tissue, or water samples. Humic acids in the water interfere with testing.
- TEM can be used for diagnosis.

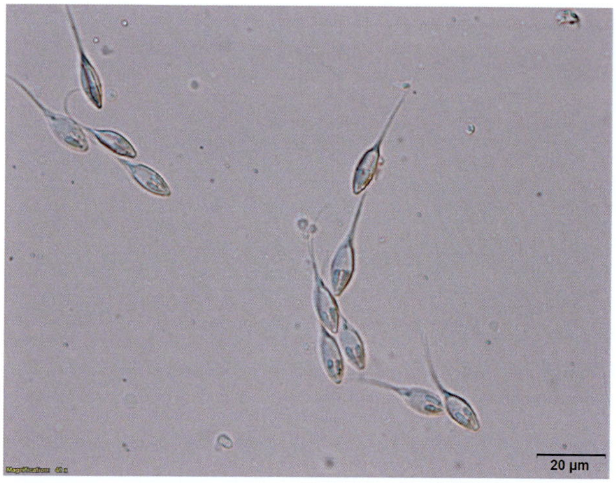

Figure C8.3 Bright-field microscopy of *Henneguya creplini* myxospores from a redfin perch (*Perca fluviatilis*). *Source*: Image courtesy of Bartolomeo Gorgoglione, University of Veterinary Medicine, Vienna.

Husbandry Management

- General husbandry management is described under C8: *Myxozoa (General).*
- Many fish will recover if removed from the source of infection and if stressors are minimized.

Medical Management

- Medical treatment is rarely effective.
- All legislation regarding medication use and disposal must be followed.

Prevention

- General preventative measures are described under C8: *Myxozoa (General).*
- Blue catfish (*Ictalurus furcatus*) may be a better choice than channel catfish where *H. ictaluri* is endemic, although they usually have less favorable production characteristics.

Zoonotic Reports

- These parasites have no known zoonotic potential.

Bibliography

Griffin, M.J., Pote, L.M., Camus, A.C. et al. (2009). Application of a real-time PCR assay for the detection of *Henneguya ictaluri* in commercial channel catfish ponds. *Diseases of Aquatic Organisms* 86: 223–233.

Griffin, M.J., Camus, A.C., Wise, D.J. et al. (2010). Variation in susceptibility of *Henneguya ictaluri* infection by two species of catfish and their hybrid cross. *Journal of Aquatic Animal Health* 22: 21–35.

Kent, M.L., Andree, K.B., Bartholomew, J.L. et al. (2001). Recent advances in our knowledge of the Myxozoa. *Journal of Eukaryotic Microbiology* 48: 395–413.

Wise, D.J., Griffin, M.J., Terhune, J.S. et al. (2008). Induction and evaluation of proliferative gill disease in channel catfish fingerlings. *Journal of Aquatic Animal Health* 20: 236–244.

Abbreviations/Acronyms

- PCR: Polymerase chain reaction
- qPCR: Quantitative polymerase chain reaction
- TEM: Transmission electron microscopy

Myxobolus spp.

Overview

- *Myxobolus* spp. are histozoic myxozoans with a predilection for cartilage. Of these, *Myxobolus cerebralis* is the most commonly reported species.
- *M. cerebralis* causes whirling disease in salmonids (*Salmonidae*). This is a serious disease of both cultured and wild populations. Transmission to wild stock from restoration and restocking programs is a particular concern.
- *Myxobolus* spp. rarely cause significant problems in aquariums.

Etiology

- Phylum *Cnidaria.*
- Class *Myxozoa.*
- Family *Myxobolidae.*
- Several species cause disease in fish, including:
  - *Myxobolus* (*Myxosoma*) *cerebralis.*
  - *Myxobolus koi.*
  - *Myxobolus albi.*

Life Cycle and Transmission

- General life cycle information is described under C8: *Myxozoa (General).*
- The myxospore and actinospore stages are known for *M. cerebralis.*
  - Salmonids are the vertebrate host.
  - Oligochaetes (*Tubifex tubifex*) are the invertebrate host. The actinospore stage is called *Triactinomyxon dubium* or *Triactinomyxon gyrosalmo*, often referred to as TAMs.
- Actinospores are only viable for three to four days in 12°C (54°F) water and for shorter periods at higher water temperatures.
- The life cycle takes months at typical temperatures.
- As well as the indirect life cycle, *Myxobolus* spp. can show direct transmission between fish; this is unusual for myxozoans.
- Transmission between infected water sources can be due to piscivorous birds and anthropogenic activity, particularly commercial stocking of infected fish.

Geographic Distribution

- *M. cerebralis* is native to the Eurasian continent. The current distribution includes freshwater and saltwater habitats around North America, Columbia, New Zealand, and South Africa.

Signalment

- *M. cerebralis* is reported in farmed and wild freshwater salmonids, particularly rainbow trout (*Oncorhynchus mykiss*); also sockeye salmon (*Oncorhynchus nerka*), cutthroat trout (*Oncorhynchus clarkii*), gila salmon (*Oncorhynchus gilae*), brook trout (*Salvelinus fontinalis*), Danube salmon (*Hucho hucho*), and grayling (*Thymallus thymallus*). Brown trout (*Salmo trutta*) and lake trout (*Salvelinus namaycush*) can be infected but rarely show clinical signs.
- *M. albi* is reported in common gobies (*Pomatoschistus microps*) and lumpfish (*Cyclopterus lumpus*).
- The disease is typically more severe in young fish, before cartilage becomes ossified.

Risk Factors

- General risk factors are described under C8: *Myxozoa (General).*
- *M. cerebralis* causes highest morbidity and mortality at ~10–15°C (50–59°F).

Signs/Clinical Findings

- Inappetence or reduced feeding, weight loss, and poor growth rates are common.
- Other signs depend on the species and target tissue.
- *M. cerebralis* affects cartilage and nerves.
  - Abnormal swimming is common in acute infections, typically rapid spiraling; this is the reason for the common name of whirling disease.
  - Dark tails, sometimes known as black-tail, are common in three to six month old salmonids during acute infections.
  - Skeletal abnormalities are seen during or following chronic infections. These include short opercula, short rostrums, and jaw and spinal deformities.
  - Exophthalmos may be seen.
- *M. koi* primarily affects gill cartilage.
  - Dyspnea and tachypnea are common.
  - White to tan nodules on the gills are common.
- *M. albi* affects cartilage of the gills, skull, or pectoral girdle.
  - Exophthalmos is the most common sign in lumpfish, with white to tan nodules on the sclera.
- Mortality is usually low and sporadic but may reach 100% in young fish or under other stressors.

Differential Diagnoses

- Full differentials are described in Section B.
- Common differentials for spiral swimming in a group of teleosts include toxin exposure or central nervous system infection, which may be bacterial (particularly *Streptococcus* and *Vibrio* spp.), viral, or parasitic (particularly *Myxobolus* spp.).

Diagnosis

- A tentative diagnosis is often based on finding spores on histology of affected tissues. Confirmation usually requires molecular testing.
- Mature spores may be in plasmodia within pseudocysts. They are broad oval spores, typically ~8 × 9 μm, with two polar capsules that are bilaterally symmetrical (Figure C8.4). The parasites are detectable on most routine stains and the polar capsules stain Gram-positive and shell valves stain acid-fast positive.
- Necropsy or coeliotomy are often unremarkable apart from the clinical signs described above.
- Histology typically shows granulomatous inflammation and characteristic spores at the tissue site (e.g. *M. cerebralis* in salmonid cartilage). Many commercial laboratories provide this diagnostic for salmonids.
- PCR and ISH tests are available commercially for *M. cerebralis* and show a higher sensitivity than histology or direct microscopy. qPCR tests allow assessment of parasite load and can be done on water samples.
- *M. cerebralis* may be reportable to local or national agencies. It is reportable in the United States.

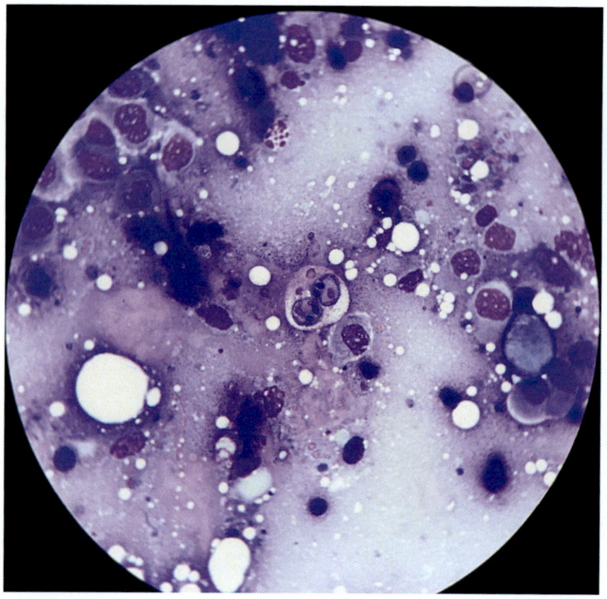

Figure C8.4 Spores from a *Myxobolus* sp. on impression smear using Dif-Quik® stain. *Source*: Image courtesy of Pierre-Marie Boitard, Fili@vet.

Husbandry Management

- General husbandry management is described under C8: *Myxozoa (General).*

Medical Management

- This parasite is often considered an incidental finding.
- Medical treatment is rarely effective, although combination treatments show more promise than single treatments.
- Reported treatments (see Chapters A12 and A13 for more details):
  - Salinomycin and amprolium orally, each at ~110 mg/kg every 24 hours for 30 days, has typically been the most effective protocol for reducing severity of clinical signs.
- All legislation regarding medication use and disposal must be followed.

Prevention

- General preventative measures are described under C8: *Myxozoa (General).*
- Monitor closely for clinical signs or routinely test for *M. cerebralis* in young salmonids.
- Brown trout and lake trout may be a better culture choice than other salmonids in systems where *M. cerebralis* is endemic.

Zoonotic Reports

- These parasites have no known zoonotic potential.

Bibliography

Arndt, R.E. and Wagner, E.J. (2004). Rapid and slow sand filtration techniques and their efficacy at filtering triactinomyxons of *Myxobolus cerebralis* from contaminated water. *North American Journal of Aquaculture* 66: 261–270.

Arndt, R.E., Wagner, E.J., Bobo, C., and St. John, T. (2006). Laboratory and hatchery-scale evaluation of sand filters and their efficacy at controlling whirling disease infection. *Journal of Aquatic Animal Health* 18: 215–222.

Athanassopoulou, F., Karagouni, E., Dotsika, E. et al. (2004). Efficacy and toxicity of orally administrated anti-coccidial drugs for innovative treatments of *Myxobolus* sp. infection in *Puntazzo puntazzo*. *Diseases of Aquatic Organisms* 62: 217–226.

Cavin, J.M., Donahoe, S.L., Frasca, S. et al. (2012). *Myxobolus albi* infection in cartilage of captive lumpfish (*Cyclopterus lumpus*). *Journal of Veterinary Diagnostic Investigation* 24: 516–524.

Hedrick, R.P., McDowell, T.S., Mukkatira, K. et al. (2008). The effects of freezing, drying, ultraviolet radiation, chlorine and quaternary ammonium treatments on the infectivity of myxospores of *Myxobolus cerebralis* for *Tubifex tubifex*. *Journal of Aquatic Animal Health* 20: 116–125.

Kent, M.L., Andree, K.B., Bartholomew, J.L. et al. (2001). Recent advances in our knowledge of the Myxozoa. *Journal of Eukaryotic Microbiology* 48: 395–413.

Wagner, E.J., Smith, M., Arndt, R., and Roberts, D.W. (2003). Physical and chemical effects on viability of the *Myxobolus cerebralis* triactinomyxon. *Diseases of Aquatic Organisms* 53: 133–142.

Abbreviations/Acronyms

- ISH: In situ hybridization
- PCR: Polymerase chain reaction
- qPCR: Quantitative polymerase chain reaction

Ceratonova and *Ceratomyxa* spp.

Overview

- *Ceratonova shasta* is a coelozoic myxozoan parasite that is still commonly known by its former name, *Ceratomyxa shasta*. It causes enteritis in freshwater salmonids (*Salmonidae*). The disease is only reported from salmonid aquaculture.
- Other *Ceratomyxa* spp. are mostly reported from the gallbladder or urinary system of marine fish.

Etiology

- Phylum *Cnidaria.*
- Class *Myxozoa.*
- Family *Ceratomyxidae.*
- The most commonly reported fish parasite in this group is *Ceratonova shasta*, the cause of ceratomyxosis. It has been reassigned to this genus because of its freshwater/brackish life cycle, sequence data, and sporulation in

the intestines rather than the gallbladder or urinary system.

- Other *Ceratonova* and *Ceratomyxa* spp. reported in fish include *Ceratonova gasterostea*, *Ceratomyxa ayami* n. sp., *Ceratomyxa synaphobranchi* n. sp., and *Ceratomyxa verudaensis* n. sp.

Life Cycle and Transmission

- General life cycle information is described under C8: *Myxozoa (General).*
- The myxospore and actinospore stages are known for *C. shasta*.
  - Salmonids are the vertebrate host.
  - Freshwater polychaetes (e.g. *Manayunkia speciosa*) are the invertebrate host.
- Mature actinospores are viable for days to weeks.
- Experimental infections are possible with a single parasite, so a low infectious dose seems likely.

Geographic Distribution

- *C. shasta* is restricted to specific freshwater river systems in western North America, particularly in Oregon and California.

Signalment

- *C. shasta* is reported in freshwater salmonids, particularly rainbow trout (*Oncorhynchus mykiss*) and Chinook salmon (*Oncorhynchus tshawytscha*). Strains are usually specific to a single host species. Fish from endemic areas are more resistant than naïve fish, although they can still show clinical signs if the infectious dose is high enough.
- *C. gasterostea* is reported in freshwater three-spine sticklebacks (*Gasterosteus aculeatus*).
- *Ceratomyxa* spp. are typically in marine teleosts and elasmobranchs but have been reported from freshwater teleosts.

Risk Factors

- General risk factors are described under C8: *Myxozoa (General).*
- *C. shasta* actinospores are released when temperatures reach >10°C (50°F).

Signs/Clinical Findings

- Lethargy may be seen.
- Inappetence, reduced feeding, weight loss, or poor growth rates may be seen.
- Coelomic distension due to ascites and granulomatous inflammation is common.
- Vent swelling and hyperemia are common.
- Skin darkening may be seen, particularly in rainbow trout.
- Gill pallor due to anemia may be seen.
- Exophthalmos may be seen.
- Mortality in juvenile salmonids is often around 40% but can reach 100%.
- Survivors may show poor growth and poor resilience.

Differential Diagnoses

- Full differentials are described in Section B.
- Common differentials for enteritis and weight loss in salmonids include chronic disease (often viral, bacterial, or parasitic), and nutritional or social factors.

Diagnosis

- A tentative diagnosis is typically from finding spores on direct microscopy, impression smears, or histology of the intestinal tract, gallbladder, kidney, or coelom. Definitive diagnosis for *C. shasta* is by PCR.
- Mature spores are arcuate (kidney-bean shaped), ~6–8 × 14–22 µm, with two polar capsules that are bilaterally symmetrical (Figure C8.5). Spores are usually seen in a variety of developmental stages and sizes. The parasites are detectable on most routine stains and the polar capsules stain Gram-positive and shell valves stain acid-fast positive.
- Necropsy or coeliotomy typically show coelomic effusion with hemorrhage and necrosis of the caudal intestines and vent. Other viscera may be pale due to anemia. Nodules are sometimes seen in adults.
- Histology can be used to confirm enteritis. Inflammation varies but is often granulomatous.
- Commercial PCR tests are available for *C. shasta*. They can be run premortem on fecal samples and potentially coelomic effusion. Water samples can also be screened.

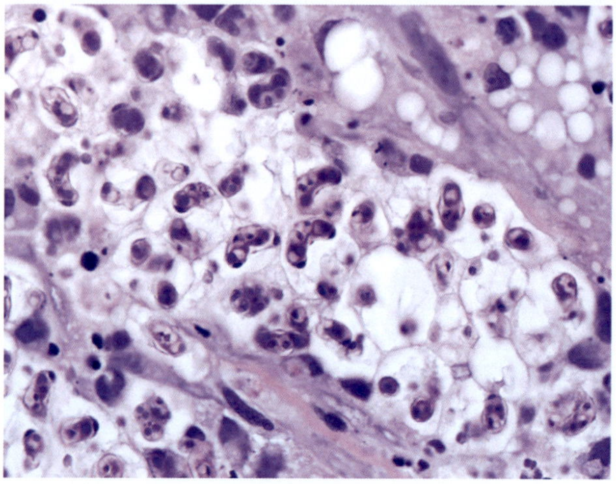

Figure C8.5 Spores from *Ceratonova shasta* on histology of the intestines of a rainbow trout (*Oncorhynchus mykiss*) showing arcuate mature spores. H&E x400. *Source*: Image courtesy of Justin Stilwell, University of Georgia.

Husbandry Management

- General husbandry management is described under C8: *Myxozoa (General).*
- For salmonids in freshwater, consider conversion to salt water to prevent further infections.

Medical Management

- Medical treatment has little effect and is not reported.
- All legislation regarding medication use and disposal must be followed.

Prevention

- General preventative measures are described under C8: *Myxozoa (General).*

Zoonotic Reports

- These parasites have no known zoonotic potential.

Bibliography

Atkinson, S.D., Foott, J.S., and Bartholomew, J.L. (2014). Erection of *Ceratonova* n. gen. (Myxosporea: Ceratomyxidae) to encompass freshwater species *C. gasterostea* n. sp. from threespine stickleback (*Gasterosteus aculeatus*) and *C. shasta* n. comb. from salmonid fishes. *Journal of Parasitology* 100: 640–645.

Bjork, S.J. and Bartholomew, J.L. (2009). Effects of *Ceratomyxa shasta* dose on a susceptible strain of rainbow trout and comparatively resistant Chinook and coho salmon. *Diseases of Aquatic Organisms* 86: 29–37.

Fiala, I., Hlavničková, M., Kodádková, A. et al. (2015). Evolutionary origin of *Ceratonova shasta* and phylogeny of the marine myxosporean lineage. *Molecular Phylogenetics and Evolution* 86: 75–89.

Kent, M.L., Andree, K.B., Bartholomew, J.L. et al. (2001). Recent advances in our knowledge of the Myxozoa. *Journal of Eukaryotic Microbiology* 48: 395–413.

Whipple, M.J., Ganam, A.L., and Bartholomew, J.L. (2002). Lack of a prophylactic effect of orally administered glucan and fumagillin on naturally acquired infection with *Ceratomyxa shasta* in juvenile rainbow and steelhead trout (*Oncorhynchus mykiss*). *North American Journal of Aquaculture* 64: 1–9.

Abbreviations/Acronyms

- PCR: Polymerase chain reaction

Hoferellus spp.

Overview

- *Hoferellus* spp. are histozoic myxozoan parasites that infect the urinary system of freshwater fish.
- *Hoferellus carassii* causes polycystic kidney disease in goldfish (*Carassius auratus*) and koi (*Cyprinus carpio koi*). The renomegaly can be severe and affected fish usually present due to coelomic distension.

Etiology

- Phylum *Cnidaria.*
- Class *Myxozoa.*
- Family *Myxobilatidae.*
- The most commonly reported fish parasite in this genus is *Hoferellus carassii* (formerly *Mitraspora cyprini*).
- Other species include *Hoferellus cyprini*, *Hoferellus gilsoni*, and *Hoferellus gnathonemi.*

Life Cycle and Transmission

- General life cycle information is described under C8: *Myxozoa (General).*
- Fish are the vertebrate host.
- Freshwater oligochaetes (maybe *Branchiura* or *Nais* spp.) are the invertebrate host.
- In fish, the mature spores are found in the kidney and urinary bladder and are passed in urine.
- A different *Hoferellus* sp. has been identified in amphibians but it is considered unlikely to play any role in the disease in fish.

Geographic Distribution

- *H. carassii* was first found in Europe and Japan and is now in freshwater habitats worldwide.

Signalment

- *Hoferellus* spp. affect freshwater fish and are usually host-specific, e.g.:
  - *H. carassii* in pond-reared goldfish and Prussian carp (*Carassius gibelio*), but not koi.
  - *H. cyprini* (the type species) in pond-reared common carp (*Cyprinus carpio*), but not goldfish.
  - *H. gilsoni* in European eels (*Anguilla anguilla*).
  - *H. gnathonemi* in elephantnose fish (*Gnathonemus petersii*).

Risk Factors

- General risk factors are described under C8: *Myxozoa (General).*

Signs/Clinical Findings

- Coelomic distension due to severe renomegaly and/or coelomic effusion is common.
- Inappetence or reduced feeding may be seen.
- Abnormal swimming or buoyancy may be seen.
- Gill pallor due to anemia may be seen.
- Mortality is usually low.

Differential Diagnoses

- Full differentials are described in Section B.
- Common differentials for severe coelomic distension in goldfish and carp include obesity, egg retention, neoplasia, bacterial or viral infection, and polycystic kidney disease.

Diagnosis

- Severe renomegaly with polycystic kidneys in goldfish and koi is highly suggestive (Figure C8.6). Diagnosis is typically confirmed following cytology of the kidney, urinary bladder, cystic fluid, or coelomic effusion, or on histology.
- Mature spores are usually shaped like a bishop's hat (miter), with a pointed anterior end and a wide posterior end with caudal filaments/bristles. Some spores may be round, bullet-shaped, or pyramidal. Spores are ~7–14 × 5–11 μm and bilaterally symmetrical with two polar capsules. The parasites are detectable on most routine stains and the polar capsules stain Gram-positive. Up to 12 spores may be within round to pyriform plasmodia up to 40 μm in length. On direct microscopy, the spores may be motile using pseudopodia.
- Histology also typically shows severe hypertrophy of renal tubules and ureters.
- PCR testing may be available.

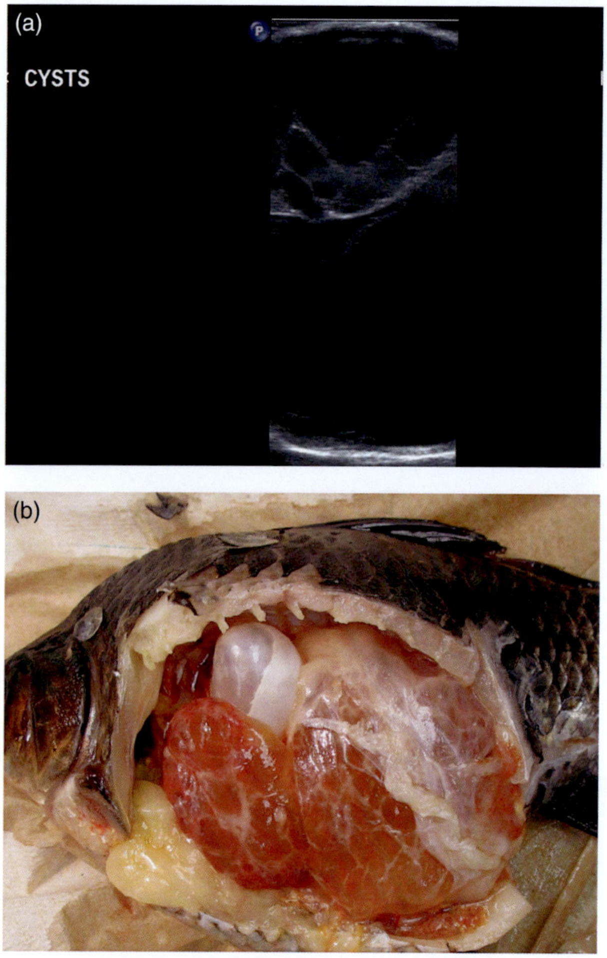

Figure C8.6 Polycystic kidneys in a goldfish (*Carassius auratus*) infected with *Hoferellus carassii* on ultrasound (a) and at necropsy (b). *Source*: Image (a) courtesy of Brittany Stevens, University of California, Davis, and (b) courtesy of Johnny Shelley, USDA-ARS Aquatic Animal Health Research Unit.

Husbandry Management

- Once clinical signs are evident, husbandry and medical management are usually ineffective.

Medical Management

- Supportive care may help.
- Euthanasia should be considered if clinical signs are severe.
- All legislation regarding medication use and disposal must be followed.

Prevention

- General preventative measures are described under C8: *Myxozoa (General).*

Zoonotic Reports

- These parasites have no known zoonotic potential.

Bibliography

Alama-Bermejo, G., Jirku, M., Kodáková, A. et al. (2016). Species complexes and phylogenetic lineages of *Hoferellus* (Myxozoa, Cnidaria) including revision of the genus: a problematic case for taxonomy. *Parasites and Vectors* 9: 13.

Kent, M.L., Andree, K.B., Bartholomew, J.L. et al. (2001). Recent advances in our knowledge of the Myxozoa. *Journal of Eukaryotic Microbiology* 48:395–413.

Abbreviations/Acronyms

- PCR: Polymerase chain reaction

Kudoa spp.

Overview

- *Kudoa* spp. are histozoic myxozoan parasites that tend to infect the striated muscle of marine fish.
- The mature spores of typical *Kudoa* spp. are distinctive with four polar capsules.
- *Kudoa thyrsites* can cause post-harvest myoliquefaction in pen-reared salmonids (*Salmonidae*).

Etiology

- Phylum *Cnidaria.*
- Class *Myxozoa.*
- Order *Multivalvulida.*
- Family *Kudoidae.*
- The most economically important species in fish is *K. thyrsites*, one of the causative agents of post-harvest myoliquefaction in cultured salmonids. Fillets become soft after processing due to the release of proteolytic enzymes by the parasites.
- Other *Kudoa* spp. generate cysts that make fillets unmarketable (e.g. *Kudoa amamiensis* in carangids, *Seriola* spp.).
- Other species reported in fish include *Kudoa carcharhini*, *Kudoa clupeidae*, *Kudoa hemiscylli*, *Kudoa lutjanus*, and *Kudoa neurophila.*
- Typical *Kudoa* spp. have four polar capsules. Myxozoans previously identified as *Pentacapsula*, *Hexacapsula*, and *Septemcapsula* due the presence of five, six, and seven polar capsules respectively have been amended to the genus *Kudoa*.

Life Cycle and Transmission

- The life cycle is poorly understood.
- It is likely that the life cycle is indirect and involves fish and marine invertebrates.
- Direct transmission has been attempted experimentally but has not been shown.

Geographic Distribution

- Saltwater and brackish water habitats, probably worldwide, with rare reports from freshwater habitats.

Signalment

- *Kudoa* spp. are mostly reported in marine teleosts and have unusually wide host ranges.
- Postmortem muscle damage by *K. thyrsites* is predominantly found in marine Atlantic salmon (*Salmo salar*) but has been reported from >18 fish families.
- Premortem clinical signs are rarely caused by kudoids but have been reported in a few cases.
  - *K. clupeidae* in wild Atlantic menhaden (*Brevoortia tyrannus*).
  - *K. lutjanus* in cultured crimson snapper (*Lutjanus erythropterus*).
  - *K. neurophila* in cultured striped trumpeter (*Latris lineata*).
- There are rare reports of *Kudoa* spp. in elasmobranchs.
  - *K. carcharhini* in wild nervous sharks (*Carcharhinus cautus*).
  - *K. hemiscylli* in wild epaulette sharks (*Hemiscyllium ocellatum*).

Risk Factors

- General risk factors are described under C8: *Myxozoa (General).*

Signs/Clinical Findings

- Fish are usually asymptomatic.
- Reduced feeding may be seen.
- Abnormal swimming may be seen.
- Where mortalities are seen, the rate is usually low and sporadic.
- Signs of infection may not be seen until after processing due to proteolytic damage following release of the spores.

Differential Diagnoses

- Clinical signs are rarely seen and nonspecific.

Diagnosis

- Diagnosis is typically by direct microscopy, impression smear, or histology of affected skeletal or cardiac muscle, but spores have also been found in other tissues.
- Mature spores are ~10–12 μm in diameter, radially symmetrical, typically with four polar capsules, although spores with five to seven polar capsules are now classified as *Kudoa* spp. Spores may be within pseudocysts or disseminated. The parasites are detectable on most routine stains and the polar capsules stain Gram-positive and shell valves stain acid-fast positive (Figure C8.7).

Husbandry Management

- Management changes have not been effective once clinical signs are seen.

Medical Management

- Medical treatment has little effect and is not reported.
- All legislation regarding medication use and disposal must be followed.

Prevention

- Effective preventative measures have not been established but limiting exposure to infected fish or invertebrates is likely important.

Zoonotic Reports

- There are no reports of zoonotic transmission through contact or inoculation.

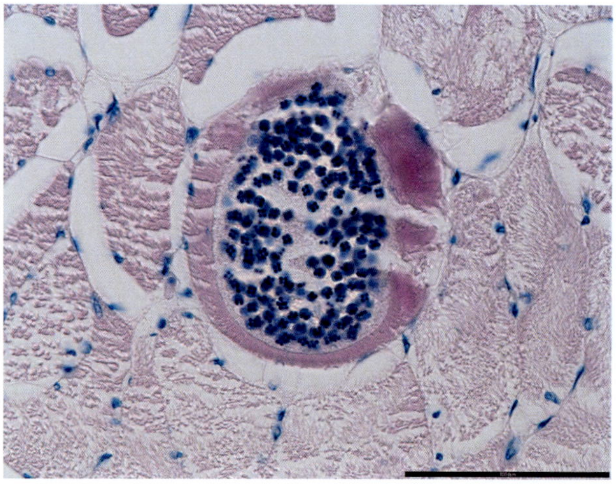

Figure C8.7 Histology image of spores from a *Kudoa* sp. in the muscle of a bullnose ray (*Myliobatis freminvillei*) on acid-fast stain; bar = 100 μm.

- There are rare reports of kudoids as potential foodborne pathogens following the consumption of raw or inadequately cooked or processed fish (e.g. *K. septempunctata* causing self-limiting diarrhea and emesis).

Bibliography

Cobcroft, J.M. and Battaglene, S.C. (2012). Ultraviolet irradiation is an effective alternative to ozonation as a sea water treatment to prevent *Kudoa neurophila* (Myxozoa: Myxosporea) infection of striped trumpeter, *Latris lineata* (Forster). *Journal of Fish Diseases* 36: 57–65.

Funk, V.A., Raap, M., Sojonky, K. et al. (2007). Development and validation of an RNA- and DNA-based quantitative PCR assay for determination of *Kudoa thyrsites* infection levels in Atlantic salmon *Salmo salar*. *Disease of Aquatic Organisms* 75: 239–249.

Gleeson, R.J., Bennett, M.B., and Adlard, R.D. (2010). First taxonomic description of multivalvulidan myxosporean parasites from elasmobranchs: *Kudoa hemiscylli* n. sp. and *Kudoa carcharini* n. sp. (Myxosporea: Multivalvulidae). *Parasitology* 137: 1885–1898.

Grossel, G.W., Dykova, I., Handlinger, J., and Munday, B.L. (2003). *Pentacapsula neurophila* sp. n. (Multivalvulida) from the central nervous system of striped trumpeter, *Latris lineata* (Forster). *Journal of Fish Diseases* 26: 315–320.

Kawai, T., Sekizuka, T., Yahata, Y. et al. (2012). Identification of *Kudoa septempunctata* as the causative agent of novel food poisoning outbreaks in Japan by consumption of *Paralichthys olivaceus* in raw fish. *Clinical Infectious Diseases* 54: 1046–1052.

Kent, M.L., Andree, K.B., Bartholomew, J.L. et al. (2001). Recent advances in our knowledge of the Myxozoa. *Journal of Eukaryotic Microbiology* 48: 395–413.

Reimschuessel, R., Gieseker, C.M., Driscoll, C. et al. (2003). Myxosporean plasmodial infection, associated with ulcerative lesions in young-of-the year Atlantic menhaden *Brevoortia tyrannus* (Latrobe) (Clupeidae) in a tributary of the Chesapeake Bay, and possible links to *Kudoa clupeidae*. *Diseases of Aquatic Organisms* 53: 143–166.

Wang, P.C., Huang, J.P., Tsai, M.A. et al. (2005). Systemic infection of *Kudoa lutjanus* n. sp. (Myxozoa: Myxosporea) in red snapper *Lutjanus erythropterus* from Taiwan. *Diseases of Aquatic Organisms* 67: 115–124.

Whipps, C.M., Grossel, G., Adlard, R.D. et al. (2004). Phylogeny of the Multivalvulidae (Myxozoa: Myxosporea) based on comparative ribosomal DNA sequence analysis. *Journal of Parasitology* 90: 618–622.

Tetracapsuloides bryosalmonae

Overview

- *Tetracapsuloides bryosalmonae* are parasites that look similar to those of the class *Myxozoa* but are now in a different class (*Malacosporea*).
- They are histozoic parasites with a predilection for the kidneys.
- They cause proliferative kidney disease (PKD, previously PKX), which is associated with significant mortality in

wild and cultured salmonids. This is an emerging disease in Northern Europe and North America.

Etiology

- Phylum *Cnidaria.*
- Unranked subphylum *Myxozoa.*
- Class *Malacosporea.*
- These parasites were historically grouped with the class *Myxozoa* but were reclassified into the *Malacosporea* due to their soft spores.
- The most commonly reported fish parasite in this group is *Tetracapsuloides* (*Tetracapsula*) *bryosalmonae.*

Life Cycle and Transmission

- The life cycle is indirect and similar to the class *Myxozoa*.
- The vertebrate hosts are salmonids (*Salmonidae*).
- The invertebrate hosts are freshwater bryozoans (e.g. *Fredericella*, *Plumatella* spp.) (Figure C8.8a).
- Spores are released through the urine.
- The spores remain infectious to fish for 12–24 hours.

Geographic Distribution

- Freshwater salmonid habitats, particularly in Europe and North America.

Signalment

- *T. bryosalmonae* is reported in freshwater salmonids, particularly rainbow trout (*Oncorhynchus mykiss*), and closely related fish such as pike (*Esox* spp.). Brown trout (*Salmo trutta*) can show disease but are often asymptomatic carriers.

Risk Factors

- General risk factors are described under C8: *Myxozoa (General).*
- Permissive water temperature is often >15°C (59°F).

Signs/Clinical Findings

- Lethargy may be seen.
- Inappetence, reduced feeding, weight loss, or poor growth rates may be seen.
- Exophthalmos is common.
- Coelomic distension is common and may be localized to the dorsocaudal coelom.
- Skin darkening may be seen; other skin lesions are usually rare.
- Edema may be seen.
- Gill pallor due to anemia may be seen.
- Morbidity and mortality are typically low but can reach 90%.

Differential Diagnoses

- Full differentials are described in Section B.
- Common differentials for renomegaly in salmonids include viruses (e.g. VHS, IPN, IHN, alphavirus, ISA), bacteria (e.g. *Renibacterium salmoninarum*, piscirickettsial-like organisms), and myxozoans.

Diagnosis

- Diagnosis is typically based on finding spores on cytology or histology of the kidneys, although parasites may be found in the gills, liver, or spleen (Figure C8.8b and c).
- Mature spores are ovoid, usually ~12–16 × 7–14 µm, with two spherical polar capsules at the anterior end. The parasites are detectable on most routine stains and the polar capsules stain Gram-positive.
- Necropsy or coeliotomy usually show renomegaly, splenomegaly, serosanguinous coelomic effusion, and pale viscera. Kidneys may be gray and mottled.

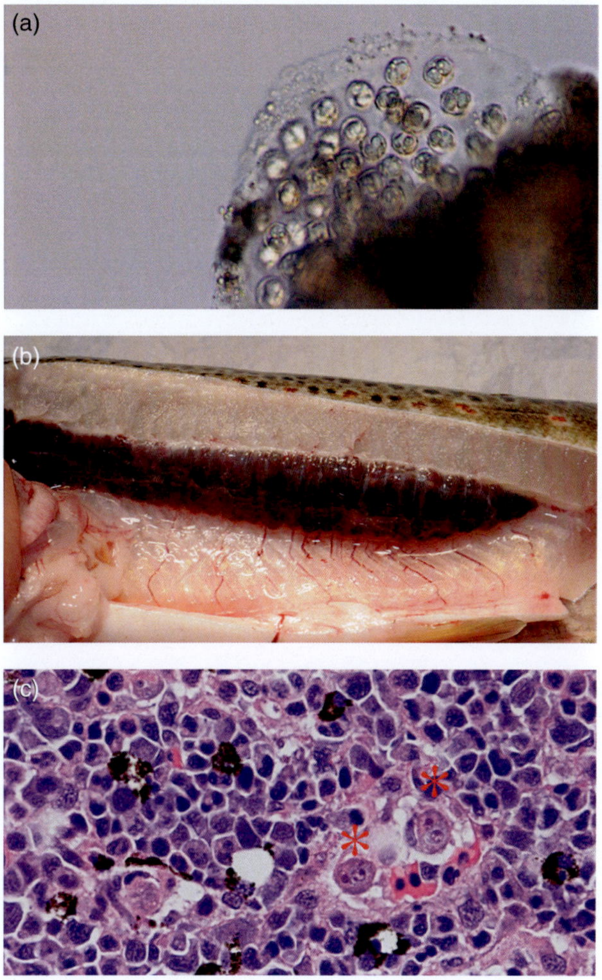

Figure C8.8 Proliferative kidney disease (PKD) caused by *Tetracapsuloides bryosalmonae* in salmonids: bright-field microscopy of *T. bryosalmonae* from a mature spore sac in the invertebrate host, bryozoan *Fredericella sultana* (a); renomegaly in a brown trout (*Salmo trutta*) affected by severe PKD (b); histology of the anterior kidney of rainbow trout (*Oncorhynchus mykiss*) – parasites are indicated by asterisks (c). *Source*: Images courtesy of Bartolomeo Gorgoglione, University of Veterinary Medicine, Vienna.

- Histology typically also shows interstitial nephritis and proliferative lesions with characteristic amoeboid-like cells.
- PCR, IHC, and ISH tests may be available for fish, bryozoans, and water samples.

Husbandry Management

- General husbandry management is described under C8: *Myxozoa (General).*
- Consider slowly reducing the water temperature to <15°C (59°F).

Medical Management

- Treatment is rarely effective.
- Reported treatments (see Chapters A12 and A13 for more details):
  - Hypersalinity immersion at 8–12 g/L for 14–21 days may reduce morbidity and mortality.
- All legislation regarding medication use and disposal must be followed.

Prevention

- General preventative measures are described under C8: *Myxozoa (General).*

Zoonotic Reports

- These parasites have no known zoonotic potential.

Bibliography

Enevova, V., Palikova, M., Blahova, J. et al. (2018). Sodium chloride treatment effects on rainbow trout suffering from proliferative kidney disease caused by *Tetracapsuloides bryosalmonae*. *Diseases of Aquatic Organisms* 131: 157–166.

Fontes, I., Hartikainen, H., Holland, J.W. et al. (2017). *Tetracapsuloides bryosalmonae* abundance in river water. *Diseases of Aquatic Organisms* 124: 145–157.

Kent, M.L., Andree, K.B., Bartholomew, J.L. et al. (2001). Recent advances in our knowledge of the Myxozoa. *Journal of Eukaryotic Microbiology* 48: 395–413.

Soliman, H., Kumar, G., and El-Matbouli, M. (2018). *Tetracapsuloides bryosalmonae* persists in brown trout *Salmo trutta* for five years post exposure. *Diseases of Aquatic Organisms* 127: 151–156.

Abbreviations/Acronyms

- IHC: Immunohistochemistry
- IHN: Infectious hematopoietic necrosis
- IPN: Infectious pancreatic necrosis
- ISA: Infectious salmon anemia
- ISH: In situ hybridization
- PCR: Polymerase chain reaction
- VHS: Viral hemorrhagic septicemia

Eimeria spp.

Overview

- *Eimeria* spp. are intracellular parasites reported from a range of marine, brackish, and freshwater fish.
- *Eimeria southwelli* is a common cause of morbidity and mortality in myliobatid rays such as cownose rays (*Rhinoptera bonasus*). Coelomic aspirates are the most useful premortem diagnostic.

Etiology

- Phylum *Myzozoa.*
- Subphylum *Apicomplexa.*
- Subclass *Coccidiasina.*
- Family *Eimeriidae.*
- *Eimeria* spp. are the most common coccidia found in fish. Some examples include:
  - *E. anguillae.*
  - *E. carpelli.*
  - *E. funduli.*
  - *E. phyllopterycis.*
  - *E. quintini.*
  - *E. southwelli.*

Life Cycle and Transmission

- *Eimeria* spp. have direct and indirect life cycles.
- The typical life cycle of *Eimeria* spp. consists of oocysts that sporulate, then release the sporocysts and sporozoites contained within. The sporozoites develop into schizonts that asexually produce merozoites to generate more schizonts. After the asexual life cycle, micro- (male) and macro- (female) gametes are produced and develop into oocysts.
- Oocysts and microgametes are the stages most commonly seen in fish.
- The method of transmission in fish is unknown.

- Oocysts can survive more than two years in salt water at 21°C (70°F).

Geographic Distribution

- Their distribution has not been determined.

Signalment

- Host ranges are usually narrow, e.g.:
  - *E. funduli* in killifish (*Fundulus* spp.).
  - *E. phyllopterycis* in weedy sea dragons (*Phyllopteryx taeniolatus*).
  - *E. southwelli* in myliobatid rays including cownose rays, spotted eagle rays (*Aetobatus narinari*), and bull-nose eagle rays (*Myliobatis freminvillei*).
  - *E. syngnathi* in blackline pipefish (*Syngnathus nigrolineatus*).
- Juvenile fish are usually more susceptible.

Risk Factors

- Risk factors are unknown, but stressors and exposure of naïve fish are likely important.

Signs/Clinical Findings

- Fish may be asymptomatic.
- Weight loss and poor body condition are common; appetite may be normal but often decreases late in the disease process.
- Regurgitation and mucoid or white fecals may be seen.
- Lethargy may be seen.
- Coelomic distension due to effusion is common.
- In cownose rays, blotchy skin discoloration and distended cutaneous lymphatics are also reported.
- Mortality is usually low but may reach 100% in cownose rays once clinical signs are seen.

Differential Diagnoses

- Full differentials are described in Section B.
- Common differentials for poor body condition and coelomic distension in fish include a variety of viral, bacterial, fungal, and parasitic infections, as well as other gastrointestinal or coelomic diseases, particularly egg retention.
- Differentials for coccidia in fish include *Eimeria*, *Cryptosporidium*, *Crystallospora*, *Calyptospora*, and *Goussia* spp.

Diagnosis

- Diagnosis is typically based on finding oocysts on direct microscopy of fecal samples, intestinal scrapings, or coelomic aspirates, or on histology of the intestine or coelomic serosal surfaces. A few species can be found within the kidney and liver.
- The most sensitive premortem diagnostic tests in myliobatid rays are coelomic aspirates and flushes. Positive samples are cloudy with abundant oocysts.
- The appearance of sporulated oocysts varies by species, e.g.:
  - *E. southwelli* oocysts are elongated (pea-pod shaped), 15–60 × 10–15 μm, with a 2 μm wall and a micropyle at one end. Mature oocysts typically have four sporocysts, each with two sporozoites (Figure C8.9).
  - *E. phyllopterycis* oocysts are spherical (like other *Eimeriidae*), 28–34 μm in diameter, with a thin wall. No micropyle is visible. A large polar granule is sometimes present. Sporocysts are ellipsoidal with circular bodies within.
- Motile biflagellated microgametes (3–4 μm in size) may be seen.
- Necropsy and histology may also show coelomic effusion and generalized serositis or enteritis.

Husbandry Management

- Management changes may not be indicated unless there are clinical signs.
- Reduce or resolve stressors.
- Consider isolation of affected animals in suitable systems.

Medical Management

- Treatment may improve clinical signs, but recurrence is common.
- Reported treatments (see Chapters A12 and A13 for more details):
  - Toltrazuril orally can resolve clinical signs for several months in cownose rays but has been associated with side effects such as regurgitation. Doses have included 10 mg/kg every 24 hours for 3–5 days, often repeated in 10 days. Dosing every 48 hours has been ineffective.

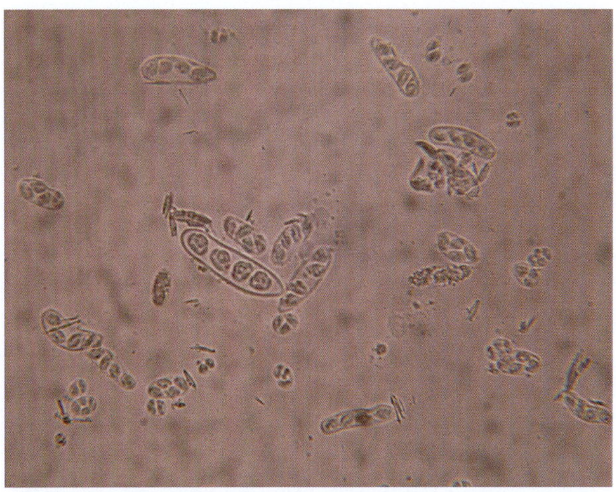

Figure C8.9 Spores from *Eimeria southwelli* sp. on bright-field microscopy of a coelomic aspirate from a cownose ray (*Rhinoptera bonasus*). *Source*: Image courtesy of Shane Boylan, South Carolina Aquarium.

  - Ponazuril orally reduced oocyst number at 50 mg/kg every seven days for four weeks in some cownose rays.
  - Copper wire particles (Copasure) at 37–2000 mg/kg orally have anecdotally improved signs in cownose rays.
- Other reported treatments have typically been considered ineffective or been associated with adverse side effects (e.g. clindamycin, sulfadimethoxine, or trimethoprim–sulfadimethoxine orally).
- All legislation regarding medication use and disposal must be followed.

Prevention
- Reduce or resolve stressors.
- Reduce exposure and transmission through good biosecurity. The risk of introducing this parasite to a naïve collection through the acquisition of myliobatid rays is high.
  - Specific pathogen-free sources of myliobatid rays.
  - Suitable quarantine of myliobatid rays with isolation, monitoring, and diagnostic testing, particularly coelomic aspirates and flushes.

Zoonotic Reports
- These parasites have no known zoonotic potential.

Bibliography

Cassle, S.E., Yanong, R.P.E., Walsh, M.T. et al. (2014). The good, the bad and the (DrUg)ly: cracking the proverbial nut on the treatment of cownose rays (*Rhinoptera bonasus*) for *Eimeria southwelli* with ponazuril. *Proceedings of the Eastern Fish Health Workshop Conference*, Shepardstown, WV.

Clarke, E.O., Grzenda, K., Murphy, D. et al. (2015). Successful treatment of *Eimeria southwelli* in a cownose ray (*Rhinoptera bonasus*) using oral copper wire particles. *Proceedings of the International Aquatic Animal Medicine Conference*, Chicago, IL.

McDermott, A., Field, C., Mejia-Fava, J. et al. (2013). Medical and surgical management of cloacal prolapses in cow nose rays (*Rhinoptera bonasus*) undergoing treatment for *Eimeria southwelli* infection. *Proceedings of the International Aquatic Animal Medicine Conference*, Sausolito, CA.

Stamper, M.A., Lewbart, G.A., Barrington, P.R. et al. (1998). *Eimeria southwelli* infection associated with high mortality of cownose rays. *Journal of Aquatic Animal Health* 10: 264–270.

Upton, S.J., Stamper, M.A., Osborn, A.L. et al. (2000). A new species of *Eimeria* (Apicomplexa, Eimeriidae) from the weedy sea dragon *Phyllopteryx taeniolatus* (Osteichthyes: Syngnathidae). *Diseases of Aquatic Organisms* 43: 55–59.

Cryptosporidium spp.

Overview
- *Cryptosporidium* spp. are obligate, intracellular coccidia that are reported sporadically in teleosts.
- In fish, the parasites are typically found in the stomach or intestinal epithelium.
- The oocysts take up acid-fast stain.
- Treatment of coccidial infections in fish has been unrewarding.

Etiology
- Phylum *Myzozoa*.
- Subphylum *Apicomplexa*.
- Subclass *Coccidiasina*.
- Family *Cryptosporidiidae*.
- Only two species from fish have been well-characterized: *Cryptosporidium molnari* and *Cryptosporidium scophthalmi*.
- Relatively little is known about *Cryptosporidium* spp. in fish.

Life Cycle and Transmission
- The typical life cycle of other *Cryptosporidium* spp. consists of oocysts that are ingested or inhaled by the host. Sporozoites are released and parasitize epithelial cells of the gastrointestinal or respiratory tracts. The sporozoites develop into schizonts that asexually produce merozoites to generate more schizonts. After the asexual life cycle, micro- (male) and macro- (female) gametes are produced and develop into thick-walled and thin-walled oocysts that sporulate in the host.
- It is likely that the life cycle of *Cryptosporidium* spp. in fish follows a similar pattern.

Geographic Distribution
- Their distribution has not been determined.

Signalment
- A variety of freshwater and marine species are susceptible.

- Examples of hosts in freshwater aquarium species include koi (*Cyprinus carpio koi*), goldfish (*Carassius auratus*), oscars (*Astronatus ocellatus*), guppies (*Poecilia reticulata*), freshwater angelfish (*Pterophyllum scalare*), red-eye tetras (*Moenkhausia sanctaefilomenae*), neon tetras (*Paracheirodon innesi*), and three-spot gouramis (*Trichogaster trichopterus*).
- Examples in marine aquarium species include orange-spine unicornfish (*Naso lituratus*) and seahorses and sea dragons (*Syngnathidae*).
- Examples in common aquaculture species include gilthead sea bream (*Sparus aurata*), European bass (*Dicentrarchus labrax*), turbot (*Scophthalmus maximus*), sea mullet (*Mugil cephalus*), and barramundi (*Lates calcarifer*).
- Juvenile fish are usually more susceptible.

Risk Factors

- Risk factors are unknown, but stressors and exposure of naïve fish are likely important.

Signs/Clinical Findings

- Fish are usually asymptomatic, even with significant histologic damage.
- If seen, weight loss and poor body condition are the most common signs; appetite may be normal or reduced.
- Regurgitation and mucoid or white fecals may be seen.
- Lethargy may be seen.
- Loss of pigmentation may be seen.
- Coelomic distension due to effusion may be seen.
- Mortality is usually low.

Differential Diagnoses

- Full differentials are described in Section B.
- Common differentials for acid-fast structures in fish include *Mycobacterium*, *Nocardia*, *Cryptosporidium* spp., myxozoans, and microsporidia.
- Differentials for coccidia in fish include *Eimeria*, *Cryptosporidium*, *Crystallospora*, *Calyptospora*, and *Goussia* spp.

Diagnosis

- Diagnosis is typically based on finding parasites on cytology or histology of the gastrointestinal mucosa. Species have preferred areas (e.g. stomach for *C. molnari* and intestines for *C. scophthalmi*). Rare cases also show dissemination to viscera.
- Oocysts are spherical or almost spherical, small (~3–5 µm diameter), with indistinct contents that consist of four sporozoites. There are no sporocysts around the sporozoites. The oocysts stain acid-fast positive (Figure C8.10).
- Histology typically shows free or intracellular oocysts, necrosis, sloughing, or villous atrophy and fusion. The inflammatory response varies; there may be a granulomatous gastritis or enteritis. Microgametes and other stages may also be seen
- In rare cases, oocysts can be found premortem on fecal acid-fast stain; this can be a useful diagnostic if the parasite has been found in one of a group of fish.
- PCR or nested PCR may be available from fecal, gastric, or intestinal samples. This should be followed by sequencing for species identification
- EM and FA tests may be available.

Husbandry Management

- Management changes may not be indicated unless there are clinical signs.
- Reduce or resolve stressors.

Medical Management

- Treatment may improve clinical signs, but recurrence is common.
- Possible treatments (see Chapters A12 and A13 for more details):
  - Supportive care is often indicated, particularly fluid and nutritional support.
  - Ponazuril orally may reduce clinical signs.
  - Metronidazole orally may reduce clinical signs.
- All legislation regarding medication use and disposal must be followed.

Prevention

- Reduce or resolve stressors.
  - Low stocking density.
  - Suitable social groups and habitats.
  - Excellent water quality and preferred water temperature.
  - Good nutrition.
  - Suitable handling and transport protocols.

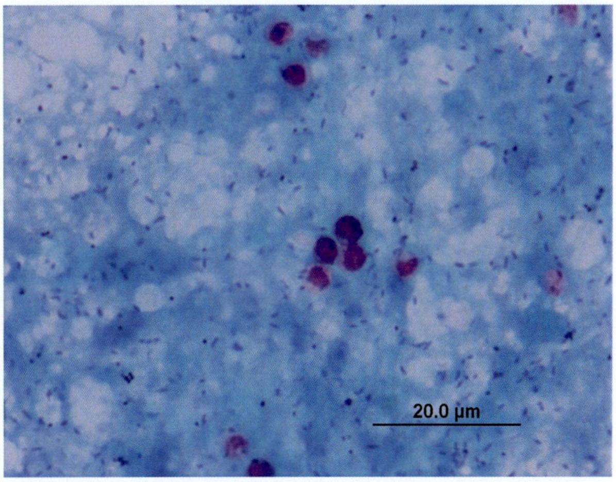

Figure C8.10 *Cryptosporidium* oocysts on acid-fast staining of the gastrointestinal contents from an emaciated lemonpeel angelfish (*Centropyge flavissima*).

- Reduce exposure and transmission through good biosecurity.

Zoonotic Reports

- There are no reports that *Cryptosporidium* species known to be pathogenic in fish are zoonotic.
- *Cryptosporidium* spp. isolated from mammals are zoonotic (e.g. *C. parvum*, *C. hominis*, *C. meleagridis*, *C. felis*, *C. canis*, *C. muris*). Transmission is typically waterborne or feco-oral.
- *C. parvum* has been identified in wild and cultured freshwater and marine fish in a variety of locations using PCR surveys. This may represent a zoonotic risk.

Bibliography

Alvarez-Pellitero, P. and Sitja-Bobadilla, A. (2002). *Cryptosporidium molnari* n. sp. (Apicomplexa: Cryptosporidiidae) infecting two marine fish species, *Sparus aurata* L. and *Dicentrarchus labrax* L. *International Journal of Parasitology* 32: 1007–1021.

Alvarez-Pellitero, P., Quiroga, M.I., Sitjà-Bobadilla, A. et al. (2004). *Cryptosporidium scophthalmi* n. sp. (Apicomplexa: Cryptosporidiidae) from cultured turbot *Scophthalmus maximus*. Light and electron microscope description and histopathological study. *Diseases of Aquatic Organisms* 62: 133–145.

Certad, G., Dupouy-Camet, J., Gantois, N. et al. (2015). Identification of *Cryptosporidium* species in fish from Lake Geneva (Lac Léman) in France. *PLoS One* 10 (7): e0133047.

Koinari, M., Karl, S., Ng-Hublin, J. et al. (2013). Novel and zoonotic *Cryptosporidium* species in fish from Papua New Guinea. *Veterinary Parasitology* 198: 1–9.

Morine, M., Yang, R., Ng, J. et al. (2012). Additional novel *Cryptosporidium* genotypes in ornamental fishes. *Veterinary Parasitology* 190: 578–582.

Reid, A., Lymbery, A., Ng, J. et al. (2010). Identification of novel and zoonotic *Cryptosporidium* species in marine fish. *Veterinary Parasitology* 168: 190–195.

Yang, R., Dorrestein, G.M., and Ryan, U. (2016). Molecular characterization of a disseminated *Cryptosporidium* infection in a koi carp (*Cyprinus carpio*). *Veterinary Parasitology* 226: 53–56.

Abbreviations/Acronyms

- EM: Electron microscopy
- FA: Fluorescent antibody
- PCR: Polymerase chain reaction

Appendix 1
Conversions

Catherine A. Hadfield

Seattle Aquarium, Seattle, WA, USA

Distance/Area

1 m = 3.28 ft
1 m = 1.09 yd
1 m = 100 cm
1 m = 39.37 in.
1 cm = 0.39 in.
1 ft = 30.48 cm
1 in = 2.54 cm
1 yard = 91.44 cm
1 acre = 4047 m^2
1 acre = 4840 yd^2

Weight

1 kg = 2.2046 lb
1 kg = 1000 g
1 kg = 1 L freshwater
1 g = 1000 mg
1 g = 15.43 grains
1 g = 0.035 oz
1 mg = 1000 μg
1 μg = 1000 ng
1 oz = 28.35 g
1 lb = 16 oz
1 lb = 453.6 g

Volume

US gallon = 3.785 L
1 US gallon = 0.134 ft^3
1 US gallon = 4 quarts
1 UK/imperial gallon = 4.55 L
1 L = 1000 mL
1 mL = 1 cc
1 mL = 1000 μL
1 mL ~ 20 drops
1 cup = 237 mL
1 tablespoon = 14.79 mL
1 tablespoon = 3 teaspoons
1 teaspoon = 4.93 mL
1 drop = 0.05 mL
1 fluid ounce = 29.57 mL
1 acre-foot = 325 851 US gallons
1 acre-foot = 43 560 ft^3
1 m^2 = 10.764 ft^2

Concentration

1 mg/L = 1 ppm
1 g/L = 1 ppt
100% = 1000 mg/mL

Temperature

T (°F) = (T in °C × 1.8) + 32
T (°C) = 0.56 × (T in °F − 32)

Energy

1 kcal = 1000 cal
1 cal = 4.18 J

Appendix 2
Common Disinfectants

Catherine A. Hadfield

Seattle Aquarium, Seattle, WA, USA

This table provides general information on common surface disinfectants. Efficiency of disinfection depends on the concentration, contact time, temperature, pH, hardness, chemical structure of the disinfectant, surface characteristics of the materials, and the amount of organic or inorganic material. Cleaning is always recommended prior to disinfection. All disinfectants have the potential for toxicity. Product labels and Safety Data Sheets must be reviewed in detail prior to use. The use of trade names is only to provide examples and does not signify endorsement of a particular product.

	Ethyl or isopropyl alcohols (70–90%)	**Biguanides**	**Oxidizing agents**	**Phenols**	**Quaternary ammonium compounds (QAC)**	**Chlorine halogens**
Examples	Ethyl alcohol, isopropyl alcohol	Chlorhexidine (e.g. Nolvasan-S, Hibistat, Virosan)	Peroxygen (e.g. Virkon-Aquatic), hydrogen peroxide (e.g. Perox-Aid), peracetic acid (e.g. Oxy-Sept 333)	Lysol, Pheno-Tek	Benzalkonium chloride, also known as alkyldimethyl ammonium chloride, and mixtures (e.g. Roccal-D, D-256, F10)	Sodium hypochlorite or bleach (NaOCl), calcium hypochlorite (e.g. HTH), chlorine dioxide (ClO_2)
Enveloped viruses (lipoviruses)	Good	Variable	Some	Variable	Variable	Good
Non-enveloped viruses	Variable	None	Variable	None	None	Some
Extracellular Gram-negative bacteria	Good	Good	Good	Good	Some	Good
Extracellular Gram-positive bacteria	Good	Good	Good	Good	Good	Good
Mycobacteria	Some	None	Variable	Variable	None	Some
Chlamydia-like bacteria	Good	Some	Good	Variable	Good	Good
Fungi	Variable	Variable	Variable	Variable	Variable	Some
Spores	Sporostatic only	Sporostatic only	Some sporicidal activity	Sporostatic only	Variable sporicidal activity	Some sporicidal activity
Effective in the presence of organic material	No	Yes	Yes	Yes	No	No
Effective in hard water	Some	Some	Yes	Yes	Variable	Yes

(Continued)

(Continued)

	Ethyl or isopropyl alcohols (70–90%)	Biguanides	Oxidizing agents	Phenols	Quaternary ammonium compounds (QAC)	Chlorine halogens
Preferred pH range	NA	Neutral/acidic (5–7)	NA	Neutral (7–7.5)	Neutral/alkaline (7–9)	Neutral (6–8)
Precautions	Irritant; flammable; may swell or harden rubber and plastic	Easily inactivated by soaps and detergents	Irritant in undiluted form; may corrode some metals (copper, brass, zinc)	Irritant; must be rinsed; may damage rubber or plastic; often formulated with soap or other detergent	Irritant; must be rinsed; inactivates iodine products	Irritant; hypochlorite must be rinsed or deactivated with sodium thiosulfate; chlorine tests can be used to check residues; never mix with acids or ammonium products; may corrode metal, rubber, and fabrics; inactivated by UV exposure and some metals
Other comments	Does not leave a residue	Good residual activity; some formulations combined with alcohol	Test strips are available for some products to check effective concentrations	Good residual activity	Good residual activity; doses can be hard to compare in the literature due to a wide variety of products	Doses can be hard to compare in the literature due to differences in reporting; commercial (undiluted) chlorine bleach typically has 5.25% NaOCl and 50 000 mg/L available chlorine; a common household dilution (1:200) = 0.025% and 250 mg/L available chlorine

NA: Not available.

Appendix 3
Fish Diagnostic Laboratories in the United States

Catherine A. Hadfield

Seattle Aquarium, Seattle, WA, USA

This appendix provides names and contact details for laboratories in the United States that provide diagnostic services for fish, organized by state. It is not an exhaustive list and does not signify endorsement of a particular laboratory.

Arkansas

University of Arkansas at Pine Bluff
Aquaculture and Fisheries Center
Pine Bluff, Lonoke, and Lake Village, Arkansas
http://www.uapb.edu/academics/school_of_agriculture_fisheries_and_human_sciences/aquaculture_fisheries/aquaculture_fisheries.aspx
(501) 676-3124, (870) 575-8137

U.S. Department of Agriculture
Stuttgart National Aquaculture Research Center
Stuttgart, Arkansas
http://www.ars.usda.gov/main/site_main.htm?modecode=60-28-10-00
(870) 673-4483

California

University of California, Davis
California Animal Health & Food Safety Laboratory System Aquaculture Service
Davis, California
https://cahfs.vetmed.ucdavis.edu/tests-and-fees/diagnostic-services/aquaculture
(916) 752-3411

U.S. Fish and Wildlife Service
California-Nevada Fish Health Center
Anderson, California
https://www.fws.gov/canvfhc/
(530) 365-4271

Colorado

Pisces Molecular
Boulder, Colorado
http://www.pisces-molecular.com
(303) 546-9300

Connecticut

University of Connecticut
Veterinary Medical Diagnostic Laboratory
Mansfield, Connecticut
http://cvmdl.uconn.edu/
(860) 486-1138

Florida

University of Florida
Fish Disease Diagnostic Laboratory
Ruskin and Gainesville, Florida
http://tal.ifas.ufl.edu and http://labs.vetmed.ufl.edu
(813) 671-5230

Georgia

University of Georgia
Infectious Diseases Laboratory
Athens, Georgia
https://vet.uga.edu/diagnostic-service-labs/infectious-diseases-lab/
(706) 542-3000

U.S. Fish and Wildlife Service
Warm Springs Regional Fisheries Center
Warm Springs, Georgia
http://www.fws.gov/warmsprings/
(706) 655-3382

Idaho

U.S. Fish and Wildlife Service
Idaho Fish Health Center
Orofino, Idaho
http://www.fws.gov/pacific/fisheries/fishhealth/index.cfm
(208) 476-9500

Kentucky

Kentucky State University
Fish Disease Diagnostic Laboratory Aquaculture Research Center
Frankfort, Kentucky
http://kysu.edu/academics/cafsss/aquaculture/division-of-aquaculture-research-areas/
(502) 597-6581

Louisiana

Louisiana State University
Aquatic Diagnostic Laboratory
Baton Rouge, Louisiana

http://www.lsu.edu/vetmed/laddl/
(225) 578-9777

Maine

Fish Vet Group
Portland, Maine
http://fishvetgroup.co.uk/
(207) 699-5901

Kennebec River Biosciences
Richmond, Maine
http://www.kennebecbio.com
(207) 737-2637

Minnesota

University of Minnesota
Veterinary Diagnostic Laboratory
St. Paul, Minnesota
http://www.vdl.umn.edu/services-fees/aquaculturefisheries/fish-submission-guidelines
(612) 625-8787

Mississippi

Mississippi State University
Thad Cochran National Warmwater Aquaculture Center
Stoneville, Mississippi
http://tcnwac.msstate.edu/
(662) 325-3432

New Jersey

New Jersey Department of Agriculture
Animal Health Diagnostic Laboratory
Ewing, New Jersey
http://jerseyvetlab.nj.gov/contact/
(609) 406-6999

New York

Cornell University College of Veterinary Medicine
Aquatic Animal Health Program
Ithaca, New York
https://www.vet.cornell.edu/departments/microbiology-and-immunology/research/aquatic-animal-health-program
(607) 253-3400

North Carolina

North Carolina Department of Agriculture
Veterinary Diagnostic Laboratory System
Raleigh, Monroe, Elkin, and Fletcher, North Carolina
http://www.ncagr.gov/vet/ncvdl/index.htm
(919) 733-3986, (704) 289-6448, (336) 526-2499, (828) 684-8188

Oklahoma

Oklahoma State University
Animal Disease Diagnostic Laboratory
Stillwater, Oklahoma
https://cvhs.okstate.edu/oaddl
(405) 744-6623

Rhode Island

Roger Williams University
Aquatic Diagnostic Laboratory
Bristol, Rhode Island
https://www.rwu.edu/academics/schools-and-colleges/fssns/ceed/adl
(401) 254-3299

Texas

Texas A&M University
Department of Wildlife and Fisheries Sciences
College Station, Texas
https://tvmdl.tamu.edu/
(979) 862-1558

University of Texas
Fungal Testing Laboratory
San Antonio, Texas
http://strl.uthscsa.edu/fungus/
(210) 567-7000

Virginia

Virginia-Maryland Regional College of Veterinary Medicine
Department of Biomedical Sciences and Pathobiology
Blacksburg, Virginia
http://www.vetmed.vt.edu/research/aquatic/
(540) 231-9586

Virginia State University
Aquaculture Program
Petersburg, Virginia
https://www.ext.vsu.edu/aquaculture-program/
(804) 524-5620

Washington

Northwest ZooPath
Monroe, Washington
http://www.zoopath.com
(360) 794-0630

U.S. Geological Survey
Western Fisheries Research Center
Seattle, Washington
http://wfrc.usgs.gov
(206) 526-6282

Washington State University
Animal Disease Diagnostic Laboratory
Pullman, Washington
https://waddl.vetmed.wsu.edu
(509) 335-9696

West Virginia

U.S. Geological Survey
Leetown Science Center
Kearneysville, West Virginia
https://www.usgs.gov/centers/lsc
(304) 724-4430

Appendix 4
Veterinary Training Programs in Aquatic Animal Medicine

Kathryn E. Seeley

Columbus Zoo and Aquarium, Powell, OH, USA

There are many options available to veterinarians interested in fish medicine and the wider field of aquatic animal medicine. While this appendix is focused on clinical medicine in the public or private sector, other important specialties include pathology, nutrition, epidemiology, and regulatory work.

A solid clinical background, as well as good communication and problem-solving skills are essential. Career development often involves several years of training following veterinary school, requiring long hours and flexibility. There is a benefit to obtaining broad training experiences, since aquatic animal veterinarians often care for a wide array of species in addition to fish.

Veterinary Schools with Aquatic Animal Courses

The amount of coursework provided by veterinary schools on aquatic animal medicine varies greatly. Where available, the courses are often elective. Schools in North America with one or more courses that teach components of fish medicine include:

- Cornell University
- Louisiana State University
- Mississippi State University
- North Carolina State University
- Ohio State University
- Oregon State University
- Tufts University
- University of California, Davis
- University of Florida
- University of Georgia
- University of Illinois
- University of Washington

Most veterinary schools require or allow students to participate in off-site rotations during their final year. These allow students to find programs that include aquatic animal medicine. Most universities will also have opportunities for students to help with wildlife studies. Many universities have clubs or groups geared toward aquatic animal medicine that can provide additional information.

Veterinary Student Programs and Volunteer Opportunities

Most aquariums, zoos, and wildlife rehabilitation centers, as well as some universities, private practices, and government agencies offer student programs and/or volunteer opportunities. These experiences allow students to meet and learn from members of the profession, help students demonstrate interest in the field, and allow students to determine if this is truly a field they want to pursue.

Although time can be spent on student programs or volunteering during undergraduate and preclinical veterinary training, more formal opportunities are provided for final-year veterinary students. The nomenclature varies, but these programs are usually called externships, preceptorships, or extra-mural studies. They are typically two to six weeks in duration. Because of the popularity of these programs and the growing interest in aquatic animal medicine, many of these positions are booked up to two years in advance. It is necessary to plan ahead and speaking with curriculum counselors early about final-year rotation schedules can help.

There are a variety of resources to explore possible externships or volunteer opportunities, including:

- www.aazv.org
- www.avma.org
- www.aza.org
- www.iaaam.org

Veterinary Internships and Fellowships

Paid internships or fellowships with a focus on aquatic animal medicine are offered at several institutions. They are usually one- to two-year programs. Successful applicants have a veterinary degree and usually already have some clinical experience, typically through a small animal or large animal internship. In North America, applications for several programs are through the Veterinary Internship and Residency Matching Program (VIRMP), but some are outside of the structured matching system. While many programs may include some exposure to aquatic animal medicine, it is the major focus of the programs listed below:

- Aquarium of the Pacific, Long Beach, California, USA
- Marine Mammal Center, Sausalito, California, USA
- Mystic Aquarium, Mystic, Connecticut, USA
- National Aquarium, Baltimore, Maryland, USA
- National Marine Mammal Foundation and SeaWorld San Diego, San Diego, California, USA
- St. Matthew's University, School of Veterinary Medicine, West Bay, Cayman Islands
- University of California, College of Veterinary Medicine, Davis, California, USA
- University of Florida, College of Veterinary Medicine, Gainesville, Florida, USA
- Vancouver Aquarium Marine Science Center, British Columbia, Canada

Veterinary Residencies

Residencies differ from internships and fellowships in that they have to meet requirements set up by the associated veterinary board (e.g. American College of Zoological Medicine, European College of Zoological Medicine, American Board of Veterinary Practitioners). They are usually three-year programs. Requirements for residency applicants vary and details can be found online; however, at least one internship is usually required and successful applicants may have two or three internships, including programs at aquariums and zoos. In North America, applications for most programs are through the Veterinary Internship and Residency Matching Program (VIRMP), but some are outside of the structured matching system. Several residencies are focused on aquatic animal medicine, but all zoological programs should provide some aquatic animal training.

Residencies that focus on aquatic animal medicine include:

- North Carolina State University, North Carolina, USA
- University of Florida, Florida, USA
- University of Georgia/Zoo Atlanta/Georgia Aquarium, Georgia, USA
- University of Illinois/Brookfield Zoo/John G. Shedd Aquarium, Illinois, USA

Residencies with aquatics in the collection or case load include:

- Columbus Zoo and Aquarium/Ohio State University/The Wilds, Ohio, USA
- Cornell University, New York, USA
- Louisiana State University, Louisiana, USA
- National Zoological Park, Washington DC, USA
- Oklahoma City Zoo/Oklahoma State University/Tulsa Zoo, Oklahoma, USA
- St. Louis Zoological Park, Missouri, USA
- Texas A&M University, Texas, USA
- Toronto Zoo/Ontario Veterinary College, Ontario, Canada
- University of California, Davis, California, USA
- Université de Montréal/Granby Zoo, Québec, Canada
- University of Wisconsin, Madison, Wisconsin, USA
- Wildlife Conservation Society, New York, USA

Not all programs are offered every year. Additional information can be found at:

- www.aazv.org
- www.aczm.org
- www.aza.org
- www.eczm.eu
- www.virmp.org

Conferences and Courses that Include Fish Medicine

There are many professional organizations for aquatic animal health practitioners. These provide online resources and continuing education through their sites or professional conferences. Some examples are listed below.

- American Association of Fish Veterinarians – www.fishvets.org
- American Fisheries Society – fisheries.org
- Aquatic Medicine Seminar – www.sharkreef.com/about/ams.aspx
- Aquamed – www.vetmed.lsu.edu/aquamed.htm#continuingeducation
- Aquavet – www2.vet.cornell.edu/education/externships-and-other-educational-opportunities/other-educational-opportunities/aquavet
- Eastern Fish Health Workshop – Facebook page
- European Association of Fish Pathologists – eafp.org

- International Association of Aquatic Animal Medicine – www.iaaam.org
- International Symposium on Aquatic Animal Health – isaah2018.com
- Marvet – www.marvet.org
- MDI Biological Laboratory – mdibl.org
- Oregon State University, salmon disease workshop – microbiology.science.oregonstate.edu/salmon-disease-workshop
- Regional Aquatic Workshop – www.rawconference.org
- SeaVet – conference.ifas.ufl.edu/SeaVet/
- University of Florida, Aquatic Animal Health – aquatic.vetmed.ufl.edu/education/courses
- University of Georgia – vet.uga.edu
- University of Prince Edward Island and Canadian Aquaculture Institute – http://www.upei.ca/programsandcourses/canadian-aquaculture-institute
- University of Wisconsin, Madison – ce.vetmed.wisc.edu/Fish_Health_Courses_for_Producers_and_Veterinarians
- US Fish and Wildlife Service National Conservation Training Center – https://training.fws.gov/
- Veterinary Information Network – www.vin.com
- Western Fish Disease Workshop – Facebook page
- World Aquaculture Society – www.was.org
- World Aquatic Veterinary Medical Association – www.wavma.org

Job Opportunities

Jobs in aquariums, zoos, wildlife rehabilitation centers, and universities are limited. Work in the private sector is available, typically for koi, goldfish, and tropical ornamental fish, but fish-only practices can be financially challenging. Aquaculture is a growing industry and experienced veterinarians are needed both from the client perspective as well as the regulatory side. Research in aquatic animal medicine is ongoing in governments, universities, and private organizations. Additionally, developing skills in other specialties, like anesthesia or radiology, may provide opportunities to serve as consultants. Keeping an open mind and exploring opportunities will provide the best prospects for finding a position in the field of aquatic animal medicine.

Salaries vary widely depending on job description, experience level, location, and institution. Internships and residencies typically have low compensation rates. Full-time salaries are higher, but they do not match salaries of veterinarians in private companion animal practice. Over the course of a career, many veterinarians move into nonclinical or managerial positions that still relate to aquatic animal medicine, which may entail increased compensation.

Index

Clinical Guide to Fish Medicine, First Edition. Edited by Catherine A. Hadfield and Leigh Ann Clayton.

C

d

e

l

m

n